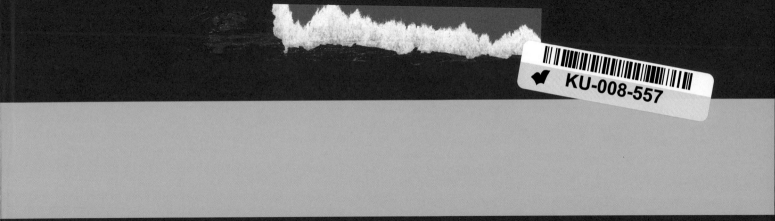

Plastic Surgery
THIRD EDITION
Volume One
Principles

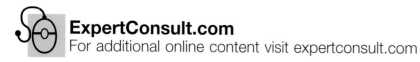

ExpertConsult.com

For additional online content visit expertconsult.com

Content Strategists: Sue Hodgson, Belinda Kuhn
Content Development Specialists: Poppy Garraway, Louise Cook, Alexandra Mortimer
Content Coordinators: Emma Cole, Trinity Hutton, Sam Crowe
Project Managers: Caroline Jones, Cheryl Brant
Design: Stewart Larking, Miles Hitchen
Illustration Manager: Jennifer Rose
Illustrator: Antbits
Marketing Manager: Helena Mutak
Technical Copyeditors: Darren Smith, Colin Woon
Video Reviewers: Leigh Jansen, James Saunders
Artwork Reviewer: Priya Chadha

Plastic Surgery

THIRD EDITION

Volume One

Principles

Editor in Chief

Peter C. Neligan
MB, FRCS(I), FRCSC, FACS
Professor of Surgery
Department of Surgery, Division of Plastic Surgery
University of Washington
Seattle, WA, USA

Volume Editor

Geoffrey C. Gurtner
MD, FACS
Professor and Associate Chairman
Stanford University Department of Surgery
Stanford, CA, USA

ELSEVIER
SAUNDERS   London, New York, Oxford, St Louis, Sydney, Toronto

ELSEVIER
SAUNDERS

Notices

Knowledge and best practice in this field are constantly changing. As new research and experience broaden our understanding, changes in research methods, professional practices, or medical treatment may become necessary.

Practitioners and researchers must always rely on their own experience and knowledge in evaluating and using any information, methods, compounds, or experiments described herein. In using such information or methods they should be mindful of their own safety and the safety of others, including parties for whom they have a professional responsibility.

With respect to any drug or pharmaceutical products identified, readers are advised to check the most current information provided (i) on procedures featured or (ii) by the manufacturer of each product to be administered, to verify the recommended dose or formula, the method and duration of administration, and contraindications. It is the responsibility of practitioners, relying on their own experience and knowledge of their patients, to make diagnoses, to determine dosages and the best treatment for each individual patient, and to take all appropriate safety precautions.

To the fullest extent of the law, neither the Publisher nor the authors, contributors, or editors, assume any liability for any injury and/or damage to persons or property as a matter of products liability, negligence or otherwise, or from any use or operation of any methods, products, instructions, or ideas contained in the material herein.

Volume 1 ISBN: 978-1-4557-1052-2
Volume 1 Ebook ISBN: 978-1-4557-4040-6
6 volume set ISBN: 978-1-4377-1733-4

ELSEVIER your source for books, journals and multimedia in the health sciences

www.elsevierhealth.com

Working together to grow
libraries in developing countries

www.elsevier.com | www.bookaid.org | www.sabre.org

ELSEVIER   BOOK AID International   Sabre Foundation

The publisher's policy is to use **paper manufactured from sustainable forests**

Printed in China
Last digit is the print number: 9   8   7   6   5   4   3   2   1

Contents

Volume Six: Hand and Upper Extremity

James Chang

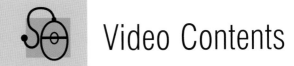

Video Contents

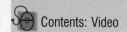

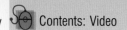

Foreword

In many ways, a textbook defines a particular discipline, and this is especially true in the evolution of modern plastic surgery. The publication of Zeis's *Handbuch der Plastischen Chirurgie* in 1838 popularized the name of the specialty but von Graefe in his monograph *Rhinoplastik*, published in 1818, had first used the title "plastic". At the turn of the last century, Nélaton and Ombredanne compiled what was available in the nineteenth century literature and published in Paris a two volume text in 1904 and 1907. A pivotal book, published across the Atlantic, was that of Vilray Blair, entitled *Surgery and Diseases of the Jaws* (1912). It was, however, limited to a specific anatomic region of the human body, but it became an important handbook for the military surgeons of World War I. Gillies' classic *Plastic Surgery of the Face* (1920) was also limited to a single anatomic region and recapitulated his remarkable and pioneering World War I experience with reconstructive plastic surgery of the face. Davis' textbook, *Plastic Surgery: Its Principles and Practice* (1919), was probably the first comprehensive definition of this young specialty with its emphasis on plastic surgery as ranging from the "top of the head to the soles of the feet." Fomon's *The Surgery of Injury and Plastic Repair* (1939) reviewed all of the plastic surgery techniques available at that time, and it also served as a handbook for the military surgeons of World War II. Kazanjian and Converse's *The Surgical Treatment of Facial Injuries* (1949) was a review of the former's lifetime experience as a plastic surgeon, and the junior author's World War II experience. The comprehensive plastic surgery text entitled *Plastic and Reconstructive Surgery*, published in 1948 by Padgett and Stephenson, was modeled more on the 1919 Davis text.

The lineage of the Neligan text began with the publication of Converse's five volume *Reconstructive Plastic Surgery* in 1964. Unlike his co-authored book with Kazanjian 15 years earlier, Converse undertook a comprehensive view of plastic surgery as the specialty existed in mid-20th century. Chapters were also devoted to pertinent anatomy, research and the role of relevant specialties like anesthesiology and radiology. It immediately became the bible of the specialty. He followed up with a second edition published in 1977, and I was the Assistant Editor. The second edition had grown from five to seven volumes (3970 pages) because the specialty had also grown. I edited the 1990 edition which had grown to eight volumes and 5556 pages; the hand section was edited by J. William Littler and James W. May. I changed the name of the text from *Reconstructive Plastic Surgery* to *Plastic Surgery* because in my mind I could not fathom the distinction between both titles. To the mother of a child with cleft lip, the surgery is "cosmetic," and many of the facelift procedures at that time were truly reconstructive because of the multiple layers at which the facial soft tissues were being readjusted. The late Steve Mathes edited the 2006 edition in eight volumes. He changed the format somewhat and V.R. Hentz was the hand editor. At that time, the text had grown to more than 7000 pages.

The education of the plastic surgeon and the reference material that is critically needed are no longer limited to the printed page or what is described in modern parlance as "hard copy". Certainly, Gutenberg's invention of movable type printing around 1439 allowed publication and distribution of the classic texts of Vesalius (*Fabrica*, 1543) and Tagliacozzi (*De Curtorum Chirurgia Per Insitionem* (1597) and for many years, this was the only medium in which surgeons could be educated. However, by the nineteenth century, travel had become easier with the development of reliable railroads and oceangoing ships, and surgeons conscientiously visited different surgical centers and attended organized meetings. The American College of Surgeons after World War II pioneered the use of operating room movies, and this was followed by videos. The development of the internet has, however, placed almost all information at the fingertips of surgeons around the world with computer access. In turn, we now have virtual surgery education in which the student or surgeon sitting at a computer is interactive with a software program containing animations, intraoperative videos with sound overlay, and access to the world literature on a particular subject. We are rapidly progressing from the bound book of the Gutenberg era to the currently ubiquitous hand held device or tablet for the mastery of surgical/knowledge.

The Neligan text continues this grand tradition of surgical education by bringing the reader into the modern communications world. In line with advances of the electronic era, there is extra online content such as relevant history, complete reference lists and videos. The book is also available as an e-book. It has been a monumental task, consuming hours of work by the editor and all of its participants. The "text" still defines the specialty of plastic surgery. Moreover, it ensures that a new generation of plastic surgeons will have access to all that is known. They, in turn, will not only carry this information into the future but will also build on it. Kudos to Peter Neligan and his colleagues for continuing the chronicle of the plastic surgery saga that has been evolving over two millennia.

Joseph G. McCarthy, MD
2012

Preface

I have always loved textbooks. When I first started my training I was introduced to Converse's *Reconstructive Plastic Surgery*, then in its second edition. I was over-awed by the breadth of the specialty and the expertise contained within its pages. As a young plastic surgeon in practice I bought the first edition of this book, *Plastic Surgery*, edited by Dr. Joseph McCarthy and found it an invaluable resource to which I constantly referred. I was proud to be asked to contribute a chapter to the second edition, edited by Dr. Stephen Mathes and never thought that I would one day be given the responsibility for editing the next edition of the book. I consider this to be the definitive text on our specialty so I took that responsibility very seriously. The result is a very changed book from the previous edition, reflecting changes in the specialty, changes in presentation styles and changes in how textbooks are used.

In preparation for the task, I read the previous edition from cover to cover and tried to identify where major changes could occur. Inevitably in a text this size, there is some repetition and overlap. So the first job was to identify where the repetition and overlap occurred and try to eliminate it. This allowed me to condense some of the material and, along with some other changes, enabled me to reduce the number of volumes from 8 to 6. Reading the text led me to another realization. That is that the breadth of the specialty, impressive when I was first introduced to it, is even more impressive now, 30 years later and it continues to evolve. For this reason I quickly realized that in order to do this project justice, I could not do it on my own. My solution was to recruit volume editors for each of the major areas of practice as well as a video editor for the procedural videos. Drs. Gurtner, Warren, Rodriguez, Losee, Song, Grotting, Chang and Van Beek have done an outstanding job and this book truly represents a team effort.

Publishing is at a crossroads. The digital age has made information much more immediate, much more easy to access and much more flexible in how it is presented. We have tried to reflect that in this edition. The first big change is that everything is in color. All the illustrations have been re-drawn and the vast majority of patient photographs are in color. Chapters on anatomy have been highlighted with a red tone to make them easier to find as have pediatric chapters which have been highlighted in green. Reflecting on the way I personally use textbooks, I realized that while I like access to references, I rarely read the list of references at the end of a chapter. When I do though, I frequently pull some papers to read. So you will notice that we have kept the most important references in the printed text but we have moved the rest to the web. However, this has allowed us to greatly enhance the usefulness of the references. All the references are hyperlinked to PubMed and expertconsult facilitates a search across all volumes. Furthermore, while every chapter has a section devoted to the history of the topic, this is again something I like to be able to access but rarely have the leisure to read. That section in each of the chapters has also been moved to the web. This not only relieved the pressure on space in the printed text but also allowed us to give the authors more freedom in presenting the history of the topic. As well, there are extra illustrations in the web version that we simply could not accommodate in the printed version. The web edition of the book is therefore more complete than the printed version and owning the book, automatically gets one access to the web. A mouse icon has been added to the text to mark where further content is available online. In this digital age, video has become a very important way to impart knowledge. More than 160 procedural videos contributed by leading experts around the world accompany these volumes. These videos cover the full scope of our specialty. This text is also available as an e-Book.

This book then is very different from its predecessors. It is a reflection of a changing age in communication. However I will be extremely pleased if it fulfils its task of defining the current state of knowledge of the specialty as its predecessors did.

Peter C. Neligan, MB, FRCS(I), FRCSC, FACS
2012

List of Contributors

Neta Adler, MD
Senior Surgeon
Department of Plastic and Reconstructive
Surgery
Hadassah University Hospital
Jerusalem, Israel
*Volume 3, Chapter 40 Congenital melanocytic
nevi*

Ahmed M. Afifi, MD
Assistant Professor of Plastic Surgery
University of Winsconsin
Madison, WI, USA
Associate Professor of Plastic Surgery
Cairo University
Cairo, Egypt
*Volume 3, Chapter 1 Anatomy of the head and
neck*

Maryam Afshar, MD
Post Doctoral Fellow
Department of Surgery (Plastic and
Reconstructive Surgery)
Stanford University School of Medicine
Stanford, CA, USA
*Volume 3, Chapter 22 Embryology of the
craniofacial complex*

Jamil Ahmad, MD, FRCSC
Staff Plastic Surgeon
The Plastic Surgery Clinic
Mississauga, ON, Canada
*Volume 2, Chapter 18 Open technique
rhinoplasty*
*Volume 5, Chapter 8.3 Superior or medial
pedicle*

Hee Chang Ahn, MD, PhD
Professor
Department of Plastic and Reconstructive
Surgery
Hanyang University Hospital, School of
Medicine
Seoul, South Korea
Volume 6, Chapter 22 Ischemia of the hand
*Volume 6, Video 22.01 Radial artery periarterial
sympathectomy*
*Volume 6, Video 22.02 Ulnar artery periarterial
sympathectomy*
*Volume 6, Video 22.03 Digital artery periarterial
sympathectomy*

Tae-Joo Ahn, MD
Jeong-Won Aesthetic Plastic Surgical Clinic
Seoul, South Korea
*Volume 2, Video 10.01 Eyelidplasty non-
incisional method*
Volume 2, Video 10.02 Incisional method

Lisa E. Airan, MD
Assistant Clinical Professor
Department of Dermatology
Mount Sinai Hospital
Aesthetic Dermatologist
Private Practice
New York, NY, USA
Volume 2, Chapter 4 Soft-tissue fillers

Sammy Al-Benna, MD, PhD
Specialist in Plastic and Aesthetic Surgery
Department of Plastic Surgery
Burn Centre, Hand Centre, Operative
Reference Centre for Soft Tissue Sarcoma
BG University Hospital Bergmannsheil, Ruhr
University Bochum
Bochum, North Rhine-Westphalia, Germany
*Volume 4, Chapter 18 Acute management of
burn/electrical injuries*

Amy K. Alderman, MD, MPH
Private Practice
Atlanta, GA, USA
*Volume 1, Chapter 10 Evidence-based medicine
and health services research in plastic surgery*

Robert J. Allen, MD
Clinical Professor of Plastic Surgery
Department of Plastic Surgery
New York University Medical Centre
Charleston, SC, USA
*Volume 5, Chapter 18 The deep inferior
epigastric artery perforator (DIEAP) flap*
*Volume 5, Chapter 19 Alternative flaps for breast
reconstruction*
*Volume 5, Video 18.02 DIEP flap breast
reconstruction*

Mohammed M. Al Kahtani, MD, FRCSC
Clinical Fellow
Division of Plastic Surgery
Department of Surgery
University of Alberta
Edmonton, AB, Canada
*Volume 1, Chapter 33 Facial prosthetics in
plastic surgery*

Faisal Al-Mufarrej, MB, BCh
Chief Resident in Plastic Surgery
Division of Plastic Surgery
Department of Surgery
Mayo Clinic
Rochester, MN, USA
*Volume 6, Chapter 20 Osteoarthritis in the hand
and wrist*

Gary J. Alter, MD
Assistant Clinical Professor
Division of Plastic Surgery
University of Califronia at Los Angeles School
of Medicine
Los Angeles, CA, USA
Volume 2, Chapter 31 Aesthetic genital surgery

Al Aly, MD, FACS
Director of Aesthetic Surgery
Professor of Plastic Surgery
Aesthetic and Plastic Surgery Institute
University of California
Irvine, CA, USA
Volume 2, Chapter 27 Lower bodylifts

Khalid Al-Zahrani, MD, SSC-PLAST
Assistant Professor
Consultant Plastic Surgeon
King Khalid University Hospital
King Saud University
Riyadh, Saudi Arabia
Volume 2, Chapter 27 Lower bodylifts

Kenneth W. Anderson, MD
Marietta Facial Plastic Surgery & Aesthetics
Center
Mareitta, GA, USA
Volume 2, Video 23.04 FUE FOX procedure

Alice Andrews, PhD
Instructor
The Dartmouth Institute for Health Policy and
Clinical Practice
Lebanon, NH, USA
*Volume 5, Chapter 12 Patient-centered health
communication*

Louis C. Argenta, MD
Professor of Plastic and Reconstructive Surgery
Department of Plastic Surgery
Wake Forest Medical Center
Winston Salem, NC, USA
*Volume 1, Chapter 27 Principles and applications
of tissue expansion*

Charlotte E. Ariyan, MD, PhD
Surgical Oncologist
Gastric and Mixed Tumor Service
Memorial Sloan-Kettering Cancer Center
New York, NY, USA
Volume 3, Chapter 14 Salivary gland tumors

Stephan Ariyan, MD, MBA
Clinical Professor of Surgery
Plastic Surgery
Otolaryngology Yale University School of
Medicine Associate Chief
Department of Surgery
Yale New Haven Hospital Director
Yale Cancer Center Melanoma Program
New Haven, CT, USA
Volume 1, Chapter 31 Melanoma
Volume 3, Chapter 14 Salivary gland tumors

Bryan S. Armijo, MD
Plastic Surgery Chief Resident
Department of Plastic and Reconstructive
Surgery
Case Western Reserve/University Hospitals
Cleveland, OH, USA
*Volume 2, Chapter 20 Airway issues and the
deviated nose*

Eric Arnaud, MD
Chirurgie Plastique et Esthétique
Chirurgie Plastique Crânio-faciale
Unité de chirurgie crânio-faciale du
departement de neurochirurgie
Hôpital Necker Enfants Malades
Paris, France
Volume 3, Chapter 32 Orbital hypertelorism

Christopher E. Attinger, MD
Chief, Division of Wound Healing
Department of Plastic Surgery
Georgetown University Hospital
Georgetown, WA, USA
Volume 4, Chapter 8 Foot reconstruction

Tomer Avraham, MD
Resident, Plastic Surgery
Institute of Reconstructive Plastic Surgery
NYU Medical Center
New York, NY, USA
*Volume 1, Chapter 12 Principles of cancer
management*

Kodi K. Azari, MD, FACS
Associate Professor of Orthopaedic Surgery
Plastic Surgery Chief
Section of Reconstructive Transplantation
Department of Orthopaedic Surgery and
Surgery
David Geffen School of Medicine at UCLA
Los Angeles, CA, USA
*Volume 6, Chapter 15 Benign and malignant
tumors of the hand*

Sérgio Fernando Dantas de Azevedo, MD
Member
Brazilian Society of Plastic Surgery
Volunteer Professor of Plastic Surgery
Department of Plastic Surgery
Federal University of Pernambuco
Permambuco, Brazil
Volume 2, Chapter 26 Lipoabdominoplasty
*Volume 2, Video 26.01 Lipobdominoplasty
(including secondary lipo)*

Daniel C. Baker, MD
Professor of Surgery
Insitiute of Reconstructive Plastic Surgery
New York University Medical Center
Department of Plastic Surgery
New York, NY, USA
*Volume 2, Chapter 11.5 Facelift: Lateral
SMASectomy*

Steven B. Baker, MD, DDS, FACS
Associate Professor and Program Director
Co-director Inova Hospital for Children
Craniofacial Clinic
Department of Plastic Surgery
Georgetown University Hospital
Georgetown, WA, USA
*Volume 3, Chapter 30 Cleft and craniofacial
orthognathic surgery*

Karim Bakri, MD, MRCS
Chief Resident
Division of Plastic Surgery
Mayo Clinic
Rochester, MN, USA
*Volume 6, Chapter 20 Osteoarthritis in the hand
and wrist*

Carla Baldrighi, MD
Staff Surgeon
Reconstructive Microsurgery Unit
Azienda Ospedaliera Universitaria Careggi
Florence, Italy
*Volume 6, Chapter 30 Growth considerations in
pediatric upper extremity trauma and
reconstruction*
*Volume 6, Video 30.01 Epiphyseal transplant
harvesting technique*

Jonathan Bank, MD
Resident, Section of Plastic and Reconstructive
Surgery
Department of Surgery
Pritzker School of Medicine
University of Chicago Medical Center
Chicago, IL, USA
*Volume 4, Chapter 12 Abdominal wall
reconstruction*

A. Sina Bari, MD
Chief Resident
Division of Plastic and Reconstructive Surgery
Stanford University Hospital and Clinics
Stanford, CA, USA
*Volume 1, Chapter 16 Scar prevention,
treatment, and revision*

Scott P. Bartlett, MD
Professor of Surgery
Peter Randall Endowed Chair in Pediatric
Plastic Surgery
Childrens Hospital of Philadelphia, University of
Philadelphia
Philadelphia, PA, USA
*Volume 3, Chapter 34 Nonsyndromic
craniosynostosis*

Fritz E. Barton, Jr., MD
Clinical Professor
Department of Plastic Surgery
University of Texas Southwestern Medical
Center
Dallas, TX, USA
*Volume 2, Chapter 11.7 Facelift: SMAS with skin
attached – the "high SMAS" technique*
*Volume 2, Video 11.07.01 The High SMAS
technique with septal reset*

Bruce S. Bauer, MD, FACS, FAAP
Director of Pediatric Plastic Surgery, Clinical
Professor of Surgery
Northshore University Healthsystem
University of Chicago, Pritzker School of
Medicine, Highland Park Hospital
Chicago, IL, USA
*Volume 3, Chapter 40 Congenital melanocytic
nevi*

Ruediger G.H. Baumeister, MD, PhD
Professor of Surgery Emeritus
Consultant in Lymphology
Ludwig Maximilians University
Munich, Germany
*Volume 4, Chapter 3 Lymphatic reconstruction of
the extremities*

Leslie Baumann, MD
CEO
Baumann Cosmetic and Research Institute
Miami, FL, USA
*Volume 2, Chapter 2 Non surgical skin care and
rejuvenation*

Adriane L. Baylis, PhD
Speech Scientist
Section of Plastic and Reconstructive Surgery
Nationwide Children's Hospital
Columbus, OH, USA
*Volume 3, Chapter 28 Velopharyngeal
dysfunction*
*Volume 3, Video 28 Velopharyngeal
incompetence (1-3)*

Elisabeth Beahm, MD, FACS
Professor
Department of Plastic Surgery
University of Texas MD Anderson Cancer
Center
Houston, TX, USA
*Volume 5, Chapter 10 Breast cancer: Diagnosis
therapy and oncoplastic techniques*
*Volume 5, Video 10.01 Breast cancer: diagnosis
and therapy*

Michael L. Bentz, MD, FAAP, FACS
Professor of Surgery Pediatrics and
Neurosurgery Chairman
Chairman of Clinical Affairs
Department of Surgery
Division of Plastic Surgery Vice
University of Winconsin School of Medicine and
Public Health
Madison, WI, USA
Volume 3, Chapter 42 Pediatric tumors

Aaron Berger, MD, PhD
Resident
Division of Plastic Surgery, Department of
Surgery
Stanford University Medical Center
Palo Alto, CA, USA
Volume 1, Chapter 31 Melanoma

Pietro Berrino, MD
Teaching Professor
University of Milan
Director
Chirurgia Plastica Genova SRL
Genoa, Italy
Volume 5, Chapter 23 Poland's syndrome

Valeria Berrino, MS
In Training
Chirurgia Plastica Genova SRL
Genoa, Italy
Volume 5, Chapter 23 Poland's syndrome

Miles G. Berry, MS, FRCS(Plast)
Consultant Plastic and Aesthetic Surgeon
Institute of Cosmetic and Reconstructive
Surgery
London, UK
*Volume 2, Chapter 11.3 Facelift: Platysma-SMAS
plication*
*Volume 2, Video 11.03.01 Facelift – Platysma
SMAS plication*

Robert M. Bernstein, MD, FAAD
Associate Clinical Professor
Department of Dermatology
College of Physicians and Surgeons
Columbia University
Director
Private Practice
Bernstein Medical Center for Hair Restoration
New York, NY, USA
Volume 2, Video 23.04 FUE FOX procedure
*Volume 2, Video 23.02 Follicular unit hair
transplantation*

Michael Bezuhly, MD, MSc, SM, FRCSC
Assistant Professor
Department of Surgery, Division of Plastic and
Reconstructive Surgery
IWK Health Centre, Dalhousie University
Halifax, NS, Canada
*Volume 6, Chapter 23 Nerve entrapment
syndromes*
*Volume 6, Video 23.01-04 Carpal tunnel and
cubital tunnel releases in the same patient in one
procedure with field sterility – local anaesthetic
and surgery*

Sean M. Bidic, MD, MFA, FAAP, FACS
Private Practice
American Surgical Arts
Vineland, NJ, USA
Volume 6, Chapter 16 Infections of the hand

Phillip N. Blondeel, MD, PhD, FCCP
Professor of Plastic Surgery
Department of Plastic and Reconstructive
Surgery
University Hospital Gent
Gent, Belgium
*Volume 5, Chapter 18 The deep inferior
epigastric artery perforator (DIEAP) Flap*
*Volume 5, Chapter 19 Alternative flaps for breast
reconstruction*
*Volume 5, Video 18.02 DIEP flap breast
reconstruction*

Sean G. Boutros, MD
Assistant Professor of Surgery
Weill Cornell Medical College (Houston)
Clinical Instructor
University of Texas School of Medicine
(Houston)
Houston Plastic and Craniofacial Surgery
Houston, TX, USA
*Volume 3, Video 7.02 Reconstruction of
acquired ear deformities*

Lorenzo Borghese, MD
Plastic Surgeon
General Surgeon
Department of Plastic and Maxillo Facial
Surgery
Director of International Cooperation South
East Asia
Pediatric Hospital "Bambino Gesu'"
Rome, Italy
*Volume 4, Chapter 19 Extremity burn
reconstruction*
*Volume 4, Video 19.01 Extremity burn
reconstruction*

Trevor M. Born, MD, FRCSC
Lecturer
Division of Plastic and Reconstructive Surgery
The University of Toronto
Toronto, Ontario, Canada
Attending Physician
Lenox Hill Hospital
New York, NY, USA
Volume 2, Chapter 4 Soft-tissue fillers

Gregory H. Borschel, MD, FAAP, FACS
Assistant Professor
University of Toronto Division of Plastic and
Reconstructive Surgery
Assistant Professor
Institute of Biomaterials and Biomedical
Engineering
Associate Scientist
The SickKids Research Institute
The Hospital for Sick Children
Toronto, ON, Canada
*Volume 6, Chapter 35 Free functioning muscle
transfer in the upper extremity*

Kirsty U. Boyd, MD, FRCSC
Clinical Fellow – Hand Surgery
Department of Surgery – Division of Plastic
Surgery
Washington University School of Medicine
St. Louis, MO, USA
*Volume 1, Chapter 22 Repair and grafting of
peripheral nerve*
Volume 6, Chapter 33 Nerve transfers

James P. Bradley, MD
Professor of Plastic and Reconstructive Surgery
Department of Surgery
University of California, Los Angeles David
Geffen School of Medicine
Los Angeles, CA, USA
Volume 3, Chapter 33 Craniofacial clefts

Burton D. Brent, MD
Private Practice
Woodside, CA, USA
Volume 3, Chapter 7 Reconstruction of the ear

Mitchell H. Brown, MD, Med, FRCSC
Associate Professor of Plastic Surgery
Department of Surgery
University of Toronto
Toronto, ON, Canada
*Volume 5, Chapter 3 Secondary breast
augmentation*

Samantha A. Brugmann, PHD
Postdoctoral Fellow
Department of Surgery
Stanford University
Stanford, CA, USA
*Volume 3, Chapter 22 Embryology of the
craniofacial complex*

Terrence W. Bruner, MD, MBA
Private Practice
Greenville, SC, USA
Volume 2, Chapter 28 Buttock augmentation
Volume 2, Video 28.01 Buttock augmentation

Todd E. Burdette, MD
Staff Plastic Surgeon
Concord Plastic Surgery
Concord Hospital Medical Group
Concord, NH, USA
*Volume 1, Chapter 36 Robotics, simulation, and
telemedicine in plastic surgery*

Renee M. Burke, MD
Attending Plastic Surgeon
Department of Plastic Surgery
St. Alexius Medical Center
Hoffman Estates, IL, USA
*Volume 3, Chapter 8 Acquired cranial and facial
bone deformities*
*Volume 3, Video 8.01 Removal of venous
malformation enveloping intraconal optic nerve*

Charles E. Butler, MD, FACS
Professor, Department of Plastic Surgery
The University of Texas MD Anderson Cancer
Center
Houston, TX, USA
Volume 1, Chapter 32 Implants and biomaterials

**Peter E. M. Butler, MD, FRCSI, FRCS,
FRCS(Plast)**
Consultant Plastic Surgeon
Honorary Senior Lecturer
Royal Free Hospital
London, UK
*Volume 1, Chapter 34 Transplantation in plastic
surgery*

Yilin Cao, MD
Director, Department of Plastic and
Reconstructive Surgery
Shanghai 9th People's Hospital
Vice-Dean
Shanghai Jiao Tong University Medical School
Shanghai, The People's Republic of China
*Volume 1, Chapter 18 Tissue graft, tissue repair,
and regeneration*
*Volume 1, Chapter 20 Repair, grafting, and
engineering of cartilage*

Joseph F. Capella, MD, FACS
Chief, Post-Bariatric Body Contouring
Division of Plastic Surgery
Hackensack University Medical Center
Hackensack, NJ, USA
Volume 2, Chapter 29 Upper limb contouring
Volume 2, Video 29.01 Upper limb contouring

Brian T. Carlsen, MD
Assistant Professor of Plastic Surgery
Department of Surgery
Mayo Clinic
Rochester, MN, USA
*Volume 6, Chapter 20 Osteoarthritis in the hand
and wrist*

Robert C. Cartotto, MD, FRCS(C)
Attending Surgeon
Ross Tilley Burn Centre
Health Sciences Centre
Toronto, ON, Canada
*Volume 4, Chapter 23 Management of patients
with exfoliative disorders, epidermolysis bullosa,
and TEN*

Giuseppe Catanuto, MD, PhD
Research Fellow
The School of Oncological Reconstructive
Surgery
Milan, Italy
*Volume 5, Chapter 14 Expander/implant breast
reconstructions*
*Volume 5, Video 14.01 Mastectomy and
expander insertion: first stage*
*Volume 5, Video 14.02 Mastectomy and
expander insertion: second stage*

Peter Ceulemans, MD
Assistant Professor
Department of Plastic Surgery
Ghent University Hospital
Ghent, Belgium
*Volume 4, Chapter 13 Reconstruction of male
genital defects*

Rodney K. Chan, MD
Staff Plastic and Reconstructive Surgeon
Burn Center
United States Army Institute of Surgical
Research
Fort Sam
Houston, TX, USA
*Volume 3, Chapter 19 Secondary facial
reconstruction*

David W. Chang, MD, FACS
Professor
Department of Plastic Surgery
MD. Anderson Centre
Houston, TX, USA
*Volume 4, Chapter 3 Lymphatic reconstruction of
the extremities*
*Volume 4, Video 3.01 Lymphatico-venous
anastomosis*
*Volume 6, Chapter 15 Benign and malignant
tumors of the hand*

Edward I. Chang, MD
Assistant Professor
Department of Plastic Surgery
The University of Texas M.D. Anderson Cancer
Center
Houston, TX, USA
*Volume 3, Chapter 17 Carcinoma of the upper
aerodigestive tract*

James Chang, MD
Professor and Chief
Division of Plastic and Reconstructive Surgery
Stanford University Medical Center
Stanford, CA, USA
*Volume 6, Introduction: Plastic surgery
contributions to hand surgery*
*Volume 6, Chapter 1 Anatomy and biomechanics
of the hand*
Volume 6, Video 11.01 Hand replantation
Volume 6, Video 12.01 Debridement technique
*Volume 6, Video 19.01 Extensor tendon rupture
and end-side tendon transfer*
*Volume 6, Video 29.01 Addendum pediatric
trigger thumb release*

Robert A. Chase, MD
Holman Professor of Surgery – Emeritus
Stanford University Medical Center
Stanford, CA, USA
*Volume 6, Chapter 1 Anatomy and biomechanics
of the hand*

Constance M. Chen, MD, MPH
Plastic and Reconstructive Surgeon
Division of Plastic and Reconstructive Surgery
Lenox Hill Hospital
New York, NY, USA
Volume 3, Chapter 9 Midface reconstruction

Philip Kuo-Ting Chen, MD
Director
Department of Plastic and Reconstructive
Surgery
Chang Gung Memorial Hospital and Chang
Gung University
Taipei, Taiwan, The People's Republic of China
Volume 3, Chapter 23 Repair of unilateral cleft lip

Yu-Ray Chen, MD
Professor of Surgery
Department of Plastic and Reconstructive
Surgery
Chang Gung Memorial Hospital
Chang Gung University
Tao-Yuan, Taiwan, The People's Republic of
China
*Volume 3, Chapter 15 Tumors of the facial
skeleton: Fibrous dysplasia*

Ming-Huei Cheng, MD, MBA, FACS
Professor and Chief, Division of Reconstructive
Microsurgery
Department of Plastic and Reconstructive
Surgery
Chang Gung Memorial Hospital
Chang Gung Medical College
Chang Gung University
Taoyuan, Taiwan, The People's Republic of
China
*Volume 3, Chapter 12 Oral cavity, tongue, and
mandibular reconstructions*
*Volume 3, Video 12.02 Ulnar forearm flap for
buccal reconstruction*

You-Wei Cheong, MBBS, MS
Consultant Plastic Surgeon
Department of Surgery
Faculty of Medicine and Health Sciences,
University of Putra Malaysia
Selangor, Malaysia
*Volume 3, Chapter 15 Tumors of the facial
skeleton: Fibrous dysplasia*

Armando Chiari Jr., MD, PhD
Adjunct Professor
Department of Surgery
School of Medicine of the Federal University of
Minas Gerais
Belo Horzonti, Minas Gerais, Brazil
*Volume 5, Chapter 8.5 The L short scar
mammaplasty*

Ernest S. Chiu, MD, FACS
Associate Professor of Plastic Surgery
Department of Plastic Surgery
New York University
New York
USA
*Volume 2, Chapter 9 Secondary blepharoplasty:
Techniques*

Hong-Lim Choi, MD, PhD
Jeong-Won Aesthetic Plastic Surgical Clinic
Seoul, South Korea
Volume 2, Video 10.01 Eyelidplasty non-incisional method
Volume 2, Video 10.02 Incisional method

Jong Woo Choi, MD, PhD
Associate Professor
Department of Plastic and Reconstructive
Surgery
Asan Medical Center
Ulsan University
College of Medicine
Seoul, South Korea
Volume 2, Chapter 10 Asian facial cosmetic surgery

Alphonsus K. Chong, MBBS, MRCS, MMed(Orth), FAMS(Hand Surgery)
Consultant Hand Surgeon
Department of Hand and Reconstructive
Microsurgery
National University Hospital
Assistant Professor
Department of Orthopaedic Surgery
Yong Loo Lin School of Medicine
National University of Singapore
Singapore
Volume 6, Chapter 3 Diagnostic imaging of the hand and wrist
Volume 6, Video 3.01 Diagnostic imaging of the hand and wrist – Scaphoid lunate dislocation

David Chwei-Chin Chuang, MD
Senior Consultant, Ex-President, Professor
Department of Plastic Surgery
Chang Gung University Hospital
Tao-Yuan, Taiwan, The People's Republic of
China
Volume 6, Chapter 36 Brachial plexus injuries-adult and pediatric
Volume 6, Video 36.01-02 Brachial plexus injuries

Kevin C. Chung, MD, MS
Charles B. G. de Nancrede, MD Professor
Section of Plastic Surgery, Department of
Surgery
Assistant Dean for Faculty Affairs
University of Michigan Medical School
Ann Arbor, MI, USA
Volume 6, Chapter 8 Fractures and dislocations of the carpus and distal radius
Volume 6, Chapter 19 Rheumatologic conditions of the hand and wrist
Volume 6, Video 8.01 Scaphoid fixation
Volume 6, Video 19.01 Silicone MCP arthroplasty

Juan A. Clavero, MD, PhD
Radiologist Consultant
Radiology Department
Clínica Creu Blanca
Barcelona, Spain
Volume 5, Chapter 13 Imaging in reconstructive breast surgery

Mark W. Clemens, MD
Assistant Professor
Department of Plastic Surgery
Anderson Cancer Center University of Texas
Houston, TX, USA
Volume 4, Chapter 8 Foot reconstruction
Volume 5, Chapter 15 Latissimus dorsi flap breast reconstruction
Volume 5, Video 15.01 Latissimus dorsi flap technique

Steven R. Cohen, MD
Senior Clinical Research Fellow, Clinical
Professor
Plastic Surgery
University of California
San Diego, CA
Director
Craniofacial Surgery
Rady Children's Hospital, Private Practice,
FACES+ Plastic Surgery, Skin and Laser Center
La Jolla, CA, USA
Volume 2, Chapter 5 Facial skin resurfacing

Sydney R. Coleman, MD
Clinical Assistant Professor
Department of Plastic Surgery
New York University Medical Center
New York, NY, USA
Volume 2, Chapter 14 Structural fat grafting
Volume 2, Video 14.01 Structural fat grafting of the face

John Joseph Coleman III, MD
James E. Bennett Professor of Surgery,
Department of Dermatology and Cutaneuous
Surgery
University of Miami Miller School of Medicine
Miami, FA
Chief of Plastic Surgery
Department of Surgery
Indiana University School of Medicine
Indianapolis, IN, USA
Volume 3, Chapter 16 Tumors of the lips, oral cavity, oropharynx, and mandible

Lawrence B. Colen, MD
Associate Professor of Surgery
Eastern Virginia Medical School
Norfolk, VA, USA
Volume 4, Chapter 8 Foot reconstruction

E. Dale Collins Vidal, MD, MS
Chief
Section of Plastic Surgery
Dartmouth-Hitchcock Medical Center
Professor of Surgery
Dartmouth Medical School
Director of the Center for Informed Choice
The Dartmouth Institute (TDI) for Health Policy
and Clinical Practice
Hanover, NH, USA
Volume 1, Chapter 10 Evidence-based medicine and health services research in plastic surgery
Volume 5, Chapter 12 Patient-centered health communication

Shannon Colohan, MD, FRCSC
Clinical Instructor, Plastic Surgery
Department of Plastic Surgery
University of Texas Southwestern Medical
Center
Dallas, TX, USA
Volume 4, Chapter 2 Management of lower extremity trauma

Mark B. Constantian, MD, FACS
Active Staff
Saint Joseph Hospital
Nashua, NH (private practice)
Assistant Clinical Professor of Plastic Surgery
Division of Plastic Surgery
Department of Surgery
University of Wisconsin
Madison, WI, USA
Volume 2, Chapter 19 Closed technique rhinoplasty

Peter G. Cordeiro, MD, FACS
Chief
Plastic and Reconstructive Surgery
Memorial Sloan-Kettering Cancer Center
Professor of Surgery
Weill Cornell Medical College
New York, NY, USA
Volume 3, Chapter 9 Midface reconstruction
Volume 4, Chapter 14 Reconstruction of acquired vaginal defects

Christopher Cox, MD
Chief Resident
Department of Orthopaedic Surgery
Stanford University Medical School
Stanford, CA, USA
Volume 6, Chapter 5 Principles of internal fixation as applied to the hand and wrist
Volume 6, Video 5.01 Dynamic compression plating and lag screw technique

Albert Cram, MD
Professor Emeritus
University of Iowa
Iowa City Plastic Surgery
Coralville, IO, USA
Volume 2, Chapter 27 Lower bodylifts

Catherine Curtin, MD
Assistant Professor
Department of Surgery Division of Plastic
Stanford University
Stanford, CA, USA
*Volume 6, Chapter 37 Restoration of upper
extremity function*
*Volume 6, Video 37.01 1 Stage grasp IC 6 short
term*
*Volume 6, Video 37.02 2 Stage grasp release
outcome*

Lars B. Dahlin, MD, PhD
Professor and Consultant
Department of Clinical Sciences, Malmö-Hand
Surgery
University of Lund
Malmö, Sweden
*Volume 6, Chapter 32 Peripheral nerve injuries of
the upper extremity*
Volume 6, Video 32.01 Digital Nerve Suture
Volume 6, Video 32.02 Median Nerve Suture

Dai M. Davies, FRCS
Consultant and Institute Director
Institute of Cosmetic and Reconstructive
Surgery
London, UK
*Volume 2, Chapter 11.3 Facelift: Platysma-SMAS
plication*
*Volume 2, Video 11.03.01 Platysma SMAS
plication*

**Michael R. Davis, MD, FACS, LtCol,
USAF, MC**
Chief
Reconstructive Surgery and Regenerative
Medicine
Plastic and Reconstructive Surgeon
San Antonio Military Medical Center
Houston, TX, USA
*Volume 5, Chapter 1 Anatomy for plastic surgery
of the breast*

Jorge I. De La Torre, MD
Professor and Chief
Division of Plastic Surgery
University of Alabama at Birmingham
Birmingham, AL, USA
*Volume 5, Chapter 1 Anatomy for plastic surgery
of the breast*

A. Lee Dellon, MD, PhD
Professor of Plastic Surgery
Professor of Neurosurgery
Johns Hopkins University
Baltimore, MD, USA
*Volume 4, Chapter 6 Diagnosis and treatment of
painful neuroma and of nerve compression in the
lower extremity*
*Volume 4, Video 6.01 Diagnosis and treatment
of painful neuroma and of nerve compression in
the lower extremity*

Sara R. Dickie, MD
Resident, Section of Plastic and Reconstructive
Surgery
Department of Surgery
University of Chicago Medical Center
Chicago, IL, USA
*Volume 4, Chapter 9 Comprehensive trunk
anatomy*

Joseph J. Disa, MD, FACS
Attending Surgeon
Plastic and Reconstructive Surgery in the
Department of Surgery
Memorial Sloan Kettering Cancer Center
New York, NY, USA
Volume 3, Chapter 9 Midface reconstruction
*Volume 4, Chapter 14 Reconstruction of
acquired vaginal defects*

Risal Djohan, MD
Head of Regional Medical Practice
Department of Plastic Surgery
Cleveland Clinic
Cleveland, OH, USA
*Volume 3, Chapter 1 Anatomy of the head and
neck*

Erin Donaldson, MS
Instructor
Department of Otolaryngology
New York Medical College
Valhalla, NY, USA
*Volume 1, Chapter 36 Robotics, simulation, and
telemedicine in plastic surgery*

Amir H. Dorafshar, MBChB
Assistant Professor
Department of Plastic and Reconstructive
surgery
John Hopkins Medical Institute
John Hopkins Outpatient Center
Baltimore, MD, USA
Volume 3, Chapter 3 Facial fractures

Ivica Ducic, MD, PhD
Professor – Plastic Surgery
Director – Peripheral Nerve Surgery Institute
Department of Plastic Surgery
Georgetown University Hospital
Washington, DC, USA
*Volume 6, Chapter 23 Complex regional pain
syndrome in the upper extremity*

Gregory A. Dumanian, MD, FACS
Chief of Plastic Surgery
Division of Plastic Surgery, Department of
Surgery
Northwestern Feinberg School of Medicine
Chicago, IL, USA
*Volume 4, Chapter 11 Reconstruction of the soft
tissues of the back*
*Volume 6, Chapter 40 Treatment of the upper
extremity amputee*
*Volume 6, Video 40.01 Targeted muscle
reinnervation in the transhumeral amputee –
Surgical technique and guidelines for restoring
intuitive neural control*

William W. Dzwierzynski, MD
Professor and Program Director
Department of Plastic Surgery
Medical College of Wisconsin
Milwaukee, WI, USA
*Volume 6, Chapter 11 Replantation and
revascularization*

L. Franklyn Elliott, MD
Assistant Clinical Professor
Emory Section of Plastic Surgery
Emory University
Atlanta, GA, USA
*Volume 5, Chapter 16 The bilateral pedicled
TRAM flap*
*Volume 5, Video 16.01 Pedicle TRAM breast
reconstruction*

Marco Ellis, MD
Chief Resident
Division of Plastic Surgery
Northwestern Memorial Hospital
Northwestern University, Feinberg School of
Medicine
Chicago, IL, USA
Volume 2, Chapter 8 Blepharoplasty
Volume 2, Video 8.01 Periorbital rejuvenation

Dino Elyassnia, MD
Associate Plastic Surgeon
Marten Clinic of Plastic Surgery
San Francisco, CA, USA
*Volume 2, Chapter 12 Secondary deformities
and the secondary facelift*

Surak Eo, MD, PhD
Chief, Associate Professor
Plastic and Reconstructive Surgery
DongGuk University Medical Center
DongGuk University Graduate School of
Medicine
Gyeonggi-do, South Korea
*Volume 6, Video 34.01 EIP to EPL tendon
transfer*

Elof Eriksson, MD, PhD
Chief
Department of Plastic Surgery
Joseph E. Murray Professor of Plastic and
Reconstructive Surgery
Brigham and Women's Hospital
Boston, MA, USA
*Volume 1, Chapter 11 Genetics and prenatal
diagnosis*

Simon Farnebo, MD, PhD
Consultant Hand Surgeon
Department of Plastic Surgery, Hand Surgery
and Burns
Institution of Clinical and Experimental
Medicine, University of Linköping
Linköping, Sweden
*Volume 6, Chapter 32 Peripheral nerve injuries of
the upper extremity*
Volume 6, Video 32.01 Digital Nerve Suture
Volume 6, Video 32.02 Median Nerve Suture

Jeffrey A. Fearon, MD
Director
The Craniofacial Center
Medical City Children's Hospital
Dallas, TX, USA
Volume 3, Chapter 35 Syndromic craniosynostosis

John M. Felder III, MD
Resident Physician
Department of Plastic Surgery
Georgetown University Hospital
Washington, DC, USA
Volume 6, Chapter 23 Complex regional pain syndrome in the upper extremity

Evan M. Feldman, MD
Chief Resident
Division of Plastic Surgery
Baylor College of Medicine
Houston, TX, USA
Volume 3, Chapter 29 Secondary deformities of the cleft lip, nose, and palate
Volume 3, Video 29.01 Complete takedown
Volume 3, Video 29.02 Abbé flap
Volume 3, Video 29.03 Thick lip and buccal sulcus deformities
Volume 3, Video 29.04 Alveolar bone grafting
Volume 3, Video 29.05 Definitive rhinoplasty

Julius Few Jr., MD
Director
The Few Institute for Aesthetic Plastic Surgery
Clinical Associate
Division of Plastic Surgery
University of Chicago
Chicago, IL, USA
Volume 2, Chapter 8 Blepharoplasty
Volume 2, Video 8.01 Periorbital rejuvenation

Alvaro A. Figueroa, DDS, MS
Director
Rush Craniofacial Center
Rush University Medical Center
Chicago, IL, USA
Volume 3, Chapter 27 Orthodontics in cleft lip and palate management

Neil A. Fine, MD
Associate Professor of Clinical Surgery
Department of Surgery
Northwestern University
Chicago, IL, USA
Volume 5, Chapter 5 Endoscopic approaches to the breast
Volume 5, Video 5.01 Endoscopic transaxillary breast augmentation
Volume 5, Video 5.02 Endoscopic approaches to the breast
Volume 5, Video 11.02 Partial breast reconstruction with a latissimus D

Joel S. Fish, MD, MSc, FRCSC
Medical Director Burn Program
Department of Surgery, University of Toronto,
Division of Plastic and Reconstructive Surgery
Hospital for Sick Children
Toronto, ON, Canada
Volume 4, Chapter 23 Management of patients with exfoliative disorders, epidermolysis bullosa, and TEN

David M. Fisher, MB, BCh, FRCSC, FACS
Medical Director, Cleft Lip and Palate Program
Division of Plastic and Reconstructive Surgery
The Hospital for Sick Children
Toronto, ON, Canada
Volume 3, Video 23.02 Unilateral cleft lip repair – anatomic subunit approximation technique

Jack Fisher, MD
Department of Plastic Surgery
Vanderbilt University
Nashville, TN, USA
Volume 2, Chapter 23 Hair restoration
Volume 5, Chapter 8.1 Reduction mammaplasty
Volume 5, Chapter 8.2 Inferior pedicle breast reduction

James W. Fletcher, MD, FACS
Chief Hand Surgery
Department Plastic and Hand Surgery
Regions Hospital
Assistant Prof. U MN Dept of Surgery and Dept Orthopedics
St. Paul, MN, USA
Volume 6, Video 20.01 Ligament reconstruction tendon interposition arthroplasty of the thumb CMC joint

Joshua Fosnot, MD
Resident
Division of Plastic Surgery
The University of Pennsylvania Health System
Philadelphia, PA, USA
Volume 5, Chapter 17 Free TRAM breast reconstruction
Volume 5, Video 17.01 The muscle sparing free TRAM flap

Ida K. Fox, MD
Assistant Professor of Plastic Surgery
Department of Surgery
Washington University School of Medicine
Saint Louis, MO, USA
Volume 6, Chapter 33 Nerve transfers
Volume 6, Video 33.01 Nerve transfers

Ryan C. Frank, MD, FRCSC
Attending Surgeon
Plastic and Craniofacial Surgery
Alberta Children's Hospital
University of Calgary
Calgary, AB, Canada
Volume 2, Chapter 5 Facial skin resurfacing

Gary L. Freed, MD
Assistant Professor Plastic Surgery
Dartmouth-Hitchcock Medical Center
Lebanon, NH, USA
Volume 5, Chapter 12 Patient-centered health communication

Jeffrey B. Friedrich, MD
Assistant Professor of Surgery, Orthopedics and Urology (Adjunct)
Department of Surgery, Division of Plastic Surgery
University of Washington
Seattle, WA, USA
Volume 6, Chapter 13 Thumb reconstruction (non microsurgical)

Allen Gabriel, MD
Assitant Professor
Department of Plastic Surgery
Loma Linda University Medical Center
Chief of Plastic Surgery
Southwest Washington Medical Center
Vancouver, WA, USA
Volume 5, Chapter 2 Breast augmentation
Volume 5, Chapter 4 Current concepts in revisionary breast surgery
Volume 5, Video 4.01 Current concepts in revisionary breast surgery

Günter Germann, MD, PhD
Professor of Plastic Surgery
Clinic for Plastic and Reconstructive Surgery
Heidelberg University Hospital
Heidelberg, Germany
Volume 6, Chapter 10 Extensor tendon injuries and reconstruction

Goetz A. Giessler, MD, PhD
Plastic Surgeon, Hand Surgeon, Associate Professor of Plastic Surgery, Fellow of the European Board of Plastic Reconstructive and Aesthetic Surgery
BG Trauma Center Murnau
Murnau am Staffelsee, Germany
Volume 4, Chapter 4 Lower extremity sarcoma reconstruction
Volume 4, Video 4.01 Management of lower extremity sarcoma reconstruction

Jesse A. Goldstein, MD
Chief Resident
Department of Plastic Surgery
Georgetown University Hospital
Washington, DC, USA
Volume 3, Chapter 30 Cleft and craniofacial orthognathic surgery

Vijay S. Gorantla, MD, PhD
Associate Professor of Surgery
Department of Surgery, Division of Plastic and
Reconstructive Surgery
University of Pittsburgh Medical Center
Administrative Medical Director
Pittsburgh Reconstructive Transplantation
Program
Pittsburgh, PA, USA
*Volume 6, Chapter 38 Upper extremity
composite allotransplantation*
*Volume 6, Video 38.01 Upper extremity
composite allotransplantation*

Arun K. Gosain, MD
DeWayne Richey Professor and Vice Chair
Department of Plastic Surgery
University Hospitals Case Medical Center
Chief, Pediatric Plastic Surgery
Rainbow Babies and Children's Hospital
Cleveland, OH, USA
Volume 3, Chapter 38 Pierre Robin sequence

Lawrence J. Gottlieb, MD, FACS
Professor of Surgery
Director of Burn and Complex Wound Center
Director of Reconstructive Microsurgery
Fellowship
Section of Plastic and Reconstructive Surgery
Department of Surgery
University of Chicago
Chicago, IL, USA
*Volume 3, Chapter 41 Pediatric chest and trunk
defects*

Barry H. Grayson, DDS
Associate Professor of Surgery (Craniofacial
Orthodontics)
New York University Langone Medical Centre
Institute of Reconstructive Plastic Surgery
New York, NY, USA
Volume 3, Chapter 36 Craniofacial microsomia
Volume 3, Video 24.01 Repair of bilateral cleft lip

Arin K. Greene, MD, MMSc
Associate Professor of Surgery
Department of Plastic and Oral Surgery
Children's Hospital Boston
Harvard Medical School
Boston, MA, USA
Volume 1, Chapter 29 Vascular anomalies

James C. Grotting, MD, FACS
Clinical Professor of Plastic Surgery
University of Alabama at Birmingham;
The University of Wisconsin, Madison, WI;
Grotting and Cohn Plastic Surgery
Birmingham, AL, USA
Volume 5, Chapter 7 Mastopexy
Volume 5, Chapter 8.7 Sculpted pillar vertical
*Volume 5, Video 8.7.01 Marking the sculpted
pillar breast reduction*
Volume 5, Video 8.7.02 Breast reduction surgery

Ronald P. Gruber, MD
Associate Adjunct Clinical Professor
Division of Plastic and Reconstructive Surgery
Stanford University
Associate Clinical Professor
Division of Plastic and Reconstructive Surgery
University of California, San Francisco
San Francisco, CA, USA
Volume 2, Chapter 21 Secondary rhinoplasty

**Mohan S. Gundeti, MB, MCh, FEBU,
FRCS, FEAPU**
Associate Professor of Urology in Surgery and
Pediatrics, Director Pediatric Urology, Director
Centre for Pediatric Robotics and Minimal
Invasive Surgery
University of Chicago and Pritzker Medical
School Comer Children's Hospital
Chicago, IL, USA
*Volume 3, Chapter 44 Reconstruction of
urogenital defects: Congenital*
*Volume 3, Video 44.01 First stage hypospadias
repair with free inner preputial graft*
*Volume 3, Video 44.02 Second stage
hypospadias repair with tunica vaginalis flap*

Eyal Gur, MD
Head
Department of Plastic and Reconstructive
Surgery
The Tel Aviv Sourasky Medical Center
The Tel Aviv University School of Medicine
Tel Aviv, Israel
Volume 3, Chapter 11 Facial paralysis
Volume 3, Video 11.01 Facial paralysis

Geoffrey C. Gurtner, MD, FACS
Professor and Associate Chairman
Stanford University Department of Surgery
Stanford, CA, USA
*Volume 1, Chapter 13 Stem cells and
regenerative medecine*
*Volume 1, Chapter 35 Technology innovation in
plastic surgery*

Bahman Guyuron, MD
Kiehn-DesPrez Professor and Chairman
Department of Plastic Surgery
Case Western Reserve University School of
Medicine
Cleveland, OH, USA
*Volume 2, Chapter 20 Airway issues and the
deviated nose*
*Volume 3, Chapter 21 Surgical management of
migraine headaches*
Volume 2, Video 3.02 Botulinum toxin

Steven C. Haase, MD
Clinical Associate Professor
Department of Surgery, Section of Plastic
Surgery
University of Michigan Health
Ann Arbor, MI, USA
*Volume 6, Chapter 8 Fractures and dislocations
of the carpus and distal radius*

Robert S. Haber, MD, FAAD, FAAP
Assistant Professor, Dermatology and
Pediatrics
Case Western Reserve University School of
Medicine
Director
University Hair Transplant Center
Cleveland, OH, USA
*Volume 2, Video 23.08 Strip harvesting the
haber spreader*

Florian Hackl, MD
Research Fellow
Division of Plastic Surgery
Brigham and Women's Hospital
Harvard Medical School
Boston, MA, USA
*Volume 1, Chapter 11 Genetics and prenatal
diagnosis*

Phillip C. Haeck, MD
Private Practice
Seattle, WA, USA
*Volume 1, Chapter 4 The role of ethics in plastic
surgery*

Bruce Halperin, MD
Adjunct Associate Clinical Professor of
Anesthesia
Department of Anesthesia
Stanford University School of Medicine
Palo Alto, CA, USA
*Volume 1, Chapter 8 Patient safety in plastic
surgery*

Moustapha Hamdi, MD, PhD
Professor and Chairman of Plastic and
Reconstructive Surgery
Department of Plastic Surgery
Brussels University Hospital
Brussels, Belgium
*Volume 5, Chapter 21 Local flaps in partial
breast reconstruction*

Warren C. Hammert, MD
Associate Professor of Orthopaedic and
Plastic Surgery
Department of Orthopaedic Surgery
University of Rochester Medical Center
Rochester, NY, USA
*Volume 6, Chapter 7 Hand fractures and joint
injuries*

Dennis C. Hammond, MD
Clinical Assistant Professor
Department of Surgery
Michigan State University College of Human
Medicine
East Lansing
Associate Program Director
Plastic and Reconstructive Surgery
Grand Rapids Medical Education and Research
Center for Health Professions
Grand Rapids, MI, USA
*Volume 5, Chapter 8.4 Short scar periareolar
inferior pedicle reduction (SPAIR) mammaplasty*
Volume 5, Video 8.4.01 Spair technique

Scott L. Hansen, MD, FACS
Assistant Professor of Plastic and
Reconstructive Surgery
Chief, Hand and Microvascular Surgery
University of California, San Francisco
Chief, Plastic and Reconstructive Surgery
San Francisco General Hospital
San Francisco, CA, USA
*Volume 1, Chapter 24 Flap classification and
applications*

James A. Harris, MD
Cosmetic Surgeon
Private Practice
Hasson & Wong Aesthetic Surgery
Vancouver, BC, Canada
Volume 2, Video 23.05 FUE Harris safe system

Isaac Harvey, MD
Clinical Fellow
Department of Paediatric Plastic and
Reconstructive Surgery
Hospital for Sick Kids
Toronto, ON, Canada
*Volume 6, Chapter 35 Free functional muscle
transfers in the upper extremity*

Victor Hasson, MD
Cosmetic Surgeon
Private Practice
Hasson & Wong Aesthetic Surgery
Vancouver, BC, Canada
*Volume 2, Video 23.07 Perpendicular angle
grafting technique*

Theresa A Hegge, MD, MPH
Resident of Plastic Surgery
Division of Plastic Surgery
Southern Illinois University
Springfield, IL, USA
*Volume 6, Chapter 6 Nail and fingertip
reconstruction*

Jill A. Helms, DDS, PhD
Division of Plastic and Reconstructive Surgery
Department of Surgery
School of Medicine
Stanford University
Stanford, CA, USA
*Volume 3, Chapter 22 Embryology of the
craniofacial complex*

Ginard I. Henry, MD
Assistant Professor of Surgery
Section of Plastic Surgery
University of Chicago Medical Center
Chicago, IL, USA
*Volume 4, Chapter 1 Comprehensive lower
extremity anatomy, embryology, surgical exposure*

Vincent R. Hentz, MD
Emeritus Professor of Surgery and Orthopedic
Surgery (by courtesy)
Stanford University
Stanford, CA, USA
*Volume 6, Chapter 1 Anatomy and biomechanics
of the hand*
*Volume 6, Chapter 37 Restoration of upper
extremity function in tetraplegia*
*Volume 6, Video 37.01 1 Stage grasp IC 6 short
term*
*Volume 6, Video 37.02 2 Stage grasp release
outcome*

**Rebecca L. von der Heyde, PhD,
OTR/L, CHT**
Associate Professor
Program in Occupational Therapy
Maryville University
St. Louis, MO, USA
Volume 6, Chapter 39 Hand therapy
*Volume 6, Video 39.01 Hand therapy
Goniometric measurement*
Volume 6, Video 39.02 Threshold testing
*Volume 6, Video 39.03 Fabrication of a
synergistic splint*

Kent K. Higdon, MD
Former Aesthetic Fellow
Grotting and Cohn Plastic Surgery;
Current Assistant Professor
Vanderbilt University
Nashville, TN, USA
Volume 5, Chapter 7 Mastopexy
Volume 5, Chapter 8.1 Reduction mammaplasty
*Volume 5, Chapter 8.7 Sculpted pillar vertical
mammaplasty*

John Hijjawi, MD, FACS
Assistant Professor
Department of Plastic Surgery, Department of
General Surgery
Medical College of Wisconsin
Milwaukee, WI, USA
*Volume 4, Chapter 20 Cold and chemical injury
to the upper extremity*

Jonay Hill, MD
Clinical Assistant Professor
Anesthesiology Department
Anesthesia and Critical Care
Stanford University School of Medicine
Stanford, CA, USA
*Volume 6, Chapter 4 Anesthesia for upper
extremity surgery*

Piet Hoebeke, MD, PhD
Full Senior Professor of Paediatric Urology
Department of Urology
Ghent University Hospital
Ghent, Belgium
*Volume 4, Chapter 13 Reconstruction of male
genital defects*
*Volume 4, Video 13.01 Complete and partial
penile reconstruction*

William Y. Hoffman, MD
Professor and Chief
Division of Plastic and Reconstructive Surgery
University of California, San Francisco
San Francisco, CA, USA
Volume 3, Chapter 25 Cleft palate

Larry H. Hollier Jr., MD, FACS
Professor and Program Director
Division of Plastic Surgery
Baylor College of Medicine and Texas
Children's Hospital
Houston, TX, USA
*Volume 3, Chapter 29 Secondary deformities of
the cleft lip, nose, and palate*
Volume 3, Video 29.01 Complete takedown
Volume 3, Video 29.02 Abbé flap
*Volume 3, Video 29.03 Thick lip and buccal
sulcus deformities*
Volume 3, Video 29.04 Alveolar bone grafting
Volume 3, Video 29.05 Definitive rhinoplasty

Joon Pio Hong, MD, PhD, MMM
Chief and Associate Professor
Department of Plastic Surgery
Asian Medical Center University of Ulsan
School of Medicine
Seoul, Korea
*Volume 4, Chapter 5 Reconstructive surgery:
Lower extremity coverage*

Richard A. Hopper, MD, MS
Chief
Division of Pediatric Plastic Surgery
University of Washington
Surgical Director
Craniofacial Center
Seattle Childrens Hospital
Associate Professor
Division of Plastic Surgery
Seattle, WA, USA
Volume 3, Chapter 26 Alveolar clefts
Volume 3, Chapter 36 Craniofacial microsomia

Philippe Houtmeyers, MD
Resident
Plastic Surgery
Ghent University Hospital
Ghent, Belgium
*Volume 4, Chapter 13 Reconstruction of male
genital defects*
*Volume 4, Video 13.01 Complete and partial
penile reconstruction*

Steven E.R. Hovius, MD, PhD
Head
Department of Plastic, Reconstructive and
Hand Surgery
ErasmusmMC
University Medical Center
Rotterdam, The Netherlands
*Volume 6, Chapter 28 Congenital hand IV
disorders of differentiation and duplication*

Michael A. Howard, MD
Clinical Assistant Professor of Surgery
Division of Plastic Surgery
University of Chicago, Pritzker School of
Medicine
Northbrook, IL, USA
*Volume 4, Chapter 9 Comprehensive trunk
anatomy*

Jung-Ju Huang, MD
Assistant Professor
Division of Microsurgery
Plastic and Reconstructive Surgery
Chang Gung Memorial Hospital
Taoyuan, Taiwan, The People's Republic of
China
*Volume 3, Chapter 12 Oral cavity, tongue, and
mandibular reconstructions*
*Volume 3, Video 12.01 Fibula
osteoseptocutaneous flap for composite
mandibular reconstruction*
*Volume 3, Video 12.02 Ulnar forearm flap for
buccal reconstruction*

C. Scott Hultman, MD, MBA, FACS
Ethel and James Valone Distinguished
Professor of Surgery
Division of Plastic Surgery
University of North Carolina
Chapel Hill, NC, USA
*Volume 1, Chapter 5 Business principles for
plastic surgeons*

Leung-Kim Hung, MChOrtho (Liv)
Professor
Department of Orthopaedics and Traumatology
Faculty of Medicine
The Chinese University of Hong Kong
Hong Kong, The People's Republic of China
*Volume 6, Chapter 29 Congenital hand V
disorders of overgrowth, undergrowth, and
generalized skeletal deformities*

Gazi Hussain, MBBS, FRACS
Clinical Senior Lecturer
Macquarie Cosmetic and Plastic Surgery
Macquarie University
Sydney, Australia
Volume 3, Chapter 11 Facial paralysis

Marco Innocenti, MD
Director Reconstructive Microsurgery
Department of Oncology
Careggi University Hospital
Florence, Italy
*Volume 6, Chapter 30 Growth considerations in
pediatric upper extremity trauma and
reconstruction*
*Volume 6, Video 30.01 Epiphyseal transplant
harvesting technique*

Clyde H. Ishii, MD, FACS
Assistant Clinical Professor of Surgery
John A. Burns School of Medicine
Chief, Department of Plastic Surgery
Shriners Hospital
Honolulu Unit
Honolulu, HI, USA
*Volume 2, Chapter 10 Asian facial cosmetic
surgery*

Jonathan S. Jacobs, DMD, MD
Associate Professor of Clinical Plastic Surgery
Eastern Virginia Medical School
Norfolk, VA, USA
*Volume 2, Chapter 16 Anthropometry,
cephalometry, and orthognathic surgery*
*Volume 2, Video 16.01 Anthropometry,
cephalometry, and orthognathic surgery*

Jordan M.S. Jacobs, MD
Craniofacial Fellow
Department of Plastic Surgery
New York University Langone Medical Center
New York, NY, USA
*Volume 2, Chapter 16 Anthropometry,
cephalometry, and orthognathic surgery*
*Volume 2, Video 16.01 Anthropometry,
cephalometry, and orthognathic surgery*

**Ian T. Jackson, MD, DSc(Hon), FRCS,
FACS, FRACS (Hon)**
Emeritus Surgeon
Surgical Services Administration
William Beaumont Hospitals
Royal Oak, MI, USA
*Volume 3, Chapter 18 Local flaps for facial
coverage*

Oksana Jackson, MD
Assistant Professor of Surgery
Division of Plastic Surgery
University of Pennsylvania School of Medicine
Clinical Associate
The Children's Hospital of Philadelphia
Philadelphia, PA, USA
Volume 3, Chapter 43 Conjoined twins

Jeffrey E. Janis, MD, FACS
Associate Professor
Program Director
Department of Plastic Surgery
University of Texas Southwestern Medical
Center
Chief of Plastic Surgery
Chief of Wound Care
President-Elect
Medical Staff
Parkland Health and Hospital System
Dallas, TX, USA
Volume 4, Chapter 16 Pressure sores

Leila Jazayeri, MD
Resident
Stanford University Plastic and Reconstructive
Surgery
Stanford, CA, USA
*Volume 1, Chapter 35 Technology innovation in
plastic surgery*

Elizabeth B. Jelks, MD
Private Practice
Jelks Medical
New York, NY, USA
*Volume 2, Chapter 9 Secondary blepharoplasty:
Techniques*

Glenn W. Jelks, MD
Associate Professor
Department of Ophthalmology
Department of Plastic Surgery
New York University School of Medicine
New York, NY, USA
*Volume 2, Chapter 9 Secondary blepharoplasty:
Techniques*

Mark Laurence Jewell, MD
Assistant Clinical Professor of Plastic Surgery
Oregon Health Science University
Jewell Plastic Surgery Center
Eugene, OR, USA
*Volume 2, Chapter 11.4 Facelift: Facial
rejuvenation with loop sutures, the MACS lift and
its derivatives*

Andreas Jokuszies, MD
Consultant Plastic, Aesthetic and Hand
Surgeon
Department of Plastic, Hand and
Reconstructive Surgery
Hanover Medical School
Hanover, Germany
*Volume 1, Chapter 15 Skin wound healing:
Repair biology, wound, and scar treatment*

Neil F. Jones, MD, FRCS
Chief of Hand Surgery
University of California Medical Center
Professor of Orthopedic Surgery
Professor of Plastic and Reconstructive Surgery
University of California Irvine
Irvine, CA, USA
Volume 6, Chapter 22 Ischemia of the hand
*Volume 6, Chapter 34 Tendon transfers in the
upper extremity*
*Volume 6, Video 34.01 EIP to EPL tendon
transfer*

David M. Kahn, MD
Clinical Associate Professor of Plastic Surgery
Department of Surgery
Stanford University School of Medicine
Stanford, CA, USA
Volume 2, Chapter 21 Secondary rhinoplasty

Ryosuke Kakinoki, MD, PhD
Associate Professor
Chief of the Hand Surgery and Microsurgery
Unit
Department of Orthopedic Surgery and
Rehabilitation Medicine
Graduate School of Medicine
Kyoto University
Kyoto, Japan
*Volume 6, Chapter 2 Examination of the upper
extremity*
*Volume 2, Video 2.01-2.17 Examination of the
upper extremity*

Alex Kane, MD
Associate Professor of Surgery
Washington University School of Medicine
St. Louis, WO, USA
Volume 3, Chapter 23 Repair of unilateral cleft lip

Gabrielle M. Kane, MBBCh, EdD, FRCPC
Medical Director, Associate Professor
Department of Radiation Oncology
Associate Professor
Department of Medical Education and
Biomedical Informatics
University of Washington School of Medicine
Seattle, WA, USA
*Volume 1, Chapter 28 Therapeutic radiation:
Principles, effects, and complications*

Michael A. C. Kane, MD
Attending Surgeon Manhattan Eye, Ear and
Throat Institute
Department of Plastic Surgery
New York, NY, USA
Volume 2, Chapter 3 Botulinum toxin (BoNT-A)

Dennis S. Kao, MD
Hand Fellow
Department of Plastic Surgery
Medical College of Wisconsin
Milwaukee, WI, USA
*Volume 4, Chapter 20 Cold and chemical injury
to the upper extremity*

Sahil Kapur, MD
Resident, Plastic and Reconstructive Surgery
Department of Surgery, Division of Plastic and
Reconstructive Surgery
University of Wisconsin
Madison, WI, USA
Volume 3, Chapter 42 Pediatric tumors

Leila Kasrai, MD, MPH, FRCSC
Head, Division of Plastic Surgery
St Joseph's Hospital
Toronto, ON, Canada
Volume 2, Video 22.01 Setback otoplasty

Abdullah E. Kattan, MBBS, FRCS(C)
Clinical Fellow
Division of Plastic Surgery
Department of Surgery
University of Toronto
Toronto, ON, Canada
*Volume 4, Chapter 23 Management of patients
with exfoliative disorders, epidermolysis bullosa,
and TEN*

David L. Kaufman, MD, FACS
Private Practice Plastic Surgery
Aesthetic Artistry Surgical and Medical Center
Folsom, CA, USA
Volume 2, Chapter 21 Secondary rhinoplasty

Lindsay B. Katona, BA
Research Associate
Thayer School of Engineering
Dartmouth College
Hanover, NH, USA
*Volume 1, Chapter 36 Robotics, simulation, and
telemedicine in plastic surgery*

Henry K. Kawamoto, Jr., MD, DDS
Clinical Professor
Division of Plastic Surgery
University of California at Los Angeles
Los Angeles, CA, USA
Volume 3, Chapter 33 Craniofacial clefts

Jeffrey M. Kenkel, MD, FACS
Professor and Vice-Chairman
Rod J Rohrich MD Distinguished Professorship
in Wound Healing and Plastic Surgery
Department of Plastic Surgery
Southwestern Medical School
Director
Clinical Center for Cosmetic Laser Treatment
Dallas, TX, USA
*Volume 2, Chapter 24 Liposuction: A
comprehensive review of techniques and safety*

Carolyn L. Kerrigan, MD, MSc
Professor of Surgery
Section of Plastic Surgery
Dartmouth Hitchcock Medical Center
Lebanon, NH, USA
*Volume 1, Chapter 10 Evidence-based medicine
and health services research in plastic surgery*

Marwan R. Khalifeh, MD
Instructor of Plastic Surgery
Department of Plastic Surgery
Johns Hopkins University School of Medicine
Washington, DC, USA
*Volume 4, Chapter 12 Abdominal wall
reconstruction*

Jae-Hoon Kim, MD
April 31 Aesthetic Plastic Surgical Clinic
Seoul, South Korea
*Volume 2, Video 10.03 Secondary rhinoplasty:
septal extension graft and costal cartilage strut
fixed with K-wire*

**Timothy W. King, MD, PhD, MSBE,
FACS, FAAP**
Assistant Professor of Surgery and Pediatrics
Director of Research
Division of Plastic Surgery, Department of
Surgery
University of Wisconsin School of Medicine and
Public Health
Madison, WI, USA
Volume 1, Chapter 32 Implants and biomaterials

Brian M. Kinney, MD, FACS, MSME
Clinical Assistant Professor of Plastic Surgery
University of Southern California School of
Medicine
Los Angeles, CA, USA
*Volume 1, Chapter 7 Photography in plastic
surgery*

Richard E. Kirschner, MD
Chief, Section of Plastic and Reconstructive
Surgery
Director, Ambulatory Surgical Services
Director, Cleft Lip and Palate Center
Co-Director Nationwide Children's Hospital
Professor of Surgery and Pediatrics
Senior Vice Chair, Department of Plastic Surgery
The Ohio State University College of Medicine
Columbus, OH, USA
Volume 3, Chapter 28 Velopharyngeal dysfunction
*Volume 3, Video 28.01-28.03 Velopharyngeal
incompetence*

Elizabeth Kiwanuka, MD
Division of Plastic Surgery
Brigham and Women's Hospital
Harvard Medical School
Boston, MA, USA
*Volume 1, Chapter 11 Genetics and prenatal
diagnosis*

Grant M. Kleiber, MD
Plastic Surgery Resident
Section of Plastic and Reconstructive Surgery
University of Chicago Medical Center
Chicago, IL, USA
*Volume 4, Chapter 1 Comprehensive lower
extremity anatomy, embryology, surgical exposure*

Mathew B. Klein, MD, MS
David and Nancy Auth-Washington Research
Foundation Endowed Chair for Restorative
Burn Surgery
Division of Plastic Surgery
University of Washington
Program Director and Associate Professor
Division of Plastic Surgery
Harborview Medical Center
Seattle, WA, USA
Volume 4, Chapter 22 Reconstructive burn surgery

Kyung S Koh, MD, PhD
Professor of Plastic Surgery
Asan Medical Center, University of Ulsan
School of Medicine
Seoul, Korea
*Volume 2, Chapter 10 Asian facial cosmetic
surgery*

John C. Koshy, MD
Postdoctoral Research Fellow
Division of Plastic Surgery
Baylor College of Medicine
Houston, TX, USA
*Volume 3, Chapter 29 Secondary deformities of
the cleft lip, nose, and palate*
Volume 3, Video 29.01 Complete takedown
Volume 3, Video 29.02 Abbé flap
*Volume 3, Video 29.03 Thick lip and buccal
sulcus deformities*
Volume 3, Video 29.04 Alveolar bone grafting
Volume 3, Video 29.05 Definitive rhinoplasty

Evan Kowalski, BS
Section of Plastic Surgery
University of Michigan Health System
Ann Arbor, MI, USA
Volume 6, Video 19.02 Silicone MCP arthroplasty

Stephen J. Kovach, MD
Assistant Professor of Surgery
Division of Plastic and Reconstructive Surgery
University of Pennsylvannia Health System
Assistant Professor of Surgery
Department of Orthopaedic Surgery
University of Pennsylvannia Health System
Philadelphia, PA, USA
Volume 4, Chapter 7 Skeletal reconstruction

Steven J. Kronowitz, MD, FACS
Professor, Department of Plastic Surgery
MD Anderson Cancer Center
The University of Texas
Houston, TX, USA
*Volume 1, Chapter 28 Therapeutic radiation
principles, effects, and complications*

Todd A. Kuiken, MD, PhD
Director
Center for Bionic Medicine
Rehabilitation Institute of Chicago
Professor
Department of PMandR
Fienberg School of Medicine
Northwestern University
Chicago, IL, USA
*Volume 6, Chapter 40 Treatment of the upper
extremity amputee*
*Volume 6, Video 40.01 Targeted muscle
reinnervation in the transhumeral amputee*

Michael E. Kupferman, MD
Assistant Professor
Department of Head and Neck Surgery
Division of Surgery
The University of Texas MD Anderson Cancer
Center
Houston, TX, USA
*Volume 3, Chapter 17 Carcinoma of the upper
aerodigestive tract*

Robert Kwon, MD
Plastic Surgeon
Regional Plastic Surgery Center
Richardson, TX, USA
Volume 4, Chapter 16 Pressure sores

**Eugenia J. Kyriopoulos, MD, MSc, PhD,
FEBOPRAS**
Attending Plastic Surgeon
Department of Plastic Surgery and Burn Center
Athens General Hospital "G. Gennimatas"
Athens, Greece
*Volume 5, Chapter 21 Local flaps in partial
breast reconstruction*

Donald Lalonde, BSC, MD, MSc, FRCSC
Professor Surgery
Division of Plastic Surgery
Saint John Campus of Dalhousie University
Saint John, NB, Canada
*Volume 6, Chapter 24 Nerve entrapment
syndromes*
*Volume 6, Video 24.01 Carpal tunnel and cubital
tunnel releases*

Wee Leon Lam, MB, ChB, M Phil, FRCS
Microsurgery Fellow
Department of Plastic and Reconstructive
Surgery
Chang Gung Memorial Hospital
Taipei, Taiwan, The People's Republic of China
*Volume 6, Chapter 14 Thumb and finger
reconstruction – microsurgical techniques*
Volume 6, Video 14.01 Trimmed great toe
Volume 6, Video 14.02 Second toe for index
*Volume 6, Video 14.03 Combined second and
third toe for metacarpal hand*

Julie E. Lang, MD, FACS
Assistant Professor of Surgery
Department of surgery
Director of Breast Surgical Oncology
University of Arizona
Tucson, AZ, USA
*Volume 5, Chapter 10 Breast cancer: Diagnosis
therapy and oncoplastic techniques*
*Volume 5, Video 10.01 Breast cancer: diagnosis
and therapy*

Patrick Lang, MD
Plastic Surgery Resident
University of California
San Francisco, CA, USA
*Volume 1, Chapter 24 Flap classification and
applications*

Claude-Jean Langevin, MD, DMD
Assistant Professor University of Central Florida
Department of Surgery MD Anderson Cancer
Center
Plastic and Reconstructive Surgeon
University of Central Florida
Orlando, FL, USA
Volume 2, Chapter 13 Neck rejuvenation

Laurent Lantieri, MD
Department of Plastic Surgery
Hôpital Européen Georges Pompidou
Assistance Publique Hôpitaux de Paris
Paris Descartes University
Paris, France
Volume 3, Chapter 20 Facial transplant
Volume 3, Video 20.1 and 20.2 Facial transplant

Michael C. Large, MD
Urology Resident
Department of Surgery, Division of Urology
University of Chicago Hospitals
Chicago, IL, USA
*Volume 3, Chapter 44 Reconstruction of
urogenital defects: Congenital*
*Volume 3, Video 44.01 First stage hypospadias
repair with free inner preputial graft*
*Volume 3, Video 44.02 Second stage
hypospadias repair with tunica vaginalis flap*

Don LaRossa, MD
Emeritus Professor of Surgery
Division of Plastic and Reconstructive Surgery
Perelman School of Medicine
University of Pennsylvania
Philadelphia, PA, USA
Volume 3, Chapter 43 Conjoined twins

Caroline Leclercq, MD
Consultant Hand Surgeon
Institut de la Main
Paris, France
*Volume 6, Chapter 17 Management of
Dupuytren's disease*

Justine C. Lee, MD, PhD
Chief Resident
Section of Plastic and Reconstructive Surgery
Department
University of Chicago Medical Center
Chicago, IL, USA
*Volume 3, Chapter 41 Pediatric chest and trunk
defects*

W. P. Andrew Lee, MD
The Milton T. Edgerton, MD, Professor and
Chairman
Department of Plastic and Reconstructive
Surgery
Johns Hopkins University School of Medicine
Baltimore, MD, USA
*Volume 1, Chapter 34 Transplantation in plastic
surgery*
*Volume 6, Chapter 38 Upper extremity
composite allotransplantation*
*Volume 6, Video 38.01 Upper extremity
composite tissue allotransplantation*

Valerie Lemaine, MD, MPH, FRCSC
Assistant Professor of Plastic Surgery
Department of Surgery
Division of Plastic Surgery
Mayo Clinic
Rochester, MN, USA
*Volume 1, Chapter 10 Evidence-based medicine
and health services research in plastic surgery*

**Ping-Chung Leung, SBS, OBE, JP, MBBS,
MS, DSc, Hon DSocSc, FRACS, FRCS,
FHKCOS, FHKAM (ORTH)**
Professor Emeritus
Orthopaedics and Traumatology
The Chinese University of Hong Kong
Hong Kong, The People's Republic of China
*Volume 6, Chapter 29 Congenital hand V
disorders of overgrowth, undergrowth, and
generalized skeletal deformities*

Benjamin Levi, MD
Post Doctoral Research Fellow
Division of Plastic and Reconstructive Surgery
Stanford University
Stanford, CA
House Officer
Division of Plastic and Reconstructive Surgery
University of Michigan
Ann Arbor, MI, USA
*Volume 1, Chapter 13 Stem cells and
regenerative medicine*

L. Scott Levin, MD, FACS
Chairman of Orthopedic Surgery
Department of Orthopaedic Surgery
University of Pennsylvania School of Medicine
Philadelphia, PA, USA
Volume 4, Chapter 7 Skeletal reconstruction

Bradley Limmer, MD
Assistant Clinical Professor
Department of Internal Medicine
Division of Dermatology
Associate Clinical Professor
Department of Plastic and Reconstructive
Surgery
Surgeon, Private Practice
Limmer Clinic
San Antonio, TX, USA
*Volume 2, Video 23.02 Follicular unit hair
transplantation*

Bobby L. Limmer, MD
Professor of Dermatology
University of Texas
Surgeon, Private Practice
Limmer Clinic
San Antonio, TX, USA
*Volume 2, Video 23.02 Follicular unit hair
transplantation*

Frank Lista, MD, FRCSC
Medical Director
Burn Program
The Plastic Surgery Clinic
Mississauga, ON, Canada
*Volume 5, Chapter 8.3 Superior or medial
pedicle*

Wei Liu, MD, PhD
Professor of Plastic Surgery
Associate Director of National Tissue
Engineering Research Center
Department of Plastic and Reconstructive
Surgery
Shanghai 9th People's Hospital
Shanghai Jiao Tong University School of
Medcine
Shanghai, The People's Republic of China
*Volume 1, Chapter 18 Tissue graft, tissue repair,
and regeneration*
*Volume 1, Chapter 20 Repair, grafting, and
engineering of cartilage*

Michelle B. Locke, MBChB, MD
Honourary Lecturer
University of Auckland Department of Surgery
Auckland City Hospital Support Building
Grafton, Auckland, New Zealand
*Volume 2, Chapter 1 Managing the cosmetic
patient*

Sarah A. Long, BA
Research Associate
Thayer School of Engineering
Dartmouth College
San Mateo, CA, USA
*Volume 1, Chapter 36 Robotics, simulation, and
telemedicine in plastic surgery*

Michael T. Longaker, MD, MBA, FACS
Deane P. and Louise Mitchell Professor and
Vice Chair
Department of Surgery
Stanford University
Stanford, CA, USA
*Volume 1, Chapter 13 Stem cells and
regenerative medicine*

Peter Lorenz, MD
Chief of Pediatric Plastic Surgery, Director
Craniofacial Surgery Fellowship
Department of Surgery, Division of Plastic
Surgery
Stanford University School of Medicine
Stanford, CA, USA
*Volume 1, Chapter 16 Scar prevention,
treatment, and revision*

Joseph E. Losee, MD, FACS, FAAP
Professor of Surgery and Pediatrics
Chief, Division Pediatric Plastic Surgery
Children's Hospital of Pittsburgh
University of Pittsburgh Medical Center
Pittsburgh, PA, USA
Volume 3, Chapter 31 Pediatric facial fractures

Albert Losken, MD, FACS
Associate Professor Program Director
Emory Division of Plastic and Reconstructive
Surgery
Emory University School of Medicine
Atlanta, GA, USA
*Volume 5, Chapter 11 The oncoplastic approach
to partial breast reconstruction*

Maria M. LoTempio, MD
Assistant Professor in Plastic Surgery
Medical University of South Carolina
Charleston, SC
Adjunct Assistant Professor in Plastic Surgery
New York Eye and Ear Infirmary
New York, NY, USA
*Volume 5, Chapter 19 Alternative flaps for breast
reconstruction*

Otway Louie, MD
Assistant Professor
Division of Plastic and Reconstructive Surgery
Department of Surgery
University of Washington Medical Center
Seattle, WA, USA
Volume 4, Chapter 17 Perineal reconstruction

David W. Low, MD
Professor of Surgery
Division of Plastic Surgery
University of Pennsylvania School of Medicine
Clinical Associate
The Children's Hospital of Philadelphia
Philadelphia, PA, USA
Volume 3, Chapter 43 Conjoined twins

Nicholas Lumen, MD, PhD
Assistant Professor of Urology
Urology
Ghent University Hospital
Ghent, Belgium
*Volume 4, Chapter 13 Reconstruction of male
genital defects*
*Volume 4, Video 13.01 Complete and partial
penile reconstruction*

Antonio Luiz de Vasconcellos Macedo, MD
General Surgery
Director of Robotic Surgery
President of Oncology
Board of Albert Einstein Hospital
Sao Paulo, Brazil
*Volume 5, Chapter 20 Omentum reconstruction
of the breast*

Gustavo R. Machado, MD
University of California Irvine Medical Center
Department of Orthopaedic Surgery, Orange,
CA, USA
*Volume 6, Video 34.01 EIP to EPL tendon
transfer*

Susan E. Mackinnon, MD
Sydney M. Shoenberg, Jr. and Robert H.
Shoenberg Professor
Department of Surgery, Division of Plastic and
Reconstructive Surgery
Washington University School of Medicine
St. Louis, MO, USA
*Volume 1, Chapter 22 Repair and grafting of
peripheral nerve*
Volume 6, Chapter 33 Nerve transfers
Volume 6, Video 33.01 Nerve transfers

Ralph T. Manktelow, BA, MD, FRCS(C)
Professor
Department of Surgery
University of Toronto
Toronto, ON, Canada
Volume 3, Chapter 11 Facial paralysis

Paul N. Manson, MD
Professor of Plastic Surgery
University of Maryland Shock Trauma Unit
University of Maryland and Johns Hopkins
Schools of Medicine
Baltimore, MD, USA
Volume 3, Chapter 3 Facial fractures

Daniel Marchac, MD
Professor
Plastic, Reconstructive and Aesthetic
College of Medicine of Paris Hospitals
Paris, France
Volume 3, Chapter 32 Orbital hypertelorism

Malcom W. Marks, MD
Professor and Chairman
Department of Plastic Surgery
Wake Forest University School of Medicine
Winston-Salem, NC, USA
*Volume 1, Chapter 27 Principles and applications
of tissue expansion*

Timothy J. Marten, MD, FACS
Founder and Director
Marten Clinic of Plastic Surgery
Medical Director
San Francisco Center for the Surgical Arts
San Francisco, CA, USA
*Volume 2, Chapter 12 Secondary deformities
and the secondary facelift*

Mario Marzola, MBBS
Private Practice
Norwood, SA, Australia
Volume 2, Video 23.01 Donor closure tricophytic technique

Alessandro Masellis, MD
Plastic Surgeon
Department of Plastic Surgery and Burn Therapy
Ospedale Civico ARNAS Palermo
Palermo, Italy
Volume 4, Chapter 19 Extremity burn reconstruction

Michele Masellis, MD, PhD
Plastic Surgeon
Former Chief
Professor Emeritus
Department of Plastic Surgery and Burn Unit
ARNAS Civico Hospital
Palermo, Italy
Volume 4, Chapter 19 Extremity burn reconstruction

Jaume Masia, MD, PhD
Professor and Chief
Plastic Surgery Department
Hospital de la Santa Creu i Sant Pau
Universidad Autónoma de Barcelona
Barcelona, Spain
Volume 5, Chapter 13 Imaging in reconstructive breast surgery

David W. Mathes, MD
Associate Professor of Surgery
Department of Surgery, Division of Plastic and Reconstructive Surgery
University of Washington School of Medicine
Chief of Plastic Surgery
Puget Sound Veterans Affairs Hospital
Seattle, WA, USA
Volume 1, Chapter 34 Transplantation in plastic surgery

Evan Matros, MD
Assistant Attending Surgeon
Department of Surgery
Memorial Sloan-Kettering Cancer Center
Assistant Professor of Surgery (Plastic)
Weill Cornell University Medical Center
New York, NY, USA
Volume 1, Chapter 12 Principles of cancer management

G. Patrick Maxwell, MD, FACS
Clinical Professor of Surgery
Department of Plastic Surgery
Loma Linda University Medical Center
Loma Linda, CA, USA
Volume 5, Chapter 2 Breast augmentation
Volume 5, Chapter 4 Current concepts in revisionary breast surgery

Isabella C. Mazzola
Milan, Italy
Volume 1, Chapter 2 History of reconstructive and aesthetic surgery

Riccardo F. Mazzola, MD
Professor of Plastic Surgery
Postgraduate School Plastic Surgery
Maxillo-Facial and Otolaryngolog
Department of Specialistic Surgical Science
School of Medicine
University of Milan
Milan, Italy
Volume 1, Chapter 2 History of reconstructive and aesthetic surgery

Steven J. McCabe, MD, MSc
Assistant Professor
Department of Bioinformatics and Biostatistics
University of Louisville School of Public Health and Information Sciences
Louisville, KY, USA
Volume 6, Chapter 18 Occupational hand disorders

Joseph G. McCarthy, MD
Lawrence D. Bell Professor of Plastic Surgery,
Director Institute of Reconstructive Plastic Surgery and Chair
Department of Plastic Surgery
New York University Langone Medical Center
New York, NY, USA
Volume 3, Chapter 36 Craniofacial microsomia

Mary H. McGrath, MD, MPH
Plastic Surgeon
Division of Plastic Surgery
University of California San Francisco
San Francisco, CA, USA
Volume 1, Chapter 3 Psychological aspects of plastic surgery

Kai Megerle, MD
Research Fellow
Division of Plastic and Reconstructive Surgery
Stanford Medical Center
Stanford, CA, USA
Volume 6, Chapter 10 Extensor tendon injuries

Babak J. Mehrara, MD, FACS
Associate Member, Associate Professor of Surgery (Plastic)
Memorial Sloan-Kettering Cancer Center
Weil Cornell University Medical Center
New York, NY, USA
Volume 1, Chapter 12 Principles of cancer management

Bryan Mendelson, FRCSE, FRACS, FACS
Private Plastic Surgeon
The Centre for Facial Plastic Surgery
Melbourne, Australia
Volume 2, Chapter 6 Anatomy of the aging face

Constantino G. Mendieta, MD, FACS
Private Practice
Miami, FL, USA
Volume 2, Chapter 28 Buttock augmentation
Volume 2, Video 28.01 Buttock augmentation

Frederick J. Menick, MD
Private Practitioner
Tucson, AZ, USA
Volume 3, Chapter 6 Aesthetic nasal reconstruction
Volume 3, Video 6.01 Aesthetic reconstruction of the nose – The 3-stage folded forehead flap for cover and lining,
Volume 3, Video 6.02 Aesthetic reconstruction of the nose-First stage transfer and intermediate operation

Ursula Mirastschijski, MD, PhD
Assistant Professor
Department of Plastic, Hand and Reconstructive Surgery, Burn Center Lower Saxony, Replantation Center
Hannover Medical School
Hannover, Germany
Volume 1, Chapter 15 Skin wound healing: Repair biology, wound, and scar treatment

Takayuki Miura, MD
Emeritus Professor of Orthopedic Surgery
Department of Orthopedic Surgery
Nagoya University School of Medicine
Nagoya, Japan
Volume 6, Chapter 29 Congenital hand V: Disorders of overgrowth, undergrowth, and generalized skeletal deformities

Fernando Molina, MD
Professor of Plastic, Aesthetic and Reconstructive Surgery
Reconstructive and Plastic Surgery
Hospital General "Dr. Manuel Gea Gonzalez"
Universidad Nacional Autonoma de Mexico
Mexico City, Mexico
Volume 3, Chapter 39 Treacher-Collins syndrome

Stan Monstrey, MD, PhD
Professor in Plastic Surgery
Department of Plastic Surgery
Ghent University Hospital
Ghent, Belgium
Volume 4, Chapter 13 Reconstruction of male genital defects
Volume 4, Video 13.01 Complete and partial penile reconstruction

Steven L. Moran, MD
Professor and Chair of Plastic Surgery
Division of Plastic Surgery, Division of Hand and Microsurgery
Professor of Orthopedics
Rochester, MN, USA
Volume 6, Chapter 20 Management of osteoarthritis of the hand and wrist

Luis Humberto Uribe Morelli, MD
Resident of Plastic Surgery
Unisanta Plastic Surgery Department
Sao Paulo, Brazil
Volume 2, Chapter 26 Lipoabdominoplasty
Volume 2, Video 26.01 Lipobdominoplasty
(including secondary lipo)

Robert J. Morin, MD
Plastic Surgeon and Craniofacial Surgeon
Department of Plastic Surgery
Hackensack University Medical Center
Hackensack, NJ
New York Eye and Ear Infirmary
New York, NY, USA
Volume 3, Chapter 8 Acquired cranial and facial
bone deformities

Steven F. Morris, MD, MSc, FRCS(C)
Professor of Surgery
Professor of Anatomy and Neurobiology
Dalhousie University
Halifax, NS, Canada
Volume 1, Chapter 23 Vascular territories

Colin Myles Morrison, MSc (Hons),
FRCSI (Plast)
Consultant Plastic Surgeon
Department of Plastic and Reconstructive
Surgery
St. Vincent's University Hospital
Dublin, Ireland
Volume 2, Chapter 13 Neck rejuvenation
Volume 5, Chapter 18 The deep inferior
epigastric artery perforator (DIEAP) flap

Wayne A. Morrison, MBBS, MD, FRACS
Director
O'Brien Institute
Professorial Fellow
Department of Surgery
St Vincent's Hospital
University of Melbourne
Plastic Surgeon
St Vincent's Hospital
Melbourne, Australia
Volume 1, Chapter 19 Tissue engineering

Robyn Mosher, MS
Medical Editor/Project Manager
Thayer School of Engineering (contract)
Dartmouth College
Norwich, VT, USA
Volume 1, Chapter 36 Robotics, simulation, and
telemedicine in plastic surgery

Dimitrios Motakis, MD, PhD, FRCSC
Plastic and Reconstructive Surgeon
Private Practice
University Lecturer
Department of Surgery
University of Toronto
Toronto, ON, Canada
Volume 2, Chapter 4 Soft-tissue fillers

A. Aldo Mottura, MD, PhD
Associate Professor of Surgery
School of Medicine
National University of Córdoba
Cordoba, Argentina
Volume 1, Chapter 9 Local anesthetics in plastic
surgery

Hunter R. Moyer, MD
Fellow
Department of Plastic and Reconstructive
Surgery
Emory University, Atlanta, GA, USA
Volume 5, Chapter 16 The bilateral Pedicled
TRAM flap

Gustavo Muchado, MD
Plastic surgeon
Division of Plastic and Reconstructive Surgery
and Department of Orthopaedic Surgery
University of California Irvine Medical Center
Orange, CA, USA
Volume 6, Video 34.01 EIP to EPL tendon
transfer

Reid V. Mueller, MD
Associate Professor
Division of Plastic and Reconstructive Surgery
Oregon Health and Science University
Portland, OR, USA
Volume 3, Chapter 2 Facial trauma: soft tissue
injuries

John B. Mulliken, MD
Director, Craniofacial Centre
Department of Plastic and Oral Surgery
Children's Hospital
Boston, MA, USA
Volume 1, Chapter 29 Vascular anomalies
Volume 3, Chapter 24 Repair of bilateral cleft lip

Egle Muti, MD
Associate Professor of Plastic Reconstructive
and Aesthetic Surgery
Department of Plastic Surgery
University of Turin School of Medicine
Turin, Italy
Volume 5, Chapter 23.1 Congenital anomalies of
the breast
Volume 5, Video 23.01.01 Congenital anomalies
of the breast: An example of tuberous breast
type 1 corrected with glandular flap type 1

Maurice Y. Nahabedian, MD
Associate Professor Plastic Surgery
Department of Plastic Surgery
Georgetown University and Johns Hopkins
University
Northwest, WA, USA
Volume 5, Chapter 22 Reconstruction of the
nipple-areola complex
Volume 5, Video 11.01 Partial breast
reconstruction using reduction mammaplasty
Volume 5, Video 11.03 Partial breast
reconstruction with a pedicle TRAM

Foad Nahai, MD, FACS
Clinical Professor of Plastic Surgery
Department of Surgery
Emory University School of Medicine
Atlanta, GA, USA
Volume 2, Chapter 1 Managing the cosmetic
patient

Fabio X. Nahas, MD, PhD
Associate Professor
Division of Plastic Surgery
Federal University of São Paulo
São Paulo, Brazil
Volume 2, Video 24.01 Liposculpture

Deepak Narayan, MS, FRCS (Eng),
FRCS (Edin)
Associate Professor of Surgery
Yale University School of Medicine
Chief
Plastic Surgery
VA Medical Center
West Haven, CT, USA
Volume 3, Chapter 14 Salivary gland tumors

Maurizio B. Nava, MD
Chief of Plastic Surgery Unit
Istituto Nazionale dei Tumori
Milano, Italy
Volume 5, Chapter 14 Expander/implant
reconstruction of the breast
Volume 5, Video 14.01 Mastectomy and
expander insertion: first stage
Volume 5, Video 14.02 Mastectomy and
expander insertion: second stage

Carmen Navarro, MD
Plastic Surgery Consultant
Plastic Surgery Department
Hospital de la Santa Creu i Sant Pau
Universidad Autónoma de Barcelona
Barcelona, Spain
Volume 5, Chapter 13 Imaging in reconstructive
breast surgery

Peter C. Neligan, MB, FRCS(I), FRCSC,
FACS
Professor of Surgery
Department of Surgery, Division of Plastic
Surgery
University of Washington
Seattle, WA, USA
Volume 1, Chapter 1 Plastic surgery and
innovation in medicine
Volume 1, Chapter 25 Flap pathophysiology and
pharmacology
Volume 3, Chapter 10 Cheek and lip
reconstruction
Volume 4, Chapter 3 Lymphatic reconstruction of
the extremities
Volume 3, Video 11.01-03 (1) Facial paralysis (2)
cross fact graft, (3) gracilis harvest
Volume 3, Video 18.01 Facial artery perforator
flap
Volume 4, Video 3.02 Charles Procedure
Volume 5, Video 18.01 SIEA
Volume 5, Video 19.01-19.03 Alternative free
flaps

Jonas A Nelson, MD
Integrated General/Plastic Surgery Resident
Department of Surgery
Division of Plastic Surgery
Perelman School of Medicine
University of Pennsylvania
Philadelphia, PA, USA
Volume 5, Video 17.01 The muscle sparing free TRAM flap

David T. Netscher, MD
Clinical Professor
Division of Plastic Surgery
Baylor College of Medicine
Houston, TX, USA
Volume 6, Chapter 21 The stiff hand and the spastic hand

Michael W. Neumeister, MD
Professor and Chairman
Division of Plastic Surgery
SIU School of Medicine
Springfield, IL, USA
Volume 6, Chapter 6 Nail and fingertip reconstruction

M. Samuel Noordhoff, MD, FACS
Emeritus Superintendent
Chang Gung Memorial Hospitals
Taipei, Taiwan, The People's Republic of China
Volume 3, Chapter 23 Repair of unilateral cleft lip

Christine B. Novak, PT, PhD
Research Associate
Hand Program, Division of Plastic and Reconstructive Surgery
University Health Network, University of Toronto
Toronto, ON, Canada
Volume 6, Chapter 39 Hand therapy

Daniel Nowinski, MD, PhD
Director
Department of Plastic and Maxillofacial Surgery
Uppsala Craniofacial Center
Uppsala University Hospital
Uppsala, Sweden
Volume 1, Chapter 11 Genetics and prenatal diagnosis

Scott Oates, MD
Professor
Department of Plastic Surgery
The University of Texas MD Anderson Cancer Center
Houston, TX, USA
Volume 6, Chapter 15 Benign and malignant tumors of the hand

Kerby Oberg, MD, PhD
Associate Professor
Department of Pathology and Human Anatomy
Loma Linda University School of Medicine
Loma Linda, CA, USA
Volume 6, Chapter 25 Congenital hand 1: embryology, classification, and principles

James P. O'Brien, MD, FRCSC
Associate Professor of Surgery
Dalhousie University
Halifax Nova Scotia
Clinical Associate Professor of Surgery
Memorial University
St. John's Newfoundland
Vice President Research
Innovation and Development
Horizon Health Network
New Brunswick, NB, Canada
Volume 6, Chapter 24 Nerve entrapment syndromes

Andrea J. O'Connor, BE(Hons), PhD
Associate Professor of Chemical and Biomolecular Engineering
Department of Chemical and Biomolecular Engineering
University of Melbourne
Melbourne, VIC, Australia
Volume 1, Chapter 19 Tissue engineering

Rei Ogawa, MD, PhD
Associate Professor
Department of Plastic
Reconstructive and Aesthetic Surgery Nippon Medical School
Tokyo, Japan
Volume 1, Chapter 30 Benign and malignant nonmelanocytic tumors of the skin and soft tissue

Dennis P. Orgill, MD, PhD
Professor of Surgery
Division of Plastic Surgery, Brigham and Women's Hospital
Harvard Medical School
Boston, MA, USA
Volume 1, Chapter 17 Skin graft

Cho Y. Pang, PhD
Senior Scientist
Research Institute
The Hospital for Sick Children
Professor
Departments of Surgery/Physiology
University of Toronto
Toronto, ON, Canada
Volume 1, Chapter 25 Flap pathophysiology and pharmacology

Ketan M. Patel, MD
Resident Physician
Department of Plastic Surgery
Georgetown University Hospital
Washington DC, USA
Volume 5, Chapter 22 Reconstruction of the nipple-areola complex

William C. Pederson, MD, FACS
President and Fellowship Director
The Hand Center of San Antonio
Adjunct Professor of Surgery
The University of Texas Health Science Center at San Antonio
San Antonio, TX, USA
Volume 6, Chapter 12 Reconstructive surgery of the mutilated hand

José Abel de la Peña Salcedo, MD
Secretario Nacional
Federación Iberolatinoamericana de Cirugía Plástica, Estética y Reconstructiva
Director del Instituto de Cirugia Plastica, S.C.
Hospital Angeles de las Lomas
Col.Valle de las Palmas
Huixquilucan, Edo de Mexico, Mexico
Volume 2, Chapter 28 Buttock augmentation
Volume 2, Video 28.01 Buttock augmentation

Angela Pennati, MD
Assistant Plastic Surgeon
Unit of Plastic Surgery
Istituto Nazionale dei Tumori
Milano, Italy
Volume 5, Chapter 14 Expander/implant breast reconstructions
Volume 5, Video 14.01 Mastectomy and expander insertion: first stage
Volume 5, Video 14.02 Mastectomy and expander insertion: second stage

Joel E. Pessa, MD
Clinical Associate Professor of Plastic Surgery
UTSW Medical School
Dallas, TX
Hand and Microsurgery Fellow
Christine M. Kleinert Hand and Microsurgery
Louisville, KY, USA
Volume 2, Chapter 17 Nasal analysis and anatomy

Walter Peters, MD, PhD, FRCSC
Professor of Surgery
Department of Plastic Surgery
University of Toronto
Toronto, ON, Canada
Volume 5, Chapter 6 Iatrogenic disorders following breast surgery

Giorgio Pietramaggiori, MD, PhD
Plastic Surgery Resident
Department of Plastic and Reconstructive Surgery
University Hospital of Lausanne
Lausanne, Switzerland
Volume 1, Chapter 17 Skin graft

John W. Polley, MD
Professor and Chairman
Rush University Medical Center
Department of Plastic and Reconstructive Surgery
John W. Curtin – Chair
Co-Director, Rush Craniofacial Center
Chicago, IL, USA
Volume 3, Chapter 27 Orthodontics in cleft lip and palate management

Bohdan Pomahac, MD
Assistant Professor
Harvard Medical School
Director
Plastic Surgery Transplantation
Medical Director
Burn Center
Division of Plastic Surgery
Brigham and Women's Hospital
Boston, MA, USA
Volume 1, Chapter 11 Genetics and prenatal diagnosis

Julian J. Pribaz, MD
Professor of Surgery Harvard Medical School
Division of Plastic Surgery
Brigham and Women's Hospital
Boston, MA, USA
Volume 3, Chapter 19 Secondary facial reconstruction

Andrea L. Pusic, MD, MHS, FRCSC
Associate Attending Surgeon
Department of Plastic and Reconstructive
Memorial Sloan-Kettering Cancer Center
New York, NY, USA
Volume 1, Chapter 10 Evidence-based medicine and health services research in plastic surgery
Volume 4, Chapter 14 Reconstruction of acquired vaginal defects

Oscar M. Ramirez, MD, FACS
Adjunct Clinical Faculty
Plastic Surgery Division
Cleveland Clinic Florida
Boca Raton, FL, USA
Volume 2, Chapter 11.8 Facelift: Subperiosteal facelift
Volume 2, Video 11.08.01 Facelift: Subperiosteal mid facelift endoscopic temporo-midface

William R. Rassman, MD
Director
Private Practice
New Hair Institution
Los Angeles, CA, USA
Volume 2, Video 23.04 FUE FOX procedure

Russell R. Reid, MD, PhD
Assistant Professor of Surgery, Bernard Sarnat Scholar
Section of Plastic and Reconstructive Surgery
University of Chicago
Chicago, IL, USA
Volume 1, Chapter 21 Repair and grafting of bone
Volume 3, Chapter 41 Pediatric chest and trunk defects

Neal R. Reisman, MD, JD
Chief of Plastic Surgery, Clinical Professor
Plastic Surgery
St. Luke's Episcopal Hospital
Baylor College of Medicine
Houston, TX, USA
Volume 1, Chapter 6 Medico-legal issues in plastic surgery

Dominique Renier, MD, PhD
Pediatric Neurosurgeon
Service de Neurochirurgie Pédiatrique
Hôpital Necker-Enfants Malades
Paris, France
Volume 3, Chapter 32 Orbital hypertelorism

Dirk F. Richter, MD, PhD
Clinical Director
Department of Plastic Surgery
Dreifaltigkeits-Hospital Wesseling
Wesseling, Germany
Volume 2, Chapter 25 Abdominoplasty procedures
Volume 2, Video 25.01 Abdominoplasty

Thomas L. Roberts III, FACS
Plastic Surgery Center of the Carolinas
Spartanburg, SC, USA
Volume 2, Chapter 28 Buttock augmentation
Volume 2, Video 28.01 Buttock augmentation

Federico Di Rocco, MD, PhD
Pediatric Neurosurgery
Hôpital Necker Enfants Malades
Paris, France
Volume 3, Chapter 32 Orbital hypertelorism

Natalie Roche, MD
Associate Professor
Department of Plastic Surgery
Ghent University Hospital
Ghent, Belgium
Volume 4, Chapter 13 Reconstruction of male genital defects
Volume 4, Video 13.01 Complete and partial penile reconstruction

Eduardo D. Rodriguez, MD, DDS
Chief, Plastic Reconstructive and Maxillofacial Surgery, R Adams Cowley Shock Trauma Center
Professor of Surgery
University of Maryland School of Medicine
Baltimore, MD, USA
Volume 3, Chapter 3 Facial fractures

Thomas E. Rohrer, MD
Director, Mohs Surgery
SkinCare Physicians of Chestnut Hill
Clinical Associate Professor
Department of Dermatology
Boston University
Boston, MA, USA
Volume 2, Video 5.02 Facial resurfacing

Rod J. Rohrich, MD, FACS
Professor and Chairman Crystal Charity Ball
Distinguished Chair in Plastic Surgery
Department of Plastic Surgery
Professor and Chairman Betty and Warren
Woodward Chair in Plastic and Reconstructive Surgery
University of Texas Southwestern Medical Center at Dallas
Dallas, TX, USA
Volume 2, Chapter 17 Nasal analysis and anatomy
Volume 2, Chapter 18 Open technique rhinoplasty

Joseph M. Rosen, MD
Professor of Surgery
Division of Plastic Surgery, Department of Surgery
Dartmouth-Hitchcock Medical Center
Lyme, NH, USA
Volume 1, Chapter 36 Robotics, simulation, and telemedicine in plastic surgery

E. Victor Ross, MD
Director of Laser and Cosmetic Dermatology
Scripps Clinic
San Diego, CA, USA
Volume 2, Chapter 5 Facial skin resurfacing

Michelle C. Roughton, MD
Chief Resident
Section of Plastic and Reconstructive Surgery
University of Chicago Medical Center
Chicago, IL, USA
Volume 4, Chapter 10 Reconstruction of the chest

Sashwati Roy, PhD
Associate Professor of Surgery
Department of Surgery
The Ohio State University Medical Center
Columbus, OH, USA
Volume 1, Chapter 14 Wound healing

J. Peter Rubin, MD, FACS
Chief of Plastic Surgery
Director, Life After Weight Loss Body Contouring Program
University of Pittsburgh
Pittsburgh, PA, USA
Volume 2, Chapter 30 Post-bariatric reconstruction
Volume 2, Video 30.01 Post bariatric reconstruction – bodylift procedure
Volume 5, Chapter 25 Contouring of the arms, breast, upper trunk, and male chest in the massive weight loss patient
Volume 5, Video 25.01 Brachioplasty part 1: contouring of the arms
Volume 5, Video 25.02 Bracioplasty part 2: contouring of the arms

Alesia P. Saboeiro, MD
Attending Physician
Private Practice
New York, NY, USA
Volume 2, Chapter 14 Structural fat grafting
Volume 2, Video 14.01 Structural fat grafting of
the face

Justin M. Sacks, MD
Assistant Professor
Department of Plastic and Reconstructive
Surgery
The Johns Hopkins University School of
Medicine
Baltimore, MD, USA
Volume 3, Chapter 17 Carcinoma of the upper
aerodigestive tract
Volume 6, Chapter 15 Benign and malignant
tumors of the hand

Hakim K. Said, MD
Assistant Professor of Surgery
Division of Plastic Surgery
University of Washington
Seattle, WA, USA
Volume 4, Chapter 17 Perineal reconstruction

Michel Saint-Cyr, MD, FRCSC
Associate Professor Plastic Surgery
Department of Plastic Surgery
University of Texas Southwestern Medical
Center
Dallas, TX, USA
Volume 4, Chapter 2 Management of lower
extremity trauma
Volume 4, Video 2.01 Alternative flap harvest

Cristianna Bonneto Saldanha, MD
Resident
General Surgery Department
Santa Casa of Santos Hospital
São Paulo, Brazil
Volume 2, Chapter 26 Lipoabdominoplasty
Volume 2, Video 26.01 Lipobdominoplasty
(including secondary lipo)

Osvaldo Ribeiro Saldanha, MD
Chairman of Plastic Surgery
Unisanta
Santos
Past President of the Brazilian Society of
Plastic Surgery (SBCP)
International Associate Editor of Plastic and
Reconstructive Surgery
São Paulo, Brazil
Volume 2, Chapter 26 Lipoabdominoplasty
Volume 2, Video 26.01 Lipobdominoplasty
(including secondary lipo)

Osvaldo Ribeiro Saldanha Filho, MD
São Paulo, Brazil
Volume 2, Chapter 26 Lipoabdominoplasty
Volume 2, Video 26.01 Lipobdominoplasty
(including secondary lipo)

Douglas M. Sammer, MD
Assistant Professor of Plastic Surgery
Department of Plastic Surgery
University of Texas Southwestern Medical
Center
Dallas, TX, USA
Volume 6, Chapter 19 Rheumatologic conditions
of the hand and wrist

Joao Carlos Sampaio Goes, MD, PhD
Director Instituto Brasileiro Controle Cancer
Chairman
Department Plastic Surgery and Mastology of
IBCC
Sao Paulo, Brazil
Volume 5, Chapter 8.6 Periareolar technique with
mesh support
Volume 5, Chapter 20 Omentum reconstruction
of the breast

Michael Sauerbier, MD, PhD
Chairman and Professor
Department for Plastic, Hand and
Reconstructive Surgery
Cooperation Hospital for Plastic Surgery of the
University Hospital Frankfurt
Academic Hospital University of Frankfurt a.
Main
Frankfurt, Germany
Volume 4, Chapter 4 Lower extremity sarcoma
reconstruction
Volume 4, Video 4.01 Management of lower
extremity sarcoma reconstruction

Hani Sbitany, MD
Plastic and Reconstructive Surgery
Assistant Professor of Surgery
University of California
San Francisco, CA, USA
Volume 1, Chapter 24 Flap classification and
applications

Tim Schaub, MD
Private Practice
Arizona Center for Hand Surgery, PC
Phoenix, AZ, USA
Volume 6, Chapter 16 Infections of the hand

Loren S. Schechter, MD, FACS
Assistant Professor of Surgery
Chief, Division of Plastic Surgery
Chicago Medical School
Chicago, IL, USA
Volume 4, Chapter 15 Surgery for gender identity
disorder

Stephen A. Schendel, MD
Professor Emeritus of Surgery and Clinical
Adjunct Professor of Neurosurgery
Department of Surgery and Neurosurgery
Stanford University Medical Center
Stanford, CA, USA
Volume 3, Chapter 4 TMJ dysfunction and
obstructive sleep apnea

Saja S. Scherer-Pietramaggiori, MD
Plastic Surgery Resident
Department of Plastic and Reconstructive
Surgery
University Hospital of Lausanne
Lausanne, Switzerland
Volume 1, Chapter 17 Skin graft

Clark F. Schierle, MD, PhD
Vice President
Aesthetic and Reconstructive Plastic Surgery
Northwestern Plastic Surgery Associates
Chicaho, IL, USA
Volume 5, Chapter 5 Endoscopic approaches to
the breast

Stefan S. Schneeberger, MD
Visiting Associate Professor of Surgery
Department of Plastic Surgery
Johns Hopkins Medical University
Baltimore, MD, USA
Associate Professor of Surgery
Center for Operative Medicine
Department for Viszeral
Transplant and Thoracic Surgery
Innsbruck Medical University
Innsbruck, Austria
Volume 6, Chapter 38 Upper extremity
composite allotransplantation

Iris A. Seitz, MD, PhD
Director of Research and International
Collaboration
University Plastic Surgery
Rosalind Franklin University
Clinical Instructor of Surgery
Chicago Medical School
University Plastic Surgery, affiliated with
Chicago Medical School, Rosalind Franklin
University
Morton Grove, IL, USA
Volume 1, Chapter 21 Repair and grafting of
bone

Chandan K. Sen, PhD, FACSM, FACN
Professor and Vice Chairman (Research) of
Surgery
Department of Surgery
The Ohio State University Medical Center
Associate Dean
Translational and Applied Research
College of Medicine
Executive Director
OSU Comprehensive Wound Center
Columbus, OH, USA
Volume 1, Chapter 14 Wound healing

Subhro K. Sen, MD
Clinical Assistant Professor
Division of Plastic and Reconstructive Surgery
Robert A. Chase Hand and Upper Limb
Center, Stanford University Medical Center
Palo Alto, CA, USA
Volume 1, Chapter 14 Wound healing
Volume 6, Chapter 4 Anesthesia for upper
extremity surgery
Volume 6, Video 4.01 Anesthesia for upper
extremity surgery

Joseph M. Serletti, MD, FACS
Henry Royster – William Maul Measey
Professor of Surgery and Chief
Division of Plastic Surgery
Vice Chair (Finance)
Department of Surgery
University of Pennsylvania
Philadelphia, PA, USA
Volume 5, Chapter 17 Free TRAM breast
reconstruction
Volume 5, Video 17.01 The muscle sparing free
TRAM flap

Randolph Sherman, MD
Vice Chair
Department of Surgery
Cedars-Sinai Medical Center
Los Angeles, CA, USA
Volume 6, Chapter 12 Reconstructive surgery of
the mutilated hand

Kenneth C. Shestak, MD
Professor of Plastic Surgery
Division of Plastic Surgery
University of Pittsburgh
Pittsburgh, PA, USA
Volume 5, Chapter 9 Revision surgery following
breast reduction and mastopexy
Volume 5, Video 7.01 Circum areola mastopexy

Lester Silver, MD, MS
Professor of Surgery
Department of Surgery/Division of Plastic
Surgery
Mount Sinai School of Medicine
New York, NY, USA
Volume 3, Chapter 37 Hemifacial atrophy

Navin K. Singh, MD, MSc
Assistant Professor of Plastic Surgery
Department of Plastic Surgery
Johns Hopkins University School of Medicine
Washington, DC, USA
Volume 4, Chapter 12 Abdominal wall
reconstruction

Vanila M. Singh, MD
Clinical Associate Professor
Stanford University Medical Center
Department of Anesthesiology and Pain
Management
Stanford, CA, USA
Volume 6, Chapter 4 Anesthesia for upper
extremity surgery

Carla Skytta, DO
Resident
Department of Surgery
Doctors Hospital
Columbus, OH, USA
Volume 3, Chapter 5 Scalp and forehead
reconstruction

Darren M. Smith, MD
Resident
Division of Plastic Surgery
University of Pittsburgh Medical Center
Pittsburgh, PA, USA
Volume 3, Chapter 31 Pediatric facial fractures

**Gill Smith, MB, BCh, FRCS(Ed),
FRCS(Plast)**
Consultant Hand, Plastic and Reconstructive
Surgeon
Great Ormond Street Hospital
London, UK
Volume 6, Chapter 26 Congenital hand II Failure
of formation (transverse and longitudinal arrest)

Paul Smith, MBBS, FRCS
Honorary Consultant Plastic Surgeon
Great Ormond Street Hospital London, UK
Volume 6, Chapter 26 Congenital hand II Failure
of formation (transverse and longitudinal arrest)

Laura Snell, MSc, MD, FRCSC
Assistant Professor
Division of Plastic Surgery
University of Toronto
Toronto, ON, Canada
Volume 4, Chapter 14 Reconstruction of
acquired vaginal defects

Nicole Z. Sommer, MD
Assistant Professor of Plastic Surgery
Southern Illinois University School of Medicine
Springfield, IL, USA
Volume 6, Chapter 6 Nail and fingertip
reconstruction

David H. Song, MD, MBA, FACS
Cynthia Chow Professor of Surgery
Chief, Section of Plastic and Reconstructive
Surgery
Vice-Chairman, Department of Surgery
The University of Chicago Medicine & Biological
Sciences
Chicago, IL, USA
Volume 4, Chapter 10 Reconstruction of the
chest

Andrea Spano, MD
Senior Assistant Plastic Surgeon
Unit of Plastic Surgery
Istituto Nazionale dei Tumori
Milano, Italy
Volume 5, Chapter 14 Expander/implant breast
reconstructions
Volume 5, Video 14.01 Mastectomy and
expander insertion: first stage
Volume 5, Video 14.02 Mastectomy and
expander insertion: second stage

Scott L. Spear, MD, FACS
Professor and Chairman
Department of Plastic Surgery
Georgetown University Hospital
Georgetown, WA, USA
Volume 5, Chapter 15 Latissimus dorsi flap
breast reconstruction
Volume 5, Chapter 26 Fat grafting to the breast
Volume 5, Video 15.01 Latissimus dorsi flap
technique

Robert J. Spence, MD
Director
National Burn Reconstruction Center
Good Samaritan Hospital
Baltimore, MD, USA
Volume 4, Chapter 21 Management of facial
burns
Volume 4, Video 21.01 Management of the
burned face intra-dermal skin closure
Volume 4, Video 21.02 Management of the
burned face full-thickness skin graft defatting
technique

Samuel Stal, MD, FACS
Professor and Chief
Division of Plastic Surgery, Baylor College of
Medicine and Texas Children's Hospital
Houston, TX, USA
Volume 3, Chapter 29 Secondary deformities of
the cleft lip, nose, and palate
Volume 3, Video 29.01 Complete takedown
Volume 3, Video 29.02 Abbé flap
Volume 3, Video 29.03 Thick lip and buccal
sulcus deformities
Volume 3, Video 29.04 Alveolar bone grafting
Volume 3, Video 29.05 Definitive rhinoplasty

Derek M. Steinbacher, MD, DMD
Assistant Professor
Plastic and Carniomaxillofacial Surgery
Yale University, School of Medicine
New Haven, CT, USA
Volume 3, Chapter 34 Nonsyndromic
craniosynostosis

Douglas S. Steinbrech, MD, FACS
Gotham Plastic Surgery
New York, NY, USA
Volume 2, Chapter 9 Secondary blepharoplasty:
Techniques

Lars Steinstraesser, MD
Heisenberg-Professor for Molecular Oncology
and Wound Healing
Department of Plastic and Reconstructive
Surgery, Burn Center
BG University Hospital Bergmannsheil, Ruhr
University
Bochum, North Rhine-Westphalia, Germany
Volume 4, Chapter 18 Acute management of
burn/electrical injuries

Phillip J. Stephan, MD
Clinical Instructor
Department of Plastic Surgery
University of Texas Southwestern
Wichita Falls, TX, USA
Volume 2, Chapter 24 Liposuction: A
comprehensive review of techniques and safety

Laurie A. Stevens, MD
Associate Clinical Professor of Psychiatry
Columbia University College of Physicians and
Surgeons
New York, NY, USA
Volume 1, Chapter 3 Psychological aspects of
plastic surgery

Alexander Stoff, MD, PhD
Senior Fellow
Department of Plastic Surgery
Dreifaltigkeits-Hospital Wesseling
Wesseling, Germany
Volume 2, Chapter 25 Abdominoplasty
procedures
Volume 2, Video 25.01 Abdominoplasty

Dowling B. Stough, MD
Medical Director
The Dermatology Clinic
Clinical Assistant Professor
Department of Dermatology
University of Arkansas for Medical Sciences
Little Rock, AR, USA
Volume 2, Video 23.09 Tension donor dissection

James M. Stuzin, MD
Associate Professor of Surgery (Plastic)
Voluntary
University of Miami Leonard M. Miller School of
Medicine
Miami, FL, USA
Volume 2, Chapter 11.6 Facelift: The extended
SMAS technique in facial rejuvenation
Volume 2, Video 11.06.01 Facelift – Extended
SMAS technique in facial shaping

John D. Symbas, MD
Plastic and Reconstructive Surgeon
Private Practice
Marietta Plastic Surgery
Marietta, GA, USA
Volume 5, Chapter 16 The bilateral pedicled
TRAM flap
Volume 5, Video 16.01 Pedicle TRAM breast
reconstruction

Amir Taghinia, MD
Instructor in Surgery
Harvard Medical School
Staff Surgeon
Department of Plastic and Oral Surgery
Children's Hospital
Boston, MA, USA
Volume 6, Chapter 27 Congenital hand III
disorders of formation – thumb hypoplasia
Volume 6, Video 27.01 Congenital hand III
disorders of formation – thumb hypoplasia
Volume 6, Video 31.01 Vascular anomalies of
the upper extremity

David M.K. Tan, MBBS
Consultant
Department of Hand and Reconstructive
Microsurgery
National University Hospital
Yong Loo Lin School of Medicine
National University Singapore
Kent Ridge, Singapore
Volume 6, Chapter 3 Diagnostic imaging of the
hand and wrist
Volume 6, Video 3.01 Diagnostic imaging of the
hand and wrist – Scaphoid lunate dislocation

Jin Bo Tang, MD
Professor and Chair
Department of Hand Surgery
Chair
The Hand Surgery Research Center
Affiliated Hospital of Nantong University
Nantong, The People's Republic of China
Volume 6, Chapter 9 Flexor tendon injuries and
reconstruction
Volume 6, Video 9.01 Flexor tendon injuries and
reconstruction – Partial venting of the A2 pulley
Volume 6, Video 9.02 Flexor tendon injuries and
reconstruction – Making a 6-strand repair
Volume 6, Video 9.03 Complete flexor-extension
without bowstringing

Daniel I. Taub, DDS, MD
Assistant Professor
Oral and Maxillofacial Surgery
Thomas Jefferson University Hospital
Philadelphia, PA, USA
Volume 2, Chapter 16 Anthropometry,
cephalometry, and orthognathic surgery
Volume 2, Video 16.01 Anthropometry,
cephalometry, and orthognathic surgery

Peter J. Taub, MD, FACS, FAAP
Associate Professor, Surgery and Pediatrics
Division of Plastic and Reconstructive Surgery
Mount Sinai School of Medicine
New York, NY, USA
Volume 3, Chapter 37 Hemifacial atrophy

Sherilyn Keng Lin Tay, MBChB,
MRCS, MSc
Microsurgical Fellow
Department of Plastic Surgery
Chang Gung Memorial Hospital
Taoyuan, Taiwan, The People's Republic of
China
Specialist Registrar
Department of Reconstructive and Plastic
Surgery
St George's Hospital
London, UK
Volume 1, Chapter 26 Principles and techniques
of microvascular surgery

G. Ian Taylor, AO, MBBS, MD, MD
(HonBrodeaux), FRACS, FRCS (Eng),
FRCS (Hon Edinburgh), FRCSI (Hon),
FRSC (Hon Canada), FACS (Hon)
Professor
Deparment of Plastic Surgery
Royal Melbourne Hospital
Professor
Department of Anatomy
University of Melbourne
Melbourne, Australia
Volume 1, Chapter 23 Vascular territories

Oren M. Tepper, MD
Assistant Professor
Plastic and Reconstructive Surgery
Montefiore Medical Center
Albert Einstein College of Medicine
New York, NY, USA
Volume 3, Chapter 36 Craniofacial microsomia

Chad M. Teven, BS
Research Associate
Section of Plastic and Reconstructive Surgery
University of Chicago
Chicago, IL, USA
Volume 1, Chapter 21 Repair and grafting of
bone

Brinda Thimmappa, MD
Adjunct Assistant Professor
Department of Plastic and Reconstructive
Surgery
Loma Linda Medical Center
Loma Linda, CA
Plastic Surgeon
Division of Plastic and Maxillofacial Surgery
Southwest Washington Medical Center
Vancouver, WA, USA
Volume 3, Chapter 4 TMJ dysfunction and
obstructive sleep apnea

Johan Thorfinn, MD, PhD
Senior Consultant of Plastic Surgery, Burn Unit
Co-Director
Department of Plastic Surgery, Hand Surgery,
and Burns
Linköping University Hospital
Linköping, Sweden
Volume 6, Chapter 32 Peripheral nerve injuries of
the upper extremity
Volume 6, Video 32.01-02 Peripheral nerve
injuries (1) Digital Nerve Suture (2) Median Nerve
Suture

Charles H. Thorne, MD
Associate Professor of Plastic Surgery
Department of Plastic Surgery
NYU School of Medicine
New York, NY, USA
Volume 2, Chapter 22 Otoplasty

Michael Tonkin, MBBS, MD, FRACS (Orth), FRCS Ed Orth
Professor of Hand Surgery
Department of Hand Surgery and Peripheral Nerve Surgery
Royal North Shore Hospital
The Childrens Hospital at Westmead
University of Sydney Medical School
Sydney, Australia
Volume 6, Chapter 25 Congenital hand 1
Principles, embryology, and classification
Volume 6, Chapter 29 Congenital hand V
Disorders of Overgrowth, Undergrowth, and
Generalized Skeletal Deformities (addendum)

Patrick L Tonnard, MD
Coupure Centrum Voor Plastische Chirurgie
Ghent, Belgium
Volume 2, Video 11.04.01 Loop sutures MACS
facelift

Kathryn S. Torok, MD
Assistant Professor
Division of Pediatric Rheumatology
Department of Pediatrics
Univeristy of Pittsburgh School of Medicine
Childrens Hospital of Pittsburgh
Pittsburgh, PA, USA
Volume 3, Chapter 37 Hemifacial atrophy

Ali Totonchi, MD
Assistant Professor of Surgery
Division of Plastic Surgery
MetroHealth Medical Center
Case Western Reserve University
Cleveland, OH, USA
Volume 3, Chapter 21 Surgical management of
migraine headaches

Jonathan W. Toy, MD
Body Contouring Fellow
Division of Plastic and Reconstructive Surgery
University of Pittsburgh
University of Pittsburgh Medical Center Suite
Pittsburg, PA, USA
Volume 2, Chapter 30 Post-bariatric
reconstruction
Volume 5, Chapter 25 Contouring of the arms,
breast, upper trunk, and male chest in the
massive weight loss patient

Matthew J. Trovato, MD
Dallas Plastic Surgery Institute
Dallas, TX, USA
Volume 2, Chapter 29 Upper limb contouring
Volume 2, Video 29.01 Upper limb contouring

Anthony P. Tufaro, DDS, MD, FACS
Associate Professor of Surgery and Oncology
Departments of Plastic Surgery and Oncology
Johns Hopkins University
Baltimore, MD, USA
Volume 3, Chapter 16 Tumors of the lips, oral
cavity, oropharynx, and mandible

Joseph Upton III, MD
Clinical Professor of Surgery
Department of Plastic Surgery
Children's Hospital Boston
Shriner's Burn Hospital Boston
Beth Israel Deaconess Hospital
Harvard Medical School
Boston, MA, USA
Volume 6, Chapter 27 Congenital hand III
disorders of formation – thumb hypoplasia
Volume 6, Chapter 31 Vascular anomalies of the
upper extremity
Volume 6, Video 27.01 Congenital hand III
disorders of formation – thumb hypoplasia
Volume 6, Video 31.01 Vascular anomalies of
the upper extremity

Walter Unger, MD
Clinical Professor
Department of Dermatology
Mount Sinai School of Medicine
New York, NY
Associate Professor (Dermatology)
University of Toronto
Private Practice
New York, NY, USA
Toronto, ON, Canada
Volume 2, Video 23.06 Hair transplantation

Francisco Valero-Cuevas, PhD
Director
Brain-Body Dynamics Laboratory
Professor of Biomedical Engineering
Professor of Biokinesiology and Physical Therapy
By courtesy Professor of Computer Science and Aerospace and Mechanical Engineering
The University of Southern California
Los Angeles, CA, USA
Volume 6, Chapter 1 Anatomy and biomechanics
of the hand

Allen L. Van Beek, MD, FACS
Adjunct Professor
University Minnesota School of Medicine
Division Plastic Surgery
Minneapolis, MN, USA
Volume 2, Video 3.01 Botulinum toxin
Volume 2, Video 4.01 Soft tissue fillers
Volume 2, Video 5.01 Chemical peel
Volume 2, Video 18.01 Open technique
rhinoplasty

Nicholas B. Vedder
Professor of Surgery and Orthopaedics
Chief of Plastic Surgery Vice Chair, Department of Surgery
University of Washington
Seattle, WA, USA
Volume 6, Chapter 13 Thumb reconstruction:
non microsurgical techniques

Valentina Visintini Cividin, MD
Assistant Plastic Surgeon
Unit of Plastic Surgery
Istituto Nazionale dei Tumori
Milano, Italy
Volume 5, Chapter 14 Expander/implant
reconstruction of the breast
Volume 5, Video 14.01 Mastectomy and
expander insertion: first stage
Volume 5, Video 14.02 Mastectomy and
expander insertion: second stage

Peter M. Vogt, MD, PhD
Professor and Chairman
Department of Plastic Hand and Reconstructive Surgery
Hannover Medical School
Hannover, Germany
Volume 1, Chapter 15 Skin wound healing:
Repair biology, wound, and scar treatment

Richard J. Warren, MD, FRCSC
Clinical Professor
Division of Plastic Surgery
University of British Columbia
Vancouver, BC, Canada
Volume 2, Chapter 7 Forehead rejuvenation
Volume 2, Chapter 11.1 Facelift: Principles
Volume 2, Chapter 11.2 Facelift: Introduction to
deep tissue techniques
Volume 2, Video 7.01 Modified Lateral Brow Lift
Volume 2, Video 11.1.01 Parotid masseteric
fascia
Volume 2, Video 11.1.02 Anterior incision
Volume 2, Video 11.1.03 Posterior Incision
Volume 2, Video 11.1.04 Facelift skin flap
Volume 2, Video 11.1.05 Facial fat injection

Andrew J. Watt, MD
Plastic Surgeon
Department of Surgery
Division of Plastic and Reconstructive Surgery
Stanford University Medical Center
Stanford University Hospital and Clinics
Palo Alto, CA, USA
Volume 6, Chapter 17 Management of
Dupuytren's disease
Volume 6, Video 17.01 Management of
Dupuytren's disease

Simeon H. Wall, Jr., MD, FACS
Private Practice
The Wall Center for Plastic Surgery
Gratis Faculty
Division of Plastic Surgery
Department of Surgery
LSU Health Sciences Center at Shreveport
Shreveport, LA, USA
Volume 2, Chapter 21 Secondary rhinoplasty

Derrick C. Wan, MD
Assistant Professor
Department of Surgery
Stanford University School of Medicine
Stanford, CA, USA
Volume 1, Chapter 13 Stem cells and
regenerative medicine

Renata V. Weber, MD
Assistant Professor Surgery (Plastics)
Division of Plastic and Reconstructive Surgery
Albert Einstein College of Medicine
Bronx, NY, USA
Volume 1, Chapter 22 Repair and grafting of peripheral nerve

Fu Chan Wei, MD
Professor
Department of Plastic Surgery
Chang Gung Memorial Hospital
Taoyuan, Taiwan, The People's Republic of China
Volume 1, Chapter 26 Principles and techniques of microvascular surgery
Volume 6, Chapter 14 Thumb and finger reconstruction – microsurgical techniques
Volume 6, Video 14.01 Trimmed great toe
Volume 6, Video 14.02 Second toe for index
Volume 6, Video 14.03 Combined second and third toe for metacarpal hand

Mark D. Wells, MD, FRCS, FACS
Clinical Assistant Professor of Surgery
The Ohio State University
Columbus, OH, USA
Volume 3, Chapter 5 Scalp and forehead reconstruction

Gordon H. Wilkes, MD
Clinical Professor and Divisional Director
Division of Plastic Surgery
University of Alberta Faculty of Medicine
Alberta, AB, Canada
Volume 1, Chapter 33 Facial prosthetics in plastic surgery

Henry Wilson, MD, FACS
Attending Plastic Surgeon
Private Practice
Plastic Surgery Associates
Lynchburg, VA, USA
Volume 5, Chapter 26 Fat grafting to the breast

Scott Woehrle, MS, BS
Physician Assistant
Department of Plastic Surgery
Jospeh Capella Plastic Surgery
Ramsey, NJ, USA
Volume 2, Chapter 29 Upper limb contouring
Volume 2, Video 29.01 Upper limb contouring

Johan F. Wolfaardt, BDS, MDent (Prosthodontics), PhD
Professor
Division of Otolaryngology-Head and Neck Surgery
Department of Surgery
Faculty of Medicine and Dentistry
Director of Clinics and International Relations
Institute for Reconstructive Sciences in Medicine
University of Alberta
Covenant Health Group
Alberta Health Services
Alberta, AB, Canada
Volume 1, Chapter 33 Facial prosthetics in plastic surgery

S. Anthony Wolfe, MD
Chief
Division of Plastic Surgery
Miami Children's Hospital
Miami, FL, USA
Volume 3, Chapter 8 Acquired cranial and facial bone deformities
Volume 3, Video 8.01 Removal of venous malformation enveloping intraconal optic nerve

Chin-Ho Wong, MBBS, MRCS, MMed (Surg), FAMS (Plast. Surg)
Consultant
Department of Plastic Reconstructive and Aesthetic Surgery
Singapore General Hospital
Singapore
Volume 2, Chapter 6 Anatomy of the aging face

Victor W. Wong, MD
Postdoctoral Research Fellow
Department of Surgery
Stanford University
Stanford, CA, USA
Volume 1, Chapter 13 Stem cells and regenerative medecine

Jeffrey Yao, MD
Assistant Professor
Department of Orthopaedic Surgery
Stanford University Medical Center
Palo Alto, CA, USA
Volume 6, Chapter 5 Principles of internal fixation as applied to the hand and wrist

Akira Yamada, MD
Assistant Professor
Department of Plastic and Reconstructive Surgery
Osaka Medical College
Osaka, Japan
Volume 3, Video 7.01 Microtia: auricular reconstruction

Michael J. Yaremchuk, MD, FACS
Chief of Craniofacial Surgery-Massachusetts General Hospital
Program Director-Plastic Surgery Training Program
Massachusetts General Hospital
Professor of Surgery
Harvard Medical School
Boston, MA, USA
Volume 2, Chapter 15 Skeletal augmentation
Volume 2, Video 15.01 Midface skeletal augmentation and rejuvenation

David M. Young, MD
Professor of Plastic Surgery
Department of Surgery
University of California
San Francisco, CA, USA
Volume 1, Chapter 24 Flap classification and applications

Peirong Yu, MD
Professor
Department of Plastic Surgery
The University of Texas M.D. Anderson Cancer Center
Houston, TX, USA
Volume 3, Chapter 13 Hypopharyngeal, esophageal, and neck reconstruction
Volume 3, Video 13.01 Reconstruction of pharyngoesophageal defects with the anterolateral thigh flap

James E. Zins, MD
Chairman
Department of Plastic Surgery
Dermatology and Plastic Surgery Institute
Cleveland Clinic
Cleveland, OH, USA
Volume 2, Chapter 13 Neck rejuvenation

Christopher G. Zochowski, MD
Chief Resident
Department of Plastic and Reconstructive Surgery
Case Western Reserve University
Cleveland, OH, USA
Volume 3, Chapter 38 Pierre Robin sequence

Elvin G. Zook, MD
Professor Emeritus
Division of Plastic Surgery
Southern Illinois University School of Medicine
Springfield, IL, USA
Volume 6, Chapter 6 Nail and fingertip reconstruction

Ronald M. Zuker, MD, FRCSC, FACS, FRCSEd(Hon)
Staff Plastic Surgeon
The Hospital for Sick Children
Professor of Surgery
Department of Surgery
The University of Toronto
Toronto, ON, Canada
Volume 3, Chapter 11 Facial paralysis

Acknowledgments

Editing a textbook such as this is an exciting, if daunting job. Only at the end of the project, over 4 years later, does one realize how much work it entailed and how many people helped make it happen. Sue Hodgson was the Commissioning Editor who trusted me to undertake this. Together, over several weekends in Seattle and countless e-mails and phone calls, we planned the format of this edition and laid the groundwork for a planning meeting in Chicago that included the volume editors and the Elsevier team with whom we have worked. I thank Drs. Gurtner, Warren, Rodriguez, Losee, Song, Grotting, Chang and Van Beek for tirelessly ensuring that each volume was as good as it could possibly be.

I had a weekly call with the Elsevier team as well as several visits to the offices in London. I will miss working with them. Louise Cook, Alexandra Mortimer and Poppy Garraway have been professional, thorough, and most of all, fun to work with. Emma Cole and Sam Crowe helped enormously with video content. Sadly, Sue Hodgson has left Elsevier, however Belinda Kuhn ably filled her shoes and ensured that we kept to our timeline, didn't lose momentum, and that the final product was something we would all be proud of.

Several residents helped, in focus groups to define format and style as well as specifically engaging in the editing process. I thank Darren Smith and Colin Woon for their help as technical copyeditors. Thanks to James Saunders and Leigh Jansen for reviewing video content and thanks also to Donnie Buck for all of his help with the electronic content. Of course we edited the book, we didn't write it. The writers were our contributing authors, all of whom engaged with enthusiasm. I thank them for defining Plastic Surgery, the book and the specialty.

Finally, I would like to thank my residents and fellows, who challenge me and make work fun. My partners in the Division of Plastic Surgery at the University of Washington, under the leadership of Nick Vedder, are a constant source of support and encouragement and I thank them. Finally, my family, Kate and David and most of all, my wife Gabrielle are unwavering in their love and support and I will never be able to thank them enough.

Peter C. Neligan, MB, FRCS(I), FRCSC, FACS
2012

I want to thank my wife Kathryn for her unfailing good cheer and support on the nights and weekends I worked on this volume. I would also like to thank my sons, Cole, Pierce and Jack, for their limitless curiosity and energy, which continually challenges my view of the world. I am grateful to my assistant, Arnetha Whitmore, for her skill in helping me juggle too many things. And I need to acknowledge the Elsevier staff, especially Poppy Garraway, for her delicate touch in ensuring that I never got too far behind.

Geoffrey C. Gurtner, MD, FACS
2012

Dedicated to the memory of Stephen J. Mathes

Plastic surgery and innovation in medicine

Peter C. Neligan

SYNOPSIS

- There is a major difference between research and innovation, though the two are often interrelated.
- Most advances in surgery come from innovation rather than basic research.
- Surgical innovation is one of the defining features of plastic surgery.
- Surgical innovation is made safe by defining principles.
- A detailed knowledge of anatomy is a major factor on which these principles are based.
- A balance between out-of-the-box thinking and conservative deliberation is the perfect milieu to effect change yet keep perspective.

Introduction

We often tell our students that the great thing about plastic surgery is that we are the last real general surgeons. We are not confined to a body area or linked to a disease, unlike almost every other medical specialty. Similarly, while there are some operations that are reasonably standardized, plastic surgery is the one specialty in which this is more the exception than the rule. We often perform operations that we've never exactly done before and will likely never do in precisely the same way again. We almost always have completed elements of the surgery before, or we may add elements from another sphere of surgery to create a new approach to a problem. Sometimes this is born of necessity, the challenge of solving a unique problem for which there is no standard or well-accepted solution. Sometimes it is born of the will to do something better, to solve a problem in such a way that is better than the accepted means of dealing with it. When I tell nonmedical people this they are usually shocked and somewhat appalled. To the uninitiated it may seem cavalier, even dangerous. However these innovations are based on principles that we learn in our training and that we come to apply in our practice. That is the magic of plastic surgery. Of course this type of surgical innovation raises ethical issues and it is something with which many institutions are struggling, not merely in the domain of plastic surgery but in the field of surgery in general. Many institutions already have processes and protocols in place to oversee and regulate innovation.[1] When is innovation in surgery ethical and when is it not? This has already been the source of much discussion in the literature.[2–4] How far can we safely push the envelope? That particular discussion is beyond the scope of this chapter. Suffice it to say that it is important to strike a balance between necessary oversight of research practices and a supportive environment where research can flourish.

Innovation and research

What is the difference between innovation and research? Wikipedia (http://en.wikipedia.org/wiki/Research) defines research as follows: "Research can be defined as the search for knowledge or any systematic investigation to establish facts." Here (http://en.wikipedia.org/wiki/Innovation) is the definition for innovation: "Innovation is a change in the thought process for doing something or 'new stuff that is made useful'."[5] It may refer to an incremental emergent or radical and revolutionary change in thinking, products, processes, or organizations. Innovation can come from research but does not necessarily need to. This is true in other fields. For example, innovations in the computer industry are often simple changes introduced to facilitate a task, only to sometimes completely change how things are done. Most of the surgical innovations we see are not the result of research. In fact, not infrequently, an innovation is subsequently subjected to more rigorous study. A surgeon may design a new operation or, for example, a new flap. This may be a variation on an old procedure or sometimes something completely new. As already mentioned, it may have been forced on the surgeon because of the circumstances of the case. There may be no other way to solve the problem. When it works the surgeon decides to design a study to explain why the procedure worked or to describe the blood supply of the flap. Though one could argue that this is not the ideal way to do things, it certainly happens[6,7] and is merely a reflection of the dynamic nature of surgical innovation. Innovation may be planned or, in the case of this example and as happens probably more frequently, be made on the fly. Research may be innovative. A researcher may design a novel experiment to probe a theory, an approach to the problem that has not been explored before. This is also innovation and is more commonly how research and innovation are linked. An innovative idea is subjected to the scientific method that research demands. What makes an innovator? It has been said that the characteristics than most major innovators have in common include: (1) the ability to recognize an idea; (2) persistence in developing the strategy; and (3) commitment to the project, and final completion of a response to the problem or problems in question.[8]

Innovation and plastic surgery

The history of plastic surgery, at least the history of modern plastic surgery, is one of constant development. We regularly devise new ways of dealing with a particular problem. We develop a technique, perfect it, and then either lose it to some other group or give it away. There are numerous examples of this, from cleft surgery to microsurgery, from hand surgery to craniofacial surgery. While some see this as a major problem, I would argue that it is the lifeblood of plastic surgery. We are constantly developing new solutions for diverse problems. Some of these problems are generated from within our own practices; some come from our interaction with other specialties. We develop solutions and frequently allow those other specialties to run with the ball while we go on to something else. The facility to adapt is important in all spheres. For example, this ability to adapt, change, and incorporate new ideas is what has made English such a dominant language. It is the reason that Apple Computers has become an industry leader. This is the essence of innovation. There are numerous examples in biology that underline how the power of adaptation is the power of survival. For plastic surgery the same holds true and, while some fear the demise of the specialty, I would argue that while we adapt and develop, there will always be a place for plastic surgery.

Composite tissue allotransplantation

In research we work with models – models of disease, models of a procedure. Animal models provide a means by which we can study the process that we are interested in addressing in our patients. Occasionally, in order to solve a problem, we move to models that are perhaps less relevant to our everyday clinical practice. For example, most people don't realize that the first kidney transplant was performed by Dr. Joseph Murray, a plastic surgeon at the Peter Bent Brigham Hospital in Boston[9] *(Fig. 1.1)*. People are generally intrigued by this snippet of information. What was a plastic surgeon doing transplanting kidneys? How could this be? His practice as a plastic surgeon raised questions in his mind surrounding transplantation. His experience treating burn patients sent back from the war during World

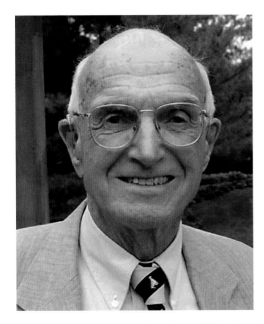

Fig. 1.1 Joseph Murray. (Courtesy of National Kidney Foundation.)

War II gave him wide exposure to skin grafting and raised issues of immune rejection that he would later find ways to address. In trying to work out the immunology of skin grafts he moved to a single-organ model, the kidney, in order to answer the question he had originally conceived. This culminated in the first successful kidney transplant performed from one twin to another by Dr. Murray at the Peter Bent Brigham Hospital in Boston in 1954. Having helped develop the specialty of transplantation, he went on to perform the world's first successful allograft in 1959 and the world's first cadaveric renal transplant in 1962. Dr. Murray ultimately returned to his roots, the practice of plastic surgery, and was awarded the Nobel Prize in Physiology or Medicine in 1990 for his contribution to the science of transplantation.

Now that wheel has turned full circle and plastic surgery is, once again, in the mainstream of transplant innovation (Ch. 34). Hand and face transplants have become a reality and, though still not in the mainstream of practice, it is likely that composite tissue allotransplantation (CTA) will become more common in the foreseeable future. In fact, even now, some would argue that hand transplantation is the standard of care (see Volume 6, Ch. 38). Face transplantation is sure to follow (see Volume 3, Ch. 20). Furthermore, it is likely that CTA will address those reconstructions that we cannot realistically achieve with conventional reconstructive

techniques. This would include transplantation of functioning eyelids, noses, ears, tongue, and other specialized organs. While total nasal reconstruction, as an example, has attained a high level of sophistication, the truth is that elegant nasal reconstructions are achieved by only a small number of expert surgeons utilizing very complex techniques in a series of operations over a period of months or years. The concept of a surgeon being able to transplant a nose in a single stage and achieve an elegant result is very attractive. Obviously many obstacles remain before we will see this in practice. CTA is a perfect example of how an innovative technical advance engenders increased research activity. The barrier to successful transplantation is not a technical one, it is an immunologic one and current interest in CTA has spawned a new wave of research activity in the field of immunology. This demands a collaborative and multidisciplinary approach, something that, again, plastic surgeons do well.

Collaboration

Plastic surgeons cannot lay claim to being the only innovators in medicine. Medicine is full of innovators. Yet it is true that the nature of the plastic surgeon's work, more than many other specialties, demands innovation. And that is what most plastic surgeons do every day of the week. Because so much of what we do, particularly in reconstructive surgery, is in collaboration with other specialties, innovation in those areas of practice often lead to innovations in our field. Most of the innovations we see are incremental. A surgeon incrementally changes how (s)he practices or how (s)he does a particular operation. Every now and again the innovation is radical. The development of craniofacial surgery is an example of radical innovation. Paul Tessier (*Fig. 1.2*) was the first to describe a combined intra- and extracranial approach for the correction of hypertelorism,[10,11] breaking the previously held taboo of exposing the intracranial environment to the upper aerodigestive tract. Going against the surgical mainstream demands unimaginable courage. It takes pioneers like Dr. Tessier to have the courage of their convictions and push the envelope beyond the general comfort level. Apart from spawning the specialty of craniofacial surgery, Dr. Tessier's advances led to advances in related fields. One such example is that

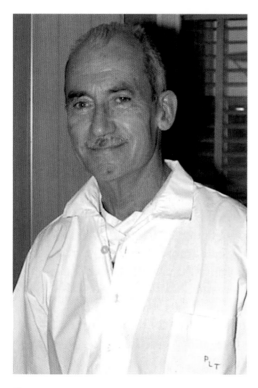

Fig. 1.2 Paul Tessier. (Courtesy of Barry M Jones.)

of skull base surgery. The craniofacial principles developed by Dr. Tessier literally opened up the field of skull base surgery. Tumors that were previously considered inoperable and inaccessible became treatable. That progress led to further innovations. So, continuing with the example of skull base surgery, the radical resections and approaches that were developed in the 1970s and 1980s[12,13] created problems such as meningitis and brain abscesses and problems related to delayed wound healing. Smaller defects could be closed with local flaps such as pericranial flaps, or galeafrontalis flaps.[14] However larger defects remained a problem until free flaps were used to close these defects.[15,16] Then the incidence of all of the complications, the brain abscesses, meningitis, and wound-healing problems, were all dramatically reduced and the surgery became safer. So microvascular surgery made skull base tumor surgery safer.

More recently, in this field we have seen innovations in the surgical approaches to the skull base facilitate the development of endoscopic skull base surgery. Large resections are now feasible through an endoscopic approach. This development has had a large impact on these patients because extensive open approaches with the associated risks of scarring and deformity are no longer necessary. However, with these large endoscopic resections, we are seeing the re-emergence of problems such as meningitis and abscess because of the difficulty in reconstructing these defects endoscopically.[17] This has led to the development of new reconstructive techniques and approaches in order to address these complications.[18–20]

This is an excellent example of how a multidisciplinary approach can advance a field. An innovation in one area can create a problem in another area that forces further innovation. Progress in surgery, regardless of specialty, demands a balance between innovators and conservatives. Innovators push the envelope and work best when they are paired with conservatives who rein them in to a degree. Thus, a balance between out-of-the-box thinking and conservative deliberation is the perfect milieu to effect change, yet keep perspective.

Drivers of innovation

Innovation is also forced in times of upheaval and change. The classic examples are war and natural disasters. More surgical advances are made in wartime than in peacetime. This is because specific problems are seen in unprecedented numbers and demand a solution. In this sort of environment it becomes reasonable to break the rules. One simply has to cope. Out of this generally comes a change in practice. Most of the advances in how we manage major trauma have come from the arena of war. The MASH units of the Korean conflict taught us that initiating treatment early, in the field, saves lives. The ultimate progression of that concept has been the development of robotic surgery, bringing high-level expertise to the field so that skilled intervention can be effected at the earliest possible opportunity. The fact that this can be achieved using robotic technology makes it feasible for a highly skilled surgeon located in some central site to treat multiple injuries in separate locations. The types of injury seen in war also lead to changes in practice. Plastic surgery, as we know it today, was born during the first world war. Sir Harold Gillies *(Fig. 1.3)* developed techniques for facial reconstruction initially at Aldershot and later at the Queen's Hospital in Sidcup, Kent, UK. (It later became Queen Mary's Hospital.) His innovative solutions for some of the

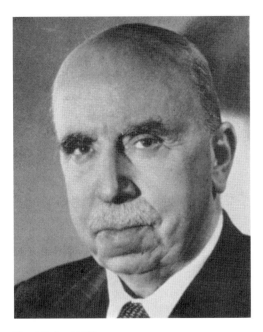

Fig. 1.3 Harold Gillies.

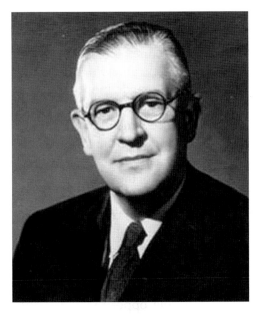

Fig. 1.4 Archibald McIndoe. (Courtesy of Blond McIndoe Research Foundation, registered charity no. 1106240.)

injuries he saw led to the development of modern plastic surgery.

During the Second World War the Plastic Surgery Unit at the Queen Victoria Hospital in East Grinstead, UK, headed by Sir Archibald McIndoe (Gillies' cousin) *(Fig. 1.4)* became famous for treating severely burned airmen. This surgery was so experimental that McIndoe's

patients formed a club known as the Guinea Pig club. The club was initially formed as a drinking club and its membership was made up of injured airmen in the hospital as well as the surgeons and anesthesiologists who treated them. Airmen had to have gone through a minimum of 10 surgical procedures before being eligible for membership in the club. By the end of the war the club had 649 members. The club itself was socially innovative because McIndoe conceived it as a way of integrating injured airmen back into society. He convinced some of the local families in East Grinstead to accept his patients as guests and other residents to treat them as normally as possible. It was very successful and East Grinstead became known as "the town that doesn't stare."

Innovation and development in other spheres have also changed the face of plastic surgery and brought further reconstructive challenges to surgeons. For example, the development of effective body armor has led to an increase in the types of injury we see in unprotected areas such as the limbs and the head and neck. It is not that these injuries didn't occur before. It is simply that before the military had effective body armor, soldiers were dying of their injuries and we did not have to deal with their devastating facial or extremity injuries. Limb amputations are surprisingly common. In the US it is estimated that there are 10 000 new upper limb amputees every year. This has led to the development of innovative prosthetics as well as innovative techniques to power these prosthetics. Use of myoelectric technology has led to innovations in the surgical approach to amputations and amputation stumps.[21,22] It is likely that CTA will change the reconstructive landscape for these devastating injuries.

Principles of innovation

I mentioned that innovations are based on principles. What are those principles and on what are they based? Obviously the specific principles will depend on the area under study. The principles on which innovation are based will be different for plastic surgeons as compared to gastrointestinal surgeons, for example. Central to everything and what I consider the core of plastic surgery is a detailed knowledge of anatomy. As a specialty and in general, plastic surgeons have a more detailed knowledge of anatomy than any other specialty. Of course the cardiac surgeon knows the heart better than anyone and the orthopedist knows bones better than anyone but neither of these specialties is likely to be in each other's domain very often. Yet, the plastic surgeon is frequently asked to cover exposed fractures or to provide vascularized cover for an infected sternotomy wound. Neither of these tasks is possible without a detailed knowledge of the anatomy of the region. Regardless of the area of subspecialty practice one is in, whether it is cosmetic surgery or hand surgery, a detailed knowledge of anatomy is the most important core understanding that is required to do the job well.

To drill down and define the single element of anatomic knowledge that is most vital to us, the answer would have to be vascular anatomy. So much of what we do involves the rearrangement of tissue, whether locally, regionally, or from afar. We have to know what keeps that tissue alive and we have to preserve that element. It is interesting to look at the advances that have been made in plastic surgery over the past 50 years. Many of them are directly related to a better knowledge of vascular anatomy. The most tangible of these is the development of flap surgery. We have come from an era when all flaps were random to the present time when we know not only which blood vessel is supplying our flap but how much of that tissue is being perfused by that blood vessel.

Innovations in imaging technology allow us the luxury of a road map to the vascular anatomy of our planned reconstruction using computed tomography and/or magnetic resonance imaging technology.[23–25] Even better, we have a surgical GPS that allows us to visualize perfusion in real time using indocyanine green.[26] Technical advances allow us to transfer the tissue and perform a microvascular anastomosis to restore its blood supply. However it goes beyond that. We can also restore function, sometimes using microsurgical techniques, other times, once again, utilizing our knowledge of anatomy, by robbing Peter to pay Paul. Tendon transfers, for example, have long been a technique for restoring function to a compromised limb.[27–29] More recently, nerve transfers have been utilized and are proving to be a valuable addition to our reconstructive armamentarium.[29] These are all examples of innovation, describing a new solution to an otherwise insoluble problem.

We have also combined our knowledge of vascular anatomy with our knowledge of genetic engineering. The science of genetics is covered in Chapter 11 of this volume. Using genetic engineering we can program cells to perform certain tasks. We can suppress certain functions and stimulate others: in other words, we can manipulate cells. This is a very powerful science and has potential applications across all of medicine. The process of transfection, whereby DNA or RNA is introduced into cells to modify gene expression, is widely used in molecular research. Geoff Gurtner, Editor of this volume of *Plastic Surgery*, introduced us to the concept of "biologic brachytherapy."[30] Using techniques of viral transfection, he has been able to design flaps that not only close a surgical defect but introduce a therapeutic element to the reconstruction by having the flap produce peptides appropriate to the disease entity being treated, producing probiotics for infected wounds, or antiangiogenic peptides for oncologic reconstructions. This innovative approach combines the best of plastic surgery with the best of genetic engineering to provide a new and better solution to an existing clinical problem. Biologic brachytherapy represents the melding of anatomic knowledge with tissue-engineering principles and is a very exciting development.

The concept of flap prefabrication is another imaginative way of providing a better solution to a clinical problem.[31] Using these techniques, the most appropriate reconstructive construct can be assembled prior to the definitive reconstruction. While flap prefabrication is an elegant approach to a complex problem, it demands a high level of expertise, imagination, and an innovative outlook. It also demands multiple stages and increased time to complete the reconstruction. In some disease states such a delay may not be feasible. Engineering body parts introduces us to the concept of "spare-parts" surgery and is yet another approach that is currently being developed. Wayne Morrison, working in the Bernard O'Brien Institute in Melbourne, Australia, has been able to grow functioning cardiac muscle[32] as well as functioning islet cells.[33] Spare-parts surgery, while still not a reality, is no longer the stuff of science fiction.

The concept of making new tissue constructs is not new and is the basis, for example, of bone distraction and tissue expansion. Tissue expansion has been around since the 1980s. In fact, like many things in medicine, it was originally described long before that,[34] but was only popularized in the 1980s.[35] It has become one of the standard ways to reconstruct a breast following mastectomy and, of course it has multiple other uses. When first introduced by Radovan, it was considered with a great deal of skepticism, like many innovations. Unfortunately Radovan did not live to see his idea become widely accepted.

Innovation also involves the application of established techniques in new areas. Bone distraction is an example of that. Devised by Ilizarov for the treatment of long bones, the technique has been adapted to the craniofacial skeleton. The applications of bone distraction in plastic surgery are more recent. Popularized by McCarthy,[36] bone distraction has changed the practice of craniofacial surgery, minimizing the extent of surgery required to treat certain conditions while improving outcomes. Such developments occur all the time and sometimes there is a disconnect between the development of the original idea and its ultimate application. An example of this is the Brava bra. This was first developed as a means of achieving breast augmentation non-surgically.[37] Applying a vacuum to the breast caused swelling and enlargement. This was somewhat of a transitory enlargement but, nevertheless, an enlargement. Several other innovations led to a rethinking of what was happening with the Brava system and ultimately led to a very innovative approach to breast reconstruction that is still in the initial stage of skeptical interest but that may well become an established technique. This association of ideas is often how innovation works. What were these different ideas? Each in its own right is a major innovation.

The first is fat grafting. This is an old idea and one with a checkered history. Dermal fat grafts have long been an accepted method of correcting small contour defects. Attempts at engrafting larger fat deposits have generally been unsuccessful. The concept of fat injection as a means of engrafting fat is another idea that was greeted with skepticism until Coleman showed us that it does work when the fat is deposited in small aliquots with a fine cannula.[38–40] This technique is now widely practiced in both aesthetic and reconstructive arenas and has become an invaluable addition to our armamentarium.

The second innovation is tissue expansion, already mentioned above. Though tissue expansion has been around for a long time, we have thought of it in terms of internal expansion, i.e., expansion produced by the implantation of an expanding device. The suction system used by the Brava bra introduces us to the concept of external expansion, i.e., expansion caused by external forces, the application of a vacuum to the skin.

The third innovation is that of vacuum-assisted closure, the VAC system. This is an idea so simple that we all wish we had thought of it. However, as with many things in medicine, it is not as simple as it first appears. Not only, it appears, does the VAC mechanically remove debris and exudate from the wound, but it also promotes angiogenesis and cell proliferation.[41–43]

Putting all these concepts together, Khouri and Del Vecchio[44] developed a system for both breast reconstruction as well as breast augmentation. The Brava system, married to the structural fat-grafting concept, is used, in the belief that the external expansion induced by the Brava vacuum produces edema, angiogenesis, and cell proliferation that permit larger volumes of fat to be deposited in a favorable matrix, thereby increasing graft take and fat retention. To date, the results of this approach are remarkable. Undoubtedly there are many unanswered questions and here, once again, we have an example of an innovation that has already found clinical application but that requires extensive research to elucidate the mechanism of the clinical picture we are seeing.

Fat grafting, as well as providing a clinical solution to many problems, both aesthetic and reconstructive, has also engaged our curiosity in another area, that of stem cell research. This again represents an association of ideas from disparate fields. Many of the changes we see as a result of fat grafting are not readily explained by the injection of fat alone. As an example, it has been reported that many of the skin changes associated with radiation seem to be reversed when fat is injected into, for example, a breast defect resulting from lumpectomy and radiation.[45] Why should this be? The answer, stem cells, may be a simplistic solution to explain something we don't understand. The answer may also be our introduction to a whole new area of development for plastic surgery. Of course, as we've seen before, not only does this innovation (fat grafting) solve a clinical problem, it raises numerous questions and opens the door to new areas of research and quite likely to even newer innovations.

External influences and innovation

In order to achieve some of our surgical results not only do we rely on our own expertise as surgeons; we also rely on our tools, our instruments and devices. Microsurgery could not have developed without the development of the operating microscope and appropriate instrumentation. One of the biggest barriers to modern microsurgery was the inability to swage an ultrafine suture to a sufficiently small needle. Similarly, the manufacture of implants of any kind demands an expertise that we, as surgeons, do not have. Bioengineers, chemists, physicists, and all manner of experts are required to help bring our ideas into clinical practice. None of these developments are possible without the partnership of industry. Of course this is a double-edged sword as it introduces other interests and possible conflicts. Nevertheless, it is a vital part of the development of any specialty.

I've already mentioned how microsuture development led to the development of reconstructive microsurgery. Once it was possible to do microanastomoses, it became possible to replant amputated digits. The new technology spurred the advance of flap surgery and our interest in vascular anatomy was again renewed. This inspired the likes of Mathes and Nahai[46] to elucidate and classify the blood supply of muscles and others to describe new myocutaneous flaps. Ian Taylor[47] started his classic cadaver injection studies that led to the development of the angiosome theory. Later, Isao Koshima and Soeda[48] described perforator flaps and that development and innovation is ongoing.

Craniofacial surgery is another subspecialty area that could not have developed without the help of industry. When Joseph Gruss recognized the importance of internal fixation for the craniofacial skeleton in the early 1980s,[49] he was using wires to piece together comminuted fractures painstakingly. This led him and others to the recognition of the concept of facial buttresses and to the development of plating systems for the face. This approach is now standard of care but could not have happened without the expertise of the engineers and implant biologists who worked with surgeons to develop the plating systems and instrumentation that make it all possible. Once again, this is an ongoing process.

Every aspect of plastic surgery has undergone such change and development. In cosmetic surgery we have also seen these changes evolve. In each area, surgeons have developed a better understanding of anatomy and function and developed, with industry, ways to improve and develop the field. Endoscopic techniques were adapted from other areas of practice and applied to the face; minimally invasive techniques led to the development of barbed sutures and suspension systems. Implant biology has brought is various injectable fillers and broadened the scope of cosmetic surgery in a way that was once unimaginable.

So innovation is a natural consequence of practice. In every sphere people strive to improve things – surgeons to do better operations, anesthesiologists to improve pain control, industry to provide better materials and instruments. These innovations occur in all specialties and, as we have seen, innovation in one specialty can influence how another develops. What about innovation itself? How can we ensure that innovation is as safe as possible and conducted in some sort of organized fashion and with some form of structure? Do we need such organization and such structure? As I mentioned at the outset, a discussion on the ethics of innovation is beyond the scope of this chapter. However there are some things that are useful to consider.

Documentation, data gathering, and regulation

It is important to document change. If one asks a surgeon how many procedures (s)he has done, the answer is usually a gross exaggeration. Similarly we tend to underestimate our complications. We're not good at remembering stuff though we think we are. It is surprising when one starts to keep a database how sobering it is to see the actual numbers. It's also surprising how much information one can glean and this information is vital if we are to change and improve. Innovation implies change and in times of change it is imperative to document results. How else can one evaluate the effects of the innovation? So documentation and data gathering are important aspects of innovation.

The difficulty with innovation arises in that gray zone between innovation and research. Small changes are easy to effect, large changes more difficult! Most institutions regulate change through the institutional review board (IRB). Regulation is necessary yet it is also restrictive. The IRB process varies from institution to institution but, in general, is becoming more and more stringent. This can have a significant effect on the development of medicine as a whole. It is widely believed, for example, that the reason the first heart transplant did not occur in the US was because of the stringent regulations governing experimental surgery in the US as compared to South Africa, where Dr. Christiaan Barnard, an American-trained cardiac surgeon, performed this operation. Institutions also grapple with the dilemma of allowing some degree of innovation, yet controlling quality and risk exposure. The latter is an important consideration for institutions and individuals alike. Apart from protecting the individual and the institution, regulation also introduces and enforces an element of objectivity. When one is involved in developing a theory, an operation, or some sort of change, it is very easy to lose objectivity and that is a serious issue.

Regulation enforces objectivity and the difficulty lies in the balance between creativity and objectivity. Just as one can become obsessed with creativity and freedom of expression, however, one can also become obsessed with objectivity and regulation. Finding a balance between the two is sometimes difficult. Added to that is the conflict of interest that is sometimes introduced to the process when a commercial value is associated with the innovation, particularly when a significant sum may already have been invested in developing it. That introduces the ethics of practice and this subject is covered in another chapter.

So we have seen that innovation is an important part of medicine. It is separate from research, though often stimulates research. It is as difficult to regulate as it is to define and, at least in some instances, may be stifled by regulation. From all of the innovations I have touched on in this chapter we can see that innovation is vital to the development of medicine in general and to the evolution of plastic surgery in particular.

Access the complete references list online at **http://www.expertconsult.com**

1. Neumann U, Hagen A, Schönermark M. Procedures and criteria for the regulation of innovative nonmedicinal technologies into the benefit catalogue of solidly financed health care insurances. *GMS Health Technol Assess.* 2008 Feb 6;3:(Doc13.).

   Because great interest in an efficient range of effective medicinal innovations and achievements has arisen, many countries have introduced procedures to regulate the adoption of innovative nonmedicinal technologies into the benefit catalogue of solidly financed healthcare insurances. This report describes procedures for the adoption of innovative nonmedicinal technologies by solidly financed healthcare insurances in Germany, England, Australia, and Switzerland.

2. McCulloch P, Altman DG, Campbell WB, et al. No surgical innovation without evaluation: the IDEAL recommendations. *Lancet.* 2009;374:1105–1112.

   This paper proposes recommendations for the assessment of surgery based on a five-stage description of the surgical development process. Achievement of improved design, conduct, and reporting of surgical research will need concerted action by editors, funders of healthcare and research, regulatory bodies, and professional societies.

3. Ergina PL, Cook JA, Blazeby JM, et al. Challenges in evaluating surgical innovation. *Lancet.* 2009;374: 1097–1104.

   Research on surgical interventions is associated with several methodological and practical challenges of which few, if any, apply only to surgery. This report discusses obstacles related to the study design of randomized controlled trials and nonrandomized studies assessing surgical interventions. It also describes the issues related to the nature of surgical procedures. Although difficult, surgical evaluation is achievable and necessary. Solutions tailored to surgical research and a framework for generating evidence on which to base surgical practice are essential.

4. Barkun JS, Aronson JK, Feldman LS, et al. Evaluation and stages of surgical innovations. *Lancet.* 2009;374: 1089–1096.

   Surgical innovation is an important part of surgical practice. Its assessment is complex because of idiosyncrasies related to surgical practice, but necessary so that introduction and adoption of surgical innovations can derive from evidence-based principles rather than trial and error. A regulatory framework is also desirable to protect patients against the potential harms of any novel procedure. In this first of three series papers on surgical innovation and evaluation, we propose a five-stage paradigm to describe the development of innovative surgical procedures.

8. Toledo-Pereyra L. Surgical innovator. *J Invest Surg.* 2011;24:4–7.

To be a surgical innovator is to be someone who has the capacity to modify established concepts in surgery. C Walton Lillehei, Owen H Wangensteen, William S Halsted, and Alfred Blalock are a few of many good examples of American surgeon innovators whose contributions can help us to discern how they thought about innovation within the surgical sciences. These four innovators readily contemplated the essence of innovation but mostly dedicated themselves to search for the appropriate answers to serious and difficult clinical tasks.

2

History of reconstructive and aesthetic surgery

Riccardo F. Mazzola and Isabella C. Mazzola

SYNOPSIS

- History shows that almost every possible local flap has been described in the past and that the ingenuity of plastic surgeons was unlimited.
- The lesson drawn from history reveals that the so-called new flaps are variations of what has already been published.
- We have to be humble and recognize that "nothing is new under the sun."

Gaspare Tagliacozzi (1545–1597), from Bologna, Italy, defined plastic surgery as the art devoted to repairing congenital or acquired defects ("to restore what Nature has given and chance has taken away"), and which has as its primary goal the aim of correcting a functional impairment, but also re-establishing an appearance as close as possible to normality ("the main purpose of this procedure – he writes – is not the restoration of the original beauty of the face, but rather the rehabilitation of the part in question").[1] The term "plastic" comes from the Greek πλαστικός (plasticós), moldable.

Origin of plastic surgery

The distant past

The ancient origin of plastic surgery relates to the healing of wounds. Management of wounds caused by stones, weapons, arrows, and animal bites goes back millions of years, when primitive humans had to face four major problems: (1) arrest of posttraumatic loss of substance; (2) bleeding; (3) infection; and (4) pain. Attempts to transform a defect that heals slowly by secondary intention into one healing quicker by primary intention may well account for the first example of a reparative procedure.

However, this must have been quite complex without appropriate tools, in the presence of hemorrhage and without anesthesia. There is no documentation of stitching of wounds among primitive people.[2] We may extrapolate from what was reported in ancient Hindu medicine, where wound edges were sewn with simple means like fibers or strips of tendon, or pinned together using insect mandibles.

In Ancient Egypt

We are well informed about Egyptian surgery thanks to the Smyth papyrus, the most ancient medical text. The papyrus is a later transcription (about 1650 BC) of an original manuscript dating from the Old Kingdom (between 3000 and 2500 BC). It describes 48 surgical cases, including wounds, fractures, dislocations, sores, and tumors, and suggests their potential management. Fresh wounds were treated conservatively with the application of grease and honey using linen and swabs. Adhesive strips of cloth, stitches or a combination of clamp and stitches were advocated to bring together the margins of the wound. A surgical knife was never mentioned, as wounds already existed in the cases presented.[2] Treatment of nasal fractures is accurately explained. First, clots should be removed from the inside of the nostrils, then the bony fragments repositioned; two stiff rolls of linen were applied externally "by which the nose is held fast" and finally "two plugs of linen saturated with grease placed into the nostrils."[3]

In Mesopotamia

Mesopotamia is the region between the rivers Tigris and Euphrates (now approximately Iraq) where Sumerian civilization was born. Medicine was well developed, although strongly influenced by astrology and divination. During excavations of the Nineveh palace, a great library containing more than 30 000 clay tablets with cuneiform inscriptions was discovered, 800 of them of a medical nature. They were written about 600 BC, although the text dates from around 2000 BC. The tablets of interest for plastic surgery are few and concern wound healing or congenital anomalies. "If a man is sick with a blow on the cheek, pound together turpentine, tamarisk, daisy, flour of Inninnu (…) mix in milk and beer in a small copper pan; spread on skin and he shall recover."[4] Another tablet suggests the use of a dressing with oil for an open wound.

Monsters (congenital malformations) were considered important in predicting future events and in determining their course. "When a woman gives birth to an infant (…) whose nostrils are absent, the country will be in affliction, and the house of the man ruined; that has no tongue the house of the man will be ruined; that has no lips affliction will strike the land and the house of the man will be destroyed."[5] Interestingly, surgery is never mentioned in clay tablets, although surgery was certainly performed. In the King Hammurabi Code,[2] dating from about 1700 BC, surgical malpractice was recognized with precise laws: "If a physician carried out a major operation on a seignior with a bronze lancet and has caused the seignior's death or he opened the eye socket of a seignior and has destroyed the seignior eye, they shall cut off his hand." "If a physician carried out a major operation on a commoner's slave with a bronze lancet and has caused [his] death, he shall make good slave for slave."

In India

The birth of plastic surgery has a close correlation with the art of reconstructing noses. This apparently curious origin has a logical explanation if one considers the common tradition of certain ancient populations of mutilating the nose of adulterers, thieves and prisoners of war as a sign of humiliation. In an attempt to improve this terrible disfigurement, surgeons invented different solutions over the centuries.

In India, amputation of the nose was rather common and repair was carried out by the Koomas, a low caste of priests, or, according to others, a guild of potters. In the *Áyurvédam*, the Indian sacred book of knowledge which deals with medicine, the missing portions of the nose were reconstructed using local flaps transposed from the cheek. An accurate description of blunt (*yantra*) and sharp (*sastra*) instruments necessary to perform surgical operations in general and rhinoplasty in particular is supplied.[6]

It is not possible either to establish the exact date of the work (it is thought to have been written about 600 BC), or to prove that Sushruta, the author, was one man. On the contrary, there is evidence that over the centuries various Indian surgeons contributed to describe the procedures included in the book. When was the forehead skin used? There is no mention of it. In the second half of the 17th century, the Venetian adventurer Nicolò Manuzzi (1639–1717) wrote a manuscript about the Moghul empire in which an account of forehead rhinoplasty is supplied. Regrettably the manuscript, kept in the Marciana Library at Venice, was not published until 1907.[7] Information on the forehead flap in nasal reconstruction only reached the western world at the end of the 18th century, thanks to a letter signed BL, addressed to Mr. Urban, editor of the *Gentleman's Magazine,* and published in October 1794 (*Fig. 2.1*).[8]

A friend of mine has transmitted to me, from the East Indies, the following very curious and, in Europe, I believe unknown chirurgical operation, which has long been practiced in India with success; namely, affixing a new nose on a man's face.

There follows the accurate description of the two-step procedure carried out on Cowasjee, a bullock driver of the English army, who fell under the disfavour of Tippoo Sultan, who had his nose amputated. It demonstrates

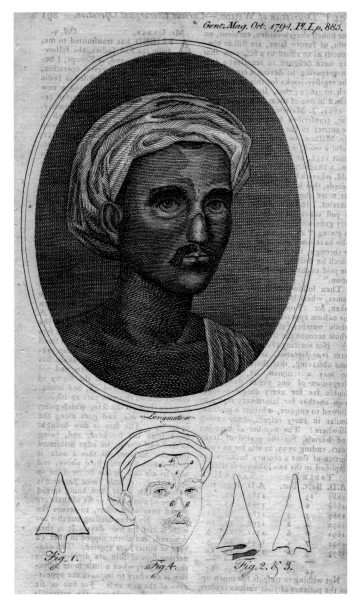

Fig. 2.1 Indian forehead flap nasal reconstruction. (Reproduced from BL. Letter to the editor. Gentleman's Magazine 1794;64:891–892.)

Asklepieion (Latin: *aesculapīum*) was a healing temple, sacred to Asklepios, the Greek god of medicine. Hippocrates rejected the views of his time that illness was due to supernatural influence, possession of evil spirits, or disfavor of the gods. He based his medical practice on the direct observation of disease and on an analysis of the human body, introducing scientific methods into medicine. Hippocrates taught and practiced medicine throughout his life, traveling in various Greek regions. He established the Great School of Medicine on the isle of Kos. He probably died in Larissa (Greece) at the age of 83 or 90.

About 70 medical treatises, assembled during the Alexandrian era (third century AD), were attributed to Hippocrates. They form the so-called *Corpus Hippocraticum*. Whether Hippocrates himself is the author of the *Corpus* and these works are authentic has been the matter of great dispute and controversy.[9] The *Corpus* contains manuals, lectures, research, philosophical thoughts, and essays on different topics of medicine, without any logical order and even with significant contradictions among them. The works of Hippocrates were true best-sellers, reprinted numerous times over the centuries. The first printed edition of the *Opera omnia* (*Complete Works*) was issued in Latin in Rome in 1525, and in Greek in Venice in 1526 by the Aldine Press.

The surgical knowledge of Hippocrates was vast. He used cauterization for the management of raw surfaces, reduced malunited fractures, and practiced cranial trephination to evacuate hematomas.

In Rome

In Rome, surgery was well developed, at least judging from the rather sophisticated bronze instruments discovered in Pompei and now kept at Naples National Museum. Many were stored in traveling kits to be used by surgeons for emergency or in the battlefields.

The two most representative figures of Roman medicine were Celsus and Galen.

Aulus Cornelius Celsus (25 BC–50 AD) was probably not a physician, but a writer from a noble family and the author, in about 30 AD, of *De Medicina* (*On Medicine*) in eight volumes. In book seven, chapter nine, vessel ligature and lithotomy as well as lip closure (cleft lip or lip tumor) by means of flaps are reported. It explains how "defects of the ears, lips and nose can be cured"

the high level of surgery reached by the Indians in carrying out an operation, without anesthesia, in a very similar way to what we perform nowadays.

In Greece

Greek medicine was influenced by Hippocrates, the greatest physician of his time. Historians consider that Hippocrates was born in the island of Kos around the year 460 BC, and probably trained in medicine at the Asklepieion of Kos. In ancient Greece and Rome, the

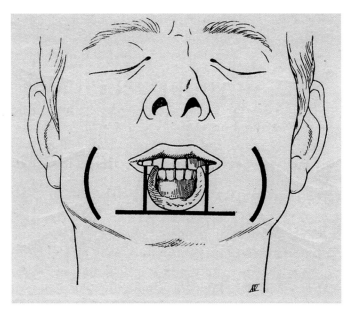

Fig. 2.2 Lip repair according to Celsus. (Reproduced from Nélaton C, Ombredanne L. *Les Autoplasties*. Paris, Steinheil, 1907.)

(*curta in auribus, labrisque ac naribus, quomodo sarciri et curare possint*), followed by a description of wound closure by advancement flap.[10] "The defect should be converted into a square (*in quadratum redigere*). Then, from the inner angles transverse incisions are made (*lineas transversas incidere*), so that the part on one side is fully divided from that on the opposite side." "After that, the tissues which have been undermined, are brought together" (*in unum adducere*). "If this is not possible two additional semilunar incisions are made at some distance from the original (*ultra lineas, quas ante fecimus, alias duas lunatas et ad piagam conversas immittere*), but only sectioning the outer skin. [...] These latter incisions enable the parts to be easily brought together without using any traction" (*Fig. 2.2*). Celsus holds a key role in the history of plastic surgery, as he is considered the earliest writer on this topic. He is responsible for introducing the four cardinal signs of acute inflammation, "redness and swelling with heat and pain" (*rubor et tumor, cum calore et dolore*). A copy of Celsus's manuscript was discovered in Milan in 1443, and printed for the first time in 1478 in Florence.[11] *De Medicina* went through more than 50 editions.

Claudius Galen (*c.* 129–201 AD) was born in Pergamon (Turkey), studied medicine at the Asklepieion (see above) in his native city and moved to Rome. He wrote about head traumas, techniques of trephination for evacuating hematomas and various types of bandaging. An excellent anatomist, he described more than 300 muscles and seven pairs of cranial nerves and contributed to neurology, demonstrating that nerves arise from the brain or spinal cord. He observed that section of the laryngeal nerve resulted in dysphonia. For management of wounds he used sutures and cautery. Numerous works of Galen were lost, but 82 survived. Originally written in Greek, many were translated into Arabic and Latin. Galen's *Opera* was first printed in Latin in Venice in 1490 and in Greek at Venice in 1525 by the Aldine Press.

Plastic surgery after the decline of the Roman Empire

Byzantine surgery

Oribasius (325–403 AD) wrote a collection of medical texts entitled *Synagogae Medicae* in which reconstructive procedures for cheek, nose, ears, and eyebrow defects are described.[12] Paulus of Aegina (625–690 AD), surgeon and obstetrician, was the author of a medical encyclopedia (*Epitome*) in seven volumes. In book 6, which deals with surgery, a description of tracheotomy, tonsillectomy, and lip repair is supplied.[13,14] "Defects [Greek, *colobomata*] of the lips and ears are treated in this way. First the skin is freed on the underside. Then the edges of the wound are brought together and the callosity is removed. Finally, stitches holding them into position are applied." This technique closely resembles that of Celsus.

The Middle Ages

Arabian surgery

Arabian medical writers came from different nations, such as Persia, Syria, and Spain. Their only common denominator was the language. The most representative figure was Abū-l-Qāsim or Albucasis (*c.* 936–1013 AD), whose famous treatise, *Al Tasrif* (*On Surgery*), was translated into Latin and first published in 1500. It was the first independent surgical treatise ever written in detail. It included more than 200 illustrations of surgical instruments, such as tongue depressor, tooth extractor, hooks, and cauteries, most invented by Albucasis himself, with an explanation of their use.[15] Like most Arabian surgeons, Albucasis was a proponent of cautery, for different clinical applications and the management of wounds and cleft lip. He was the first to use a syringe with a piston.

The rise of the universities

The founding of the universities is one of the most important events in the Middle Age and a key factor in the development of modern culture. Originally, *universitas* denoted an aggregation of masters (*magistri*), students, or both, and the primary goal was teaching philosophy and theology. Lessons were practiced in the house of the masters or in small rooms. Students sat on the floor, whereas the professor was in the chair. The oldest university, at least in Europe, was Bologna, established in 1088, followed by Paris, Oxford, and Montpellier. In Bologna medicine was taught and cadaver dissection was accepted, thus significantly contributing to the development of anatomy. Mondino de' Luzzi (1270–1326) was the first anatomist to lecture directly in front of the cadaver (*Fig. 2.3*). As anatomists were also surgeons, such as Henry of Mondeville (1260–1320) or Guy of Chauliac (1300–1368), surgery was part of the teaching of anatomy.

The discovery of printing

The invention of printing around 1440 by Gutenberg spread medical knowledge and considerably enlarged the libraries of universities and monasteries.

The first printed textbook on surgery was *La Ciroxia* (*On Surgery*), by William of Saliceto (1210–1277), issued in Venice in 1474. This text has particular relevance in the history of surgery, because it reintroduced the use of the surgical knife to replace cautery, strongly advocated by Arabian surgeons. The first printed textbook on anatomy was *Anatomia* by Mondino de' Luzzi, issued in Padua about 1476, which remained the reference text for numerous years. The printed works of Hippocrates, Galen, Celsus and Arabian writers served to educate medical students.

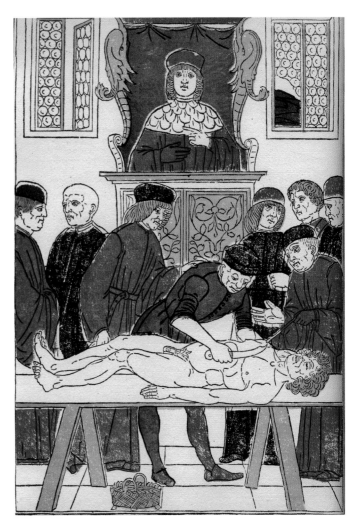

Fig. 2.3 Mondino in the chair supervising a cadaver dissection. (Reproduced from Ketham J. *Fasciculo de Medicina*. Venice, Gregorio de' Gregorii, 1493.)

The Renaissance

Renaissance surgery

One of the greatest surgical figures of the Renaissance was the Frenchman Ambroise Paré (1510–1590) (*Fig. 2.4*). A humble but very talented barber surgeon, Paré amassed considerable experience from his tireless work in the battlefields. He disputed the common belief that gunshot wounds were poisoned and required the barbaric practice of wound-cleansing using hot cautery or pouring boiling oil into the wound. He applied a paste of egg yolk instead, mixed with oil of roses and turpentine, to patients' great relief. In 1545, he published a treatise on gunshot wounds, demonstrating that the use

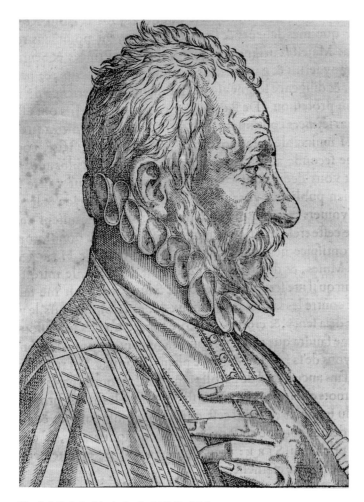

Fig. 2.4 Portrait of Ambroise Paré (1510–1590).

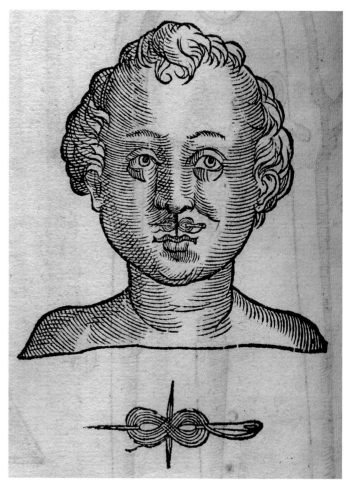

Fig. 2.5 Cleft lip repair. (Reproduced from Paré A. *Les Oeuvres*. Paris: Buon, 1575.)

of cautery was unnecessary (*La méthode de traicter les playes*). He wrote extensively on surgery and his works are collected in *Les Oeuvres*, published in 1575.[16] To demonstrate relationships between anatomy and surgery, he borrowed images from *De Humani Corporis Fabrica*, issued a few years earlier, in 1543, by Andreas Vesalius (1514–1564). He sutured cleft lip, whereas he closed the cleft of the palate using obturators (*Fig. 2.5*). To approximate scars he stitched adhesive on the outside of the wound margins (*Fig. 2.6*), and supported Tagliacozzi's work on nasal reconstruction.

Nasal reconstruction in the western world

In the western world the first attempt to restore the nasal pyramid dates back to the first half of the 15th century. It was performed by members of the Branca family from Catania (Sicily). Gustavo (early 15th century) used skin taken from the cheek. His son, Antonio, made considerable improvements to the operation. He selected the arm as the donor site, to avoid further scars on the face. About 1460, at Antonio's death, the Branca method, which was kept as a family secret and passed on by word of mouth, was discontinued in Sicily.

In the late 15th century, nasal reconstruction was resumed by Vincenzo Vianeo in Calabria (southern Italy). His sons Pietro (about 1510–1571) and Paolo (about 1505–1560) established a flourishing clinic for rhinoplasty in Tropea (Calabria). Evidence of their reconstructive work comes from the Bolognese army surgeon Leonardo Fioravanti (1517–1588) (*Fig. 2.7*), who assisted in Vianeo's operations and published an accurate report in *Il Tesoro della Vita Humana* (*Treasure of Human Life*) issued in Venice in 1570.[17]

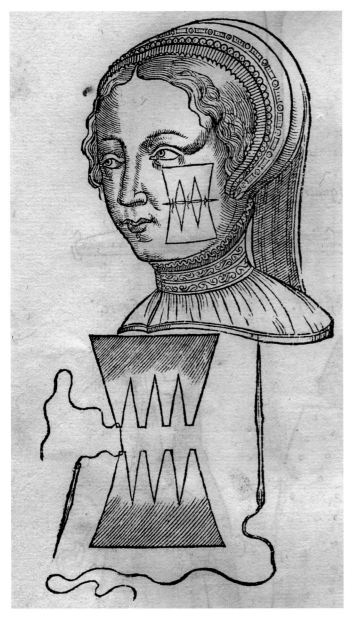

Fig. 2.6 Facial wound suture. A piece of linen is stitched to the skin to facilitate wound edge approximation. (Reproduced from Paré A. *Les Oeuvres*. Paris: Buon, 1575.)

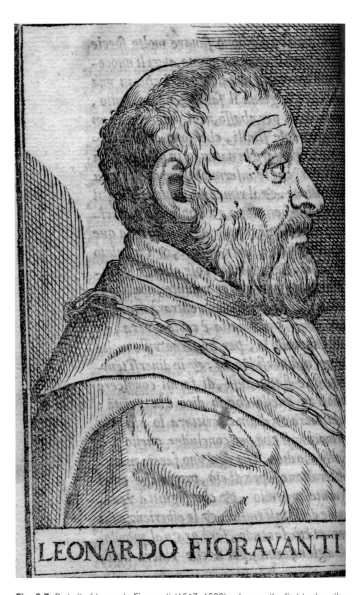

Fig. 2.7 Portrait of Leonardo Fioravanti (1517–1588), who was the first to describe the arm flap procedure for nasal reconstruction. (Reproduced from Fioravanti L. *Il Tesoro della Vita Humana*. Venice: Sessa, 1570.)

I moved to Tropea where at that time there were two brothers Pietro and Paolo, who made a nose for anyone who had lost his by some accident [...]. I went every day to the house of these surgeons, who had five noses scheduled for repair and when they wanted to perform these operations they called me to watch and I, pretending I had not the courage to look at, I turned my face away, yet my eyes saw perfectly. Thus, I observed the whole secret from top to toe, and learned it.

Then follows the description of the arm flap procedure.

Possibly Fioravanti's book came under the eyes of Gaspare Tagliacozzi (1544–1599) from Bologna, Professor of Surgery at Bologna University, who successfully applied the technique on some patients. In 1597, he published in Venice a textbook *De Curtorum Chirurgia per Insitionem* (*On the Surgery of Injuries by Grafting*),[1,18] in which the nasal reconstruction operation is shown

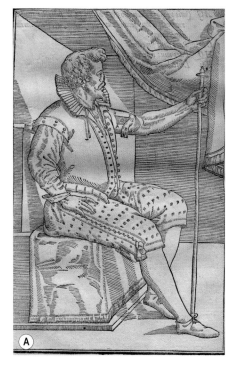
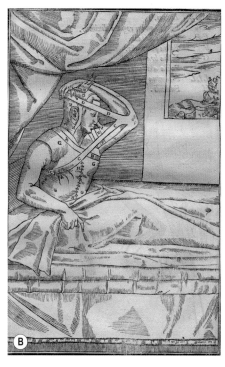
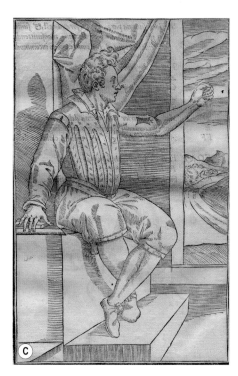

Fig. 2.8 Nasal reconstruction with the arm flap. **(A)** Preoperative view of the patient. The missing nose and flap are outlined; **(B)** the flap sutured into position; **(C)** final result. (Reproduced from Tagliacozzi G. *De Curtorum Chirurgia per Insitionem*. Venice: Bindoni, 1597.)

step by step and skillfully illustrated. The instruments necessary for the operation are presented first, followed by the indications, flap outlined on the arm, flap inset, the bandage necessary to secure the arm into position, flap severed, trimmed, outcome of nasal repair, as well as different clinical applications for lip and ear (*Fig. 2.8*). The book was well received and was reprinted in a pocket edition at Frankfurt the following year, directed specifically at military surgeons who were often confronted with the problems of nasal repair in the battlefields.

Although Tagliacozzi was not the discoverer of rhinoplasty, and the arm flap operation is now rarely performed, he deserves credit for being the first to make a work of art out of a surgical practice, for systematizing and promulgating nasal reconstruction. He is rightly considered the founder of plastic surgery.

The decline of plastic surgery

After Tagliacozzi's death, apart from his pupil GB Cortesi (1554–1634), who published a book on nasal reconstruction in 1625,[19] the operation, which was difficult to perform, became obsolete for almost two centuries. Sporadic cases were reported in 17th- or 18th-century literature. Instead of recommending autologous tissue for restoring a missing nose, surgeons like Fallopio (1523–1562), Heister (1683–1758), Camper (1722–1789), and others advocated the application of an epithesis, convinced that noses made out of wood or silver were far superior to those of skin.

The rebirth of plastic surgery

The 1794 letter to the editor of the *Gentleman's Magazine* (see above) holds a key position in the revival of plastic surgery. The English surgeon Joseph Constantine Carpue (1764–1846) read it and made practical and successful use of its contents. In 1814, he carried out the first forehead flap rhinoplasty of modern time at St. Bartholomew's Hospital, London, on an officer of His Majesty's Army, who had his nose amputated during a battle. The operation lasted 35 minutes, "it was no child's play, extremely painful – the officer said – but it was no use complaining." At the end he exclaimed: "my God, there is a nose!"

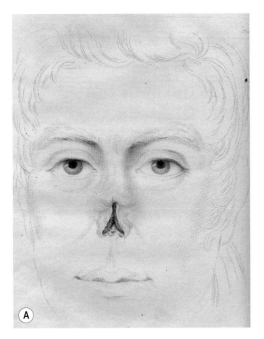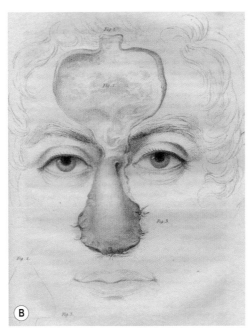

Fig. 2.9 Nasal reconstruction with the forehead flap. **(A)** Preoperative view; **(B)** the flap transposed into position. (Reproduced from Carpue J.C. An Account of two Successful Operations for Restoring a Lost Nose from the Integuments of the Forehead, in the Case of two Officers of his Majesty's Army. London: Longman, Hurst, 1816.)

In 1816, Carpue issued an account of nasal reconstruction, which marks the prelude to the rebirth of modern plastic surgery (*Fig. 2.9*).[20]

The 19th century

The golden age of plastic surgery

Carpue's work was immediately translated into German, and Carl Ferdinand von Gräfe (1787–1840), Professor of Surgery at Berlin University, promptly initiated the operation. In 1818, he published *Rhinoplastik oder die Kunst den Verlust der Nase organisch zu ersetzen* (*Rhinoplasty: or the Art of Reconstructing the Nose*), where he compared the Italian and Indian procedures.[21] Von Gräfe supported the arm flap, as he was unhappy about forehead donor site scar morbidity.

The publications of Carpue and von Gräfe stimulated the interest of European surgeons to carry out nasal and other reconstructions. In Germany, Johann F Dieffenbach (1794–1847), head of surgery at La Charité Hospital in Berlin, performed rhinoplasty, facial restorations, and cleft palate and cleft lip repairs. He reported his contributions in *Chirurgische Ehrfahrungen* (*Surgical Experiences*), issued in 1829.[22] In France, Jacques Mathieu Delpech (1777–1832), chief surgeon at Montpellier, wrote *Chirurgie Clinique de Montpellier* in 1828, with a detailed section on rhinoplasty.[23] Outstanding works on the rediscovered art were presented by Pancoast (1805–1882)[24] in the US, Balassa (1814–1868)[25] in Hungary, and Sabattini (1810–1864)[26] in Italy. A review of the state of the art of nasal reconstruction in Europe in the mid 19th century was published by Nélaton and Ombrédanne in 1904,[27] and more recently by McDowell,[28] Rogers,[29] and Mazzola.[30]

With the advent of anesthesia (1846) and the possibility of closing the donor site primarily, leaving a scar that was often unnoticeable, forehead rhinoplasty became the procedure of choice due to its simplicity, good color match, and excellent results.

The first attempt to close a cleft palate goes back to the second decade of the 19th century. The priority is shared between Carl Ferdinand von Gräfe[31] and Philibert Roux (1780–1854) from France.[32] However, the greatest advance was made in 1862 by Bernard von Langenbeck (1810–1887), who outlined two mucoperichondrial flaps obtaining a more reliable closure.[33] Refinements in cleft lip repair were published by the Frenchmen Joseph Malgaigne (1806–1865)[34] and Germanicus Mirault (1796–1879) in 1844.[35]

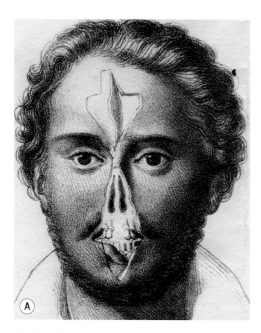
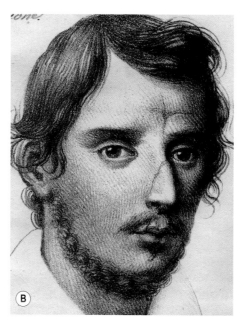

Fig. 2.10 The lip switch technique for upper lip repair: **(A)** flap outlining; **(B)** final result. (Reproduced from Sabattini P. Cenno storico dell'origine e progressi della Rinoplastica e Cheiloplastica seguita dalla descrizione di queste operazioni praticamente eseguite sopra un solo individuo. Bologna: Belle Arti; 1838.)

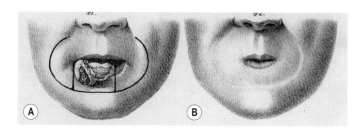

Fig. 2.11 (A, B) The double lateral flaps for lower lip repair. (Reproduced from von Bruns V. *Chirurgischer Atlas.* Tübingen, Laupp, 1857.)

Reconstructive procedures for lip[36] were reported by Pietro Sabattini in 1838, using the lip switch technique[26,37] (*Fig. 2.10*), and by Victor von Bruns (1812–1883) in 1857, using double lateral flaps for oral sphincter restoration[38] (*Fig. 2.11*), whereas eyelid repair was reported by Johann Fricke (1790–1841) in 1829, who described a pedicled skin flap from the ipsilateral temporal or cheek region to correct upper or lower eyelid defects respectively[39] (*Fig. 2.12*).

One of the greatest advances in 19th-century surgery was the demonstration that a piece of skin, fully separated from its original site, might survive when transplanted to another part of the body to cover a granulating raw surface.[40] This became possible through the pioneering work of Giuseppe Baronio (1758–1811) from Milan, who performed the first autologous skin graft in a ram in 1804 (*Fig. 2.13*).[41,42] Sixty-five years later Jacques Reverdin (1842–1929) carried out the first successful epidermic graft on a human being at Hôpital Necker in Paris, opening a new era in wound-healing management.[43] The route for skin grafting was traced. A few years later, Louis Ollier (1830–1900) transferred a large piece of split-thickness skin, which included the superficial layers and underlying dermis.[44] Carl Thiersch (1822–1895)[45] and John R Wolfe (1824–1904)[46] made further advances in the procedure. In the late 1800s, skin grafting became the preferred solution for the management of chronic and granulating wounds.

The 20th century

The origin of modern plastic surgery

Trenches played an important role during World War I. Created for shielding purposes, they actually only protected soldiers' lower body and trunk, whereas the head and neck remained exposed to enemy weapons. As they returned home, soldiers with major maxillofacial mutilations found it impossible to step back into society, and this constituted a new social problem.

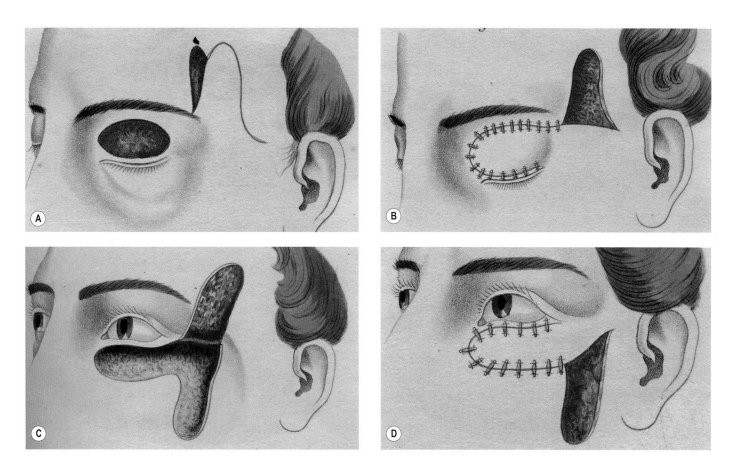

Fig. 2.12 (A–D) Upper and lower eyelid repair with a temporal and cheek flap respectively, according to Fricke. (Reproduced from Fritze HE, Reich OFG. *Die plastische Chirurgie*. Berlin, Hirschwald, 1845.)

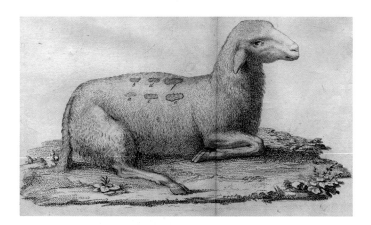

Fig. 2.13 First autologous skin graft in a ram. (Reproduced from Baronio G. *Degli innesti Animali*. Milan: Stamperia del Genio, 1804.)

Treatment of these devastating facial wounds urged the development of a new discipline, plastic surgery. The first plastic surgeons came from general surgery, otolaryngology, or orthopedics during the first 20 years of the 20th century.

Associations were created all over the world to help these poor individuals. The most famous was *Les gueules cassées* (The Facial Cripples), founded in France in 1921, by Colonel Picot. In addition to these associations, France, the UK, Germany, Italy, and Czechoslovakia established specialized centers to manage these injuries that had never been seen before. The key to success was the cooperation between plastic surgeons, trained in soft-tissue defect management, and oral surgeons, expert in stabilizing bone fractures using dental appliances.

Hippolyte Morestin (1868–1919), who worked with the dentist Charles Auguste Valadier (1873–1931) at Hôpital Val-de-Grâce (Paris), first realized the importance of such a team approach. For this he is considered the pioneer in facial reconstructive surgery.

In 1915, the New Zealand otolaryngologist Harold Gillies (1882–1960), at that time working in France on behalf of the Red Cross, visited Val-de-Grâce military hospital. He was much impressed by the work of

Hippolyte Morestin and Valadier pushed him to take care of facial disfigurements. In 1917, upon his return to the UK, Gillies established a center for the management of face and jaw injuries at Queen's Hospital, Sidcup. It became the referral center in Europe. Treatment was provided to British and allied soldiers wounded in the battle of the Somme (July 1, 1916), where Britain suffered almost 500 000 casualties with an enormous number of dramatic facial mutilations (*Fig. 2.14*). Gillies operated among a multidisciplinary team with William Fry (1889–1963) and Henry Pickerill (1879–1956) as dental surgeons, and a qualified group of anesthesiologists. He systematized new reconstructive procedures, like the tubed flap, described by the Russian Vladimir Filatov (1875–1956),[47] which allowed the coverage of large skin defects, but also skin flaps, bone, cartilage, and skin grafts (*Fig. 2.15*). Gillies reported his experiences in *Plastic Surgery of the Face*, issued in 1920.[48]

In Germany Erich Lexer (1867–1937), one of the founders of maxillofacial surgery, built up a vast experience on the repair of the face, mandible, and eye socket using cartilage, bone, skin, and fat graft. He published a book on reconstructive surgery in 1920.[49]

The Dutch surgeon Johannes Esser (1877–1946) was active at Tempelhof Hospital, Berlin, and in Vienna. Between 1916 and 1918 Esser codified some of the flaps currently used today: cheek rotation[50] (*Fig. 2.16*), bilobed, island, and arterialized flaps, which he called biological flaps.[51] In Italy, Gustavo Sanvenero Rosselli (1897–1974)

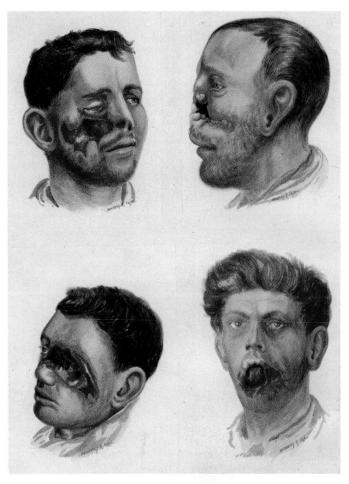

Fig. 2.14 Dramatic facial mutilations from World War I. (Reproduced from Pickerill HP. *Facial Surgery*. Edinburgh, Livingstone, 1924.)

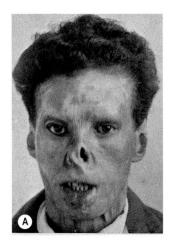 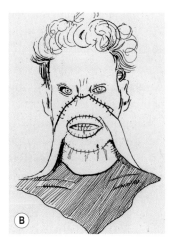 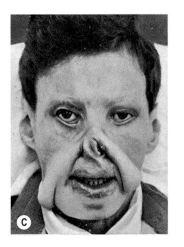 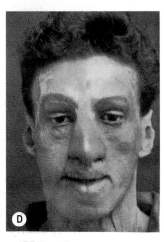

Fig. 2.15 Sequelae of facial burn from World War I. Repair using the tubed flap: **(A)** preoperative view of the patient; **(B)** outlining of the tubed flap; **(C)** the flap in position; **(D)** final result. (Reproduced from Gillies H. *Plastic Surgery of the Face*. London: Frowde, Hodder and Stoughton, 1920.)

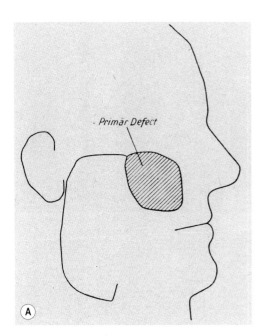
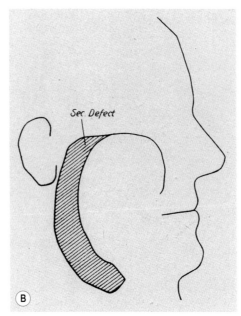

Fig. 2.16 Cheek flap transposition for closing of an orbitopalpebral defect. (Reproduced from Esser JFS. *Die Rotation der Wange.* Leipzig: Vogel, 1918.)

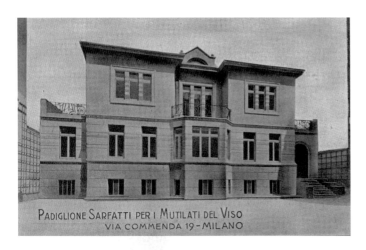

Fig. 2.17 The Pavilion for Facial Cripples in Milan, headed by G. Sanvenero Rosselli (1897–1974).

complex maxillofacial injuries at Walter Reed Hospital. Other renowned reconstructive surgeons were Robert Ivy, Truman Brophy, John Staige Davis, and the Armenian Varaztad Kazanjian.

The training programs

By the end of World War I, reconstructive techniques had achieved surprising results. Transfer of skin flaps (tubed or pedicled) and use of grafts (skin, cartilage, bone, fat) became routine procedures. New units were established all over the world. Thus, the need for training programs, where young doctors could become familiar with reparative methods, was essential. Queen's Hospital at Sidcup, headed by Sir Harold Gillies, was probably the most famous for the management of facial injuries. Anesthesia improved considerably thanks to Ivan Magill, who developed nasal and endotracheal intubation. Other training programs in the UK were organized by Sir Archibald McIndoe, Rainsford Mowlem, and Pomfret Kilner.

In Paris, the otorhinolaryngologist Fernand Lemaître (1880–1958) established a residency at the International Clinic of Oto-Rhino-Laryngology and Facio-Maxillary Surgery, having Eastman Sheehan (1885–1951), Professor of Plastic Surgery at Columbia University New York,

was appointed head of the *Padiglione per i Mutilati del Viso* (Pavilion for Facial Cripples) in Milan (*Fig. 2.17*). It became a European referral center for reconstructive surgery and was visited by surgeons from all over the world.

Frantisek Burian (1881–1965) headed an important plastic surgery unit in Prague, Czechoslovakia.

In the US the specialty only grew after World War I. Vilray Blair (1871–1955), trained at Sidcup, established the first independent unit in the US for the care of

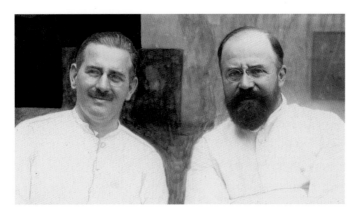

Fig. 2.18 Fernand Lemaître and Eastman Sheehan at the International Clinic in Paris, in 1927.

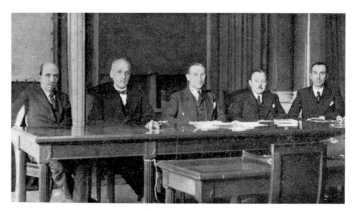

Fig. 2.19 Executive Council members of the Société Européenne de Chirurgie Structive, Brussels, 1936. From left to right: Sir H Gillies, JFS Esser, M Coelst, P Kilner, G Sanvenero Rosselli.

as course director (*Fig. 2.18*). The 2-year fellowship included an intense program of lectures and practical surgical demonstrations. Attendees from various parts of Europe and the US were numerous. Among them was the Italian Gustavo Sanvenero Rosselli, later appointed head of the Plastic Surgery Clinic in Milan. In the US the first training program was organized by Vilray Blair at Washington University in St. Louis.

The birth of the scientific societies

The aim of the scientific societies was to improve the scientific level of the specialty and to defend the public from charlatans. The first society was the American Association of Oral and Plastic Surgeons, established in 1921 by Truman Brophy (1848–1928), who strongly supported close cooperation between oral and plastic surgeons. Initially membership required the MD and DDS degrees.

In Europe, the first society was the Société Française de Chirurgie Réparatrice Plastique et Esthétique, established in 1930 by Charles Claoué (1897–1957) from Bordeaux and Louis Dartigues (1869–1940) from Paris. It only lasted 2 years.

In 1931, Jacques Maliniak (1889–1976) founded the American Society of Plastic Surgeons.

The first supranational society was the Société Européenne de Chirurgie Structive, created in 1936 by the Belgian Maurice Coelst (1894–1963) (*Fig. 2.19*), with the aim of gathering annually all those specialists interested in the new discipline.[52] The term *structive* was

coined by Johannes Esser, as he considered it more appropriate than "plastic" to emphasize the repairing concept.

In 1937, Vilray Blair organized the American Board to certify real plastic surgeons.

The scientific journals

At the time of the foundation of the American Society (1931), the Belgian Maurice Coelst established and edited the *Revue de Chirurgie Plastique* (*Fig. 2.20*). The journal, the first one on this topic, played an important role in the history of plastic surgery between the two wars. Thanks to an international editorial board, which included the most important plastic surgeons, the journal published high-quality papers written by Gillies, Maliniak, and Rethi, the proceedings of the American Society of Plastic Surgery and those of the Société Française de Chirurgie Réparatrice Plastique et Esthétique.[53] Papers appeared in the author's preferred language and were summarized in English, French, and German.

In 1935, the *Revue de Chirurgie Plastique* changed its name into *Revue de Chirurgie Structive*, becoming the official journal of the Société Européenne de Chirurgie Structive. The *Revue* lasted until the end of 1938 (8 years), when it ceased publication, due to the advent of World War II.

In 1946, the *Plastic and Reconstructive Surgery Journal* was established and Warren B Davis was appointed as editor.

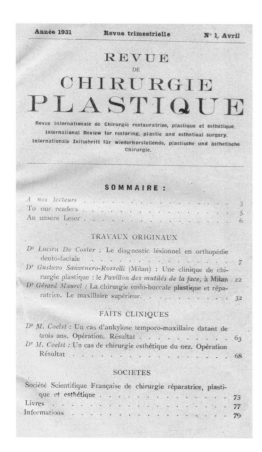

Fig. 2.20 The first issue of the *Revue de Chirurgie Plastique*, established by M Coelst in 1931.

The bases for the official recognition of plastic surgery as an independent specialty were settled.

Postwar plastic surgery

Recent history sees an incredible development of new reconstructive procedures, initiated in the 1960s with the recognition of arterialized flaps, continuing with the clinical definition of the cutaneous vascular territories nourished by a single vessel, previously identified by Carl Manchot (1866–1932) in 1889[54] (*Fig. 2.21*), and culminating with their microvascular transfer. The application in surgical practice of musculocutaneous flaps, originally described by the Italian Iginio Tansini (1855–1943)[55] (*Fig. 2.22*), the introduction of craniofacial techniques, developed in the late 1960s by Paul Tessier (1917–2008),[56] the systematization of breast reconstruction, the use of fat grafting for numerous aesthetic and reconstructive indications, and even the most recent face transplantation, constitute further achievements of our fascinating specialty.

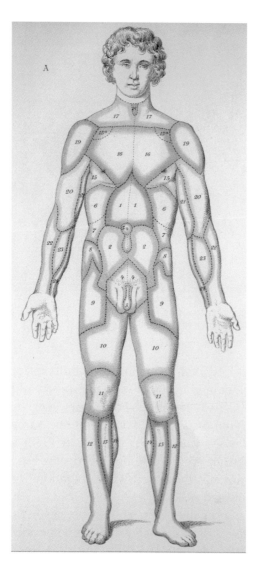

Fig. 2.21 The cutaneous vascular territories nourished by a single vessel. (Reproduced from Manchot C. *Die Hautarterien des menschlichen Körpers*. Leipzig: Vogel, 1889.)

Aesthetic surgery

The origin

The end of the 19th century marks the beginning of aesthetic surgery. Correction of prominent ears, performed in 1881 by the New York surgeon Edward Ely (1850–1885), is considered the first purely aesthetic procedure,[57] followed by modifications of nasal appearance.

In 1887, John Orlando Roe (1848–1915), an otolaryngologist from Rochester, showed members of the New

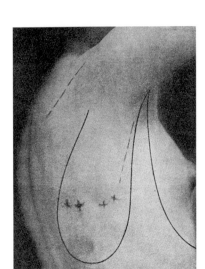
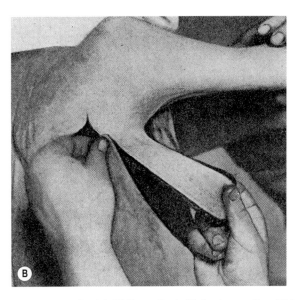
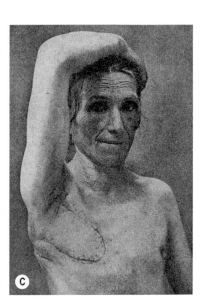

Fig. 2.22 The latissimus dorsi musculocutaneous flap according to Tansini. **(A)** Flap outlined; **(B)** flap transposition; **(C)** final result. (Reproduced from Tansini I. Sopra il mio nuovo processo di amputazione della mammella. *Gazz Med It* 1906;57:141.)

York Medical Society that reduction of a bulbous or "pug nose," as he named it, under local anesthesia and on outpatient basis, was feasible.[58] Four years later, he presented hump removal using scissors at the same society.[59] The following year, Robert Weir (1838–1927), a general surgeon from New York, described alar base excision, now eponymically named "Weir operation," to lower an overprojected nose.[60]

On the other side of the ocean, in Europe, aesthetic rhinoplasty started in Berlin, in about the same period, with Jacques Joseph (1865–1934), who codified the steps of the technique in a rigorous sequence, still used today after almost 100 years, with minimal variations (*Fig. 2.23*). For at least 20 years, Joseph directed rhinoplasty in Europe, receiving the most famous patients from every part of the world. His experience was included in a monumental work, *Nasenplastik und sonstige Gesichtsplastik (Rhinoplasty and other Facialplasties)*, published in 1931, which remained an unsurpassed text for several decades.[61]

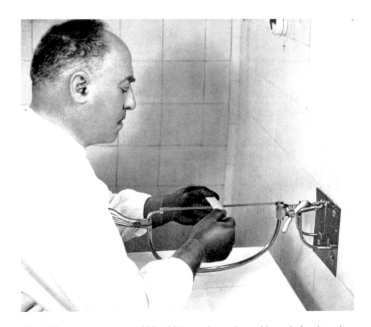

Fig. 2.23 Jacques Joseph (1865–1934), carving a piece of ivory, before inserting it into the nasal dorsum. (Reproduced from Joseph J. Nasenplastik und sonstige Gesichtsplastik nebst einem Anhang über Mammaplastik. Leipzig: Kabitzsch, 1931.)

Development

The problem of the beauty doctors

However, the real explosion of aesthetic surgery took place in Europe and in the US between the two world wars.

The importance given to personal appearance produced, in the early 20th century and especially during the interwar period, a horde of quacks, charlatans, and beauty doctors often working in beauty salons, exclusively on a commercial basis. They advertised in newspapers, women's magazines, and yellow pages as cosmetic surgeons. They appealed to popular imagination by promising a more attractive look with simple, fast procedures on an outpatient basis, at relatively high cost and by insisting on how beautiful faces and noses were crucial in creating a favorable first impression for finding a job, or expanding social relationships.[62]

For this reason trained surgeons practicing reconstructive as well as aesthetic procedures established plastic surgical societies in the interwar period (see above) in an attempt to isolate purely cosmetic surgeons. The idea was to draw a separating line between "beauty doctors" and "true plastic surgeons." However, it was not an easy task because the general public was more interested in the successes of cosmetic surgery than in the outcome of reconstructive procedures.

An example is given by Charles C Miller (1880–1950), regarded as an "unscrupulous charlatan" by some or "the father of modern cosmetic surgery" by others for having published in 1907 *The Correction of Featural Imperfections*, a pioneering work on aesthetic procedures, where facial operations, such as double-chin excision and eyelid and nasolabial fold modification, were illustrated.[63] Miller made extensive use of paraffin injections, considered the panacea for improving saddle nose. When paraffin was abandoned because of devastating local (paraffinomas) and systemic sequelae (pulmonary embolism, phlebitis), he replaced it with crude rubber mixed with gutta-percha and ground in a mill.[64]

Another borderline cosmetic surgeon was Henry J Schireson (1881–1949), who knew a moment of fame in the US having successfully operated on a British actress. Apart from this episode, he faced a series of lawsuits for malpractice which culminated in having his licence revoked for a period of time. In 1944, *Time* defined him as the "king of quacks."

Trained surgeons made considerable efforts to create a positive view of plastic surgery. Their talent contributed to transform a field regarded with suspicion into an accepted branch of surgery. Eastman Sheehan (1885–1951), Jacques Maliniak (1889–1976), Jerome P Webster (1888–1974), Vilray Blair (1871–1955), Ferris Smith (1884–1957), and others all played important roles in forming plastic surgery's professional and public image during the specialty's organizing years as a recognized medical branch. Sheehan, course director at Lemaître's International Clinic in Paris, was elected President of the American Association of Plastic Surgeons in 1935, despite the controversial view of him of many of his American colleagues, who regarded him as a publicity-seeking skilled operator. Maliniak is best remembered as the founding member of the American Society of Plastic Surgeons in 1931. He was a prolific writer, publishing *Sculpture in the Living* (1934)[65] and *Rhinoplasty and Restoration of Facial Contour*, (1947)[66] and had an important aesthetic surgical practice in New York, mainly for nose and breast. Webster was one of the founding fathers of US plastic surgery and a talented surgeon in the reconstructive as well as aesthetic field. Smith was course director at Lemaître's International Clinic in Paris, and author of *Reconstructive Surgery of the Head and Neck*, issued in 1928 with a section devoted to aesthetic rhinoplasty.[67]

In Paris, Suzanne Noël (1878–1954) established a successful solo practice in the very exclusive 16th *arrondissement*. Her operations were simple, but effective, mainly related to facial rejuvenation and entirely performed on an outpatient basis (*Fig. 2.24*). Major surgery, such as abdominoplasty or mammoplasty was executed in a private clinic. In 1926, she published *La Chirurgie Esthétique. Son Rôle Sociale,* one of the first textbooks on this topic and the first written by a woman.[68] Raymond Passot (1886–1933), a leading Parisian aesthetic surgeon, added innovative techniques for breast ptosis and abdomen and facial rejuvenation. His book *La Chirurgie Esthétique pure*, dating from 1931, shows a wide range of operations in the field of aesthetic surgery[69] (*Fig. 2.25*). Julien Bourguet (1876–1952), another Parisian cosmetic surgeon, became renowned for having first presented the transconjunctival approach for baggy eyelid correction in 1929 at an international meeting. The detailed description was published sometime later.[70]

In Berlin, in addition to Joseph, who carried out cosmetic operations other than rhinoplasty, such as facelift or reduction mammoplasty,[61] Eugen Holländer (1867–1932) practiced. Holländer was known for the first account of a facelift done in 1901 at the request of a noble lady, who urged him to perform an elliptical excision of skin in front of her ear, believing that youth could be retained through surgery.[71] In the same paper, Holländer shows two cases of facial atrophy he had treated with fat injection, the first report of this type of procedure.

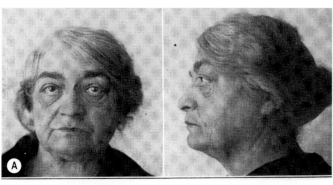

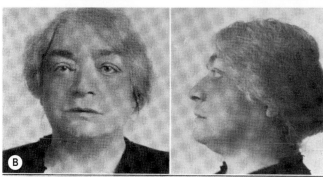

Fig. 2.24 Result of a facelift carried out by Suzanne Noël (1878–1954) about 1925. (Reproduced from Noël S. *La Chirurgie Esthétique. Son rôle sociale*. Paris: Masson, 1926.)

Postwar aesthetic surgery

After World War II and in more recent years, aesthetic surgery grew significantly. The number of plastic surgeons around the world increased and generated support for expansion of the specialty. The quality of the established techniques for the correction of noses, faces, necks, eyelids, ears, chins, breasts, and abdomens improved considerably. A series of new cosmetic operations for solving a myriad of problems developed. A typical example is management of the hypoplastic breast. Over the years it was treated with paraffin, sponge implants, fat grafts, and liquid silicone, with

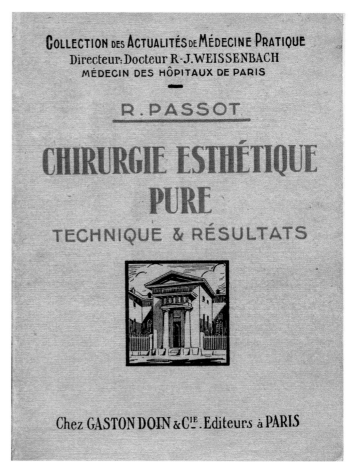

Fig. 2.25 The book on aesthetic surgery by Raymond Passot (1886–1933), published in 1931.

poor or dramatic results. In the mid-1960s the silicone mammary prosthesis was offered in clinical practice, representing the first convincing solution. Liposuction, introduced in the mid-1980s, soon became one of the most popular interventions. Fillers, botulinum toxin, and fat injection favorably improved a wide range of aesthetic problems, with minimally invasive procedures.

Access the complete reference list online at **http://www.expertconsult.com**

2. Majno G. *The Healing Hand. Man and Wound in the ancient World*. Cambridge: Harvard University Press; 1982.

   Written by an internationally renowned pathologist, who dedicated his life to the study of the fibroblast and its role on inflammation, The Healing Hand is one of the most extraordinary textbooks ever published on how different

   civilizations faced the problem of managing wounds and infections. It is an amazing journey on the difficulties encountered by peoples to survive injuries through centuries.

5. Ballantyne JW. The teratological records of Chaldea. *Teratologia*. 1894;1:127–142.

18. Gnudi MT, Webster JP. *The Life and Time of Gaspare Tagliacozzi*. New York: Reichner; 1950.

An account on the life of the Renaissance Bolognese surgeon Gaspare Tagliacozzi, who wrote the first textbook on plastic surgery in 1597. Besides all the documents concerning Tagliacozzi, his life and technique for nasal reconstruction, the work brings together a detailed history of plastic surgery from the remote ages to the 19th century.

29. Rogers BO. Nasal Reconstruction 150 Years ago: Aesthetic and other Problems. *Aesth Plast Surg*. 5:283–327, 1981.

   Blair Rogers acquired an international reputation as the historian of plastic surgery. He wrote numerous papers on this topic during his life. The present work highlights the history of nasal reconstruction in the early 19th century.

30. Mazzola RF. Reconstruction of the Nose. A historical Review. *Handchir Mikrochir Plast Chir* 2007;39:181–188.

   It is well known that plastic surgery started as the art of reconstructing noses. The present paper traces the history of nasal reconstruction from its remote origin in India through the 19th century. A complete overview of the different techniques available.

56. Tessier P, Guiot G, Rougerie J, et al. Ostéotomies cranio-naso-orbito-faciales. *Hypertélorisme Ann Chir Plast*. 1912:669–712.

57. Rogers BO. A Chronologic History of Cosmetic Surgery. *Bull NY Acad Med*. 1971;47:265–302.

   Originated at the end of the 19th century, cosmetic surgery developed rapidly in the US and in Europe. Blair Rogers traces the birth of this new branch of surgery by quoting the pioneers in this field like Miller, Joseph, Passot, Noel, and others, and highlighting their contributions.

62. Haiken E. *Venus Envy. A History of Cosmetic Surgery*. Baltimore: Hopkins University Press; 1997.

   The author describes the quest for perfection through surgery from the beginning of the 20th century until the present time in the US. Supervised by the late Robert Goldwyn, the book offers a brilliant overview about perception of the different cosmetic surgery procedures in American culture.

65. Maliniak JW. *Sculpture in the living*. New York: Pierson, 1934.

66. Maliniak JW. *Rhinoplasty and Restoration of facial contour*. Philadelphia: Davis, 1947.

67. Smith F. *Reconstructive Surgery of the Head and Neck*. New York: Nelson, 1928.

70. Bourguet J. La véritable Chirurgie Esthétique du visage. Paris: Plon; 1936:56.

3

Psychological aspects of plastic surgery

Laurie A. Stevens and Mary H. McGrath

SYNOPSIS

- Plastic surgeons deal with the psychological needs and responses of their patients on a daily basis.
- To determine whether a person is a suitable candidate for the requested surgical procedure, plastic surgeons must have a keen eye and intuitive sense, know the right questions to ask, and have the good judgment to learn from their past experiences, especially those in which errors were made.
- The aim of this chapter is to provide the plastic surgeon with tools to determine the appropriateness of the patients' requests, to assess their capacity to tolerate the requested procedure, and to predict the likelihood that they will be satisfied with the surgical results.
- For a plastic surgeon to understand how psychological processes may affect a patient's reactions to plastic surgery, the foundation lies in understanding the psyche – how it is formed and how it works.
- Personality structure affects a patient's experience of surgery and its accompanying alterations in body image; awareness of this is essential to good communication and rapport with a patient.

Body image and plastic surgery

Defining body image

Although it is mentioned casually and widely, the term *body image* actually describes a complex psychological abstraction. Real physical appearance is only a part of it, and body image has been defined as the mind–body relationship, the subjective perception of the body as seen through the mind's eye, or the psychological effects of what a person looks like.[1] In 1935, Schilder, one of the first to study body image, described it as a tri-dimensional scheme of one's own body involving interpersonal, environmental, and temporal factors.[2] Within his construct, body image is a result of what our bodies look like, what people say about how we look, our reactions to this input, the circumstances and community in which we grow up, and when key life events occur. Within this frame of reference, consider two examples:

In the first instance, there is a large muscular girl with small breasts. If she also has a championship tennis serve and is part of an active, close-knit, sports-minded family that celebrates her triumphs, her feelings about her breasts may be quite different from those of a girl of the same age who stands out as the least feminine and shapely member of her socially prominent, appearance-conscious family.

In a second example, an individual is told continually that he has his grandfather's rather large and prominent nose. This may be welcome news if he was a legendary fellow known for his charisma and respected for his business and political successes. The feeling might be different if he was a solitary, ill-tempered failure, disliked and avoided by his children.

Thus, the possession of certain physical characteristics is colored by feelings about their value, and a person's reaction to having familial, ethnically normative, or culturally popular features is influenced by personal perceptions. Because of this, body image is necessarily subjective. We cannot know someone else's feelings about his or her body by an external evaluation of his or her actual appearance. It follows that changing someone's appearance for the better is a positive event, only if the person considers it an improvement.

Body image determines emotional response and behavior

Perceptions of body image affect emotional response and drive behavioral changes. Let us look at how this important sequence occurs and then consider how this cause and effect make plastic surgery a profound and life-altering event for many patients.

When a person looks and thinks about himself or herself, a body image is formed. Individuals appraise themselves on the basis of this image, of their physical and mental abilities, and their relative success in the environment. This produces a psychological effect, with varying amounts of confidence or anxiety. These feelings of self-confidence or inadequacy will then influence their ability to perform. Thus, in dealing with other people and with life's challenges and problems, one's body image influences the amount of success that can be realized. Repeating this process over and over on a daily basis, we learn what can be accomplished and then use this information to direct our behavior. Goal-oriented patterns develop as we learn to avoid situations in which we are not effective and seek out those that reward our efforts. As we do this, others learn our strengths and weaknesses, and this further determines their response and behavior toward us.[3]

Four stages of body image development

Early childhood

Beginning in the earliest months, children learn how to think about themselves from those around them. As a child's parents proffer approval and love or, alternatively, show a lack of attention or disapproval, the child learns about his or her attractiveness and value to others. In a warm and loving environment, a child will develop feelings of self-worth, and these become the foundation of a positive body image.

Starting school

The second stage of body image development begins at the age of 5 or 6 years, when the child leaves the security of the family to begin school and encounters outside competition with peers. If the child is attractive to others and capable of projecting qualities desirable to the other children, the child will be well accepted. Reinforced by positive feedback, the child will grow in confidence and be ready to invest further in rewarding behaviors, and patterns of thinking about himself or herself will be further established.

Adolescence

With puberty, the child's physical appearance changes dramatically. There are changes in height; facial features enlarge; secondary sex characteristics develop; and the adolescent must deal with body hair, acne, and odor. The changes are not equal among adolescents in terms of when they occur or the endpoints they reach, and with all of this, comes great vulnerability to the opinions of others. As physical changes occur, the teenager will respond to the objective changes with impressions that will be tested repeatedly against the opinion of peers. In gauging the reactions of others, a self-picture will emerge and engender an unusually strong emotional response in this age group. Assaulted with feelings of insecurity, inadequacy, or depression, the adolescent may respond with behavioral changes that alter social interaction and introduce a negative pattern of body image development.

Aging

With the passage of time and concomitant changes in physical appearance, body image again undergoes adaptation. Now, as one appears less vigorous and fresh, competitors respond by granting less authority to the older individual. Faced with this response, the physically older person starts to show weakening of body image and retreats from situations in which he or she was previously comfortable.

How plastic surgery changes body image

Plastic surgery is effective and useful to many patients because it changes body image. As long as this change is perceived by the patient as an enhancement, there will be resultant positive changes in his or her emotional life and behavioral patterns and, thus, improved quality of life. It is significant that plastic surgery tends to be undertaken at the time of one of the four stages of body image development discussed in the preceding section.[4–6]

Plastic surgery may be undertaken in the child with a congenital deformity or a physical defect that could cause others to withdraw emotional or physical contact with the child. Even if the deformity is of trivial proportions, its correction will eliminate a factor that might cause early rejection. The second period, when a child enters school, is the usual time to correct protruding ears, webbed toes, scars, small hairy nevi, and other problems that will mobilize the attention of and draw comments and criticisms from the child's peers. The teenage years are a time for correction of recently developed unattractive features, such as a large nasal hump, or humiliating conditions, such as gynecomastia. The aging person seeks plastic surgery to correct deficiencies associated with maturation (e.g., wrinkling, a worn and tired appearance).

Given that the motivation to have aesthetic and reconstructive plastic surgery may often be psychological and involves body image, the key to achieving success is selection of patients. The core value of the surgery lies not in the objective beauty of the visible result but in the patient's opinion of and response to the change. Recognition and understanding of psychological issues begin with identification of the personality traits that determine human interactions.

Personality and character formation

Much has been written about how personality or character develops in human beings. We all have personality traits that characterize who we are and how we interact with the world. These traits govern how we perceive and relate to our environment and ourselves. These traits are consistent and stable, despite outside stimuli and influences.

The ego is the chief executive of the mind, in charge of balancing the internal and external influences that confront it. These influences include memories, drives, anxieties, perceptions, and external needs. To function

smoothly, the ego has to have a set of automatic operations that deal with these influences. These operations are called defense mechanisms.

Defense mechanisms

We use defense mechanisms to cope with the stresses of our internal and external worlds. These mechanisms are not under our conscious control and develop in response to our early life experiences. Our repertoire of defenses contributes to our character formation and enables us to forget painful experiences, to minimize or deny anxiety-provoking situations, and to evade unwanted impulses (sexual and aggressive).[7] For purposes of understanding plastic surgical patients and their response to surgery, the defense mechanisms of regression, denial, projection, repression, distortion, somatization, intellectualization, rationalization, and sublimation are discussed.

Regression is a return to a previous stage of functioning or development to avoid anxiety or conflict.[7] Regression may be seen in both healthy and unhealthy adaptations to illness. Patients have to undergo some degree of regression to allow themselves to be cared for when they are ill and to be in a dependent position. However, regression may get to a pathologic level when the patient acts in an infantile and helpless manner and is unable to participate as a partner in the medical care.

Denial is being consciously unaware of a painful aspect of reality. Through denial, patients invalidate unpleasant or unwanted bits of information and act as though they do not exist.[7] Denial, like regression, can be adaptive or maladaptive in the medical setting. For example, a certain degree of denial can function to allow a patient to cope with an overwhelming feeling of helplessness or hopelessness in response to a diagnosis of terminal cancer. Denial becomes maladaptive when it interferes with a patient's ability to participate in medical care. Denial need not be confronted when a patient is accepting appropriate medical treatment and participating in care. Denial can reach psychotic proportions in psychiatrically ill individuals.

Projection is when one attributes one's unacknowledged feelings to others.[7] Projection may be displayed by falsely attributing or misinterpreting attitudes, feelings, or intentions of others (e.g., "I'm not angry at her; she's angry at me.").

Repression involves keeping unwanted memories, thoughts, or feelings from conscious awareness.[7] The patient who "forgets" unpleasant news that the physician tells her or him is likely to be repressing the disturbing thoughts or feelings.

Distortion occurs when patients grossly reshape external reality to suit their inner needs, including magical beliefs and delusional thinking.[8]

Somatization is when patients convert their psychic conflicts and conflicted feelings into body symptoms.[8] The most common presentation of somatization is hypochondriasis.

Intellectualization is when the patient controls anxieties and impulses by excessively thinking about them rather than experiencing them.[8] These thoughts are devoid of affect or feeling.

Rationalization is when the patient justifies his or her attitudes, beliefs, or behavior that might be unacceptable by inventing a convincing fallacy.[8]

Sublimation is the transformation of drives, feelings, and memories into healthy and creative outcomes.[8]

Perioperative psychological reactions

Even when the surgeon has preoperatively considered a patient to be a suitable candidate for surgery, it does not mean that he or she should cease to look for signs of psychological disturbance in the patient in the postoperative period. Transient episodes of anxiety or depression that last days to weeks after surgery have been reported in studies by Edgerton et al.[9] and Meyer et al.[10] A patient may experience psychiatric side-effects to various medications used preoperatively, intraoperatively, and postoperatively. The sudden onset of a new psychiatric symptom should suggest a medication-induced psychiatric side-effect. Perhaps one of the most profound reactions seen is lidocaine-induced delirium after regional limb surgery, in which a local anesthetic block was used. This can happen if there is an inadvertent intravenous injection of the anesthetic agent.

Mood improvement has been reported in a variety of cosmetic surgery patients postoperatively.[11–20] Even the so-called high-risk patients, those thought most likely to have a poor psychological outcome, may show benefit after cosmetic surgery.[21] These findings have led to the conclusion that cosmetic surgery can be psychologically beneficial even to patients with psychiatric conditions, assuming that they are properly managed by their physician and psychiatrist.[22]

In the discussions that follow, different personality styles and disorders are discussed relative to how they respond to surgery and recovery.

The physician–patient relationship

Surgeons are invested with strong emotions by patients who are entrusting them with their bodies and lives. Patients may develop special feelings for their surgeons that are similar to those associated with figures of authority from their past.[23] This may account for the idealization of the surgeon as the "miracle worker" or "savior", as well as for some of the unwarranted angry feelings toward the surgeon. This is a phenomenon known as transference. The nature of the physician–patient relationship is extremely important to the success of the treatment of the seriously ill patient. Although many physicians are uncomfortable with the patients who develop feelings about them, it is important to recognize the phenomena of transference, counter-reaction, and counter-transference.

Transference can be described as recreating, in the physician–patient relationship, a conflicted relationship with a childhood figure. The transference may be of a paternal or a maternal nature, but this is not necessarily the case. Grandparent, aunt or uncle, and sibling transferences can also occur. When transference is present, the patient will react to the physician as if the physician were the transferential figure; in other words, feelings about that figure become "transferred" onto the physician. If the transference is positive, it generally does not need to be addressed. However, if the transference is negative, it does need evaluation.

An example of negative transference is the patient who treats the physician as if he or she were sadistic, uncaring, cold, and heartless, when the physician is trying his or her best to be empathic, warm, and caring. The patient is acting in an overly exaggerated fashion out of proportion to the real interaction. Often, the transference is not a total distortion of the real relationship between the physician and patient; the patient may have picked up on some aspect of the physician's personality or behavior that has served as the foundation for the development of transferential feelings.

The physician's emotional reaction to the patient's expression of transferential feelings is termed counter-reaction. For example, when the patient becomes angry with the physician, the physician wishes to withdraw or may feel anger in response. Instead, the physician should try to figure out how best to respond to the patient's feelings and behavior without personalizing them. This is not easy, as physicians, like their patients, are only human, and are prey to their own feelings and those of others towards them. Counter-reaction, which is a common or "normal" response to the patient's emotions or behaviors, needs to be differentiated from counter-transference.

Counter-transference is the physician's reaction to the patient based not on the real circumstances but on issues or conflictual relationships in the physician's own life – if you will, a "neurotic" response to a patient's transference. When these feelings occur, they may be intense for both the patient and the physician. Recognition of these feelings and their origins is an important insight and a good tool to have to improve relationships with patients and to avoid pitfalls in the treatment relationship, including the selection of specific interventions.

Personality styles and personality disorders

There are various personality types or styles that all physicians treat in clinical practice. This section focuses on the personality styles and disorders most commonly encountered by the plastic surgeon, the typical reactions to surgery or alterations of body image, and the medical management of these.

When personality traits become inflexible and maladaptive and cause either significant impairment in social or occupational functioning or subjective distress, they constitute a personality disorder.[24] Personality disorders are generally apparent by late childhood or adolescence, continue throughout most of an individual's adult life, and may become exaggerated in the older years.

There are four characteristics that all personality disorders share. They are: (1) an inflexible and maladaptive response to stress; (2) a disability in working and loving that is generally more serious and always more pervasive than that found in neurosis; (3) elicitation by interpersonal conflict; and (4) a peculiar capacity to "get under the skin" of others.[25] Patients with personality disorders see the rest of the world, rather than themselves, as having a problem. They have little insight into their own behavior or its impact on others around them.

Obsessive-compulsive personality and personality disorder

Many individuals with an obsessive-compulsive personality are highly successful and productive members of the community. This personality style lends itself to efficiency, effectiveness, and goal-directed behavior. These individuals tend to deal with feelings by using intellectualization; are preoccupied with details, organization, and schedules; tend to be perfectionistic; are scrupulous about matters related to morality and ethics; have trouble delegating tasks to others; and can be rigid, stubborn, and miserly.[26]

When obsessive-compulsive patients become anxious, they can quickly decompensate and become overly invested in routines or seemingly trivial information. These patients can overwhelm the physician with questions and occupy enormous physician and staff time, leading to resentment by caretakers. It is important to reassure these patients and to address their fears and anxieties; sometimes the surgeon should try to determine what may be making them anxious or fearful and provide appropriate comfort. These patients are often unaware of their feelings, and providing them with detailed medical explanations can be helpful to them. Giving them tasks to perform makes them feel like a partner in their therapeutic treatment and in decision-making. This could take the form of having them change dressings, measure their fluid intake and output, or care for scars with topical moisturizers. Even if these measures are not strictly necessary, they will help these patients manage their anxiety.

Patient example

Ms A. is an overly neat 43-year-old successful business executive who underwent a blepharoplasty. After surgery, she barraged the surgeon's office with endless questions and details and occupied excessive amounts of staff time on the telephone. The surgeon, Dr B., had Ms A. come in for an extra postoperative visit and instructed her to prepare, in advance, a list of questions she needed answered. After answering her questions, Dr B. addressed her anxiety about the eventual outcome, reassuring her that this was a normal concern, and tried to determine how best to continue to reassure her. She was given a scheduled daily call-in time, limited to 5 min, during which she could ask her questions and receive support and reassurance.

Narcissistic personality and personality disorder

Narcissistic patients have an excessive need for admiration, an exaggerated sense of self-importance, and grandiose notions of their beauty and power. They have a sense of entitlement; can be exploitative of others to achieve their own ends; lack empathy towards others; can be envious of others or feel that others are envious of them, and may be arrogant and haughty in their behaviors and attitudes.[26]

Because these patients place such value on their physical appearance, surgery to alter their appearance will naturally generate some anxiety. They generally find the physical effects of aging on their appearance unacceptable. Similarly, they find distressing any surgical complication or even the typical swelling and bruising that are the sequelae of surgical procedures. These patients need to be educated as much as possible about the process of healing and recovery and offered reassurance along the way about common postoperative events. They respond to being treated like equal, independent partners in their care.

Plastic surgeons should take care not to be taken in by the narcissistic patient's idealization of them (e.g., "You're the best plastic surgeon in the country."). These patients can quickly switch to profound devaluation of the surgeon if the surgeon displeases them or causes them discomfort. These patients tend to become demanding when they are physically uncomfortable and anxious, and they respond best to empathic reassurance.

Dependent personality and personality disorder

These patients exhibit clinging and submissive behavior, seemingly needing endless reassurance and support.

They have great difficulty making daily decisions without an excessive amount of advice and reassurance. They want others to assume responsibility for their major decisions. They experience difficulty initiating actions because of a lack of self-confidence in their judgment and abilities. They often find it difficult to disagree with others because they fear rejection or disapproval. Dependent personalities have great discomfort when they are alone and are fearful that they cannot take care of themselves.[26]

This translates in the surgical situation to the dependent patient's becoming clinging and fearful after surgery, in part facilitated by the regression initiated by being taken care of while ill. This behavior can sometimes alienate healthcare providers and bring about the very thing the dependent personality fears, to be alone and abandoned. The physician should try to recognize these fears and provide reassurance to the patient that he or she will not be abandoned. Warm support should be offered, but firm limits must be set on undue neediness and manipulativeness.

Paranoid personality disorder

Paranoid patients have a pervasive mistrust and suspicion of others.[26] They fear that motives are ill-intentioned and they suspect, with an insufficient basis in fact, that others are trying to harm, exploit, or injure them. They may attribute a malevolent intent to innocent remarks. They are unforgiving and bear grudges, even to seemingly benign slights. They perceive others as attacking their character or reputation and may respond angrily and with vindictiveness.

These patients experience surgery as an "intrusion" and attack on their bodies. They find it difficult to establish a therapeutic alliance with healthcare providers. Their lives sometimes appear to be without direction, i.e., "drifters." They have few friendships and few social interactions. Their occupational choices are most successful when they choose professions in which they have little contact with others and can work in relative isolation.

Under stress, paranoid individuals can develop brief psychotic episodes. It is preferable not to perform elective cosmetic surgery on such an individual. If the paranoid patient requires reconstructive surgery or other nonelective cosmetic surgery, it is important to respect the patient's distance and interact with the patient in a professional manner, not attempting to get too close or friendly, because this behavior may be viewed with suspicion. The surgeon should be direct and answer questions in a candid and honest fashion. Any distortions by the patient that are noted by the surgeon should be addressed and discussed openly. Accusations should be neither disputed nor confirmed but explained as coming from illness rather than from any attempt to injure the patient.[27]

Histrionic personality and personality disorder

Histrionic[26] patients tend to be excessively emotional and exhibit attention-seeking behavior. Although they are often lively, flirtatious, and dramatic, they continually demand to be the center of attention. If they feel the spotlight move away from them, they may do something dramatic to refocus attention on themselves (e.g., make a scene on the floor; call patient relations). They are highly suggestible and easily influenced by others and current fads. The plastic surgeon should take care in assessing this patient to ascertain the real reasons for seeking surgery.

Histrionic persons may be overly trusting, especially of physicians, whom they see as magically solving their problems. They tend to view the therapeutic relationship as more intimate than it actually is and may develop romantic fantasies about their physicians. Individuals with histrionic personality disorder are at an increased risk for suicidal gestures and may make threats to get attention and coerce better caregiving.

The surgeon should adopt a professional manner with these patients and give the appropriate amount of attention to them. The surgeon must be very careful not to become too friendly or to be drawn into their seductive behavior. Certainly, one should not be flirtatious or seductive in response. Firm limit setting with regard to the nature of the therapeutic relationship and the physician's role in the patient's life is necessary.

Borderline personality disorder

Borderline patients[26] have a pattern of unstable interpersonal relationships. They may have an identity disturbance characterized by shifting and changing senses of self, goals, values, and aspirations. Likewise, feeling states or moods can also show wild swings and variability. Borderline patients can be impulsive and often have trouble controlling their anger and emotions. Their behavior can be self-destructive and manipulative. They may engage in gambling, excessive money spending, binge eating, substance abuse, unsafe sex, or reckless driving. At the extreme, they may perform self-mutilating acts (cutting or burning), or suicidal behavior. Completed suicide occurs in 8–10% of such patients. During periods of extreme stress, transient paranoid ideation or dissociative symptoms (e.g., depersonalization) may occur but generally do not persist.

Such patients are best handled with strict limit setting. The physician should make every attempt to be consistent and attentive but not respond to manipulative behavior. The patient should be given a schedule for visits and follow-up plans to limit fears of abandonment.

These patients generally respond best to the corrective experience of developing a trusting, stable relationship with the physician who does not retaliate in response to their angry and disruptive behaviors.[28] Use of the resources of other healthcare providers, such as a psychiatric consultant for psychotherapy and psychopharmacotherapy or a nurse practitioner to "spread the transference," can help make these patients feel adequately attended to and cared for. However, it is important for the surgeon to continue to care for them in the usual fashion because these other relationships are not a substitute for the surgeon's relationship with them.

Strategies for management of the difficult patient

The hateful patient

The "hateful patient" is a term coined by James E. Groves in his seminal article in the *New England Journal of Medicine*.[29] These are patients who often inspire dread in their physicians when they see their names on the appointment schedule. These patients often make a provider feel angry and helpless, leading to possible retaliation or confrontation. Who are these individuals? It is helpful to recognize these patients, to understand why they inspire negative feelings, and to manage their treatment on the basis of specific principles. One cannot pretend that negative feelings do not exist because failing to acknowledge these feelings can lead to suboptimal medical care.

The dependent clinger

Dependent clingers[29] range from having mild requests for reassurance to demanding requests for many different forms of attention (such as analgesics, long explanations, caring, affection). These patients may be experienced as "bottomless pits" of neediness, and avoidance behaviors on the part of the physician may ensue.

The warning signs of the dependent clinger are the overly grateful patient who idealizes the physician, professes undying "love" and admiration, and behaves in a seductive manner. The physician becomes "the inexhaustible mother"; the patient becomes the "unplanned, unwanted, unlovable child."[29]

Patient example

Ms T., a 24-year-old woman who is seeking augmentation mammaplasty, places several telephone calls before her surgery, asking for more information and needing reassurance about the upcoming surgery. Her plastic surgeon gives her the time she seems to need to make her feel comfortable about the procedure. Several days postoperatively, she starts to place telephone calls to the office, escalating in frequency and urgency. She is requesting office visits, despite little objective need for a visit outside of the usual postoperative follow-up. She also starts to ask for analgesic medications and to request reassurance about her breast size and her discomfort. The plastic surgeon stops answering her calls and lets his nurse field the questions and calls. As a result of not being able to reach the surgeon directly, she starts to page him in the evenings, telling his service that it is an emergency.

The best management of this patient is to set firm limits relative to appointments and telephone contacts. The physician needs to kindly but clearly state to the patient that he/she has human limitations and cannot be an inexhaustible resource to the patient, available at any time of day or night. Regular office visits should be scheduled, during which time the patient can see the physician and ask questions. The surgeon's nurse can also schedule visits in between visits to the physician to provide reassurance. These actions should give the patient the contact needed without disrupting the office and the physician's life. Enlisting the help of a psychiatric consultant can be helpful in providing additional support to the patient and spreading the transference.

The self-destructive denier

All physicians have patients who deny their illnesses.[29] Denial is pathologic when it interferes with the patient's ability to accept proper medical care for the illness. Otherwise, denial can be adaptive in coping with the illness.

However, there is a group of patients who are self-destructive deniers. Unlike the adaptive deniers, these patients are fundamentally dependent on others and seem to revel in their self-orchestrated destruction. They appear to their physicians as taking great pleasure in putting obstacles in the path to delivery of optimal care.

Patient example

Mr B., a 49-year-old man, is an intravenous drug abuser. He has a long history of drug-related medical problems and hospitalizations. Despite multiple attempts to get him to pursue drug treatment, he has resisted attending any programs. He was admitted to the hospital with bacterial endocarditis and given intravenous antibiotics for 6 weeks. Shortly after discharge, he was readmitted with cellulitis from a fresh intravenous heroin injection site. The plastic surgeon was consulted to provide skin flaps for coverage after skin loss followed the cellulitis. After that treatment and discharge, he was readmitted with recurrence of the endocarditis and required additional skin grafting for breakdown due to new soft tissue infections. Two months later, he was admitted with sepsis and died in the hospital.

Self-destructive deniers make their physicians feel angry, helpless, used, and abused. They engender rescue fantasies, especially in younger physicians, but may also lead their physicians to have negative feelings toward them. Physicians often feel guilty about their hateful feelings towards such patients.

The best management is to see the patient's pattern of self-destructive denial and to set realistic expectations relative to the patient's ability to get well. It may be helpful to think of the patient as having a degenerative or terminal illness, for which there is no medical treatment and to set the goal of providing supportive care and alleviating suffering.

The entitled demander

The entitled demander[29] is fundamentally similar to the dependent clinger in neediness; however, the presentation is quite different. These patients are demanding, devaluing, and intimidating. These are the patients who threaten lawsuits or contact patient relations representatives when the medical staff does not fulfill their demands as they require.

Their primary feeling state is one of entitlement. This is actually a defense against fears of loss of control and helplessness. However, when a physician is at the other end of the angry demands and entitled behavior, it is easy to understand how one could become enraged with this patient. They also make the physician feel fearful of their threats. The usual reaction to these patients is to let them know, in no uncertain terms, how undeserving they are of what they demand. This usually does not work with this population.

Groves[29] speaks eloquently about how to handle such a patient, as follows:

> I know you're mad about this ... and at the other doctors. You have reason to be mad. You have an illness that makes some people give up and you're fighting it. But you're fighting your doctors too. You say you're entitled to repeated tests, damages for suffering and all that. And you are entitled – entitled to the very best medical care we can give you. But we can't give you the good treatment you deserve unless you help. You deserve a chance to control this disease; you deserve all the allies you can get. You'll get the help you deserve if you'll stop misdirecting your anger to the very people who are trying to help you get what you deserve – good medical care.

This strategy allows the patient to fulfill the underlying wish to receive "the best" medical care and, it is hoped, will enlist the individual as an ally in the treatment. It enables the physician to tactfully address the entitled, demanding behavior in a constructive way, rather than to respond with rage or retaliation.

Manipulative help-rejecting complainers

No matter to what lengths the physician may go to help them, this is the group of patients who will try to thwart the help.[29] They express their hopelessness that any physician can help them. They return to the physician's office week after week to affirm that the recommended treatment failed once again. When one physician "fails" them, they shop for the next.

Like the dependent clinger and the entitled demander, they tend to have no limits to their need. They do not seem to wish to get well; instead, they seem to wish an "undivorceable marriage" with their healthcare provider. When one symptom resolves, another appears to replace it. These patients often suffer from undiagnosed and untreated depression.

Patient example

Ms S. is a 30-year-old sales associate with intractable hand pain. She has gone for consultations all over the country and has received numerous diagnoses, including causalgia, reflex sympathetic dystrophy, and carpal tunnel syndrome. She has had hundreds of diagnostic procedures, but (fortunately) she has refused to have surgery when it was recommended. She had a 14-day hospitalization at a pain treatment center, during which time her hand pain diminished with a combination of antidepressants, relaxation therapy, behavioral therapy, and occupational and physical therapy. However, after discharge, she failed to follow any of the recommendations, and the pain recurred. She is now angry that the pain center failed to cure her and is determined to find a physician who can find the "real cause" of her pain.

This group of patients makes physicians worry that they may have overlooked a correctable illness and makes them feel anxious and uncertain about their clinical skills. It is usually not constructive to confront this patient with his or her behavior or neediness. It is important to realize that the ultimate goal of the patient is to never be abandoned and to always be connected to the physician. However, he or she is fearful of real closeness with the physician.

A good strategy for the physician is to communicate to these patients that he or she may not be able to help them and to share their pessimism that they can be "cured." Instead, the physician could suggest treatments that may provide "some" relief (but not enough that the patient will be cured, thereby engendering fear in the patient of losing the physician). This technique was used by Ms S.'s physician, who also treated her depression and offered behavioral strategies to alleviate her pain, while telling her that he did not think that the techniques could be more than 50% helpful. Ms S. was satisfied with this approach, which allowed her to hold onto her symptom and to her relationship with her physician simultaneously but also permitted her to become more functional in her daily life. Psychiatric consultation can be helpful but not as a replacement for the primary physician; it must be presented as an adjunctive treatment.

Surgical procedures and related psychological issues

Aesthetic facial surgery

Our society seems to value youth and to associate the physical changes of aging with weakness and loss of worth. Surgery to rejuvenate the face can be of enormous benefit to the person with an aging appearance. It may allow the person to feel better and acquire acceptance, to feel sexually attractive to others, and to be viewed as more vibrant, strong, and youthful. There are clear economic, psychological, and social benefits to having a more youthful appearance.

Surgery of the aging face is done for the purpose of restoring a previously existing appearance or preexisting image of the face. This type of surgery seems to require no dramatic body image readjustment[30] because the aging face does not appear to be fully incorporated into the body image over time. This operation is generally successful and psychologically beneficial to the individual.

Procedures to rejuvenate the face are generally performed in the middle to later ages of life. This is a time of potential loss – of loved ones, of career, of friends and family, menopause, baldness, the empty nest left by children's emancipation. In a study of facelift patients older than 50 years, Webb et al.[11] found that 90% had lost an important person in the 5 years before surgery. Dunofsky[31] found the study population of women who had facial cosmetic surgery to be more narcissistic and to have more problems with separation-individuation

than the control group but to have no differences in self-esteem and social anxiety. Edgerton et al.[32] found that 74% of facelift patients had been diagnosed with a psychiatric disorder.

Sarwer and Crerand[33] looked at the various preoperative studies in the literature and found that clinical interview-based investigations identified a higher incidence of psychopathology in the cosmetic surgery population. However, when preoperative studies using standardized psychometric testing as part of the assessment were evaluated, little psychopathology was uncovered.

There have been various studies that alluded to greater psychological difficulties in male than in female facelift patients.[32,34] However, the percentage of men having facelifts has increased during the past 20 years, with no clear increase in psychological difficulties postoperatively.

In Goin et al.'s study,[35] the motivations for facelift surgery were related to feelings about aging in 70% of the patients, and most were satisfied with the results, even when they had some unrealistic expectations. Friel et al. also reported a similarly high satisfaction rate.[36] The study of Leist et al.[37] revealed that about 13% of patients were dissatisfied with their surgical results.

Postoperatively, facelift patients may experience some hypoesthesia or paresthesias of the face and neck. They may experience some sleep disturbance caused by physical discomfort. Those individuals who particularly prize their autonomy and independence may find it difficult to manage the postoperative period of physical discomfort and incapacity. However, psychological reactions are usually short-lived, and patients are generally satisfied with their results, experiencing a sense of enhanced attractiveness and self-esteem.

Aging face patients who seek facelift surgery appear to be motivated by the desire to restore their previous youthful visage. Rhinoplasty patients, on the other hand, are seeking to change their basic appearance.

Rhinoplasty

The literature is filled with articles and studies about the patients who seek rhinoplasty. In general, older studies of this group of patients suggested a great deal of psychopathology. In 1975, Gibson and Connolly[38] studied rhinoplasty patients 10 years postoperatively and found a high level (38%) of psychopathology, including schizophrenia. They compared this group with a trauma and disease group, in which they found only 8% with a psychological disorder. Wright and Wright[39] found a high level of psychopathology based on psychological testing measures (Minnesota Multiphasic Personality Inventory) in their controlled study of rhinoplasty patients. Compared with the control group, patients seeking rhinoplasty were more self-critical, more sensitive to others' opinions of them, and more restless. The most consistent personality diagnosis was "inadequate personality," which probably translates into "dependent personality" by today's diagnostic nomenclature. Hay and Heather's 1973 study[16] of 45 rhinoplasty patients demonstrated psychological disturbance in about 58% of the study group. Micheli-Pellegrini and Manfrida's study[40] as well as Linn and Goldman's study[41] also revealed a high incidence of psychopathology. Zahiroddin *et al.*, however, found no significant difference in the rate of psychiatric disturbance and the decision to undergo rhinoplasty.[42]

There has been much focus in the plastic surgery literature on the so-called minimal defect rhinoplasty patient. The 1960 study of Jacobson *et al.*[43] looked at 20 consecutive men requesting cosmetic surgery for "minimal defects." The most requested procedure was rhinoplasty. All but two of the patients (those two refused psychological evaluation) were found to have psychiatric diagnoses. Seven were found to have psychosis; four were found to be neurotic; seven had personality disorders. Half of the patients underwent the procedure, and more than 50% of these surgical patients had postoperative psychological problems, including one suicide attempt.

However, not all studies have supported a link between rhinoplasty and psychopathology, and in actual practice, a great majority of rhinoplasty patients seem to benefit from the surgery. The patients described by Linn and Goldman[41] reacted with "elation" after the surgery and shortly afterwards, were no longer preoccupied with their nose and were pleased with the cosmetic results. They found an overall improvement in the patient's level of adjustment. They hypothesized that the anatomic changes made to the nose and subsequent change in others' behavior toward the patient led to a release of the psychic energy attached to the nose. Goin and Goin's study[44] of rhinoplasty patients who were simultaneously in psychotherapy, supported Linn and Goldman's hypothesis. Goin and Goin asserted that the loss of self-consciousness achieved after the rhinoplasty led to greater self-confidence, which led others to behave differently toward the patient, enabling the patient's self-esteem to grow with this reinforcement. In this group, 33% showed no detectable psychological changes postoperatively, and most were happy with their surgical results. On balance, a substantial number of studies seem to demonstrate psychological and psychosocial benefit from rhinoplasty surgery.

Several studies during the last decade have shown that the psychological benefits of rhinoplasty surgery are greater in female than in male patients.[45,46] Slator and Harris[47] found that male patients show more symptoms of anxiety and depression than do their female counterparts preoperatively, but they found no evidence to support earlier suggestions that requests for rhinoplasty may be early symptoms of severe psychiatric illness.

Several writers have urged plastic surgeons to be cautious about drastically altering the appearance of the patient. Some patients experience a sense of a "loss of identity."[7] In a series of more than 5000 rhinoplasty patients, Bruck[48] reported that older patients often poorly tolerate drastic changes in their appearance. He warns against "type changing" rhinoplasty in patients older than 35 years. Other authors looking at dissatisfaction of the patient in the setting of multiple rhinoplasty procedures may have been seeing cases of body dysmorphic disorder, which at the time of the papers was not a recognized psychiatric entity.

Rhinoplasty patients, especially men, may experience some concerns relative to their sexual identity in the postoperative period. These concerns appear to be connected to feelings about the size and shape of their nose. Consequently, to avoid psychiatric disturbances in the postoperative period, the plastic surgeon needs to try to ferret out the presence of sexual identity disturbances before deciding to operate. Likewise, psychotic patients should be identified and surgery avoided in this population because their psychotic thinking or delusions may be exacerbated by the surgery.

Augmentation mammaplasty

In general, augmentation mammaplasty patients are happy with their plastic surgical result. Even in the presence of scarring and capsular contractures, most augmentation mammaplasty patients are satisfied with their aesthetic appearance and the psychological benefits derived from the surgery.[20,49] The groups of women most commonly seeking augmentation mammaplasty are small-breasted women who have always been unhappy with the appearance of their breasts and seek the surgery for psychological reasons, women whose breasts have undergone involution postpartum or with nursing and who wish to restore their previous size and appearance, and those who seek the surgery for occupational reasons (such as actresses, models, and nude dancers).

In general, the first group is the least psychologically healthy group before surgery. There appears to be a higher than normal incidence of depressive disorders,[50–52] with one study by Edgerton et al.[50] reporting the percentage to be up to 60%. These patients often have poor self-esteem and feelings of inadequacy. They may feel a diminished sense of femininity and sexual attractiveness. Sexual functioning may be impaired by inhibitions about not wanting their breasts viewed or fondled during sexual play.

After augmentation mammaplasty, patients will report enhanced self-esteem, greater feelings of attractiveness and femininity, fewer inhibitions during sexual activity, and improved mood. Studies by Kilmann et al.[53] and Schlebusch and Mahrt[54] have reported improvement in body image after breast augmentation. The patients rapidly integrate their augmented breasts into their body image. Druss[51] explained this remarkable change in behavior, outlook, and self-esteem from a psychoanalytic perspective. He stated that a woman seeks augmentation mammaplasty in an effort to repair chronic and deep-seated intrapsychic conflicts. In his study group, he found that the patients had problematic identification with their mothers, secondary to the mother's being emotionally unavailable. This failure of identification led to poorly formed self-images as women and doubts about femininity. Druss' observations may help explain why not all small-breasted women seek augmentation mammaplasty and many seem content with their breast size.

Interestingly, in light of the breast implant controversy and litigation during the 1990s, many women with augmented breasts chose to have explantation of their silicone implants because of their fears. Although many of these women felt less fearful after explantation, many also felt depressed when they had to return to their original breast size. Some chose to be reimplanted with saline implants to restore the positive feelings captured by the original augmentation procedure.

Reduction mammaplasty

Many women who seek reduction mammaplasty experience significant physical discomfort from their heavy and pendulous breasts and report restrictions in activities, especially sports. Finding clothing that fits properly is a problem. They describe feelings of unease wearing bathing suits. Many feel self-conscious about the size of their breasts and state that people, especially men, look at their breasts before looking at their faces. They may avoid social interactions and sexual encounters because of their discomfort and wear bras and clothing that minimize their breast size.

Studies of the psychological issues in breast reduction surgery are not numerous. Goin et al.[15] showed preoperative evidence of depression in a small sample; Hollyman et al.[55] also found a higher incidence of depression and anxiety compared with control subjects, also in a small sample. Sarwer et al.[56] reported that breast reduction patients experience greater dissatisfaction with their overall body image, worry and embarrassment about their breasts in public and social situations, and avoidance of physical activity.

Postoperatively, this is a satisfied group of patients. They quickly integrate their smaller breasts into their body image. They are often more self-confident and feel more feminine and sexually attractive. On occasion, patients are more satisfied with their surgical results than are their surgeons. Despite visible aesthetic problems postoperatively with scarring, and the frequency of some loss of nipple-areola sensibility, patients are generally satisfied.

Jones and Bain[57] reviewed the literature of outcome studies that demonstrated a high degree of satisfaction of patients (78–95% being very or moderately satisfied) and improvement in body image and psychological wellbeing. Chadbourne et al.[58] performed a review of the literature and meta-analysis of published studies and found that although quality of life parameters of physical function were statistically improved, measures of psychological function were not. Other studies did document psychological and emotional benefits after reduction mammaplasty.[59-63] However, one study by Guthrie *et al.*[64] described this population of patients, compared with a control group of large-breasted women not seeking reduction surgery, as having greater psychological and physical difficulties, with higher levels of anxiety and depression as well as poorer self-esteem, body image, and interpersonal functioning.

Patients may occasionally experience a sense of loss and require readjustment to their new body. There may be some social and sexual disturbances now that they no longer feel the need to isolate themselves because of their self-consciousness. They may need encouragement to become more socially active and less withdrawn.

Trauma: acquired defects

Hand transplantation

Accompanied by much media interest and public debate, the first hand transplants were reported in 1998 and 1999. It was clear that the transplantation of cadaver hands to the forearm amputation stumps of living patients was technically possible. What was less clear was the appropriateness of consigning the recipients to a lifetime of immunosuppressive therapy for a nonlife-threatening condition.[65]

In the discussions that followed, it was mentioned frequently that for the patient who has lost a hand, transplantation offers the potential psychological benefit of restoring body image, as well as improving function. This consideration was used to defend the level of risk accompanying transplantation, but it has not yet been established. Of the original four recipients of a hand transplant, three are reported to be pleased with the results at 2 years and to have incorporated the transplanted hand into their self-image. The fourth patient was enthusiastic initially, but the hand was later amputated at his request.[66]

Whereas the psychological status of the patients themselves remains to be studied over time, information has come forward from the discourse of these cases about the psychology of decision-making.[67] Those physicians and patients alike, struggling with the advisability of performing hand transplantation and looking at the risk-to-benefit ratio can come to very different

conclusions. Work from the field of decision-making analysis has shown that physicians and patients proceed from different frames of reference and prioritize values differently in making medical decisions. Patients tend to show a large preference for a risky alternative that has a chance of erasing a loss and of return to the previous status quo, and they tend to think of immediate rather than long-term risks (e.g., immunosuppression).[68] These and other irrational factors, such as denial of the possibility that they will have a severe complication, need to be made explicit in the decision-making process, particularly with a procedure as uncertain as hand transplantation.

Burns

Burn patients must initially face the issues concerning survival, the pain caused by the burn itself, and the need to often undergo multiple procedures (e.g., skin grafts, dressing changes). They are then faced with issues concerning scarring caused by the burn and the deforming nature of these scars. The anatomic location of the scarring is relevant because those scars that are more obvious to others (e.g., on the face) lead to discomfort in their presence and increased self-consciousness. Often, plastic surgical procedures are performed in stages during a protracted period, which delays the return to preinjury functioning. The chronicity of treatment can pose psychological difficulties, as is true with any chronic illness.

Psychological difficulties seen in the burn population include depression, helplessness, frustration, hopelessness, diminished self-image, self-consciousness, social isolation, and despair. There is a greater likelihood that burn patients will discontinue treatment and lose contact with their physicians and other caretakers.[69] This avoidance may be reflective of anxiety with repeated surgeries, permanent scarring, and loss of hope that their disfigured appearance can ever be changed.

In general, a multidisciplinary approach is the most helpful in the burn population. The team should include the surgeon, primary care physician, mental health professional, nursing staff, physical therapist, occupational therapist, and support group therapy. Family members may also benefit from supportive therapy, individually or in a group. Close attention should be paid to the patient's mental state, mood, and degree of demoralization. Medical personnel sometimes make the mistake of dismissing a clinical depression. Pain management is extremely important, and mood stabilizers and antidepressants may also be helpful. Staff should try to look past the disfigured appearance to see the person inside. Having a normal conversation with the patient about daily life, sports, or current events will be reassuring as it indicates the person is still intact internally and can be interesting to others and accepted by them. Staff can empathize with the patient's self-consciousness, but it is important to emphasize the person's strengths and assets and help him or her return as soon as possible to activities that previously gave pleasure and self-esteem.

Cancer and reconstruction

Breast cancer: lumpectomy, mastectomy, and reconstruction

The treatment of breast cancer has undergone a remarkable evolution during the past 20 years, both from a medical standpoint and from the psychological perspective. Cancer treatment has been revolutionized by new chemotherapeutic agents and surgery sparing the breast and nipple, which have enhanced the psychological wellbeing of women with breast cancer. The survival rates have also improved with early detection and improved treatment.

A woman's reaction to loss of her breast is related to how she felt about her breasts and their role in her sexuality and self-image before the diagnosis of cancer. Common reactions after mastectomy are depression,[70,71] diminished self-esteem,[72–75] feelings of being "less of a woman," and fears related to recurrence.[76,77]

When post-mastectomy breast reconstruction became accepted in the 1970s, it was hypothesized that a woman would have to live for a time without a breast to be happy with an imperfect, reconstructed breast. However, various researchers showed that immediate reconstruction at the time of mastectomy offers the patient with breast cancer a higher quality of life after mastectomy[76,78] and better integration of the "new" breast into the body image.[79–81] In addition, regardless of timing, breast reconstruction offers the opportunity to minimize feelings of disfigurement, deformity, mutilation, sexual unattractiveness, and loss of femininity.

Reconstruction does not interfere with the grieving process initiated by mastectomy. Women are able to properly mourn the loss of the breast while feeling "whole," "symmetric," and feminine after reconstruction. They still have to face the fact that they have cancer and need appropriate follow-up treatment and care. Reconstruction sometimes gives women who had been dissatisfied previously with their breast size the opportunity to reduce or augment their breasts. Nipple-areola reconstruction completes the cosmetic result.

Many women with breast cancer choose lumpectomy, a breast-sparing surgery, rather than mastectomy for aesthetic and psychological reasons. Not all lumpectomy patients are happy with their surgical results, related to the quantity and location of the tissue excised. The breast sometimes looks misshapen, causing distress for the patient and interfering with her comfort with her sexuality and being unclothed with her sexual partner or in locker rooms. Even though the defect may not be readily apparent to others, some patients will later request reconstructive breast surgery. They wish to restore the symmetry and shape of their breasts to minimize feelings of disfigurement and to benefit their self-image and psychological and sexual functioning.

Head and neck cancer

Head and neck cancer precipitates a loss of function and loss of form of the face and oral cavity that can be devastating to both the patient and the family. Facial expression (controlled by the facial muscles), speech, and ability to eat and drink in a socially acceptable fashion with one's friends and family are of vital importance.[82] Any disfigurement of the face may lead to social, interpersonal, and occupational handicaps.

In the preoperative period, patients must prepare themselves for the likely disfigurement and dramatic change in their face. In the early postoperative period, the patient experiences a great deal of anxiety. This results from a difficulty with communication and speech, especially if there is a tracheostomy or nasogastric tube in place, and the need for frequent lengthy dressing periods for wound and flap care.[83] Many patients have a severe reactive depression during this time. They often feel fearful, abandoned, and intensely alone because of their inability to speak or difficulty with communication.

Pain management may be necessary. The combination of analgesic agents and antidepressant medication is often effective. Because overuse of alcohol may be a factor in this population of patients, the surgeon should be alert for signs of alcohol withdrawal. Later in the recovery period, the patient next has to grapple with the change in appearance and body image. Simultaneously, the patient is also becoming aware of difficulties with swallowing, speech, and dribbling.

In addition to functional changes, there are reactivity and adjustment to the diagnosis as well as consideration of the prognosis of cancer, which may include the potential need for adjuvant cancer treatment. All of these experiences may engender chronic depression, social withdrawal, loss of self-esteem, anxiety, and feelings of loss and grief in the patient. Family relationships may be disrupted, leading to further distress. Patients may not be able to return to their previous occupation, and this may be devastating, especially if their career was an important factor in their self-esteem. When they are out in public, strangers may stare at their disfigured face, fostering hurt and humiliation. Discharge planning should include the initiation of important treatment services, such as speech, physical, and occupational therapy, as well as education concerning wound care and psychological support for the patient and caregivers.

Plastic surgery in childhood

Acquired and congenital defects: general considerations

An overt physical defect does not have a direct relationship to the degree of a person's response to a handicap.[84] Some patients cope well with a major deformity, whereas others decompensate psychologically when they are faced with a minor scar. Castelnuevo-Tedesco[85] remarked, "when an individual acquires a defect in contrast to someone who is born with one, he always feels a sense of loss; loss of hope, loss of his future, loss of normality and the rich experiences that go with it." However, when a defect is perinatal or congenital, the individual grows up maintaining lower expectations about what he or she will expect in life, and the sense of loss is hardly present as a psychological issue.[86]

Children born with congenital defects do have an awareness of having had an experience that is out of the ordinary, different from that of others.

Craniofacial anomalies

Anecdotal reports have led to the impression that children with craniofacial deformities are either shunned or overprotected by family and others. Clifford[87] described negative initial maternal reactions after the birth of a deformed child. However, good clinical studies have not borne out initial impressions and anecdotal reports in the literature.

Pertschuk and Whitaker[88] studied 51 patients several months before reconstructive surgery for craniofacial deformities. They reported that on the whole, the younger children were remarkably well adjusted. They were often outgoing and had regular friends. Their appearance did not, according to the children, pose great difficulties in their daily lives. Although they did report teasing at school, they seemed to manage adequately in the school setting. These children were being referred for surgery by their parents, who were concerned about future problems with vocational pursuits and teenage socialization. The most frequently reported problems in this younger group were in the behavioral realm. A small minority were socially isolated, inhibited, or aggressive. The authors suggest that whatever psychological trauma these children may experience from the deformity, it is manifested in behavioral rather than in personality problems. In contrast, older patients with craniofacial deformities do not cope well with their deformities. There are problems with dating and sexual relationships, although there does not seem to be substantial difficulty with same-gender friendships. Self-esteem and self-image are adversely affected in this older group, and they are self-conscious about their defect.

As a result, the younger population seems to function better than the older one, presumably because they use the defense mechanism of denial to cope. It also seems that facing dating and sexual situations produces anxiety, fear, self-consciousness, and self-doubt in the older child.

These data have a bearing on the question of timing of reconstructive surgery in this population of patients. The results support the contention that there are psychological advantages to performing surgery earlier in life, definitely before the onset of adolescence. Pertschuk and Whitaker's postoperative results show that a younger group has better behavior, reduced anxiety, and perhaps improved socialization, even allowing for their better psychosocial adjustment preoperatively.[88] In both younger and older groups, the majority of patients and parents express satisfaction with the surgical results. The satisfied patients experience a positive impact on their behavior, personality, and self-esteem. In disappointed patients and parents, there is little psychosocial change noted postoperatively. Their work generally confirms Macgregor's finding that patients with more major deformities are more satisfied with whatever surgical changes can be effected, even if they are slight.[89]

Often in craniofacial reconstructive surgery, the procedure can only hope to transform a grossly unattractive person into a milder, less conspicuously unattractive person. Patients need to be carefully counseled about what to expect postoperatively to minimize disappointment. It may sometimes be better to under-estimate potential gain to avoid arousing unrealistic expectations; when the gains are more than expected, the patient and family are likely to be happier with the surgical results.

The best measure of the success of craniofacial surgery is the psychosocial adjustment of the patients after surgery. Are they less fearful in social or dating situations? Do they feel free to pursue their occupational goals and leisure activities? Do they take pleasure in their friendships and relationships? Are they able to participate in daily life without significant self-consciousness or inhibition? Allam's study, with greater than 15-year follow-up, reports encouraging levels of social function in patients treated for severely stigmatizing Apert syndrome.[90]

Aesthetic surgery in teenagers

Body image development occurs in stages, and puberty stands out as a particularly sensitive time as the teenager undergoes major changes in his or her physical appearance and does this at a time of heightened vulnerability to the opinion of others. Physical change occurs in almost every area of the body. The mouth widens, the nose becomes prominent, and the chin is the last to increase in size. Body hair appears and darkens, breasts develop, sweat glands become active, voice quality changes, and complexion and acne problems arise.

As these physical changes are occurring, the adolescent's cognitive abilities expand. Thinking becomes more abstract, multidimensional, complex, and subtle. Adolescents become more self-aware and develop the capacity for self-reflection and reflection on the thoughts of others, using others as an audience to validate and evaluate themselves. They depend heavily on what others think, are vulnerable to peers for validation, and respond with complex emotional reactions.[3]

In this context, plastic surgery to correct a truly unattractive feature can be remarkably successful in changing the teenager's body image in a positive way. By making what the adolescent and his or her peers see as an improvement in appearance, self-perception is altered, and the youngster grows in comfort and confidence and feels a greater sense of wellbeing. Plastic surgery is remarkably free of conflict in this population, and teenagers undergo a rapid reorganization of self-image after plastic surgery with subsequent positive changes in behavior and interpersonal interactions.

In 2002, teenagers represented about 3% of the total number of patients having plastic surgical procedures in the United States (*Table 3.1*).[91] For these patients, plastic surgery is taking place when they have the greatest concerns about becoming attractive, competent, and acceptable to other people. Compared with other age

Table 3.1 **Plastic surgery procedures on patients 18 years and younger**

Procedure name[a]	Patients ≤18 years old (*n*)
Rhinoplasty	40 696
Otoplasty	3919 (age 13–18 only)
Suction-assisted lipectomy	3002
Male breast reduction (gynecomastia)	2008
Breast augmentation	3095
Mastopexy	497
Chin augmentation	1316

[a]Numbers for reduction mammaplasty were not included in the statistics. (Data from the American Society of Plastic Surgeons. National Clearinghouse of plastic surgery statistics report. American Society of Plastic Surgeons; 2003. Online. Available at: www.plasticsurgery.org)

groups, plastic surgery in teenagers produces very little anxiety and emotional conflict, and this is different from their response to other invasive procedures, such as intra-abdominal surgery or repair of facial lacerations. Studies investigating this apparent lack of conflict have looked at teenage rhinoplasty, which is by far the most frequently performed operation in this group. It has been suggested that this event, when it is affirmed by parental acceptance, represents an area of agreement and common thinking between parent and child at a time when almost every other issue has become a source of conflict. Some of the affirmation may flow from the parent's own narcissistic wish for a more beautiful child or from parental guilt; the teenager may be relieved that the narcissistic aspirations are shared. For the youngster, a plastic surgery operation is a gift and requires no effort at a time when he or she is being challenged to achieve in academic, athletic, and social realms. There may also be undertones of magical transformation, as in the childhood stories in which the ugly duckling becomes a beautiful swan rising above its critical peers – again through no effort on the part of the duckling.[10,92]

Teenage patients seem to undergo rapid reorganization of their self-image after rhinoplasty. A previous overawareness of the body part disappears; they tend to forget what they used to look like, and the fact of the surgery itself is recalled only casually. The patients harbor little sense of invasion and in general tend to be more pleased and satisfied than are older patients having the same operation. Feelings of inferiority may be replaced with self-confidence, and anxiety and self-consciousness in social situations tend to diminish. Gifford[92] comments on the "major changes in behavior, body awareness, or identity" after rhinoplasty.

Patient example

A 16-year-old boy felt that his large, beaked nose made him look ugly, mean, humorless, and unathletic. His family reassured him that he looked fine, but he continued to feel insecure and self-conscious with his classmates and considered himself unattractive to girls. After much discussion, he underwent a rhinoplasty in which the dorsum was lowered and the hump eliminated. He was happy with the result, went to college, and did well. Ten years later, he was studied with in-depth psychiatric

interviews and expressed pleasure that he had gone forward with the surgery and given himself an "edge." He recognized the surgery as positive and useful and said it freed him from a preoccupation with his appearance, which let him then focus on working on other issues in his life.

For this patient, as for most plastic surgery patients, the surgery was successful, not because the plastic surgeon did a nice job on the nose but because the surgery was done on a patient who then felt more positive about himself. The surgery treated a body image discomfort that lay at the heart of the young man's sense of identity.[93]

Not every teenager who seeks surgery is well suited for an operation. Emotional maturity is required to understand the limitations of plastic surgery and the complications that can occur. In addition, the teenager needs to have reached certain growth milestones or physical maturity, depending on the surgical procedure. The American Society of Plastic Surgeons developed a position statement about surgery in teenagers, and this cites important characteristics of the teenage patient.[94]

- The adolescent must initiate and reiterate his or her own desire for the plastic surgery improvement.
- There must be realistic goals and appreciation of the benefits and risks.
- There must be sufficient maturity to tolerate the discomfort and temporary disfigurement of a surgical procedure.

The position statement cautions against plastic surgery in teens who are prone to mood swings or erratic behavior, who are abusing drugs or alcohol, or who are being treated for clinical depression or other mental disease.

Selection of patients: danger and pitfalls

General risk factors

It is generally known that patients with major psychiatric illnesses or with vague, unrealistic expectations of plastic surgical procedures are more likely to be dissatisfied with their surgical results. However, there are no definable criteria by which to distinguish the patients

Important questions to ask the patient and information for the surgeon to ascertain during a plastic surgical evaluation include the following:

- The patient's ability to be realistic about expectations regarding the surgical results: Are the expectations unrealistic? Can education make them more realistic?
- The objective assessment of the identified defect and a realistic appraisal of the deformity by the surgeon: Is the patient's complaint out of proportion to the nature of the defect ("minimal" defect)?
- History of prior cosmetic procedures and degree of satisfaction: How does the patient feel about previous surgeons? Is the patient a "doctor shopper"?
- If the patient is satisfied or dissatisfied, did the focus shift to a new body part?
- Is the patient seeking a "perfect" result? Will the patient be able to tolerate a scar?
- Indication of an ulterior motive, e.g., expecting that the surgery will result in a job promotion or magical improvement of a troubled marriage: Does the patient place the success of the surgery on the realization of that motive?
- History of whether the patient has prior psychiatric illness or treatment: Is there a history of depression, anxiety, substance abuse, obsessive-compulsive disorder, social phobia, or impulse control disorders?
- Is there a history of litigation?
- The degree of functional impairment: What is the patient's occupational, social, and interpersonal functioning and marital status?
- Is there a history of hair or skin pulling/picking? How much time is spent daily thinking about the "defective" body part or mirror gazing? How much time is spent daily on grooming?
- History of eating disorder symptoms (anorexia, bulimia, binging and vomiting, laxative abuse): Does the patient have a body image disturbance (such as thinking he or she is too fat when objectively not overweight)?
- Is there any avoidance behavior? Does the patient avoid situations that would expose or exacerbate the perceived defect? Is the patient housebound?
- Is there a history of suicidal behavior or self-mutilation?
- Is the patient being pressured by others to have the requested surgery?
- Do significant others (spouse, family, close friends) think that the requested surgery is unwarranted or do they disagree with the decision?
- Is there any evidence of post-traumatic stress syndrome (especially in the reconstructive population)? Did the patient experience a profound physical and psychological trauma, such as a life-threatening injury (e.g., burn)?

who will be satisfied with their postoperative results and those who will be dissatisfied. Careful assessment during initial evaluation should be conducted to ascertain the patient's viability as a surgical candidate (*Box 3.1*).

There are populations of patients, such as those with body dysmorphic disorder, who, after objectively successful cosmetic surgery, may be dissatisfied, bring litigation against the surgeon, commit suicide, or even present a danger to the surgeon with homicidal ideas and impulses. Plastic surgeons and psychiatrists have the unhappy distinction of being the victims of homicide and assault more often than physicians in other specialties.

Psychiatric syndromes of concern to plastic surgeons

Depression

Why is it important to obtain a history of mood disorders and to determine whether the patient is depressed or has suffered from depression? Studies in psychoneuroimmunology have shed light on the negative effects of depression on the course of healing and postoperative recovery and on its impact on morbidity and mortality. Natural killer cell activity, helper (CD4) and suppressor (CD8) cell activity, numbers of T lymphocytes, and lymphocyte mitogen response have been shown to be negatively affected by depression.[95] Similarly, these changes are found in patients with a significant life stress, such as work-related stress, divorce, bereavement, or caring for a patient with Alzheimer disease.[95] As a consequence, the plastic surgeon should attempt to avoid performing an elective procedure on a depressed individual.

The prevalence of all depressive disorders is between 9% and 20% of the US population (*Box 3.2*). The incidence of major depression is higher in medically ill patients and in separated or divorced individuals compared with the general population.[96] Major depression is present in up to 18% of preadolescents and approximately 5% of adolescents, although there have been reports of depressive symptoms, if not full-blown depression, in up to one-third of adolescents in this country.[97] Depression is associated with an increased use of medical services.[98]

As many as 50% of depressions may be "masked," that is, not obvious or easily recognized.[26] A masked depression is suspected if the patient is having a higher level of marital or family conflicts, increased alcohol use, problems with job performance or excessive absenteeism, truancy from school or poor school performance, social withdrawal, or a seeming lack of motivation.

Box 3.2 **Major depressive episode: DSM-IV diagnostic criteria**

A. Five (or more) of the following symptoms have been present during the same 2-week period and represent a change from previous functioning; at least one of the symptoms is either (1) depressed mood or (2) loss of interest or pleasure.
Note: Do not include symptoms that are clearly due to a general medical condition, or mood-incongruent delusions or hallucinations.
   1. Depressed mood most of the day, nearly every day, as indicated by either subjective report (e.g., feels sad or empty) or observation made by others (e.g., appears tearful)
   Note: In children and adolescents, can be irritable mood
   2. Markedly diminished interest or pleasure in all, or almost all, activities most of the day, nearly every day (as indicated by either subjective account or observation made by others)
   3. Significant weight loss when not dieting or weight gain (e.g., a change of more than 5% of body weight in a month), or decrease or increase in appetite nearly every day
   Note: In children, consider failure to make expected weight gains
   4. Insomnia or hypersomnia nearly every day
   5. Psychomotor agitation or retardation nearly every day (observable by others, not merely subjective feelings of restlessness or being slowed down)
   6. Fatigue or loss of energy nearly every day
   7. Feelings of worthlessness or excessive or inappropriate guilt (which may be delusional) nearly every day (not merely self-reproach or guilt about being sick)
   8. Diminished ability to think or concentrate, or indecisiveness, nearly every day (either by subjective account or as observed by others)
   9. Recurrent thoughts of death (not just fear of dying), recurrent suicidal ideation without a specific plan, or a suicide attempt or a specific plan for committing suicide.
B. The symptoms do not meet criteria for a mixed episode.
C. The symptoms cause clinically significant distress or impairment in social, occupational, or other important areas of functioning.
D. The symptoms are not due to the direct physiological effects of a substance (e.g., a drug of abuse, a medication) or a general medical condition (e.g., hypothyroidism).
E. The symptoms are not better accounted for by bereavement, i.e., after the loss of a loved one, the symptoms persist for longer than 2 months or are characterized by marked functional impairment, morbid preoccupation with worthlessness, suicidal ideation, psychotic symptoms, or psychomotor retardation.

Reprinted with permission from the *Diagnostic and Statistical Manual of Mental Disorders*, © 2000 American Psychiatric Association.

Box 3.3 **Generalized anxiety disorder: DSM-IV diagnostic criteria**

A. Excessive anxiety and worry (apprehensive expectation), occurring more days than not for at least 6 months, about a number of events or activities (such as work or school performance).
B. The person finds it difficult to control the worry.
C. The anxiety and worry are associated with three (or more) of the following six symptoms (with at least some symptoms present for more days than not for the past 6 months).
   Note: Only one item is required in children.
   1. Restlessness or feeling keyed up or on edge
   2. Being easily fatigued
   3. Difficulty concentrating or mind going blank
   4. Irritability
   5. Muscle tension
   6. Sleep disturbance (difficulty falling or staying asleep, or restless unsatisfying sleep).
D. The focus of the anxiety and worry is not confined to features of an Axis I disorder, e.g., the anxiety or worry is not about having a panic attack (as in panic disorder); being embarrassed in public (as in social phobia); being contaminated (as in obsessive-compulsive disorder); being away from home or close relatives (as in separation anxiety disorder); gaining weight (as in anorexia nervosa); having multiple physical complaints (as in somatization disorder); or having a serious illness (as in hypochondriasis), and the anxiety and worry do not occur exclusively during post-traumatic stress disorder.
E. The anxiety, worry, or physical symptoms cause clinically significant distress or impairment in social, occupational, or other important areas of functioning.
F. The disturbance is not due to the direct physiological effects of a substance (e.g., a drug of abuse, a medication) or a general medical condition (e.g., hyperthyroidism) and does not occur exclusively during a mood disorder, a psychotic disorder, or a pervasive developmental disorder.

Reprinted with permission from the *Diagnostic and Statistical Manual of Mental Disorders*, © 2000 American Psychiatric Association.

Increased irritability or exaggeration of the usual personality traits may sometimes be a clue to this possibility.

If the surgeon suspects a depressive disorder, he or she should refer the patient for a psychiatric consultation, explaining to the patient how healing and recovery could be adversely affected by the presence of depression. The patient is advised that after appropriate treatment and recovery from the depression, surgery can be reconsidered.

Generalized anxiety and panic disorders

Anxiety disorders are the most common psychiatric illnesses (**Box 3.3**). When assessing a patient, the surgeon must try to distinguish between the typical anxieties that patients experience in anticipating surgery and an anxiety disorder. Typical anxieties are worries about the anesthesia, concerns about the degree of pain, and fears regarding loss of control.[99]

Anxiety reaches pathologic proportions when there is excessive worrying that the patient finds difficult to control. The worrying may be accompanied by easy fatigability, difficulty concentrating, irritability, sleep disturbance, restlessness, and generalized muscle tension.[26] The anxiety or associated physical symptoms may be interfering with occupational, social, or interpersonal functioning.

Panic attacks, a form of anxiety disorder, are described as discrete periods of intense fear or discomfort, developing suddenly and peaking in a 10-min period. Patients will report any or all of the following physical sensations: palpitations, sweating, shaking, sensation of shortness of breath, chest pain or discomfort, nausea or abdominal distress, light-headedness, derealization (feeling unreal) or depersonalization (feeling outside of one's body), fear of losing control or dying, numbness and tingling, and chills or hot flushes.

If the surgeon identifies anxiety symptoms, it is important to address them and treat them in advance of the surgery. The typical anxieties previously discussed can usually be allayed with explanation and reassurance. When an anxiety disorder exists, psychiatric consultation should be obtained, and the psychiatrist can partner with the plastic surgeon in making a decision about the timing of surgery and observe the patient postoperatively if surgery is undertaken.

Eating disorders

Eating disorders are illnesses characterized by disturbances in eating behavior and perceptions about food and eating. Anorexia nervosa is an illness characterized by refusal to maintain a minimally normal body weight and a significant disturbance in an individual's perception of the body's shape or size (*Box 3.4*).[26] These patients usually accomplish weight loss through reduction in total food intake but may also purge (self-induced vomiting or the misuse of laxatives or diuretics) or engage in increased or excessive exercise. Some anorexic patients will have the physical signs and symptoms of semistarvation or starvation, including amenorrhea, constipation, abdominal pain, cold intolerance, lethargy or excess energy, hypotension, hypothermia, bradycardia, and skin dryness. Some will develop lanugo, a fine downy body hair on the trunk. Bulimia nervosa is characterized by binge eating and inappropriate compensatory methods to prevent weight gain (*Box 3.5*).[26] The binging usually occurs in secrecy and continues until the individual is physically uncomfortable. Individuals with bulimia nervosa may employ self-induced

---

Box 3.4 **Anorexia nervosa: DSM-IV diagnostic criteria**

A. Refusal to maintain body weight at or above a minimally normal weight for age and height (e.g., weight loss leading to maintenance of body weight less than 85% of that expected; or failure to make expected weight gain during period of growth, leading to body weight less than 85% of that expected).

B. Intense fear of gaining weight or becoming fat, even though underweight.

C. Disturbance in the way in which one's body weight or shape is experienced, undue influence of body weight or shape on self-evaluation, or denial of the seriousness of the current low body weight.

D. In postmenarchal females, amenorrhea, i.e., the absence of at least three consecutive menstrual cycles. (A woman is considered to have amenorrhea if her periods occur only following hormone, e.g., estrogen, administration.)

Specify type:

Restricting type: during the current episode of anorexia nervosa, the person has not regularly engaged in binge-eating or purging behavior (i.e., self-induced vomiting or the misuse of laxatives, diuretics, or enemas).

Binge-eating/purging type: during the current episode of anorexia nervosa, the person has regularly engaged in binge-eating or purging behavior (i.e., self-induced vomiting or the misuse of laxatives, diuretics, or enemas).

Reprinted with permission from the *Diagnostic and Statistical Manual of Mental Disorders*, © 2000 American Psychiatric Association.

Box 3.5 **Bulimia nervosa: DSM-IV diagnostic criteria**

A. Recurrent episodes of binge eating. An episode of binge eating is characterized by both of the following:
   1. Eating, in a discrete period of time (e.g., within any 2-h period), an amount of food that is definitely larger than most people would eat during a similar period of time and under similar circumstances
   2. A sense of lack of control over eating during the episode (e.g., a feeling that one cannot stop eating or control what or how much one is eating).

B. Recurrent inappropriate compensatory behavior in order to prevent weight gain, such as self-induced vomiting; misuse of laxatives, diuretics, enemas, or other medications; fasting; or excessive exercise.

C. The binge eating and inappropriate compensatory behaviors both occur, on average, at least twice a week for 3 months.

D. Self-evaluation is unduly influenced by body shape and weight.

E. The disturbance does not occur exclusively during episodes of anorexia nervosa.

Specify type:

Purging type: during the current episode of bulimia nervosa, the person has regularly engaged in self-induced vomiting or the misuse of laxatives, diuretics, or enemas.

Nonpurging type: during the current episode of bulimia nervosa, the person has used other inappropriate compensatory behaviors, such as fasting or excessive exercise, but has not regularly engaged in self-induced vomiting or the misuse of laxatives, diuretics, or enemas.

Reprinted with permission from the *Diagnostic and Statistical Manual of Mental Disorders*, © 2000 American Psychiatric Association.

vomiting, laxatives, and diuretics to compensate for the binging. Patients with bulimia nervosa are typically in the normal weight range, although they may be slightly underweight or overweight. In both syndromes, there may also be mood disorders. In those who induce vomiting, dental enamel may be eroded. Electrolyte imbalances and hematologic abnormalities can also be found.

The overwhelming majority of patients with eating disorders are female, and when they seek plastic surgery, they usually inquire about breast surgery or suction-assisted lipectomy. However, by virtue of their body image disturbance, patients with eating disorders usually do not benefit from plastic surgery. The surgery can never match the body image they fantasize will be the cosmetic result. For the sake of these patients, it is appropriate to defer aesthetic surgery and refer them to a psychiatric consultant.

Substance abuse

Information about substance abuse is not elicited routinely by physicians, especially when there is no explicit evidence to suggest a problem. In addition, there are varying opinions about what constitutes "abuse." The three-martini lunch may be alarming to some physicians but not to others.

There are several good reasons why the plastic surgeon should make an inquiry about the patient's use of drugs and alcohol. Most important, the patient could develop signs of alcohol or drug withdrawal in the postoperative period; if the physician does not have the information or index of suspicion to consider withdrawal, diagnosis and treatment would be delayed, which carries its own morbidity and mortality. Second, substances like alcohol can have a negative impact on the recovery and rehabilitation process.[100–102] Third, substance dependence, especially drugs such as opiates, has a direct impact on pain management postoperatively. Finally, the dependency may be a symptom of an underlying psychiatric condition, such as depression or anxiety.

Body dysmorphic disorder: "imagined ugliness"

Body dysmorphic disorder (BDD)[103] is a psychiatric disorder in the spectrum of obsessive-compulsive disorders (**Box 3.6**). Afflicted individuals perceive

> **Box 3.6 Body dysmorphic disorder: DSM-IV diagnostic criteria**
>
> 1. A preoccupation with a slight or imagined defect in appearance. If a slight physical anomaly is present, the person's concern is markedly excessive.
> 2. The preoccupation causes clinically significant distress or impairment in social, occupational, or other important areas of functioning.
> 3. The preoccupation is not better accounted for by another mental disorder (e.g., dissatisfaction with body shape or size characterizing anorexia nervosa).
>
> Reprinted with permission from the *Diagnostic and Statistical Manual of Mental Disorders*, © 2000 American Psychiatric Association.

themselves to be ugly, despite having a normal appearance, and present to plastic surgeons for aesthetic surgery without perceiving the psychological underpinnings of their concerns. They perform repetitive, compulsive behaviors, such as frequent mirror checking, excessive grooming, and skin picking.[104] Patients with BDD often have little or no insight into their illness, and some are frankly delusional, convinced that the imagined defect is real.[105] The imagined body defects are focused mostly on the face but may also be focused on the hair, hands, feet, and sexual body parts.

The preoccupation, anxiety, and self-consciousness connected to BDD may lead to interference with daily functioning (occupational, social, and interpersonal), and a significant percentage of patients with BDD may become housebound.[106] These patients may have excessive preoccupation with their imagined physical defects to the level of delusional or psychotic thinking; some of these patients may have suicidal ideation or may have attempted suicide in the past.[107,108]

There is strong evidence that patients with BDD do not benefit from aesthetic surgery. Phillips and Diaz[109] reported in their study that 83% of procedures performed on patients with BDD led to an exacerbation or no change in BDD symptoms. A study by Veale[110] revealed that 76% of patients with BDD who underwent cosmetic surgery reported dissatisfaction with the postoperative result.

With repeated cosmetic surgeries, patients with BDD may actually become worse, often developing a rather grotesque surgically altered appearance. This fosters the vicious circle of seeking more surgery. With estimates that between 50% and 88% of patients with BDD have undergone cosmetic procedures,[111] it is enormously important to detect signs of BDD. Whether a prospective plastic surgery patient has BDD is not always clear. Judgments about beauty and ugliness and whether a defect should be categorized as "slight" are inherently subjective. Only if the preoccupation with the slight or imagined defect is excessive compared with the objective appearance is the diagnosis of BDD easily made.

There has been some work attempting to differentiate the patient with BDD from other cosmetic surgery patients. A study by Aronowitz et al.[112] looked in a controlled fashion at the differences between patients with BDD and other plastic surgery patients. They found patients with BDD more likely to report preoccupation for longer than 1 h daily; greater associated anxiety, depression, and obsession; greater disagreement with others regarding the defect; greater associated functional impairment; and greater fixed belief in the reality of the defect. The patients tended to seek multiple consultations with plastic surgeons and dermatologists until they found one to provide the treatment they requested.

As well as considering their defects more serious, patients with BDD worry about a larger number of body defects than do other cosmetic surgery patients and feel less satisfaction with past surgeries. After cosmetic procedures, patients with BDD may shift preoccupation to other body parts or aspects of their appearance or even increase their preoperative level of dissatisfaction, since it may not match their idealized image of how they think their revised body part should look. Because there is a gross distortion of the body image to begin with, a cosmetic change is unlikely to correct this distortion. Even when there is an objectively satisfactory outcome, the patient with BDD may introduce a lawsuit or become violent toward the surgeon or harmful to himself or herself. Some patients with BDD may self-mutilate to try to alter their appearance.

If the surgeon evaluating a patient suspects that he or she may have BDD, psychiatric consultation should be sought and strongly encouraged. The surgeon may confront great resistance in suggesting psychiatric consultation; the surgeon should not perform the requested surgery on the patient.

Psychiatric treatment is available for the patient with BDD. Psychotherapy, especially cognitive-behavioral techniques,[113] may be helpful, and it is often used in conjunction with psychopharmacotherapy. These techniques attempt to restructure distorted thinking. Clomipramine, a potent serotonin reuptake inhibitor, has been shown to be effective and superior to desipramine, a selective norepinephrine reuptake inhibitor, in ameliorating the symptoms of BDD.[114] In addition, other serotonin reuptake inhibitors like fluoxetine, citalopram, fluvoxamine, sertraline, and paroxetine may be helpful, but they may need to be administered at higher doses and for longer duration than is typical in the treatment of depression.

BDD in men is an under-recognized disorder.[115,116] A study by Garner[117] found that the percentage of men who are dissatisfied with their overall appearance is 43%, a number that has tripled during the past 25 years, and that men appear to be similar to women in their levels of dissatisfaction with how they look. Likewise, BDD appears to affect men as well as women. Mayville et al.[118] found that 2.8% of females and 1.7% of males in a community sample of 566 adolescents fulfilled the criteria for BDD. Some investigators have found a higher proportion of men than of women with BDD, and the largest published sample of patients with BDD revealed 51% to be male.[109]

Muscle dysmorphia is a newly described disorder characterized by a preoccupation with the idea that one's body is not sufficiently lean and muscular.[119] It involves a body image disturbance similar to that seen in anorexia. This preoccupation can interfere with important areas of functioning; the patients often have a compulsive need to maintain their workout and diet schedule, may use performance-enhancing substances, despite knowledge of adverse psychological or physical consequences, and often shy away from showing their bodies in public. In a 1997 study of 156 unselected weightlifters, 10% perceived themselves to be less muscular than they were objectively.[120] Another study in 1997 of 193 men and women with BDD demonstrated that 9.3% had muscle dysmorphia.[121]

Violent behavior

Violence is something that all physicians correctly fear. The ability to predict that a patient is or will be violent is not ensured. The role of psychopathology and violence is a subject of long debate. There is evidence that certain categories of psychiatric patients are over-represented in groups of violent patients. Patients with psychotic disorders, like paranoid schizophrenia, pose a higher risk of violent behavior.[122] However, non-psychotic disorders are also often associated with violent behavior,[123] particularly borderline and antisocial personality disorders.

Alcohol and drugs are often associated with violence. The violence may be purposeful: for the purpose of procuring drugs or money. It may be related to the lowering of inhibitions against violent or antisocial behavior caused by the substances or decreased cognitive alertness, resulting in impaired judgment. For this reason, screening for the presence of substance abuse as well as for severe personality and psychotic disorders should be an essential part of the plastic surgical evaluation of a potential patient.

Strategies for management of the dissatisfied patient

There are many discussions in the literature about why patients may be dissatisfied with the results of their plastic surgery. Hoopes and Knorr[124] concluded that patients whose chief motivation is to resolve difficulties in interpersonal relationships and whose chief expectation is that others will change their behavior toward them have the greatest dissatisfaction with their surgery and the highest incidence of postoperative problems.

Linn[125] asserts that the "chief preoperative problem with these patients is not a psychiatric one," but rather that the surgeon has made a poor decision about whether a correctible deformity exists. Certainly, as the syndrome of body dysmorphic disorder has been better understood, it is likely that many dissatisfied patients may have suffered from this disorder that has slipped by, undiagnosed by the plastic surgeon.

Gifford[92] wonders "why there are so many favorable results even in patients with neurotic motivations and severe psychopathology, and why there are such emotionally malignant reactions in the rare failures." He opines that "all serious emotional sequelae cannot be predicted and prevented without refusing operation to many patients who would probably have an uneventful course." He also suggests that severe character

> Box 3.7 **Psychological contraindications to plastic surgery**
>
> - The patient is uncertain as to which aspect of the appearance he or she would like to change.
> - The patient is unable to contemplate an imperfect result.
> - The patient has an unstable personality disorder or an untreated major psychiatric illness.
> - The patient has unrealistic expectations about the surgery that are not modifiable by education.
> - The patient is under emotional stress during the consultation or at the time of the planned surgery.
> - The patient complains of the opposition of others in his or her life, such as family members, to the planned surgery.
> - The patient is motivated to have the surgery at the request of or because of pressure by others.
> - In the case of a revision of a previous surgery, the surgeon thinks the previous result is reasonable despite the patient's vocal complaints and dissatisfaction about the result.
> - The patient is a "doctor shopper" and dissatisfied with the results of prior multiple procedures.
> - The patient pins the success of the surgery on realization of a particular goal (e.g., the resolution of marital problems or a job promotion).

pathology (e.g., borderline personality disorder) is often present in the dissatisfied patient.

Reich[126] found that the existence of psychopathology is not a contraindication to plastic surgery but that it should be viewed in relation to two criteria: (1) whether the expectations for the surgery are realistic and (2) the ability of the patient to tolerate an imperfect result.

One of the most significant decisions the plastic surgeon makes is whether to perform the requested surgical procedure. Satisfaction of the patient is not necessarily predictable, even by a careful psychiatric examination.[127] However, several psychological factors that often present at initial evaluation should be considered contraindications to plastic surgery (*Box 3.7*). The feature underlying most dissatisfaction in plastic surgery is a breakdown in rapport and communication between patient and surgeon. Breakdown in communication between patient and surgeon can lead to a vicious circle, described by Gorney.[128] A patient's disappointment, anger, or frustration generates the surgeon's reactive hostility, defensiveness, and arrogance, which deepens the patient's anger, leading to eventual litigation. The dissatisfied patient must be handled carefully to avoid this circle (*Box 3.8*).

Box 3.8 **Managing the dissatisfied patient**

- Remember that the patient's dissatisfaction is often transitory and related to postoperative psychological changes. Be supportive and understanding and let the patient vent his or her feelings.
- See dissatisfied patients frequently and offer concern and compassion. Allow the patient to see that you are an ally in resolving the problem.
- Do not get angry with the patient. Anger will create an adversarial situation and make the patient feel abandoned and isolated. The patient will respond with angry defensiveness, and this may increase the likelihood of litigation.
- Consider an offer to revise an operation if you concur with the patient's complaints and dissatisfaction, but only if you think that you can better the appearance.
- Suggest a "waiting period" before performing any additional surgery to allow the patient to live with the current appearance and integrate it more fully into the body image.
- Sit with the patient and have a frank discussion of the complaints. Respond to them, one by one, and express the problems you are experiencing with caring for the patient, including what obstacles you think he or she may be placing in the way of receiving optimal care. Always take the position of being an ally and partner in obtaining satisfaction but acknowledge when you cannot meet expectations. If you conclude that the expectations are unrealistic, try patiently to educate the patient, using photographs and whatever data you think will accurately portray a reasonable surgical result.
- If the patient is terminally enraged with you or you with him or her, and there does not seem to be any positive working relationship, simply state that the relationship can no longer be productive for the patient and refer the patient to several of your colleagues for consultation, offering to help the patient make the transition to the new surgeon as smoothly as possible.

Conclusion

The need for a thoughtful interview with the patient who requests a plastic surgical procedure, whether for aesthetic or reconstructive reasons, cannot be overstated. The plastic surgeon can be guided to make sound decisions about whether to offer a requested surgery to a patient by being attentive to psychological motivations and body image concerns and alert for psychiatric disorders and warning signs of a problem patient. Failing to pay attention to potential pitfalls and one's intuitive sense about a patient may result in a dissatisfied patient. Calling on a psychiatric consultant to help evaluate the patient and to work collaboratively through the preoperative and postoperative period (if the decision is made to operate) is often helpful. Presenting the psychiatric consultant as a member of the surgical team to assist with body image adjustment and other psychological issues may encourage compliance and allow the patient to feel more comfortable with the consultation. Even if the patient is lost by the suggestion of a psychiatric referral, it is better not to operate on a patient who may not be satisfied with the results.

 Access the complete references list online at **http://www.expertconsult.com**

17. Moss TP, Harris DL. Psychological change after aesthetic plastic surgery: a prospective controlled outcome study. *Psychol Health Med.* 2009;14:567–572.

    Although aesthetic surgery is performed to address self-image, which is intimately tied to one's emotional state, the psychological response to these procedures is seldom rigorously assessed. This prospective study addresses this relative void in the literature.

18. Dayan SH, Arkins JP, Patel AB, et al. A double blind, randomized, placebo-controlled health-outcomes survey of the effect of botulinum toxin type a injections on quality of life and self-esteem. *Dermatol Surg.* 2010;36(Suppl. 4):2088–2097.

19. Murphy DK, Beckstrand M, Sarwer DB. A prospective, multi-center study of psychosocial outcomes after augmentation with natrelle silicone-filled breast implants. *Ann Plast Surg.* 2009;62:118–121.

20. Sarwer DB, Infield AL, Baker JL, et al. Two-year results of a prospective, multi-site investigation of patient satisfaction and psychosocial status following cosmetic surgery. *Aesthet Surg J.* 2008;28:245–250.

36. Friel MT, Shaw RE, Trovato MJ, et al. The measure of face-lift patient satisfaction: the Owsley Facelift Satisfaction Survey with a long-term follow-up study. *Plast Reconstr Surg.* 2010;126:245–257.

42. Zahiroddin AR, Shafiee-Kandjani AR, Khalighi-Sigaroodi E. Do mental health and self-concept associate with rhinoplasty requests? *J Plast Reconstr Aesthet Surg.* 2008;61:1100–1103.

63. Iwuagwu OC, Stanley PW, Platt AJ, et al. Effects of bilateral breast reduction on anxiety and depression: results of a prospective randomised trial. *Scand J Plast Reconstr Surg Hand Surg.* 2006;40:19–23.

    This prospective trial was designed to examine the psychological benefits of breast reduction in patients with macromastia. The authors report significant improvements in depressive symptoms.

90. Allam KA, Wan DC, Khwanngern K, et al. Treatment of Apert syndrome: a long-term follow-up study. *Plast Reconstr Surg.* 2011;127:1601–1611.

　　A long-term assessment of results after surgical management of Apert syndrome is presented. The authors report positive psychosocial outcomes in this population.

102. Akinbami F, Askari R, Steinberg J, et al. Factors affecting morbidity in emergency general surgery. *Am J Surg.* 2011;201:456–462.

108. Bjornsson AS, Didie ER, Phillips KA. Body dysmorphic disorder. *Dialogues Clin Neurosci.* 2010;12:221–232.

4

The role of ethics in plastic surgery

Phillip C. Haeck

SYNOPSIS

- Ethics as seen by professional associations.
- Ethical relationships with patients.
- The ethics of advertising.
- The role of ethics in the outpatient office.
- Ethics in the operating room.
- Ethical relations with other providers and third-party payers.
- The ethics of expert witness testimony.
- Summary.

The subject of ethics pervades the specialty of plastic surgery. Ethical decisions are highly prevalent in its practitioners yet few realize they confront these choices regularly, almost daily. Behaving in a morally responsible fashion, maintaining high personal codes of conduct, and remaining competent in the operations is a non-cognitive function for the vast majority of surgeons; it is deeply ingrained in the psyche. It also serves the surgeon well in presenting an overall highly regarded and deserved reputation amongst colleagues and the public.

Who to operate on and, more importantly, who not to operate on can in many instances be dilemmas that require moral choices. But many times the rationale is played out in the surgeon's subconscious, one more decision out of dozens made daily, with just a few moments to evaluate the alternatives. Plastic surgeons do not go home to their spouses every night and claim they made a number of highly ethical choices today. Yet in reality the effects of not making the right choices can set up traps and entanglements. Breaching unwritten and written moral codes may bring consequences in this specialty. The harm may be done to others. The fallout is usually the surgeon's predicament.

Consider this common scenario. A patient consults the plastic surgeon for a rhinoplasty, complaining of poor breathing and an old fracture. She also doesn't like the shape of the tip of her nose. She claims she has no money for any private payment of the fees involved. But she also claims to have over a half-dozen friends who want their noses changed and states she will take them to meet the surgeon on each of her subsequent visits. The surgeon agrees to charge her insurance company for the entire procedure, hoping in the end to capture more business from the friendly and social patient, deciding it is a justifiable prevarication. Is this an ethical dilemma?

The moral issues of this story become a web of further entanglement when the insurance company suspects it paid for a portion of the surgery that was cosmetic and not functional. A few months later the patient receives a denial of payment from the company for what they have determined is the cosmetic portion of her anesthesia charges, the facility fee and surgeon's fees. She is suddenly required to pay a sizable amount of money and in turn begs the surgeon to write off the balance since she still cannot afford to make up the difference.

Did the surgeon commit fraud? Was his decision to further his practice by committing a deception immoral? If he refuses to let the patient off the hook financially, will this affect his reputation with her friends who are by now signing up for their own surgery? Even if he made the very first decision that led to this predicament casually he cannot easily make this last choice without some degree of moral calculation.

Consider another situation. A 65-year-old uninsured diabetic is hit by a bus and suffers a compound tibia-fibula fracture and degloving injury of one-third of his lower leg. He is a smoker and is insulin-dependent. After the fracture is stabilized the plastic surgeon is asked to consult on the case for soft-tissue coverage of the sizable defect. Knowing that the zone of crush injury is extensive and there is compromised blood flow to the lower leg the surgeon must decide if a long and expensive operation with a modest but very real chance of being unsuccessful is worth the effort and cost. With an amputation below the knee the chances this man will ambulate in a prosthesis are good, but not guaranteed. Will prolonged recovery from a valiant limb salvage operation be the better choice? The surgeon knows he will not be reimbursed well for his efforts. His decision, if made on high standards, is based on what is right for the patient, not the surgeon.

These types of choices are encountered in similar situations on a daily basis by plastic surgeons all over the country. How one deals with these types of scenarios is multifactorial, complex and requires sophisticated decision trees. It is not immoral or unethical to say no in these situations.

Highly ethical persons have a well-developed internal moral code. They conduct themselves accordingly and believe that to do anything less would make them guilty of immorality. Contrast this with a sociopath who has no capacity for guilt, makes choices that he knows will deliberately harm others and then denies responsibility for the consequences. People living at the opposite extremes of this spectrum are rare. Most of us fall somewhere in between, the angel on one shoulder and the devil on the other.

Surgeons are themselves no different even though they have all supposedly taken the oath of Hippocrates to "above all else, do no harm." The training of surgeons results in behavior that is consistent with the moral character of the role models the surgeon learned from, in both a positive effect and a negative one, sometimes full of awe, other times full of loathing. The behavioral end result of this training is a hybrid of choices, instincts, and internal codes that is rarely monolithic. More often the surgeon who has trained hard for a subspecialty designation is a complex, principled individual with a great capacity for a wide variety of mostly predictable and virtuous behaviors.

The specialty of medical ethics comprises a wide range of subjects that is considered valuable for physicians to consider and be knowledgeable about. It also takes into account the effects surgeons can have on society and vice versa. This includes controversial issues such as whether or not society should allow late-term abortions, death with dignity, or rationing of expensive treatments, to name a few. In general, the literature in medical ethics contains very little on the subject of plastic surgery.

In the lay literature, the ethics of having one's appearance altered is a somewhat more common, but still rare, subject. Feminists weigh in on this topic most frequently, as do PhD candidates in the fields of sociology and behavioral psychology.[1-3] Yet these dialogues do not take into account the possibility that the surgeon has high moral standing. Instead the plastic surgeon is cast as a villain, forcing his or her susceptible patients into paying more than they can afford for quite frivolous reasons. The patients are defined as foolishly chasing an impossible-to-obtain god-like appearance, involuntary victims of society's fascination with attractiveness. A further subtheme of these publications is the speculation that widespread alteration of homely persons into attractive ones will in the long term breed out common sense in our society.

The specialty journals in reconstructive or cosmetic surgery rarely, if ever, contain purely ethical articles of interest to the plastic surgeon.[4-6] There are, for now, no ethical courses one can take at medical symposia, and forums on the subject of ethical plastic surgery are unheard of.

Yet the fact remains that ethical decisions are quite common in the lives of plastic surgeons, in some cases occurring even on a daily basis.

Ethics as seen by professional associations

The American Society of Plastic Surgeons (ASPS), the largest membership organization in the specialty, was formed in 1935. The association's attempt at a written Code of Ethics was first published in 1980. Members in good standing are expected to be familiar with this code and to adhere in their daily practice of surgery to the standards espoused within it. Failure to adhere to the guidelines can result in disciplinary action, including expulsion.

The expectations for ethical behavior on the part of members of the professional association are strongly worded and very specific. At times the code has been modified to meet new challenges such as those posed by the internet, charity raffles, and expert witness testimony. All realms of the specialty are covered within its dictums. The code also clearly spells out how a member will be dealt with if there is perceived to be a violation of the rules of the code.

Other members, patients, and lay persons can all lodge a written or verbal complaint with the ASPS Ethics Committee, stating what they think may be unethical behavior on the part of the member, actions that fall outside the proscriptions of the code. The member is then investigated by his or her peers and if it is decided that a violation did take place, the information is then passed along to the Judicial Council. The Council, comprised of members voted into that position, holds hearings to determine if sanctions should be placed on the member. Personal appearances before the Council are welcomed and the decisions made after a hearing are binding. Appeals of these decisions can be made to the Board of Trustees of the organization but are done infrequently. Plastic surgeons who are members of the American Society of Aesthetic Plastic Surgery (ASAPS) are subject to the same Code of Ethics and discipline. Members in good standing of both organizations may be elected to hold positions on the Ethics Committee and the Judicial Council for a period of 2–3 years.

Table 4.1 is a compilation of the data available from a review of the ASPS Ethics Committee's activities over the 4 years from 2006 to 2009.

While fewer complaints have been lodged lately, down to 81 in 2009 from 139 in 2006, the number of

Table 4.1 American Society of Plastic Surgeons Ethics Committee's activities, 2006–2009

Ethics complaints	2006	2007	2008	2009
New complaints	139	131	114	81
Complaints dismissed	101	77	54	36
Cases reviewed	38	54	60	45
Referred to judicial	10	15	18	15
Cases disciplined	5	9	8	8
Complaints closed	153	129	108	84

Table 4.2 Average complaints by category per year, 2006–2009

Advertising	50
Medical board discipline	20
Contest	11
Standard of care	12
Expert witness testimony	10
Professional misconduct	6
Exorbitant fees	3
Criminal charges	2
Expert report	2
Total	116

complaints that are reviewed after a committee investigation remained stable over this same period. Likewise the number of reviews that led to a hearing stayed at the same level, as did the number of hearings that resulted in disciplinary action.

Table 4.2 reveals the average number of complaints by category over the 4-year average. Advertising interpreted to violate the Code of Ethics has remained the complaint with the highest frequency over many years. The second highest category remains the investigation of those members who have been sanctioned by their state medical boards. The third category, unethical behavior while participating in a contest where the prize is free surgery, remains controversial. Some members feel that promoting themselves over nonmembers who are self-designated cosmetic surgeons is necessary to compete for potential patients and that this portion of the code is too restrictive. Still others feel it adequately reduces the number of violations of the code and reduces behavior that besmirches the reputation of all plastic surgeons. This controversy is unlikely to end soon.

Plastic surgeons overall have a highly visible position in the medical profession. Reactions to unethical behavior can thus be intense and scathing. For this reason members of the ASPS and ASAPS are reminded from time to time to review their Code of Ethics. While the vast majority of members will never in their careers be accused of violating it, pleading that you had no idea your actions were directly opposed to the body of rules for conduct in the code never works well as a defense when confronted by this system.

Ethical relationships with patients

In an ideal world plastic surgeons would only meet patients for consultations that were precisely matched to their skills, with the perfect indications for only the operations they preferred to perform. The surgeon would immediately comprehend the correct desires of the patient, infallibly interpreting that person's own unique ability to deal with a complication or a less than desirable result. The surgical results would always heal immediately with no complications. The adoring patient would then refer many more patients just like themselves.

In reality things are rarely clear and perfect. Patients fret about what they will look like after cosmetic surgery; they worry hopelessly before reconstructive surgery that they will still end up looking deformed and disfigured. They fritter away the surgeon's time with endless questions about whether or not they should have the surgery. Then they present impossible impediments to surgery scheduling and are often unrealistic about their recovery, postoperative pain, and activity restrictions. In a busy, demanding practice how surgeons take control of these situations, occasionally to their own advantage, can sometimes lead to unethical decision-making. Taking the high moral ground, while always the best choice, can sometimes seem impractical and intrusive when demands on the surgeon are almost overwhelming.

When a surgeon's compensation is determined solely by the number of surgeries he or she can be perform in a week, a month and a year, operating on a person ill suited to the surgery can possibly, perhaps eventually,

occur. Some surgeons claim only to operate on patients with whom they feel comfortable. Obviously they have the luxury of dismissing patients they don't like and have a practice of truly elective procedures only. Being financially rewarded from performing surgery on people with unrealistic expectations, who may be ill suited emotionally for the end result, is not the norm in this specialty. Yet it does occur, perhaps too often.

The consequences of this, an upset patient who abhors the result and threatens lawsuits or reports to the media, will in most cases lead to regret, the surgeon ruing the day he or she laid the scalpel to that person's skin. But it does not necessarily guarantee the surgeon has learned to be more careful from the experience.

In the training of plastic surgeons, being grilled over and over from the elder surgeon as to the correct indications for surgery is common. The master surgeon feels he or she is there to teach future surgeons the unwritten rules, the pitfalls of making the wrong choice, and the integrity required to succeed in the specialty. Once in practice, however, new surgeons no longer have to answer for their every action. The guidance for making the right, not the wrong, choice is up to them alone, and the consequences can lead to an unhappy patient, a profound effect on their reputation, disciplinary action or, most unfortunately, malpractice litigation.

So it is that surgeons are ultimately judged by the "standard of care," what a reasonably prudent surgeon would do with similar training in similar circumstances. Moral and ethical behavior is one facet of the standard of care.

Truly ethical surgeons choose their patients based on a thorough evaluation that includes many factors, compensation being the least important. Patients with unrealistic expectations or obsessive behavior are dismissed appropriately. Patients who need reconstruction are chosen on the surgeon's ability to match the correct operation to the problem. Patients with needs beyond the surgeon's own particular skills are referred to others who have more expertise in that area.

Society expects that conventional and virtuous surgeons spend time teaching their patients what their expectations should be both for the less than perfect result and for unfortunate but rare complications. The option to dismiss the surgeon or seek another one once patients know the risks and alternative treatments should always be allowed. This is accompanied by a disclosure of how much financial responsibility the patient must bear for reoperations when things do not go as planned and another operation is needed.

In reconstructive surgery patients' ability to pay or the type of insurance coverage they have does not affect the ethical surgeon's decisions to operate. The complete lack of insurance is balanced by the ability to find some type of payment coverage through social services or simply accept a very reduced fee in exchange. The need for the operation should not be altered by the compensation that will result, especially if it is little to nothing at all.

The ethics of advertising

Advertising was considered completely unethical for plastic surgeons well into the 1980s. A few who tried it were considered outlaws and often expelled from their national or state and local plastic surgery associations. Many felt it "cheapened the specialty" and that reputation was all that should be needed to attract more patients.

Along came the 1990s and the social attitudes of the specialty changed. Television discovered plastic surgery and shows like Extreme Makeover thrust plastic surgery into the homes of millions, making "mommy makeovers" a household word. But it was the internet that tore down the last bit of reluctance to make promotion a major part of the everyday practice of plastic surgery.

Advertising in the specialty, when done in good taste and without hyperbole, will now be around for a long time. Unfortunately unethical advertising, done in poor taste with mind-numbing self-promotion, is also here to stay (*Fig. 4.1*).

The ASPS Code of Ethics has been modified several times in the last dozen years to keep up with the changing relaxation of social mores to physician advertising. But complaints from members about other surgeons' unethical promotions continue to rank as the most frequent complaints each year to the ASPS Ethics Committee (*Table 4.2*).

Examples abound. *Figure 4.2* is exactly what the Code of Ethics was meant to prevent with a rather tacky approach that cheapens and sullies the specialty regardless of the origin. The public lumps all plastic surgeons into one category, whether they are Board-certified or self-designated.

Showing misleading before-and-after photos, then implying this to be a typical result that can be obtained by any patient, is considered unethical as well (*Fig. 4.2*). In addition the temptation to airbrush imperfections or scars out of the photos can be hard to resist when software applications abound that make this an easy task. Any altering of before-and-after photos is considered by the ASPS ethics process to be false and misleading advertising, subject to sanctions.

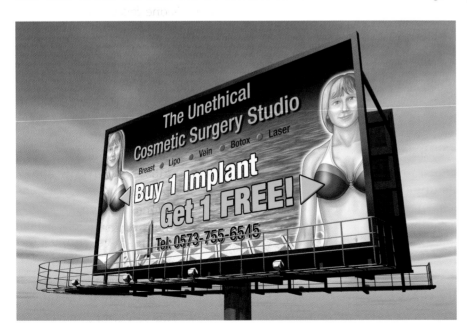

Fig. 4.1 Unethical advertising: billboard photo: "two for one."

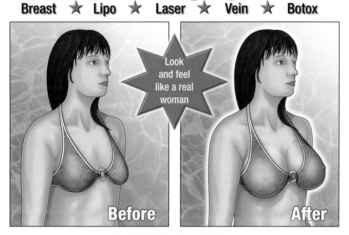

The Unethical Cosmetic Surgery Studio

Breast ★ Lipo ★ Laser ★ Vein ★ Botox

Look and feel like a real woman

Before   After

Tel: 0573 755-6545

Fig. 4.2 Unethical advertising where a single image is used for both before and after figures through the magic of digital alterations.

Other behaviors considered to be unethical include the trading of surgery *quid pro quo* for media exposure in a high-profile person. Examples unfortunately exist of television figures such as news reporters undergoing surgical treatment in return for free testimonials about the surgeon, on air or at public appearances. While the media industry doesn't consider this out of the ordinary, plastic surgery associations maintain that it is in fact unethical.

The role of ethics in the outpatient office

Building and maintaining relationships with patients and staff can occupy a good deal of the plastic surgeon's time. The temptation to extend those relationships outside the office or the practice and outside a professional nature will always be present. Grateful patients wish to offer favors in exchange for their surgeon's success. Adoring staff members want to know more about what their boss is like outside the clinic. It is only natural for attractions such as these to take place. How the surgeon handles this can make him or her more successful, but can also lead to situations that can become unconventional, complicated, and entangling.

While it is not considered unethical to socialize with one's staff, establishing sexual relationships with staff and patients violates general standards for professional conduct, and can end with unfortunate consequences, including charges of sexual harassment or other civil charges. Lecherous behavior, physical advances, and the creation of a sexually harassing environment are grounds for dismissal from professional organizations, civil lawsuits, and can even at times be considered criminal in nature.

Conventional behavior sets limits on these situations. But the unique situation in plastic surgery, where the female patient may be both physically and emotionally exposed, can create powerful forces that test the limits of decency, honesty, and virtue in male plastic surgeons. To a lesser extent the opposite gender roles can also occur, as women are becoming plastic surgeons at record rates.

Personal standards of conduct vary tremendously in the specialty, but television shows depicting sleazy, illegal, and unconventional behavior by plastic surgeons may have some element of truth. The malevolent, licentious, and perverse personality in some surgeons may in fact be portrayed in these situations. Hopefully this will remain rare and only in the purview of television. Brazen behavior may eventually be reported to some type of authority. The potential personal damage that can be done in these situations by and to surgeons should be deplorable to all.

Attorneys experienced with workplace lawsuits always recommend that, if a romantic relationship develops between a patient and a single physician, the patient must be given the choice of terminating either the doctor–patient relationship or the personal relationship. If the first choice is made the patient should submit to being discharged from the surgeon's care to another physician. Likewise, if a romantic relationship arises with staff members it is considered ethical and wise to discontinue the employee–employer relationship immediately, though the evidence suggests this happens infrequently.

The plastic surgery practice with multiple physicians presents the possibility for competitive economic and unprofessional behaviors amongst surgeons and staff. Manipulation of the staff to hinder the success of partners or to direct more business to oneself is considered unethical. Hiding income from expense-sharing agreements, contributing to rumors and lies about other partners, and other obtrusive and malevolent behaviors towards them ignore the rules of decency and virtue.

Ethics in the operating room

The outcomes of any surgery depend on the correct application of principles, decisions, and treatments, all of which require multiple informed and decent choices. How the surgeon conducts himself, resisting the temptation to blame others and even the instruments when things do not go as planned, affects his reputation amongst staff and colleagues. Each correct or incorrect decision made during surgery can be a reflection of the character and mores of each surgeon.

Cutting corners for economic reasons, covering up mistakes, and delivering different outcomes than planned may be fundamental indications of a dishonest character. Surgery is not immune to the effects of personality flaws.

The analogy of the old fairy tale by Hans Christian Anderson, The Emperor's New Clothes, to the potential for deceitful behavior occasionally exhibited by plastic surgeons can be illustrative. In the story, the weaver promises to make the emperor a set of clothes invisible to those ignorant or unfit for their positions, completely fooling him into wearing nothing. It is a classic case of "mind over matter."

To the extent this can be applied to plastic surgery, the limited effects of some surgery may depend on the extent to which the surgeon built up the patient's expectations, knowing full well that the patient had paid for something possibly requiring more time and effort or that might have had a more clearly effective result. While this is rarely as brazen as in the old fairytale, it can slip into various parts of surgery, especially with the more common use of treatment machines the patients know little about. The happiness of the patient depends on the expectations for beauty woven into the sales presentation by the surgeon. Results will vary of course.

Certain energy-dependent skin treatments whose effects take many months to be appreciated parallel this story. Is it dishonest to promise fewer wrinkles when it is known the effects won't be as plainly evident as other treatments or as a more expensive surgery? When the frequently pricey payments on the machine need to be met, the temptation to oversell it can be enormous. The ethical dilemma is not just to sign reluctant patients up but also then to deny that the outcome was less effective and did not meet their expectations.

Conventionally moral surgeons recognize this trap and avoid it, choosing to defer income for traditional effectiveness. Others, who might still consider themselves to have mainstream values, nonchalantly overlook the issues for the sake of keeping busy, building their reputation and impressing other surgeons with the size of the practice. Willful and malevolent deception may not be in the forefront; mostly it is hidden, buried in this specialty behind layers of complex situations. But it certainly exists in many forms.

Ethical relations with other providers and third-party payers

The ASPS Code of Ethics is very specific about the pitfalls in monetary relationships that can exist in referral networks. Brazen kickbacks for referring a patient for whom the surgeon will be rewarded financially are considered illegal in most states. Fee splitting is as well. With Medicare it can become a federal offense. More subtle alignments and *quid pro quos* with the referring physician may not constitute civil violations but nonetheless should be considered carefully as a possible ethical violation before being carried out.

Correctly applying Current Procedural Terminology codes which accurately and adequately depict the procedure that was performed is presumed to be the norm in surgery. Yet constant tension with third-party payers over what can be interpreted as their unjustified decreased reimbursement for procedures requiring high levels of skills creates a negative attitude that can pervade the business side of the profession.

When it is assumed the insurance company "cheated" the surgeon on the last payment, the temptation to overbill the next procedure is difficult to resist. Is it justifiable to "unbundle" codes, upcode, and overbill when one knows that the insurance company has the upper hand anyway? Who is really harmed by this? It is situational ethics in play: the seemingly acceptable deception that is justified because everyone else, including the payers, is playing the same game.

Much has transpired over the past 5 years as several large insurance companies have been taken to court in class-action lawsuits for unlawful changes to the billings of physicians. Their reply is that fraudulent surgical billing is rampant and they have to protect their bottom line. The truth may lie somewhere in between. Nevertheless, the real world seems to forgive physicians tempted to push the envelope of honor and conduct for now, given the intense fiscal realities. Patients may abhor what they hear about hospital billing, but forgive their own surgeon if he seems honest and caring. The more personal this becomes, the less patients consider it greed if it seems to be in favor of a surgeon who did a successful procedure on them.

On the other hand, in university teaching hospitals, where an attending surgeon is expected to supervise the training of many residents, there were in the past submissions of surgeon's fees for being in two places at once, or even not present at all. The explanation was that as a teaching surgeon the physician was ultimately responsible for all of the outcomes and therefore justified in receiving the compensation. Some well-publicised record fines from the Centers for Medicare and Medicaid in the last decade have led to very strict rules for supervision and billing. Unethical billing is now scrutinized more closely than ever and the plastic surgery team may not be an exception. Obtrusive rules may have constrained the system and possibly gone beyond reason. Unfortunately they now exist because of the past abuse of the system by a very few.

The ethics of expert witness testimony

As in other sections of this chapter, once again, the issues outlined in the ASPS Code of Ethics are applicable here as well. Usually one of the most frequent complaints brought against a surgeon by another member of the ASPS is for testifying either in deposition or at trial in a manner that can mislead the jury or simply be out and out contrived of false statements of fact. Many of these complaints center around the expert declaring that the standard of care was to do the surgery in a specific fashion. In fact, however, many surgeons may not adhere to those same principles and perform the surgery differently, but not necessarily outside the standard. Condemning one way or the other as not in alignment with accepted principles when in fact it may very well be, can swing the jury or judge to rule against the other member. Regardless of the outcome the member who has a legitimate issue can submit the testimony he or she feels was false or misleading to the ASPS Ethics Committee who will review the situation and arrive at a conclusion.

The Code of Ethics is also very specific about the expert's reasonable experience with the surgery that was performed. The phrase "recent and substantial experience" needed to be more carefully defined because of retired surgeons' declarations of the standard of care when in fact they may have not performed any surgery, let alone the one in question, for over a decade. As the code is written now this means within the last 3 years. Testifying about a procedure the surgeon has not performed then in 4 or more years can be considered misleading testimony.

Overall, these issues became such frequent complaints that multiple other modifications to the Code sections on testifying have had to be made. This now includes a declaration that all experts may be asked to sign, certifying they will be truthful in their testimony. The submission of the signed statement is voluntary but can be used as evidence in the courtroom, especially when a plaintiff's expert is another member of the ASPS and has been known to have made misleading statements in other trials.

Summary

The practice of medicine is complex, requiring constant decisions, discussions, and testing. How this plays out in the daily lives of plastic surgeons depends on their background, training, personal mores, and interpersonal skills. Unethical behavior can range from pushing the envelope in insurance coding and billing, all the way to fraud, sexual deviation, and the cover-up of surgical misadventures. It is a pervasive issue that can be seen as either business as usual or a moral stance always to behave ethically. Human nature being what it is, the give and play between highly ethical behaviors and the alternative will always be a part of the specialty.

References

1. Goering S. The Ethics of Making the Body Beautiful. Lessons for Cosmetic Surgery For a Future of Cosmetic Genetics. *Centre Study Ethics Soc* 2001;13:20.

   The author uses a discussion of the ethics of cosmetic surgery to broach the less familiar territory of potential ethical dilemmas surrounding "cosmetic genetics." If a practice used to enhance one's own self-image reinforces negative conceptions of normality, this practice is discouraged.

2. Miller FG, Brody H, Chung KC. Cosmetic Surgery and the Internal Mandate. *Cambridge Q Health Ethics*. 2000;9: 353–364

   The "internal morality" of medicine is described as the physician's duty to adhere to certain clinical virtues. The ethics of cosmetic surgery are discussed in this context.

3. Scott K. Cheating Darwin: The Genetic and Ethical Implications of Vanity and Cosmetic Plastic Surgery. *J Evol Technol* 2009:20:1–8

   This paper describes the ethics of cosmetic surgery in the context of evolution. The argument is advanced that cosmetic surgery uncouples the phenotype and its role in attracting a mate from the genotype, and may therefore have ethical implications.

4. Constantine M. The Confusing Ethics of Mismanaged Care. *Ann Plast Surg* 1995;35;2:222–223

   This essay begins with a vignette in which the author, a plastic surgeon, is asked to determine whether certain procedures are "cosmetic" or "reconstructive." What follows is a deft discussion of the difficult position modern physicians find themselves in when asked to participate in resource allocation.

5. Krizek T. Surgical Error: Ethical Issues of Adverse Events. *Arch Surg* 2000;135:1359–1366

   This paper addresses the ethical questions surrounding adverse events. Specifically, issues inhibiting efforts to reduce the frequency of such occurrences are discussed.

6. Reisman NR. Ethics and Legal Issues of Injectible Treatments. *Clin Plast Surg*. 2006;33;4:505–570

5

Business principles for plastic surgeons

C. Scott Hultman

SYNOPSIS

- This chapter provides a broad overview of the essential principles that characterize what a business does and how a business does its work.
- The ability to apply business concepts is of paramount importance if plastic surgeons are to become and remain leaders in healthcare.
- Plastic surgeons should understand and use strategy, accounting, finance, economics, marketing, and operations to help guide decisions about their practice.
- Innovation, entrepreneurship, and human resource management are three areas where plastic surgeons can add value to their practice and distinguish themselves from their competition.

Introduction

Not only is healthcare business, it is big business.

The healthcare–industrial complex incorporates multiple sectors to deliver health and depends on an expanding group of interdisciplinary teams, services, and institutions to achieve this value proposition. Business sectors involved in the delivery of healthcare include not only professionals such as doctors, nurses, and administrators, but also hospitals, nursing homes, and home healthcare groups; drug manufacturers and developers; manufacturers of medical equipment and instruments; diagnostic laboratories; biomedical research; and biotechnological entrepreneurs.

Current estimates by the Office of Economic Cooperation and Development place healthcare spending at 16.0% of US gross domestic product, with that percentage expected to increase to 19.5% by 2017.[1] For every dollar spent in the US on healthcare, 31% goes to hospital services, 21% to physicians, 10% to pharmaceuticals, 8% to nursing homes, and 30% to other categories, such as diagnostics laboratories, medical equipment, and medical devices. Of note, 7% of total spending is assigned to administrative overhead costs.

If healthcare provided by physicians is not business, then physicians are certainly surrounded by business; they must navigate a complex environment that is full of paradoxes, inefficiency, and bureaucracy. Unfortunately, physicians receive no formal education in business but must learn on the job, through mistakes and successes, often one patient and one business problem at a time. Although many critics argue that healthcare has been tainted by the intersection with big business, which places the bottom line at the top and undermines the physician–provider relationship, many other thought leaders contend that healthcare needs business, to help solve problems of inconsistent quality, sporadic access, and rising costs. Indeed, business thinking and business processes are desperately needed to transform our current system, so that healthcare can be available to all people, at fair-market prices, to improve the health of our community.

Why should plastic surgeons care about the business of healthcare? From an individual perspective, every plastic surgeon must either run a business or be part of a business, if the surgeon's practice is to thrive, grow, change, and continue to provide high-quality care. Whether one works for oneself, for a hospital or health maintenance organization, for an academic institution, for a nonprofit or nongovernmental organization, for a free community clinic, or for an overseas volunteer mission trip, plastic surgeons are involved with organizations that utilize business principles and interface with business entities.

From a broader perspective, however, plastic surgeons are uniquely situated to serve as leaders of healthcare systems and healthcare businesses. Given our extensive training, our collaboration with multiple specialties, our diverse portfolio of services that we provide, our problem-solving skills, and our entrepreneurial spirit, plastic surgeons have the leadership skills, influence, and positioning within the healthcare system to effect real change. Just as the Greek word *plastikos*, which means to shape or to mold, was chosen to describe what we do as surgeons, this word could also impart upon us the ability to shape or mold our systems of healthcare delivery.

The knowledge and application of business principles are of paramount importance if plastic surgeons are to become and remain leaders in healthcare. The purpose of this chapter is to provide a broad overview of the essential principles that characterize what a business does and how a business does its work. Each section offers a very superficial view, and readers are strongly encouraged to explore in more depth the following components of this chapter:

1. Strategy
2. Accounting
3. Finance
4. Economics
5. Marketing
6. Operations
7. Innovation
8. Entrepreneurship
9. Sustainable enterprise
10. Human resource management
11. Legal and regulatory considerations
12. Negotiation
13. Ethics
14. Leadership.

At the very least, plastic surgeons must learn the language of business, so that we can have meaningful interactions with hospital administrators, insurance carriers, salespeople, and marketing firms. Hopefully, though, plastic surgeons can utilize the principles of business to improve the care that we provide, and in the end, to transform the industry in which we practice our science, and our art.

Strategy

Competitive advantage begins and ends with strategy. Nearly all of the components of business are affected by strategy, from finance to operations, from marketing to managing human capital, and therefore a review of business principles should commence with an understanding of how strategy guides decision-making within an organization.

Strategy can be characterized as the art of inducing your competitor to do something else, while you focus on doing what you do well. In more academic terms, strategy is the process of forming, implementing, and evaluating decisions that enable an organization to achieve its long-term goals. Strategy is dictated by (and in turn, can influence) the organization's mission, vision, and values, which serve as a foundation to guide policy, projects, and programs. Furthermore, strategy is about competing on differentiation – creating a value proposition, in which a firm provides the consumer with a product or service of greater quality or at less cost than its competitor, deliberately choosing a different set of activities to deliver a unique mix of outputs.

Before examining specific strategic principles, one should become familiar with how the business environment affects the flow of inputs to outputs, along the supply chain. Because value is added at various points along this process, the entire axis, from supplier to consumer, is called the value chain. Primary activities of the company, which include inbound logistics, operations, outbound logistics, marketing and sales, and ultimately

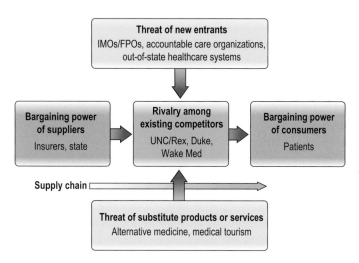

Fig. 5.1 Strategy: Porter's 5-Forces model. HMOs, health maintenance organizations; PPOs, preferred provider organizations.

customer service, each create value that manifests in the final product; these processes are guided by strategic priorities and are coordinated by support activities that include technological development, human resource management, and firm infrastructure.

The most established and respected model of the business environment is Michael Porter's 5-Forces model of competition (*Fig. 5.1*).[2] Each industry contains: (1) previously established competitors; (2) the potential for new entrants; (3) the threat of substitute rivals, who often compete on price; (4) suppliers, who can have significant bargaining power; and (5) buyers, who create demand for the outputs. Understanding the environment of a specific industry, such as healthcare, can strengthen decision-making and help with strategic planning. For example, how should an academic plastic surgery practice respond to the influx of recently graduated residents into the community? How should the solo private practitioner attract new patients in a fixed market, when a group practice dominates the landscape? How should surgeons challenge scope of practice with nonsurgeon physicians and nonphysician providers? What is the optimal portfolio of services, specifically the mix of reconstructive surgery, cosmetic procedures, and skin care, to achieve the goals of the organization?

Once the dynamics and landscape of the business environment are defined, specific decisions can be made regarding change in operations, marketing, investment in new assets, alliances, or supply chain.[3–5] Most mature industries, such as the automotive industry or the personal computer industry, settle into a competitive scenario in which one firm dominates with 60% market share, while a second firm contains 30% of the market share, and the remaining competitors occupy 10%. Because of barriers to entry, new entrants may not be able to compete successfully, unless disruptive technology lowers production costs or the market shifts, due to cultural, social, economic, or political forces. In fact, significant competitive advantage is conferred to small, nimble firms that focus their product line or services and offer a unique selling proposition to a targeted segment of the market. When executed correctly, this activity, termed judo strategy, has the power to undermine dominant businesses and increase market share substantially.

A major limitation of competitive strategy is that most efforts deal with gaining a larger portion of a fixed market or attracting new customers via the "rising tide" of a slowly growing market. If companies in search of sustained, profitable growth compete with multiple rivals, then differentiation becomes difficult, price wars may ensue, and the total profit pool shrinks. Instead, companies may pursue a "blue-ocean strategy," in which uncontested but related market space is discovered, rendering rivals obsolete and generating new demand. Previous "settlers" will "migrate" to this new market space and become "pioneers." Apple has done this over and over with the personal computer market, introducing new devices that expand the functionality of their operating system and hardware, evidenced by the transition from desktop to laptop to iPhone to iPad.

True value innovation comes when a company jumps out of its industry and creates an entirely new market, often in a different industry.[6,7] This foray into uncharted territory, which is referred to as "white space," typically occurs when a company develops a disruptive technology that permits the use of core competencies to produce a radically different product or service. Apple was successful in capturing the dominant position in the digital music market by designing and offering iTunes, despite being a computer company. Inherent to this success was the fact that Apple also changed the business model for purchasing music; consumers could buy singles or albums, listen to samples, and of course, use the website for free.

In summary, strategy involves the following steps:

1. Industry analysis – assess industry profitability today and tomorrow.
2. Positioning – identify sources of competitive advantage.
3. Competitor analysis – study current competitors, future entrants, and substitutes.
4. Assessment of current strategy – predict effectiveness and sustainability.
5. Option generation – search for new customers, new segments, new markets.
6. Development of capabilities – planning now for future opportunities.
7. Refining strategy – assess uniqueness, trade-offs, compatibility with vision and values.

Accounting

Business management must be based upon a common language that is used to communicate objectively information related to the quantitative metrics of an organization. That language is accounting. This section will review the tools that accountants use to assess the financial health of a business: income statement, balance sheet, summary of cash flows, and financial ratios.[8-10] The nuances of accounting are beyond the scope of this overview, but healthcare providers must have a basic comprehension of these instruments and how they represent the financial standing of their practice, their hospital, and their healthcare system. Furthermore, these instruments are used in budgeting to construct pro forma predictions of future performance.

The field of accounting is governed by generally accepted accounting principles, also known as GAAP, which are rules used to prepare, present, and report financial statements for various entities, such as nonprofit organizations, publicly traded companies, and privately held firms. Although the government does not set these standards, the US Securities and Exchange Commission does require that public firms follow these rules. Managerial accounting, which is used to allocate cost and assign overhead, does not follow GAAP and is dependent upon institutional culture and practice.

Income statement

The income statement, also known as the profit/loss statement, describes financial transactions within a defined period of time, which may be quarterly or annually. Revenue refers to the gross income that a company receives from normal business activities, typically the sales of goods or services, but may also include rent, dividends, or royalties. In accrual accounting, revenue occurs at the time of the transaction, not when receipts are collected. Net income is expressed as a profit or loss, after deducting expenses, which usually include operating expenses (cost of goods sold (COGS), variable overhead expenses), depreciation of assets and amortization of leases, fixed overheads (selling and administrative expenses, research and development), interest expenses, and taxes.

Revenue
  less operating costs =
Gross profit
  less fixed overhead
  less depreciation (assets) and amortization (leases) =
Operating income (earnings before interest and tax: EBIT)
  less interest expenses =
Pre-tax income
  less income taxes =
Net income

Balance sheet

The balance sheet is a snapshot of what the company owns and owes, at a single point in time. On one hand, the balance sheet summarizes the cumulative impact of all transactions, but the balance sheet does not provide much useful information on the operational performance of the firm. The net worth of the company, referred to as owners' equity, is defined as the difference between the assets and the liabilities. Reframed another way, the following equation must always balance:

Assets = liabilities + equity

The actual worth of a company is difficult to ascertain, but one method to calculate value is market capitalization, which is (share price) × (shares outstanding); this represents the public consensus of the value of the firm's equity.

Assets are defined as resources with probable future economic benefit, obtained or controlled by the entity, as a result of past transactions, that are expected to contribute to positive net cash flows. Examples of assets include cash and cash equivalents (prepaid expenses, bonds, stock), accounts receivable (the money that is owed but has not been collected), inventory (raw materials, work in process, and finished goods), property/plant/equipment (purchase price less depreciation), goodwill (intangible value of brand), and intellectual property.

Liabilities refer to what a company owes, or from a different perspective, how the assets were obtained. Liabilities include short-term loans (credit lines), current portion of long-term debt, accounts payable (the money a company owes its vendors), and long-term debt.

Owners' equity – the difference between assets and liabilities – can be allocated into several categories: preferred shares (which usually receive periodic dividends), common stock, and retained earnings (accumulated earnings that have been reinvested into the business, instead of being distributed as dividends).

Summary of cash flows

An assessment of a company's cash flows is critical in determining the financial viability of the firm, because profit is not the same as cash. This disconnect is due to multiple reasons: (1) cash may be coming in from investors or loan; (2) revenue is booked at time of sale, not collection; (3) expenses are matched to revenue, not when they are actually paid; and (4) capital expenditures do not count against profit (because only the depreciation is charged against revenue) but require cash or debt to pay for the assets. As a result of this discrepancy between when a good or service is provided and when cash is exchanged, following the flow of cash can be very complicated. Fortunately, we have accountants. For mature, stable, and well-managed companies, cash flow does approximate net profit. But for younger, growing, and poorly managed companies, profit can occur without gaining cash (resulting in bankruptcy, because bills cannot be paid) or cash can accrue without being profitable (which bodes poorly for long-term success, if expenses cannot be controlled).

Overall cash flows are further subdivided into three categories – operations, investing, and financing – based upon the conduit for the flow. Cash flows from operating activities (CFO) indicate how much cash was generated from operations: selling goods and services. Cash flows from investing activities (CFI) indicate how much cash the company spent (or received) from buying and selling businesses, property, plant, and equipment (PPE). Finally, cash flows from financing activities (CFF) indicate how much cash the firm borrowed, received from selling stock, or used to pay down debt or repurchase stock.

Total cash flow represents the true flow of money through a firm and is a composite of the operations, investing, and financing, represented by the following equation:

$$\text{Total cash flow} = \text{CFO} + \text{CFI} + \text{CFF}$$

Many financial analysts believe that total cash flow myopically focuses on earnings while ignoring "real" cash that a firm generates and retains for future investments. Therefore, another measure of the ability of a firm to create value is free cash flow (FCF), which is defined numerically as:

$$\begin{aligned}\text{Free cash flow} &= \text{CFO} - \text{capital expenditures}\\ &= \text{Net income} + \text{amortization} + \\ &\quad \text{depreciation} - \text{change in working}\\ &\quad \text{capital} - \text{capital expenditures}\end{aligned}$$

In other words, free cash flow represents the total cash that a company is able to generate after laying out the funds required to maintain or grow its asset base. Free cash flow is very important to investors because this allows a firm to pursue opportunities that increase shareholder value. This is the best source of capital for development of new products and services, acquiring new companies, paying stock dividends, and reducing debt. Cash really is king, and this is why.

Financial ratios

Because companies even within a single industry can vary in size and maturity, such instruments as the income statement, balance sheet, and summary of cash flows may not permit a valid comparison of those companies. Instead, financial ratios – the numerical relationship between two categories – can provide powerful insight into the financial health of a company. Jonathan Swift observed that "vision is the art of seeing what is invisible to others," and financial ratios provide that vision.

Four types of ratios help managers and stakeholders analyze a company's performance: profitability, leverage, liquidity, and efficiency. These ratios can be used to follow the performance of a firm over time or to compare several firms across related industries.

Profitability ratios

Gross margin = gross profit/revenue
Operating margin = operating profit/revenue
Net margin = net profit/revenue
Return on assets = net profit/total assets
= (net income/revenue) × (revenue/assets)
Return on equity = net profit/shareholders' equity
Contribution margin = revenue – variable direct costs
(technically not a ratio, but loved by CFOs
everywhere)

Leverage ratios

Debt-to-equity ratio = total liabilities/shareholders' equity
Interest coverage = operating profit/annual interest
charges

Liquidity ratios

Current ratio = current assets/current liabilities
Quick ratio = (current assets – inventory)/current
liabilities

Efficiency ratios

Days in inventory = average inventory/(COGS/day)
Inventory turns = 360/days in inventory
Days sales outstanding = accounts receivable/(revenue/
day)
Days payable outstanding = accounts payable/(COGS/
day)
PPE turnover = revenue/PPE
Total asset turnover = revenue/total assets

Figures 5.2–5.4 demonstrate the income statement, balance sheet, and cash flows for a proposed aesthetic and laser center that offers patient consultations, skin care, and office-based procedures. Pro formas are typically estimated for 3–5 years and include many assumptions about revenue streams, costs, and growth. Such planning is important to the success of the venture, so that real-time performance can be compared to the expected results, and changes can be implemented if necessary. *Figure 5.5* demonstrates the time to breakeven, when revenue exceeds expenses, and income becomes positive.

Finance

The goal of finance is to maximize corporate value while minimizing the firm's financial risks.[11] If accounting is the language and grammar of business, then finance is a combination of poetry and theoretical physics, with some rock'n'roll added to keep the mix interesting. The central thesis of finance is that risk can be managed successfully, in such a way that wealth is created, by combining the variables of cash, assets, supply chain, and human capital, to produce a good or service that is more valuable than the cost of production. The consumer, however, is the final arbiter who decides if the good or service is more valuable than the cost of the inputs, and if the output is more valuable than the price the consumer is willing to pay. If so, the consumer exchanges money for the good or service.

Risk can be measured statistically and therefore, given assumptions that are known with certainty, the outcome of decision-making can be predicted with specific probability. Thus, the decision to make an investment in a new piece of equipment, a new employee, a new product line, or to purchase another company, can be made with a certain level of confidence. However, when some variables are unknown (ambiguity) or when no variables are known (true uncertainty), sound financial management may not be possible, to the point that flipping a coin may provide more insight regarding outcomes.

This section will introduce common tools used by financial managers when analyzing a financial scenario, to determine go/no-go decisions about acquiring and allocating assets. While understanding the mechanics of such calculations is not essential, understanding the logic behind the decision-making is critical, as well as understanding the significance of the results. We will review the following concepts: time value of money,

Pro Forma Income Statements — **Overhead Applied to Net Income**

	capacity/yr	capacity/d	operating breakeven/day			Y1	Y2	Y3	Y4	Y5	TOTAL
UTILIZATION					mean	22%	53%	73%	80%	80%	
				55%	maximum	40%	60%	80%	80%	80%	
ENCOUNTERS New patient consults	2560	10.67	5.87			563.20	1356.80	1868.80	2048.00	2048.00	
Surgical procedures	1297	5.40	2.97			285.34	687.41	946.81	1037.60	1037.60	
Non-operative procedures	1975	8.23	4.53			434.47	1046.67	1441.65	1579.89	1579.89	
Aesthetician visits	1920	8.00	4.40			422.40	1017.60	1401.60	1536.00	1536.00	
REVENUE New patient consults						$69,334.72	$168,003.36	$232,004.64	$256,005.12	$256,005.12	$981,352.96
Surgical procedures						$1,054,805.44	$2,555,874.72	$3,529,541.28	$3,894,666.24	$3,894,666.24	$14,929,553.92
Non-operative procedures						$187,939.44	$455,391.72	$628,874.28	$693,930.24	$693,930.24	$2,660,065.92
Aesthetician visits						$33,280.00	$80,640.00	$111,360.00	$122,880.00	$122,880.00	$471,040.00
Skin Care Product Sales						$9,204.00	$22,302.00	$30,798.00	$33,984.00	$33,984.00	$130,272.00
TOTAL Revenue						$1,354,563.60	$3,282,211.80	$4,532,578.20	$5,001,465.60	$5,001,465.60	$19,172,284.80
Less Physician Revenue (40% of Total Revenue)						$541,825.44	$1,312,884.72	$1,813,031.28	$2,000,586.24	$2,000,586.24	$7,668,913.92
(subject to UNC overhead @ 26%)						$140,874.61	$341,350.03	$471,388.13	$520,152.42	$520,152.42	$1,993,917.62
TOTAL Facility Revenue						$812,738.16	$1,969,327.08	$2,719,546.92	$3,000,879.36	$3,000,879.36	$11,503,370.88
Less Variable Costs (COGS)						$248,659.45	$602,520.98	$832,052.78	$918,127.20	$918,127.20	$3,519,487.60
GROSS MARGIN						$564,078.71	$1,366,806.11	$1,887,494.15	$2,082,752.16	$2,082,752.16	$7,983,883.28
Less Total Operating Expenses (includes SGA, personnel)						$1,019,507.96	$1,191,508.04	$1,277,908.04	$1,285,108.04	$1,285,108.04	$6,059,140.12
OPERATING INCOME (EBIT)						-$455,429.25	$175,298.07	$609,586.11	$797,644.12	$797,644.12	$1,924,743.16
Less interest	buildiing upfit					73845	72142	70305	68321	66181	$350,794.00
	laser suite					30727	24877	18543	11682	4252	$90,081.00
	TOTAL interest					$104,572.00	$97,019.00	$88,848.00	$80,003.00	$70,433.00	$440,875.00
TOTAL COSTS (variable, operating, interest)						$1,372,739.41	$1,891,048.02	$2,198,808.82	$2,283,238.24	$2,273,668.24	$10,019,502.72
NET INCOME						-$560,001.25	$78,279.06	$520,738.11	$717,641.12	$727,211.12	$1,483,868.16
Less UNC overhead	26%					$0.00	$20,352.56	$135,391.91	$186,586.69	$189,074.89	$531,406.05
NET INCOME after overhead assessment (NIAOA)						-$560,001.25	$57,926.51	$385,346.20	$531,054.43	$538,136.23	$952,462.11

Income Statement Analysis

		Y1	Y2	Y3	Y4	Y5	TOTAL
Gross Margin (%)	gross profit/sales	69.40%	69.40%	69.40%	69.40%	69.40%	69.40%
Operating Margin	operating income/sales	-56.04%	8.90%	22.41%	26.58%	26.58%	16.73%
Return on Sales	net income/sales	-68.90%	3.97%	19.15%	23.91%	24.23%	12.90%

note: **SALES** = total facility revenue=total revenue less physician revenue

Fig. 5.2 Accounting. Sample pro forma: profit/loss statement.

opportunity cost, net present value (NPV), discounted cash flows (DCF), weighted average cost of capital (WACC) and the hurdle rate, return on investment (ROI), and internal rate of return (IRR).

Time value of money

Money increases in value over time, and such appreciation is actually logarithmic (although it takes a while to get going!). Even Einstein conceded, "The most powerful force in the universe is compound interest." Essentially, a dollar today is worth slightly more tomorrow and a lot more in 10 years. A dollar invested in a money market account with an annual return of 2% will yield 2 pennies next year, increasing the value of this investment to $1.02, which is future value of today's dollar. The formula for the time value of money is:

$$\text{Present value (PV)} = \text{future value}/(1 + \text{interest rate})^{\text{number of periods}}$$

Why does money have a time value? Economists attribute this to two factors: postponement of consumption and expectations of inflation. Interest rates are a hedge against this type of depreciation. As risk of an investment increases, then the reward to the investor needs to increase, to convince the investor to part with $1 today, in the hopes of having possibly $1.20 next year (which would be a 20% return). The actual rate that money can appreciate is determined by multiple factors, such as the risk of the specific investment, the performance of the stock market, the return on US Treasury bonds, and the monetary policy established by the Federal Reserve, which sets the overnight lending rates to commercial markets.

Consequently, obtaining capital costs money. If one borrows money from the bank, this loan creates risk for

Balance Sheet — Overhead Applied to Net Income

				YEAR UTILIZATION	Y1 40%	Y2 60%	Y3 80%	Y4 80%	Y5 80%
ASSETS	Liquid Assets	Cash			$0.00	$0.00	$0.00	$17,123.30	$647,593.68
		A/R (estimated at 17% of annual revenue: 60 days)			$230,275.81	$557,976.01	$770,538.29	$850,249.15	$850,249.15
		Inventory			$5,000.00	$5,000.00	$5,000.00	$5,000.00	$5,000.00
	Total Liquid Assets				$235,275.81	$562,976.01	$775,538.29	$872,372.46	$1,502,842.83
	Fixed Assets--PPE	Plant			$975,000.00	$926,250.00	$877,500.00	$828,750.00	$780,000.00
		less depreciation (20y)			-$48,750.00	-$48,750.00	-$48,750.00	-$48,750.00	-$48,750.00
		Equipment			$605,480.00	$518,982.86	$432,485.71	$345,988.57	$259,491.43
		less depreciation (7y)			-$86,497.14	-$86,497.14	-$86,497.14	-$86,497.14	-$86,497.14
		Lasers			$415,920.00	$332,736.00	$249,552.00	$166,368.00	$83,184.00
		less depreciation (5y)			-$83,184.00	-$83,184.00	-$83,184.00	-$83,184.00	-$83,184.00
	Net fixed assets				$1,777,968.86	$1,559,537.71	$1,341,106.57	$1,122,675.43	$904,244.29
	TOTAL ASSETS				$2,013,244.67	$2,122,513.72	$2,116,644.87	$1,995,047.88	$2,407,087.11
LIABILITIES	Debt	Current	Credit line		$668,803.92	$819,657.46	$536,124.41	$0.00	$0.00
		A/P							
		Long-term							
			Plant	$975,000.00	$953,515.00	$930,327.00	$905,302.00	$878,293.00	$849,144.00
			principal paid		$21,485.00	$23,188.00	$25,025.00	$27,009.00	$29,149.00
			Lasers	$415,920.00	$345,447.00	$269,124.00	$186,467.00	$96,949.00	$1.00
			principal paid		$70,473.00	$76,323.00	$82,657.00	$89,518.00	$96,948.00
		Total long-term		$1,390,920.00	$1,298,962.00	$1,199,451.00	$1,091,769.00	$975,242.00	$849,145.00
	TOTAL DEBT				$1,967,765.92	$2,019,108.46	$1,627,893.41	$975,242.00	$849,145.00
	Equity	Capital contributed from Department of Surgery			$605,480.00	$605,480.00	$605,480.00	$605,480.00	$605,480.00
		Reserves			$0.00	$0.00	$0.00	$300,000.00	$300,000.00
		annual net income (post-tax)			-$560,001.25	$57,926.51	$385,346.20	$531,054.43	$538,136.23
		Retained earnings			-$560,001.25	-$502,074.74	-$116,728.54	$414,325.88	$952,462.11
		Net retained earnings (after building reserve)			-$560,001.25	-$502,074.74	-$116,728.54	$114,325.88	$652,462.11
	TOTAL EQUITY				$45,478.75	$103,405.26	$488,751.46	$1,019,805.88	$1,557,942.11
	TOTAL LIABILITIES				$2,013,244.67	$2,122,513.72	$2,116,644.87	$1,995,047.88	$2,407,087.11
	NOTES:	A/R will approach zero for cosmetic cases but could be substantial for recon cases (>60 days)							
		A/P will be relatively small compared to overall debt and will be paid within 30 days							
		Retained earnings will be applied to reserves, until 3 months' of operating costs are covered (3/12 * 1.2M)							
		All shares will be held by the Department of Surgery							
		total annual revenue			$1,354,563.60	$3,282,211.80	$4,532,578.20	$5,001,465.60	$5,001,465.60
		A/R @ 17% (60 days)			$230,275.81	$557,976.01	$770,538.29	$850,249.15	$850,249.15

Fig. 5.3 Accounting. Sample pro forma: balance sheet.

that institution, so the bank will need to collect more money from the borrower, when the debt is repaid, at some point in the future. But here is the catch: Banks need to charge not only for the time value of money, which is their expected rate of return (also called the discount rate), but the bank must also hedge against your riskiness as a borrower, driving up the cost of capital and increasing the interest rate that you must pay. In fact, if the bank can make a safer investment, with a possibly higher rate of return, then the bank should not pursue the loan.

Opportunity cost

When considering a new project or purchasing a piece of equipment, one should proceed if the intrinsic value of the asset equals or exceeds its cost. What one must also consider, though, is the opportunity cost of tying up precious time, money, and energy in that project or asset, when those resources could be invested elsewhere. The definition of opportunity cost is the potential benefit forgone from not following the financially optimal course of action. Rather than thinking in

Cash Flows				Overhead Applied to Net Income				
			YEAR	Y1	Y2	Y3	Y4	Y5
			UTILIZATION	40%	60%	80%	80%	80%
Cash flows from operating activities	**CFO**							
net income				-$560,001.25	$57,926.51	$385,346.20	$531,054.43	$538,136.23
A/R	starting A/R			$0.00	$230,275.81	$557,976.01	$770,538.29	$850,249.15
	ending A/R			$230,275.81	$557,976.01	$770,538.29	$850,249.15	$850,249.15
	change in A/R			-$230,275.81	-$327,700.19	-$212,562.29	-$79,710.86	$0.00
depreciation	plant	15 yr		$48,750.00	$48,750.00	$48,750.00	$48,750.00	$48,750.00
	equipment	7 yr		$86,497.14	$86,497.14	$86,497.14	$86,497.14	$86,497.14
	lasers	5 yr		$83,184.00	$83,184.00	$83,184.00	$83,184.00	$83,184.00
payment for inventory				-$5,000.00				
NET CASH: CFO				-$576,845.92	-$51,342.54	$391,215.05	$669,774.71	$756,567.37
Cash flows from investing activities	**CFI**							
payment for purchase of PPE				-$1,390,920.00				
NET CASH: CFI				-$1,390,920.00	$0.00	$0.00	$0.00	$0.00
Cash flows from financing activities	**CFF**							
notes payable borrowings				$1,390,920.00				
principal payment on long-term debt		BUILDING		-$21,485.00	-$23,188.00	-$25,025.00	-$27,009.00	-$29,149.00
		LASERS		-$70,473.00	-$76,323.00	-$82,657.00	-$89,518.00	-$96,948.00
NET CASH: CFF				$1,298,962.00	-$99,511.00	-$107,682.00	-$116,527.00	-$126,097.00
NET CHANGE IN CASH from cash flow calculations				-$668,803.92	-$150,853.54	$283,533.05	$553,247.71	$630,470.37
Net change in cash = CFO + CFI + CFF								
NET CHANGE IN CASH from balance sheet and income statement				-$668,803.92	-$150,853.54	$283,533.05	$553,247.71	$630,470.37
CASH AT BEGINNING OF YEAR				$0.00	-$668,803.92	-$819,657.46	-$536,124.41	$17,123.30
CASH AT END OF YEAR				-$668,803.92	-$819,657.46	-$536,124.41	$17,123.30	$647,593.68

NOTE: negative cash flows in Y1/Y2 will be covered by a combination of short term debt and credit lines from the Department of Surgery

Fig. 5.4 Accounting. Sample pro forma: summary of cash flows.

yes/no parameters, investors should make either/or decisions, searching for other opportunities, until they can compare the proposed course of action with the next best alternative. In the world of surgery, where most physician revenue is generated from procedures, any activity that takes the surgeon out of the operating room (OR) should be carefully compared to what the surgeon could accomplish by staying in the OR.

Net present value and discounted cash flows

The decision to pursue a project, when economic considerations are important, involves determining the NPV of that opportunity. NPV is calculated by adding a time-series of cash flows, both incoming and outgoing, that the project is expected to produce, over a series of future periods. This calculation would include the initial cost of purchasing the asset, at DCF_0, plus the anticipated revenue that the asset would generate, from DCF_1 to DCF_n. Each future cash flow must be discounted back to its present value.

$$NPV_{0-n} = DCF_0 + DCF_1 + DCF_2 + \ldots + DCF_n,$$
where $n =$ number of periods

If the NPV is > 0, then the investment would add value to the firm, and the project may be accepted. If the NPV is < 0, then the investment would subtract value from the firm, and the project should be rejected. The discount rate selected is often the firm's WACC, which blends the cost of debt (borrowing money) with the cost of equity (shareholders' expected returns on their stock). Another approach in selecting the appropriate discount rate is to determine the rate that another investment would yield, if this capital were used in a different project. This required rate of return is often referred to as the hurdle rate, which is higher for riskier projects

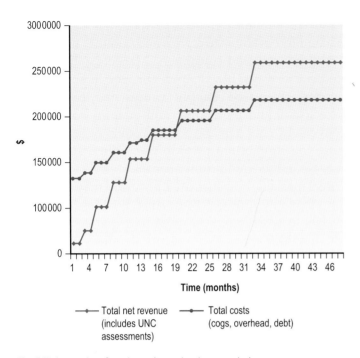

Fig. 5.5 Accounting. Sample pro forma: breakeven analysis.

and lower for safer ones. The hurdle rate represents the expected rate of return for risk-free projects (tied to the US Treasury bill) plus the potential rate of return for risky projects.

Return on investment

After one has projected future cash flows for an investment, how can one evaluate these future cash flows, in terms of the value of this investment? Several approaches are helpful in deciding the potential value of future ventures and in retrospectively examining the actual value of past ventures. These methodologies include: formal ROI or yield, the payback method, the IRR, and the NPV/DCF model. The most rigorous and powerful technique is NPV/DCF analysis, but limitations include multiple assumptions regarding future cash flows, selecting the appropriate discount rate, and complexity of the calculation. As a result, predictions using NPV tend to be conservative, but at least they incorporate the time value of money, so that the investor can make decisions based on the value of today's dollars.

A much simpler approach to calculating ROI is yield, which is represented by the following formula:

Yield = (gain from investment – cost of investment)/
cost of investment

Yield, however, is expressed as a percentage, and therefore gives little information about the magnitude of the value of the investment. Furthermore, yield can be easily manipulated by using varied metrics to define "gain" and "cost." Yield is helpful when comparing similar products or services, within a market or industry.

The payback method, which measures the time required for the cash flow from the project to pay for the original investment, is also quite popular with mid-level managers, who need to justify the purchase of capital equipment and predict time to breakeven.

Payback time = cost of investment/annual cash flow

What payback period does not take into account is depreciation of the equipment, useful lifespan of the asset, and residual value of the asset at the end of the period. Furthermore, cash flows for a project or asset usually change from year to year, and therefore the payback period only estimates when the project or asset reaches breakeven. If the useful life of the investment is greater than the payback time, then the investment should be pursued, at least for financial reasons.

Another technique used to assess ROI is IRR. Instead of assuming a particular discount rate for an investment and calculating the NPV, the IRR method determines the actual return projected by the cash flows. The IRR is then compared with the firm's hurdle rate, which may vary for different projects, depending upon the risk, the time horizon for the returns, and the cost of capital for the firm or WACC. Another way of understanding this method is that IRR represents the hurdle rate necessary to make NPV = 0. Problems with using IRR include not quantifying the overall value of the project, as well as how long the company can anticipate the length of the return. Nevertheless, IRR, payback method, and yield are helpful when communicating potential ROI to stakeholders, because of their simplicity and ease of understanding.

Economics

The sheer enormity of the field of economics prohibits a detailed review in this setting, but nevertheless, key concepts can be outlined. The entire discipline ranges from macroeconomics to microeconomics, from normative economics to behavioral economics, from heterodox economics to game theory.

Like other branches of economics, healthcare economics deals with decision-making in the setting of uncertainty, limited resources, and variable demand.[12–14] However, healthcare economics is distinctly different from other branches of economics, because healthcare is an industry that includes extensive government intervention and regulation; asymmetry of information between provider, patient, and payer; lack of precise metrics, with regard to patient outcomes; and considerable externalities, which are the downstream effects on other entities, outside the healthcare system.

Demand for a good or service is based upon a buyer's willingness to pay, which in turn is influenced by the buyer's tastes or needs, the consumer's income or wealth, and the availability of substitute and complementary goods. Demand curves can then be constructed to describe an individual's or population's willingness to purchase: as price increases, demand decreases. Price elasticity represents the change in quantity demanded as a function in change of price and is crucial to the way that markets adjust. Goods or services with close substitutes, such as Botox and Dysport, have a flat, elastic curve, in which small changes in price produce large changes in demand. Other goods and services may have steep, inelastic demand curves, in which large changes in price may have minimal effects on demand; this is the case for necessities with few substitutes, as well as some luxury items. Price elasticity for a given good or service may also vary, based upon the specific segment of the market targeted, and may be influenced by macroeconomic forces.

Supply of a good or service depends on a firm's short-term and long-run strategic goals. Decisions about supply are based initially on marginal costs, which vary with level of production. As production increases, so do marginal costs. However, average fixed costs decrease with increasing volume. These curves are combined to produce a U-shaped curve of average total cost, the nadir of which is the lowest price that the firm can charge and break even. A company can offer a good or service, as long as the market price remains above the average total costs. An aggregate market supply curve demonstrates that, as price increases, more firms are willing and able to produce outputs.

Market equilibrium occurs when the supply and demand forces adjust to a price and quantity that satisfy both producers and consumers. Markets will move in predictable ways, based upon changes in supply and demand. Increased supply causes the equilibrium price to fall and the equilibrium quantity to increase. Conversely, new demand for a product or service will cause the equilibrium price to rise, with a subsequent increase in the equilibrium quantity.

Real markets, however, are messy and may behave in ways that only approach these rules. For these economic models to work, markets must have perfect competition, in which products are identical, sellers and buyers do not engage in strategic manipulation of supply and demand, players make rational choices, entry and exit barriers are nonexistent, and participants are fully informed. Such a market does not exist. Predicting how economic forces shape the healthcare market is a considerable challenge, given that such competition is far from perfect.

Firms can gain strategic advantage, then, by exploiting the inefficiencies of the market. Ethical approaches include product differentiation, segmentation of the market, responding to new cultural, social, and political shifts, and using technology and innovation to create new value propositions. Unethical tactics would involve maintaining an asymmetry of information between consumer and producer, taking advantage of irrational decision-making, artificially creating demand or limiting supply, collusion with other players, and creating impassable barriers of entry for new participants. In the healthcare industry, providers must remain cognizant of these opportunities – both ethical and unethical – and maintain a level of responsibility that ensures professionalism at all times.

In summary, markets strive for equilibrium, but adjustments in supply and demand may not lead to productive efficiency, which by itself is not a guarantee of the fair distribution of wealth in society. A final quandary to ponder: not all of the costs and benefits of a transaction accrue to the buyer and the seller. These externalities – downstream effects on society – may be beneficial (new technology that extends life), but are too often detrimental (production of medical waste products). How can we incorporate these externalities into our decision-making, so that we increase the total social value of our actions?

Marketing

Business could not exist without the customer, and marketing is the process that enables business to connect with the customer.[15,16] Marketing strategy identifies, attracts, satisfies, and retains customers. Seeking to build more than a single exchange between the producer and the consumer (or in healthcare, the provider and the patient), marketing is first and foremost driven by customer needs and desires. The ideal approach in marketing is initially to understand the customers in the context of their environment, which includes not only assessment of market size but also competitive forces, barriers to entry, and market structure. Next, marketing seeks to develop a specific product or service offering, based upon anticipated customer needs that may or may not be adequately met, or may not even be appreciated. Finally, marketing strives to deliver customer value, in the form of price point, quality, and distribution.

Although marketing strategy has often oversimplified by focusing on the "4Ps" – product, price, promotion, placement – this is a good starting point for our review. Product refers to the characteristics and defining features of a good or service. Price is determined by factoring in cost of production with what additional value can be extracted by the producer, based upon value-added features and the demand for the good or service. Calculating breakeven volume is important to determine if a pricing strategy is reasonable. The formula for finding out how many units a company must sell, so that its costs are covered, is represented as follows:

Breakeven unit volume = fixed costs/(sales price – variable costs)

To achieve a specific profit target, the formula can be modified as follows:

Volume = (fixed costs + total profit)/ (sales price – variable costs)

Promotion involves the channels that will be necessary through which the company can communicate its message and may involve advertising, use of a sales force, or incentives (bundled pricing, discounts, rewards, and frequent buyer benefits, for example). Placement is arguably the most important of these variables;

marketing experts segment a general market to determine what types of people (young versus old, male versus female, high-income versus low-income) desire what types of products. Segmentation allows for better allocation of a company's finite resources, enables the firm to target specific high-yield groups, and improves positioning of the product for higher market penetration. In fact, a company can offer related but slightly different products if marketing research demonstrates that multiple segments have slightly different needs. Instead of pursuing a one-size-fits-all philosophy and missing segments of the market, a firm can employ marketing analysis to justify, with confidence, multiple offerings of related products.

Over the past two decades, in which consumers have been empowered by the internet (online auctions, availability of product reviews, and easy comparison of prices), marketing has shifted from a supply-side model to a demand-based one, in which customers' perspectives are factored into the supplier-centric approach of the 4Ps. Products are now viewed as solutions for the customer, promotion now includes transfer of information, price has been replaced by consumer value, and placement is viewed as access.

To identify market segments that might purchase a product or service, and to determine what qualities that segment would find most valuable, marketing research utilizes complex analytical tools such as regression analysis, conjoint analysis, perceptual maps, and scenario planning to make decisions. *Figure 5.6* demonstrates the

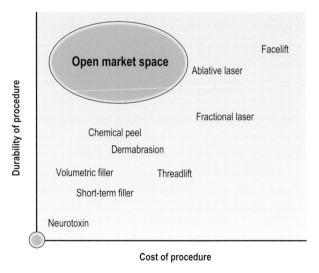

Fig. 5.6 Marketing. Perceptual map.

crowded landscape of facial rejuvenation, in which patients may choose from a number of interventions, based upon such parameters as price, durability, invasiveness, and time to recovery. Marketing seeks to identify which customers want what procedures and to target that group specifically. Occasionally, uncontested market space is discovered, based upon changing customer preferences, or opens up, due to advances in technology.

The act of connecting customer to product or service is central to the charge of marketing and can reap tremendous returns, in terms of revenue, branding, and goodwill. As such, marketing is viewed as an investment by the company, similar to research and development, in which ROI is predicted and carefully studied, along with other metrics such as market share, customer attrition, customer satisfaction, exchanges and returns, and size of accounts receivable. Other research tools include customer focus groups, demographic data, and customer questionnaires.

In addition to using such strategies as segmentation, targeting, and positioning, marketing also can utilize branding as a powerful tool to communicate the qualities of a new offering. In many ways, a strong brand serves, albeit not legally, as a promise that the new product or service will be similar to previous offerings. Branding can include a logo, phrase, image, or feeling that serves as a placeholder for the company and its reputation. One strategy that is not particularly effective but must be mentioned, to warn against, is that of perceptual shifting. This occurs either when promotion attempts to shift the needs and desires of a targeted group, so that they believe that they need or desire the product or service, or when promotion shifts the perceived qualities of the offering, so that these features more closely correspond with the needs and desires of the targeted group. Such a strategy will produce a very short-term effect, which may temporarily improve sales, but will have disastrous long-term effects on the relationship with the customer. This strategy is employed when firms do not desire repeat transactions with their customer or when a product is reaching obsolescence and the entire industry is shrinking.

With the recent decline in print media and other traditional communication outlets such as radio and network TV, marketing has turned to the internet to promote goods and services, provide information to the consumer, and match the appropriate offering with the correct group. Many economists arguably contend that in our new digital age, the cost of storing information is approaching zero and the value of information may creep toward infinity. Despite whether or not this can be proven, it is clear that digital information has completely changed the rules of marketing. Companies can gather specific information about consumers, based upon their shopping habits at Amazon, their friends on Facebook, what they write on blogs in the Huffington Post, and what articles they read at CNN.com. For a fraction of the cost of traditional media, firms can reach out to their customers through direct e-mail or via search engines. Marketing departments now focus on search engine optimization and search engine marketing. As some companies experiment with new revenue streams, both online and offline, some products may be offered for free, while related services may cost a premium.

Operations

Operations can be defined as matching supply with demand.[17,18] Although economists can describe how prices change with alterations in supply and demand, managers responsible for production of inventory or for coordination of services have an entirely different perspective: excess demand is lost revenue, and excess supply is wasted resources. How the manager balances supply and demand determines not only potential revenue from goods and services but also operating costs, which together yield operating income for the firm.

Operational effectiveness is critical to the firm's success; in fact, this can be a source of competitive advantage. Companies that get more from their inputs, or use fewer inputs, to produce higher-quality outputs will be able to offer goods or services at lower costs than their competitors or extract more financial value from these goods and services. This flow of inputs to outputs is also called the supply chain, and when managed well, adds value to the final product, before this is passed on to the consumer.

To optimize the flow of this value chain, the field of operations utilizes elements of queuing theory to predict and control demand, as well as the theory of constraints, to predict and control supply. Perhaps the greatest challenge in determining demand for a good or service is variability. In medicine, for example, long clinic waits to see a physician are often due to variability in patient arrival times, which is compounded by a variability in service times by the provider. This is why patients of a certain type are often scheduled in batches, to minimize the variability on both sides of the equation. In the service industry, key metrics that should be tracked, in an effort to improve operational effectiveness, include:

Capacity = maximum supply a process can generate

Capacity utilization = arrival rate/service rate

Throughput time = wait time + service time

Flow time = (1/service rate)/(1 − capacity utilization)

Inventory = average flow rate ×
           average flow time (Little's law)

Inventory turns = 1/flow time = COGS/inventory

Bottlenecks in the production process (for goods) or delivery process (for services) occur when the demand at a specific station in the flow process is greater than the outputs produced at that station. At any given point, a process has technically only one bottleneck, which is defined as the resource with the lowest capacity. Flow through a station can be measured to identify the bottleneck, but this point of constraint is often evident by high utilization, no slack or buffer, piled-up inventory, and complaints from workers and consumers.

Principles used to match supply with demand include:

1. Since the limiting resource defines capacity, focus on improving output at the bottleneck (this, of course, creates a new bottleneck somewhere else in the system).

2. Maintain enough inventory and work in process to keep the pipeline flowing, to prevent stock-out, and to anticipate variability in demand, but not too much that capital is overinvested on unfinished goods or unused services.

3. Systems or stations operating at close to 100% capacity are not sustainable; 80% utilization is considered to be a reasonable target.

4. Plan carefully, as variability and uncertainty can propagate along the supply chain, creating a bull-whip effect of increasing impact that yields far too much or far too little output.

5. Prevention costs less than inspection and correction; never add value to a part that is defective.

6. Never allow the cause of the problem to persist by working around it.

7. High quality is not free, but it can be a great investment.

8. Forecasts are always wrong, sometimes more so than others.

9. Service industries face unique challenges that involve customization of the output and a high degree of labor interaction.

In an effort to improve operational efficiency, a number of methods have been developed to reduce defects, increase throughput, and improve quality. Lean manufacturing is a production process in which any expenditure or resource that does not add value to the customer is a target for elimination. Originally developed by Toyota, lean manufacturing attempts to "work smarter, not harder" by reducing or eliminating seven sources of waste: overproduction, unnecessary transportation, inventory, motion, defects, overprocessing, and waiting. Although this approach yields only incremental improvements in operations, the system itself was an innovation that provided competitive advantage over other firms in the automobile production industry.

Another methodology that provides incremental improvements, through reduction in defects and quality improvement, is Six Sigma, originally developed by Motorola. Using the DMAIC model of define, measure, analyze, improve, and control, experts (known as black belts, green belts, and yellow belts, depending upon level of training and responsibility) attempt to improve the quality of process outputs by minimizing variability in the production line and reducing defects or errors to less than 3 per million (6 standard deviations from the desired target, thus Six Sigma). Quality management tools used to identify areas needing improvement include business process mapping, cost–benefit analysis, critical to quality trees, Pareto charts, and SIPOC analysis (suppliers, inputs, process, outputs, and customers). After determining the root cause of defects or inefficiencies, Six Sigma experts apply and test such interventions as contingency planning, parallel processing, and workflow redesign to reduce defects, improve quality, and maximize throughput. Although the methodology of Six Sigma provides only incremental improvement to inefficient systems and may, in fact, stifle "outside-the-box" innovation, improvements in operational productivity and quality may yield substantial financial rewards, in terms of cost savings, company goodwill and branding, and customer and employee satisfaction.

In service industries, the value chain can be strengthened by focusing on not only quality but also stakeholder happiness. In *Putting the Service-Profit Chain to Work*, Heskett *et al.* describe a model of stakeholder satisfaction, in which internal service quality yields employee retention and productivity, which in turn drives up external service value, securing customer loyalty and retention, which has a direct impact on revenue growth and profitability.[19] Employees and consumers can move from a zone of indifference to zones of affection or defection, depending upon their level of satisfaction. In fact, Jones and Sasser argue, in *Why Satisfied Customers Defect*, that complete customer satisfaction is the key to securing loyalty – intent to repurchase – and generating superior long-term financial performance.[20] Different industries have different loyalty/satisfaction curves, creating a mixture of consumers that includes apostles, loyalists, mercenaries, defectors, hostages, and terrorists. Companies should direct efforts at achieving complete satisfaction to retain the loyalists and attract the mercenaries (the apostles will stay), while the terrorists should not be pursued and hostages should be let go. In healthcare, patients who are not completely satisfied or mostly satisfied will find other providers.

Case study 5.1

At the University of North Carolina, we hypothesized that implementation of a Six Sigma program in perforator flap breast reconstruction could improve operational, financial, and clinical outcomes, by reducing variation, improving quality and efficiency, and optimizing throughput. A successful program in microsurgery requires the complex coordination of diverse teams, resources, and processes, and as such, improvements in efficiency and performance can be difficult.

Using the DMAIC model (define, measure, analyze, improve, control) of process improvement, we utilized SIPOC analysis (suppliers, inputs, process, outputs, customers), VOC (voice of the customer) questionnaires and focus groups, cause/effect trees, and workflow/critical pathway analysis to identify inefficiencies in the process. With the primary goal of decreasing operative times (preop-to-arrival in OR, arrival-to-cut, and cut-to-close), we implemented the following interventions: reducing redundant anesthetic and surgical steps, eliminating nonessential nursing tasks, having consistent personnel with adequate training, frequent in-servicing of microscope and flap-monitoring devices, rearrangement of OR bed and equipment, and creation of a microsurgery supply cart. We compared Six Sigma patients ($n = 27$) with a control group of patients before Six Sigma ($n = 39$), focusing on operational, financial, and clinical outcome measures.

From 2006 to 2009, 66 patients (median age 48.4, body mass index 29.3) underwent 98 breast reconstructions with deep inferior epigastric perforator (DIEP) and/or superficial inferior epigastric artery perforator flaps, by fellowship-trained microsurgeons. Total OR time decreased from 714 to 652 minutes ($P = 0.08$), with preop-to-cut time falling from 73 to 65 minutes ($P = 0.03$). The greatest drop in total OR time came with unilateral cases (672 to 498 minutes, $P = 0.001$), with less substantial gains noted in bilateral, immediate, or delayed cases. Length of stay decreased from 6.3 to 5.6 days ($P = 0.05$). Complication and take-back rates did not change, with only 1 total flap loss and 3 partial flap losses. Physician revenue increased modestly from $4490 to $4949 per case. More impressively, physician revenue/ minute jumped from $6.28 to $7.59 ($P = 0.02$). Hospital revenue increased minimally from $14676 to $15418 per case, but facility revenue/minute had more impressive gains, from $21.84 to $25.11. Contribution margin (revenue less variable costs) increased by $1264 per case, due to reduction in OR time and length of stay.

We conclude that a Six Sigma initiative in perforator flap breast reconstruction improves operational, financial, and clinical outcomes, evidenced by decreased operative time, reduced length of stay, reduction in variable costs, improved physician revenue, and increased contribution margin to the healthcare system. Maintaining these gains in efficiency, defect reduction, and quality will be critical and may prove to be quite challenging.

Innovation

Whereas the field of operations provides value through incremental improvement, innovation produces radical or revolutionary changes in thinking, design, products, processes, and even organizations.[21-24] Operations serves to exploit existing inefficiencies, with the goal of lower costs, faster production, and higher quality, via interventions such as tighter supply chain coordination, lean manufacturing techniques, and zero-defect policies. Innovation, on the other hand, disrupts the current paradigm and not only expands the existing market but may also create entirely new markets. Thomas Krummel, a pediatric surgeon who directs the Stanford Biodesign Program, describes a sequence of discovery, invention, innovation, and entrepreneurship that is the blueprint for translational medicine.[23] More importantly, he asks, "why should innovation be left to chance?" and provides a cogent argument for studying, understanding, and teaching innovation. Medical knowledge can be utilized directly in patient care, but training other physicians, developing new solutions, and applying new technologies can increase the impact of surgeons exponentially.

A reasonable question, which has a surprising answer, is "why do we need to innovate?" Peter Drucker, in fact, wrote that the two essential functions of a company are innovation and marketing, because these create real value; all other processes are costs.[21] Since the business environment is always changing, the position of a company, relative to its competition, new entrants, substitutes, suppliers, and consumers, is also in flux. A company that enjoys dominant market share today could become easily displaced tomorrow. Apart from innovation, the only competitive advantage that a company can maintain is based upon incremental improvements in price, quality, and access – until a new company introduces an innovation that dramatically affects these qualities, significantly expands the size of the market, or actually changes customer needs and preferences. Innovation is actually most effective and needed during periods of stability, whereas process improvement is most valuable to a company during periods of growth.

Successful innovation requires discipline and hard work, in addition to creativity. Companies that have mastered the process of innovation, such as Apple, Mayo Clinic, and the design firm Ideo, follow a roadmap that consists of four phases: breakthrough or discovery, platform development, derivative changes, and maintenance. Through a carefully orchestrated plan, in which these phases overlap, project managers allocate resources (time, money, people) based upon the importance of each phase, level of uncertainty, and location in the critical pathway. Apple may introduce a new product, such

as the iPod, iPhone, and iPad, every few years, but each of these devices undergoes an iterative process of improvement and value-added upgrades in technology. By having a diverse portfolio of new products, Apple is ensuring the success of its company, similar to a mutual fund with multiple investments. Occasionally, such innovation is disruptive, displacing some products, increasing competition with a company's own products, and creating new markets for other entrants. Such is the case with digital music: Apple changed from a computer company to an information and communications company, within a decade. Apple was able to apply breakthrough technology to create new products. If Apple had focused on incremental improvements in its operating system or software, as Microsoft has done, then such spinoff applications as e-books, online newspapers, and of course iTunes might not yet exist. The real challenge will come from Google, which started as a search engine but now intends to dominate the landscape of cloud computing.

Three drivers of successful innovation are understanding the consumer, "crossing the chasm," and managing failure. To succeed over a long-term horizon, companies need to serve and retain their existing customers and acquire new ones by applying incremental and disruptive technologies. The focus of any commercial venture should start with the voice of the customer – listening to what the customer wants – and should finish with what the customer needs. Good marketing may be able to identify needs that do not yet exist, or segments of the population that have not been identified. Second, anticipate who will need the product or service, and when. Prototypes and early versions (think iPhone v1.0) are critical in attracting the innovators (our medial students) and early adopters (our residents), who will demonstrate product viability and create an early buzz. ROI, however, will not occur until the early majority (me) and late majority (my boss) adopt this technology. Even laggards, who usually resist new technology, may be an attractive group to target, as they may become the early adopters of the next technology. Crossing this chasm, from early adoption to market penetration, is where most companies fail. The third component of successful innovation, then, is learning from failure and managing failure. Just as lean manufacturing and Six Sigma permit incremental improvement in production systems, controlled experimentation increases the yield of innovation efforts. Measures to minimize risk include separation of invention from execution, maintaining a diverse and deep pipeline of ideas and projects, and collaborating with people outside your area of technical expertise or "comfort zone."

Case study 5.2

The core competency of plastic surgery is innovation. As surgeons, the moment we stop innovating, we become irrelevant. Other providers can replicate almost everything that we do, from reconstructive to aesthetic procedures. Plastic surgeons have sought solutions to surgical problems and pioneered the development of new fields, such as hand surgery, transplantation, and microsurgery, but other disciplines have appropriated these techniques and incorporated them into their scope of practice. If plastic surgeons cannot compete on differentiation, then we must compete on some combination of quality, price, or service. This is reasonable for most healthcare providers, whose practices depend on reducing variability and improving throughput, but our heritage has been defined by our willingness to take on new problems, improve standards of care, and embrace the uncertainty of what our next patient will need.

Such is the case with breast reconstruction. Until the late 1970s, women with mastectomy defects had few options other than delayed reconstruction with implants, yielding results that were unpredictable, highly variable, and of marginal quality. With the introduction of vascularized, autologous tissue, however, the paradigm for reconstruction quickly shifted to immediate reconstruction with pedicled flaps. An interesting side note is that the omentum was proposed as an early source of tissue to solve the problem of durability and quality, before the introduction of the transverse rectus abdominis myocutaneous (TRAM) or latissimus flaps. Surgeons recognized a market need – breast reconstruction without prosthetic materials – but had not yet identified a solution. With the advent of microsurgery in the 1980s, predictions were made that the field would again shift to "free" TRAMs, but this did not happen until much later. What did occur, in the 1990s, was the convergence of economic and technological forces that shifted the pendulum back toward implant-based reconstruction. More favorable reimbursement and improved outcomes with sentinel lymph node dissection, skin-sparing mastectomies, and the reintroduction of silicone gel implants by the Food and Drug Administration guided this change, despite the fact that reconstruction with living tissue was a superior technology. During the first decade of this century, we have again witnessed a shift back to autologous flaps, namely perforator flaps that spare muscles, reduce donor site morbidity, and may improve the final outcome.

The driver for this most recent change has arguably come not from a refinement in technique, which certainly did occur, but from the market. Women with mastectomy defects, with the breast cancer gene, with complications from previous aesthetic breast surgery, have identified the DIEP flap as the standard of care and have created unprecedented and unpredicted demand for this procedure. Interestingly, such market segmentation was not the product of targeting efforts by surgeons but was largely self-generating, as more women used the internet to gain information, in the form of blogs, access to PubMed, and other electronic media. New technologies, like fat grafting and tissue engineering, will certainly change the field of breast reconstruction, again.

Entrepreneurship

Whereas technology is the way that you do things and innovation is the way you do new things, entrepreneurship is the way that you increase the value of what you do.[25] Entrepreneurship is a way of thinking, as well as a process, that increases the impact of innovation. An entrepreneur articulates a vision and develops a system that assembles inputs, creates a product, service, or information, and captures new value from the outputs. Entrepreneurial leaders act to bring a future business possibility into existence, with a sense of urgency, not constrained by limitations in capital, personnel, or productions. Instead, the entrepreneur utilizes his or her imagination, drive, passion, and networking, to gain the support of investment bankers, suppliers, and customers. Perhaps the most important resource to an entrepreneur, though, is an asymmetry of knowledge. Entrepreneurs may be aware of: (1) macroeconomic forces yielding change in demographic, social, and cultural norms; (2) new technologies without defined applications; and (3) existing inefficiencies embedded within current industries. Such incongruities, in the setting of new technology and changing markets, represent tempting opportunities for entrepreneurs. Good entrepreneurs find opportunities; great entrepreneurs make opportunities.

What is the process, then, for turning a challenge into an opportunity? The first and single most important act is to establish a value proposition, which can be defined as that core competency which makes your product or service unique and valuable. The value proposition presents a problem and solution, describes what you do and how you do it, and serves to differentiate you from the competition – all in one sentence. From this value proposition, the entrepreneur next develops a business model, which must then be translated into a business plan.

With details carefully thought out and available to potential stakeholders, the entrepreneur must seek support for this plan through different types of communication. The elevator pitch, which is a 30-second distillation of the new venture, is designed to attract interest and pique the listener's curiosity. The executive summary is a one-page summary of the business plan, whereas the business plan is a highly detailed document, ranging from 20 to 60 pages, designed to address specific questions, as investors look further into the venture. A 10-minute overview, typically delivered as a PowerPoint talk, is also necessary to get investors actually to read the business plan.

At every stage, the entrepreneur seeks to increase the interest of potential stakeholders and actively listens to feedback, so that the business plan can be revised, rewritten, and refocused, as often as needed. If the entrepreneur can gain the commitment of the stakeholders, then begins the process of raising capital, carefully managing cash, and coordinating logistics. Entrepreneurs typically bootstrap for as long as they can, utilizing human, intellectual, and social capital, rather than borrowing money or seeking outside funding. Entrepreneurs know that the worst time to raise money is when they absolutely need it, because they must cede control and ownership of the company each time investors are brought on board with an influx of capital. Venture capital is particularly challenging to accept, because these investment bankers demand a five to seven times return on their investment, within a time horizon of several years, and because their exit strategy is ultimately about sale of the company, not necessarily growth of the company. Angel investors, friends and family, philanthropy and endowments, academic and community grants, small-business loans, and even credit cards are more attractive (but limited) sources of capital, permitting the entrepreneur to retain control as long as possible. Finally, the cost of capital is highest at the beginning of the venture, because the risk is greatest, and borrowing costs decrease as the venture becomes more successful.

Writing a business plan is an art that entrepreneurs must master. *Figure 5.7* depicts a model that can be used when designing the elements of a new venture. Much like writing abstracts and journal articles, repetition

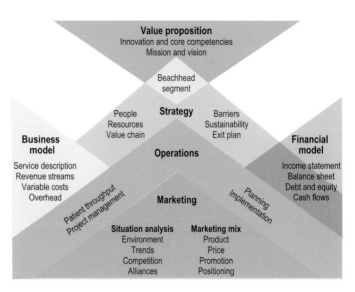

Fig. 5.7 Entrepreneurship: new-venture model.

improves the quality of the product. But unlike scientific papers, which are published once and do not change, business plans are living documents that are constantly in flux and mandate frequent update. Nevertheless, a typical business plan follows an established model and contains the following components:

1. Executive summary
2. Value proposition
3. Vision, mission, values statement
4. Marketing analysis
    a. Situation analysis
        i. Environment
        ii. Trends
        iii. Company analysis
        iv. Competition
        v. Alliances
    b. Target market and segmentation
    c. Positioning and differentiation
    d. Channels
    e. Branding
    f. Sales tools
    g. Marketing budget
5. Business model
    h. Description of service or product
    i. Revenue streams
    j. Variable costs
    k. Overhead and fixed costs

6. Strategy
   l. Beachhead segment
   m. Value chain
   n. Growth
   o. Response to competitors, new entrants, substitutes
7. Governance and management teams
8. Financial pro formas
   p. Income statement
   q. Balance sheet
   r. Cash flows: operations, financing, investments
9. Debt and equity structures
10. Operations
    s. Planning – Gantt chart
    t. Implementation
    u. Throughput assessment
    v. Continuous improvement plans
11. Legal and regulatory issues
12. Sustainability practices (triple bottom line of people, planet, profit)
13. Barriers and roadblocks
14. Contingency plans
15. Exit strategy.

Eventually, the chief executive officer (CEO) entrepreneur, having built a successful company, must make some major decisions, beyond resource allocation and management of revenue streams. In the short run, the leader will need to delegate operational decisions, while focusing on setting strategy, team building, establishing culture, and reinforcing vision and values. Ultimately, however, the entrepreneur may recognize an internal calling to cede control, in order to begin the process again, with a new idea, perhaps in a new industry, with a new market. Others, however, remain with the company as a technical advisor or may serve on the Board of Directors, content with knowing that, despite great odds, they created something of value. To paraphrase Steve Jobs, they "put a ding in the universe."

Sustainable enterprise

Sustainable enterprise is a well-established concept that has recently caught the attention of academics in organizational behavior, business executives, supply chain managers, shareholders, and even consumers.[26–33]

The importance of sustainable enterprise is so great that specific companies, as well as entire industries, are reassessing their vision and values, so that organizations can meet a new triple bottom line of "people, planet, and profit." Green business, or sustainable enterprise, produces no or little negative impact on global or local environments, the community, society, or the economy, with specific attention to progressive human rights and environmental policies.

Previous efforts toward "reduce, reuse, recycle, repair, and redistribute" have been replaced by more aggressive attempts to minimize the carbon footprint of a business, search for renewable energy sources, and lessen the impact of waste materials on the environment, with the goal of establishing a business that meets the needs of the present, without compromising the ability to meet the needs of the future. Specific examples of sustainable business practices include telecommuting, having a paperless office, minimizing shipping and packing material, leasing equipment that can be returned and refurbished, lean production methods which utilize less raw materials and produce less inventory, continuous improvement processes in the supply chain, and conducting business in Leadership in Energy and Environmental Design (LEED)-certified buildings, which have lower energy requirements and are made of post-consumer materials. Products of service are durable goods that the manufacturer plans to reprocess (thus the term "cradle to cradle," when describing the responsibility of the manufacturer), and products of consumption are short-lived materials that are nontoxic and biodegradable.

These sustainable business practices have coalesced into the more formal principle of corporate social responsibility, in which self-regulation is integrated into the overall business model of a company or industry. Businesses have discovered that sustainable practices can generate lasting value to shareholders and stakeholders, in terms of quality, access, and cost of services and goods. Leaders such as Ikea, Nike, Ford, and even Walmart have been able to reduce expenses, minimize risk, increase revenues, and create stronger brands by building environmental and social thinking into their business strategies. Most large companies now have a chief sustainability officer and publish an annual sustainability report that corresponds to the annual financial report.

What can we do in healthcare, and specifically plastic surgery, to leverage green practices and improve our triple bottom line? Interestingly, plastic surgery has been a leader in social justice for decades. Mission trips to developing nations, in which specialized services are provided and reusable equipment is donated, has been a focus of many plastic surgeons, who could have spent more time in their private practices and generated more money for their businesses. What is especially admirable, in terms of sustainability, is the effort to teach these surgical techniques to providers in developing nations, so that infrastructure is developed and continuity of care is established, between visiting groups and the local communities. For surgeons who do not travel outside the US, multiple opportunities exist within our borders to establish similar exchanges, which can include work done at Native American reservations, in underserved areas like Appalachia, or at a community clinic. Even maintaining on-call emergency department privileges, performing lower-reimbursing reconstructive surgery, and assuming some indigent care all count as sustainable efforts, as the surgeon is contributing to a triple bottom line that does not neglect the needs of his or her local community. Such volunteerism is sustainable enterprise and should be a goal for all who practice this craft.

Healthcare, in general, has lagged behind other industries, in terms of sustainable business practices. One definition for sustainable medicine is the improvement of health within the natural life cycle, which seeks to avoid strain on social, environmental, and economic systems, so that new technologies can benefit all people within a community, not just those who can afford it. Extending this definition to the entire population of our planet, we have a moral obligation to provide basic healthcare to all, in the form of clean water, food, vaccinations, and preventive medicine. Jeffrey Sachs, a progressive economist at Columbia University, and Muhammad Yunus, winner of the Nobel Peace Prize for his work on microfinance in India, both contend that we have the resources and technology to end extreme poverty during our lifetime. Part of the answer to eradicating extreme poverty is improving the health of those 2.5 billion people who exist at the "bottom of the pyramid" (individuals who live on less than $2.50/day). Optimizing global health is possible with improved water purification systems, agricultural alliances to improve supply chain logistics, regulation of markets to eliminate corrupt middlemen in local markets, access to medical supplies such as antibiotics and antiretrovirals, and establishing microcredit and microloans. Once again, sustainable health endeavors are not only desirable from an ethical perspective, but such ventures can open new markets and new opportunities for investment.

Human resource management

Perhaps one of the most important, least appreciated, and often neglected components of business administration is human resources management (HRM), which can be defined as that component of an organization that strategically manages the value chain of human capital.[34] Although employees cannot be considered an asset of a company, workers at all levels provide the critical steps of adding value to the product or service, as inputs are converted to outputs. Furthermore, employees, as well as customers, can be an incredible reservoir of innovation, if this resource is managed appropriately, in terms of recruiting, developing, retaining, and promoting talent. HRM is so critical to the success of an organization that HR practices often dictate the culture of that business and provide competitive advantage in and of itself, by attracting people of the highest quality and best fit. At Google, for example, employees are encouraged to spend 20% of their time on projects outside their line of responsibility; such an environment fosters controlled experimentation and is directly responsible for that company's rapid ascent in the world of information technology.

Managing people is a daunting responsibility and, when done correctly, looks effortless, but when not done well, creates a workplace that stifles creativity, undermines quality, and detracts from the value proposition of the company. As complex as managing human capital is, several best practices have emerged that can be shared:

1. Leadership starts with self-awareness.
2. Communication with employees is a central role of the manager.
3. Effective managers can articulate their own values and vision.
4. Effective managers foster an environment that brings out the best in others.

5. Effective managers are willing to engage in difficult conversations about difference.

6. Effective managers understand how groups work and focus on creating a culture of performance, with defined metrics, that enhances teamwork and collaboration.

7. Effective managers are change leaders.

8. Effective managers learn, reflect, and renew.

In healthcare, HRM is often focuses on "workforce development," which refers to the continuing education and training of employees for current, new, and changing jobs. What a nurse does today may be very different from what he or she will do in the future, and employees must be able to adapt to the changing models of healthcare delivery. Not only must healthcare providers deal with changing technology and evolving systems of healthcare, but also these employees must be able to work well with people of different educational backgrounds, different generations (traditionalists, baby boomers, generation Xers, and millennials), and different work/life balances. Diversity in the workplace no longer refers to people of different cultures, but recognizes different values, work styles, and needs.

What HRM leaders have discovered in healthcare is that investing in the organization's people has a far greater ROI than trying to recruit superstar candidates for specific jobs. Furthermore, treating employees like customers, as well as customers as employees, is the key to retaining both providers and patients. Provider and patient satisfaction is very important, not only in the rankings of healthcare systems, but also in future revenue streams. Very satisfied patients will continue to seek healthcare with their same providers and will refer their friends and family. Such marketing is priceless. This practice of stakeholder fulfillment is not only good business, but also great medicine.

Case study 5.3

Like many other public institutions, employee satisfaction and retention at the University of North Carolina Healthcare System are particularly difficult, as many high-potential, high-performing workers are often recruited to private, smaller medical practices, where salaries are higher and benefits more extensive. Recognizing that workforce development would be critical to increasing employee job satisfaction, which in turn is linked to patient satisfaction, senior leaders in HRM created the equivalent of a corporate

university. Companies like IBM, Cisco, and Disney offer educational resources for employees who need or desire new skill sets, who want to acquire new knowledge, and who wish to advance their careers. These educational programs vary from 1-hour didactic sessions to year-long courses and projects, during which time employees are granted the flexibility to pursue this training, solve real-time challenges, and apply this learning to future work within the company.

In 2008, with the support of the Dean and CEO of the Hospital, UNC Healthcare System created the Learning Institute, which consists of four components: the College of Leadership Excellence, the College of Quality and Service, the College of Workforce Development, and the College of Clinical Excellence. The College of Leadership Excellence, in turn, contains four Academies: Emerging Leaders, New Leaders, Operational Leaders, and Strategic Leaders. Resources and programs for the participants include online learning via podcasts and vodcasts, a quarterly book club on leadership and healthcare, participation in Six Sigma quality and efficiency initiatives, access to mentors and professors in the Schools of Public Health and Business, and a formal CEO challenge, in which participants learn about and solve actual operational and strategic problems, as identified by senior administrators.

Since the program was initiated, employee satisfaction regarding professional fulfillment has increased from the 33rd to 72nd percentile, voluntary attrition within the first year has dropped from 22.1% to 11.8%, and, most importantly, very few employees who leave do so after the 6-month probation period. The UNC Healthcare System estimates that these efforts toward employee development and retention have saved the institution $13 million, by reducing employee turnover to below industry standards. Such a cost savings obviously makes senior leadership happy, but a far-reaching effect is improved patient satisfaction scores, as measured by Press-Gainey.

Legal and regulatory considerations

As might be expected, the legal and regulatory components of healthcare are so labyrinthine that these considerations could easily occupy the contents of an encyclopedia. Nevertheless, plastic surgeons must be aware of the broad categories that affect their practice, and most importantly, and have a low threshold to seek legal counsel, when needed. In addition to knowing about malpractice law, healthcare providers must have some familiarity with contract law, labor relations, corporate structure and liability, rules of emergency medical treatment, scope of practice by nonphysician providers, certificate of need for and accreditation of outpatient facilities, and protection of patient confidentiality. A comprehension of these issues is not only recommended but is necessary, as providers must comply with state and federal regulations or face investigation, legal expenses, fines, court time, or prison, depending upon the degree of culpability, intent, and involvement.

This purpose of this section, however, is to examine how regulatory and legal changes in the business world have recently impacted healthcare as a business.[35-37] Understanding the macroeconomics of and market changes in healthcare, as a result of government intervention, will hopefully assist the healthcare provider in making more informed decisions when delivering healthcare. This section will not debate the benefits or detrimental effects of regulation, but will rather present the changes that have occurred, as objectively as possible.

Before discussing how recent regulation has affected the business of healthcare, it is important to review the basic forms of business ownership. A sole proprietorship is an entity owned by one person, who assumes personal liability for debts incurred by the business. A partnership is a type of business in which two or more individuals agree to share profits but also liabilities; the advantage of such a structure, like that of a proprietorship, is that net income is taxed only once. A corporation is a business with a distinct and separate identity from its members; for-profit and not-for-profit corporations must be owned by multiple shareholders and are overseen by a board of directors, which manages the executive team. Most hospitals follow this model, while many physicians in private practice may function as a proprietor or as the head of an S-corporation. Finally, a cooperative is a type of corporation with limited liability whose members, in contrast to shareholders, share decision-making capabilities. One disadvantage of corporations and cooperatives is that profit is subject to double taxation: first on net income of the entity, after operating and indirect expenses are deducted, and second on the returns to the stakeholders, in the form of personal income, dividends, and other capital gains, such as stock that is sold.

Sarbanes–Oxley Act, 2002

In response to corporate and accounting scandals such as Enron, Tyco, and WorldCom, as well as the "dotcom" bubble that burst and cost investors billions of dollars,

both the House and the Senate overwhelming supported and passed the Sarbanes–Oxley Act (SOX).[38] Public confidence in the nation's securities markets had been greatly undermined, and this legislation attempted to restore the stability of these markets, through oversight and control. In addition to creating a Public Company Accounting Oversight Board, SOX mandated that: (1) auditors could not provide consulting services to the same clients; (2) senior executives must take individual responsibility for the accuracy and completeness of their corporate financial reports; and (3) financial disclosures of public companies must include enhanced reporting of off-balance sheet transactions, assumptions for pro formas, and stock transactions of corporate officers. Although SOX did not have provisions directly dealing with healthcare, this act affected the healthcare industry, as every publicly held company involved with healthcare would have to undergo significant restructuring of their accounting practices. Proponents contend that such legislation was essential to strengthen accounting controls and restore investor confidence, while opponents cite the overly complex oversight necessary for compliance, leading to reduced competitiveness with foreign businesses.

American Recovery and Reinvestment Act, 2009

As the US headed into the worst recession since the Great Depression, Congress passed the American Recovery and Reinvestment Act, in an attempt to create jobs, promote investment, and induce consumer spending.[39] Because the Federal Reserve had already decreased interest rates to zero, with little effect on the credit markets, fiscal policy was chosen over monetary policy as a plan to stimulate the economy, and therefore an infusion of government capital – $787 billion – was utilized to bridge the output gap created by a fall in consumer spending. Although the majority of the capital was used to fund projects and programs in energy, communications, education, and transportation, healthcare received $151 billion, with the vast majority of this money used to support Medicare. In the wake of this stimulus package, the national economy has remained volatile but appears to have stabilized, and the demand for healthcare services has not decreased, as many economists predicted.

Patient Protection and Affordable Care Act, 2010

In a bitterly fought, highly publicised partisan struggle, Congress eventually passed the Patient Protection and Affordable Care Act, which in summary is a healthcare reform bill that focuses on health insurance reform.[40] An estimated 32 million people who currently do not have health insurance will be able to obtain coverage. Benefits of this legislation include expanded Medicaid eligibility, subsidized insurance premiums, incentives for small businesses to provide healthcare coverage, prohibition of denials by insurance companies, establishing a market of health insurance "exchanges," and financial support of medical research and information technology, such as the electronic medical record. Critics insist that the proposed deficit reduction of $143 billion, over the first decade, will be neither achievable nor maintainable. The cost of this plan is offset by fees on pharmaceutical companies and on medical devices, new taxes on high-income brackets, improved efficiencies from information technology, and reduced administrative expenses.

Dodd–Frank Wall Street Reform and Consumer Protection Act, 2010

Already considered the most sweeping change to financial reform since the Great Depression, the Dodd–Frank Wall Street Reform and Consumer Protection Act is designed to fix permanently the economic problems that the Stimulus Act helped to stabilize.[41] The aim of the bill is as follows: "To promote the financial stability of the United States by improving accountability and transparency in the financial system, to end 'too big to fail', to protect the American taxpayer by ending bail-outs, [and] to protect consumers from abusive financial services practices." The impact on the financial regulatory system will certainly be far-reaching, with significant restructuring of the flow of capital within our economy. Specific targets of reform include hedge funds and other investment banking instruments, the Federal Reserve, Wall Street transparency and accountability, mortgage and commercial lending institutions, and consumer and investor protection programs. The question for the healthcare industry is not if the Dodd–Frank Act will affect healthcare delivery, but how.

Negotiation

Negotiation can be defined as "a dialogue intended to resolve disputes, to produce an agreement upon courses of action, to bargain for individual or collective advantage, or to craft outcomes to satisfy various interests."[42] Whenever a decision is made, negotiation occurs. If a surgeon decides to start a laser practice, he or she must examine the opportunity cost in pursuing that service and negotiate, with the stakeholders of his or her practice – receptionists, nursing staff, patients – how this change will impact the practice. If a junior partner wants to develop a microsurgical breast reconstruction practice, he or she must negotiate with the hospital for more operative block time, carve out with insurance companies a more favorable reimbursement schedule, and gain the blessing of the senior partners, who will have to cover these patients when the primary surgeon is not available and absorb these low-margin cases into their revenue stream. If an academic plastic surgery practice wishes to develop and build an outpatient aesthetic center with procedural rooms, the division chief must perform a complex negotiation with multiple parties (the Dean, Chairs, hospital administrators), over multiple iterations, regarding multiple issues.

Although some individuals are blessed with excellent empathic and communication skills and can negotiate successfully, negotiation is a discipline that can be learned. Practice and preparation are the keys to success. The field of negotiation, as an academic discipline, is a rich body of work that incorporates game theory, auction strategies, psychology, and behavioral economics. Perhaps the seminal work in this field is *Getting to Yes: Negotiating Agreement Without Giving In*, by Fisher *et al.*[43] The two overriding principles are: (1) knowing what you want versus want you need; and (2) knowing what your opponent wants and needs. Negotiating begins with considerable preparation, not just predicting what your opponent will do, as if in a chess match, but what your opponent requires to improve his or her position. In fact, both opponents in a two-party negotiation may not even know what their best position is or why a certain solution may be favorable for each other. Creativity and communication are critical for success.

Negotiation, then, begins by developing and articulating your BATNA: your best alternative to a negotiated agreement. This is the walk-away position if no agreement can be reached, or "the lowest you will go," which should be ascertained before the negotiation begins. After deciding that you will not bargain over these positions, utilize the following four principles: (1) separate the people from the problem; (2) focus on interests and not positions; (3) invent options for mutual gain; and (4) insist on using objective criteria.[44–48]

These concepts of "principled" negotiation work most of the time. Occasionally, however, negotiation reaches an impasse, and breakthrough can be achieved by reframing the problem. Specifically, avoid escalation by not reacting, arguing, rejecting, or pushing. Step out of the situation, help the other side view the problem objectively, and reframe the problem from their perspective. Determine what options will provide mutual gain, or at the very least, minimize losses. In other words, pick your battles wisely. Concession is not failure, but often resets the parameters of the problem, so that future iterations of the "game" may yield an outcome in your favor.

Particularly difficult negotiations involve those individuals or groups who will not compromise over their demands, who have an asymmetry of information, who are unwilling to view the problem from your perspective, or who threaten to use power to enforce their solution. People who fall into this category are the school-yard bully, an impaired physician, sociopaths, terrorists, and sometimes the "difficult patient," who may have an underlying body dysmorphic disorder. One option is not to negotiate – step away from the situation – and use other means to resolve a dispute, such as legal action. However, skilled negotiators can still deal with these challenging situations effectively, by using uncertainty, chaos, and ambiguity to disarm opponents and neutralize their position. Successful negotiators can translate little gains into positive momentum, by focusing on future rounds of the negotiation and setting up more effective positions for the future.

Ethics

In healthcare, we are faced with multiple challenges that test our ethical grounding. Healthcare providers must make numerous decisions regarding patient care every day, and society rightfully expects these providers to behave ethically. Competency in patient care and medical knowledge is required but not sufficient; providers must also demonstrate competency in interpersonal and communication skills, systems-based practice, practice-based learning, and professionalism, all of which involve a firm commitment toward ethical practice. So important are these competencies that medical education, residency training programs, state licensure, board certification and maintenance of certification, and hospital credentialing incorporate these elements in evaluating healthcare providers.

John Canady, past president of the American Society of Plastic Surgeons and former chair of its Ethics Committee, observed, "Plastic surgeons who are aware of competing interests that influence their decision-making processes stand a greater chance of achieving ethical outcomes. Nevertheless, with the growing volume of nonreimbursed care and expectations of perfect outcomes, achieving uniformly ethical decisions without burdensome self-sacrifice is difficult at best."[49] Competing factors that influence decision-making for plastic surgeons include personal finances (ownership of surgery centers, selection of procedures, pricing), regulatory forces (Emergency Medical Treatment and Active Labor Act (EMTALA), Joint Commission on Accreditation of Healthcare Organizations (JCAHO), American Association for Accreditation of Ambulatory Surgery Facilities (AAAASF)/Accreditation Association for Ambulatory Healthcare (AAAHC), Occupational Safety and Health Administration (OSHA), and Health Insurance Portability and Accountability Act (HIPPA) – to name just a few), and professional duty (informed consent, discussion of error).

When faced with a dilemma, healthcare providers must incorporate intuition and reasoning into making a decision. Resolution of an ethical question often requires careful consideration of culture, infrastructure, leadership/governance, and personal integrity. Ethical intelligence can be developed. In his book *Strengthening Ethical Wisdom*, Jack Gilbert argues that intentions, manifest by vision, mission, values, strategy, and goals, directly impact performance.[50] In healthcare, this translates into patient safety, quality of care, productivity and throughput, patient and employee satisfaction, reputation, and financial health. Medical ethics is practical, case-based, and relative to the context of the situation.

Just as ethics helps to guide decision-making in healthcare, so too should ethics play a major role in the choices made by business entities. The history of ethics and capitalism is quite fascinating. Adam Smith, who published *The Wealth of Nations* in 1776, argued that markets were guided by "the invisible hand" to produce the right amount of goods for society, but that such a force was intimately tied to our ethical obligations to each other.[51] Andrew Carnegie and other industrialists from the 1800s articulated the need for business to pursue charity and steward-ship, both forms of social philanthropy, because with power comes responsibility. Even Milton Friedman, the Nobel-winning economist from the University of Chicago, who believed that the only ethical obligation of business is to maximize profits, emphasized that business efficiently creates and allocates wealth in society if the stakeholders are honest, transparent, and just.

Today, business ethics is just good business. A new paradigm for delivering stakeholder value has replaced the previous model of maximizing shareholder returns. Because suppliers, customers, employees, competitors, and communities are all affected by the decisions of a business, a stakeholder approach to organizational structure maps out these relationships and attempts to align competing interests, to maximize value creation of the networks, products, services, and information. Most business leaders are aware that values, rights, duties, and responsibilities must inform decision-making, much like these principles affect medical ethics. Consequences may not only have legal ramifications but may also impact the bottom line. Values-based capitalism strives to maximize stakeholder wealth by trying to humanize the institution of business and encourage stakeholders to perform at their best, not their worst. Key principles of values-based capitalism include: stakeholder cooperation, shared responsibility, recognition of complexity, continuous creation, and emergent competition.

In response to recent, highly publicised business scandals involving fraudulent accounting, Ponzi schemes, excessive executive compensation, business–government collusion, and illegal derivative trading, academic leaders in business management have come forward to develop the MBA oath *(Box 5.1)*.[52] Similar to the Hippocratic oath for physicians, this pledge

> **Box 5.1 The MBA oath**
>
> **As a business leader I recognize my role in society:**
> - My purpose is to lead people and manage resources to create value that no single individual can create alone
> - My decisions affect the well-being of individuals inside and outside my enterprise, today and tomorrow
>
> **Therefore, I promise that:**
> - I will manage my enterprise with loyalty and care, and will not advance my personal interests at the expense of my enterprise or society
> - I will understand and uphold, in letter and spirit, the laws and contracts governing my conduct and that of my enterprise
> - I will refrain from corruption, unfair competition, or business practices harmful to society
> - I will protect the human rights and dignity of all people affected by my enterprise, and I will oppose discrimination and exploitation
> - I will protect the right of future generations to advance their standard of living and enjoy a healthy planet
> - I will report the performance and risks of my enterprise accurately and honestly
> - I will invest in developing myself and others, helping the management profession continue to advance and create sustainable and inclusive prosperity
>
> In exercising my professional duties according to these principles, I recognize that my behavior must set an example of integrity, eliciting trust and esteem from those I serve. I will remain accountable to my peers and to society for my actions and for upholding these standards.
>
> This oath I make freely, and upon my honor.

acknowledges that management is a profession bound by ethical principles.

Leadership

The most concise answer to the question "what defines a leader?" is "someone who has followers." The real question, though, should be framed as follows: "what defines a great leader?" This answer is quite elusive, depending upon the leader, the context, and the constituents.[53]

In business, leaders must first and foremost be effective managers *(Fig. 5.8)*. "The manager is the dynamic, life-giving element in every business. Without leadership, the 'resources of production' remain resources and never become production. In a competitive economy, above all, the quality and performance of its managers determine the success of the business, indeed they determine its survival. For the quality and performance of its managers is the only effective advantage an enterprise in a competitive environment can

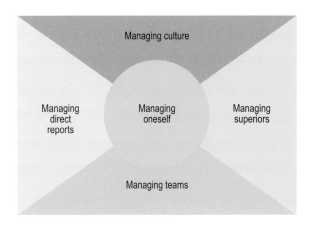

Fig. 5.8 Leadership: integrating the components.

have." So begins *The Practice of Management*, published in 1954 by Peter Drucker, considered the defining, seminal work on modern management theory and practice.[54,55]

Although managers differ from leaders along many parameters, the skill sets of both are complementary and, when combined, provide synergy that enhances the strength of an organization[56–61]:

Managers administer	Leaders innovate
Managers ask how and when	Leaders ask what and why
Managers imitate	Leaders originate
Managers focus on systems	Leaders focus on people
Managers maintain	Leaders develop
Managers rely on control	Leaders rely on trust
Managers accept the status quo	Leaders challenge the status quo
Managers look at the bottom line	Leaders look toward and past the horizon
Managers do things right	Leaders do the right thing
Managers operate	Leaders strategize
But, managers often lead	Leaders often manage

Drucker continues, "To succeed in this new world, we will have to learn, first, who we are. Success in the knowledge economy comes to those who know themselves – their strengths, their values, and how they best perform." Individuals must determine where they belong and what they should contribute. In this age of discontinuity, when information has become as valuable as capital, and communication is critical to the flow of adding value, individuals must manage their own careers, carving out discrete niches, keeping themselves engaged, and knowing when to change course.

For leadership to be effective, the individual uses social influence to gain the support of followers, through positional, personal, and relational power, to accomplish a common goal. Many theories have been proposed to describe exactly how leadership works, but ultimately leaders must be responsible for a number of functions, such as delegation, empowerment, negotiation, conflict resolution, innovation, inspiration, and guiding change. Through a variety of leadership styles – forcing, avoiding, compromising, accommodating, and collaborating – leaders must also learn how to "manage from the middle." Serving as a conduit for transfer of information, knowledge workers today must manage up and down, both their supervisors and their direct reports. Those who can effect change in such an environment are incredibly effective and influential, adding value to the human capital of an organization.

Perhaps the most critical function of a leader is the building of high-functioning, high-performing teams. Teamwork has become increasingly important in business, because of several factors: environmental complexity and pace, the dependence upon internal and external partners, the need for multiple sources of information, and the desire to have varied perspectives and diverse thought. The smartest of us is not as smart as all of us. Teams, however, do not automatically form and function smoothly. An effective leader builds collaborative teams that deliver results by establishing the following characteristics: goal compatibility, trust and commitment, interdependence and accountability, open communication and acceptance of ideas, and converting conflict into creativity. The leader also serves as the team's advocate, gaining support from senior executives, providing the necessary resources to solve the problem, and keeping stakeholders informed. It turns out that being an effective team leader has less to do with technical knowledge and more to do with emotional intelligence and communication skills.[60]

Kouzes and Posner offer a simple but extremely helpful model of leadership in which credibility serves as the foundation for all future success. Having studied hundreds of leaders across many types of disciplines, they provide these recommendations for becoming a great leader: (1) model the way – clarify values and set the example; (2) inspire a shared vision – envision the future and enlist others; (3) challenge the process – search for opportunities, experiment, and take risks; (4) enable others to act – foster collaboration and strengthen others; and (5) encourage the heart – recognize contributions and celebrate the values and victories.[59] This model dispels the myth that "it is lonely at the top," because the goal of leadership should be to bring everyone to the top.

Leadership at the very top – CEOs of large, complex organizations – no doubt requires social influence to achieve goals, but this type of leadership also contains unique challenges that require unique skills, to deliver effective direction and strategy, organizational structure, selection of people, and appropriate incentives. Nohria and Khurana examined 110 newly appointed CEOs from mostly public companies, with median revenue of $3.7 billion.[53] Average age at appointment was 49.7 years, and average time with the company had been 14.1 years. Seventy-five percent of these CEOs had been inside candidates, and 64% had a graduate-level degree. The findings were surprising. Challenges specific to their new role as CEO included broader scope than anticipated, placating the Board of Directors, constraints in power, difficulty obtaining reliable information, maintaining visibility, having to produce within a limited time horizon, and expectations of change by the stakeholders. These CEOs discovered, however, that indirect levers could be quite powerful, by shaping context so that members of the organization could make good decisions, take appropriate action, and advance the mission of the company. Other interesting findings included:

- Time spent working on issues internal to the company: 69%
- Time allocated to core agenda items: 52%
- Time spent in face-to-face communication: 81%
- Time spent with constituents other than direct reports: 42%
- Time spent communicating with groups: 63%.

Based upon these findings, specifically that indirect levers of influence may be more important than direct levers, Porter and Nohria recommend that CEOs pay special attention to allocating their most limited, yet crucial resource: their presence. CEOs – and perhaps all leaders – can manage their presence by setting a clear personal agenda, communicating relentlessly, gathering information continuously, leveraging symbolism, and harnessing the power of a strong management team. Establishing legitimacy, through competence, fairness, results, and integrity, instills confidence in the stakeholders, who are then empowered to do their best.

The ultimate challenge of all leaders is to take their organization from "good to great." Jim Collins identified 11 publicly traded, stable companies that experienced substantial, sustained growth, as defined by financial performance several multiples better than the competitors in their industry.[57] Collins identified specific factors responsible for helping transition from "good to great": focusing on core competencies, forging a culture of discipline, finding the right people to figure out where to go, confronting the brutal facts while maintaining hope, using technology accelerators, and creating momentum from the additive effect of small initiatives. What all of these companies had in common, though, was level 5 leadership: CEOs who had personal humility and professional will. The most effective leaders were not outspoken and charismatic, but rather humble, selfless individuals who displayed fierce resolve in delivering the company's value proposition. Integrity and vision matter; these qualities confer upon the leader the ability to transform an organization from good to great.

Acknowledgments

This work was supported, in part, by the Ethel B and James A Valone Plastic Surgery Research Endowment, at the University of North Carolina – Chapel Hill. The author wishes to thank his wife, Suzanne, for her inspiration, insights, and unending support. She is an angel, the light of my life.

Access the complete reference list online at **http://www.expertconsult.com**

7. Kim C, Mauborgne R. *Blue Ocean Strategy*. Boston, MA: Harvard Business Press; 2005. 238 pages.

   This highly original work describes why thinking outside the box, and creating space outside of the box, is preferable to competing in the red waters of a fixed market.

8. Berman K, Knight J, Case J. *Financial Intelligence: A Manager's Guide to Knowing What the Numbers Really Mean*. Boston, MA: Harvard Business Press; 2006.

   In my opinion, this is the most concise, readable, and applicable text on accounting and finance. I found this book after getting my MBA. If you want to understand the numbers of business, read this book now!

36. Christensen C, Grossman JH, Hwang J. *The Innovator's Prescription: A Disruptive Solution for Healthcare*. NY, NY: McGraw Hill; 2009.

    These experts in innovation approach healthcare as an industry that must be disrupted and rebuilt. Results pending.

37. Porter ME, Teisberg EO. *Redefining Healthcare: Creating Values-Based Competition on Results*. Boston, MA: Harvard Business Press; 2006.

    Healthcare is a business that exists in a highly competitive environment. The reform that we currently need may come from restructuring our competitive models to create new value, for patients and providers.

43. Fisher R, Ury W, Patton B. *Getting to yes: Negotiating agreement without giving in*. 2nd ed. NY, NY: Penguin Books; 1991.

    Almost everything that we accomplish requires negotiation. This work remains the best book on negotiation, decades later.

53. Nohria N, Khurana R. *Handbook of Leadership Theory and Practice*. Boston, MA: Harvard Business Press; 2010.

    This gargantuan "handbook" on leadership covers almost everything you need to know: who leaders are, what they do, and why they matter.

57. Collins J. *Good to Great: Why Some Companies Make the Leap … and Others Don't*. NY, NY: Harper Business; 2001.

    Over-hyped, over-quoted, and over-referenced, this book is not just good, but great.

61. Dr. Seuss. Oh! The Places You'll Go, 1990. Random House, 56 pages.

    Reading level: age 4–8; applicability: all ages. Very few authors match Dr. Seuss' creativity, innovation, and vision. The genius of this book is that the storyteller combines the inevitability of change with the need to embrace it. "You'll be on your way up! / You'll be seeing great sights! / You'll join the high fliers / who soar to high heights." There is fun to be done, indeed.

6

Medico-legal issues in plastic surgery

Neal R. Reisman

SYNOPSIS

- Plastic surgeons will have a significant interaction with attorneys as they care for the injured, abused, and possibly negligently treated.
- Informed consent is a process, not merely a signed document.
- An express warranty may be established by including in the record a photo the patient believes will be the result.
- Fraud and abuse claims have NO statute of limitations and are not covered by liability insurance.
- HIPAA is created to protect patient privacy and covers medical records and photography.
- Agency Law places responsibility for employee negligence when performing work related duties on the employer.
- Divulging patient information in a blog or social media web site is a HIPAA violation.
- It is critical to notify your liability carrier as soon as possible if you receive notice of a lawsuit against you.
- Physicians who basically share an office may each be exposed to liability in caring for patients.
- Patient selection, when proper and appropriate is the best method to avoid a negligence claim against you.

Introduction

Plastic surgeons have many interactions with the legal system. While medicine has many nuances and inferences, the law is steeped in legal doctrine, and the written word. An impression causing considerable concern is that if something is not recorded and written, it never occurred. The practice of medicine is filled with usual actions that may not be specifically documented, leading to a major conflict between medicine and the law. This chapter will focus on the interactions between plastic surgeons in the legal system and also methods of reducing medico-legal risk and improving patient safety. Areas of the law will be presented and its impact on plastic surgical practice will be emphasized.

Interactions with attorneys and the legal system

Plastic surgeons can have a significant interaction with the legal system through their care of patients, which through injury and disease, may lead to legal representation. The work-related injury, auto-accident, animal bites, and domestic abuse often will initiate a lawsuit. The physician will participate in documenting injury, future medical expenses, and commenting on disability and scarring usually through a deposition and occasionally live testimony at trial. There are those who abhor any interaction with attorneys, but realistically many feel it appropriate to participate in the legal system and certainly represent and assist their patient. There are some guidelines and rules to follow. The Health Insurance Portability and Accountability Act (HIPAA) now requires written consent before you can discuss any patient information with anyone outside of the medical treatment area. An attorney acting within ethical guidelines will provide you with an authorization by their client and your patient to discuss the patient's care and treatment. You are prohibited from discussing the patient's information without such authorization. Do not be fooled by legal-appearing or court-initiated papers that seem to override written approval. Ask the attorney for authorization and confirm with your patient as necessary. If a deposition is required, assure that you have proper written authorization.

It has also been suggested if you are hired as an expert, that you seek advanced payment for your time and establish a written agreement that if the deposition is canceled more than 2 weeks from the scheduled date, you will refund the payment. If the deposition is canceled in the second week, then one half of the payment will be refunded, and if it is canceled closer to the scheduled time, the payment will be forfeited. Establish an hourly rate and seek 2 hours in advance. It is also wise to schedule a deposition at the end of the day and not in the middle, which could significantly interfere with patient scheduling.

Legal interactions: depositions and narratives

Much of the correspondence between the plastic surgery practice and an attorney may be in their request for an official narrative outlining care, past treatments, future concerns, and specific questions the attorney might pose. The medical narrative should be factual and list what sources are used and what the report is based on. One should be honest in describing past and future concerns and not be too overreaching or inadequate in description. It is common to cite that your opinions are based on a review of certain documents, discussions with the patient, and the conclusions are based on training and experience. Depending on state law, there is usually a customary fee for such a narrative, which should be collected in advance of any dictation to the record. It is important to cite when references are used, for it is not uncommon to be given certain documents to help influence your opinion. When all these documents are subsequently reviewed, opinions may differ from the original narrative, which can now be explained by specific lists of information reviewed.

Areas of the law

There are many areas of the law that have an impact on plastic surgical practice. Most will include a claim of negligence, which initiates your malpractice insurance. Other claims either strengthen the malpractice claim or add additional claims that are not covered by your malpractice insurance; all are intended to add additional pressure to settling the suit.

Tort law: negligence, malpractice

Tort law is the basic area of the law covering negligence and malpractice. There are four requirements of the negligence action. The first area is a duty to provide care and acts in question. The second is that duty is breached, usually in a sub-standard way. The third requirement is that the breach is directly responsible for whatever damages occur. This is called proximate cause. And the fourth requirement is that there are damages as the result of the prior three requirements. The proof and arguments surrounding these four elements comprise a malpractice claim. Other legal interactions will also involve your testimony establishing these four elements. An example would be a dog bite resulting in a lawsuit. You have surgically repaired the laceration and now must testify that this injury is from the dog and the damages that you describe are directly the result of the bite. While this may appear ridiculous, as these questions are posed to you, you can now see that the three elements of this tort case can be established. The first element of that duty might be to protect people from the dog.

Informed consent

The doctrine of informed consent is a necessary part of both legal interactions and patient care. There are two standards utilized for informed consent. A few states utilize the reasonable "doctor standard", which states that information a reasonable physician thinks is important must be presented to a patient for their informed consent. More commonly, a reasonable "patient standard" is used. The standard states that all information a reasonable patient would want and need to know should be presented as they make their informed choice.

There is much confusion about how much information should be outlined and in what fashion. There are those who believe the informed consent process should be videotaped as there is always a question after-the-fact about what was discussed or presented. This is usually unnecessary as documentation should include the process of information presented, questions asked and answered, and finally an understanding of what the physician can and cannot do. There are many styles of learning and current thinking is to include three styles during the informed consent process. There are visual learners, auditory learners, and kinesthetic learners. The visual learner would want to see a picture, photograph, or some demonstrative example of what is being proposed. The auditory learner wants to listen very carefully to recommendations, the surgical procedure, pre-and postoperative instructions, reasonable expectations, alternatives to care, and inherent risks and complications. The kinesthetic learner is looking for how all of this affects them personally. The goal of informed consent is reaching high levels of understanding, which may be reached by combining all three learning styles throughout the process of informed consent. It is not a signed document itself, but the process of understanding documented by the consent. I believe the surgeon has a responsibility to outline the risks and hazards of the proposed procedure. It is also suggested to develop a team of surgeon, nurse, coordinator, and others to achieve this goal. There are some patients who never reach a complete understanding of the informed consent process and it is recommended that surgery then should not proceed. It is also recommended that multiple visits and discussions be utilized allowing appropriate time for discussions at home, reflection on goals, and adequate questions to be answered before proceeding with a nonemergent procedure.

Privacy law

Privacy law is intended to protect patient information. This includes their medical information, photographs, lab results and correspondence. HIPAA covers many protections for the patient. The practice has an obligation to explain and document the patient's understanding and acceptance. There is a duty to secure their information, and even pursue those who violate such protections. The practice will have an obligation under new "red flag rules" to check identity of patients with their coverage, further protecting the patient against identity theft. The plastic surgery office must be careful when using patient information or photography in a commercial way, such as on a website, advertisement or patient outcome booklet, shown to prospective patients. A breach of privacy is not covered by your malpractice insurance and any judgments as a result of this breach must come from you alone and not your insurance company. It is not unusual to have a claim joined to a negligence claim that patient information was not protected. This often adds to the stress of a lawsuit and may add incentives to settle the claim. If you have patient permission to show such information, a specific written consent for commercial use must be signed by the patient. You can help yourself and your practice by adopting HIPAA rules,[1] identifying a "red flag" office employee who can safeguard patient identity, and being very diligent about obtaining consent forms for treatment, release of information, specific commercial use and photographic consents. Areas of concern are thus social networks and blogs, such as Facebook and Twitter. There is risk of a surgeon or practice describing "a day in the life of a plastic surgeon" on a blog, but that day's patient may recognize him or herself, even though no name is mentioned.

Warranty law

Warranty law involves two specific types of warranty issues; "express warranty" and "implied warranty". You should understand that warranty issues are not covered by your malpractice policy. An express warranty utilizes a demonstrative part of the record to create a guarantee towards a result. This can be accomplished by including a photograph that the patient brings of a result they seek, or it may change created results that are made a permanent part of the business record. It is well accepted among physicians that there are no warranties or guarantees towards a result, since healing can be so specific and usually out of the physician's control. While the visual aids are important in educating the patient about procedures and expectations, the practice should be very careful not to establish a guarantee of a certain result. Patients seemingly have unrealistic expectations, as the media and other factors portray certain social appearances. Utilize all educational tools including imaging to help the patient understand the procedure and the results but make sure you have both a disclaimer and documented discussions concerning realistic expectations.

The implied warranty can be more difficult. This is not based on something added to the chart that is tangible but rather an understanding that the patient presents to you that you must consider and address. Examples might be the fact that 2 weeks after a major surgery, the patient is expecting to travel to a family or business retreat. There is a possibility that the patient reasonably may be able to attend such a function, but are you willing to guarantee they will heal appropriately to do so? This becomes the main issue of these implied warranties. The patient discloses a requirement that they present. You should be careful to disclose and document the many reasons that might interfere with their requirement. Possibly changing the date of surgery or other considerations should be addressed. If nothing is discussed or documented, and the patient misses their major event, it could be judged as your fault and you would be responsible for any financial losses they incur. This is becoming more common, as patients seek and demand quicker recoveries, adding procedures at the last minute, all within a shorter and shorter timeframe. Implied warranties could arise from time issues, financial estimates and costs, future care and treatments, and issues concerning results and expectations. Make sure the entire office team discusses patient comments and interactions because it is not uncommon to have a patient disclose varied demands to a receptionist or coordinator and never mention them to the surgeon. Include a paragraph in your informed consent document as well as your financial agreement that no warranties express or implied are present and that the patient understands and agrees with this.

Product liability

Product liability issues cover the increasing number of products we distribute, utilize or prescribe. There are many areas within product liability that would expose the practice. Those arising from negligent use of a product may have claims falling within their malpractice policy. Other misuse of a product or altering a product by placing on your private-label may elicit additional claims not covered by your malpractice policy. Any device, product, or prescription that is given to a patient should include full instructions, risks, hazards, and alternatives. A key factor in this area is that liability is created in the foreseeable stream of commerce. That is when you give a sample of a skin care product to your patient; it is foreseeable that they might share that with family members and friends. It therefore becomes important to provide good safety instructions as to its use, allergies if any, and concerns of treatment, and document those in the record. When their friend uses the product and has a reaction, you may be responsible, even though you have never seen the friend as a patient. Adding private-labels to the product may hide important ingredients and instructions. You should be careful to maintain such important information. Altering the product, even as simply as putting your name on it, may eliminate the manufacturer's responsibility to defend you for using it appropriately. Be careful and investigate what are FDA approved uses for the product and/or device. Be cautious when industry reps suggest a different use without providing you with written approval. A physician has the ability to prescribe off-label but some precautions are necessary. The three necessary elements for off-label use are: (1) that the product is approved by the FDA for use; (2) that the proposed use is not experimental, and (3) there should be written confirmation of the patient accepting and understanding the off-label use.

Fraud and abuse

Fraud and abuse can definitely turn a winnable malpractice case into one that has to settle or is lost. Fraud is defined as the intent to deceive and abuse is defined as the intent to confuse. There are multiple ways in which fraud and abuse can be a part of a plastic surgery practice. Not only can fraud and abuse have a very negative effect on the outcome of a malpractice case, but in many states, a fraud conviction can both jeopardize your medical license and involve criminal activity. One way of avoiding the perception of fraud is to assure your medical billing and coding conforms to your operative record and treatment notes. It is generally understood that the codes used for billing can be changed as an ongoing process. You must be consistent when adjusting the billing codes to reflect ethically on the procedures and treatments performed. Another area of exposure to fraud is the medical record. Altering a medical record can also expose you to both civil and criminal penalties. There are many ways to disclose an altered record that you should be aware of.

One technique involves an ESDA test, which measures pressure indentations on a page. An ESDA (electrostatic detection apparatus), is a piece of equipment commonly used in questioned document examination, to reveal indented impressions on paper, which may otherwise go unnoticed. It is a nondestructive technique (will not damage the evidence in question), thus allowing further tests to be carried out. It is a sensitive technique, and has been known to detect the presence of fresh fingerprints. When writing is fashioned on a sheet of paper resting upon other pages, the impressions produced are indented onto those below. It is these indentations which are detected using ESDA, thus allowing a match of the original document to its source (such as a ransom note, or a threat to extort) to the offender's notepad.

Where two or more handwriting styles can be found mixed into a single document, and features of one handwriting style depart from the features of the other, ESDA can help reveal the differences in pressures employed between the individuals responsible for the writing samples, otherwise unified on a single exemplar. An indention on the page below can be evaluated to show corrections, additions, and other information about writings. A hospital chart has the most recent chronology on the top with past recordings on the bottom. When the patient is discharged, the chronology is reversed with the earlier dates on top and later dates on the bottom. Consequently, if there is a pressure indentation on a later date's page, that entry was made after the patient was discharged, which is altering a record.

Another method of documenting record alteration is analysis of the inks used. Each ink is dated and it is possible to confirm suspicions by testing the date of a questionable record entry. Records are changed appropriately based on misstatements and incorrect entries. The proper method of correcting a medical record is to draw a thin line through the misstatement allowing readability in addition to making an entry contemporaneous to the correction date and time in the record.

Both entries should be initialed and date and time confirmed.

A further example of potential concern occurs when multiple procedures are performed necessitating two operative reports. The patient has a carpal tunnel and is seeking liposuction. Her insurance through her business is self-insured and the employee health representative is a gossip, so she asks you to not disclose the liposuction to her company. The appropriate course would be to dictate two operative notes and make reference about each within each. The hand surgery operative note would make reference to an additional surgery to be dictated separately. The liposuction operative note would confirm prior hand surgery occurred and this procedure followed. A question of fraud or abuse that is deceiving or confusing, would be to have no reference of both procedures, possibly suggesting the total operative time was for the hand surgery alone.

Fraudulent concealment is yet another type of fraud that can plague the practice. If false or misleading information is given to a patient that they have been relying on, a fraudulent concealment claim may be generated. The significance of this is that it still is fraud, there is no malpractice insurance coverage, and it tolls, or extends the statute of limitations. That means if there is a 2-year statute of limitations after which an allegation claim is not valid, a fraudulent concealment issue can remove the statute's affect and render the claim still valid. An example where this may occur is in a lesion that is excised on the back with frozen sections showing removal of a squamous cell cancer with margins free of disease. The permanent section however, and the final pathology report, show tumor at the superior margin. This information is not disclosed to the patient who develops a recurrence; files a lawsuit 1 year after the statute of limitations would have prohibited such a lawsuit. A fraudulent concealment claim allows the lawsuit to proceed.

"Qui Tam", part of the False Claims Act,[2] has the federal government rewarding fraud whistleblowers. Basically, a disgruntled employee files a false claim lawsuit against you, the employer, citing fraudulent claims, and the US government joins the lawsuit, allowing the whistleblower to collect a percentage of any judgment or settlement. This emphasizes the need for appropriate, ethical billing and coding, as well as eliminating disgruntled employees from the workplace.

Contract law

Contract law should have a limited role in plastic surgical practice. It is suggested to have a work employment contract with independent contractors, physicians in the practice, and aestheticians. Such an agreement would cover work-related requirements, ethical and legal standards, confidential and HIPAA requirements and other safeguards to the workplace. It is not uncommon for an aesthetician, employed by the practice, to quit and take all of the confidential patient information to her next place of employment. This is a direct HIPAA violation and there is a duty to retrieve and protect such information. Having a protective clause in your employment agreement prohibiting such an act is a further safeguard. Some states such as California and Colorado, allow arbitration clauses as part of their state-wide tort reform. It can be attractive to establish such an arbitration required agreement in advance of surgery but it would not be legal to remove the patient's right to bring suit. One can argue further that the more a contract is established with a patient, the more likely a breach of the contract can be claimed when the results do not equal the patient's expectation. Contract law would be more of a problem in descending results and care than tort or negligence law. The patient merely has to prove that the contract was breached and their expected results failed, to collect money, whereas in a negligence action the physician must be proven to have acted negligently, which is usually more difficult to establish. A breach of contract merely requires that a contract be established and a party failed to fulfill their end of the agreement. damages are paid to fulfill the contract. A negligence claim, however, requires a party to be negligent as to a duty of care, and damages are paid to compensate for the negligent act. Develop an office policy manual outlining appropriate and expected care, as well as restricted and prohibited acts. Utilize an updated employment agreement for staff similarly outlining required and prohibited behavior.

We are observing an increase in "contract" personnel, often in the form of aestheticians, or personnel, etc. The practice should be careful here in establishing guidelines for such individuals. This should be covered in an office policy manual. Contract personnel are not employees, and should have their own liability, not falling under agency law. This means you cannot totally manage their daily work, or cover them with insurance like the other employees. The issue of "control" over their work product is an important factor is labeling them as contract personnel or an employee; not the language used in their agreement. You should continually check on their licenses, malpractice history, and quality. You can provide them with the tools to perform their work, but not control their work such as you would with an employee. The issue is whether you will be responsible for their alleged negligence should a claim be made. The independent contractor is liable for their own negligence, while the employee through Agency law is your responsibility.

Regulatory issues within the law

There are many regulatory agencies overseeing a plastic surgical practice. The HIPAA is established to protect patient privacy and medical information. The patient should sign an acknowledgment of their privacy protection, and this is kept in the patient's file. There are obligations to safeguard against identity theft, known as "red flag rules".[3] The practice must identify an individual to record each patient's identity and inspect for procedures, billing, and insurance correspondence, to assure appropriateness throughout. This can include possibly copying the patient's ID, such as a driver's license or passport, including a photograph of the patient, and checking the above documents so they match the practices care and treatment.

The Occupational Safety and Health Administration (OSHA)[4] covers office supplies and equipment assuring safety in the workplace. All supplies should be labeled with appropriate precautions marked, as well as a log of emergency treatment, should an accident occur. The FDA controls manufacturers of devices and products and although does not directly oversee physicians, there are requirements necessary for off-label use. Off-label use involves the nonexperimental use of an approved FDA device or product in a nonapproved fashion. Such use should have a specific consent documenting off-label usage and acknowledging patient acceptance. The practice should be very careful to only purchase FDA approved supplies and avoid the temptation from frequent internet and mail solicitation for supplies that are "just like" those approved. Such a purchase would be illegal and could make the purchaser and practice subject to civil and criminal charges. State medical boards as well as state nursing and other regulatory agencies outline appropriate care in the office. It would behoove the practice to inquire about new standards and guidelines that apply. Ignorance is no excuse for inappropriate behavior. State board actions described who can do what in an office environment and with what degree of supervision. It is very important for all staff and physicians in the practice to understand and comply with these rules. It is unwise to ask an employee to care for a patient when it violates state rules. An example would be an aesthetician who was asked to inject Botox when the state prohibits anyone but a physician, nurse practitioner or physician assistant to perform such an injection. Another example is to have your laser technician treat patients with you, the physician, out of the office and the state requires direct supervision of such treatments by a physician. If there is a bad outcome of such treatment, or anything that would trigger an investigation; it severely damages any defense raised and could void malpractice liability coverage. The practice must be vigilant in keeping-up with the each state board rule and regulation, and decisions that affect a medical practice, nursing practice and others who participate in a plastic surgical endeavor.

Agency law

Agency law encompasses those in the workplace and their interactions. It is a doctrine that the employer is responsible for negligent acts of the employee during the scope of employment or in furtherance of the business. Any negligent acts by an employee are attributable to the employer. It therefore becomes important for the employer to outline what is acceptable and unacceptable behavior, usually in an "office policy manual". Supervision becomes important, as claiming that one was unaware of risky or negligent behavior is no excuse and will not defer blame. You should have been aware of risky or negligent activity. However, violating the office policy manual that clearly defines what should not occur may help protect the practice against a liability claim. The practice should make attempts to avoid harassment in the workplace while developing a good team for communication with patients. Problem employees should be addressed promptly following the office policy manual as to counseling, disciplinary action, and termination. There should be documentation as how these issues are addressed so if and ex-employee challenges their dismissal, the practice can support the decision.

There are many employee issues such as embezzlement, disruptive employees, employees who "steal" patient information, and have disagreements about hours, vacation and daily routines. All should be covered in the manual. Embezzlement can be potentially avoided by having a dual system of checks, say accounts payable and receivables matched against bank statements. One employee responsible for both sides may be a formula for theft. Develop written policy for hours, telephone, smoking, vacation days, and patient interactions that everyone agrees with, and sign a kept copy. Have a confidentiality clause that forbids theft of patient information describing HIPAA violations and the requirement of the practice to pursue those who violate this clause. A common example is the aesthetician employee who leaves for another job and takes all of your patient data to the next job. HIPAA requires you to protect such data and make attempts to retrieve it.

Internet and "blog" defamation law

The internet has dramatically influenced the practice of plastic surgery. Patient's e-mail us from multiple states and seek information about care. It seems that patients share their experiences on many of the social networks. Generally, the internet can bring us additional exposure and patients, while adding significant risk and potential problems. Some basic guidelines concerning e-mails are not to answer out-of-state inquiries with any specificity that the perspective patient can rely on. Failure to follow this guideline may expose you to practicing in the state in which you have no medical license – a crime. This only applies to prospective patients with whom you have not yet entered into a doctor–patient relationship. The practice should develop generic answers concerning basic information to respond to the out-of-state resident. It is usually recommended to include a disclaimer, e.g., if your symptoms and condition worsen you should seek help immediately in your community. The ongoing correspondence between the practice and the patient should be copied and recorded in the patient's chart. Telephone texting should have a similar documentation in the patient's file. Much of ongoing communication today involves internet messaging and it behooves the practice to establish policies which make such communication a necessary part of the medical record.

Many practices wish to enter the social networking community such as Facebook or Twitter, establishing blogs and plastic surgery updates. One has to be very careful not to violate patient confidentiality by disclosing private information about procedures. One has to take care and not even mention what procedure you are doing on a specific day, as friends of the patient's who might believe that day is reserved for their friend, are now aware of the specifics about the procedure, which is a violation. One way around such exposure is to utilize generic procedures that are not specifically tied to a given day and include patient safety issues, general patient instructions, and current trends of plastic surgery. The practice must maintain a high level of professionalism complying with the HIPAA and other privacy issues. The use of photographs for commercial education and internet website usage require a specific written consent acknowledging their use. This is separate from the general photography consent considered as a part of diagnosis and treatment. The same considerations are given for office photographs, books, and references displayed to other patients.

A recent troubling trend is blogging by patients against the practice. A patient may have a perceived problem and begins to write on a website or a blogging page their interpretation of the negative. This is clearly one-sided and may in fact not be accurate. Despite this, the practice cannot respond due to the HIPAA, without a specific written authorization. This one-sided attack poses great concern. There are attempts to control patient's speech through copyright law, but many believe this to be either unethical or restrictive. It may be suggested to develop a nonpatient specific practice blog outlining complications, noncompliance, and high risk procedures, as a balance to these attacks. The first inclination would be to attack the blogger legally, however, First Amendment speech permits such opinions. The attacker who creates a fake website mimicking the practice is confusing and misrepresenting to the public, and may be subject to a lawsuit if you can identify and find them. Another suggestion is to utilize the internet search engines to place their blogging page on the second or third internet page, thereby reducing visibility. This will often lead to "games" where each attempts to manipulate the other, resulting in an extortion demand for money to remove the blog. These actions by disgruntled patients have damaged many practices and threatened more. Attempts are being made to better control blogging sources in an effort to make this more fair and balanced.

Basic actions of a malpractice lawsuit (a guide)

There are many stages of a malpractice lawsuit. They include notice, discovery, pretrial motions, trial, and aftermath. Notice of the intent to file a lawsuit is controlled by each state with a required timely response by the physician or practice. Notice is usually provided certified for by a delivery service and must be taken seriously. As soon as notice is received, secure the medical records, and notify your malpractice carrier. Fight the urge to add to the medical record or alter it in any way. Obtain copies of the medical record from hospital facilities as well as your own office record. It may be wise at this point in time to ask employees as well as yourself to write a recollection of the patient's care and treatment with key words used prior to such writing, on advice of counsel and on anticipation of litigation. A life of a lawsuit may be over five years, and remembrances get lost over time as well as employees leaving. It is therefore suggested that "On advice of counsel", each employee and physician in contact with the plaintiff write what they remember and keep these writings separate from the medical record. Keep these writings privileged and available only as an attorney–client work product, which the other side should not obtain. Keep these recollections separate from the medical record and under lock and key. There will be requests for medical records from the plaintiff and your malpractice carrier. You should have meetings with your carrier's agent and the assigned law firm. Usually notice is not the actual lawsuit but the intent to file a lawsuit should a settlement not be reached. Your carrier, attorney and you will discuss the case in depth evaluating the facts, standards of care, and defensibility. Once a lawsuit is filed, your team will develop an answer within the timed requirement and the process begins. Follow your hospital and facility by-laws, which might require notification of such a lawsuit.

The next stage is discovery. Discovery includes responding to written questions called interrogatories, and depositions to record testimony for future use. This process may take a number of years. You should remember to never respond to any such request without your attorney's input. You will have noticed your deposition well in advance and utilize the time to prepare at length with your attorney. All parts of discovery, such as depositions, require advance written notice of time and place. This allows one to prepare, collect information from the record, and seek consultation with legal counsel before actually providing the deposition. I would recommend you prepare with a senior attorney rather than the most junior associate. While you are quite comfortable in operating room, the attorney is more comfortable taking your deposition. You must prepare by expecting certain questions, disclosing all concerns to your attorney, and understanding the process of the deposition. Once all the facts are gathered, a trial date is scheduled and make sure you block your calendar and devote the appropriate amounts of time for preparation. The pre-trial stage includes demands from each side for exclusions, expert testimony, and other concerns about your case. Frequently, arbitration or mediation is recommended by the court. A failure to reach settlement brings the trial date to schedule. The trial itself may take 1–2 weeks, depending on the complexity of the case and the court's schedule. You should plan on being there every day, following the advice of your counsel, being extremely respectful of the process and visibly concerned and gracious. The defense has two experts, while usually the plaintiff only one. You are your case's best expert and an additional expert is hired. Work with the expert and your attorney to win your case. It may be wise to travel with your attorney when taking the deposition of the plaintiff's expert as you may provide valuable on-site information to assist in their deposition. You will not be reimbursed for such travel, but the value to your case may far exceed your expenses. The last stage may involve appeals and other judicial and legal maneuvering, pending the outcome the trial.

Aesthetic practice liabilities

The aesthetic plastic surgery practice has specific risks inherent to this area. Patient expectations are paramount to achieving desired goals and limiting risk. A disturbing trend is the lack of patient accountability combined with an unrealistic set of goals. It appears that any inherent risk or complication generates a legal concern even if fully disclosed in an informed consent document. More than ever, patient selection and appropriateness of procedure is important. Patients often demand certain procedures and the practice should be careful to assure the proposed procedure is an appropriate fit for this specific patient. Many believe it safer to create a more specific informed consent document listing the additional risks of such patient demands. The problem with this is that you may create additional risks by outlining such in a consent document. The ultimate responsibility of patient acceptance is yours and no document will protect you against an inappropriate decision. Smoking continues to be a major source of liability, as it affects healing as well as scarring and overall recovery. Adding additional risks to the consent is a good example of not avoiding liability where a better choice would have been not to accept the patient. Trends toward more mini procedures, while desirable for the patient, may not achieve the desired goals. Breast surgery continues to be the lead of malpractice claims, with augment mastopexy the majority. Any delay in healing, poor scar, or shape often leads to a lawsuit. Other trends concern where the surgery occurs, as questions arise after lengthy surgery in an outpatient setting. The balance between appropriate procedures, facility and anesthesia versus cost continues to remain an issue.

Cosmetic medicine has assumed a lead in number of procedures performed and must follow general guidelines for risk prevention. Each skin care treatment, toxin injection, and filler injection should have a consent document. Additional concerns about who provides the treatment should follow state law, be it the medical board of the state, nursing board of the state, or skin care aesthetician governing body of the state in question. Establish patient care guidelines and follow them throughout the practice. An example might be: a patient for IPL treatment who, despite being told not to get a suntan, comes in for a treatment with a tan. It is wise not to treat the patient, despite their anger or demands. It is suggested that you see prospective patients at least twice preoperatively allowing time for questions and procedure refinement. Include financial agreement discussions about costs of the proposed procedure as well as future costs, especially if a complication occurs. Develop a team to both address the patient's needs as well as discuss appropriate procedures and treatment plan. Recognize today's social pressures and media influences to present options to the patient that are realistic for the physician to achieve their goals. Try and avoid gimmicks and competing with unrealistic choices to keep the patient in your practice.

Managed care liabilities

The distance between aesthetic surgery and managed care/reconstructive surgery is narrowing. Patients have as many demands and unrealistic expectations for reconstructive surgery as they may exhibit in aesthetic surgery. The practice should present realistic options and procedures to the patient and after a clear understanding and acceptance, proceed with treatment. Additional concerns may arise with managed care coverage, and these should be addressed with the patient with good documentation. Your authorization letter should be honest, complete, and represent the facts and why treatment is medically necessary and appropriate. As you know, it is not uncommon to receive a denial, but remain a patient advocate and appeal as appropriate and necessary. The practice should be careful in not discussing fees with competitors, as this could violate antitrust laws. If you provide service through an emergency room, and not on the patient's managed-care panel, attempt to see the patient postoperatively without charge and document their satisfactory progress.

Liability carrier's issues

The choice of carrier providing your malpractice insurance is a critical one. Inquire as to their financial stability, track record, coverage inclusions, claims made or occurrence type, opportunity for purchase of a tail, and

contractual decisions about settling claims. There is an increase in state board complaints and ask whether if representation is included in their coverage. Check on which law firms represent physicians through the carrier and how responsive they are to the physician. It is not only the premium that should affect your choice. Many physicians have paid a very low premium only to subsequently find out the company is bankrupt and they have no coverage at all. There are carriers common to plastic surgery that are active within our societies as well as understand the nuances of a plastic surgical practice. Determine your limits of coverage based on your practice, hospital privilege, and risks and exposures. The level should be appropriate to maintain hospital and facility privileges, yet not excessive, helping to make you a target. Evaluate companies that encourage discussion about problem patients while not considering each inquiry a claim. Look at their rating and past record in a plastic surgery arena.

Legal issues in physician partnerships

A higher percentage of physicians are associating with partners than in the past. It becomes important to understand the legal implications of such arrangements. There are many types of associations from full partnerships, office-sharing arrangements, limited liability partnerships, single specialty groups, and multi-specialty groups. One considering such an association should seek input from their accountant, attorney, estate financial planner, family, and compliance with their business plan. Spend considerable time with the individual you seek to join or associate with. It is amazing how often what started as a great idea of like minds ends up with exasperation in being so different in goals and style. Make sure you complement each other, and can retain some of your autonomy and individualism, important to a plastic surgery mindset.

Whatever format you choose, establish a communication mechanism, as well as a conflict resolution format. The best of intentions can rapidly go downhill without continuing to "make it work". Have legal counsel work with your business plan to make it equitable and yet protective to both/all parties. All aspects of the arrangement must be considered, especially financial issues, and termination issues. The agreement is a binding contract and must reflect *all* considerations agreed upon. There should be no verbal or handshake addendums that are not included within the pages of the agreement.

Issues to consider and resolve are:

1. Ownership – office, equipment, other investments, and the right to make decisions about new and past expenditures

2. Duration of the agreement, including renewals, termination, and adjustments

3. Duties and expectations of each party should be carefully defined and described

4. Financial allocation of expenses – fixed (rent, employees, leases, personal expenses, e.g., pager, etc.), variables based on collections (medical supplies, office supplies, etc.)

5. Ethics – defining standards (ASPS, ACS, state board, federal), malpractice requirements

6. Termination process – who gets what, staff issues, costs involved, e.g., to copy records, etc.

7. Hold harmless clause: adding staff and physicians decisions, management of office

8. Accounts receivables (always difficult) – possibly a trust established by senior associate keeping funds collected by junior associate, but in name of junior associate, only released when agreement and liabilities are resolved

9. Financial considerations – bonuses, salary, advances, etc.

10. Confidentiality clause

11. Marketing; advertising

12. Ownership of telephone number, name, etc.

13. Restrictive covenants – can and will be enforced as long as "reasonable" as to time, description, and distance. So, a restriction for the practice of medicine for a period of 5 years in the entire city will probably not be enforced. However, a restriction for the practice of plastic surgery for a period of 1 year within 5 miles of every office location currently used probably will be enforceable. Another option is to consider a "liquidated damages clause". This acknowledges the difficulty in enforcing such restrictive covenants, and in advance, arrives at a money settlement (e.g., $150 000) that the leaving doctor must pay the other doctor for breaching restrictive covenants. This amount may be withdrawn from accounts receivables due to the leaving doctor or other arrangements that are enforceable.

There are many more considerations necessary for a successful association, despite the legal structure. The most important is perceived fairness and ongoing attempts to keep it positive, efficient, and responsive to the many changes and challenges affecting the plastic surgery practice.

Patient selection

Patient selection has become the most important part of risk protection as well as practice building. There is a disturbing trend of less accountability in the patient and an approaching "must be perfect" expectation for the practice. Lawsuits have been filed by patients who develop a known inherent risk of a procedure, despite having good documentation about such risks in advance. Lawsuits have been filed even with poor patient compliance, even when discussed in advance of how important this is. It approaches a mindset that any inherent risk or complication must have been the result of "something done wrong".

The key to limiting this is to choose patients you feel you can trust and those for whom you can realistically reach their expectations. It is wise to see the patient more than once pre-treatment to assess their goals and expectations, as well as how they interact with you and your staff. In tough economic times, it is difficult to say "no" to a patient, but "no" is much preferable to defending a malpractice lawsuit. Be realistic in approaching your choices of procedures. Patients are becoming more specific-procedure driven, rather than issue driven. They might come in asking for a facelift, when in fact other choices might be more beneficial and appropriate. We should educate them and understand we are responsible for the choices made, not the patient. We are the experienced physicians and our role is to protect and guide the patient, sometimes protecting them from themselves. It is not appropriate to grant the patient's desires unless they are appropriate and achievable.

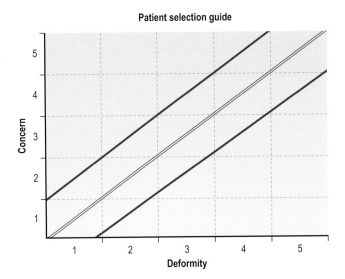

Fig. 6.1 Dr Mark Gorney developed a "GorneyGram" that helps physicians assess realistic goals of the patient.

There is a difficult defense in a malpractice suit when the defendant physician states "the patient wanted this procedure and signed all the informed consent documents indicating greater risk". The physician has the task of approving procedures, not the patient. The patient cannot appropriately consent to an inappropriate procedure. The surgeon should have either rejected accepting the patient or suggested an appropriate procedure. There is distinct added liability from not following this principle.

Dr Mark Gorney developed a "GorneyGram" that helps physicians assess realistic goals of the patient *(Fig. 6.1)*. It balances the deformity present against the affect such a deformity has on the patient. For example, Quasimodo, the hunchback of Notre Dame seeks contour corrective surgery. He states anything you can do to improve things would be great. Quasimodo would be on the bottom right of the Gorneygram; a good place to be. Another patient with a minimal small 1 cm scar on her lower cheek from chickenpox cannot leave the house without covering it to extreme. This patient is in the upper left area of the Gorneygram; a most dangerous place. Likely, nothing you can do will help the patient to her acceptable level. There should be an assessment of all patients to see where they lie on this scale. Some areas will change over time, but it is amazing how accurate this is overall in helping to define which patients are better candidates for your care.

Summary

There are many legal interactions and risks within a plastic surgical practice. One should be aware of these risks and develop standards of protecting the patient, practice, and physician. I would suggest attempting to keep up with the changing medico-legal environment by attending risk courses; explore state medical board rule changes, and the plastic surgery society's panels. Establish relationships within the legal community as your practice grows. This will become a useful resource for questions that arise and have a positive impact on the medical malpractice arena. Understanding all of the above is important, but the most important risk protection is appropriate patient selection. Choose patients you like and feel you can trust, and develop a relationship. Match the chosen procedure with their expectations and follow them as you would want to be seen if you were the patient. Develop a team that reflects your attitude and caring for the patient.

References

1. The Health Insurance Portability and Accountability Act (HIPAA) of 1996 (Public Law 104–191). Privacy and Security Rules.
2. The Federal False Claims Act (31 USC ss. 3729–3733). False Claims.
3. The Fair and Accurate Credit Transactions Act of 2003. Identity Theft Red Flags and Address Discrepancies. *Federal Register*. 72:217 (9 November 2007) p. 63718.
4. *Occupational Safety and Health Administration*. Online. Available at: http://www.osha.gov

Further reading

Federal Food, Drug, and Cosmetic Act (FD&C Act). *Medical device safety business associate contracts. Sample business associate contract provisions.* FR 67 No.157; 2002:53182, 53264.

Gorney M. Ten years' experience in aesthetic surgery malpractice claims. *Aesthet Surg J*. 2001; 21(6):569–571.

Nora PF, ed. *Professional liability/risk management: a manual for surgeons*, ed 2. Chicago, Ill: The Professional Liability Committee, American College of Surgeons; 1997.

An update on subjects in the area of professional liability and risk management that have changed since the 1st edition was published in 1991.

7

Photography in plastic surgery

Brian M. Kinney

SYNOPSIS

- Photography is not only useful, documentary, collaborative, didactic, medical-legal, a research tool and even promotional – it is standard of care and a *sine qua non* for proper practice in plastic surgery.
- Our specialty is highly visual and relies on accurate representation of form, as well as function, to diagnose, plan, treat, evaluate, and track patient surgical outcomes.
- The photographic record contains much more information than can be easily be documented in words, including color, tone, texture, shape, vascularity, bulk, spatial relationships of anatomic structures, global aesthetics, aging, and historical changes, to name only a few.
- The value of images increases with time.
- It is difficult to imagine our specialty without the incredible utility of photography, as it is intrinsic to the visual nature of what we do.

Purpose

The first principle of photography as a medical record is to document the pre- and postoperative condition of the patient, serving as an accompaniment and function analogous to radiography, CT scans, nuclear imaging, or magnetic resonance imaging. Preoperatively, the record is a guide in evaluating the patient's condition, highlighting relationships of the anatomy, and demonstrating aspects of physiologic function for tissues like the nose, eyes, mouth, and hand. Postoperatively, images record changes for patient teaching, self-evaluation for retrospective review, and assessment of results *vis-à-vis* planned outcome. Intraoperative imaging may feature key aspects of the surgical procedure.

Much of plastic surgery rests in an unusual setting in medicine. The core and history is reconstructive in nature, largely born from efforts to rebuild injuries sustained by First World War soldiers. Whether reconstructive or aesthetic, its essence is to restore form and function, and today, a great portion is neither urgent nor critical to immediate health. Instead, much is elective and focused on quality of life, especially in the aesthetic arena. Reviewing photographs with a patient may transform the preoperative planning from an interaction tilted one way from the doctor *to* the patient. Instead, the effort may be collaborative and consultative, an interaction between the doctor *and* the patient.[1,2] Various scenarios can be examined and evaluated with digital imaging, modeling and morphing. Care must be taken when showing potential postoperative results, to avoid the implication of an implied or guaranteed result.[3] One popular software program (Mirror Image)[4] contains an important default disclaimer at the bottom of the morphing screen, "Simulation only: Actual results may differ."

The didactic nature of medical photography cannot be underestimated. Decades ago, sketches were used, followed by black and white photography, color transparencies and film, with the modern progression to digital images in the last 15–20 years. For all practical purposes, analog photography is a niche market and digital imaging reigns supreme. Between the consultation and the operative procedure, planning requires good recall and representation of the anatomy. The image serves to refresh the memory of the surgeon. In addition, it is critical for patients to understand excesses or deficiencies of tissues, issues of symmetry.[3] Features of their anatomy may facilitate or hinder surgical planning, influence choices in surgical approach, affect risks of complications, compromise or augment patient satisfaction. Patient teaching requires proper photographic representation of the preoperative condition and explanation of the changes achieved with surgical intervention. The evolution of a surgical practice can be tracked most easily over a period of years through systematic inspection of imaging of the patients' condition through the course of their diseases or conditions. A particularly common phenomenon is for a patient to not recall how she looked before surgery when critically viewing the postoperative result. Occasionally in reconstructive procedures and more often in aesthetic ones, the patient's psychological "set point" is re-established at the her current condition, and the desire for further enhancement leaves her considering that not enough progress was achieved as a result of the surgery. Photos are indispensable in this setting and may provide reassurance that goals have been reached.

Maintaining proper images and consistently evaluating them postoperatively systematically can only improve awareness of surgical choices and outcomes. Properly preserved analog images may last decades with original fidelity and 100 years of more with mild degradation. Technology has evolved rapidly with digital imaging largely supplanting color film and transparency image storage. Digital images may not last much longer. Challenges in the evolution of technology lead to viewing problems (incompatibilities in hardware), scrambling issues (changes in compression algorithms), inter-relation limitations (expired webpages or hyperlinks), custodial problems (where the data resides), translation issues (how to read old storage with new technology) to name a few. If digital concerns are solved, images could last centuries or more.[5] Building a digital database and engaging in periodic data mining is a core component of self-improvement in clinical care. The advent of digital photography eliminates or ameliorates concerns about lack of space, difficulties in storage like degradation of image quality, the ability to compare past and present results over large series and related issues. However, they are subject to their own vagaries. Old retrieval technologies (floppy disks, CDs , etc.) may be difficult to obtain in the near future. They are subject to catastrophic failure. For example, a scratch on a transparency may slightly degrade the quality of the image, while the same event in a digital image may make it unreadable. Digital images must be backed up and the methodologies rapidly change necessitating continual hardware upgrades. The best storage methods have changed 5–10 times in the last 20 years from floppy disk to magneto-optical disks, magnetic tape back-up, compact discs (CDs), digital video disks (DVDs), DVD RAM disks, USB flash drives, portable hard drives, network attached storage drives, and more recently, "in the cloud," that is to say, online in a remote data storage center on the internet. Much like the evolving standards in business and research regarding storage of e-mail and digital documents for potential legal cases, our *de facto* standards dictate that photographs must be preserved, organized, properly referenced and identified, while easily retrievable.

Informed consent is a key part of medical record-keeping, and photography is essential to proper medical records. Almost every patient understands that photographs are part of the medical records. In fact, many insist on seeing "befores and afters" in their initial consultation, the best time to establish the necessity of accurate documentation. Some patients have a strong need for privacy; however, most surgeons will refuse to operate on a patient who refuses medical photography. Patients understand they have control and options on how their pictures will be used. Some practices allow only internal records in their private chart, others may permit sharing with other patients in consultation without identifying data, and some are comfortable with unrestricted use on the internet, in print, and television advertising. A thorough, detailed consent form specifically for the use of images is necessary for a proper medical legal record.[1] Consent forms from the American Society of Plastic Surgeons are available for member surgeons.[6] An additional method developed in our clinic allows granularity in designating permission of use with check boxes and a grid to supplement the verbiage in the signed form.[7]

Photography's utility as a research and interpretative tool in our field is without question.[8] Comparison of how our journals have progressed from the first decade of the 20th to the 21st century shows that our journals have gone from black and white to color photographs, to online digital images in low and high resolution, to online video. Three-dimensional simulations that allow a "fly through" of the anatomy have been available in recent years. Information density in images is an order of magnitude greater than the written word. With decreasing costs in the digital era, increasing use of imaging improves learning and documentation. In coming years, and perhaps even before the end of the decade, widespread use of artificial intelligence for image processing will likely allow for digital data mining of the image content itself. This would be a major advancement beyond assigning database attributes to digital files like age, preoperative, and postoperative photograph dates, type of procedure, etc. Instead, we may begin to see digital reference to quality of outcomes, conditions of anatomy on validated grading scales, etc. Even now, consumer digital cameras have "face finders," automated red-eye reduction and similar tools. Professional systems have capabilities like automatic pore evaluation on the skin and cell counters for microscopic work. One could imagine many future potential applications like automatic color detection, evaluation of cutaneous vascularity, flap perfusion and others.

Since the mass "migration" to the internet by the general population, the public has turned online to research plastic surgery, compare results, investigate complications, nurture special interest groups and procedures, and engage in promotion and marketing. There are many egregious examples of excess, manipulation and deception; however, there are even more beneficial opportunities for patient education, practice marketing, advocacy and public health outreach. In addition, surgeons often disregard photographic documentation standards of care.[9]

Standards in capturing images

Little has changed for the framing and composition of images since Morello et al.[10] and Zarem[11] and many

Key principles

- The same camera should be used. Changing a digital camera (and therefore the color and white balance) essentially alters the pixel resolution, photonic sensitivity and hardware image processing.
- Shutter speed and aperture must remain the same. Positioning of the patient and photographer in the room should not vary.
- Guide marks on the floor may be required; flash equipment and lighting should not vary.
- Adequate lighting is essential. Shutter speed should be at 1/60 of a second or faster.
- On digital cameras, keep the magnification factor the same that is comparable with a 35 mm camera 100 mm lens for essentially all images except full body views, where a view comparable to a 50 mm lens may be used.
- Focus by moving the camera closer or farther from the patient and note the position of the mechanized zoom lens barrel in relation to the camera body.
- Do not change the white balance and keep it in synch with the lighting used (often flash or fluorescent) on a medium blue background.
- While modern cameras often contain 10 megapixels or more, generally more than five are not required.
- Space for digital images is not an issue in this era of terabyte hard drives, and the speed is easily adequate for rapid access of data.
- More images than will likely be used in a career can be stored on light, portable drives.

before them specified these aspects of photographic standards in plastic surgery. However, many other factors have evolved in the transition to the digital world.[12] Key principles (see above) must be followed.[13] Consistency in results is affected by numerous factors.[8,10,11,13] Facial photographs are taken at the 100 mm lens digital 35 mm camera equivalent, while body images are taken at the 50 mm lens equivalent.[14] Shadows are to be avoided. Colors must be natural. Lighting should be unobtrusive and consistent. Standards must be obeyed.[15,16]

Digital image characteristics

Many variables affect images, and many are in control of the plastic surgeon. Parker et al.[8] have documented four basic ways in which inconsistency is introduced into photography: (1) photographer-based; (2) publisher-based; (3) combined; and (4) patient-based. Category 1 in their scheme includes view (composition), background and zoom and are generally consistent in a variety of journals. Publisher-criteria, size and image labeling are less problematic. Combined criteria, color, brightness, contrast, and resolution vary in published journals. Category (4) criteria: clothing, accessory apparel, make-up, facial expression, and hairstyle, are designated as patient-based, but are substantially under the control of the photographer. A dark colored drape can be used over the shoulders for facial photographs. Accessory apparel should be removed, as make-up, false eyelashes, and similar accoutrements of fashion may interfere. Hairstyle can be mitigated by using standardized hairbands or ties.

Galdino categorizes factors into direct and indirect.[12,13] Direct variables include lens, viewfinder, digital chip, resolution, compression and software algorithms of the camera. Indirect are listed as lighting, metering, depth of field, color temperature of lighting and output method. Both categories are easily controlled by remaining consistent techniques from visit to visit.

Background

Medium blue or 18% gray backgrounds provide the best skin tones and affect exposure least. White or black backgrounds affect exposure on the most commonly used camera setting (matrix metering), so the mode must be changed to spot mode metered on the skin in the center of the field. However, the sharp contrast will not create a natural skin coloring. Standard blue towels used in surgery are close enough to ideal to be used without problems, but green surgical towels are not.

White balance

Accurate, lifelike color reproduction is dependent on neutrality, an equal distribution of colors in the white, gray and black in the image to ensure accuracy of hue. A color balanced image contains all hues in equal proportions of illuminating white light. Unfortunately, different types of reference white points exist in various environments. Indoor scenes lit by incandescent lamps are distinctly different from daylight. Fluorescent lights come in various shades of blue. Operating room lighting is variable in color, temperature, angle, and distance from the patient. The white balance adjustment attempts to capture neutral colors by compensating for these changes. Modern digital cameras have numerous settings like daylight, fluorescent 1 and 2 (or high and low), and auto white balance, among others. The auto white balance setting is often misled by the pulsations of overhead fluorescent lights and may produce variations from image to image. Ideally, a multiple flash system in a dedicated photography room is used to eliminate these problems. Single on-camera flash is inadequate due to shadowing effects in all backgrounds except black.

Composition and positioning

Full face

In the anterior-posterior (AP) view, the superior border of the head must be framed by a small amount of background, about 10% of the vertical height of the image. The inferior border of the image should stop near the level of the suprasternal notch. In the lateral view, the patient's body and head should be facing 90° from the focal plane of the camera. While some cropping of the occipital region is acceptable, in general, lateral views should include the full view. Oblique views should be taken at 45° and, in this view; the tip of the nose should protrude slightly beyond or rest just at the contour of the distal malar eminence. Five standard views are taken, an AP, two oblique and two lateral, right and left for each of the latter two (*Fig. 7.1*). When indicated, the malar eminence may be imaged, generally the bird's eye view is preferred over the worm's eye view, unless a particular feature of anatomy is involved.

Musculature should be relaxed in all photographs unless otherwise specified.

Eyes

The same five image views (anterior, two laterals and oblique views) are part of the basic set for the eyes. Close-up images of the eyes should include a small border of forehead skin above the eyebrows and extend inferiorly to the upper lip at the nasal spine. For the lateral and oblique views, positioning is similar to the views of the head honoring the superior and inferior borders herein. Additional views are essential and include the following at a minimum: (1) closed eye view

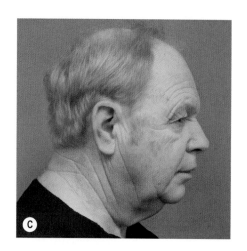

Fig. 7.1 Full face. Five standard views: **(A)** Anterior-posterior; **(B)** right oblique; **(C)** right lateral; **(D)** left oblique; and **(E)** left lateral.

to highlight the superior tarsal sulcus and fold, and (2) upward gaze to highlight inferior orbital fat pockets and the lower lid margin. A squinting view consists of open eyelids with contracting of the superior and inferior orbicularis oculi to feature the impact of muscle action on eyelid shape and function. Occasionally, a view with tightly-closed eyelids to highlight the orbital orbicularis, zygomaticus muscles and others is required for certain surgical procedures *(Fig. 7.2)*.

Glabella

Images of the corrugator muscles may be taken at rest and on full contraction to document wrinkling on the validated four-part glabellar rhytid scale *(Fig. 7.3)*. Full face images are often used; however, the superior border is best cut off at the location (or former location in baldness) of the anterior hairline and the inferior border is often positioned midway between the radix and the tip of the nose on a horizontal line through the lower margin of the malar eminence. The closer view provides more detail of pore size, eyebrow position and skin texture. Oblique and lateral views are generally not necessary.

Nose

The superior margin of the nasal view is essentially the same as for the eyes – just above the eyebrows. However, the inferior margin is at the upper lip or between the closed lips. In addition to the five basic views, worm's eye view or chin-up view is included *(Fig. 7.4)*. The superior and inferior borders are the anterior scalp line and the mentum, respectively. When muscular release at the dorsum or nasal spine is contemplated, dynamic pictures of contraction should be included.

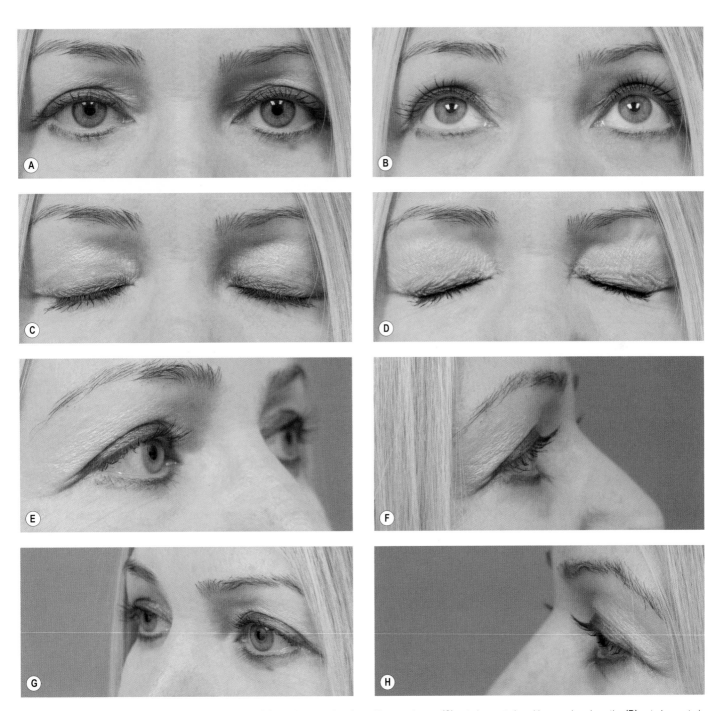

Fig. 7.2 Eyes. Standard views: **(A)** Anterior-posterior view; **(B)** anterior-posterior view with upward gaze; **(C)** anterior-posterior with eyes closed gently; **(D)** anterior-posterior with eyes closed tightly; **(E)** right oblique in forward gaze; **(F)** right lateral in forward gaze; **(G)** left oblique in forward gaze; and **(H)** left lateral in forward gaze.

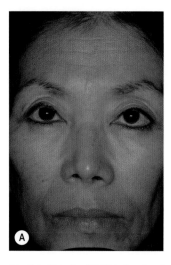 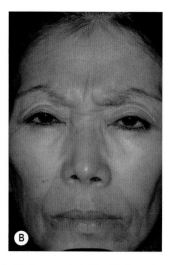 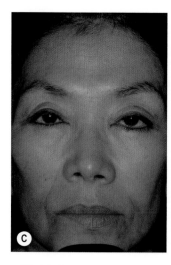 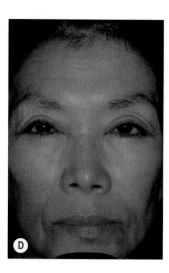

Fig. 7.3 Glabella. **(A)** Glabella relaxed; **(B)** glabella contracted; **(C)** glabella post relaxed; **(D)** glabella post contracted.

Lips, nasolabial folds, and mentum

The superior border is on a line just above the nasal tip and includes the alar base, while the inferior border allows a small amount of background to show below the chin *(Fig. 7.5)*. The lips should be slightly parted to detect features in the mucosal surfaces near the intersection of the upper and lower borders. When injections into vertical lip lines are performed, the pursed lip or orbicularis-contracted view is added. Additional views may include contraction of the mentum when toxins or soft tissue fillers are part of the therapeutic intervention.

Dental occlusal views

When intraoral or two-jaw surgery is considered, dental occlusal views are required and cheek retractors must be utilized.

Ears

Adequate visualization of the ears requires that the hair must be out of the way. Anterior and posterior views should include the full head and supplemental mid-range views should extend from the upper neck to above the occipital ridge to bring the ear more fully into the image. Lateral images should include close-up composition with the vertical height roughly twice the height of the ear itself.

Chest and breast

Variations in the configuration of the trunk dictate that the principle of bordering the image based on regional anatomy is critical in these images *(Fig. 7.6)*. Vertical borders should range from above the suprasternal notch in the lower third of the neck to below the mid-costal margins. There are three basic variations in arm positioning on the lateral view of the breast: (1) arms at side; (2) arms on hips; and (3) arms behind the lower back. The most common in the author's experience, is the former. Oblique views may be taken in positions one and two above, while occasionally AP views are taken with arms taken above the head.

Lower trunk, abdomen, and buttocks

The five standard views are supplemented with a posterior view *(Figs 7.7, 7.8)*. When the buttocks are the focus of the image, no panties are used. It is essential to use disposable, blue paper photographic panties to standardize the clothing, color and white balance. Almost invariably otherwise, a patient would arrive on a subsequent visit with different color, contour and texture of undergarments. In addition, sometimes patients will arrive with a distracting, different dark-light tan line in summer climes. Legs should be slightly apart to allow viewing of the groin against the light background.

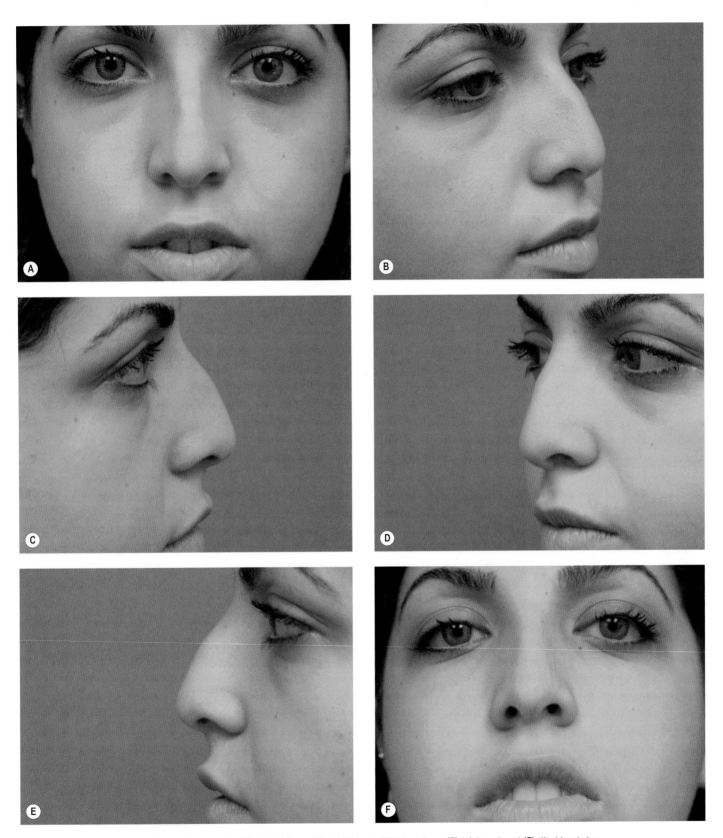

Fig. 7.4 Nose. Standard views: **(A)** anterior-posterior; **(B)** right oblique; **(C)** right lateral; **(D)** left oblique; **(E)** left lateral; and **(F)** tilted head view.

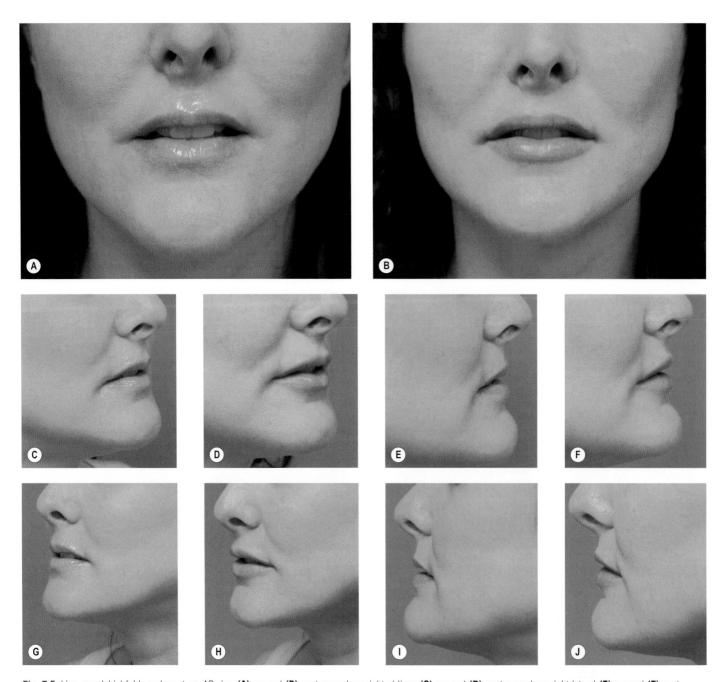

Fig. 7.5 Lips, nasolabial folds and mentum. AP view **(A)** pre and **(B)** post-procedure; right oblique **(C)** pre and **(D)** post procedure; right lateral **(E)** pre and **(F)** post procedure; left oblique **(G)** pre and **(H)** post procedure; left lateral **(I)** pre and **(J)** post procedure.

Lower extremity

The five standard views should also be supplemented by a posterior view *(Fig. 7.9)*. For a full view, the upper margin should be found at the level of the umbilicus and the lower margin inferior to the toes or heel depending on the view. For the half upper or lower view, the lower or upper margin respectively should be just below the knee at the level of the inferior popliteal fossa or just above the patella. The photographic background must extend onto the floor, all the way out of the frame for the lower view.

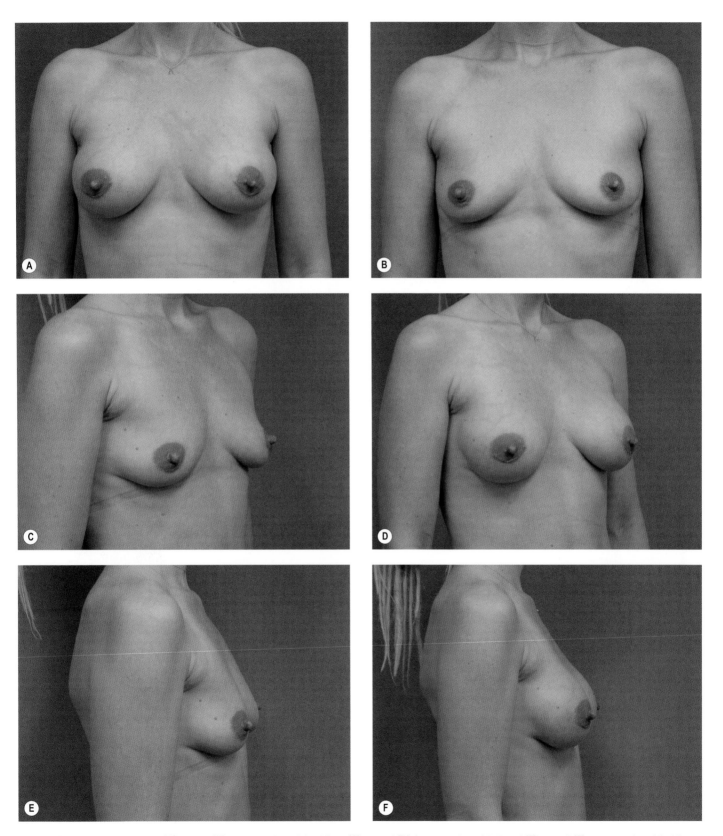

Fig. 7.6 Chest and breast. AP view **(A)** pre and **(B)** post-procedure; right oblique **(C)** pre and **(D)** post procedure; right lateral **(E)** pre and **(F)** post procedure; left oblique **(G)** pre and **(H)** post procedure; left lateral **(I)** pre and **(J)** post procedure.

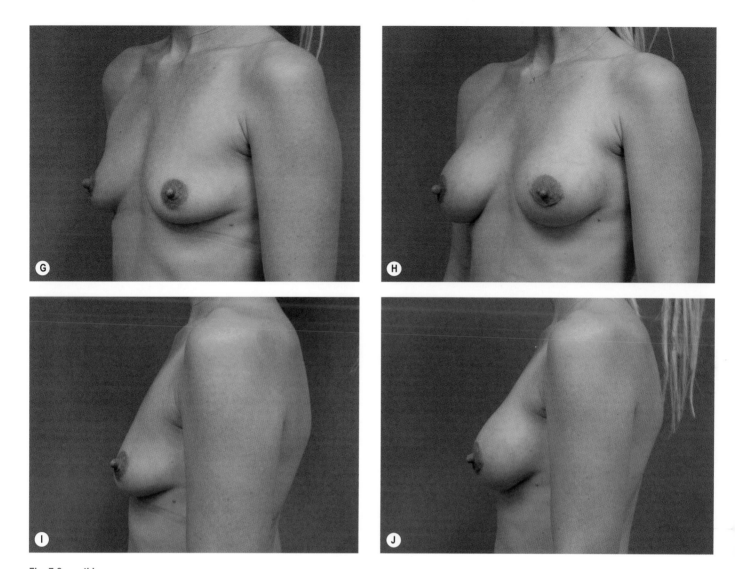

Fig. 7.6, cont'd

Hands and feet

A full dorsal and volar view is required. In some patients, oblique views are required as well. Dynamic views in flexion and extension are an essential component of the complete medical record *(Fig. 7.10)*.

Specialty views

Other regions of anatomy follow the same principles: (1) clear margins of background or adjacent anatomy;

(2) AP, lateral and oblique views; (3) dynamic views as indicated; and (4) macro-views when required to demonstrate features of anatomy.

In the hospital and operating room

The compact digital camera has largely supplanted the 35 mm film camera in the emergency department and on the go. Results are excellent and convenience is high. However, when expense is not an issue, many surgeons prefer SLR-like full-frame (35 mm diagonal) digital

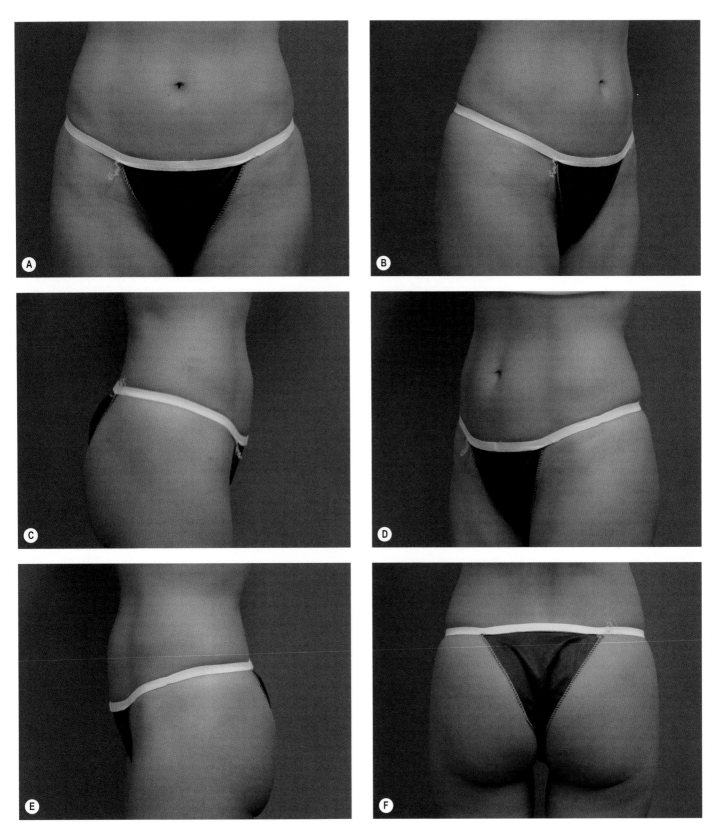

Fig. 7.7 Lower trunk, abdomen and buttocks. Standard views: **(A)** anterior-posterior; **(B)** right oblique; **(C)** right lateral; **(D)** left oblique; **(E)** left lateral; and **(F)** posterior view.

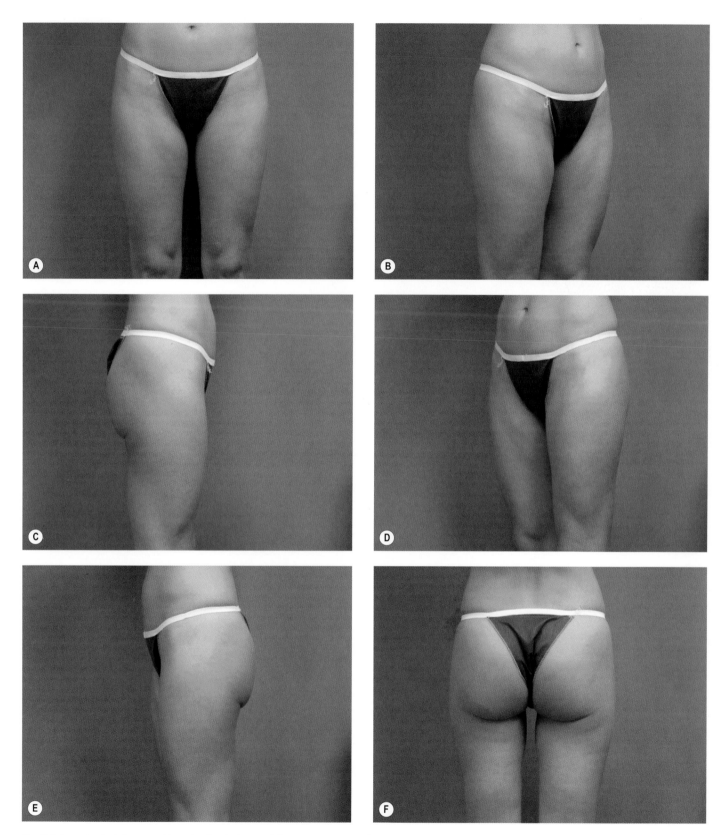

Fig. 7.8 Lower trunk, abdomen and buttocks. Standard views: **(A)** anterior-posterior; **(B)** right oblique; **(C)** right lateral; **(D)** left oblique; **(E)** left lateral; and **(F)** posterior view.

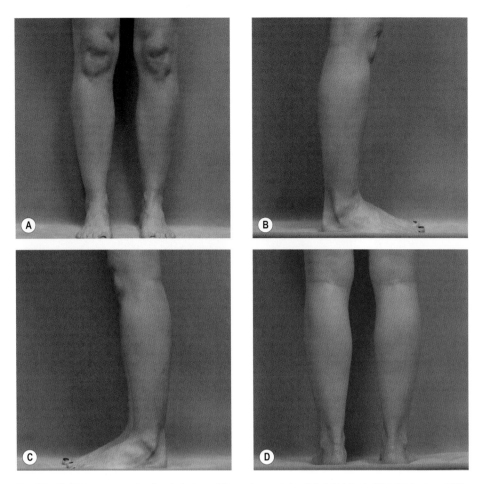

Fig. 7.9 (A–D) Lower extremity. Standard views: **(A)** anterior-posterior; **(B)** right lateral; **(C)** left lateral; and **(D)** posterior view.

cameras in the operating room. Operating room lights vary from hospital to hospital and even from room to room. On-camera hot shoe flashes for large format cameras are of much higher quality than built-ins for compact cameras. This allows for consistency in color balance, as ambient light does not provide the illumination for the exposure. Standardized use of auto white balance without a flash in a compact camera is a close second. Macro-mode or close-up focusing may put sterility of the operative field at risk and is more problematic. Automatic exposure reliably creates an image with proper lighting in the operating room.

The need for proper composition of the picture remains in the operative setting or emergency department and may be overlooked amidst other priorities. The framing principles already discussed should be followed to the extent allowed by the sterile field and drapes. Anatomic landmarks should be included at the borders of the frame. Shiny instruments, stained surgical drapes, gauze or glare from overhead lights must be eliminated or covered. Often the lighting is harsh and must be removed from the field to prevent oversaturation of the image.

Archiving and image management

Cameras

There are many excellent resources in the literature for discussions on film photography. The era of light

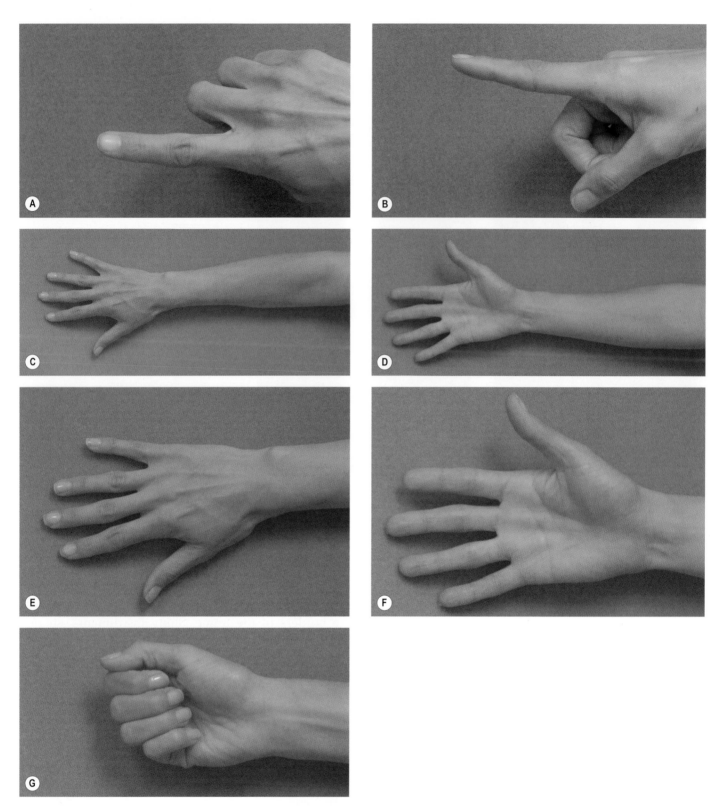

Fig. 7.10 (A–G) Hands.

sensitive silver halides suspended in a gelatinous emulsion in film photography is largely over and resides in niche markets, essentially outside the field of plastic surgery.[17] Film or analog photography had an amazing 160-year run from the 1840s, before being supplanted by digital, around the new millennium.[18] Because the overwhelming majority of cameras in use today are digital, we will concentrate here on digital. Like a film, digital imagers generally consist of red, green, and blue filters. Film has continuous stacked emulsions or layered films of colors, while digital uses variations on a checkerboard pattern of cells to filter light. In the Bayer pattern, most commonly found in digital cameras, every other pixel is green, while one in four is either red or blue. A few cameras like those from Canon use a complementary metal oxide semiconductor (CMOS) sensor, but most use charged couple devices (CCDs). In the former, each element contains its own transistor and circuitry providing for independent reading of data. When photons strike a CCD, charges propagate down each row of the checkerboard pattern and this limits the speed with which they can propagate. Newer CCDs have triple-stacked sensors (red, green, and blue, RGB) that lower resolution, but increase sensitivity. Well-designed cameras of either type will capture excellent images.

Choosing a digital camera can be overwhelming due to the myriad of choices available. Even a simple point and shoot can take good pictures due to unrelenting commercial competition among manufacturers and the decreasing cost of components. However, the plastic surgeon will require something more capable, albeit a large format, 35 mm size digital camera is not truly essential for adequate pre- and postoperative photographs in the proper setting. Cell phone cameras are inadequate, as are entry-level compact devices. Lifestyle and fashion cameras are not suitable.

There were "resolution wars" in marketing cameras 10 years ago, but gladly those are over. Resolution is most often used to describe how many pixels are in the array. Minimum sizes now are >3000 × 2000 or 6 megapixels. Actually, most cameras are capable of ≥10. The number of pixels sets the upper limit of image quality, but not the lower limit. Another more important gauge of resolution is how sharply an image resolves fine detail, often depicted by extremely small, narrow lines. This is a more functional definition, though less commonly used.

The enthusiast compact category is generally adequate for plastic surgeons to use on a daily basis, if the additional expense of a prosumer or professional digital camera is not within the budget. Numerous features are available: high pixel count, an advanced hardware algorithm for interpreting the light image that strikes the chips, zoom and video capability are highly valued. Perhaps most important is the quality of the glass and the design of the optics in the lens itself. Features such as rapid shutter speed, geotagging, or very large aperture are not so critical in the patient-care setting. However, enthusiast cameras are capable of capturing images almost indistinguishable from higher end models in a controlled setting such as the plastic surgeon's photographic room or the operating theater. Prosumer cameras have many of the features of a digital single lens reflex (dSLR), but generally without interchangeable lenses, a staple of the professional model. In essence, a plastic surgeon only requires a 50 mm equivalent and a 100 mm equivalent lens setting. Advanced computer design of camera zoom lenses has allowed for excellent shooting characteristics with compact cameras in both the 50 and 100 mm range, with minimal degradation of image quality. In other words, it is possible to get along with an enthusiast or prosumer camera in most situations.

Professional dSLRs are larger, heavier, machined to precise specifications, resistant to moisture, impact and sturdy with full-frame 36 × 24 mm sensors that can potentially capture up to 25 megapixels in one image. Medium format cameras with pixel counts up to 60 million are rarely found or required in our specialty. While many professional cameras do not have video capability, almost all enthusiast cameras allow for recording video of 30 s to 1 min. This is entirely adequate for documenting repeated key steps in an operative procedure, while not reaching the standards of a cinematographer.

Format

Storage

Digital memory cards come in a variety of types. The most common are compact flash, which are large, sturdy, and found in larger or pro models. They are capable of transferring data at up to 30 Mb/s for high resolution video, or HDTV. Resolution may be 720p, horizontal lines scanned progressively without interlacing, 1080i or 1080p, which contains 1920 pixels wide by 1080 pixels high, either interlaced (i) or progressively (p) scanned. Progressive scanning at this resolution is not yet commonly found, nor required for most situations without a professional photographer.

Secure digitals come in a regular or high capacity format (SD or SDHC). Recently, 64 GB and even 128 GB models are available with speed adequate to capture video at high resolution. Micro-SD cards are generally relegated to cell phone cameras and data storage.

Memory card readers are widely available and very inexpensive, like memory cards. Data can be uploaded to a computer via a cable attached to the camera from the computer, usually USB. However, it is quite common to remove the card, insert a spare into the camera and read the data from a card reader.

With the advent of the multi-terabyte hard drive, both desktop and portable, storage of thousands or tens of thousands of pictures is no longer an issue. Maintaining a disciplined, regular back-up program, however, is as essential as any record-keeping in the practice. At least two copies should be maintained onsite, and another offsite at a remote location to obviate water, fire, or earthquake damage.

File formats

There are dozens of data structures or architecture, also known as file formats. We will only concentrate on a couple of the most commonly used: tiff, jpg (or jpeg for joint photographic experts group), Photoshop, gif and raw. Fortunately, almost any software will convert one still image type to another. However, it is important to understand their advantages and disadvantages.

TIFF is best used for print reproduction because it is a bit-mapped (like a printer) or raster Tag Image File Format. It supports 24-bit color depth per pixel, dimensions and color look-up tables "tagged" to the header of the data file. The way the tag specification is written gives rise to various version of a TIFF file. Lossless compression with the LZW algorithm makes compression safe for data quality.

JPEG (jpg) is perhaps the most common file type and it is "lossy." Compression can be chosen from a 12-part scale from none to as much as 90%, while data quality diminishes accordingly. For quick exchange of images via email this is ideal. Minimal compression almost retains original image fidelity. There is almost no software that cannot easily read this format and with wide latitude in software storage parameters there is great flexibility.

Photoshop is a proprietary format of Adobe Systems Corporation, San Jose, CA, but is so commonly used as to almost be a standard. Color management, 48-bit color and layers are supported. The file suffix is ".psd."

Raw format varies from camera to camera because it is dependent on the hardware interface with the light capturing chip (CCD or CMOS) inside the camera. It is the truest image as there is no white balance, color processing, compression, sharpening, or other manipulation of the data. Because the data is unprocessed, capture rates can be much faster with higher throughput.

Video, unfortunately, is plagued by numerous incompatible standards. Even file formats with identical suffixes may be unreadable by other software or hardware, e.g., mp3 or mp4 (motion picture experts group 3 or 4) are often not readable unless the original software used to create the file is available. A software codec (coder-decoder) is required and often is not cross-platform for PC or Mac. That rigorous discussion awaits another setting. Apple ".mov" (QuickTime) movies are a very popular format. So is Windows ".wmv" (Microsoft Windows Media Video). Others advanced file types can be used. On the web, Adobe ".flv" (Adobe Flash Video) is very commonly used, especially in the YouTube video setting, where millions of videos are published.

Image attributes, metadata, and retrieval

As the images are safely transferred to storage media, critical new information must be attached to the data. Up-to-date cameras use a format called EXIF for recording camera type, lens, date, time, shutter, aperture, and many other items. Even more critical for plastic surgery is information like, patient age, sex and weight, ICD9 diagnostic codes, CPT operative codes, type of implant used, pre- or postoperative status, date of original surgery and other critical pieces of medical data. These are proprietary to individual software packages and make changing platforms difficult after even a few months or a year of use. Data fields are usually stored in custom Microsoft Access or SQL Server format. What once was a demanding and difficult exercise is now made transparent and easy by improved software interface designs.

There are several companies in our specialty (NexTech, Tampa, FL; Canfield Imaging Systems, Fairfield, NJ; Crisalix, Lausanne, Switzerland) that specialize in image database creation and storage, simulation of surgical results and patient management.

The Health Insurance Portability and Accountability Act of 1996 (PL 104–91) was enacted in 1996, which resulted in a major increased emphasis on patient privacy among other concerns. In Title II, one of the five rules is known as the Privacy Rule, effectively enacted April 14, 2003, before the main Act. One of its many functions is to regulate the use and disclosure of Protected Health Information (PHI). The broad interpretation of this law includes any part of the medical record. The American Recovery and Reinvestment Act of 2009 extended Privacy and Security Provision of HIPAA to business associates of covered entities and provides for stiff civil and criminal penalties for violation. Additional provisions cover electronic health records (EHR) and compel compliance no later than January 1, 2013. Loss or dissemination of digital images can be much more serious than film photographs, with the risk of electronic data "going viral" over the internet to thousands, or even millions of people.

Digital image processing

Measurement and analysis

Orthognathic surgery has rested on the principles of image measurement and analysis since the early days of film photography. Measurements were made directly on photographs or transparencies and taken to the operating room to guide surgical osteotomies. Now these measurements can be made directly on the digital image. A well-developed model of cleft lip repair has been incorporated into the training program for a large charitable organization prior to surgeons going overseas on mission work.

Identifying and highlighting anatomic landmarks for the medical record in breast augmentation surgery increasingly has become a part of the preoperative consultation.[19] It is the first step in building a predictive model for planning pocket dissection, choosing implant size, evaluating postoperative size and may lead over time to reduced rates of reoperation.

Planning and simulation

The term surgical simulation has been broadly defined to include anything from computer-assisted tutorials to interactive learning to engaging in mock surgery with haptic feedback and complete with unexpected complications.[20] Surgical planning is more easily achievable, requires less computer power and complexity in programming. Organized medicine was challenged by the Institute of Medicine Report, *To Err Is Human: Building a Safer Health System* in 2000.[21] It has been estimated that 44 000 deaths occur yearly, the seventh leading cause of death, due to medical errors. Many of these occurred during surgery, as a result of surgical planning or postoperative care.

Computer-based surgical planning is generally available in plastic surgery from commercial companies (NexTech, Canfield, and Crisalix); however, the more elaborate mannequin-based systems are rare.

The future

Three-dimensional imaging

3D technology began almost at the same time as photography itself, when David Brewster invented the Stereoscope in 1844. It was refined by Louis Jules Duboscq when he took a picture of Queen Victoria and displayed it at the Great Exhibition in 1851, where it became very well known throughout the world. Stereoscopic cameras started being more common tools, even for personal use, by the Second World War.

Several commercial techniques for 3D visualization in movies were later developed, from "Natural Vision" in the 1950s; "Space-vision" in the 1960s; "Stereovision" in the 1970s; polarized glasses in the 1980s, and later in the 1990s using IMAX 3D technology, until the last boom of 3D movies culminating in the release of the movie Avatar in 2010.

The X-ray, discovered by Dr Roentgen in 1895, caused a sensation in the medical world as it enabled doctors to see through the human body without surgery. The next breakthrough improvement in medical imaging occurred in 1972 with the development of 3D computed tomography (CT), which employs tomography created by computer processing. 3D imaging technology greatly increases surgical precision. Previously, doctors had to imagine the 3D image of the human body while looking at plane delineations or 2D pictures. Thanks to volumetric visualization of the images, doctors can now visualize internal structures and enhance diagnosis.

In conventional medical procedures, diagnosis, treatment, and outcome are typically judged by objective criteria. The patient's subjective feelings are of relevance, but of a secondary nature. In plastic surgery, on the other hand, the healthcare model is often one of wellness and enhancement, the patient is not ill or diseased and therefore the diagnosis, treatment, and outcome may be dominated by the patient's subjective assessment of an elective surgical procedure. Consequently, even the most technically perfect surgical procedure can lead to patient dissatisfaction, should the result not meet aesthetic and psychological expectations. Failure to meet these expectations can lead to the need for re-operation, increased medico-legal risk and additional costs directly to the surgeon. Furthermore, the market dynamics of cosmetic surgery are strongly driven by patient referrals, which again are based upon patient satisfaction. In breast augmentation surgery, for example, it can be advantageous that the patient is collaboratively involved in the process of implant selection, supported by the surgical team, and that the patient 'buys-in' to the selection process with enthusiasm, confidence and conviction. One of the major reasons to undergo plastic surgery is to change the external appearance of the patient, a central question that all patients have in common is "how should I look like after my operation?" One way to answer this is through 3D imaging.[22]

Today, 3D physics-based finite element analysis (FEA) technology can provide patients with a simulated view of their anatomy in a postoperative condition. While other methods to show the patient a probable outcome, such as: specials bras and sizers; computer slide shows with various before/after photographs of previous patients; collecting photographs from magazines, and morphing software based on photographs, all have limitations. All these methods require realistic imagination by the patient. State of the art technology allows patients to see themselves from varying angles in 3D before the operation, increasing communication with the surgeon by interacting collaboratively with the image, and simulating the outcome of the surgical procedure.

Techniques for 3D modeling include, on one hand, expensive, space-limited and obsolescence sensitive hardware scanners, and on the other hand, those based on the physical reconstruction of the body from 2D photographs. The former requires a large upfront investment amortized over time. The latter method functions on a pay-as-you-go basis and takes advantage of ease of use, simplicity, and minimal interference with the way the surgeon performs a consultation. When no special hardware is required, photographs are coupled with anatomical measures and physiologically-based data processing and simulation. Whatever technique employed, 3D and virtual reality is the future.[23–26]

Video

Much of what has been said of 3D technology can be said of video medical records, other than the simulation aspects. Motion picture film has been a part of medicine for decades for surgical education, while digital video as a part of a medical record is a very recent and evolving innovation, not yet a standard of care. Almost every modern digital camera has the capability of capturing video in short duration clips. However, the lenses are not specifically designed for professional quality where heavy, expensive equipment is required and far more computer power and capability is mandatory. Creation and routine use of detailed video is beyond the scope of most busy plastic surgery practices, except in special circumstances with outside consultants. It obligates a commitment to production values, editing, composition, and a host of skills residing in the professional medical videographer. Short videos (under 1 min) can document features like range of motion, bulk strength and tone, elasticity and even aesthetic contours in motion. However, long compositions require expert direction, videography and editing. The future will certainly increasingly incorporate digital video in the practice of plastic surgery.

Access the complete references list online at **http://www.expertconsult.com**

1. Reed ME, Feingold SG. Ethical consideration. In: Nelson GD, Krause JL, eds. *Clinical photography in plastic surgery*. Boston: Little, Brown; 1988:129–153.

3. Chávez AE, Dagum P, Koch RJ, et al. Legal issues of computer imaging in plastic surgery: a primer. *Plast Reconstr Surg*. 1997;100(6):1601–1608.

   Medical simulation adds a new dimension to patient consultation. While potential legal concerns accompany this technology (such as the potential to enter into an "implied contract"), the savvy practitioner can responsibly employ this technology and minimize legal risk.

4. Mirror Image Software Suite, Canfield Imaging Systems, 253 Passaic Avenue, Fairfield, NJ 07004–02524 USA.

   "Mirror" is a powerful and user-friendly clinical imaging suite. Capable of tasks from image manipulation to advanced database functionality.

8. Parker WL, Czerwinski M, Sinno H, et al. Objective interpretation of surgical outcomes: is there a need for standardizing digital images in the plastic surgery literature? *Plast Reconstr Surg*. 2007;120(5):1419–1423.

11. Zarem HA. Standards of Photography. *Plast Reconstr Surg*. 1984;74:137–144.

13. Galdino GM, Vogel JE, Vander Kolk CA. Standardizing digital photography: it's not all in the eye of the beholder. *Plast Reconstr Surg*. 2001;108(5):1334–1344.

The intricacies of selecting a digital camera ideal for patient photography are considered.

14. DiBernardo BE, Adams RL, Krause J, et al. Photographic standards in plastic surgery. *Plast Reconstr Surg*. 1998; 102(2):559–568.

15. Plastic Surgery Educational Foundation/Clinical Photography Committee. *Photographic standards in plastic surgery*. Arlington Heights: Plastic Surgery Educational Foundation, Clinical Photography Committee; 1991.

   A very practical guide to achieving high quality, standardized patient photographs is presented. A compact PDF is available for download.

23. Smith DM, Oliker A, Carter CR, et al. A virtual reality atlas of craniofacial anatomy. *Plast Reconstr Surg*. 2007;120(6):1641–1646.

   An interactive 3D computer graphics model of craniofacial anatomy is described. Methods of creation and future applications are discussed.

26. Smith DM, Aston SJ, Cutting CB, et al. Applications of virtual reality in aesthetic surgery. *Plast Reconstr Surg*. 2005;116(3):898–906.

8

Patient safety in plastic surgery

Bruce Halperin

SYNOPSIS

- Modern medicine has greatly reduced the risk of surgery.
- Identifying which patients are at greatest risk for surgery starts the risk reduction process.
- Identification of medical factors leading to complications helps prevent untoward outcomes.
- Specialized care for the liposuction patient.
- Specialized care for the patient having facial aesthetic surgery.
- Avoiding fire in the operating room.
- Protocol-based systems for risk reduction.
- Reducing patient risk through optimal patient care.
- Do it better, do it safer.

The risk of having surgery

The decision to perform surgery to correct a defect or medical condition begins a cascade of decision-making and, by necessity, a series of compromises. It is the underlying desire of the medical profession to prolong and enhance the lives of patients who seek attention. Since the beginning of the practice of medicine it has been understood that undesired outcomes may occur. The acceptance by the patient of undesired outcome has changed over the course of medical history. As medical science has progressed, the expectations of patients and the medical profession have risen. As medical science understands ever-increasing levels of human biologic complexity, the expected outcome from medical intervention may change yet again. It is not yet clear to the practicing physician or public as to the fundamental cause of undesired medical outcomes.

It is clear that many of the undesired outcomes we now see are a result of failure to implement knowledge we already possess. We must further question whether it is our healthcare delivery system that is in fact responsible for many of the undesired outcomes that our patients face. When we decide to perform a surgical procedure we accept the risk of undesired outcome. Using the knowledge of scientific studies we select what we believe to be the "best" path to resolution of the patient's condition. The question in our minds must always be: What is the "best" pathway in this particular surgical case?

Prior to the introduction of anesthesia the surgical experience was a decidedly unpleasant one for the patient. The success of a surgical procedure (read: survival) was often based on the speed at which the procedure was accomplished. If nothing else, the introduction of anesthetic techniques brought the ability of the surgical team to take more time in accomplishing the procedure. The introduction of an additional medical intervention (anesthesia) on the patient brought additional undesired effects and perioperative death.[1,2] Since the introduction of general and regional anesthesia as part of normal surgical practice, surgical and anesthetic complication rates have been analyzed using a variety of clinical criteria. It is this wide variety of criteria that has led to confusion in the medical literature and in the mind of practicing clinicians of the actual risk attributable to anesthesia care during a surgical intervention. Do we consider in our complication rate only events that happened during the actual surgical procedure? Do we only consider events attributed solely to providing anesthesia or do we consider the contribution of surgery to the untoward outcome?[3] The time course for evaluation of surgical and anesthetic complications remains controversial and almost certainly is related to the nature of the surgical procedure and type of anesthesia, if any, that was used during surgery. The wide variety of time indices that are used in the medical literature for the study of perioperative complications makes comparison of studies very difficult. Definitions of the time period for study of perioperative mortality range from 48 hours, as defined by the Joint Commission on Accreditation of Healthcare Organizations, to 30 days, as defined by the American College of Surgeons. Similarly, the inability to compare clinical studies adds to the confusion in defining clinical risk to the patient from a given surgical or anesthetic technique. For anesthetic risk we need to consider not only cases where anesthesia is deemed the sole cause of complication and mortality but also cases where anesthesia is a significant contributing factor of complications and mortality.

It remains extremely difficult, even with review of the extensive body of medical literature, to predict accurately the risk for any given patient who is about to undergo any given surgical procedure. We can safely claim that complications from anesthesia have been greatly reduced since the widespread acceptance of anesthesia techniques. Beecher and Todd published in 1954 that, where anesthesia was a very important contributing factor, death occurred in 1:1560 surgeries.[4] Today, patients want to know the current state of the art of medical science in regard to perioperative risk and complication. One of the most useful and popular ways to assess risk in the surgical patient population is by the American Society of Anesthesiologists (ASA) physical status. This classification system was originally designed in the early 1940s and updated in 1961 (*Table 8.1*).

The ASA classification system has been shown to correlate with surgical and anesthetic outcome.[5] Lagasse's study[5] concluded that the incidence of anesthesia-related mortality within 48 hours of surgery was 1:13 000

Table 8.1 **ASA classification**	
ASA I	Normal healthy patient without active disease
ASA II	Patient with mild systemic disease (e.g., hypertension under medical control)
ASA III	Patient with severe systemic disease
ASA IV	Patient with severe systemic disease that is a constant threat to life
ASA V	Patient who is moribund and is not expected to survive without surgery
ASA VI	Patient who has been declared brain-dead for organ donation
ASA, American Society of Anesthesiologists.	

procedures, when evaluating all patients coming for a surgical procedure. Of great interest, but of little surprise to the practicing anesthesiologist, was that anesthesia-related deaths increased with increasing ASA classification. Other reports dating as far back as 1987 report anesthesia-related mortality rates at 1:185 000.[6] The study by Buck et al.[6] was performed before the widespread acceptance of new technology monitoring systems (pulse oximetry and capnography) that serve as early-warning systems for respiratory compromise. More recent studies have shown even better safety outcome results for patients having surgery. A 2004 study performed in France again showed that mortality rates increased with increasing patient ASA status, at a rate of 4 deaths per million surgeries for ASA category I patients and with 554 deaths per million in ASA category IV patients.[7] The effect of medical progress on improved clinical outcome is often difficult to detect when the incidence of maloccurrence is infrequent. Significant changes in daily anesthesia practice began in the mid-1980s with the introduction of the Harvard Standards of Practice I – minimal monitoring. These anesthesia standards required the use of monitoring devices to detect and prevent impending disaster during surgery.[8] The 1986 ASA standards for basic intraoperative monitoring encourage both capnography and pulse oximetry during conduct of anesthesia and surgery. The incidence of accident and death rate in ASA status I and II patients was studied before and after the adoption of the new monitoring standards at Harvard hospitals (*Table 8.2*). The implementation of these standards, along with the introduction of new monitoring techniques, has greatly reduced the incidence of

Table 8.2 Incidence of intraoperative anesthesia complications

Dates	ASA status I and II patients (n)	Intraoperative accidents (n)/incidence		Death (n)/incidence	
1/1976–6/1985	757 000	10	1/75 700	5	1/151 400
7/1985–6/1988	244 000	1	1/244 000	0	0/244 000

Monitoring standards instituted 7/1985,
ASA, American Society of Anesthesiologists.

unrecognized hypoventilation and hypoxemia leading to intraoperative complication and death.[9–11]

The implications of these findings for current clinical practice in the operating room are clear. Monitoring equipment for electrocardiogram, blood pressure, pulse oximetry, capnography, inspired concentration of oxygen on anesthesia machines, and temperature must be available in the operating room, functioning and used in all appropriate situations. The proper use of monitoring devices during surgery improves safety during surgery. Nonfunctioning monitoring equipment postpones surgery.

It is the experience gained from in-hospital surgery and advances in medical care that have allowed the development of outpatient surgery. Recent data show that upwards of 60% of surgery at community hospitals in 2005 was performed in an outpatient setting.[12] It is almost certain the percentage of patients undergoing cosmetic and reconstructive surgery on an outpatient basis is even higher. In the mid-1970s there were two free-standing outpatient surgery centers in the US. There are now over 5000. The success of outpatient surgery done outside a hospital operating room is based on the cost-efficient ability of these centers to meet the medical needs of the patient and the medical staff safely. It has been shown repeatedly that outpatient surgery can be performed with a safety standard equal to or exceeding that available in an inpatient hospital-based environment. The spectrum of settings for performance of surgery continues to expand with the development of office-based surgical facilities.[13] The American Society of Plastic Surgery through the Patient Safety committee has published an outstanding series of articles outlining advisory principles for safety in ambulatory surgery.[14] These reports, based on the medical literature combined with the general principles described above, set an educated guideline for conduct of outpatient plastic surgery. A primary area of concern for the plastic surgeon is patient selection for surgery and whether or not to perform the surgery on an outpatient basis. We have previously described the data that demonstrate that complications increase with an increase in a patient's ASA status. Prospective stratification of 17 638 patients by age found that patients over the age of 65 years were 1.4 times as likely to have an untoward intraoperative event and twice as likely to experience an intraoperative cardiovascular event as patients under 65.[15]

Obese patients/sleep apnea patients having plastic surgery

Multiple studies have demonstrated an increase in perioperative risk associated with obesity. Complications during surgery associated with patient obesity include increased rates of failed regional anesthesia, unplanned hospital admissions, and an increased incidence of deep venous thrombosis.[16] It is also unreasonable to expect medical care providers to be able to manage the obese patient physically without assistance from other healthcare assistants. Unless an ambulatory center is prepared to have the help the obese patient will require, the patient should have surgery in a facility with the necessary staff available. Setting a weight limit for patients, based on the ability of the staff of the center to manage the patient, avoids uncomfortable situations when the patient arrives for surgery and the facility is unable to take care of him or her. Proper planning at the surgical facility reduces surgical cancelations. Obese patients have a higher incidence of sleep apnea than patients of normal body habitus. Physical characteristics that predispose patients to having obstructive sleep apnea include body mass index over 35, neck circumference of 17 inches (43 cm) in men or 16 inches (41 cm) in women, craniofacial abnormalities affecting the airway, nasal obstruction, and tonsil hypertrophy.[17]

Table 8.3 Criteria for determining the severity of sleep apnea after sleep study

Severity of obstructive sleep apnea	Adult apnea–hypopnea index	Pediatric apnea–hypopnea index
None	0–5	0
Mild	6–20	1–5
Moderate	21–40	6–10
Severe	>40	>10

The 2006 report by the ASA taskforce on perioperative management of patients with obstructive sleep apnea is a valuable reference for conduct of care of this classification of patients.[17] The severity of sleep apnea, as determined by a formal sleep study, is seen in *Table 8.3*. The severity of oxygen saturation depression during apnea events and the number of apneic events per hour should be considered in evaluating the patient for surgery.

Proper perioperative clinical management of patients with sleep apnea is of critical importance. Airway management of the obese patient, with or without sleep apnea, may be difficult. Careful airway evaluation preoperatively with notation of mouth opening, mental–hyoid distance, submandibular compliance, range of motion of the cervical spine, and Mallampati score may indicate potential difficulties in airway maintenance and intubation.[18] Conduct of the actual anesthetic for patients having sleep apnea and having plastic surgery depends on many factors. Certainly the type of surgery, the severity of airway disease, and the desires of the patient are major components in the decision-making process. The need for intubation or airway manipulation during surgery should not be an automatic exclusionary criterion for outpatient surgery in a patient with a history of sleep apnea. Appropriately selected patients with a history of sleep apnea who are observed and monitored for extended periods of time after surgery may do well on an outpatient basis. Patients with sleep apnea requiring large amounts of postoperative narcotics or sedatives and those who are noted to have decreased oxygen saturation levels on room air or inadequate ventilation will require admission and continued monitoring in an acute care setting. Monitoring of the sleep apnea patient after surgery and after hospital admission includes continuous oxygen saturation. Monitoring of oxygen saturation levels on an every 4–6-hour basis makes no sense given the fact that obstructive apneic events are more likely after surgery and hypoxic brain injury may occur in a matter of minutes.

In addition, it may be unwise to attempt to complete a surgical procedure on a patient with sleep apnea using local anesthesia with deep levels of sedation. Commonly used medications for sedation during surgery, including narcotics and benzodiazepines, may exacerbate apneic episodes leading to hypoxia and hypoventilation. Performing procedures on a patient with sleep apnea with the patient in the prone position and limited airway access without first securing the airway may be particularly hazardous. It is often difficult to monitor ventilation accurately in a nonintubated patient. New technologies to detect hypoventilation will need to be developed to monitor ventilation accurately in nonairway-controlled patients. Development of continuous arterial CO_2 using a noninvasive format will further improve patient safety during surgery.[19] Patients using continuous positive airway pressure (CPAP) as a therapeutic modality for sleep apnea should be instructed to bring the CPAP equipment to the surgical center. The center should have personnel knowledgeable in the application of CPAP devices available to assist in the respiratory care of the patient. Similarly, patients who use CPAP at home should use their CPAP while resting or asleep at the hospital.

Despite careful attention to airway evaluation, clinical experience and prospective studies have demonstrated a relatively poor ability of the medical practitioner to predict which patients will have a difficult airway. Upwards of 3% of patients deemed to have "normal" airways may have difficulty with intubation. The implications of our inability to predict which patients will have a difficult airway include the need to have an extensive selection of airway management tools available in the surgical setting where airway complications may arise. In addition to the traditional array of laryngoscopes and blades, airways, and endotracheal tubes of many sizes comes the need for fiberoptic laryngoscopes, laryngeal mask airways, and the personnel who can readily use these tools. Newer technologies, including video laryngoscopes, should be available to those trained in these techniques. It is not a question of how much equipment you can purchase, but which equipment you are skilled at using during an emergency to establish an airway. Every surgical facility should be capable of performing a surgical airway (tracheostomy) in the rare case of failed airway management.

Review of large databases evaluating the safety of surgery has shown that surgery and anesthesia are very safe. The risk of anesthesia as the cause of death in ASA I and ASA II category patients is in the range of $1:150\,000–1:300\,000$ patients.[20,21] Therefore, it should be no surprise when medical publications are presented with a small series of patients undergoing outpatient surgery in an office-based surgery center that the reported complication and death rates are very low.[22] In a study on office-based surgery, 84.3% of patients were ASA class I, 15.6% ASA II, and only 0.1% ASA class III. It would require a very large data collection of ASA I and II patients to provide evidence of increased risk or an improved outcome in a particular surgical setting or using a specific anesthesia technique in this subset of patients.

Similar publications have documented the highest levels of safety in the office surgery environment using general anesthesia. Hoefflin *et al.* published a series of 23 000 consecutive surgical patients over an 18-year period. The advantages of general anesthesia with airway control during surgery are also presented.[23] Again, given the relatively low incidence of complications in this patient population and the small number of patients studied, it will be difficult to show statistically significant change in clinical complication rates. The American Association for Accreditation of Ambulatory Surgery Facilities study of 400 675 patients concluded that patient safety in accredited office-based surgical facilities was equal to or exceeded the safety level of surgery in a hospital.[24] As these articles propose, there are tangible benefits to office-based surgery, including cost containment, convenience, and ease of scheduling. There is little doubt that patients prefer the quieter, gentler ambience of the office/outpatient surgery center than a busy hospital environment. The office-based surgery/outpatient surgical environment can provide a superb surgical environment for patient, physician, and staff as long as the quality of care equals or exceeds that of the full service hospital in all regards.

Intraoperative management of the plastic surgery patient

Both the medical literature and nonpeer-reviewed publications extol the virtues of a variety of anesthesia techniques for plastic surgery, particular aesthetic surgery. The general public would like to believe that a less invasive and seemingly simpler anesthesia technique will be safer. Physicians who are not knowledgeable of the medical literature may contribute to this misconception. As we have seen in the case of patients with sleep apnea, local anesthesia with deep levels of sedation may not be an appropriate anesthetic choice and may put the patient at substantial risk of airway compromise. Both local anesthesia and general anesthesia produce a similar incidence of complications in patients having oral surgery on an outpatient basis.[25,26] The 2006 closed claims analysis from the ASA Closed Claims database demonstrated that, relative to the incidence of the anesthesia technique, death during monitored anesthesia care and general anesthesia was twice as common as in patients undergoing a regional anesthetic.[27] The primary complication leading to death in this study was inadequate oxygenation and ventilation. In this closed claim study, respiratory insufficiency was found to have occurred in 15% of patients who had monitored anesthesia care versus 7% of patient who had general anesthesia. Other factors in this group, such as patient age and ASA classification, may have contributed to the findings. Randomized studies comparing anesthesia technique for a given surgical procedure must be performed before declaring a winner in the category of anesthesia technique for patient safety. Very large patient populations will need to be evaluated so that appropriate conclusions can be drawn.

Some anesthesia techniques used during surgery appear to have been poorly evaluated for possible complications. Epidural anesthesia for patients undergoing liposuction appears to expose the patient to large doses of local anesthetics when used in both the delivery of epidural anesthesia and as a component of the tumescent solution. Vasodilation by regional anesthetic blockade of the sympathetic nervous system seems to conflict with the application of dilute solutions of epinephrine for vasoconstriction during liposuction. Again, heavy sedation of a patient in the prone position with a high dermatome level of regional anesthetic seems unwise for patients undergoing liposuction because of concerns with airway compromise and respiratory insufficiency. Despite these considerations, numerous publications have supported regional anesthesia use in this setting. A well-thought-out anesthetic plan that is coordinated with the surgeon and operating room staff will add to patient safety.

Advances in medical technology and medical practice have allowed the development of outpatient surgery to be performed in both a free-standing surgical center and in the medical office-based surgery setting. The American Society of Plastic Surgery commissioned a taskforce on patient safety in office-based surgical facilities and published a taskforce statement.[28] This taskforce statement provides conservative judgments on the nature of surgical procedures appropriate for the office-based setting and the appropriate magnitude of these same surgeries. Of particular interest to the practicing physician was the recommendation for limiting the volume of liposuction to a total of 5000 cc of total aspirate volume (fat and fluid). A large study looking at the clinical outcome of 631 large-volume liposuction patients showed a high degree of safety and extremely low complication rates with much larger total aspirate volume.[29] Our current clinical policy limits aspirate volume to 5000 cc of supernatant fat in the outpatient setting and allows aspiration of an additional 1000 cc of fat for patients admitted to the hospital after surgery for continued monitoring. The medical literature provides very little basis for the taskforce recommendations and the medical literature and clinical experience suggest that larger aspirate volumes may be safely performed at a single operation. The physiologic injury of liposuction depends on the surgical technique employed and the body surface area of the patient. Removing 5000 cc of fat from a 100-lb (45-kg) patient will have very different physiologic consequences than the same type of surgery performed on a much larger patient.

Recommendations for limits on liposuction aspiration should be based on appropriate medical and physiologic considerations. Suggestions have been made to limit the duration of a plastic surgery procedure as a method of establishing safe medical practice. Perioperative clinical risk increases with longer surgical duration. Bringing the patient back to the operating room for a second surgery also involves exposing the patient to additional risk. The decision to perform one longer surgery or two shorter surgeries involves many factors.

The American Society of Plastic Surgery Patient Safety Committee published *Evidence-Based Patient Safety Advisory: Liposuction* in 2009.[14] The use of lidocaine as a component of the wetting solution injected into the fat prior to aspiration has been well discussed in the medical literature. Local anesthetic in the wetting solution is used for two purposes. The first is to reduce the level of additional anesthesia (general or sedation) that is needed to complete the procedure and keep the patient comfortable during surgery. The second purpose is to provide postsurgical analgesia in the body areas where surgery has been performed. Death from local anesthetic overdose has occurred during liposuction. Mistakes have been made in the compounding of the wetting solution used during liposuction surgery. Bottles of 2% lidocaine have been added to the wetting solution when 1% lidocaine was prescribed for compounding. Bupivacaine 0.5% has been added to wetting solutions when lidocaine 0.5% was prescribed for compounding. Catastrophic outcomes have occurred from these errors. The compounding of wetting solutions must be confirmed by two individuals to insure accuracy and prevent error. Limitation of lidocaine dosing must be conservative because of erratic and unpredictable serum levels of local anesthesia from any given wetting solution administration.[30,31] Multiple studies have documented that plasma lidocaine levels peak 10–12 hours after wetting solution containing dilute concentrations of epinephrine is injected in the adipose tissue prior to liposuction. For patients undergoing liposuction on an outpatient basis, peak lidocaine levels will occur after discharge from the surgical facility. Following tumescent injection into highly vascular areas of the body such as the neck, peak lidocaine levels occur more rapidly (6 hours) and at higher serum levels.[32] In liposuction surgery with large volumes of tumescent injection, sources of additional local anesthetic administration, such as laryngeal tracheal anesthetics, should be avoided by the anesthetic provider. Epinephrine levels peak after tumescent injection at about 3 hours postinjection.[30] It has been postulated that elevated epinephrine levels post tumescent injection may contribute to renal blood flow changes, leading to decreased urine output during larger-volume liposuction.[29] Perioperative fluid management for the patient undergoing liposuction has been a topic of great debate. Clinical studies and clinical experience have shown that approximately 30% of injected wetting solution is aspirated during liposuction with 70% of the injected tumescent volume remaining in the adipose tissue and subsequently absorbed into the central circulation.[33,34]

Deep venous thrombosis/pulmonary emboli in the liposuction patient

The prevention of venous thromboembolism in the perioperative period should be part of the surgical strategy for every patient. The use of prophylactic therapy for prevention of venous thromboembolism during surgery has been well established in the medical literature.[35] However, determining an appropriate therapeutic program for venous thromboembolism prevention remains confusing for many surgical practitioners, especially when the surgical procedure is deemed "minor," the duration of surgery is deemed short, and the patient is discharged home after recovery from surgery and anesthesia.

The primary concern with chemoprophylaxis for venous thromboembolism prevention is postoperative bleeding, particularly after facial cosmetic surgery, surgery that may affect patency of the airway, and liposuction where large areas of tissue have been disrupted and blood collection may be extensive. As a result of these concerns, prophylactic therapy for ambulatory plastic surgery has focused on the use of graduated compression stockings and the use of intermittent pneumatic compression devices fitted for the foot or leg. The use of these techniques has been shown to reduce the incidence of venous thromboembolus.[36] It remains to be demonstrated whether these nonpharmacologic techniques prevent pulmonary embolism or death following outpatient plastic surgery. Compressive stockings must be properly fitted for them to be effective, and ill-fitted stockings may lead to venous occlusion or arterial compromise of the lower extremity.

The use of intermittent pneumatic compressive devices for the leg or foot increases venous flow and is thought to reduce pooling of blood in the veins. Once again, proper fitting of the device is mandatory and use of the pneumatic compressive device should start before beginning anesthesia and continue through the recovery period in the postanesthesia care unit. The development of venous thromboembolism may extend well into the postoperative period following discharge from the medical care facility. In selected cases it may be wise to continue mechanical prophylaxis at home, after discharge from surgery, for the high-risk patient. Patients who have undergone circumferential liposuction of the thigh or calf where the venous flow of the lower extremity may be compromised may benefit from extending the duration of mechanical prophylaxis. Mechanical prophylaxis is contraindicated in patients with lower-extremity edema, a history of peripheral vascular disease of the lower extremity, or wounds or ulcers of the feet or legs.

Patients at high risk for venous thromboembolism include those with a history of prior venous disease, obesity (body mass index >30), postoperative immobility, diabetes, history of tobacco use, history of cancer, advanced age, long duration of surgery, and the use of general anesthesia.[37] This subset of high-risk patients may benefit from a combination of mechanical and pharmacologic prophylactic measures to reduce the incidence of venous thromboembolism. Patients who are thought to be hypercoagulable (e.g., protein S deficiency or factor V Leiden) may also warrant both mechanical and pharmacologic therapy for thromboprophylaxis during outpatient ambulatory surgery.[38] Pharmacologic prophylaxis is contraindicated in patients with active bleeding, recent or anticipated regional anesthesia (epidural or spinal), infective endocarditis, proliferative retinopathy, and in patients with thrombocytopenia. Patients undergoing surgery with epidural anesthetics and the use of an indwelling epidural catheter should have the catheter removed before starting anticoagulant therapy. In patients with an indwelling catheter in whom anticoagulation therapy has been instituted, the catheter should be removed at the low point of clinical effectiveness of anticoagulation therapy; that is, just before the administration of the next dose of medication. The international normalized ratio should be <1.5 at the time of catheter removal. The use of heparin and low-molecular-weight heparin is contraindicated in patients with a history of heparin-induced thrombocytopenia. Fondaparinux may be an appropriate prophylactic therapy for patients with heparin-induced thrombocytopenia. Aspirin as a sole modality for venous thrombosis prophylaxis is generally not recommended. Aspirin may be indicated in a small subset of patients at high risk for venous thrombosis and with specific contraindications for other mechanical and pharmacologic therapies.

Intermittent pneumatic compression devices are routinely used for all liposuction patients because of concern with venous stasis, vascular endothelial injury, and/or activation of the coagulation pathway secondary to tissue trauma during surgery. Anticoagulation therapies started prior to or immediately following liposuction surgery pose substantial bleeding risk to the patient. During liposuction, large areas of tissue are disrupted during surgery and visualization of bleeding sites may be difficult. Patients who develop pulmonary thromboemboli in the early postoperative period and given aggressive anticoagulant therapy have experienced a great amount of bleeding in the body areas having liposuction. Anti coagulated liposuction patients will experience severe bleeding, even with aggressive compressive garment therapy in the regions of recent surgery. Venacaval filters have been successfully placed in postliposuction patients experiencing pulmonary emboli. For postliposuction patients experiencing these life-threatening complications, consultation with critical care medicine and vascular surgery specialists is mandatory.

Care of the liposuction patient during surgery

Coordination of patient care during liposuction by the operating team is mandatory. Strategies for tumescent solution dosing, fluid management, patient positioning, and maintenance of the patient's body temperature during surgery should be planned prior to the start of the surgical procedure. Liposuction patients frequently have large portions of their body surface area exposed to cold operating room temperatures. Maintaining body temperature for the patient during surgery may become a complex problem for the surgical team. Anesthetics routinely cause blood flow redistribution, antagonizing the body's normal mechanisms for temperature regulation. Warmed intravenous fluids and tumescent solutions for liposuction will aid in temperature preservation. Water-based operating table heating pads have been

shown to have little benefit for temperature preservation. Routine use of two forced air heating blankets, one over the upper part of the body and the second over the lower part of the body, have almost eliminated concern over hypothermia during liposuction. Changes in body positioning during liposuction surgery must be performed expeditiously, with reapplication of the forced air blankets as soon as is possible to maintain body temperature.

The most common postoperative complication after liposuction is skin and body contour irregularity. Of course, the most serious outcome after liposuction is death. Abdominal wall and vital organ perforation has been reported to occur in 14.6% of 95 fatalities following 496 245 liposuction procedures.[39] Patients with previous abdominal surgery or known to have a ventral hernia appear to be at increased risk of abdominal wall perforation. Careful preoperative abdominal examination will identify many patients with abdominal wall hernias. Advanced imaging by computed tomography scan may be necessary to help identify patients with abdominal wall defects that could lead to severe complications after abdominal liposuction. Meticulous surgical technique is required to reduce the incidence of vital organ injury. Perforation of the posterior flank, leading to retroperitoneal injury, thoracic perforation, and spinal cord injury, has been reported during liposuction. Delay in diagnosis of an abdominal wall perforation may lead to peritoneal spillage, necrotizing fasciitis, sepsis, and death.[40] The only thing worse than such a catastrophic complication is the failure to diagnose such a condition. Physician denial that a complication has occurred is a strong component in the pathway leading to a devastating clinical outcome after surgery.

Facial aesthetic surgery

Hematoma formation after facial rejuvenation surgery can have serious consequences. Small hematomas may be treated with conservative techniques such as external pressure to the affected area or require percutaneous aspiration with a needle and syringe. Large hematomas, expanding hematomas, or blood collections causing pressure on the patient's airway are more likely to require surgical intervention. Surgical studies have identified perioperative hypertension with systolic blood pressure greater than 150 mmHg and diastolic blood pressure greater than 90 mmHg as a prime marker for postoperative hematoma formation after facial surgery. Recommendations for aggressive blood pressure control surrounding the time of planned rhytidectomy have been proposed by many authors. Whether preoperative prescription of antihypertensive medications such as clonidine should be used to reduce the incidence of postoperative facial hematoma, as opposed to intraoperative titration of antihypertensive medications, is as yet unanswered. As with any such critical question, randomized studies will need to be performed. The administration of oral or intramuscular medications around the time of surgery should be carefully evaluated. The perioperative use of thorazine to control intraoperative and postoperative blood pressure during rhytidectomy needs to be questioned. Thorazine has a long half-life and a long clinical duration of action. It has numerous undesired drug interactions, including potentiation of narcotic analgesics, and a variety of side-effects. Given that we now have better, titratable antihypertensive medications, more potent antiemetics, and better perioperative sedative medications, thorazine in the surgical setting is a drug best relegated to history.

Airway management of the patient with a postoperative facial hematoma may be frightening. Facial and neck hematomas may significantly distort the airway making direct laryngoscopy and intubation impossible. Careful evaluation of the patient's airway and anatomy distortion should be performed prior to administration of sedative medications or induction of general anesthesia in a patient with facial or neck hematoma. Deviation of the trachea by a neck hematoma or swelling of the base of the tongue or pharynx can cause airway obstruction. Traditional airway rescue techniques such as the laryngeal mask airway may not be effective because of anatomical distortions caused by the hematoma. Securing the airway with an endotracheal tube with the patient awake and spontaneously breathing may be the safest technique prior to induction of general anesthesia in patients with distorted anatomy from a postoperative hematoma. Opening a suture line with evacuation of a small area of hematoma may relieve pressure on the airway and restore a more normal airway anatomy. In this clinical setting preparations should be made for performing a surgical airway prior to attempts at fiberoptic or awake intubation. Preparation for an airway crisis will help avoid a clinical disaster should airway complications develop. Massive neck swelling may also make performance of a surgical airway or cricoid thyroidotomy difficult.

Evacuation of a small postoperative facial hematoma after rhytidectomy may be an appropriate procedure for an office-based surgery center or free-standing surgery center. In a case with possible airway compromise following facial surgery, a hospital-based operating facility may provide the greatest level of safety for the patient. It may be necessary for the patient to remain intubated after hematoma evacuation because of continued swelling in the neck, pharynx, and base of tongue. Again, preparation for rapid deterioration of the patient's airway is mandatory.

Complications from breast surgery

The incidence of pneumothorax following breast augmentation and breast reconstructive surgery is very low – less than 1% of cases. The incidence of a pneumothorax following primary breast augmentation is fortunately very rare, but must be considered in a patient with otherwise unexplained postoperative respiratory complications. Pneumothorax after secondary breast surgery and breast reconstruction has been reported at a higher incidence but remains infrequent. Severe postoperative respiratory distress after breast surgery may require positive-pressure respiratory assistance and intubation along with needle aspiration of the chest for evacuation of a pneumothorax. Chest tube insertion for continued management of a pneumothorax is rare, but may be required for a persistent air leak. Keeping this potential complication in mind will allow recognition of the disorder when it presents itself clinically.

Fire in the operating room

The development of thermal injury secondary to a fire in the surgical field can lead to devastating consequences. As many as 200 operating room fires involving patients undergoing surgery may be occurring every year. The concept of the fire triad helps to explain the development of a fire during surgery. The fire triad includes: (1) an oxidizer, which in an operating room setting includes oxygen and nitrous oxide; (2) an ignition source, which may be an electrocautery-type device or laser; and (3) a fuel source such as drapes, gauze, prepping solutions, or a patient's body tissue. Prevention of fires in the operating room during surgery starts with physician and staff awareness of the possible contributing factors to an operating room fire. The ASA Taskforce on Operating Room Fires has developed specific recommendations to reduce the incidence of operating room fires.[41] Oxygen-enriched environments readily promote ignition of a combustible material. The contour of the surgical drapes around the patient's face may allow oxygen to accumulate and promote combustion. Allowing free air flow around a surgical area may reduce the incidence of ignition of combustible material. Minimizing the delivery of supplemental oxygen (nasal cannula or face mask) to the surgical region may reduce the incidence of combustion. For patients receiving supplemental oxygen via nasal cannula or face mask while undergoing facial surgery, minimizing the oxygen concentration in the surgical field is mandatory. This may be achieved by using the lowest possible oxygen flow to the patient that produces satisfactory oxygen saturation levels, and by suctioning in the surgical field to reduce oxygen accumulation in the surgical area. It may be necessary to secure the airway for high concentration of oxygen delivery to the patient to reduce the risk of fire of the face or airway.

Surgical sponges should be moistened when used near an ignition source. Flammable skin-prepping solutions should be allowed to dry before draping to reduce the risk of accumulation of potentially flammable gases. The lowest possible cautery and laser settings should be used to limit ignition potential. Treatment of a facial or airway fire includes stopping the flow of delivered gases to the patient, removal of burning material as soon as possible, including an enflamed endotracheal tube if it has caught on fire, and extinguishing flames with saline as rapidly as possible. Concerns with airway thermal injury must be thoroughly evaluated with laryngoscopy and bronchoscopy if necessary. Airway management after facial fire or airway thermal injury will require additional medical consultation and intensive care unit monitoring of the patient.

Protocol-based systems for reducing wrong patient and wrong-sided surgery

Much of this chapter has discussed techniques for improving patient safety during surgery based on our knowledge of the pharmacology and physiology of the surgery being performed. Other portions of the chapter have sought to educate the medical practitioner through review of the medical literature of surgical and anesthetic risk. Other portions of this textbook seek to educate the medical practitioner on surgical technique and improving clinical outcome through better surgery. Most physicians strive to improve clinical outcome by advancing their knowledge of the scientific literature that is the basis of medical practice. However, poor patient outcome during surgery is often due to failure of the medical system to meet the needs of the patient. Medical facilities should have mechanisms in place to insure that patients receive the correct surgical procedure. Following this concept, the Joint Commission under the National Patient Safety Goals has adopted the Universal Protocol for Preventing Wrong Site, Wrong Procedure and Wrong Person Surgery.[42] The Universal Protocol is founded on the concept that performing the wrong surgery must be prevented and that aggressive strategies must be implemented for successfully protecting the patient. Verification of patient identity is performed multiple times by multiple individuals involved in the medical care and surgical care process. This verification process begins with preoperative patient verification and confirmation of medical conditions. This preoperative verification includes patient identity confirmed verbally with the patient and with checking the patient's arm band. Confirmation of the surgical site and surgical procedure along with proper surgical site marking by the physician or designee is performed. Verification of the surgical permit, appropriate history, and physical examination documentation along with laboratory studies and plans for blood transfusion are included in this preoperative review. Which members of the surgical team should be allowed to perform surgical site marking remains highly controversial in the medical community. These debates will continue, but it is safe to state that the surgical site must be marked preoperatively, meeting the National Patient Safety Goals and good perioperative medical judgment.

Box 8.1 Confirm the following information with the patient prior to induction of anesthesia

Patient identity
Site marking by surgeon
Surgical consent
Current history and physical
Allergy band
Special needs or instrumentation, i.e., continuous positive airway pressure machine for after surgery for a patient with sleep apnea

Box 8.2 Confirm with anesthesia care provider

Anesthesia safety check completed
Pulse oximeter in place and functioning
Anticipated difficult airway or pulmonary aspiration risk
Risk of blood loss greater than 500 cc in an adult or greater than 7 mL/kg in a child
Need for blood typing and crossmatch
Special anesthesia equipment needs

The World Health Organization has adopted a surgical patient safety checklist to reduce the incidence of medical errors.[43] This checklist includes procedures to be performed prior to the induction of anesthesia (*Boxes 8.1 and 8.2*).

Performance of the "time-out" procedure ensures that the correct patient is about to undergo the correct surgery on the correct surgical site. The "time-out" procedure requires that the entire operative team focus on the identification process and participate in performing the "time-out." The operative team includes the surgeon and surgical assistants, the anesthesia care provider, the nurse in the operating room, the surgical technician, and other individuals in the operating room who will be participating in the surgical procedure (i.e., radiology personnel). When more than one procedure is to be performed on the same patient by different surgeons, a "time-out" is performed before the start of each portion of the surgery. The "time-out" procedure must confirm:

1. The patient's identity is correct.
2. The surgical site is correct.
3. The surgical procedure that is planned.
4. Surgical consent is complete and accurate.
5. The surgical site has been properly marked and is visible in the surgical field.

6. Imaging studies and implantable devices are available (if indicated).
7. Prophylactic antibiotics (if indicated) have been given.
8. Deep venous thrombosis prophylaxis has been instituted (if indicated).
9. Implementation of aseptic technique has been reviewed.
10. Procedure duration and anticipated blood loss are checked.
11. Other areas of concern during surgery by any member of the surgical team are noted.

After completion of the procedure a post surgical evaluation is performed by the surgical team. This portion of the surgical safety checklist includes:

1. Sponge and needle counts are correct.
2. Review of the surgical consent confirms completion of all planned procedures.
3. Pathology specimens will be properly sent to the lab.
4. Plans for postanesthesia recovery have been made and personnel have been notified of the patient's forthcoming arrival.

All team members must be full participants in the "time-out" procedure. Failure to perform these well-established procedures puts the patient at risk for grave error and brings into question the quality of care being provided to the patient.

The sociology of the plastic surgery operating room

The American Society of Plastic Surgery and the American Society for Aesthetic Plastic Surgery have promoted a "patient-first" initiative in advocating for safety in the operating room. Advances in surgical technique and perioperative medical management have allowed improved clinical outcomes. As much as our medical knowledge increases, we sense a great disappointment when the clinical outcome is not as good as expected. Attempts at regulation of the surgical environment, with accreditation of surgical facilities, have certainly increased the quality of documentation during surgery, but have they improved outcome? Accreditation of a surgical facility includes reviewing processes and systems but may not actually observe the performance of a single surgery. The accreditation process taking 1, 2, or 3 days evaluates a surgical facility at a point in time. The actual conduct of that facility going forward may not come under scrutiny for another 1–3 years. Compromise in standards by a physician or by the surgical facility may occur slowly and yet soon be so substandard as to put the patient at unnecessary risk. Ultimately, the decision to practice plastic surgery safely will rest with the physician.

The standard of clinical practice in a surgery center or office-based surgical facility must meet or exceed that of an accredited hospital. A series of 10 core principles was published in 2004 advocating the fundamentals of practice for aesthetic surgery.[44] These same principles are as valid today as when they were first published and should apply to all practitioners and all surgical specialists. Patients should be selected for surgery based on the established criteria set by the ASA classification system. Physicians performing office-based surgery must have admitting privileges at a nearby hospital and a transfer agreement with that hospital facilitating patient transfer and admission when needed. Physicians performing office-based surgery must show competency by maintaining surgical privileges at an accredited licensed hospital or ambulatory surgery center for the same procedures being performed in the office setting. Serious peer review of surgical performance and medical management in an outpatient surgical center or a private surgical facility should be mandatory for the benefit of the patient. Is it appropriate that a physician who is denied privileges at a hospital to perform surgery has the right to open a private facility without peer review and perform those same procedures? Should a privately owned surgical facility function as a hiding place for a physician to escape peer review? The same rules that apply to a practicing surgeon should also apply to the practicing anesthesiologist. No medical practitioner should be above answering to his or her medical peers during a clinical review.

We must begin to question the conduct of clinical practice in the operating room during surgery. A patient can reasonably expect that the focus of the surgical team will be dedicated to performing their jobs to deliver the best possible surgical outcome. Surgical team members (nurses, scrub technicians) who have gone through great effort to maximize the quality and safety of the surgical outcome are not interchangeable with other individuals who have not familiarized themselves with the medical facts of the case. The risk for error increases and the quality of care for the patient decreases when surgical team members change during surgery. No matter how complete the medical "handoff" from one team member to another, no handoff can be as complete as having been in the case from the beginning. Having several different operating room nurses and surgical technicians during a single surgery increases the risk of error and should be discouraged. Continuity of care by the anesthesia care team also improves patient safety. Plastic surgery cases may take a long time and some change in personnel may be necessary during the procedure, but should be minimized. It should not need to be said, but surgery should be performed by the attending surgeon and designated assistants and not by unlicensed minimally trained individuals deemed "qualified" by the surgeon. A lack of operating room oversight can lead to poor practice quality that may not be detected by a chart and documentation review by a certifying agency.

Best of intentions, not the best of results

Despite the best of intentions on the part of physicians and the healthcare system, errors occurring during hospitalization may cause upwards of 98 000 deaths per year and over 1 million significant injuries. Recent publication of a study showing a failure of new hospital policy and procedures to improve patient safety in a hospital setting is disappointing. Chart review of 2341 randomly selected hospital admissions from 10 randomly selected hospitals between 2002 and 2007 was performed.[45] In this review, patients were deemed to have been harmed during their hospitalization in 588 instances, about 1 in 4 patients. In 50 of these cases the harm was considered to have been life-threatening, 17 cases resulted in permanent injury and 14 deaths were deemed in part due to medical error. Despite implementation during the study period of policies and procedures to reduce medical error, the error rate remained steady at 25 harms per 100 hospital admissions.[46]

Access the complete references list online at **http://www.expertconsult.com**

5. Lagasse RS. Anesthesia safety: model or myth? A review of the published literature and analysis of current original data. *Anesthesiology*. 2002;97:1609.

   This paper presents an excellent review of literature comparing a variety of indicators that measure patient safety during anesthesia. Different measurement techniques illustrate several perspectives on the current state of surgical safety. By understanding the literature we may be better able to advise patients of the relative risk of their planned surgical procedure.

8. Eichhorn JH. Prevention of intraoperative anesthesia accidents and related severe injury through safety monitoring. *Anesthesiology*. 1989;70:572–577.

   This paper describes the statistics behind the claims of improved safety during anesthesia with the use of state-of-the-art monitoring techniques. The Harvard experience before and after the introduction of monitoring standards.

13. Iverson RE, the ASPS Task Force on Patient Safety in Office-based Surgery Facilities. Patient safety in office-based surgery facilities: procedures in the office-based surgery setting. *Plast Reconstr Surg*. 2002;110, 1337–1344.

    This paper presents the safe performance of office-based surgery. The ASPS taskforce report on patient safety. Guidelines and thought processes for safe outpatient surgery including recommendations for intraoperative management of the patient and the need for office-based surgical facility accreditation.

17. American Society of Anesthesiologists. Task force on perioperative management of patients with obstructive sleep apnea. *Anesthesiology*. 2006;104 No. 5.

    This paper remains a cornerstone for the perioperative management of patients with a history of sleep apnea and who are having anesthesia and surgery. An evidence-based set of recommendations for perioperative management of the sleep apnea patient. A more specific set of recommendations published in the literature will be helpful after additional clinical experience with this subset of patients.

22. Bitar G, Mullis W, Jacobs W, et al. Safety and efficacy of office-based surgery with monitored anesthesia care/ sedation in 4778 consecutive plastic surgery procedures. *Plast Reconstr Surg*. 2003;111:150–156.

    This paper describes a large series of patients undergoing plastic surgery using monitored anesthesia care as the anesthetic of choice. However, the low incidence of complications in this patient subset does not allow the paper to conclude that one anesthetic technique is safer than another technique.

23. Hoefflin SM, Bornstein JB, Gordon M. General anesthesia in an office based plastic surgical facility: a report on more than 23 000 consecutive office based procedures under general anesthesia with no significant anesthetic complications. *Plast Reconstr Surg*. 2001;107:243.

    This paper describes a very large clinical experience of patients undergoing plastic surgery using general anesthesia in an office-based setting. Again, because of the low incidence of complications in this patient population, no conclusion as to the superiority of this technique compared to other techniques can be made.

29. Commons GW, Halperin BD, Chang CC. Large volume liposuction: a review of 631 consecutive cases over 12 years. *Plast Reconstr Surg*. 2001;108:1753.

    This paper describes a series of patients who underwent large-volume liposuction and the associated very low complication rate associated with the procedure. A description of the surgical technique and the pharmacology and physiology behind the medical approach to the patient is presented. A demonstration that larger volumes of fat aspirate may be performed with a high degree of patient safety.

34. Kenkel JM, Lipschitz AH, Luby M, et al. Hemodynamic physiology and thermoregulation in liposuction. *Plast Reconstr Surg*. 2004;114:503–513.

    This paper presents the results of invasive hemodynamic monitoring studies performed during liposuction. The results are particularly helpful for understanding the physiologic effects of the wetting solution used for liposuction. Understanding the physiologic changes during surgery is mandatory for the proper management of the liposuction patient. The importance of maintaining normothermia during liposuction is also described and the factors leading to intraoperative heat loss are outlined for the benefit of the clinician.

41. Caplan RA, Barker SJ, Connis RT, et al. Practice advisory for the prevention and management of operating room fires. *Anesthesiology*. 2008;108(5):786–801.

    This paper is the most comprehensive publication on the subject of fire in the operating room during surgery. An explanation of the causation of operating room fire helps the practitioner to understand the recommendations made to reduce the incidence of this terrible complication. Failure to follow the standards put forward in this paper puts the patient at additional risk of an intraoperative ignition event.

45. Landrigan CP. Temporal trends in rates of patient harm resulting from medical care. *N Engl J Med*. 2010;363: 2124–2134.

9

Local anesthetics in plastic surgery

A. Aldo Mottura

SYNOPSIS

- Local anesthesia is widely used for minor surgery.
- Local anesthesia use can be extended to incorporate larger surgeries.
- The benefit to the patient is to avoid general anesthesia while breathing spontaneously.
- Using bupivacaine in the anesthetic solution, four to six hour surgeries are also possible and bupivacaine provides some hours of postoperative pain relief.
- In each region, an intelligent infiltration anesthesia technique is preferable to tumescent technique.
- For large procedures, the assistance of the anesthesiologist provides better sedation as well as the benefit of shared responsibility.

 Access the Historical Perspective section online at
http://www.expertconsult.com

Introduction

For aesthetic surgery and short or superficial operations, such as rhino-otoplasties or facelifts, some surgeons have been using local anesthesia with great success. Lately, larger aesthetic surgeries have been performed with the use of local anesthesia under superficial or deep sedation.

While general anesthesia released the surgeon from the responsibility of caring for a sleeping patient, some others prefer to use sedation and local anesthesia because of their advantages: the use of gases, muscle relaxants, and tracheal intubation are avoided, sedation can be regulated, there is less bleeding during surgery, and postoperative analgesia may be easier to manage. Furthermore a smooth and easy recovery with early discharge helps to diminish costs and improve efficiency as well as safety.

When the surgeon decides to use local anesthesia and sedation, four steps should be considered: (1) selection of the patient; (2) selection of sedation-analgesia; (3) selection of anesthetic drugs; and (4) selection of infiltration techniques.

Patient selection

There are patients for general, epidural, and local anesthesia. If you fail to select the ideal anesthesia for the patient, problems can arise during surgery.

Preoperative evaluation of the patient should pay particular attention to issues such as age, general physical condition, personality, preference for local anesthesia, drug history, and the extent of surgery.

Once these issues are considered, the surgeon can make a decision on whether or not the patient is a suitable candidate. One factor that has to be considered is cost. In general, having a procedure done under local anesthesia is cheaper than the same procedure under general anesthesia. For this reason, the surgeon may be tempted to treat a patient under local anesthesia when general anesthesia would be a better choice for that patient. Such a "borderline" case is fraught with potential problems and making the decision purely on economic grounds should therefore be avoided.

The borderline patient can be termed thus because (s)he usually has abnormal fears, and possibly a labile personality. One other very important factor is the confidence of the surgeon in his/her ability to perform the particular operation under local anesthesia.

In my experience, fear is one of the most important obstacles to this kind of anesthesia because it is a reaction that appears when a person thinks that something is threatening him or her, and the person's responses become exaggerated and somewhat unpredictable.

Age is important. In general, teenagers may sometimes be difficult since they lack maturity and experience and may sometimes, as a consequence, behave unpredictably. Patients who are ignorant of the procedure may also fear the unknown and may be less suitable candidates. Sometimes, despite extensive explanation, patients cannot grasp the essence of the procedure and may therefore be less than ideal candidates for local anesthesia. Sometimes these fears and exaggerated responses may be related to such diverse issues as ethnicity, life experiences, and personality.

Patients with abnormal or exaggerated fears should not be accepted for local anesthesia, but others who are afraid of only some aspects of the surgery can be deemed suitable and placed in the group of ideal candidates, following a very good explanation of how the surgery is performed. This explanation should include a description of the level of anesthesia, and perhaps a visit to the operating room before surgery with someone who can answer the patient's questions and help to ease anxiety and nervousness.[15]

Choice of sedation

Sedation means depressed consciousness and, indirectly, decreased discomfort during surgery. In general, this allows the patient to tolerate a procedure by relieving anxiety, discomfort, and pain.

There are several ways to sedate a patient. There are also different levels of sedation. Some surgeons use only a mild sedative, choosing to perform operations with the patient awake. Others have the patient under moderate sedation but maintaining verbal contact, while others prefer to have the patient completely asleep, that is, in deep sedation. Deep sedation may be accompanied by a partial or complete loss of protective reflexes and may include the inability to maintain a patent airway. Planned deep sedation should be administered preferably by an anesthesiologist or certified registered nurse anesthetist under the direction of an anesthesiologist or an operating physician.[16]

Premedication

Sedation-analgesia begins with premedication. Very nervous patients should be medicated some days prior to surgery; otherwise it can be very difficult to calm them down once they are in the operating room.

Lorazepam has been demonstrated to be a very effective drug. It is usually administered the night before surgery and again when the patient wakes up on the morning of surgery. In this way anxiety as well as gastric secretions are reduced.[17] Premedication should also vary according to each patient.

Sedation

The ideal situation is to receive a sedated patient in the operating room. Midazolam is the most common drug administrated in the operating room. It can be administered intramuscularly (IM) or intravenously (IV) 15–30 minutes before surgery. For more extensive procedures a combination of narcotics and anticholinergics, like scopolamine or atropine, can be used for each patient depending on degree of nervousness, blood pressure, and other physiologic indicators. For short procedures and for the beginning of longer ones, the most common combination is midazolam–fentanyl. Thirty minutes after this injection, the patient arrives at the operating room very calm, relaxed, or sleepy, so that he or she is not very aware of what occurs during the preoperative preparations. Sometimes this premedication is sufficient, but if the patient needs more profound medication, then the surgeon has several options.

Drugs used for sedation include diazepam, midazolam, or propofol, while for analgesia ketamine and fentanyl can be used. Some surgeons like Thomas Baker[18] or Charles Vinnik[19-22] use a combination of midazolam–ketamine. This is referred to as dissociative anesthesia. Ketamine is a short-acting drug that provides a rapid dissociative anesthesia lasting 45 minutes IM and 10–15 minutes IV. It has a short recovery time and is especially indicated for hypotensive patients. According to Ersek,[23,24] it also decreases platelet aggregation.

The initial decision is whether the patient needs sedation, analgesia, or both.

For sedation, the effects of diazepam and midazolam are similar but their duration differs: 3–4 hours or sometimes less for midazolam and 6–12 hours for diazepam.

For analgesia, ketamine is a very safe neuroleptic drug that does not depress the central nervous system (CNS). On the contrary, it stimulates it (not recommended for nervous or hypertensive patients); while fentanyl is a narcotic that depresses the CNS (not recommended for hypothyroid or hypotensive patients).

Intraoperative administration of drugs should be IV and in small doses using short intervals of some minutes, in order to titrate the minimal doses and not to administer unnecessary overdoses.

The effect of ketamine and fentanyl lasts 10–20 minutes but all medication wears off faster when the patient is nervous or has tachycardia, because the metabolism of the drugs is accelerated.

In the operating room, if the surgeon is alone, a nurse or another person should monitor the patient's vital signs, in spite of the convenient alarms of the pulse oximeter or cardioscope monitors.

If the local anesthesia has been correctly infiltrated and the patient wakes up during surgery, the anesthesiologist or the surgeon has to evaluate whether the patient needs further sedation, intravenous analgesia, or complementary local anesthesia.

Propofol is a hypnotic drug with a very short effect that needs repetitive administration or a continuous infusion that must be monitored by an anesthesiologist.

For sedation and analgesia, the surgeon has to study the effect of a few drugs he/she will use and combine, along with the optimal doses, metabolism, and side-effects. Under superficial sedation the patient may wake up and secrete epinephrine, which activates hepatic and renal metabolism, raises blood pressure, and increases the metabolism of anesthetic and sedative drugs. For this reason some surgeons prefer deep sedation.

If the surgeon wants to operate under deep sedation, it is preferable to have an anesthesiologist monitor the patient. This shared responsibility eases the stress of the procedure and makes for a safer environment for the patient.

Selection of local anesthetics

The effect of local anesthesia is achieved by four mechanisms: (1) chemical nerve blockade; (2) compression of the nerves; (3) distension of the nerves; and (4) ischemia of the nerves produced by vasoconstrictors. The effect of the anesthetic depends on the concentration of the drugs, the use of epinephrine, the blood supply of the area injected, and the thickness of the nerves.

There are several different anesthetic drugs, but each one should be considered according to the duration of its effect. The author's experience in infiltrative anesthesia is with lidocaine and bupivacaine.

Anesthetic drugs

Lidocaine is a very old and safe anesthetic drug that allows 90 minutes of numbness. Its standard dose is 500 mg for a 70-kg person, or 7 g/kg, or 25 mL of lidocaine 2%, but it is known that these doses can be augmented many times (some papers mention up to five times the maximum recommended dose) *(Fig. 9.1)*.

Bupivacaine is a long-lasting anesthetic that is largely used in block anesthesia and, in plastic surgery, is mainly used for postoperative pain relief. Its dose is 1.25 mg/kg, 25 mL of 0.50% bupivacaine for a 70 kg person without ephinephrine. In the author's experience, 3.3 mg/kg can be used safely when it is very diluted and with the addition of ephinephrine. This drug has an onset of 15–30 minutes and profound conduction blockage that lasts around 6–12 hours.

Vasoconstricting agents

Vasoconstriction can be achieved in different ways. The main and more popularized drug is epinephrine.

The standard concentration of epinephrine is 1:1000 and it can be diluted in 100/500/1000 mL, obtaining a

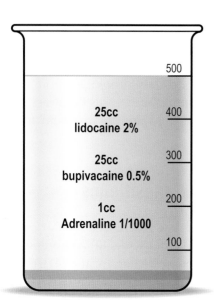

Fig. 9.1 Anesthetic solution with 25 mL lidocaine 2%, 25 mL bupivacaine 0.5%, epinephrine (adrenaline) 1/1000 1 mL and saline solution up to 500 mL.

dilution 1:100 000, 1:500 000 or 1:1 000 000. This drug's vasoconstrictive action lasts 1–6 hours and causes central effects such as tachycardia and hypertension.

Ornipressin is a vasoconstrictive agent without central action (it does not raise the blood pressure nor alter the cardiac rhythm). Its vasoconstrictive effect lasts 4–6 hours. One milliliter can be diluted in 250, 500, or 1000 mL of saline solution and can be combined with any anesthetic. All vasoconstrictors have the capacity to produce ischemia in the peripheral nerves that blocks the conduction of stimulus. As long as the vasoconstriction lasts, so does the anesthesia. The trade name for omnipressin was Por-8 (Sandoz) but for the moment, it has been discontinued.[25]

Carbonated anesthesia

Anesthetic pH is usually 6.4, which produces some pain at the time of infiltration. To avoid this, it has been advocated to add sodium bicarbonate to raise the pH to 7.4. The duration of local anesthesia when using bupivacaine and carbonated anesthesia is unknown.

There are many formulae that combine different anesthetics and vasoconstrictors.

For large aesthetic surgeries Mottura's formula[26–33] is to combine 20 mL lidocaine 2% (7 mg/kg), 20 mL bupivacaine (1.5 mg/kg), and 1 mL epinephrine 1:1000.

These drugs can be diluted in 400–1000 mL saline solution or lactated Ringer's (*Fig. 9.1*).

Selection of technique

Infiltration of large amounts of local anesthetics for liposuction is called tumescence. This implies massive inflation into the fat. This produces a balloon effect with a hard palpable surface. To perform proper local anesthesia, the anesthetic solution has to be infiltrated throughout the surgical field in a consistent way, blocking all the nerve branches.

Infiltration should begin on the side the surgeon thinks is less painful. (S)he should proceed with a very fine needle, injecting slowly, because rapid distension of tissues is painful. Once the skin is anesthetized, the fine needle is changed for a longer one or for a cannula. The inner side of an Abbocath no. 16 or a spinal needle is very useful.

For facelift

Using 400 mL of the same solution, the scalp is infiltrated first with a long needle in the subdermis, underneath the incision line and 2 cm behind the marked line, to assure a better vasoconstriction effect. Then the forehead is infiltrated always deeply, up to the orbital rim and the nasal dorsum, continuing afterwards with the cheeks and the neck.

In general, the infiltration extends 2 cm beyond the whole marked area of the face and neck because the dissection can cross premarked limits (*Fig. 9.2*).

The medial part of the neck, including skin as well as the deeper tissues to incorporate the posterior aspect of the central fat, is also infiltrated to facilitate dissection. When the infiltration is finished, 15 minutes have already elapsed and surgery can start on the scalp that was infiltrated first. Then the face is dissected and finally the neck. Before superficial musculoaponeurotic plane dissection, this layer is infiltrated for vasoconstriction and for hydraulic dissection and separation of the planes. During the duration of the surgery, which may include blepharoplasty, anesthetic generally does not have to be reinjected. Some surgeons use a progressive infiltration. This means that they incrementally inject anesthetic to different areas as the surgery progresses. This is also a useful technique.

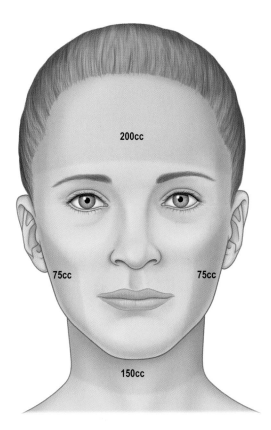

Fig. 9.2 Distribution of infiltration in the face.

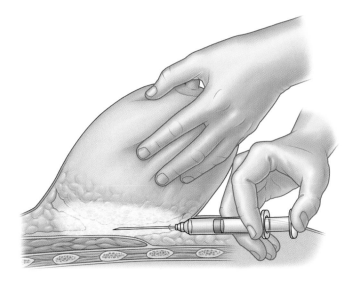

Fig. 9.3 Infiltration in the retroglandular plane.

For breast reduction

The total amount of anesthetic solution used varies according to the volume of the breast. Thus, for minor hypertrophies 400 mL is used, for large hypertrophies 400–500 mL, and for gigantomastias, over 600 mL.

Infiltration begins in the submammary fold with 20–40 mL of the solution. The entire breast is then held firmly with one hand and pulled away from the chest wall to present the retroglandular space for infiltration. This maneuver reduces the surfaces to be anesthetized *(Fig. 9.3)*.

Using a forward and backward movement and an 8-cm-long needle, I search the middle fingertip of the left hand which is holding the gland, infiltrating with the right hand in a fan-shaped manner from the submammary crease upward. The skin is jabbed at three points: (1) the medial side, to block the anterior branches of the intercostal nerve; (2) the lateral side, to block the lateral perforans; and (3) the medial retroglandular space, to block the anterior perforators that are always

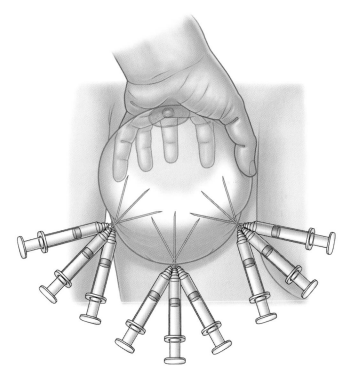

Fig. 9.4 At the submammary fold, three points for the irradiated distribution of the anesthesia.

at the chondrosternal spaces. The retroglandular space is easy to find because the needle slides in without effort. When the gland is entered, it can be appreciated because of resistance of the parenchyma. In this maneuver 60–80 mL of the solution is used *(Fig. 9.4)*.

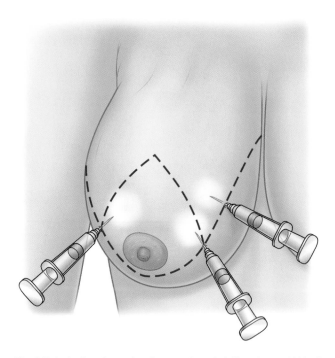

Fig. 9.5 At the line of resection, the parenchyma is infiltrated to avoid bleeding.

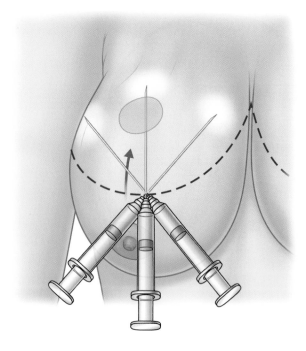

Fig. 9.6 For the nonvertical technique, the deep subcutaneous plane is profusely infiltrated.

The subcuticular space following the incision lines and the place where the areola will be placed are filled with anesthesia using 20–60 mL of the solution. No epinephrine is used under the areola, especially when a pedicle is planned. The parenchyma is infiltrated transversely to the skin in a progressive way, where the scalpel will pass *(Fig. 9.5)*.

The remaining anesthesia is kept in the container for further infiltration during the operation, in case it is necessary.

For breast hypertrophy requiring up to a 1000-g resection on each side, both breasts are anesthetized simultaneously, using less than 500 mL for each one. After that, the first breast is operated and the main stitches are placed at the key points to rebuild the gland. When the first resection is completed, a considerable amount of the anesthesia is lost. Then surgery is performed on the other breast using the same method. After the resection, a similar amount of anesthesia is also gone. Therefore, less than the maximum dose remains. After the resection and rebuilding of both breasts, the surgeon and the assistant simultaneously complete the suturing of the subcutaneous layer, the areola, and the skin. When the hypertrophy is over 1000 g per side, one side can be anesthetized, the surgery performed, and

subsequently the entire procedure repeated on the contralateral side. This avoids the possibility of massive absorption and overdose.

The prepectoral fascia should not be injured as no anesthesia is placed beneath it. Since bleeding is minimal, the time taken to secure hemostasis is short. The minimal bleeding is due to the wide infiltration of anesthesia as well as the use of vasoconstrictors that constrict the vessels before entering the gland. Intraoperative monitoring (pulse, blood pressure, electrocardiograph, Po_2 monitoring) is similar to that in other major surgeries.

Due to minimal blood loss, recovery is very fast and, in general, the patient can be discharged in the afternoon. This procedure can be applied to different reduction techniques by modifying the superficial infiltration according to the area to be incised and resected *(Fig. 9.6)*.

For breast augmentation

When the implant is placed in the prepectoral space, the anesthetic solution and the technique of infiltration are similar to those applied in breast reductions.

In case of subpectoral augmentation or in transaxillary augmentation, special attention should be

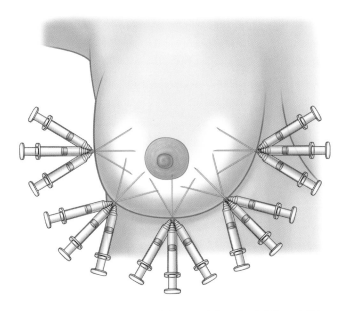

Fig. 9.7 For breast augmentation, all the area of dissection is infiltrated. This infiltration could be subglandular or subpectoral.

placed to the axilla so as to anesthetize the subpectoral space.

For the axillary approach, the site of the skin incision is first infiltrated. Then with a 10–12-cm needle, the subcutaneous area around the submammary sulcus is infiltrated. Then the needle tip is directed up to the anterior surface of the sixth rib where it begins to touch and infiltrate this surface in a fan-shaped manner, progressing medially to the sternum and laterally to the anterior axillary line. The same is done on the fifth and fourth rib. From the submammary crease and at the sternum's lateral border, the needle tip is moved horizontally over the anterior fourth, fifth, and sixth rib surfaces. On the lateral side, by holding up the pectoral muscle with the left hand, the needle is directed from the anterior axillary line to the anterior surface of the sixth to the second rib toward the medial part of the breast.

The whole area of the two breasts to be dissected is now anesthetized (with vasoconstrictor effects). The surrounding 2–3 cm outside the premarked lines should also be infiltrated, since the dissector sometimes crosses the demarcation line. The hydric dissection of the anesthetic also facilitates the disruption of muscle insertions *(Fig. 9.7)*. Special attention should be paid not to penetrate inside the thorax. This is especially important in very lean women where the intercostal muscles are thin and especially when there are irregularities in the ribs of the chest wall.

For the submammary approach, without infiltration of the axilla, the technique of infiltration is the same. For the subareolar approach, the areola and the parenchyma are infiltrated together with the submammary space.

In small patients, 500 mL of prepared anesthetic solution is normally used, while in bigger patients or in adenomastectomies and breast reconstruction patients, where different spaces (subcutaneous, retroglandular, and retropectoral) are infiltrated, 600–800 mL is administered.

For abdominoplasties

Around 600–800 mL of anesthetic solution is prepared. Once the patient is on the operating table, the anesthesia is injected deeply over the fascia (not into the adipose tissue). With the left hand the adiposity is grasped, trying to separate the fat from the fascia, where the anesthesia has to be injected. A fine needle is used to jab the skin at strategic points so that the anesthesia radiates from them to cover a larger area. This avoids having to infiltrate twice in the same place or to leave areas without anesthesia. A larger needle or a cannula can also be used. Special attention is paid to previous abdominal scars where residual fibrosis of the fascia could have involved some nerves, proving to be, therefore, more demanding. During the operation and dissection of the flap, the assistant is advised to manipulate it gently because excessive traction could produce nerve elongation and pain. In some cases, complementary anesthesia is injected around the great perforating nerves beneath the fascia, since very diluted anesthesia does not always affect large nerves. The fascia can be infiltrated all along the rectus abdominis before or after the suturing with a solution composed of 20 mL bupivacaine and 100 mL saline solution that will allow 6–8 hours of postoperative pain relief. Although different types of abdomen can be treated using this technique, it is especially indicated for small, limited, or standard abdominoplasties *(Fig. 9.8)*. Other authors have reported similar successes.[34,35]

For liposuctions

I prepare more diluted anesthesia, since almost all the fat needs to be injected. Using this technique the drugs are the same but the dilution is larger. Once the

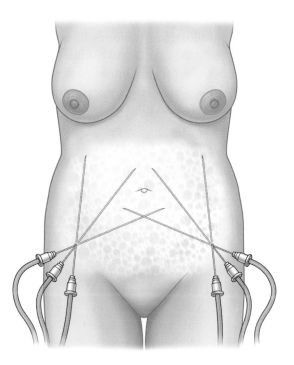

Fig. 9.8 For liposuction, the infiltrated abdomen.

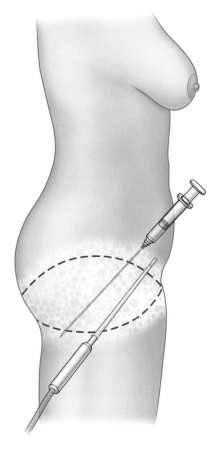

Fig. 9.9 For ultrasonic and laser liposuctions, all the fat layers should be infiltrated.

infiltrated regions are aspirated, then other areas are infiltrated with more anesthetic solution. Using this technique, I have infiltrated up to 3000 liters of anesthetic solution with no intraoperative complications. Attention should be paid to the amount of epinephrine used as excessive epinephrine injection can cause CNS problems.

Areas of similar extension were anesthetized as described above, e.g., two trochanteric areas with an infraumbilical adiposity and several small regions, combined in different ways. The infiltration of the area had to be made deep over the fascia and in the subdermal layer, but it also had to surpass the premarked adiposity limits because the cannula often passes beyond the demarcation. There are areas such as knees, trochanters, or flanks where anesthetics spread easily, while there are others with more fibrous or trabecular tissues, like the supraumbilical area, where anesthetics remain inside each trabecular compartment and therefore infiltration should be performed more accurately. For ultrasonic and laser liposuctions, all the fat layers should be infiltrated. Sometimes during liposuction these regions need supplemental IV ketamine or fentanyl.

This procedure is especially indicated for minor or moderate adiposities or secondary liposuction, when there is some residual fat to be treated *(Fig. 9.9)*.[36–41]

Problems or complications

Respiration

During surgery, an intranasal cannula helps to assure good oxygenation. The main advantage of the pulse oximeter has been the alarm that alerts the drop in the percentage of oxygenation, allowing for timely correction. If the patient is conscious, (s)he is told to take a deep breath. In very sedated patients, the most common cause of airway obstruction is posterior displacement of the tongue. In order to correct this, the mandible is pushed forward and the head is tilted back, which advances the tongue and opens the airway. If opening the mouth does not improve respiration, a plastic airway laryngeal or tracheal tube is inserted into the mouth.

If the patient is not yet breathing on his/her own, a face mask attached to an Ambu bag is placed firmly over the nose and mouth, and then the patient is given four breaths in rapid succession, allowing one exhalation. This, fortunately, is a rare occurrence.

Hypertension

Sometimes the cause of hypertension is intraoperative medication with epinephrine, ketamine, or both. In these cases, sedation is recommended with the usual sedatives but, in cases of severe hypertension, hydralazine 5 mg or chorpromazine IV can be administered.

Hypotension

Hypotension can occur when the patient is under heavy sedation. If systolic blood pressure is less than 70 mmHg, it is below a safe limit. Saline solution or lactated Ringer's injection is infused rapidly and at intervals. Vasoconstrictors or atropine are the indicated drugs to use.

Bradycardia

Courtiss and Kanter[42] stated that a pulse underneath 50 beats/min can be observed in athletes. Atropine should be sufficient to raise this level. Cases of bradycardia are rarely observed because the administration of epinephrine and ketamine produces the opposite effect: tachycardia.

Tachycardia

Tachycardia generally occurs after the administration of ketamine and epinephrine; the heart rate is accelerated but conduction is normal. Treatment with beta-blockers using propranolol is indicated to counteract this effect.

Nonsinus tachycardia is divided into supraventricular and ventricular.

Supraventricular tachycardia is controlled by vagotonic stimulation, such as carotid sinus massage. If this fails, verapamil (Isoptin) should be administered. If the patient has ventricular tachycardia and the general condition is satisfactory, lidocaine is administered. If the general condition is poor, treatment consists of electrical countershock. In patients with certain cardiovascular diseases, it is recommended that cardiologists be present in the operating room.

Reversal effect of oversedation

Flumazenil is the antagonist that reverses the effects of diazepam and midazolam, while naloxone reverses the respiration depression and hypotension caused by the opioids. However, it is seldom needed.

In some sensitive patients, sedation effects last longer than expected. To enhance the metabolism of drugs, it is advisable to give small doses of atropine and glucose solution IV with vitamin C. This medication has a rapid effect and the patient can be discharged 1 hour later.

Adverse drug interactions

Certain interactions of drugs can be seriously harmful to patients. Hypotensive agents like beta-blockers, propranolol, cimetidine, tricyclic antidepressants, and monoamine oxidase inhibitors should not be administered with epinephrine. Monoamine oxidase inhibitors interact with narcotics. To prevent problems, basal medication should be interrupted two days before surgery, or epinephrine should be replaced by ornipressin.

Nausea and vomiting

Both symptoms can be a consequence of: (1) the collateral effects of opioids; (2) a digestive problem; or (3) a combination of these two.

Opioids cause two reactions: in the CNS stimulating the vomiting center, and a spasmogenic effect in the abdomen. Patients with gastric or biliary pathologies are more sensitive to these side-effects. The objective is to prevent them. Gastric acidity has to be neutralized before surgery with aluminum hydroxide, ranitidine, or glycopyrrolate; spasmogenic reactions with antispasmodic medication (scopolamine); and the central action can be treated with metoclopramide or ondansetron before finishing surgery.

Allergic reaction to local anesthetics

Allergic reactions to these local anesthetics are rarely observed. Methylparaben is used as a preservative compound that is added to the solution of local anesthetic. If a patient has an allergic history related to local anesthetics (at the dentist's, for example), some tests are performed, and eventually pure anesthetics without preservatives are used.

Two organs can be affected by overdoses of absorption of local anesthetics: the brain and the heart. High doses of concentrated anesthetics can be accidentally injected intravenously or intra-arterially. The brain is more susceptible than the myocardium; consequently, the early symptoms of toxicity are related to CNS and later to myocardial dysfunction.

Central nervous system toxicity

Signs and symptoms range from mild to severe. In increasing order of severity, the following sequence of signs and symptoms may occur: numbness of the mouth and tongue, tinnitus, lightheadedness, visual disturbance, slurred speech, muscle twitching, unconsciousness, generalized convulsions, apnea, and coma. CNS toxicity is enhanced by acidosis and hypoxia because of a rapid oxygen consumption after convulsions.

Cardiovascular toxicity

Cardiovascular toxicity is due to slowing of the conduction in the myocardium, myocardial depression, and peripheral vasodilation. It can be seen after 2–4 convulsant local anesthetic doses have been injected. Toxicity of this drug is rare and related to massive overdose absorption or intravascular injection. Reaction to bupivacaine toxicity in the CNS is similar to the experimental reaction described for lidocaine, but after intra-arterial administration, the cardiovascular effects of ventricular arrhythmias or fibrillation can lead to a fatal outcome. Special care should be taken in selecting this drug in patients with severe cardiac insufficiencies. It should not be used in association with tocanide, an antiarrhythmic, since toxic effects are added. The lethal dose of this drug was tested in dogs. Looking for the dose limit, the dogs were intra-arterially injected with a lethal dose. When cardiac arrest appeared it could not be reversed

> **Box 9.1 Early diagnosis of toxicity**
>
> 1 Oxygenation by bag, mask, or intubation
> 2 Anticonvulsants: diazepam 10–20 mg IV or thiopental 100–150 mg IV
> 3 If hypotension occurs: epinephrine 15–30 mg IV
> 4 If the heart stops:
> - Energetic cardiopulmonary resuscitation
> - Epinephrine 1 mg IV or intercardiac
> - Ventricular fibrillation by high conversion energy
> - Bretylium 80 mg as an antiarrhythmic

as when lidocaine was used. Since then, this concept has been repeated over time. In the case of intra-arterial or intravenous injection of pure concentrated bupivacaine, cardiac arrest can occur, as in the case reported by Ersek.[43]

Treatment of toxicity

If effective treatment is desired, early diagnosis must be established (*Box 9.1*).

As Baker and Gordon once stated: "give oxygen, stop convulsions."[18]

Discussion

Different actions of local anesthesia

Using a large infiltration of solution with anesthetic drug, anesthesia is achieved by different physiopathologic mechanisms. The oldest one was described by Halstead[2] in 1885. He suggested that, even after the injection of water, the distension of the cell membrane of nerves produces an alteration in nerve transmission, obtaining some kind of anesthesia. This was a brilliant observation 100 years before the advent of tumescence. Then Vishnevsky[44,45] describing an infiltration of 1–2 liters of very diluted novocaine solution 0.25%, coined the phrase "massive creeping infiltration."

How long the action of the anesthesia lasts depends not only on the chemical component of the drug but also on the addition and concentration of epinephrine. If the patient is asleep during surgery, the blood pressure remains low and the vasoconstriction lasts longer. Once the patient is awake, blood pressure rises, the capillaries and arteries open, the absorption of local anesthetic accelerates, and then the liver accelerates the hepatic metabolism of the drugs.

Absorption of local anesthetics

Not all tissues have the same rate of absorption of anesthetics. According to an experimental study in pigs, published in 2001,[33] three areas were studied: (1) the abdomen; (2) the face and neck; and (3) the pectoral areas. In the first part of the study, it was demonstrated that, during an abdominoplasty, a considerable amount of anesthetic is lost (around 50%) in the incision, dissection, and removal of tissues. That is in keeping with our personal clinical experience. In the second part of the study, in which three different areas were injected, the highest absorption levels were found in the thoracic study, where the pectoral muscle was infiltrated. That was very possibly due to the anesthetic distribution into the muscular fibers and at the axilla, where there is a very rich blood supply. The lowest absorption was found in the abdominal study, where the infiltration was performed in the subcutaneous layer. Face and neck absorption levels were in the middle, greater than the abdomen and less than the thorax, perhaps because the tissue involved had a higher blood supply than the abdominal tissue, but less than the pectoral muscle. According to Kenkel et al.,[46] all lipoaspirate analyses showed that 9.1–10.8% (mean, 9.7%) of the infiltrated dose was removed during liposuction. Tissue lidocaine levels below 5 µg/mL were demonstrated in a 4–8-hour microdialysis study.

Vasoconstrictive effect of epinephrine

In small capillaries, after 15 minutes of vasoconstriction, intravascular coagulation occurs. Big vessels bleed, but weakly, then hemostasis is easier and faster. Bleeding rebound is not observed. According to my personal observation, the vasoconstriction of the skin lasts 2–6 hours, depending on the patient's blood pressure.

Toxicity of anesthetics

Toxicity of local anesthetic is related to overdose and intravascular administration. Lidocaine can be used in doses 5 times higher than 7 mg/kg, recommended by the manufacturer when it is used in large dilutions. A solution consisting of 20 mL lidocaine 2% in 800 mL saline solution has a lidocaine concentration of 0.04%. In blood tested during breast reduction surgeries, the highest peak was 0.67 µg/mL[29]; that is because the large dilution of the drug and the vasoconstrictor effect of the epinephrine delay absorption. The peak concentration of lidocaine varied between 0.9 and 3.6 µ/mL and occurred between 6 and 12 hours postoperatively.[47] Epinephrine (1 : 1 000 000) significantly delays the absorption of lidocaine administered by the tumescent technique.[48]

As an alternative to the concept of the tumescent technique, Fodor[49] described the super wet technique that consists of the infiltration of 1 mL of anesthetic solution per 1 mL of aspirated fat, thereby decreasing the total amount of infiltration.

In plastic surgery, we use bupivacaine, usually in the subcutaneous space, mainly diluted and with the addition of epinephrine. Therefore the absorption of diluted bupivacaine in this situation is slow. It has also been argued that, using sedation, the symptoms of toxicity of anesthetic do not appear.

In an attempt to test bupivacaine in blood during large aesthetic surgeries, I sent blood samples to be studied. The lab made several attempts to find this drug in blood, but although the method used can test bupivacaine levels above a level of 35 mg/mL, they were not able to find any trace of the drug in my patients. This is most likely because the large dilution of the drug and the vasoconstrictor effect of the epinephrine delay absorption. Farley et al.[50] also reported that using bupivacaine in the wet solution for liposuction is safe. Frushstorfer et al.[51] and Tolbet Wilkingson (personal communication) reported a mixture of lidocaine–bupivacaine using 50% of the maximum dose of each drug, in this way avoiding overdosing. Tolbet Wilkingson reported having experience in rhytidectomies, breast augmentation, and breast reduction with 6–12 hours of patient comfort without any sign of toxicity of the drug.

In 1997 Joseph Hunstadt[52] reported his experience in injecting the abdominal wall before surgery in a tumescent technique with a very diluted Marcaine solution. Just before the final suturing of the flap, he injected into the areolar and subfacial tissue, at the periphery of the entire dissection, observing that this way is more effective than when injected laterally to the fascial placation. In subpectoral breast augmentation, after completion of the augmentation, through a red Robinson catheter, he administered a dilute Marcaine–epinephrine solution that permeates pocket and literally acts as a regional block. He uses a solution of 30 mL, 0.25% bupivacaine and 100 mL saline solution, using half of the solution in the pocket of each breast. Other surgeons reported similar experiences and results. It was also reported by Jim Carraway (personal communication) that, in abdominoplasty, injecting Marcaine laterally to the medial facial plication provides many hours of pain relief after surgery. Bupivacaine has also been used for some other surgeries, such as pediatric surgery and neurosurgery.[53]

In my experience of more than 4000 cases of major aesthetic procedures using bupivacaine and lidocaine in large dilutions, I have not observed a single case of toxicity of these drugs. When general anesthesia is used, I infiltrate in the same way. The vasoconstriction facilitates the prolongation of the anesthetic effect. I do not think that laying bupivacaine in the layer of the surgical field has the same postoperative analgesic effect than when all tissues are infiltrated with this drug.

Epinephrine

Epinephrine 1:1000 is added to almost all anesthetic solutions. It is always used very diluted and infiltrated in the subcutaneous layer. In liposuction 1/1 000 000 is used. It seems that in liposuction 7.5 mg[54] or 10 mg[55] can be safely used.

The highest peak of absorption is 1–4 hours after infiltration. Because the signs of ephinephrine toxicity are tachycardia, hypertension, and cardiac arrhythmias, patients with a history of tachycardia, hypertension, or cardiac arrythmias should not be infiltrated with this anesthetic solution. Epinephrine peaks are comparable with major physiologic stress or major abdominal surgery. In a study by Brown et al.,[54] the mean epinephrine infiltration was 7.5 mg and the peak of absorption was at 1–4 hours after infiltration local vasoconstriction prolonged the time of absorption.

Carbonated anesthesia

Anesthetic pH is usually 6.4, which produces some pain at the time of infiltration. To avoid this, it has been advocated to add sodium bicarbonate to elevate the pH to 7.4.

The alkaline anesthetic solution was described at the beginning of the past century when Läwen[5,6] and Grös[4] determined that the addition of bicarbonate prolonged the effects of the anesthetic by a factor of 2. If one wants to prolong the anesthetic effect an alkaline anesthetic solution can be used. The effect of the addition of bicarbonate to bupivacaine is unknown.

The pre-emptive effect of local anesthetics

This concept means that the pain can be prevented before it starts. Anticipation of the pain reflex reduces postoperative analgesic medication. Once the spinal reflex of pain starts, even when the patient is under general anesthesia, the incision starts the pain reflex. The infiltration of local anesthetics under the incision lines avoids the initiation of this reflex. Bourget et al.,[56] in a study of 200 consecutive patients undergoing elective laparotomy, were unable to corroborate this theory and concluded that pain was no better controlled with preincisional infiltration than with postincisional infiltration of bupivacaine. This raises the question of the benefit of pre-emptive anesthesia at the local level in long-term postoperative care. Leaving bupivacaine in the area of the dissection seems also to be successful in the control of postoperative pain. The anesthetic action could be produced as a consequence of a single administration of bupivacaine at the end of the procedure, as advocated by Hunstadt[52] and Mahabir et al.,[57] or by an infusion pump, as described by Losken et al.,[58] Baroody et al.,[59] Lu,[60] Pacik et al.,[61] Azmier et al.,[62] and McCarthy et al.[63] The preoperative infiltration and the postoperative administration of bupivacaine are effective in the control of the postoperative pain but it is not clear which of these three procedures provides more effective pain relief/control and better cost-effective patient satisfaction.

The effect of local anesthetic is the consequence of several mechanisms of action: (1) the chemical action in the axon transmision; (2) hydrolic distension of the nerves when some kind of tumescence is injected; and (3) the vasoconstrictor effect of the epinephrine that produces ischemia in the nerves and thus anesthesia and retards the absorption of the anesthetics injected.

The ability to perform abdominal cosmetic surgery in an ambulatory setting provides a more comfortable environment for the patient, eases scheduling for the

physician, and decreases costs. Avoiding the use of general anesthesia allows for quicker recovery, shorter length of hospital stay, and decreased rate of postoperative complications.

Conclusions

For operations using sedation and local anesthesia, patient selection, the selection of appropriate sedation, the anesthetic formula, and the technique of administration as well as the usual dose toxicity of each drug should be carefully considered.

The main concepts used in the administration of local anesthesia are large dilution of drugs, half of the anesthesia is lost during surgery, profuse infiltration facilitates surgery and brings some hours of postoperatory analgesia. Perhaps it takes time to learn but it is highly convenient when the surgeon can avoid the use of myorelaxants, opioids, and the gases of general anesthesia.

With local anesthetic infiltration, surgeries are less demanding, there is less bleeding, and the immediate postoperative period is painfree, which is quite rewarding.

 Access the complete reference list online at **http://www.expertconsult.com**

16. Iverson R. Sedation and analgesia in ambulatory settings. *Plast Reconstr Surg.* 1999;104:1559–1564.

    This is a clinical practice guideline for anesthesia in the setting of outpatient plastic surgery procedures. A practical primer is provided that covers topics ranging from pharmacology to postoperative management.

17. Colon GA, Gubert N. Lorazepam (Ativan) and fentanyl (Sublimaze) for outpatient office plastic surgical anesthesia. *Plast Reconstr Surg.* 1986;78:4.

    This is a clinical practice guideline for anesthesia in the setting of outpatient plastic surgery procedures. A practical primer is provided that covers topics ranging from pharmacology to postoperative management.

21. Vinnik CA. Is there a place for the use of ketamine in plastic and reconstructive surgery? *Ann Plast Surg.* 1980;4:85–87.

    A series of brief correspondence is presented outlining arguments for and against the use of ketamine in outpatient plastic surgery procedures. These pieces highlight the key points a practitioner must consider in deciding whether or not to employ this potent agent.

30. Mottura AA. Local infiltrative anesthesia for transaxillary subpectoral breast implants. *Aesth Plast Surg.* 1995;19:37–39.

    A case series is presented to illustrate the effectiveness of local anesthesia for breast augmentation, and selected breast reconstructive procedures. Technical details of the block are provided, followed by a summary of outcomes.

32. Mottura AA. Local anesthesia for abdominoplasty, liposuction and combined operations. *Aesth Plast Surg.* 1993;17:117–124.

    This report details a technique for local anesthesia in abdominoplasty and liposuction. As most of the infiltrated anesthesia was removed, and the solutions were quite dilute, higher total doses could be safely administered.

52. Hunstadt J. Marcaine induces clinically beneficial analgesia in the inmediate postoperative period. *Aesth Surg J.* 1997;17:269–270.

    This is an essay on the appropriateness of marcaine for use in outpatient plastic surgery procedures. The agent is found to be very effective when used under carefully controlled circumstances, but the possible complications of an IV bolus are quite dire.

10

Evidence-based medicine and health services research in plastic surgery

Carolyn L. Kerrigan, E. Dale Collins Vidal, Andrea L. Pusic, Amy K. Alderman, and Valerie Lemaine

SYNOPSIS

The key take-home messages from this chapter are how to:

- gather existing evidence on outcomes
- interpret evidence on outcomes
- design new studies to add evidence on outcomes
- identify and analyze existing sources of data to create new evidence on outcomes
- capture the patients' perspective on outcomes
- recognize the importance of an essential dimension of evidence: the patients' perspective
- consider the cost dimension in achieving outcomes
- understand the challenges and approaches in translating good evidence into daily clinical practice.

Physicians must make complex decisions in situations of uncertainty – often with incomplete, inaccurate, or outdated information. The goal of outcomes research is to improve the information available to make these complex decisions. It is important to understand that measuring outcomes is not just about the final result of our interventions. More importantly, it is a means by which we gather evidence to improve decision-making, the processes of care, and the systems in which we work. Maximizing patient care and surgical outcomes requires continuous efforts to identify information needs and to produce the best evidence to fulfill these needs.

The best evidence – where do we find it?

There are two ways to obtain best evidence for decision-making to improve the quality of care *(Fig. 10.1)*. The first is to evaluate existing data and identify those reports that are convincing based on a good study design and clinically meaningful outcomes. When the current evidence is inadequate, the second choice is to produce new credible evidence. This section will describe a structure for evaluating existing evidence and then introduce methods for producing best evidence.

Evaluating existing literature

Best evidence requires three things: (1) a good study design; (2) an appropriate statistical analysis; and (3) clinically meaningful outcome measures. In a thorough review, Offer and Perks[1] have enumerated the challenges that plastic surgeons face when trying to practice evidence-based medicine. They cite the lack of quality evidence in our literature as a major factor. Even a superficial perusal of our journals makes it clear that they are replete with descriptions of procedures by individual surgeons and the "outcomes" of those procedures in that surgeon's hands. These studies, known as case reports or case series, have limited applicability to other practices, and are not structured, not compared,

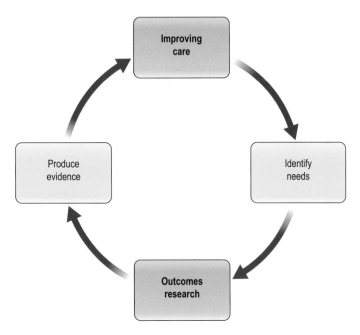

Fig. 10.1 Improved care is linked to better evidence.

and not randomized. This is not only weak evidence on which to make medical decisions, but it is not an acceptable way to make such decisions in this era of healthcare reform and pay for performance (P4P).[2] As shown in Figure 10.1, the stronger the evidence, the better the care one is able to deliver.

Literature search strategies

Practicing evidence-based medicine involves searching for the best available research, appraising the relevant studies for validity, and then translating the evidence to optimize patient care.[3] Many clinical questions remain unanswered because of problems formulating relevant questions, insufficient access to information resources, and a lack of search skills.[4] Today, there are a variety of strategies and web-based resources that allow searches of the relevant literature to answer many clinical questions.[4] Some examples are provided below.

PubMed

The US National Library of Medicine provides access to more than 16 million citations through PubMed, accessing references from MEDLINE and directly from journals.[4] Information from PubMed searches has been shown to improve both patient care and health outcomes significantly.[4]

Clinical Queries

Clinical Queries is a feature of PubMed that can help identify citations with the study design of interest. It is able to link the type of question (e.g., intervention, diagnosis, natural history, and outcome) to a search strategy that specifies the desired study design.[4]

PICO

The critical first step in the pursuit of evidence-based medicine is to ask a well-formulated question.[4] Without sufficient focus and specificity, an otherwise relevant and important clinical question can be mired in irrelevant evidence.[4] When the PICO framework is used with the PubMed Clinical Queries (see above), it has been shown to improve the efficiency of the literature search.[4] The acronym PICO stands for patient problem, intervention, comparison, and outcome, and is a strategy to pose a well-formulated question.[4] In a literature search for evidence in plastic surgery, for example, a question framed using the PICO approach might be expressed this way: In patients undergoing breast reduction (P), preoperative antibiotic prophylaxis (I) versus no prophylaxis (C), what is the rate of postoperative infections (O)?

Meta-analysis

Conceptually, a meta-analysis is the summation of multiple qualitative studies in order to increase the sample size, thus strengthening the conclusions over that which can be drawn from an individual article. This analysis allows researchers to reach a more reliable conclusion when there are conflicting results from multiple studies.[5] Ideally, a meta-analysis is conducted using the highest level of evidence, such as randomized controlled clinical trials. Although meta-analysis can also be conducted on cohort studies and even case series, the quality of the evidence and, therefore, the conclusions are weaker.

Meta-analysis has some disadvantages. First, meta-analysis has been criticized for both overly broad inclusion criteria and, conversely, for overly strict inclusion criteria. Either may result in degradation of the results. Inclusion criteria that are overly broad may lead to inclusion of studies of lesser quality or with less reliable results. Very strict inclusion criteria may mean that the studies that are included have limited generalizability. Another disadvantage is that meta-analyses are costly

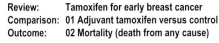

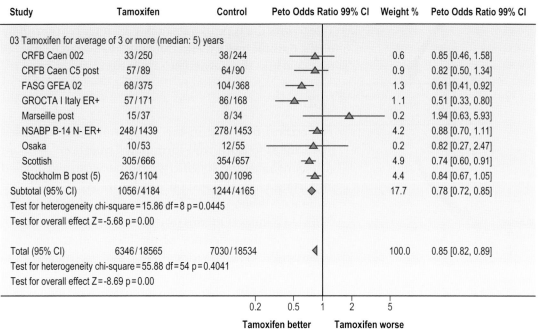

Fig. 10.2 Meta-analysis of randomized controlled trials evaluating the impact of adjuvant tamoxifen on survival risk among women with early breast cancer.[6] Multiple studies have been included, with the findings of each plotted on the central axis. Data are represented as an odds ratio. (Odds ratio, similar to relative risk, reports the proportion of an occurrence to a nonoccurrence.) The summary analysis, which incorporates data from these studies, appears at the bottom of the vertical axis and suggests a benefit for the use of adjuvant tamoxifen in early breast cancer.

and require a significant time commitment from the research team.

The technique of meta-analysis may have limited applicability in plastic surgery, where there are few randomized trials and the metrics from one study to another may vary considerably. An example of a meta-analysis can be seen in *Figure 10.2*.[6] This figure demonstrates an analysis of randomized trials evaluating the impact of tamoxifen on survival. As the reader can observe, there are multiple studies, with the findings of each plotted on a central axis. The summary analysis, which incorporates data from these studies, appears at the bottom of the vertical axis and suggests a benefit for the use of tamoxifen in early breast cancer. As can be seen, the 95% confidence interval for that summary measure is quite narrow. This implies a better point estimate of the true benefit of tamoxifen. Also note that the quality of the individual study is used to determine its weight in computing the summary score.

More recently, researchers conducted a meta-analysis of randomized controlled trials comparing rates of capsular contracture using either smooth or textured

implants. These authors identified seven randomized controlled trials that addressed this issue. Individually four of the seven studies did not find a statistically significant decrease in the rate of contracture with textured implants. However, when the results of the studies were pooled, the meta-analysis suggested that textured implants had lower rates of contracture.[7] To see further examples of good-quality meta-analyses, the reader is referred to the online Cochrane reviews.[8]

Systematic reviews

Systematic reviews are evaluations of the literature conducted according to clearly stated, scientific research methods that are designed to minimize the risk of bias and the errors associated with traditional literature reviews. The review process includes a comprehensive search based on defined criteria and includes a thorough evaluation of the quality and validity of the studies identified in the search process.[9]

The best-known source for systematic reviews is the Cochrane Database of Systematic Reviews, which

contains over 3600 completed reviews.[8] The Cochrane Group also provides a handbook for systematic reviews of interventions which prescribes seven steps for preparing a review:

1. structuring the question
2. identifying possible studies for inclusion
3. evaluation of selected studies
4. data collection and synthesis
5. analyzing results
6. discussion of the findings
7. updating reviews.

Systematic reviews are influential tools in supporting evidence-based practice and some consider them to provide stronger evidence than randomized controlled trials. Moreover, they are essential for summarizing existing data, thereby avoiding the wasted effort that would result from unnecessary duplication of previous studies.[9] To see further examples of good-quality systematic reviews, the reader is referred to the online Cochrane reviews.[8]

Study design and levels of evidence

Broadly, study designs can be divided into experimental and observational studies. Experimental studies, which include randomized controlled clinical trials, patient preference trials, and large, multicenter trials, test a hypothesis by examining the impact of an intervention on the outcome. In contrast, observational studies, which include cohort studies, case-control studies, case series, and case reports, describe the natural history or incidence of disease or analyze associations between risk factors and the outcomes of interest. As one might expect, there is generally a direct correlation between the complexity of a study design and the quality of the resulting data (*Table 10.1*).

Experimental studies

Randomized controlled clinical trials

The randomized controlled clinical trial is perhaps the most complex of the experimental study designs and is the standard to which all others must be held. The design of the randomized controlled trial evolved over

Table 10.1 Levels of evidence

Level of evidence	Type of study	Key features
Level I	Randomized controlled trial	Two randomly selected groups, one serving as a control, with a blinded comparison of outcomes of an intervention
Level II	Prospective and retrospective cohort studies	A single group followed over time and evaluated for risk factors relative to outcome or incidence of disease
Level III	Case-control study	Two groups, one with and one without disease, with a comparison of risk factors relative to outcomes
	Well-designed clinical study	Experimental study design with an intervention and a control arm compared for outcomes
Level IV	Cross-sectional cohort study	A single group evaluated at a single point in time for disease prevalence or risk factors
	Case series	A single group of consecutive cases identified by a disease or condition and followed over time
Level V	Expert opinion	Opinion based on experience and review of literature
	Case reports	A small group identified by a disease or condition and followed over time

Adapted from the American Society of Clinical Oncology.

the course of many years and each component of the design attempts to minimize the influence of study bias and confounders on the results. The ultimate goal is to create a sample population that is truly representative of the whole. In this way, the results of a limited trial can be generalized to the population at large with confidence.

According to the National Institutes of Health, clinical trials are conducted in four phases, each serving a different purpose and helping researchers answer different questions (*Table 10.2*). In phase I, an experimental drug or intervention is evaluated in a small number of test subjects (20–80) to evaluate its safety, determine a dose–response curve, and identify potential side-effects. In phase II, the experimental drug or intervention is given to a larger group of subjects (100–300) to test its effectiveness and further evaluate its safety profile. In

Table 10.2 Four phases of clinical trials	
Phase	Purpose
I	To test an experimental drug or treatment in 20–80 people to evaluate safety, determine a safe dosage range, and identify side-effects
II	To test the experimental drug or treatment in 100–300 people to determine effectiveness and evaluate its safety
III	To test the experimental drug or treatment in 1000–3000 people to confirm effectiveness, monitor side-effects, compare it to commonly used treatments, and collect information to allow for its safe use
IV	Postmarketing studies to learn more about the drug's or treatment's risks, benefits, and optimal use

phase III, the experimental drug or intervention is given to a much larger group of subjects (1000–3000) in order to "confirm its effectiveness, monitor side-effects, compare it to commonly used treatments, and collect information that will allow the experimental drug or treatment to be used safely". In phase IV, postmarketing surveillance is continued to identify additional information on the risks, benefits, and optimal use of the intervention.[10]

Unfortunately, randomized controlled trials are expensive and often impractical to answer questions that compare one surgical intervention to another.[11,12] While patients are often willing to be randomized to take a pill versus a placebo, few are willing to be randomized to one of two surgical procedures or to a sham procedure. Further, surgeons often have a strong preference for one type of surgery over another and are therefore unwilling to randomize patients.[13]

Although the randomized controlled clinical trial is considered the "gold standard," it is not without limitations.[11] For example, the underlying assumptions of randomized controlled clinical trials may be invalid.[11] The preferable treatment between two alternatives may be unclear; evidence of treatment effects from other sources may be insufficient; only specific effects resulting from the intervention are therapeutically valid; and only when the trial's inclusion and exclusion criteria match the characteristics of an individual patient can the outcome of the study be fully transferred to clinical practice.[11] In addition, randomized controlled clinical trials are inadequate to study infrequent or delayed adverse events; they are difficult, if not impossible, to

conduct for the study of rare diseases; and although the benefits and harms of an intervention may be well recognized, its extent or significance is not always well assessed.[12]

Alternatives to randomized controlled clinical trials

In practice randomized controlled clinical trials often pose logistical challenges and ethical problems, which limit sample sizes.[14,15] Therefore, alternatives to randomized controlled clinical trials are needed.

Patient preference trials

When patients or surgeons have strong treatment preferences and refuse randomization, patients may be willing to participate in a preference trial. A preference trial is a trial in which the patient is offered the treatment options rather than random assignment. Patients who have a clear preference are given their preferred treatment while patients without a preference are randomized.[16–18] Thus both randomized and non-randomized patients are studied together under the same protocol other than the treatment assignment.

There are a range of opinions as to the validity and usefulness of this study design. Some researchers believe they complement, rather than replace, randomized controlled clinical trials.[17] Preference trials have been criticized for results that may not be generalizable due to the inherent bias in allowing patients with a strong preference to select their own treatment. Patients who prefer a specific treatment may be more compliant than others who have no such preference. This, and other potential impacts of a patient's preference on actual outcome, is not yet a well-understood bias that can be accounted for. In addition, particularly in small studies, there is the inability to control fully for potential confounders that may differ significantly between treatment groups.[17] Proponents of preference trials believe that subjects who choose their treatment may be more representative of patients in actual clinical practice and that they can provide insights into the patient decision-making process.[16]

Large multicenter trials

When an insufficient number of patients are enrolled in a randomized controlled clinical trial, researchers may choose to use large multicenter trials to increase the sample size.[16] A multicenter controlled clinical trial carries the same requirements as a single-center trial and each site must follow the same protocol, with identical inclusion and exclusion criteria, randomization strategies, interventions, and methods for collecting and evaluating the outcomes.[14] Nevertheless, some researchers have found variability in surgery and surgical techniques in multicenter trials.[16]

Observational studies

Given the difficulty of executing a randomized controlled trial, the next best level of evidence is produced by a good experimental study or well-designed cohort study, with the former having some, but not all, the features of a randomized controlled trial. Although there is widespread belief that observational studies are less valid, often overestimating the magnitude of treatment effects, there are at least several reports suggesting that good observational studies can provide the same level of internal validity as randomized trials.[19,20]

Cohort studies

Cohort studies evaluate a group or cohort at risk for disease. The evaluation may occur over time or at a single point in time. The latter is further described as a cross-sectional cohort study and is often used to collect data on the prevalence of disease. The second common use of cohort studies is to analyze the exposures that put subjects at risk for disease or interventions that reduce that risk. This requires an evaluation of the cohort at a minimum of two points in time. The study may be designed prospectively *(Fig. 10.3)* or retrospectively *(Fig. 10.4)*. In the prospective cohort study, the investigator develops a hypothesis about variables that may impact the outcome under investigation, collects data about those risk factors, and then follows the cohort for development of the outcome of interest. For example, when the association between smoking and lung cancer was suspected, a prospective study design increased the strength of that causal association.

While prospective studies lend credence to causal associations, they are expensive and generally require years of follow-up. Retrospective studies have similar goals, but identify the cohort at risk in the present and investigate the risk factors or exposures that occurred in

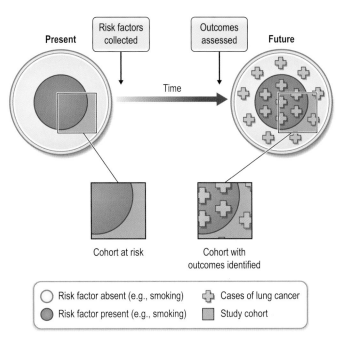

Fig. 10.3 In the prospective cohort study, the investigator develops a hypothesis about variables that may impact the outcome under investigation, collects data about those risk factors, and then follows the cohort for development of the outcome of interest. For example, when the association between smoking and lung cancer was suspected, a prospective study design increased the strength of that causal association. While prospective studies lend credence to causal associations, they are expensive and generally require years of follow-up.

the past. This is often done by subject recall or chart analysis, both of which are flawed when compared to prospective data collection. Data collected in this manner are more likely to be incomplete, inaccurate, inconsistent, or subject to recall bias. On the other hand, the major advantages of retrospective studies are that they can be done in a relatively short timeframe and are much less costly than prospective studies.

Case-control studies

Case-control studies *(Fig. 10.5)* differ from cohort studies in that two distinct groups of subjects are investigated. The first group (case) is selected by the presence of disease and the second (control) by its absence. In contrast, a single population at risk for disease is studied in a cohort design. Like cohort studies, the case-control design may be prospective or retrospective. The major strength of the case-control study is in the investigation of rare conditions or outcomes. Its weakness lies in the inability to assess incidence or prevalence of disease and

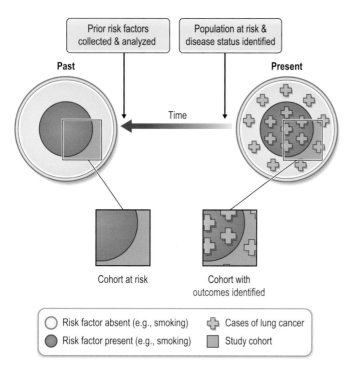

Fig. 10.4 In the retrospective cohort study, the investigator identifies a cohort, collects data about those exposures or risk factors that occurred in the past, and then examines the association between risk factors and outcomes. For example, when the association between smoking and lung cancer was suspected, a retrospective study design supported the hypothesis but failed to show a causal association. In retrospective studies, data collection is often done by subject recall or chart analysis, both of which are flawed when compared to prospective data collection. The major advantages of retrospective studies are that they can be done in a relatively short timeframe and are much less costly than prospective studies.

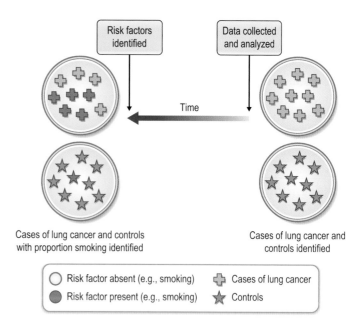

Fig. 10.5 Case-control studies differ from cohort studies in that two distinct groups of subjects are investigated. The first group (case) is selected by the presence of disease and the second (control) by its absence. Like cohort studies, the case-control design may be prospective or retrospective. The major strength of the case-control study is in the investigation of rare conditions or outcomes. Its weakness lies in the inability to assess incidence or prevalence of disease and its increased susceptibility to bias.

its increased susceptibility to bias. Controls may be concurrent or historic, matched (on key variables such as age and sex) or unmatched.

Case series and case reports

As defined above, cases are simply a collection of subjects that have been identified by the presence of a disease or condition. In our literature, these are frequently reported based on a specific intervention. If the collection of subjects is large and consecutive (case series), it may provide valuable information about indications and contraindications for surgery and expected outcomes. If the cases are nonconsecutive (case reports), it raises concerns about sampling bias, such as patient self-selection or surgeon's recall bias, that may dilute the ability of the study to capture the true indications and outcomes. The value of case reports lies in their

ability to report on a new idea, a new surgical approach, and refinement of existing surgical techniques and to communicate rare adverse events.

Large-database analysis

Population-based research

Effectiveness versus efficacy

Evaluating surgical outcomes is necessary to provide high-quality care, patient safety, and informed patient choice. Surgeons must have reliable information about surgical risks and outcomes that can be transferable to their own patient population. Surgical outcomes data from single-surgeon or single-center studies demonstrate the efficacy of a procedure performed by a particular surgeon but do not provide data on the effectiveness of a procedure performed by different surgeons in diverse patient populations.

Clinicians need to have information on an intervention's outcomes under real-world conditions, not just in

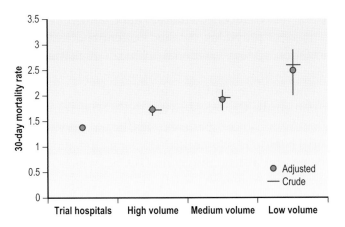

Fig. 10.6 Mortality rates following carotid endarterectomy in patients enrolled in a randomized controlled trial (trial hospitals) compared to those not enrolled in a study and operated on at hospitals with high, medium, and low volumes of endarterectomy cases. (Adapted from Wennberg DE, Lucas FL, Birkmeyer JD, *et al.* Variation in carotid endarterectomy mortality in the Medicare population: trial hospitals, volume and patient characteristics. JAMA 1998;279:1278–1281.)

Table 10.3 Understanding the relationship between sample size and statistics

	Sample size	Number of complications	Complication rate (%)
Large physician group	48 500	1500	3
Plastic surgeons	46	4	8
Difference is not statistically significant			
Large physician group	48 500	1500	3
Plastic surgeons	46	0	0
Difference is not statistically significant			
Large physician group	48 500	1500	3
Plastic surgeons	100	0	0
Difference is not statistically significant			

the optimal setting.[21,22] As we discussed in the prior section, case series and clinical trials performed across a few academic centers are at risk for selection bias, and the results represent outcomes under optimal conditions. National databases, on the other hand, include patients and physicians from all types of healthcare settings, allowing assessment of outcomes in the "real world." This was demonstrated with the randomized clinical trials for carotid endarterectomy procedures *(Fig. 10.6)*.[22] The clinical trials reported a very low mortality rate for these procedures. However, after the clinical trials concluded, the mortality following carotid endarterectomy was substantially higher than that reported in the trials, even among those institutions that participated in the randomized studies. Mortality with carotid endarterectomy was also found to be inversely proportional to a center's volume. Thus, clinical trials generally do not represent real-world surgical outcomes.[22] An alternative, research using a national database, is a population-based approach that provides information on a procedure's effectiveness under real-world conditions rather than just its efficacy in ideal situations.

The importance of power

Adequate sample size is another key component to outcomes research. True differences in outcomes can only be detected when research studies are adequately powered through a large-enough sample size.[23,24] Plastic surgery faces the challenge of being a relatively low-volume group of providers compared to other specialties, such as those treating cardiovascular disease. Outcomes studies with small patient samples are often underpowered and at risk for a type II, or B, error. This statistical error happens when a study does not find a statistically significant difference between treatment groups when a difference truly exists.[25] Chung *et al.* found more than 80% of "negative studies" in the *Journal of Hand Surgery* had powers of less than 0.80 to detect a 25% difference between treatment groups.[26] There is a greater than 20% risk of missing a true difference between treatment groups when a study has less than 0.80 power. The primary reason for the low power among these studies was insufficient sample size.[26] Large-database analyses can provide sufficient sample size to avoid an underpowered study.

Table 10.3 illustrates the importance of an adequate sample size in outcomes research. In this theoretical example, imagine a large group of physicians having performed a cosmetic procedure on 48 500 patients with 1500 complications (3% complication rate). Imagine a small group of plastic surgeons having performed the same procedure on 46 patients, and 4 had a complication (8% complication rate). This is not a statistically significant difference due to the small number of procedures performed by the plastic surgeons. Imagine, in a similar example, the complication rate for the large group of physicians remains at 3% (1500 patients with a complication) and, due to a slight change in sampling, the plastic surgeons had no complications on 46 patients (0% complication rate). This is also not a statistically significant difference because the study was underpowered in regard to the number of patients treated by plastic surgeons. In fact, the study sample could increase to 100 patients for the plastic surgeons with no complications and still there would not have been a statistically significant difference between provider groups.

Data sources

Clinical registries

Large databases in healthcare can be generally described as either a clinical registry or administrative claims data (*Table 10.4*). Clinical registries are designed for the purpose of collecting clinical data and have the advantage of providing detailed patient and treatment information. Many national clinical registries are disease-specific, such as Surveillance Epidemiology and End Results (SEER) registry and the National Comprehensive Cancer Network (NCCN) that monitor outcomes in cancer patients. Plastic surgery has a national clinical registry called Tracking Operations and Outcomes for Plastic Surgeons (TOPS), which is supported by the American Society of Plastic Surgeons and the American Board of Plastic Surgery. The primary purpose of TOPS is to facilitate monitoring the quality of surgical care in plastic surgery. These types of clinical registries can be invaluable to researchers who are interested in studying patient populations that may not be captured in claims data, such as younger patients not captured in Medicare or the self-pay cosmetic patients. Researchers should be aware of the potential limitations

Table 10.4 Examples of clinical registries and administrative claims data

Data source	Description
Clinical registries	
Surveillance, Epidemiology and End Results (SEER) registry	Sponsored by the National Cancer Institute and collects data on cancer incidence and survival for approximately 26% of the US population[146]
National Comprehensive Cancer Network (NCCN)	Alliance of the leading cancer centers in the US that are dedicated to improving the quality of cancer care[147]
National Surgical Quality Improvement Program (NSQIP)	Program is sponsored by the American College of Surgeons and includes academic and private-sector hospitals which desire to participate. Data include inpatient and outpatient visits among patients undergoing major surgical procedures[148]
Tracking Operations and Outcomes for Plastic Surgeons (TOPS)	Program is sponsored by the American Society of Plastic Surgeons, the Plastic Surgery Educational Foundation, and the American Board of Plastic Surgery. Board-certified plastic surgeons may participate. Inpatient and outpatient data are collected[149]
Administrative claims data	
State–federal partnerships	State healthcare organizations submit datasets to the Agency for Healthcare and Research Quality[150]
State Inpatient Database Nationwide Inpatient Sample Kids Inpatient Database State Ambulatory Surgery Database	
Medicare[151]	
Part A Part B	Inpatient hospital discharge abstracts Outpatient claims data
Veterans Affairs (VA) data	
Patient Treatment File (PTF) Outpatient Care Files (OCF)	Inpatient hospital discharge abstracts Outpatient visits at VA-based clinics
CosmetAssure[152]	Insurance company that covers complications related to cosmetic surgery

of data sources. For example, the SEER registries only capture information within the first 4 months of initial treatment, and the TOPS database relies on voluntary physician-reported data. However, a recent study supports the validity of the TOPS database.[27]

Administrative claims data

Administrative data, also known as "claims data" or "discharge data," are collected for billing purposes and lack detailed patient information found in clinical registries. The data are available from several different sources, including hospitals, states, and payers. The content usually represents only one episode of care, unlike a clinical registry. The data are commonly in a uniform format called a hospital discharge abstract, which includes: a patient identifier, hospital identifier, demographic information (age, gender, race, payer), admission acuity (emergent, urgent, elective), length of stay, hospital charges, discharge status (death, transfer, extended care, home), primary/secondary diagnoses and procedures. Outcomes data from administrative sources are generally limited to mortality, length of stay, and charges. Data accuracy is better for primary procedure codes, diagnosis codes, demographics, and outcomes and less accurate for secondary diagnoses, which makes risk adjustment difficult.

It is not possible to use claims data to evaluate cosmetic procedures since these procedures are self-pay. Researchers have used information from CosmetAssure to evaluate cosmetic surgery outcomes.[27] CosmetAssure is an insurance policy sold nationally that covers medical and surgical complications from cosmetic surgery. There is a financial incentive to report a covered complication. However, clinical outcomes collected in the database are limited.

How to use large databases for research

Administrative data can be a good starting point for a research project since the data are readily available and often inexpensive. The data source can also provide a large sample size that can help when studying a rare event or condition. The research question must take advantage of the strengths of the data for the project to be successful. Advantages of administrative data include population-based data that can be used to assess regional variations in care, real-world outcomes, and epidemiological trends.

Small-area variation

Prior to the 1970s, the rate of surgery for a population could not be determined, and data were limited to the number of cases performed at a given institution or by a specific surgeon. In 1973, Wennberg and Gittelsohn published a method for estimating the population served by a medical center, which allowed for the first time the calculation of procedure rates (e.g., the number of tonsillectomies per 100 000 people served).[28,29] We now know that certain surgical procedures demonstrate wide and unexplained variations in regional and national rates (e.g., hysterectomy, prostatectomy, cesarean section) whereas other procedures are performed at similar rates (e.g., appendectomy, cholecystectomy). In general, those procedures whose risks and benefits are well established exhibit the least variability. Procedures with high variability suggest that the optimum management has yet to be established or adopted. Although small-area variations allow us to make observations about differences in procedure rates, they do not help explain these variations or tell us which rate is right. What it does suggest is that a more definitive evaluation needs to be undertaken to identify the optimal treatment strategy.[30] The Dartmouth Atlas of Health Care is one of the best examples of how to use administrative data to examine variations in the rates of surgery in the US using data from the national Medicare database, provider files, and American Hospital Association.[31]

Volume–outcome analysis

Another field of investigation that falls under the broad heading of large-database analysis is the area of volume–outcome studies. There is growing evidence to suggest that surgical outcomes are better at high-volume institutions.[32] The reason may in part be due to the skill of the surgeon but also reflects the hospital and systems that support a given population of patients. A landmark paper by Birkmeyer et al.[33] described a significant correlation between surgeon volume and operative mortality in the US using Medicare data. Another example is the work by Roohan et al.[34] on the 5-year survival of patients with breast cancer treated at low-, moderate-,

Table 10.5 Volume–outcome association for 5-year survival after breast cancer treatment

Hospital volume	Breast cancer cases/year	5-year survival risk ratio
Very low	1–10	1.60
Low	11–50	1.30
Moderate	51–150	1.19
High	>150	1.00

(Adapted from Roohan PJ, Bickell NA, Baptiste MS, et al: Hospital volume differences and five-year survival from breast cancer. Am J Public Health 1998;88:454–457.)

and high-volume centers (**Table 10.5**). This work shows that there is as much as a 30% difference in the 5-year survival between low- and high-volume hospitals.

Large cohort studies

Large-database analysis has played a key role in cohort studies. This allows relatively rare events to be analyzed with a large sample size, giving greater statistical significance and power to the analysis. It often involves linking multiple databases to examine risk factors or exposures relative to outcomes. The outcomes measured most often are mortality and cancer, as both are frequently tracked through various regional and national registries.

Epidemiology

Large databases are also useful tools to evaluate trends over time in surgical utilization and outcomes for a population. For example, the Nationwide Inpatient Sample was used to document a dramatic increase in the use of bariatric surgery in the US.[35] The national SEER database has been used to assess sociodemographic differences in receipt of postmastectomy breast reconstruction[36] and assess trends in the use of breast reconstruction after the Women's Health and Cancer Rights Act.[37] These studies found that the overall use of breast reconstruction across the US is low, that race/ethnicity is a significant predictor of receipt of postmastectomy reconstruction, and that the use of reconstruction did not increase significantly after the passing of the federal law that mandated insurance coverage of these procedures.

Examples of large-database analyses in plastic surgery

Many large national and state databases have had limited applications for plastic surgeons.[38,39] The most obvious reason is that many of the procedures performed by plastic surgeons are not captured in these databases. For example, the Medicare database captures only patients older than 65 years who use Medicare as the primary payment mechanism.

Two authors have made an effort to use these databases to garner information on small-area variations useful to plastic surgeons. Gittelsohn and Powe used data from the state of Maryland to compare rates of elective surgery, such as septoplasty, rhinoplasty, reduction mammoplasty, and blepharoplasty.[40] Significant variations were noted in rates of surgery. Explanatory variables were explored, and the authors concluded that income and race were significant predictors of surgery. Keller et al. have looked at variations in the rate of surgery for carpal tunnel syndrome in the state of Maine.[41] They were able to identify a 3.5-fold difference in rates, and the authors concluded that the major driving factor is physician decision-making. We do not know the "right" rate of carpal tunnel surgery, but the data provided by studies such as this will enable us to begin to ask the appropriate questions.

Large databases have provided the source for cohort investigations on the relationship between breast reduction and a reduced risk for development of breast cancer. Boice et al.[42] identified breast reduction patients in Sweden using hospital discharge data and linked with Swedish registries for cancer, death, and emigration and compared results with expected breast cancer incidence in the general population using the Swedish Nationwide Cancer Registry. The investigators found that women 7.5 years after reduction mammaplasty were at a statistically significant 28% decreased risk of cancer. The NCCN database has been used to evaluate the association between postmastectomy breast reconstruction and the delivery of adjuvant chemotherapy for breast cancer patients.[43] The authors found that immediate-postmastectomy breast reconstruction does not appear to lead to omission of chemotherapy, but it is associated with a modest, but statistically significant, delay in initiating treatment. For most, it is unlikely that this modest delay has any clinical significance. Regarding cosmetic

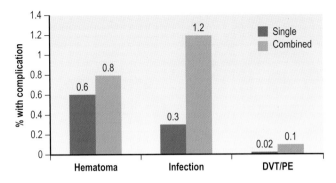

Fig. 10.7 The graph displays differences in overall complications for breast augmentation between single and combined procedures in the Tracking Operations and Outcomes for Plastic Surgeons database. Complications for combined procedures represent overall rates of a complication and cannot be assigned to a particular procedure. The rates of all the complications between single and combined procedures were significantly different ($P < 0.01$) using Pearson chi-square. DVT, deep venous thrombosis; PE, pulmonary embolism.

procedures, the TOPS and CosmetAssure databases have been used to assess outcomes with abdominoplasty and breast augmentation procedures.[27] The low complication rates found in this study support the safety of these procedures when performed by plastic surgeons. However, the authors stress that surgeons should be aware of the overall higher complication rates associated with combining breast augmentation with other procedures *(Fig. 10.7)*. In summary, these represent just a few examples of the potential use of large databases in plastic surgery research.

Patient-reported outcomes research

Definition of terms

In plastic surgery research, attention is increasingly being placed on understanding the patient's perception of the surgical result and the impact that surgery has on quality of life (QoL). To appraise and demonstrate the benefits of a chosen surgical technique or alternate treatment adequately, it is important for plastic surgeons to understand the available approaches to measurement of patient-reported outcomes (PRO).

Patient satisfaction and QoL may be measured using specially designed questionnaires, known as PRO measures. This term applies specifically to a questionnaire used in a clinical or research setting where responses are collected directly from patients. These questionnaires quantify QoL and/or significant outcome variables

(e.g., patient satisfaction, symptoms) from the patient's perspective. PRO instruments provide a means of gaining insight into the way patients perceive their health and the impact treatments have on their QoL. A good PRO measure should evaluate the impact of disease, trauma, surgical or nonsurgical intervention on various aspects of a patient's day-to-day life in a manner that is scientifically sound and clinically meaningful.[44]

In plastic surgery research, many of the PRO measures frequently employed in studies to evaluate surgical outcomes have not been developed and validated using acknowledged guidelines.[44–47] Such PRO measures are considered *ad hoc* questionnaires, and although they may pose clinically reasonable questions, one cannot be confident about their reliability (ability to produce consistent and reproducible scores) or validity (ability to measure what is intended to be measured). The use of such measures, however, has been extensive in plastic surgery. As an example, in a systematic review to identify PRO measures developed for use with breast surgery patients, our team identified 65 *ad hoc* measures.[45]

PRO measures that can be used in any patient group regardless of their health condition are called "generic questionnaires," which allow direct comparisons across disease groups, or between sick and healthy groups. These measures can provide important information for health policy decisions. For example, research using the Short Form 36 (SF-36) – the most widely used generic measure in the world[48] – with breast reduction patients shows that women report clinically important differences in QoL compared with women in the general population.[49–52] In the US, breast reduction is a procedure for which health insurance companies frequently dispute payment; it is thus useful to place the health burden experienced by women with breast hypertrophy into the context of patients with other medical conditions (e.g., women with hip or knee osteoarthritis seeking joint replacement).

However, there are limitations associated with the use of generic measures. Given their generic nature, they sometimes lack sensitivity to the particular concerns of a patient group. For instance, the SF-36, which measures physical, emotional, and social functioning, does not include questions about sexuality, body image, or satisfaction with breast appearance, which are clearly important concerns of breast reduction patients.[53]

Generic measures, like the SF-36, may then not evaluate the most important issue for a particular patient group. Disease- or condition-specific questionnaires address problems specific to a single disease or treatment group. Such measures, when developed through indepth patient interviews, can help to identify issues of importance to a specific group of patients. As these measures include content areas that are more relevant to a given patient group, they are more likely than generic measures to be sensitive to measuring changes in specific aspects of health. However, in general they cannot be used to make comparisons across different patient groups.

An additional challenge is that, in plastic surgery, there are many areas for which condition-specific instruments have been either inadequately developed or not developed at all.[45–47] This situation is rapidly being remedied with the development of new plastic surgery-specific questionnaires. As an example, the BRAVO study,[54] which evaluated the effectiveness of breast reduction surgery, was conducted in 2001 using the Breast Reduction Symptoms Questionnaire. This questionnaire only provided an evaluation of symptom relief. Since then, the science of PRO measurement has evolved and new measures, such as the BREAST-Q,[55] provide a comprehensive appraisal, including satisfaction with breast appearance and psychosocial well-being.

Essential elements for PRO measures

PRO measures must be clinically meaningful and scientifically sound. A questionnaire that is clinically meaningful addresses those issues considered important to patients and their surgeons. Scientific soundness refers to the demonstration of reliable, valid, and responsive measurement of the outcome of interest. A reliable measure yields consistent and reproducible results of the same measure. Reliability is an important property of a PRO measure because it is essential to establish that any changes observed between patient groups are due to the intervention or disease, and not to problems in the measure *(Fig. 10.8)*. Test–retest reliability may be evaluated by having individuals complete questionnaires on more than one occasion over a time period when no changes in outcome are expected to have occurred. The degree to which individual responses

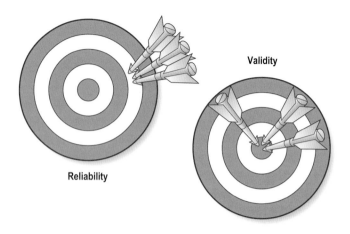

Fig. 10.8 Reliability and validity. The quality of any standardized survey is judged by its reliability and validity. The reliability is traditionally measured by test–retest; the validity is a measure of accuracy. Looking at it simplistically, reliability is the ability to hit the same spot repeatedly on the target, whereas validity is the ability to hit the bull's eye repeatedly.

remain the same is reported statistically as Cronbach's alpha[56] and intraclass correlation coefficients.[57]

Validity is the ability of an instrument to measure what is intended to be measured *(Fig. 10.8)*. The distinction between reliability and validity is important because, just as reliability does not imply validity, the inverse is also true. That is, a reliable measure will always yield the same score, but it may not be valid, as it may not necessarily measure what it is meant to be measuring. Establishment of validity may be considered an ongoing process. The measure is looked at from various perspectives, including an assessment of the development process, consideration of known group differences, evaluation of internal consistency and of convergent and discriminant validity relative to other existing measures.

Responsiveness is defined as the ability of a measure to detect significant change accurately. If a PRO measure is used to evaluate changes as the result of a surgical procedure or to follow patients over time, the measure must be sensitive to change. Responsiveness is examined by measuring outcomes before and after an intervention, and evaluating the measure's sensitivity to change.

Overview of PRO measure development

To choose a QoL measure for use in a study or in clinical practice, prospective users should take into account the process used to develop PRO measures. Knowing how a PRO measure was developed is crucial to choosing an appropriate measure. Not infrequently, researchers choose questionnaires based simply on whether or not they have been "validated" and ask few questions about how the items for the questionnaire were constructed and tested. A poorly constructed or *ad hoc* questionnaire may be deemed "validated" simply because it has been used in various studies and some basic statistical evidence has been supplied. Frequent use of a questionnaire does not equate with quality nor improve its psychometric properties. Rather, to ensure that a PRO measure will ultimately prove to be a reliable, responsive, and valid measure, a rigorous step-by-step development process is essential. During the development process, careful qualitative work is necessary to conceptualize, map out, and operationalize the variables most relevant to patients. PRO measures that are developed based on expert opinion alone cannot be expected to address all satisfaction and QoL issues that patients find relevant. Thus, while expert opinion is clearly valuable, patient interviews and focus groups are essential sources of information.

Since the early 1990s, there has been increasing international consensus regarding appropriate methods for the development and validation of QoL measures, culminating with the 2002 report by the Scientific Advisory Committee of the Medical Outcomes Trust[58] and more recently with the US Food and Drug Administration recommendations.[59] Cano *et al.*[44] summarized these guidelines in a three-step approach to PRO measure development that involves procedures for item generation, item reduction, and psychometric evaluation. We have added a fourth step representing the ongoing process of instrument improvement *(Fig. 10.9)*.

In the first step, the conceptual model to be measured is formally defined, and a pool of items is generated. These items for a PRO measure are developed through the following three sources: review of the literature, qualitative patient interviews, and expert opinion. The item pool is developed into a questionnaire which is pretested or pilot-tested on a small sample of patients in order to clarify ambiguities in item wording, confirm appropriateness, and determine acceptability and completion time.

In the second step, the PRO measure is field-tested using a large sample of patients. The questions that represent the best indicators of outcome are then

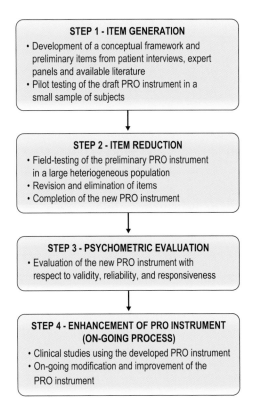

Fig. 10.9 Four steps of patient-reported outcome (PRO) measure development.

retained in a shortened version of the PRO measure based on their performance against a standardized set of psychometric criteria. The research team's objective is to choose the best items from the field test measure for inclusion in the final measure. Items are eliminated according to tests of item redundancy, endorsement frequencies, missing data, factor analysis, and scaling assumptions. The item reduction process completes questionnaire development.

In the third step, a psychometric evaluation study is performed. This step involves the administration of the item-reduced questionnaire to a large population of patients to determine acceptability, reliability, validity, and responsiveness.

The fourth and final step involves the ongoing modification and improvement of the instrument. As an example, building upon the existing four modules of the BREAST-Q, a new procedure-specific module is currently being developed for breast-conserving therapy (BCT) patients. This module will facilitate comparisons between treatment groups (e.g., BCT versus mastectomy and reconstruction) and evaluations of new surgical approaches (e.g., oncoplastic surgery, fat grafting).

Our research group's development of the BREAST-Q illustrates how new PRO measures can be constructed.[55] In phase I, a conceptual framework to understand patient satisfaction and QoL in breast surgery patients was developed and included six domains: satisfaction with breasts, overall outcome, and process of care, and psychosocial, physical, and sexual well-being. Our team developed this conceptual framework and set of items to measure each component of the framework using indepth interviews and focus groups with patients, expert panels with plastic surgeons, and a review of the literature.[55] We then performed pilot testing and cognitive debriefing to ensure that our PRO measure addressed all relevant issues and that the items were acceptable to patients and easily understood. In phase II, we performed an extensive multicenter field test with 1950 patients. Based on these data, item reduction and scale development were performed using modern psychometric methods. In this process, approximately 60% of the items were deleted. In phase III, the item-reduced measure (BREAST-Q) was completed by a large sample of breast surgery patients ($n = 1283$), and the data were examined to determine how the measure performed. More specifically, targeting, reliability, convergent validity, discriminant validity, and responsiveness were examined.

Modern psychometric methods

The science underpinning the testing of the attributes of reliability, validity, and responsiveness is known as psychometrics. The most commonly used form of scale evaluation, and the one most familiar to surgeons, is based on traditional psychometric methods.[58] However, in recent times, researchers have become aware of the limitations of these methods and are now moving to newer techniques. As such, modern psychometric methods such as Rasch measurement[60] and item response theory (IRT)[61] are increasingly being used in the development of PRO measures. Rasch and IRT methods were first developed for use in educational testing. While traditional psychometric techniques provide ordinal-level data, Rasch analysis provides interval-level data.[60] Ordinal-level data provides only a rank order (e.g., first, second, third). In contrast, with interval-level data, one unit on the scale represents the same magnitude measured across the whole range of the scale (e.g., degrees Celsius). This improves the accuracy with which we can measure clinical change. In addition, these methods provide estimates for patients (and items) that are independent of the sampling distribution of items (and patients). Among other benefits, this allows for accurate estimates suitable for individual-person measurement. This can help to inform patient monitoring, management, and treatment directly. Other advantages include item banking, scale equating, computerized scale administration, and the handling of missing data.[62,63]

In the coming years, one may expect that these newer, more clinically amenable techniques will supersede traditional approaches to developing and testing PRO measures. Additionally in the near future, one may anticipate that electronic capture of PRO data will become widespread. As web access becomes more prevalent throughout the world, it will be possible for patients to complete questionnaires via the internet, which will allow for real-time reports. This has important implications for how PRO data may be used to inform clinical care. For research studies, the collection of ePRO data is also attractive as costs per patient are potentially reduced.

Utilities and preference-based measures

Key concepts

While PRO measures can provide valuable information on the way patients perceive their health and the impact treatments have on their QoL and other significant outcome variables, these measures do not incorporate patient preferences in their scoring systems.

"Preference" is a broad term used to describe the concept of desirability of a set of outcomes.[64] Values and utilities are two different types of preferences, depending on which method is utilized to measure the preferences: values are measured under conditions of certainty (rating scale, time tradeoff method), whereas utilities are measured under conditions of uncertainty (standard gamble method).[64] Hence, a value or utility is a measure of preference for a particular health state or health service: the more preferable an outcome, the more value or utility is associated with it. The most common

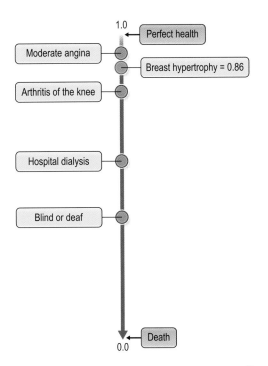

Fig. 10.10 Comparison of health states on a common utility scale. Utilities range from 0 to 1, where 0 represents death and 1 represents perfect health. Utilities differ from standard questionnaires in that they quantify quality of life with a single measure that encompasses the physical, psychological, and cultural preferences of the patient. This permits comparison between patients and across different diseases on a common scale.

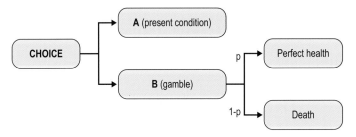

Fig. 10.11 Utility assessment with the standard gamble technique. In standard gambles, patients are asked to make a choice between two alternatives. One alternative is to remain in their current health, and the other is to accept a gamble with a chance of success and failure. The chances of success and failure are varied systematically until the point of indifference between the two choices is reached. The probability of success at this point of indifference is the utility value. Typically, the worse the perceived health of the patient, the lower the utility.

preference metric used is quality-adjusted life years (QALYs).

QALYs represent a measure of the dollar cost of a year of life if a person suffers one or more limitations of various kinds and degrees, taking into account both QoL and life expectancy.[65] QALYs can be estimated using a variety of evaluation tools such as the standard gamble, the time trade-off, or visual analog scales.[65,66] Preference-based measures incorporate the strength of patients' preference for the condition or disease, and the units of measurement range from 0.0 (i.e., death) to 1.0 (i.e., perfect health), the idea being that a year in perfect health is worth more to the patient than a year spent with a disability (*Fig. 10.10*). Importantly, some health states may be considered worse than death and thus have negative scores. Preference-based instruments thus take into account values and/or utilities in addition to QoL, and can be used in economic evaluations to aid resource allocation decisions.[67]

There are two general approaches to measuring values and utilities. The first involves use of preference classification systems in which responses to a generic health status instrument are converted to a value or utility. This conversion is computed by an algorithm developed from population-based responses. Widely used preference classification systems include the Quality of Well-Being Scale,[68,69] the McMaster Health Utilities Index,[70–72] and EuroQol.[73,74] Whereas preference classification systems are useful to study general health status and population health, they may not capture adequate information about specific conditions or individual patient preferences.

The second approach to measuring values and utilities is to assess them directly. Several techniques may be used, including a visual analog scale, time trade-off, and standard gamble.[66] The standard gamble is considered to adhere most closely to the von Neumann–Morgenstern utility theory. In this technique, patients are asked to make a choice between two alternatives. One alternative is to remain in their current health state, and the other is to accept a gamble with a chance of success or failure (*Fig. 10.11*). The chances of success and failure are varied systematically until the point of indifference between the two choices is reached. The probability of success at this point of indifference represents the value or utility estimate. Typically, the worse the perceived health of the patient, the lower the value or utility score (*Fig. 10.10*). Whereas the concept of preference assessment holds great promise for plastic surgery,[75,76] measurement of values and utilities is an evolving science. Controversy exists as to the gold-standard technique for measurement, and alternative techniques may give slightly different results.[77,78]

Comparative effectiveness analysis

Definition

The primary purpose of comparative effectiveness research (CER) is to facilitate value-based medicine, which is the practice of medicine based on the value conferred by a healthcare intervention. Depending on the definition used, CER may or may not have a cost component in the analysis.[79] The total value or utility gained is measured in QALYs and calculated by multiplying the years of utility gain by years of benefit duration. This total gain, or comparative effectiveness, can be compared with that of any healthcare intervention, no matter how disparate. The concept of CER in healthcare is similar to the consumer rating reports by Zagats for restaurants and consumer reports for cars.[80]

There is currently no standard definition for CER. Most researchers use the following definition for comparative effectiveness by the Institute of Medicine: "Comparative effectiveness research is the generation and synthesis of evidence that compares the benefits and harms of alternative methods to prevent, diagnose, treat and monitor a clinical condition, or to improve the delivery of care. The purpose of comparative effectiveness research is to assist consumers, clinicians, purchasers, and policy makers to make informed decisions that will improve healthcare at both the individual and population levels."[81] The analytic tools for data collection can include systematic reviews of evidence, modeling, retrospective analyses of databases, and prospective trials.[80] Controversy surrounds the use of randomized controlled trials for CER because the research setting should demonstrate an intervention's outcome under "real-world" situations rather than under optimal conditions (as demonstrated in *Fig. 10.6*).[80] However, the Institute of Medicine's definition of CER does not reject the inclusion of randomized controlled trials.[80,82]

National research priority

Reforming the national health system is a top priority for health policy leaders and the key aim is to control healthcare costs without impairing quality. Regional variations in treatment patterns and cost growth support the need for more informed medical decision-making.[82] Many believe that this goal will only be reached if we have better evidence to inform healthcare decisions. Better evidence can improve quality, safety, and the effectiveness of healthcare by providing both patients and providers with the information needed to make healthcare choices.[82] As a result, Congress has allocated $1.1 billion as a down payment for a national program of CER. As of this writing, the House of Representatives and the Senate Finance Committee have proposals supporting a national program of CER.[83]

Complexities

Whose perspective to take?

A variety of perspectives can be taken when examining the value of a healthcare procedure, ranging from the individual to society. The four most common perspectives evaluated are societal, patient, employer, and payer.[80] The societal perspective includes all of the benefits and costs associated with a treatment for the whole of society, rather than for just one individual patient. This type of analysis includes societal components such as work productivity and caregiver costs.[80,84] The patient perspective only includes the costs and benefits of a treatment that impact the individual patient. Any increased productivity that would benefit a company or workplace situation would not be included. Productivity that directly benefited the individual would be counted. Costs included would be those paid out of pocket by the individual and costs related to travel and time off work.[80,84]

An employer perspective only includes the benefits and costs of a treatment that impacts the employer. Any benefit from increased productivity by the employee is included. In addition, any tangential increased productivity is included, such as decreased sick leave from the other employees as a result of a vaccination. Costs included are out-of-pocket costs for the employer and lost productivity as a result of employee absenteeism.[80,84]

The payer perspective includes the benefits and costs of a treatment that impact a payer only. Benefits to the individual are not included. Increased productivity to the individual or society is not included. The time horizon used to calculate the benefits and costs is the expected length that the individual will participate in the insurance plan.[80,84]

Types of economic studies

CER may or may not include cost when comparing treatments. However, there are five primary economic analyses in healthcare that compare treatments by costs and outcomes and differ primarily by how outcomes are measured. Firstly, cost–benefit analysis compares the net costs and net benefits of two treatments. Outcomes must be converted to monetary units, such as willingness to pay. The results are typically expressed as dollars expended for dollars gained.[84,85] Secondly, cost-effectiveness analysis (CEA) measures the cost associated with two or more medical interventions for a given health state to determine the relative value of one intervention over the other. With CEA, the healthcare provider is looking to answer the following question: "what are the costs associated with the different treatment options available to achieve this goal?"[65] In a CEA, the health effects are measured in natural units directly related to the goal of interest associated with the intervention. For example, the measure of primary effectiveness can be expressed in terms of "cost per unit of effect," where the effect can be the cost of life-years saved by kidney transplantation compared to dialysis,[80,84,85] the average blood pressure decrease in mmHg, or the number of successful replantations.[86] Thirdly, cost–utility analysis (CUA) was developed to address the limitations of CEA. It has emerged in recent years as the preferred method for economic evaluations in healthcare because both the QoL and length of life must be assessed.[65,80,84–87] Overall, CUA and CEA share similarities from the cost analysis perspective. However, they differ in terms of outcomes: in CEA, outcomes are single and specific to the medical intervention under study; in CUA, outcomes can be single or multiple, and, most importantly, consider the notion of preference.[64] The analysis produces a cost per QALY for the intervention that can be compared to other procedures. Fourthly, cost consequence analysis does not convert outcomes to a common metric but instead lists all of the consequences of the treatment.[80,84] Lastly, cost minimization analysis is used to compare the costs of procedures when the outcomes are identical. This approach is rarely performed because two procedures usually have something different in regard to issues such complication rates, pain, and time of recovery.[80,84,85]

A controversial issue is whether costs are appropriate outcomes in CER. The primary justification for including costs is that the overall value of an intervention can be easily understood in economic terms.[82] However, CER may conclude that the more expensive treatment has the best value. An example is breast cancer screening in patients with BRCA genetic mutations. In a study by Plevritis et al., magnetic resonance imaging screening was found to be cost-effective relative to mammography.[88] CER looks at the benefits, not just the costs, and therefore identifies the treatment with the best value, not necessarily the one with the lowest cost.[82]

Study design

As previously discussed, there are two broad categories of research design: experimental and observational studies. Observational research has many advantages, such as speed, real-world decision, large sample sizes, and low cost. Experimental studies, such as randomized clinical trials, can overcome some of the limitations of observational studies by randomly assigning patients to different interventions, thereby controlling for known and unknown confounding factors. The Institute of Medicine's recommendations are for the national CER program to develop large-scale, clinical and administrative data networks to facilitate the use of observational and experimental data to inform CER.[83]

Limitations

There are several potential limitations to the implementation of CER in healthcare. For one, there is no standard definition for comparative effectiveness. It is also unclear what impact this type of research will have on healthcare since many providers do not incorporate this type of information into medical decision-making. Population-based study results may not be applicable to individual patient needs. Patient treatment self-selection may also affect comparative effectiveness results. A study that finds no statistically significant difference in treatment outcomes does not necessarily mean that there is no difference in outcomes. The lack of statistical significance may be due to a design flaw, such as an underpowered study or flaws in the study design. Furthermore, different perspectives such as societal, patient, and employer may have different results. It is important to understand that CER helps to inform a medical decision but does not provide a simple "one size fits all" answer.[80]

Summary

The primary reason for the interest by patients, providers, and health policy leaders in CER is the belief that better information will translate into better decisions and improved health outcomes. The long-term impact of these efforts will depend on healthcare reform legislation, the medical profession's ability to encourage physicians to change practices, and patients' willingness to participate in shared medical decision-making.[83]

Future trends

Multicenter clinical trials network

When choosing a treatment option for their patients, plastic surgeons use many sources of information to determine best practice. Understandably, surgeons tend to rely in large part on their training and personal experience. Outcome studies reporting "single-surgeon experience" have traditionally predominated in the plastic surgery literature. While such series are of some value, their findings are not necessarily generalizable to other settings (e.g., lower-volume practices).

One of the more powerful forces in shaping best practice is the randomized clinical trial. However, in certain settings, single-center trials may be difficult to conduct because of limitations in sample size and resources. One way of preserving the clinical relevance of a trial is to have multiple institutions enroll, treat, and follow patients under a common study protocol. This approach also increases the heterogeneity of the population, which may ultimately lead to study findings that are more generalizable and relevant. This heterogeneity may however make it more difficult to detect treatment differences. Compared to a single-center trial, a treatment effect may be more difficult to detect in a multi-center trial. However, those effects that are detected are likely to be more convincing than those found in a single, homogeneous population.

To facilitate such studies, the Plastic Surgery Education Foundation has recently established the Clinical Trials Network. While still in its infancy, this initiative provides a mechanism by which plastic surgeons across the country may collaborate and contribute to the advancement of clinical knowledge. The most compelling example of the value of multicenter clinical trials in plastic surgery is the Venous Thromboembolism Prevention Study. In this study, performed under the direction of the Network, five high-volume plastic surgery centers have adopted a common protocol for perioperative chemoprophylaxis of deep venous thrombosis. The incidence of venous thromboembolism is being prospectively evaluated and will be compared with the incidence of events occurring in a retrospective cohort of patients who did not receive prophylaxis. Data from this study will inform national recommendations for chemoprophylaxis, support the practice of evidence-based medicine and, ultimately, improve patient safety. One important barrier to multicenter trials in plastic surgery is the cost.

Knowledge translation

As clinical research in plastic surgery continues to advance rapidly, information overload is a constant challenge for surgeons. Incorporation of research findings into plastic surgery practice currently relies on publications in peer-reviewed journals and educational activities such as continuing medical education (CME) and continuing professional development (CPD). Because of their passive nature, CME and CPD have had limited effects on modifying physicians' practice. Discrepancies or care gaps remain between what is recognized as evidence-based practice and the care provided in everyday plastic surgery practice. Moreover, patients may be receiving potentially harmful or unproven medical and surgical interventions. In a 2001 report entitled, *Crossing the Quality Chasm: A New Health System for the 21st Century*,[89] the Institute identified three main gaps in quality of care: medical error, overuse, and underuse. As an example, despite evidence that the risk of deep venous thrombosis is particularly high for patients undergoing combined abdominoplasty and liposuction, only 60% of plastic surgeons report use of thromboprophylaxis all the time.[90]

The Canadian Institutes for Health Research (CIHR) is responsible for coining the relatively new term "knowledge translation" (KT) and defines it as "a dynamic and iterative process that includes synthesis, dissemination, exchange and ethically sound application of knowledge to improve the health, provide more effective health services and products and strengthen the health care system."[91] KT has been proposed as a solution to reduce care gaps, ensuring collaboration between the public, patients, clinicians, managers, and policy-makers to inform health-related policy and practice.[92,93]

A model for understanding KT

The CIHR elaborated a Knowledge To Action model, further subdividing KT into two categories: (1) end-of-grant KT and (2) integrated KT.[93,94] In end-of-grant KT, strategies are developed to match research findings to the needs of the appropriate individuals and organizations after research activity is completed. This approach is also known as diffusion and dissemination of research findings. Conversely, integrated KT engages individuals and organizations in every step of the research process, from establishing the research question to interpretation and dissemination of the findings. The goal of this approach is to produce research findings that are more likely to be relevant to, and used by, the stakeholders, including patients, clinicians, managers, and policy-makers.[95,96]

A variety of models exist to improve quality of healthcare through KT. One of the most common is the 4T model (*Fig. 10.12*).[97] The first strategy, referred to as T1

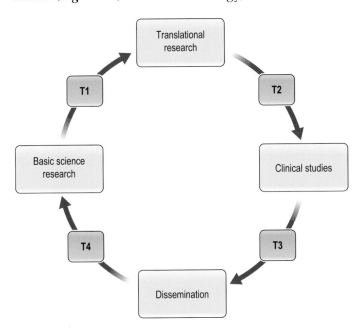

Fig. 10.12 4T Model of knowledge translation. (Reproduced from Dougherty D, Conway PH. The "3Ts" road map to transform US health care: the "how" of high-quality care. JAMA 2008; 299: 2319–2321.)

(translation 1), focuses on transforming basic science findings into translational research. Next, T2 (translation 2) comprises all activities directed at producing clinical studies based on translational research findings. Activities under T3 (translation 3) center on the dissemination and delivery of healthcare interventions to all patients, in every setting of care. Finally, T4 (translation 4) activities focus on translating dissemination experiences into new basic science investigations.

Barriers to uptake

The healthcare system currently falls short in its ability to translate knowledge into clinical practice. A study comparing medical care in the US with established national guidelines, medical literature, and existing indicators of quality demonstrated that, overall, patients received 54.9% of recommended care.[98] In fact, it takes an average of 17 years for new knowledge generated by research, such as randomized controlled trials, to be integrated into widespread practice.[99,100] In a systematic review of the literature by Cabana *et al.*, the sequence of behavior change in a physician's clinical practice has been divided into three domains: knowledge, attitude, and behavior.[101] Each domain may encounter opposing forces to the application of evidence-based knowledge. Firstly, physician knowledge acquisition may encounter barriers such as lack of familiarity and lack of awareness (e.g., increasing volume of new literature, time invested to stay informed).[101,102] Secondly, physician attitudes that favor behavior change may be deterred by the lack of outcome expectancy, self-efficacy, and motivation (e.g., mistrust regarding the validity of clinical research, skepticism about the applicability of evidence to clinical practice, discomfort regarding modification of previous practice).[101,102] Lastly, factors hindering the practical application of behavior change reflecting new research-based knowledge may be external (e.g., patient refusal, conflicting research evidence, lack of resources, organizational constraints).[101,102] Other factors influencing successful implementation of evidence-based interventions include miscommunication between the organization and the healthcare providers, preventing identification of factors hindering compliance with recommended practices. Successful implementation of evidence-based practice has thus far depended on the adoption of a comprehensive program that incorporates methods to improve culture, teamwork, and communication.[103,104]

Learning collaboratives

In a quest to improve healthcare delivery, the Institute for Healthcare Improvement developed a learning collaborative model in 1995, called the Breakthrough Series model. It is an ongoing learning process in which groups of practitioners from different healthcare organizations work in a structured environment to improve a chosen area of their practice.[105]

While clinical trials networks are designed to test an intervention (e.g., drug, surgical procedure, medical device, screening approach), quality improvement learning collaboratives focus on the best way to adopt, implement, and adapt evidence-based practice to real-life environments. These collaboratives often identify ways to improve quality and reliability and to decrease healthcare costs by meticulous comparisons of variation in care processes, culture, and systems between organizations.[106] Many successful collaboratives have come together around diverse health conditions such as cardiac care,[107] cystic fibrosis,[108] infant care,[109] central line infection,[103] and a whole host of topics sponsored by the Institute for Healthcare Improvement.[110]

In collaborative endeavors, the ultimate goal is to promote the dissemination and adoption of evidence-based practice to help organizations and healthcare professionals close the gap between actual and best practice in healthcare. Using adult learning principles, learning collaborative allows practitioners to collaborate and learn from their collective experience and challenges. By bridging together practitioners with different roles in the same organization[103] and from different organizations,[111] information is shared on best practice, quality methods, and experiences while implementing systematic improvements to the overall system of care.

In their systematic review, Schouten et al.[112] reported on the impact of quality improvement collaboratives and concluded that the evidence is "positive but limited" and that further study is warranted to understand the most effective models.

What does this mean for plastic surgeons? Within plastic surgery, a pilot learning collaborative has been launched using TOPS[113] as a central data repository. The collaborative's focus is on sharing practices around abdominal procedures and resultant seroma rates. A challenge for the plastic surgery community is that a high percentage of surgeons practice alone in a private practice setting and may lack the resources needed to participate in such endeavors. In addition, the practice of plastic surgery takes place in a highly competitive marketplace where a culture of collaboration, rather than competition, may be a difficult, but not impossible, shift to enable. It is possible that outside forces such as changing reimbursement strategies will nudge our community towards recognizing the value in collaborative learning and improvement.

Role of electronic medical records/integrating data collection into flow of usual care versus research

To have truly effective KT and continuous improvement in the quality, safety, and value of healthcare, an infrastructure that supports data use in clinically intelligent ways is paramount. Current systems are limited by use of paper and by lack of interoperability, even when electronic data is available, thus making the majority of clinical data relatively inaccessible in practical terms. Where clinical data are currently used (e.g., Surgical Care Improvement Project (SCIP)[114] measures and National Surgical Quality Improvement Program (NSQIP)[115]), full-time employees must be hired to abstract data manually from paper or electronic records and re-enter them in a different format for submission. Due to these high labor costs, only a small sample of surgical cases and data points can be included. When clinical research trials are performed, much of the data collection is done on paper, duplicating information already present in the medical record, which again represents a very labor-intense process. Furthermore, when patient-reported data are collected, patients may be asked to answer questions similar to those already asked during the clinical encounter, thus adding significant redundancy to patients as well. In addition, it can be challenging or even impossible to score paper-based questionnaires at the bedside, thus depriving the patient–provider relationship of data that could otherwise have a significant impact on their decision-making.

Several specialty societies, including the American Society of Plastic Surgeons, have hired consultants to design data collection web sites such as TOPS. However, this typically requires practitioners to abstract data manually and re-enter it into the national database, thus creating a significant barrier to participation by many. Few groups, other than the Cancer Trialists Collaborative Group, which receives national funding, have been successful at carrying out and sustaining such efforts.

Possible solutions: generic

With the evolution of computer technology and the internet, the feasibility of turning data into meaningful information for activities such as decision-making at the bedside, physician feedback, benchmarking, improvement of care, credentialing, certification, and research is becoming much more affordable, practical, and realistic. Although information technology has much to offer in enabling the transformation of healthcare delivery, it has been slow in adoption and effectiveness compared to other industries. To stimulate growth, the federal government has developed a 5-year plan to phase in and define "meaningful use" of electronic medical records (EMRs).[116] The hope is that this will increase meaningful adoption of health information technology (HIT) by both providers and hospitals.

Standards for PRO measures have not yet been included in the current and future proposed definitions of "meaningful use." However, decision support rules and best practice alerts may well benefit from inclusion of these measures. For instance, a PRO instrument for depression could generate a best-practice alert for referral to a mental health professional.[117] Likewise, a PRO measure for domestic abuse could generate a best-practice alert for referral to social services professionals. Having such PRO measures integrated into the flow of care electronically, thus enabling immediate scoring and reporting to the healthcare team, advances our ability to provide high-quality care. This reaches beyond what we have been able to achieve in the past with paper-based and research measures administered and scored well after an office encounter, and often never reported back to the care team.

The gradual adoption of EMRs by more and more health systems, practices, and individual practitioners provides a growing opportunity to capture structured data at the point of care. Not only can these systems facilitate the systematic capture of data, but they also allow systematic analysis and reporting. This reporting can be done with several purposes in mind, such as instantly providing decision support and best-practice evidence to providers at the time of patient encounter. The reporting can be "rolled" up to a cohort of patients with similar health conditions (e.g., all breast cancer patients), similar procedures (e.g., all free flaps), or on a provider's panel (e.g., all surgical cases performed by the same surgeon). These reports could also be aggregated at the practice level, departmental level, or at the national level.

Possible solutions: plastic surgery and PRO measures

It is often a challenge for plastic surgeons to mobilize the resources within their clinical environment to develop and program the tools to collect field-defined data specific to the specialty. However, several innovative centers have begun to do just that with PRO measures. Just as we have easy access to timely and standardized laboratory results, so should we have similar availability of timely and standardized PRO at the bedside. In many cases, particularly in the specialty of plastic surgery, PRO measures may provide us with better decision-making information, or may add an important dimension to more traditional biometric measures. For instance, the Levine score[118] for carpal tunnel patients, when available during an encounter, is very helpful to individual patients and their surgeons in quantifying the impact of the symptoms and in tracking the effect of a particular treatment. Likewise, the BREAST-Q[55] has been developed to provide useful bedside information as well as valuable research information.

At Dartmouth, we have been able to integrate electronic patient-reported intake and outcomes into routine care for the purpose of improving the quality and efficiency of care, reporting, and research. This has been operationalized across 14 specialty programs, including comprehensive breast care and hand care. At Memorial Sloan-Kettering, the BREAST-Q is routinely administered at the point of care. Plastic surgeons participating in TOPS can sign up to have the BREAST-Q sent to their breast patients for longitudinal postoperative tracking. A common sentiment expressed by practitioners who have access to these measures at the time of an encounter is that they cannot imagine ever returning to a practice style where this information was not available.

As we become more sophisticated at measurement, it becomes important that, as a community, we endorse and use the same measurement tools so that we can make meaningful comparison of the data through our national registry. There is no doubt that these measures will continue to improve through an ongoing iterative process. The more plastic surgeons participate, the more they can help shape the design of these data systems to make them even more practical at the bedside, and more effective at answering important clinical questions through well-designed research studies and learning collaboratives.

What do we do with the outcomes?

EMRs and HIT have the potential to improve the quality of healthcare and support the transformation of the way medicine is practiced and provided to patients. Computerized continuous quality assessment from data found in EMRs should facilitate ongoing monitoring and improvement of healthcare quality as well as clinical decision-making. Numerous national initiatives are currently assessing ways to measure care systems with the goal of collecting and comparing data on the structure of healthcare systems, care interventions, and patient outcomes. These data are valuable to many stakeholders: patients, providers, healthcare payers, and government agencies. Thus, there is currently an unprecedented focus on quantifying healthcare quality, as improving the outcomes of care is an important and pressing challenge.

The first model summarizing factors influencing patient outcomes was developed by Donabedian in 1966.[119] This framework is still relevant today, and hypothesizes that care structures (e.g., dedicated microsurgical care team) and care processes (e.g., standard limb replantation care pathway) play a role in patient outcomes. In this type of model, outcomes can take any form appropriate to one's practice, for example, mortality, health status, functional status, satisfaction, QoL, and cost.

The creation of clinical practice guidelines has become a strategy frequently used to improve healthcare quality and outcomes. They represent a way of outlining evidence-based practices through a review and synthesis of the literature in an attempt to guide patient care

better. However, although extremely useful, guidelines alone are not sufficient to produce improvements in the quality of care. The strategy of publication and dissemination of practice guidelines has failed to guarantee their implementation. Today, performance measures, public reporting, P4P, and patient decision aids are increasingly used to improve clinical quality. Embedded in all of these initiatives are a variety of measures of patient outcomes.

Performance measures

In the process of facilitating the measurement of healthcare quality, performance improvement measures serve as a vehicle for translating the strongest clinical evidence into practice more rapidly. Measures typically go through many iterations before they are widely endorsed as being meaningful and reliable. In the earlier stages of maturation, it has been proposed that the measures be called "quality metrics."[120] These metrics can be used to assist providers, hospitals, or the healthcare system in self-assessment, enhancing both quality of care and patient outcomes. With repeated improvements in the measures themselves, they may rise to the exacting standards of organizations such as the National Quality Forum[121] and be endorsed as formal "performance metrics"[120] and used for public reporting, comparison of care between institutions or healthcare providers, P4P initiatives, and soon for meaningful use initiatives. The credentialing and financial incentives behind compliance with performance metrics encourage healthcare providers and organizations to offer the strongest evidence-based quality of care.

One of the main examples of a process-driven quality initiative is SCIP.[114,122,123] This national quality partnership of organizations was initially a voluntary collaborative to improve surgical care by reducing surgical complications. It transitioned to a mandatory publicly reported system in 2005.[124] The ultimate goal of this program was to reduce the incidence of preventable surgical morbidity and mortality nationally by 25% by the year 2010 through collaborative efforts. This program has four preventable complication modules: (1) surgical site infections[114]; (2) venous thromboembolism[125]; (3) cardiovascular events; and (4) respiratory complications. The withholding of a pro-rated Medicare payment was used as a financial incentive to guarantee participation in SCIP. However, at present, studies evaluating the effect of SCIP process measures following colorectal surgery on surgical site infection rates have mixed results.[126,127] Of note, these studies have relatively small sample size at each participating institution. Furthermore, SCIP measures of performance target a limited set of surgical procedures, none of which pertains to plastic surgery. Such measures are primarily useful at the organizational level, but not at the level of the individual provider. However, collection of SCIP measures from a data-rich EMR will make reporting at the individual provider level much more feasible.

The American College of Surgeons' NSQIP[115] is another initiative that is gaining increased traction amongst surgical specialties and hospitals to track and improve surgical outcomes. Although in the past NSQIP has not included data on plastic surgical cases, discussions with the American Society of Plastic Surgeons are currently underway. For participating hospitals, and the surgeons they represent, clinical data rather than administrative data can be used to compare outcomes across organizations and support improvement efforts.

To date, the only study addressing performance measures in plastic surgery was conducted in the UK. The British Association of Plastic Surgeons, following a requirement of National Health Service clinicians to take part in clinical audits, has taken the initiative to identify surgical procedures that could be used as markers of performance across the specialty.[128] In their pilot study, a national performance assessment for pedicled and free-flap survival was completed. When comparing four plastic surgery units, the overall outcome achieved was 89% total flap survival.

The Maintenance of Certification Program of the American Board of Plastic Surgery is venturing into this arena of physician performance measurement. They have recently launched the Practice Assessment in Plastic Surgery (PA-PS) modules for 20 of the most common plastic surgical procedures. Although far from being as robust as what will be needed in the future, these modules will likely undergo frequent upgrades to improve their usefulness to the practicing clinician and will undoubtedly include PRO in the future.

On another front, the Joint Commission, that accredits healthcare organizations, has created a standard around evaluation of professional practice at the individual provider level.[129] Like other initiatives, preliminary measures will be derived largely from process data and perhaps surgical complications and we will await future iterations to integrate patient-reported outcomes.

Public reporting and P4P

Despite limited evidence on their benefits, public reporting of hospital quality data and P4P are the two most advocated strategies to accelerate improvements in healthcare quality and safety.[130] Measuring and publishing information about quality of hospitals, health plans, and physicians are driving P4P programs. Public accountability of quality measures has proved an excellent motivator for healthcare providers and hospitals to invest efforts in quality activities, as performance measures are open to the public for review.[131,132]

P4P is a compensation model used by private payers that links financial incentives to the quality of healthcare provided.[133] While the P4P concept is gaining momentum as a means of improving overall quality of care by reducing gaps between clinical practice and evidence-based guidelines, it is also viewed as a way of encouraging efficient use of healthcare resources. P4P initiatives can take various forms, encompassing different payment models, various stakeholders (e.g., hospitals, group practices, private practitioners), and diverse clinical conditions. The available evidence regarding the impacts of P4P has been mixed.[134–136] Some large-scale studies report moderate enhancements in process-of-care measures, but to date, no impact has been reported on patient outcomes or efficiency of care.[130,137–139]

Recently, the federal government has introduced its own Pay for Reporting (P4R) program: the Physician Quality Reporting Initiative. This initiative offers financial incentives to Medicare providers who participate in quality reporting. Unlike P4P programs, the P4R model compensates physicians regardless of their performance on process and outcome measures.[140]

In 2002 and 2003, a natural experiment occurred, involving thousands of American hospitals participating in a national public reporting initiative, with more than 200 organizations engaged in a simultaneous P4P initiative. Lindenauer et al.[130] observed that hospitals participating in both public reporting and P4P programs showed modestly greater improvements in healthcare quality than hospitals engaged in public reporting alone.

Some critics argue that little evidence links performance measures to patient outcomes.[132] One explanation for this may be found in the realization that current measures focus on a very small number of processes of care out of the total interventions that characterize the patient's experience in the hospital.[131] Also, results of randomized controlled trials with homogeneous study samples may not be generalizable to all patients.[132] Besides, outcomes in daily practice are influenced by various amalgamations of patient and treatment variables, which are seldom replicable in randomized controlled trials. In addition, many of the studies that failed to demonstrate an improvement in outcomes did not assess outcomes occurring at longer intervals after the delivery of the process of care to the patient. Moreover, the present burden of comprehensive data collection limits investigators' ability to capture patient information between care settings over time. Data collection should be facilitated by the widespread use of electronic medical records, allowing researchers to evaluate long-term outcomes readily.[131]

Decision aids for patients

Making an informed decision about the best treatment can be difficult for patients, especially when there is more than one medically reasonable option. Over the last 30 years, the field of evidence-based decision-making in healthcare has grown rapidly. Patient decision aids aim to support this process and help patients arrive at informed value-based choices. According to the International Patient Decision Aids Standards collaboration, decision aids are evidence-based tools designed to prepare patients to contribute actively to the decision-making process when choosing among healthcare options, according to their preferences and values.[141–143] They differ from conventional patient education materials in that they are more detailed, specific, and deliberated, and they provide a more personalized focus on options and outcomes, with the goal of helping patients make informed choices.[142] Decision aids for patients do not replace the patient–physician encounter; instead, they supplement the provider's counseling about healthcare options.[142] They can be used before, during, or after an interaction with a practitioner.

A recent Cochrane systematic review of patient decision aids reported that they improve patients' knowledge regarding their options, and reduce decisional conflicts from feeling uninformed or confused about personal values.[142] After using decision aids, fewer patients are ambivalent about their treatment choice. Importantly, more patients participate actively in the decision process. However, randomized controlled trials have failed to demonstrate that these tools improve patient outcomes such as decision uncertainty, satisfaction, anxiety, or QoL.[144] Moreover, there is scarce evidence on the effects of decision aids on patient compliance with treatment, decisional regret, litigation rates, healthcare costs, and resource use.[142]

Evidence supporting the use of decision aids in clinical practice is substantial.[142,144,145] A good decision aid should meet the needs of its target population, and be acceptable to both patients and providers who wish to incorporate them in their clinical practice. Barriers to successful implementation are the lack of effective systems for delivering decision support. Further research is needed to assess the effects of decision aids on congruence between patients' values and their chosen options.

Designing and building high-quality decision aids is greatly enhanced when the available evidence base, including patient-reported outcomes, is robust. There is much opportunity for the plastic surgery community to add to this evidence base.

Conclusions

This chapter would be incomplete without emphasizing the key take-home messages. A clinician cannot make good decisions without good evidence and cannot generate good evidence without good study design and good data. Maximizing patient care and surgical outcomes will require continuous efforts to identify information needs and to produce the best evidence to fulfill these needs. Outcomes research offers a broad spectrum of methods by which to obtain good evidence, and these have been insufficiently leveraged by our specialty. In particular, measuring the patients' perspective on outcomes is a crucial dimension of research and clinical care that is underdeveloped and underutilized.

Measuring outcomes is not just about the final result of our interventions but a means by which we gather evidence to improve decision-making, the processes of care, and the systems in which we work. Collaborative data collection through clinical trials and quality improvement initiatives is essential to the generation of clinically meaningful information in our specialty. Our decisions need to be based on the highest-quality evidence and not the accumulated experience of a single surgeon, even if that surgeon is truly expert in the field. Equally important to generating clinically meaningful information is to translate that information into practice by providing surgeons with mechanisms to implement and monitor new standards.

Access the complete references list online at **http://www.expertconsult.com**

11. Walach H, Falkenberg T, Fonnebo V, et al. Circular instead of hierarchical: methodological principles for the evaluation of complex interventions. *BMC Med Res Methodol.* 2006;6:29.

   Walach and coauthors discuss the widely held assumption around the hierarchy of evidence which places randomized controlled trials (RCTs) at the top – which are in turn trumped only by meta-analyses of multiple RCTs. However, this hierarchy is based on a pharmacological model of therapy. When generalized to other interventions such as integrative medical management, wound healing, and surgery, the hierarchical model is valid for limited questions of efficacy. RCTs are strong in the arena of internal validity (minimization of bias), but not as much so in regard to external validity or generalizability of the findings. Rather than an "evidence hierarchy", they propose a "circular model" of evidence that would include multiple methods, with different research designs, balancing strengths and weaknesses to arrive at the best clinical evidence

22. Wennberg DE, Lucas FL, Birkmeyer JD, et al. Variation in carotid endarterectomy mortality in the Medicare population: trial hospitals, volume, and patient characteristics. *JAMA.* 1998;279:1278–1281.

   This paper assessed the perioperative mortality among Medicare patients undergoing carotid endarterectomy (CEA). The study found that the risk of preoperative mortality following CEA was significantly higher than reported in the clinical trials, even among the institutions that participated in the trials. This study demonstrates the caution that one should have when translating the efficacy of clinical trials to effectiveness in everyday practice.

26. Chung KC, Kalliainen LK, Hayward RA. Type II (beta) errors in the hand literature: the importance of power. *J Hand Surg [Am].* 1998;23:20–25.

   This manuscript describes how many papers in the Journal of Hand Surgery had insignificant sample size and power to provide an adequate assessment of therapeutic efficacy. The authors found that 82% of "negative" studies had a power less than 0.80 to detect at 25% treatment effect. Researchers and clinicians should be aware of the importance of adequate sample size and statistical power in order to avoid making a type 2 or beta error, which is the erroneous conclusion that the null hypothesis is correct.

44. Cano SJ, Klassen A, Pusic AL. The science behind quality-of-life measurement: a primer for plastic surgeons. *Plast Reconstr Surg.* 2009;123: 98e–106e.

   The authors provide an overview of the key principles underlying the development of patient-reported outcomes instruments. They provide definitions of the terminology pertaining to this field of study, along with explanations of relevant concepts. The authors also provide a description of the essential elements to assess the quality of an instrument, along with a summary of the latest developments in psychometric methods of quality-of-life measurement.

106. Ayers LR, Beyea SC, Godfrey MM, et al. Quality improvement learning collaboratives. *Qual Manag Health Care.* 2005;14:234–247.

   The authors interviewed individuals who had developed and implemented highly successful learning collaboratives and describe the key characteristics that made these initiatives successful and sustainable. For those interested in knowing how to succeed, the authors' description of the importance of building trust, appreciating and dealing with differences in organizational cultures and rallying around a passion for quality improvement are very helpful.

11

Genetics and prenatal diagnosis

Daniel Nowinski, Elizabeth Kiwanuka, Florian Hackl, Bohdan Pomahac, and Elof Eriksson

SYNOPSIS

- Gene expression is mainly regulated at the level of gene transcription. Cells respond and adapt with changes in gene expression to soluble factors, cell–cell, and cell–matrix contacts.
- Epigenetic regulation of gene expression is preserved through cell division and is mainly determined by the three-dimensional organization of chromatin.
- In gene therapy the expression of individual genes is modified or abnormal genes are corrected. The delivered transgenes may be categorized as gene inhibitors, gene vaccines, or gene substitutes.
- Nonbiological or biological methods are used to deliver transgenes to cells. The most common nonbiological method is delivery by cationic liposome vectors. The predominating type of biological gene delivery is through viral vectors.
- Gene therapy approaches are being developed to improve tissue repair and regeneration. The most common approach is to deliver genes coding for growth factors. Gene therapy can be combined with cell therapy and biomaterial scaffolds to induce and direct tissue regeneration.
- Based on the main mechanism of pathogenesis, congenital anomalies may be categorized as malformations, deformations, disruptions, or dysplasias.
- About 70% of cleft lip and palate cases are nonsyndromic. They are usually sporadic (noninherited) and have multifactorial etiologies involving different genes and environmental factors.
- Most craniosynostosis syndromes are caused by gain of function mutations in fibroblast growth factor receptors (FGFRs). These syndromes are inherited as autosomal-dominant disorders; however most cases arise as a result of de novo mutations.
- Ultrasonography can be used to detect craniofacial malformations, such as facial clefts and craniosynostosis. Prenatal diagnosis of congenital anomalies with known genetic mutations can be confirmed with invasive testing.

 Access the Historical Perspective section and Figure 11.1 online at **http://www.expertconsult.com**

Introduction

The last half-century has seen a tremendous expansion of knowledge in genetics. The contribution of this progress to plastic surgery has already been substantial. Various methodologies to explore gene structure, function, and regulation are widely utilized in research on wound healing and tissue regeneration. The elucidation of the genetic basis for various syndromes has increased our understanding of pathogenesis and improved our diagnostic possibilities. Moreover, the tools for prenatal diagnosis have been improved. Few would argue that ongoing and future advances in genetics will bring new and improved therapies for patients with conditions treated by the plastic surgeon.

This chapter is a review of genetics relevant to plastic surgery. The first section about the human genome will provide the reader with the basic concepts to understand genetics as a basis for disease. Next follows a section on gene therapy. Current methods for modification of gene expression and examples of possible therapeutic applications in plastic surgery have been described. We have included a short account of the moral and ethical aspects of genetics in medical research and practice.

The remaining part of the chapter is dedicated to different aspects of genetic and prenatal diagnosis. A section on the genetic etiology and pathogenesis of craniofacial anomalies is followed by a brief description of prenatal diagnosis. Lastly, there is a short discussion on future prospects.

Human genome

Basic molecular biology

DNA

Genes are made of the molecule deoxyribonucleic acid, or DNA *(Fig. 11.2)*. The DNA molecule is a long polymer of units called deoxyribonucleotides, or nucleotides. Each nucleotide is in turn composed of the phosporylated sugar phospodeoxyribose, and one of the four nucleotide bases adenine (A), guanine (G), cytosine (C), and thymine (T). Two such polymers form a two-stranded double helix with the sugar phosphates as hydrophilic backbones on the outside, and the hydrophilic bases on the inside. The bases of one strand bind to the bases of the other, so that A pairs with T and G pairs with C. As a consequence, the DNA chain is complementary and the sequence of one strand generates the sequence of the other. At one end the DNA chain starts with a sugar phosphorylated at its 5′ carbon and at the other end the chain ends with a 3′ hydroxylated carbon. The two chains are in antiparallel orientation with the 3′ end of one chains binding to the 5′ end of the complementary chain.

Upon cell division DNA is synthesized in the process of replication. The complementary matching of nucelotide bases creates the basis for this process.

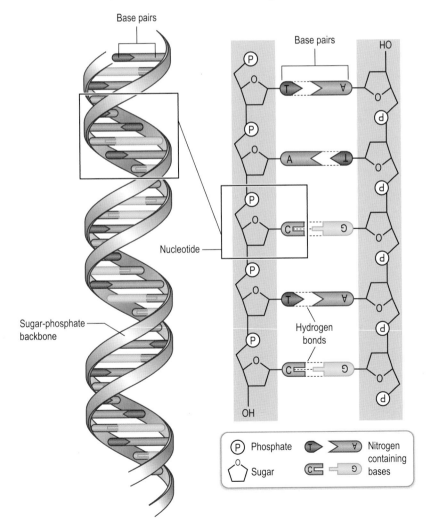

Fig. 11.2 Structure of the DNA molecule: the ladder-like double helix with the hydrophilic, phosphorylated sugar backbone on the outside and the hydrophobic nucleotide bases on the inside (left). The two strands of the molecule are complementary so that A binds with T and G with C (right). A, adenine; T, thymine; G, guanine; C, cytosine; P, phosphate.

Each DNA strand thus constitutes the template for the synthesis of an identical daughter DNA molecule. In eukaryotes, replication starts at multiple sites along the DNA molecule. Several DNA-binding proteins act to unwind the DNA double helix and separate the two strands, thereby opening up the molecule for replication. Synthesis starts with the formation of a RNA primer by the enzyme primase. The primer is a short complementary stretch of RNA that primes DNA synthesis by the enzyme DNA polymerase III. This enzyme creates phosphodiester bonds between the 3′ hydroxyl group of one sugar residue and the 5′ phosphate group of another. The sequence of the DNA template dictates the addition of nucleotides to the newly synthesized molecule. DNA polymerase has a built-in proofreading mechanism that removes nucleotides that have been incorrectly inserted during synthesis. Furthermore, DNA excising and repairing enzymes work to detect and correct DNA that has been damaged by various factors, such as oxygen radicals, radiation, and certain chemicals.

Organization of genomic DNA

One DNA molecule makes up one chromosome and each human chromosome contains about 1.3×10^8 basepairs. Human germ cells are haploid, which means they have one set of 23 different chromosomes, and somatic cells are diploid and contain 23 pairs, or 46 chromosomes. The autosomes are the 22 pairs that are not either of the two different sex chromosomes, X or Y. The 46 DNA molecules that make up the genome must be packed into the confined space of the somatic cell nucleus. This is accomplished with the help of DNA-binding proteins, or histones, and the consequent formation of chromatin (*Fig. 11.3*). Two of each histones 2A, 2B, 3, and 4 form a protein complex called the nucleosome. The DNA molecule winds around the

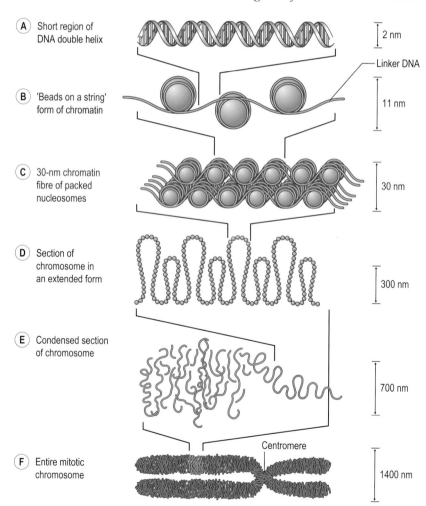

(A) Short region of DNA double helix — 2 nm

Linker DNA

(B) 'Beads on a string' form of chromatin — 11 nm

(C) 30-nm chromatin fibre of packed nucleosomes — 30 nm

(D) Section of chromosome in an extended form — 300 nm

(E) Condensed section of chromosome — 700 nm

Centromere

(F) Entire mitotic chromosome — 1400 nm

Fig. 11.3 Organization of genomic DNA. **(A)** The unfolded structure of the DNA double helix makes up the linker DNA, with short stretches of DNA in between nucelosomes. **(B)** The DNA molecule wraps around the histone structures called nucleosomes to form a structure viewed as "beads on a string" in the electron microscope. **(C)** The unfolded chromatin is packed to form the 30-nm chromatin fiber. **(D–F)** There is increased condensation from euchromatin to heterochromatin by the process of supercoiling. The mitotic chromosome is the most condensed form of chromatin.

nucleosomes and each nucleosome is separated by a piece of linker DNA. In this unfolded state this structure is viewed as "beads on a string" in the electron microscope. The nucleosomes are brought together by another histone, H1, to form the 30-nm chromatin fiber. Nonhistone proteins further condense the chromatin in a process called supercoiling. The condensed chromatin visible under the light microscope is called heterochromatin and the less compacted chromatin is called euchromatin. The chromosomes are most condensed just before mitosis. At this stage the cell is about to divide, the DNA has been replicated, and each chromosome is therefore composed of two chromatids. Each chromosme has a long (q) and a short (p) arm separated from each other by the centromere.

Gene expression

A gene is a portion of the DNA molecule that contains information for the synthesis of gene products, which may be proteins or RNA molecules. In the diploid organism there are two alleles or copies of each gene, occupying the same locus, one on each chromosome. When the alleles are identical the organism is homozygous for that particular gene. Conversely, heterozygosis refers to different alleles at a particular genetic locus. The DNA sequence of the gene contains coding regions, exons, and noncoding regions, or introns. The information kept in the DNA molecule is transferred to an RNA molecule in the process of transcription. There are three major classes of RNA, messenger (m)RNA, transfer (t)RNA and ribosomal (r)RNA, and they all have different functions in the synthesis of proteins. The DNA sequence of genes encoding for a protein is transcribed into mRNA, which in turn forms the template for protein synthesis. This flow of information from DNA to protein is called the central dogma.

The RNA molecule has a similar chemical structure to DNA, albeit with a few differences. The sugar backbone in RNA is composed of ribose instead of deoxyribose, and the nucleotide base thymine (T) is replaced by uracil (U). Moreover, the RNA chain is a single-stranded molecule as opposed to the double-stranded DNA. When RNA is synthesized the sequence of bases depends on the sequence of DNA being transcribed. The DNA bases T, A, G, and C specify the bases A, U, C, and G, respectively, in RNA. Thus, the newly synthesized RNA molecule is complementary to the DNA template. The DNA/RNA sequence of a gene is composed of triplets of nucleotides called codons. Each codon specifies one amino acid and the way these triplets are read to specify the amino acid sequence of a polypeptide is called the reading frame. Start and stop codons constitute the initiation and terminations sites respectively for polypeptide chain synthesis. The enzyme RNA polymerase that recognizes the beginning of the gene sequence and creates phosphodiester bonds between the individual nucleotides catalyzes the transcription process. The nucleotide of the DNA template at the beginning of transcription is designated +1 and transcription is said to proceed downstream from this point, towards the 5′ end of the DNA strand. However, the RNA molecule is normally used as a reference and transcription is said to proceed from 5′ to 3′. Upstream nucleotides, designated with a negative number, form the DNA sequence up to the beginning of transcription. The DNA sequence just upstream of the gene is called the promoter. This sequence binds the RNA polymerase and various transcription factors upon initiation of transcription.

At termination of transcription the RNA strand is separated from the DNA template. In eukaryotes this process involves polyadenylation in the 3′ end of the RNA molecule. The mechanism, which separates the RNA from the DNA at termination of transcription in prokaryotes, is either a formation of a G–C-rich hairpin loop (Rho-independent), or the binding of a peptide factor called Rho (Rho-dependent).

In eukaryotes, mRNA transcripts undergo several modifications. The 5′ end is methylated to form the 7-methyl guanosine cap, while the 3′ end is altered by the above-mentioned polyadenylation to form the poly-A tail. Both the capping and the addition of the poly-A tail increase the stability of mRNA molecules towards degradation. Before the mRNA molecule can be used as a template for protein synthesis it undergoes the process of splicing, in which the parts of the mRNA sequence that correspond to introns, or noncoding regions, are removed. In alternative splicing, exons are rearranged in different ways to create different splice variants, or isoforms, of the protein in question. This constitutes an important regulatory mechanism by which cells can synthesize different variants of a peptide at different time points. However, alternative splicing to produce aberrant proteins is also highly

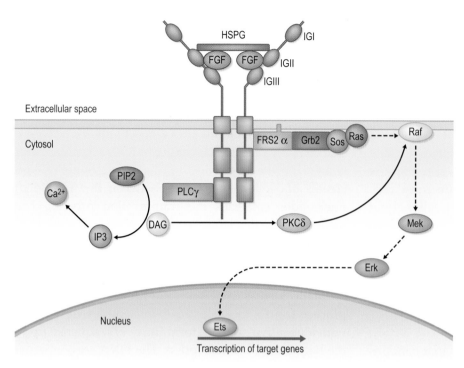

Fig. 11.4 Fibroblast growth factor receptor (FGFR) signal transduction pathways. The FGFRs are composed of an extracellular and an intracellular part. The extracellular part has three immunoglobulin domains (IGI, IGII, IGIII). FGF ligands linked to heparin sulfate proteoglycan (HSPG) bind to the FGFR which activates the receptor and leads to receptor dimerization. The activated receptor docks fibroblast receptor substrate 2 alpha (FRS2α), which leads to FRS2α phosphorylation at tyrosine residues. The next step is the activation of Grb2 and Sos. The Grb2–Sos complex activates Ras, which in turn phosporylates and activates Raf. Raf activates ERK, which enters the nucleus to phosphorylate and activate Ets transcription factors. FGFR activation also leads to activation of phospholipase C-γ (PLCγ). PLCγ hydrolyzes phosphatidyl-inositol-4,5-diphosphate (PIP_2) to inositol-1, 4, 5-triphosphate (IP_3) and diaglycerol (DAG). IP_3 causes Ca^{2+} release while DAG activates Raf through activation of protein kinase c-δ (PKC δ). This in turn leads to Ras-independent MEK-ERK activation.

implicated in disease. In syndromic craniosynostosis, mutations in the gene coding for FGFR2 may produce splice sites that lead to the synthesis of aberrant receptor protein.[11]

Gene regulation

The control of gene expression is an extraordinarily complex process. The entire genome, with all its genes, is present in every somatic cell. However, the phenotype and behavior of cells during development, tissue repair, and homeostasis are directed by a differential and highly selective pattern of gene expression. The moment-to-moment alterations in gene expression are mainly regulated at the level of gene transcription. Cells respond and adapt with changes in gene expression to a wide range of stimuli from the external microenvironment, such as soluble factors, cell–cell contacts, or cell–matrix contacts. The effect of these stimuli on gene expression is in turn mediated by intracellular signal transduction mechanisms. Upon extracellular stimulation, complex cascades of intracellular enzymatic reactions are activated which ultimately result in the activation of a specific set of transcription factors *(Fig. 11.4)*. Transcription factors bind to the promoter sequence and together with the RNA polymerase they form the preinitiation complex. Other transcription factors bind to so-called enhancer sequences, located upstream or sometimes downstream of the gene. The transcription factors encoded by homeobox-containing genes are particularly important for the developmental process.[12] A homeobox is a DNA sequence of about 180 basepairs that encodes for a so-called homeodomain, an amino acid sequence that binds DNA. Complicated molecular pathways involving several different growth factors regulate the timely and coordinated expression of genes during embryogenesis. Two growth factor families with particular importance in this regard are the transforming growth factor-β (TGF-β) superfamily and the fibroblast growth factors (FGF).[13] Bone morphogenic proteins (BMP) are members of the TGF-β superfamily and modulate transcription of homeobox-containing genes, such as *MSX1* and *MSX2*. *MSX1* and *MSX2* have both been implicated in the formation of orofacial clefts.[14] Mutations in *FGFR* genes that lead to an increase in receptor signaling are the principal mechanisms behind FGFR-related craniosynostosis syndromes.[15] The role of these factors in craniofacial development is elaborated below.

Epigenetic mechanisms

Stable variations in gene expression may be governed by other mechanisms than by actual variations in the primary DNA sequence. A number of so-called epigenetic mechanisms may modify the expression of genes and cause alterations in cellular phenotype. These mechanisms are preserved through cell division and are believed to be important for the stable tissue and cell-type-specific gene expression in differentiated cells. Moreover, epigenetic mechanisms may be inherited to affect the expression of phenotype. The investigation of epigenetic mechanisms has become a rapidly growing field of research with important implications for developmental biology as well as various disease processes. The so-called epigenotype is mainly formed by the three-dimensional organization of chromatin.

The three-dimensional architecture of chromatin regulates gene expression.[16] Unfolding of the chromatin structure exposes the DNA sequence to transcription. Protein-encoding genes are as a consequence expressed in an environment of euchromatin and, conversely, the highly condensed heterochromatin inhibits transcription. The physical three-dimensional arrangement of chromatin is in turn regulated by different biochemical epigenetic mechanisms that may be transferred through cell division. The histones may be modified by methylations or acetylations. The pattern of methylation and acetylation of the histones in turn directs the binding of other chromatin-binding proteins that regulate gene transcription. Another mechanism is methylation of CpG dinucleotides of the DNA molecule by enzymes called DNA methyl transferases. DNA methylation generally silences gene transcription and the pattern of DNA methylations acts in concert with histone modifications to determine chromatin structure and regulate transcription *(Fig. 11.5)*.

The epigenetic mechanisms give rise to so-called epigenetic phenomena.[17] X-inactivation is the phenomenon by which one of the X chromosomes in females is randomly inactivated. The inactivated X chromosome can be visualized as a highly condensed chromatin structure, the Barr body. By inactivating one of the two

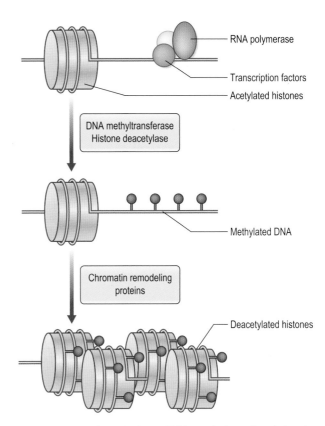

Fig. 11.5 Epigenetic mechanisms of DNA organization and restriction of gene transcription. The unfolded chromatin exposes the DNA molecule to the enzymes of gene transcription (top). Gene transcription is restricted by covalent modifications of DNA and histones. Bases in the DNA molecule are methylated by DNA methyltransferases. Methylated DNA restricts transcription by preventing transcription factors from binding to the DNA. Histone deacetylases modify histone proteins so that they become positively charged, which leads to binding to the negatively charged DNA and more compacted chromatin (middle). DNA methylation promotes binding of chromatin remodeling proteins that interact with histones to fold the chromatin into a more condensed state (bottom).

X chromosomes in the somatic cells of females, the transcription of genes on the X chromosome, and consequent protein synthesis, is kept at the same level in males and females. During embryonic life paternal and maternal X chromosomes are inactivated in a random fashion. Therefore in any tissue there will be an equal number of cells with the active X chromosomes from either parent. This explains why most X-linked diseases are not expressed in females. Nonrandom X inactivation is an epigenetic abnormality that may lead to the occurrence of X-linked disease in females.

Gene regulation may depend on the sex of the parent from which the gene was inherited. Genomic imprinting is an epigenetic phenomenon that promotes the expression of only one parental allele. This is primarily accomplished by differential DNA methylation of alleles

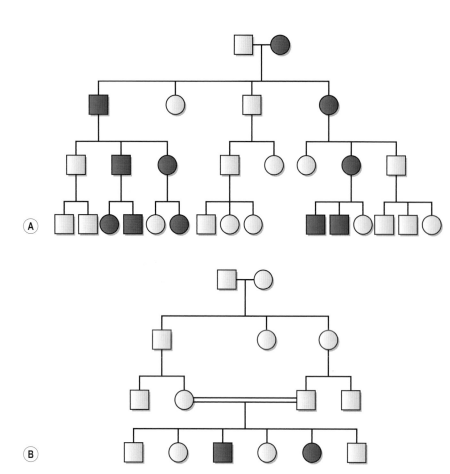

(A)

(B)

Fig. 11.6 (A) Autosomal-dominant pattern; **(B)** autosomal-recessive inheritence pattern. (Reproduced with permission from Cohen MM. Dysmorphology, syndromology, and genetics. In: McCarthy JG (ed.) Plastic Surgery. Philadelphia: WB Saunders, 1990:105, 106.)

in a pattern specific to the parent of origin. Thus, an imprinted inherited gene is not expressed, which results in a departure from the unifactorial, mendelian pattern of inheritance for the trait directed by that gene. Uniparental disomy is a nonmendelian pattern of inheritance where there are two copies of a genomic sequence from one parent, and none from the other. If uniparental disomy occurs for imprinted genes, it may result in loss of function and disease.

Inheritance

Mendelian patterns of inheritance

Phenotypic traits determined by a single genetic locus are inherited according to the laws of unifactorial or mendelian inheritance. The inheritance of these traits may be either autosomal or sex-linked.

Autosomal inheritance

Autosomal inheritance refers to the transmission of traits directed by genes on any of the 22 pairs of autosomes. Autosomal inheritance may be either dominant or recessive *(Fig. 11.6)*. Dominant traits are expressed in heterozygous states, while recessive traits are only expressed in individuals homozygous for that particular genetic locus. Thus, in autosomal-dominant disease the risk for the offspring to an affected individual is 50%. In autosomal-recessive disease, two parents, both heterozygous for the disease-causing gene, will have a 25% risk of having an affected child. Importantly, autosomal-dominant disease may arise as a result of inheritance, or from *de novo* gene mutation. A and B blood group antigens are both autosomal-dominant, but may be simultaneously expressed, a phenomenon referred to as codominance. Phenotypes determined by inherited or *de novo* mutated genes may be expressed

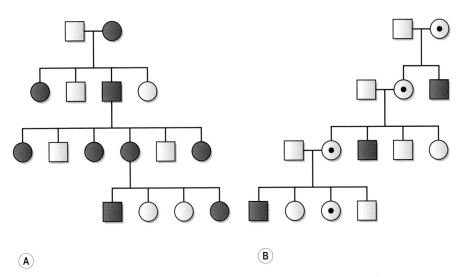

Fig. 11.7 (A) X-linked dominant pattern; **(B)** X-linked recessive pattern. (Reproduced with permission from Cohen MM. Dysmorphology, syndromology, and genetics. In: McCarthy JG (ed.) Plastic Surgery. Philadelphia: WB Saunders, 1990:105, 106.)

to a varying degree. Thus, the same disease, caused by mutations in the same gene, may present with anything from very mild to severe manifestations. The explanation for this variable expressivity may be caused by different mutations in the same gene, other modifying genetic and molecular mechanisms, or environmental factors. Nonpenetrance refers to the situation when individuals heterozygous for an autosomal-dominant trait do not express the corresponding phenotype. This explains why autosomal-dominant disease may skip generations to reappear in coming generations.

Sex-linked inheritance

The genes on the X and Y chromosomes are inherited according to a pattern of sex-linked inheritance. X-linked dominant traits may be expressed in both males and females, but will never be transmitted from affected father to son *(Fig. 11.7)*. Daughters with affected fathers will on the other hand have a 100% risk of inheriting the trait. Affected mothers will have a 50% risk of transmitting an X-linked dominant trait to both daughters and sons. X-linked recessive traits are much more common and are almost exclusively expressed in males, as the two copies of the X chromosome in females, one from each parent, will usually ascertain heterozygocity. Examples of X-linked recessive disease are Duchenne's muscular dystrophy, Becker's muscular dystrophy, and hemophilias A and B. Y-linked inheritance affects only males, exemplified by inheritance of the H-Y histocompatibility antigen.

Nonmendelian patterns of inheritance

Nonmendelian inheritance refers to specific patterns that do not follow the principles of mendelian inheritance. One example is the inheritance governed by the epigenetic phenomenon of imprinting described above. Other patterns are uniparental disomy and mitochondrial inheritance.

Uniparental disomy

In uniparental disomy the individual has inherited both chromosomes, or part of a chromosome, from a single parent. Thus, the corresponding genomic sequence from the other parent will be missing. Normally this does not affect phenotype; however, if combined with imprinting, as described above, disease may occur. Illustrative examples are the syndromes of Prader–Willi and Angelman.[18] About 75% of patients with Prader–Willi syndrome have deletion in the proximal portion of the long arm of chromosome 15, and in the majority of cases this occurs on the paternally derived chromosome. Patients with Angelman syndrome have the same deletion, but on the maternal chromosome. The deleted segments contain the disease-causing genes and the disease develops due to imprinting of these genes on the chromosome-derived form the other parent.

Mitochondrial inheritance

In addition to the nuclear set of 46 chromosomes, mitochondria have their own DNA, the so-called mtDNA that constitutes the mitochondrial genome. The mitochondrial genome is inherited from the mother and mainly contains genes that code for proteins with roles in the electron transport chain. Mutations in the mitochondrial genome may lead to a number of disorders, for example, chronic progressive ophthalmoplegia and aminoglycoside-induced deafness.

Genetic causes for disease

Any disorder where the etiology is totally or partially traced to genetic abnormalities may be considered a genetic disease. This definition creates a wide spectrum, including diseases linked to mutations in a single gene, inherited according to the laws of unifactorial inheritance, as well as conditions of complex etiology, where increased susceptibility to environmental factors is created by polymorphisms or mutations in several different genes. However, the link between genetic abnormality and disease phenotype in monogenic disease is not always as straight as dictated by mendelian laws. Mutations in the same gene may give rise to different syndromes. This may be exemplified by the mutations in the FGFR2 receptor giving rise to the various forms of craniosynostosis syndromes, such as Crouzon, Pfeiffer, Apert, and Jackson–Weiss. Furthermore, the presentation of Crouzon syndrome caused by FGFR2 mutations may range from pansynostosis, severe exorbitism, and midfacial retrusion in infancy, to subtle craniofacial dysmorphism detected in adulthood. This plasticity in the relationship between genotype and phenotype may be due to different mutations in the same gene, environmental factors, or due to modifiers, other molecular mechanisms that alter the pathophysiologic effects of the disease-causing gene mutation. Mutations in different genes may give rise to the same disorder. The term "oligogenic" is sometimes used to describe disease caused by mutations in any of a few genes, illustrated by mutations in either FGFR1 or FGFR2 as a cause of Pfeiffer syndrome. The vast majority of human genetic diseases are however polygenic, multifactorial disorders. The term "polygenic" refers to inheritance dictated by the expression of several or many genes, each with a small contribution to the phenotypic trait. Common conditions such as hypertension and diabetes are caused by complicated mechanisms dictated by the expression of many genes and environmental factors.

Mutations

Most interindividual differences in the genetic code do not cause disease. In fact, the DNA sequence is highly variable between any two individuals. This variability is created by so-called polymorphisms, variations in the genetic code that in themselves normally do not give rise to disease. However, certain patterns of polymorphisms may be related to increased risk of disease and variable response to environmental factors. The most common form of polymorphism is single nucleotide polymorphism, or SNP. SNPs are nucleotide substitutions that occur in 1 out of approximately 300 nucleotides in coding and noncoding DNA. The SNPs can be used as markers for specific regions of the genetic code and so-called SNP maps have been extremely useful in genetic studies and diagnosis.

The most common forms of genetic mutations are single nucleotide substitutions. Other examples are deletions or insertions of several nucleotides. Mutations may result in amino acid substitutions (missense mutation). The altered amino acid sequence may in turn cause structural or functional modifications of the protein. These modifications may cause disease by several different mechanisms. The physiologic activity of the protein may be abolished (loss of function) or increased (gain of function). Alternatively, structural modifications may alter target functions for other proteins or create dysfunctional polypeptide complexes. Gene mutations may alter gene expression at various levels. Mutations in gene promoters or other sequences that bind transcription factors may increase or decrease transcription, while mutations in introns may affect the splicing of mRNA transcripts. Other mutations may alter the stability of the mRNA molecule, leading to increased degradation or accumulation of transcripts. Mutations may also affect protein synthesis by interfering with initiation and termination of translation. The so-called nonsense mutations introduce a stop codon, which prematurely terminates protein synthesis and leads to a truncated protein product. Frameshift mutations alter the reading frame and may lead to the synthesis of abnormal polypeptide chains. Such malformed proteins are frequently susceptible to proteolytic degradation.

Inherited chromosomal abnormalities

Errors in disjunction of chromosomes during meiosis or mitosis may cause an abnormal number of chromosomes, or a numerical abnormality. The most common abnormality seen in human disease is aneuploidy, or a number of chromosomes that is not a multiple of the haploid set of chromosomes. Aneuploidy in humans is most often due to an abnormal number of sex chromosomes. Supernumerary X chromosomes may lead to increased dosage of gene products from the X chromosome. However, if all but one of the X chromosomes are inactivated, the effect on phenotype may be very slight. Monosomy for X chromosome, or 45X, is the most common of all numerical abnormalities. However, 45X usually leads to abortion in the first trimester. Autosomal numerical abnormalities are usually in the form of trisomy. The most common of all chromosomal conditions is Down syndrome, caused by trisomy 21. Certain chromosomal sites are prone to various rearrangements that produce structural chromosomal abnormalities. Segments of chromosomes may be deleted or duplicated. CATCH 22 (see below) is a syndrome that may include abnormalities of the palate and is caused by deletion of locus 22q11.[19] Other types of structural abnormalities are translocations, where there is an exchange of segments between chromosomes, and inversions, referring to a situation when a chromosomal segment is detached, inverted, and reinserted.

The gene as a focus for therapy

The methodology of transfection, whereby DNA or RNA is introduced into cells to modify gene expression, is widely used in molecular research. Transfection and overexpression of genes in specific cell types can be used to study the function of proteins. Gene regulation can be investigated by introducing DNA constructs composed of gene promoters linked to reporter genes. Gene expression can be silenced by the introduction of antisense oligonucleotides that bind complementary to specific DNA sequences to block transcription.

The development of the various methodologies for gene transfection opened up for the prospect of therapeutic modification of gene expression. The first phase I clinical gene therapy trials for adenosine deaminase deficiency and malignant melanoma were reported in 1990.[20,21] In gene therapy the introduction of DNA or RNA into cells is utilized for curing disease or altering gene expression to achieve transient advantage of tissues in processes such as tissue repair and regeneration. The expression of individual genes can be modified or abnormal genes can be corrected. The delivered DNA or RNA may be categorized as gene inhibitors, gene vaccines, or gene substitutes. Gene inhibitors, such as siRNA, inhibit the expression of defective genes. Gene vaccines encode for specific pathogens that activate cell-mediated and humoral immune responses. Gene substitutes are complete genes that substitute for absolute or relative deficiency of a specific gene product. There are currently about 1500 approved clinical trial protocols worldwide. In all, 64.5% of all ongoing trials concern cancer disease, 8.7% are for cardiovascular disease, and 7.9% concern monogenetic disease.[22]

Gene therapy often refers to stable transformation, where the introduced gene is integrated into the target cell genome to cause a permanent modification of gene expression. Inherited monogenic disorders are the best candidates for this kind of therapy. Examples are hemophilia A and B, cystic fibrosis, and Huntington's disease. Stable transformation has however so far only been achievable in therapy directed at the modification of germ cells, which is widely practiced in agriculture and which is used to generate clones of genetically modified laboratory animals. Germ cell gene therapy raises complex moral and ethical issues and has so far not been practiced in humans. Transient transformation is more appropriate to enhance tissue function during a limited therapeutic period in conditions such as wound healing and cancer. Regardless of the therapeutic aim, gene therapy relies on methodology to deliver genes effectively to cells and tissues. Gene therapy may be combined with cell therapy, where transfection is performed *ex vivo* followed by transplantation of the transformed cells to the patient *(Fig. 11.8)*. The *ex vivo* cell therapy approach caries several advantages such as more efficient transfection, reduced risk for undesired local and systemic reactions to vectors, and improved possibility of targeting specific cell types. Despite the

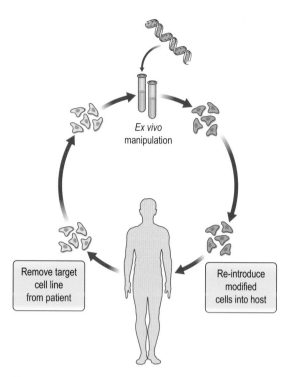

Fig. 11.8 *Ex vivo* gene therapy. Target cells, such as bone marrow-derived mesenchymal stem cells, endothelial progenitor cells, or skin fibroblasts, can be recovered from the patient for *ex vivo* gene therapy. Gene delivery may be performed by various biological or nonbiological methods. The genetically modified cells are reimplanted to the patient at the site of the tissue defect or disease.

Ex vivo manipulation

Remove target cell line from patient

Re-introduce modified cells into host

establishment of various methods for gene delivery and transgene expression in humans, there has been limited success with genetic therapy in clinical praxis thus far. Significant challenges directly related to gene transfer technology include achievement of sufficient transgene levels, appropriate duration of transgene expression, and increased therapeutic specificity. In addition, treatment of multifactorial, polygenetic disease requires further identification of appropriate target genes.

Gene delivery

Gene delivery is achieved through physical, chemical, and biological approaches.[23] All these approaches can be used *in vivo* or *ex vivo*. Transgene delivery in the form of naked DNA is often less efficient mainly due to rapid degradation by nucleases. Therefore, various specialized technologies have been developed to increase transfection efficiency. The ideal gene delivery approach should: (1) allow for delivery of appropriate

transgene size; (2) evade immunologic/toxic reactions or other detrimental effects; (3) allow for target cell specificity; (4) produce efficient delivery; and (5) provide gene modification of appropriate duration.

There are nonbiological and biological methods for gene delivery. The nonbiological methods may in turn be divided into needle injection of naked DNA, physical and chemical methods.[24] Physical approaches, such as microseeding, electroporation, ballistic, ultrasound or hydrodynamic delivery, employ a physical force to deliver the transgene into the cell through the plasma membrane. Chemical approaches use synthetic or naturally occurring chemical compounds as transgene carriers. The predominating type of nonbiological method is chemical, through delivery by cationic liposomes. The liposomes are synthetic vectors composed of positively charged cationic lipids and co-lipids, which may be noncharged phospholipids or cholesterol. These liposomes are mixed with transgene-containing plasmids to form particles called lipoplexes. The DNA bound in these particles is resistant against degradation by nucleases. Cellular uptake is presumed to occur through endocytosis and the DNA exits the intracellular vesicles before degradation in lysosomal compartments *(Fig. 11.9)*.

Liposomes have been of limited value for *in vivo* gene therapy mainly due to a risk of toxic reactions and rapid plasma clearance. Other examples of chemical methods are receptor-mediated and cationic polymers. Viral gene delivery is the predominating form of biological gene delivery.[25] Commonly used viruses are adenoviruses, herpes simplex viruses, and retroviruses. Viral gene delivery is based on the natural ability of viruses to infect host cells with genetic material. In order to be used as vectors, viruses first have to be genetically modified. The genes required for viral replication are deleted and replaced by the gene of interest. To compensate for this inability to replicate, the viral vectors are propagated in packaging cell lines that provide the genes encoding for the structural proteins for the viral particle. In general, the viral approaches are associated with higher transfection efficiency and more stable transformations. The main concerns with biological methods are the risks of transmitting disease, inducing insertional mutations, or evoking immunological or toxic reactions. In retroviral vectors, the retroviral single-stranded RNA genome is reverse-transcribed into

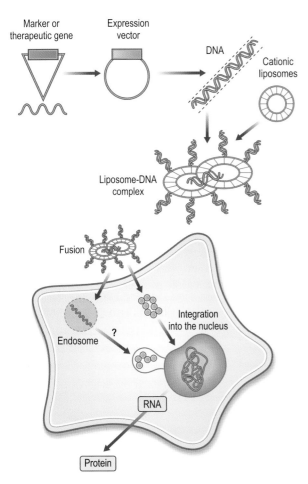

Fig. 11.9 DNA delivery to cells using cationic liposomes. Cationic liposomes form complexes (lipoplexes) with negatively charged DNA through electrostatic interactions. The particles enter the cells through the process of endocytosis. The endosomal membrane is destabilized in the cytosol and the DNA molecule enters the nucleus.

double-stranded DNA and the transgene is integrated into the genomic DNA of host cells. This offers the possibility of stable transfection, however, with a risk for insertional mutations *(Fig. 11.10)*. The risks of toxicity of viral gene therapy were clearly demonstrated by the tragic death of an 18-year-old male patient treated for ornithine transcarbamylase deficiency.[26]

Immunosuppression has been used to reduce immunological responses to viral vectors. However, this strategy considerably increases the risks and side-effects of the treatment. Nonviral biological vectors such as bacterial, bacteriophages and virus-like particles may become valuable delivery tools in certain gene therapy niches.[27] Today, about two-thirds of clinical gene therapy trials are based on viral vectors, and merely 5–10% deploy

lipofection as a mode of gene delivery.[22] Features of the various techniques for gene delivery are summarized in *Table 11.1*. There is a need for more efficient and safer methods for gene delivery, and ongoing research aims at the development of improved technologies for delivery.

Gene therapy in tissue repair, reconstruction, and regeneration

Gene therapy has become an important area in the search for new therapies to improve wound healing and promote regeneration of tissues.[28] The increased understanding of the molecular mechanisms that govern the differentiation and proliferation of cells during the various stages of the wound-healing and regenerative processes has provided candidate factors for therapy. Application of peptide factors to the wound environment is often inefficient due to sequestration by the matrix, degradation, and clearance. Therefore, gene therapy to achieve sustained localized and modification of gene expression for these factors is highly attractive. Gene therapy has been experimentally used to improve repair in skin, bone, cartilage, and tendon. Moreover, genetic modification of stem cell populations can be used to stimulate regeneration in tissue defects, or to facilitate the *in vitro* generation of composite tissues. An interesting development is the use of microvascular flaps as carriers of cells genetically modified to suppress recurrence of malignancy.

Gene therapy combined with biomaterial scaffolds as carriers of genetically modified cells can be used to stimulate new tissue formation. These scaffolds are composed of various natural or synthetic materials. The scaffolds serve several purposes. Conduction refers to the supportive effect on the formation of new tissue. Cells attain a proper three-dimensional phenotype and utilize the scaffold for migration and formation of extracellular matrix. Induction refers to the function as carrier and reservoir for molecules that stimulate the generation of new tissue. Vectors can be delivered to the transfection site by scaffolds. Alternatively the scaffolds can be populated by *ex vivo* genetically modified cells. The scaffolds have several important potential advantages in gene therapy. The biomaterial may increase transfection efficiency by protecting against transgene degradation and providing more sustained delivery.

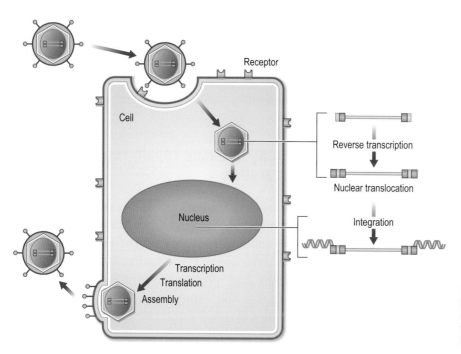

Fig. 11.10 Retroviral gene transfer. The retroviral single-stranded RNA genome is reverse-transcribed into double-stranded DNA and the transgene is integrated into the genomic DNA of host cells. Retroviruses offer the possibility of stable transfections.

Table 11.1 **Common techniques for gene delivery**

Gene delivery technique	Advantages	Disadvantages
Direct injection of naked DNA/plasmid DNA	Simple, local delivery, unlimited gene size, nontoxic and nonimmunogenic	Only direct injection, very low transfection efficiency, transient gene expression only
Gene gun	Can deliver large amounts of DNA; technically simple	Nonspecific, physical damage to cell required for DNA uptake, low transfection efficiency, potential foreign-body reaction
Microseeding	Can deliver large amounts and different types of DNA	Low transfection efficiency, cellular damage, limited experience
Electroporation	Large transgene size, nontoxic	Nonspecific, complex equipment, damage to cell membrane required for DNA uptake
Cationic liposomes	Technically simple, can transfect any cell type, large transgene size, local delivery, low immunogenicity	No targeting, toxicity, low transfection efficiency, transient transfection, rapid plasma clearance *in vivo*
Retrovirus	Tranduces many different cell types, high efficiency of *ex vivo* transduction, long-term gene expression	Transduces mainly dividing cells, inefficient transduction *in vivo*, risk of insertional mutagenesis, limited transgene size, difficult to propagate in culture
Adenovirus	Transfects virtually all cell types, dividing and nondividing cells, good transfection efficiency *in vitro* and *in vivo*, no integration into host genome, large transgene size	Immune response, lack of permanent expression, pre-existing antibodies are common, potential wild-type breakthrough infection
Adeno-associated virus	Transduces dividing and nondividing cells, integrates to specific site at chromosome 19, long-term gene expression, low immunogenicity	Difficult to grow to high titers, risk of insertional mutagenesis, limited transgene size, pre-existing antibodies, complex and expensive to manufacture
Hepres simplex virus 1	Transduces wide variety of cell types, neurotropism, large transgene size, long-term expression feasible, low immunogenicity	Pre-existing antibodies, difficult to manipulate due to complex life cycle, risk of wild-type breakthrough infection

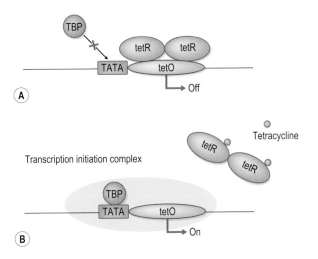

Fig. 11.11 A likely model of tetracycline repressor (tetR)-mediated transcription repression switch on the tetracycline operator (tetO)-bearing human cytomegalovirus (hCMV) major immediate-early promoter. **(A)** Binding of tetR to the tetO inserted at 10 bp downstream of the last nucleotide of the TATATAA element prevents TATA-binding protein (TBP) from binding to the TATA element, thus leading to the blockade of transcription initiation complex assembly on the target promoter and the repression of the expression. **(B)** In the presence of tetracycline, the ability of tetR to interact with tetO is abolished, which leads to the interaction of TBP with the TATA element that signals the transcription initiation.

Furthermore, local containment of vectors may prevent inflammatory reactions.

The expression of growth factors during tissue repair is spatially and temporally tightly regulated. Thus, ideally any methodology for gene therapy in wound healing should be cell-type-specific and provide temporal control over transgene expression. The combination of cell and gene therapy enables targeted delivery of transgenes *ex vivo* to specific cells recovered from the organism before local or systemic readministration. Another approach utilizes the possibility of designing DNA constructs with promoters that will only be expressed by certain cells.[29–31] DNA constructs can also be used to mediate pharmacologically induced transgene expression.[32–35] Our group developed the tetracycline repressor system, a DNA construct that enables the regulation of both the onset and level of transgene expression by the administration of tetracycline[36,37] *(Fig. 11.11)*.

Tissue repair

The skin is for several reasons a highly suitable target organ for gene therapy. The accessibility of the cutaneous surface facilitates *in vivo* gene delivery and

monitoring for any side-effects. Cells from the dermis and epidermis can be harvested for *in vitro* gene delivery and reapplied to the organism. Scaffolds can be used to deliver transgene-containing vectors or genetically modified skin cells to the wound. Skin grafts can be easily obtained and treated *ex vivo* before wound coverage. The limited time span of the wound-healing process makes it a suitable condition for transient gene modification. Furthermore, the expression of growth factors and cytokines is characterized by transient up- and downregulations, making short-term effects on gene expression more appropriate. The constant epidermal renewal by keratinocyte differentiation and exfoliation has nevertheless been regarded as a safety mechanism against any prolonged harmful effects. The rapid turnover of epidermal cells, as well as clearance of wound fibroblasts through apoptosis at the conclusion of wound healing, reduces the risk for tumor induction by insertional mutagenesis when viral delivery is utilized.

A number of gene therapy protocols have been used to improve healing in animal skin wound-healing models. The most popular approach used so far has been to deliver growth factors that are known to promote healing. Our group has described delivery of growth factors in a porcine wound-healing model. Epidermal growth factor (EGF) delivered directly to wounds by gold particles accelerated by an electric arc resulted in EGF overexpression and increased the rate of re-epithelialization.[38] The feasibility of *in vitro* transfection of keratinocytes, followed by grafting and transgene overexpression in the wound environment, was demonstrated with delivery of human growth hormone (hGH) by a retroviral approach.[39] Cultured keratinocytes were transfected with EGF using cationic liposomes *ex vivo* and regrafted to the wound. EGF overexpression and improved healing compared to nontransfected keratinocytes were observed.[40]

Other groups have mainly used rodent models to develop gene therapy protocols for wound healing. Insulin growth factor-1 (IGF1) delivered by local injection of cationic liposome vectors improved wound healing and weight gain in thermally injured rats.[41] A similar protocol was then used for the delivery of keratinocyte growth factor (KGF).[42] In a more recent study the same group demonstrated that liposomal transfection of IGF1 and KGF in combination, increased neovascularization and wound expression of vascular endothelial growth factor (VEGF) more than the transfection of either factor alone.[43] Platelet-derived growth factor-B (PDFG-B) was retrovirally delivered to mouse dermal fibroblast *ex vivo* before reapplication to wounds in a polyglycolic acid scaffold.[44] The growth factors PDGF, TGF-β, placenta growth factor and KGF, have all been delivered by adenoviruses to stimulate wound healing in experimental models.[45–48] Several research groups have used adenovirally delivered VEGF to improve healing in diabetic as well as nondiabetic rodent models.[49–52] We treated wounds in an aged pig model with adenoviral VEGF delivery without any effects on neovascularization or rate of wound healing.[53] However, we used wound chambers for optimal wound healing in a wet environment, and most probably VEGF overexpression was unable to improve healing further. This illustrates that a strategy aimed at growth factor overexpression usually presupposes a state of impaired healing and relative deficiency of the gene of interest. Recently, the results of a phase I clinical trial for treatment of diabetic foot ulcers with delivery of PDGF-B showed that periulcer injection with replication-incompetent adenoviral vector was well tolerated and improved wound healing.[54] The effect appeared to be mediated by enhanced vasculogenesis and the authors concluded that the protocol should be considered for further studies in humans.

Adenoviral delivery of different growth factors has been deployed in experimental settings to stimulate tendon repair. BPM12 and BMP14 and growth differentiation factor 5 have been successfully used to improve the healing of tendons in rat or chicken models of tendon repair.[55–57] Recently it was demonstrated that bone marrow-derived mesenchymal stem cells (BMSC) transfected with TGF-β₁ and applied to injured rat Achilles tendon improved a number of tendon-healing parameters with no additive effect from cotransfection with VEGF.[58]

There is a great need for therapies to induce bone formation. Gene therapy using osteoinductive factors has been experimentally utilized to improve fracture healing and increase bone mass around implants. Fracture healing in rodents has been stimulated by direct application of adenoviral vectors carrying BMP2.[59–64] A similar approach was used to increase vascularization and bone formation by delivery of VEGF-A.[65] A hybrid gene composed of a BMP4 transgene linked to a BMP2 secretory signal, delivered by direct application of retroviral vector to fracture periosteum, augmented the bone mass in a rat femur fracture model.[66] Degradable scaffolds loaded with naked plasmid DNA were used to deliver BMP4 and a fragment of parathyroid hormone to improve bone formation in bony defects in rat and canine models.[67,68] Liposomal vectors carrying BMP2 in degradable scaffolds composed of collagen and autologous bone increased bone mass around dental implants placed in calvarial defects in a pig model.[69] Mesenchymal stem cells genetically modified *ex vivo* to overexpress BMP2 improved repair in mouse radial segmental bone defects.[70] Muscle cells were recovered and *ex vivo* modified with a retroviral vector to express BMP4, before reimplantation to critical size rat femur defects.[71] Healing with restoration of the medullary canal and functional bone strength was achieved.

Tissue reconstruction and regeneration

Factors that promote neovascularization can be used to augment the blood supply of flaps. Several groups have demonstrated that *in vivo* delivery of VEGF enhances cutaneous and musculocutaneous flap viability in rats.[72–74] Using an *ex vivo* approach, flap viability was enhanced by VEGF overexpression in a rabbit model, where endothelial cells were genetically modified and delivered in a fibrin scaffold.[75] The mechanism of VEGF-enhanced flap viability was found to involve endothelial nitric oxide synthase.[76] Adenoviral delivery of TGF-β₁ was shown to increase the viability of epigastric artery flaps in a rat model.[77] Delivery of plasmid vectors containing PDGF-B increased the expression of VEGF and basic FGF (bFGF) and enhanced the viability of rat dorsal flaps.[78] Recently, the adeno-associated viral delivery of bFGF enhanced the viability of random pattern flaps in rats.[79]

Recovery of committed progenitor cells for combined gene and cell therapy has several potential applications in wound therapy as well as tissue-regenerative medicine. The ability of endothelial progenitor cells (EPC) to home into sites of tissue repair or ischemia and stimulate vascularization has been experimentally exploited for combined cell and gene therapy. EPCs were genetically modified *ex vivo* to overexpress VEGF and administered systemically to nude mice with hind-limb ischemia.[80] An increase of neovascularization and blood flow and drastically reduced frequency of amputation were observed. Increased viability of random flaps has been demonstrated after treatment with EPCs genetically modified to overexpress VEGF.[81]

The methodologies described above to induce bone formation in fractures and around implants have also been utilized experimentally to generate bone for reconstruction of craniofacial defects. Locally delivered adenoviral vector, containing BMP2, increased bone formation during the consolidation phase in a rat model for mandibular distraction.[82] The chemical vector polyethylenimine was used to deliver BMP4 in a polylactic-co-glycolic acid scaffold to critical-size rat calvarial defects.[83] This treatment augmented bone formation in the central region of the defects as compared to empty scaffolds. Bone marrow stromal cells were retrovirally transfected with BMP7 *ex vivo* and redelivered in a gelatin scaffold.[84] Adenoviral vector was used to transfect bone marrow stromal cells *ex vivo* with BMP2 to generate bone in maxillary and cranial defects in pig.[85,86] Skin fibroblasts genetically modified to overexpress osteogenic factors have the ability to form components of bone matrix. This feature has been utilized to generate bone in calvarial defects in rats.[87,88]

Microvascular free flaps are used to reconstruct defects after tumor-ablative surgery. The separation of the flap from the body before reimplantation creates an opportunity for *ex vivo* gene modification of cells in the flap. The delivery of transgenes that suppress any remaining tumor cells at the resection site constitutes an interesting therapeutic approach against recurrence and metastasis of malignant disease. In an experimental rodent model the afferent artery of a microvascular flap was perfused with adenoviral vectors carrying the lacZ reporter gene.[89] High regional transgene expression was observed in different cell types of the flap and no expression was found outside the flap.

Ethical issues of genetic discovery and gene therapy

The ever-growing knowledge from genetic discovery, and the possibility for therapeutic gene modification, raises several ethical issues.[90,91] The genetic database generated from the Human Genome Project raises questions of who should have access to such information and how it should be used. Should the data be classified alongside medical records and subject to the same confidentiality laws, or should employers and insurance companies have a right to access? Should the data be used to inform patients about their possible future disease patterns, even if there is no cure or available prophylaxis? The knowledge of gene structure and function is used to develop diagnostic tools and therapies. But can a gene be any one person's invention? Is it right that researchers or companies patent genes? A number of commercially available testing kits have been developed for people to do their own genetic screening, diagnosis, and even prediction of prognosis. However many questions remain to be answered about the pathogenesis of common mulitfactorial conditions such as diabetes and hypertension, and the scientific community has heavily criticized these testing kits for not providing meaningful information. Moreover, receiving genetic information without input from a medical doctor may lead to misinterpretation of results.

The possibility of finding a permanent cure for severe or life-threatening disease by gene therapy would be of great benefit for many patients. Moreover, such progress would be highly rewarding for individual scientists, institutions, and companies. Thus, there is no lack of incentives in the search for these therapies. At the same time, the development of gene therapy requires clinical trials, with a risk of severe, even life-threatening, side-effects from vector administration or from the genetic modification itself. This creates a field of tension where the basic principles of medical ethics, such as the principles of autonomy, nonmaleficence and beneficence, may be challenged. The prospect of germline gene therapy and cloning raises particularly complex moral and ethical issues. Fetal therapy could be used to prevent life-threatening disease or dangerous postnatal surgery. However, the same technologies could also be used for eugenic purposes, i.e., for genetic enhancement with the aim of maximizing well-being for individuals or societies.

In an attempt to address these concerns many regulatory bodies have been established to overlook the process involved and enforce some basic principles. The Recombinant DNA Advisory Committee was one such initiative drawn up by the National Institutes of

Health (NIH), and the Food and Drug Administration (FDA) focuses on the safety and efficacy of genetically altered products.[92] Regulations were established whereby research proposals went through a review process consisting of preliminary approval by the home institution's institutional biosafety committee and institutional review board before final approval from the Recombinant DNA Advisory Committee.

The American Society of Gene and Cell Therapy was established in 1996 and has provided a policy for ethical standards involving gene therapy clinical studies.[93] The guiding principle is that the clinical investigators must be able to design and carry out clinical research studies in an objective and unbiased manner, free from conflicts caused by significant financial involvement with the commercial sponsors of the study. In March 2000, as part of ongoing efforts to ensure patient protection in gene therapy trials, the FDA and NIH announced two new initiatives to strengthen further the safeguards for individuals enrolled in clinical studies for gene therapy: Gene Therapy Clinical Trial Monitoring Plan and the Gene Transfer Safety Symposia.[94] The ultimate aim of all societies concerned with ethical issues is to ensure that clinical trials are conducted maintaining the principles in the constitution of the United Nations Educational, Scientific, and Cultural Organization of the "dignity, equality and mutual respect of men."

Genetic disease and diagnosis

The term "genetic disease" includes all disorders where the etiology can be traced back to genetic or chromosomal abnormalities. In monogenetic disease the cause can be found in mutations of a single gene causing aberrant, malfunctioning protein. Most diseases are however complex and multifactorial, caused by many genes acting in concert with environmental factors.

Congenital anomalies

The rapid progress in genetic science has increased our knowledge about the etiology and pathogenesis of congenital anomalies commonly treated by the plastic surgeon. This progress has already enhanced our possibilities for prenatal diagnosis with importance for patient counseling and family planning.

Nomenclature

Congenital anomalies are defects in the structure of tissues, organs, or body parts, present at birth. Based on the main mechanism of pathogenesis, anomalies can be categorized into the categories of malformation, deformation, disruption, and dysplasia.[95]

Malformations are anomalies caused by an aberrant developmental process, intrinsic to the affected tissues. Orofacial clefts are representative of such abnormal morphogenesis. Fusion of the facial processes is an important step of facial embryogenesis and is dependent on timely and highly regulated proliferation, migration, differentiation, and apoptosis of cells. These cellular events are in turn regulated by molecular mechanisms, most notably by growth factors and intracellular molecules involved in cell–cell signaling. Disturbances in the molecular mechanisms may thus lead to aberrant cellular behavior, and ultimately to a malformation of involved facial tissues.

In deformations, a mechanical force causes the anomaly. Breech presentation, large fetal weight, tumor masses, unicornuate uterus, and oligohydroamnios are examples of factors that may cause mechanic fetal constriction. Developmental dysplasia of the hip is related to mechanical fetal constriction.[96] Clubfoot has traditionally been categorized as a deformation-related intrauterine compression during the third trimester. However, more recent data have failed to support this hypothesis and current knowledge suggests it is rather a congenital malformation with direct genetic causes.[97] Various deformations and contractures may occur secondary to oligohydroamnios and the severity of these deformations is correlated with its duration.[98,99] As a consequence the most severe deformations are associated with pulmonary hypoplasia and perinatal death. The oligohydroamnios, or Potter, sequence was initially described in cases of renal agenesia and is characterized by facial compression, broad flat hands, pulmonary hyopoplasia, and asymmetric positional deformities of the extermities.[100]

Disruption describes a process whereby normal development from embryologic tissues with normal developmental potential is hindered or broken down by extrinsic factors. In amniotic band sequence (ABS) fibrous tissue bands may constrict fingers or whole extremities, which may cause necrosis and even amputation. Amniotic membrane rupture, loss of amniotic fluid, and subsequent entanglement of body parts in the amniotic membrane are believed to cause the fibrous tissue bands. However, an association of ABS with cleft lip and palate and polydactyly suggests that amniotic banding may also be the result of intrinsic disturbances of morphogenesis on a genetic basis.[101]

The term "dysplasia" refers to aberrant development of embryonic tissues and includes disorders like Marfan's syndrome and osteogenesis imperfecta. In these conditions there is often widespread involvement with anomalies in several anatomic structures derived from the involved tissue.

The distinction between the different categories described above is not always clear. Some anomalies are the result of combinations of two or three of these mechanisms and the same type of anomaly may result from different mechanisms. In a study of 27 145 consecutive infants with congenital defects, 97.94% had malformations, 3.12% had deformations, and 1.65% had disruptions. In 3.51% the cause was a combination of two or three mechanisms, with malformation with deformation by far the commonest combination.[102] The described sequence of events in the oligohydroamnios sequence exemplifies the combination of renal malformation with deformation of the face and extremities. Further, the above-mentioned genetic basis for amniotic bands implies a combination of malformation and disruption. Indeed, as knowledge about the genetic ethiology of congenital anomalies expands, conditions previously believed to be pure deformations or disruption may prove to be events secondary to abnormal morphogenesis. The Pierre Robin sequence (PRS) is described as a series of events where glossoptosis secondary to micrognathia prevents palatal fusion and results in the formation of cleft palate. According to this prevailing theory, the cleft palate is a deformation caused by the mechanic force of the tongue. The etiology of PRS is however unknown. There is no scientific evidence to support intrauterine fetal constriction as a cause for micrognathia. The fact that PRS is found in several syndromes rather points towards primary genetic causes behind the mandibular growth disturbance. Candidate genetic loci and candidate genes for PRS have been

identified.[103] Thus, PRS may be another example of a malformation–deformation sequence.

Selected congenital anomalies

Orofacial clefts

Orofacial clefts include the more common cleft lip and/or palate as well as rare forms of facial clefts. Clefts are formed when embryonic facial processes fail to fuse. By the fourth week of embryonic development, the frontonasal prominence, the paired maxillary processes, and paired mandibular processes surround the primitive oral cavity. The formation of the nasal placodes then divides the frontonasal prominence into paired medial and lateral nasal processes. The upper lip and primary palate form at the end of the sixth week of development by the fusion of the bilateral medial nasal processes with one another and the maxillary processes on each side. The secondary palate develops from the maxillary processes as vertically growing palatal shelves that rise to a horizontal position during the seventh week of development and fuse in the midline. It has been demonstrated that fusion of the lip and primary palate is controlled by a different set of genes than formation of the secondary palate.[104] Clefts may occur as isolated malformations or as parts of a syndrome. Studies in mice and chicks have been of central importance for the elucidation of the genes and molecular mechanism behind the development of orofacial clefts.[105] The search for the genetic and molecular mechanisms involved in clefting combines different approaches such as: studies of genes involved in cleft syndromes, genomewide searches for genetic linkage in families with multiple cases of nonsyndromic clefts, linkage analysis, and allelic association studies of candidate genes. A comprehensive list of candidate genes known or suspected to be involved in orofacial clefting was recently published in a comprehensive review by Jugessur et al.[106]

Nonsyndromic cleft lip and palate

Cleft lip and/or palate occurs as nonsyndromic, isolated malformations in about 70% of cases, while cleft palate is nonsyndromic in half of cases.[107] Nonsyndromic clefts are usually sporadic and have multifactorial etiologies involving different genes and environmental factors. However, familial clustering and concordance in twins point towards a genetic susceptibility for orofacial clefting.[108,109] The observed concordance rates are 40–60% for monozygotic twins and 3–5% for dizygotic twins. Population studies have shown that the occurrence of cleft lip/cleft lip and palate in a family normally does not increase the risk for isolated cleft palate, and vice versa, which is in accordance with the notion that these conditions have different genetic etiologies.[107,110] Moreover, it was found that the risk for recurrence was stronger for cleft palate than for cleft lip/cleft lip and palate and that the anatomical severity of the cleft does not increase the risk of recurrence.[110] The relative risk for recurrence in first-degree relatives was 32 for any cleft lip and 56 for cleft palate only. The risk for the offspring was similar whether the affected first-line relative was the father, mother, or sibling, which points towards a major contribution from autosomal genes expressed during fetal life.

Recent discoveries from experimental animal models have increased the knowledge about the cellular and molecular mechanisms in facial embryogenesis. Growth factor signaling and activation of transcription factors regulate the cellular events behind outgrowth and fusion of facial processes. Interactions between epithelium and mesenchyme are of particular importance in this context.[111] Genes found to be involved in lip and primary palate formation are the extracellular signaling molecules bone morphogenetic proteins (*Bmp*), fibroblast growth factors (*Fgf*) and sonic hedgehog (*Shs*), the homeobox transcription factors encoded by distal-less homeobox-containing genes (*Dlx*), *Barx1*, *Msx1* and *Msx2*, and the transcription factor *Tp63*, which is implicated in the development of epithelial tissues.[112–116]

The initiation and vertical growth of the shelves of the secondary palate involve a partially different set of growth and transcription factors. These include *Osr2*, *Lhx8*, *Msx1*, *Fgf10*, *Fgfr2*, and *Tgfbr2*.[117] It has been demonstrated that *Fgf10* secreted from the palatal mesenchyme activates *Fgfr2* in the epithelium which in turn maintains epithelial SHH expression.[118] Disruption of this mechanism was demonstrated to cause cleft palate. Another mechanism for epithelial–mesenchymal interactions during palatal shelf growth involves *Bmp2* and *Bmp4*, *Shh* and the transcription factor *Msx1*. Msx1 activity regulates epithelial expression of *Bmp4* and *Shh* in the epithelium and of *Bmp2* and *Bmp4* in the

mesenchyme. Shh from the epithelium upregulates mesenchymal *Bmp2* expression, which in turn drives palatal growth.[119]

Palatogenesis is dependent on a switch from adhesion incompetence of the tissues during vertical growth to adhesion competence during horizontal growth. This switch is regulated by the membrane-bound signaling molecule Jaged-2 and by the transcription factor interferon-regulatory factor 6 (IRF6).[120–122] The process of palatal shelf fusion starts with formation of the midline epithelial seam followed by epithelial breakdown by apoptosis to allow for establishment of mesenchymal continuity. Formation of the midline epithelial seam involves the activity of adhesion factors, desmosomes, growth factors, and proteolytic enzymes.[123–125] Tgf-α is expressed in proximity to the midline seam during fusion and was the one of the first factors to be associated with orofacial clefts.[126] Tgf-β₃ secreted from the medial-edge epithelium has been found to be of particular importance in this process.[127–132] *Tgf-β₃* knockout has been demonstrated to produce cleft palate and this was rescued by exogenous administration of Tgf-β₃.[133,134] There is evidence that Irf6 is a downstream mediator of Tgf-β₃ in the medial-edge palatal epithelium.[135,136]

PDGF-C is another signaling peptide implicated in palatogenesis. *Pdgf*–/– mice die perinatally due to respiratory and feeding failure secondary to complete clefting of the secondary palate.[137] It has been shown that PDGF-C signaling is necessary for proper migration of neuroectodermal cells and it was proposed that deficient cellular migration in the palate of *pdgf*–/– mice was the mechanism behind cleft formation. SNPs linked to cleft lip and/or palate were found to be associated with decreased activity of the *Pdgf-C* promoter.[138]

The genes found to cause the various syndromes with clefts have provided clues in the search for genes involved in nonsyndromic clefts. Examples are IRF6 of Van der Woude syndrome (VWS), FGFR1 of Kallman's syndrome, Tp63 and PVRL1 of ectodermal dysplasia syndromes, TBX2 of X-linked clefting and ankyloglossia, and PTCH1 of Gorlin's syndrome.[139–149]

Syndromic cleft lip and palate

About 200 different syndromes that may include cleft lip and palate have been described. Cleft palate has been identified as a component in approximately 400 different syndromes. VWS, CATCH 22, and different types of ectodermal dysplasia belong to the more common syndromes seen in patients with orofacial clefts. All three of these syndromes may be inherited as autosomal-dominant diseases. However, 30–50% of cases with VWS and 90% of cases with CATCH 22 are caused by *de novo* gene mutations. Ectodermal dysplasia has been reported as both familial and sporadic.

VWS is characterized by cleft lip and/or palate and lower lip pits and is related to popliteal pterygium syndrome (PPS), which also includes varying degrees of popliteal webbing, pterygia, oral synychiae, adhesions between the eyelids, syndactyly, and genital anomalies. VWS/PPS is caused by mutations in the gene encoding for IRF6, *IRF6*.[150] IRF6 is a transcription factor with a highly conserved DNA-binding domain and a more variable protein-binding domain. A correlation between genotype and phenotype has been demonstrated where VWS is caused by missense mutations in both the DNA and protein-binding domains, while popliteal pterygium syndrome is mainly caused by mutations in the DNA-binding domain.[150] Furthermore, nonsense and frameshift mutations were found to be significantly more common in VWS than in PPS. CATCH 22 is a collective acronym for overlapping and phenotypically heterogeneous syndromes of common genetic etiology. CATCH 22 stands for cardiac abnormality/abnormal facies, T-cell deficit due to thymic hypoplasia, cleft palate, and hypocalcemia due to hypoparathyroidism resulting from 22q11 deletion. In total, 69–100% of patients with this deletion have palatal abnormalities, such as cleft, velopharyngeal insufficiency, bifid uvula, and submucous cleft.[19] The 22q11 deletion contains about 35 different genes. The most important of these genes for the development of the various anomalies is *TBX1*. *TBX1* belongs to the group of so-called T-box genes, a group of genes coding for transcriptional regulators, which are expressed in the pharyngeal mesenchyme and endodermal pouch in mice. However, the high variability of symtoms in CATCH 22 patients suggests that other genetic loci may be involved. FGF8 and CRKL have both been demonstrated to enhance the effect of *TBX1* mutations.[151,152] More recently, chordin was found to be a modifier of *TBX1* for the craniofacial phenotype in a murine model of CATCH 22.[153]

Ectodermal dysplasia is characterized by dysplasia of ectoderm-derived structures such as hair, teeth, nails, and sweat glands. Ectodermal dysplasia is however a group of syndromes with varying phenotypes, that in addition to the ectodermal dysplasia may include malformations such as orofacial clefts. The orofacial cleft may be of any type in the cleft lip and palate/cleft palate spectrum, and variable expressivity is seen within the same ectodermal dysplasia families. Accordingly, defects in many different genes have been associated with this group of syndromes. Interestingly, mutations in different genes may cause the same type of ectodermal dysplasia and, conversely, mutations in one gene may give rise to different types of the syndrome. Several forms of ectodermal dysplasia with orofacial cleft are caused by mutations in the TP63 gene, encoding for a transcription factor important for the development of epithelial tissues.[146]

Craniosynostosis

Craniosynostosis may be a primary or secondary condition. Primary craniosynostosis is a group of malformations caused by errors intrinsic to the developmental process of the cranial skeleton, causing fusion of the cranial vault sutures. Secondary craniosynostosis develops postnatally due to inhibited brain growth or metabolic disturbances. In 80–90% of cases, primary craniosynostosis is a nonsyndromic congenital malformation due to fusion of typically one, but occasionally several, sutures of the cranial vault. The resulting malformation depends on the suture(s) involved. About 100 different syndromes with craniosynostosis have been described. The most common are the ones related to mutations in the FGFRs such as the syndromes of Crouzon and Apert.

The bones of the cranial vault develop by intramembraneous ossification between the overlying dermal mesenchyme and the meningeal mesenchyme beneath.[154] The individual bones are formed by radial growth from condensations of ossifying mesenchymal tissue. Postnatally the sutures constitute the principal growth centers for the neurocranium, allowing for the rapid growth of the brain during the first 2 years. The activity of these growth centers is believed to be dependent on interactions between the different tissues that are juxtaposed at the suture. Sutural mesenchyme, underlying dura mater, and covering pericranium are believed to interact to regulate cellular differentiation and proliferation at the suture. Various studies have demonstrated the dura mater to be of particular importance for sutural patency and fusion.[155–158] These tissue interactions are mediated by various growth factors, receptors, and transcription factors involved in intercellular signaling. The importance of the FGFRs has been mentioned and is detailed in the section on syndromic craniosynostosis, below. Different members of the TGF-β family of growth factors have been found to be important for development of the craniofacial skeleton and for cranial suture biology. *TGF-β2* knockout mice died perinatally with a wide range of malformations, including craniofacial malformations with micrognathia and reduced size and ossification of cranial bones.[159] Mice with conditional inactivation of the Tgf-β2 receptor gene, *tgf-β2r*, in the cranial neural crest were born with complete clefts of the secondary palate and calvarial defects.[160] The balance in activity of the different TGF-β isoforms has been shown to regulate suture fusion.[161] High expression of *Tgf-β1* and *2* in relation to *Tgf-β3* was found to promote physiologic fusion of the posterior frontal suture in rats, while the opposite relation of isoform expression was related to patency of the coronal suture. More recently, evidence was presented that the effect of Tgf-β2 on suture fusion is mediated by the EGF signaling system.[162] Other members of the TGF-β family have been found to be involved in suture biology. *Bmp2* and *Bmp4* were expressed in the osteogenic front of sutures, and *Bmp2* and *Bmp4* in the mesenchyme of cranial sutures and adjacent dura mater.[163] Furthermore, it has been demonstrated that the gene for Bmp antagonist, Noggin, is expressed in the mesenchyme of patent sutures and that its expression is suppressed by Fgf2.[164] Another Bmp antagonist, Bmp3, is downregulated during physiologic fusion of the posterior frontal suture.[165] Strong support for a role of the TGF-β family in suture biology came from the discovery of a syndrome with craniosynostosis caused by different mutations in TGF-β receptors 1 or 2.[166]

Syndromic craniosynostosis

The first genetic abnormality ever found in craniosynostosis was a P148H misense and gain-of-function mutation in the transcription factor muscle segment homeobox-2 (*MSX2*).[167] This mutation was identified in a family with an autosomal-dominant syndrome, with high penetrance and variable phenotypic expressivity, that was named Boston-type craniosynostosis. Another transcription factor gene implicated in craniosynostosis is TWIST1. The Saethre–Chotzen syndrome is caused by several different *TWIST1* mutations that cause loss of transcription factor function.[168,169] This syndrome is characterized by mild and asymmetrical synostosis, low-set frontal hairline, nasal septum deviation, parrot-beaked nose, external ear abnormalities, tear duct stenosis, eyelid ptosis, canthal dystopia, and brachydactyly. The syndrome is highly heterogeneous in its phenotype and often subtle in its phenotypic expression, which reflects the pleiotropy of TWIST and the presence of other modifying molecular mechanisms. MSX2 induces bone formation and, if overexpressed, sutural fusion, by increasing the number of osteogenic cells.[170] Loss of MSX2 function has been identified in a genetic condition with parietal bone defects.[171] TWIST on the other hand has a negative effect on differentiation of osteprogenitor cells into osteogenic cells.[172] TWIST is involved in the FGF signaling pathway and appears to be a negative regulator of *FGFR* gene expression.[173] Thus, loss of TWIST function and gain of FGFR function may be components of a common molecular pathway in the pathogenesis of craniosynostosis.

The biggest group of craniosynostosis syndromes, including Crouzon, Apert and Pfeiffer, is caused by mutations in genes coding for different isoforms of *FGFGR*. Common to these syndromes, also called faciocraniosynostosis or craniofacial dysostoses, is the combination of calvarial synostosis with growth restriction of the skull base and the mid facial skeleton. The faciocraniosynostosis syndromes belong to a wider group of syndromes called the skeletal dysplasias, which also include the dwarfing chondrodysplasias. Furthermore, several of the FGFR-related craniosynostosis syndromes include limb malformations. Thus, the FGFRs are involved in the development of both the craniofacial and the appendicular skeleton.

The FGFR-related syndromes may be inherited as autosomal-dominant diseases; however most cases are sporadic and noninherited, and caused by new gene mutations. Mutations that cause craniosynostosis syndromes have been identified in *FGFR1, -2 or -3*, with *FGF2* mutations being the most common.[15] The genetic loci are 8p for FGFR1, 10q for *FGFR2*, and 4p for *FGFR3*. The FGFRs are transmembrane receptors with an extracellular domain, a transmembrane domain, and an intracellular region.[174] The ligand-binding extracellular domain consists of three immunoglobulin-like loops (Ig1, 2 and 3) and the acidic box that separates Ig2 from Ig3. The intracellular region has tyrosine kinase activity as well as other regulatory sequences.

Ligand binding is facilitated by heparin sulfate proteoglycan (hspg). Binding of hspg–ligand complex to the receptor leads to receptor dimerization and activation of intracellular pathways of signal transduction (*Fig. 11.4*). The different FGFR isoforms show great amino acid sequence homology, especially in the immunoglobulin-like loops of the extracellular domain. However, the *FGFR* gene structure allows for the synthesis of many different forms of the receptor. Alternate splicing produces a diversity of receptor isoforms with highly variable extracellular sequence compositions, which mainly serves to produce isoforms that differ in ligand-binding specificity. *FGF3* mutations in achondroplasia were reported in 1994.[175] In that same year the gene behind Crouzon was mapped to 10q25-q26 and in a subsequent paper a mutation in *FGFR2* was identified.[176] *FGFR2* mutations have since been identified in the syndromes of Crouzon, Apert, Pfeiffer, Jackson–Weiss and Beare–Stevenson (*Table 11.2*). More than 30 different *FGFR2* misense mutations have been identified.[15] Most are dispersed in the sequence encoding the extracellular domain of the receptor; however, a few mutations have been identified in the transmembrane

as well as the intracellular catalytic regions (*Fig. 11.12*). Syndromic craniosynostosis may also be caused by mutations in *FGFR1* and -3. A rare form of Crouzon syndrome with acanthosis nigrans is caused by a mutation in *FGFR3* and Pfeiffer syndrome may be caused by mutation in *FGFR1*.

Muenke syndrome is unusual in that it was defined based on its genetic abnormality, an *FGFR3*-P250R mutation.[177] The phenotype of this syndrome, first described by Glass *et al.* and then by Lajeunie *et al.*, includes coronal synostosis, hypertelorism, mild midface hypoplasia, brachydactyly, and characteristic bulging of the temporal fossae.[178,179]

Common to the FGFR mutations in syndromic craniosynostosis is that they lead to gain of function. The mutations may cause increased FGFR signaling through various mechanisms.[180] Destruction of cysteine residues may cause formation of intermolecular disulfide bonds in the extracellular domain of the receptor, resulting in ligand-independent and constitutive receptor activation. Other mutations may cause constitutive receptor activation through conformational changes of the extracellular domain. Mutations found in Apert syndrome cause alterations in receptor signaling through changes in ligand specificity. There is a great variation in the

Table 11.2 Craniosynostosis syndromes and involved genes

Syndrome	Chromosomal location	Mutated gene	OMIM entry
Crouzon	10q26	FGFR2 FGFR3	123500
Apert	10q26	FGFR2	101200
Pfeiffer	10q26 8p11	FFR2 FGFR1	101600
Jackson–Weiss	10q26	FGFR2	123150
Boston-type craniosynostosis	5q34	MSX2	123101
Beare–Stevenson	10q26	FGFR2	123790
Muenke	4p16	FGFR3	602849
Saethre–Chotzen	7p21	TWIST	101400

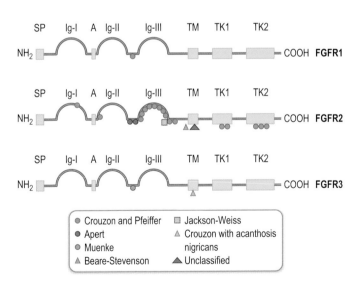

Fig. 11.12 Mutations in syndromic craniosynostosis. Schematic of mutations found in fibroblast growth factor receptor (FGFR) 1, 2, and 3, causing craniosynostosis syndromes. The extracellular region contains a signal peptide (SP), immunoglobulin (Ig)-like domains I, II, and III, and an acidic box (A). The tyrosine kinase (TK) domain has two subdomains, TK1 and TK2. The transmembrane (TM) domain spans the cell membrane.

dysmorphology within and between these syndromes, and also between affected individuals of the same family. This variation is most probably due to phenotypic effects of different mutations, tissue-specific expression of different FGFR isoforms during development, other modifying factors, and possibly environmental factors.

The increased understanding of the genetic and molecular mechanisms behind craniosynostosis may have a direct impact on clinical decision-making. The reoperation rate for intracranial hypertension was found to be considerably higher in Saethre–Chotzen as well as Muenke syndrome compared to nonsyndromic cases of bicoronal synostosis.[181,182] This implies that particularly close monitoring is warranted for the group of patients with confirmed syndromic diagnosis. Patients with unilateral frontal plagiocephaly and gene mutations have more pronounced dysmorphology compared to patients without mutations.[183,184] Accordingly, the presence of mutations is associated with higher frequency of surgical revisions and may require more extensive primary surgical procedures.

Prenatal diagnosis

The evolution of ultrasonographic technology and the increased knowledge about the genetic and molecular basis for disease have enhanced the possibilities for prenatal diagnosis of congenital anomalies. Prenatal diagnosis may either be a result of targeted investigation based on known increased risk for a particular anomaly, or may be an unexpected finding during routine screening. The diagnostic arsenal includes ultrasonography, maternal serum screening tests, transcervical retrieval of trophoblast cells, invasive tests to obtain fetal DNA, and fetoscopy.

There are several reasons for obtaining a diagnosis prenatally. The information can be used to prepare scheduled delivery in conditions with increased perinatal risk or to prepare for timely medical or surgical management after delivery. Parents may decide to have an abortion based on prenatal diagnosis. The information may also be used to prepare the parents psychologically for any congenital disease or stillbirth. A rare option after reaching a prenatal diagnosis is to perform a fetal intervention. A comprehensive description of prenatal diagnosis and screening is beyond the scope of this chapter. The following section focuses on prenatal diagnosis of facial clefts and craniosynostosis.

Ultrasound

Ultrasonography is normally performed around 20 weeks' gestation to assess fetal anatomy and can be used to visualize the dysmorphology of craniofacial malformations. Cleft lip with or without cleft palate may be detected prenatally by ultrasound.[185] Reported detection rates are in the range of 25–50% and few false-positive cases have occurred. The presence of a palatal cleft cannot be assessed with today's technology. The prenatal diagnosis of a facial cleft should be followed by a referral to a cleft lip and palate center for a consultation on postnatal management.

Syndromic and nonsyndromic craniosynostosis can be detected by ultrasonography.[186] The diagnosis is made by detection of either a dysmorphic head or other associated extremity malformations. Abnormal head shape is however found with routine scanning in about 2–3% of pregnancies and other causes such as spina bifida and trisomy 18 should be excluded. Measurements obtained that can facilitate diagnosis are the biparietal diameter and occipitofrontal diameter and from them the cephalic index (CI) is calculated. A CI <75% signifies dolicocephaly and a CI >85% is considered brachycephalic.

Head malformations secondary to synostosis are usually not seen until the third trimester. A number of nonsyndromic cases are reported; most are detected during the third trimester in conjunction with examinations performed for polyhydramnios.[187–189] Severe craniofacial manifestations such as cloverleaf skull, or extremity manifestations of craniosynostosis syndromes, are usually detectable during the second-trimester examination. Detection of the mitten-like hands of Apert syndrome in early second trimester was reported.[190] Apert diagnosis based on skull anomalies has been reported at 16 and 19 weeks' gestation.[191,192] In cases of unexpected craniosynostosis the parents should be referred to a clinical geneticist for counseling. Once the diagnosis of craniosynostosis has been confirmed the parents should be referred to a unit specializing in congenital craniofacial disorders for a discussion of prognosis and treatment.

Invasive testing

When there is a known parental genetic mutation or suspected congenital disease with known mutations, fetal DNA may be obtained through amniocentesis or chorionic villus sampling (CVS). Amniocentesis can usually be performed from gestational week 14 to 20 and has a risk for miscarriage of about 1%. CVS may be performed at about week 11, but has a somewhat higher risk for fetal loss of about 1–2%. The fetal cells collected by amniocentesis may have to be expanded in culture before DNA analysis is performed. However, if the precise mutation is known, PCR amplification of the mutated DNA segments may be used for direct diagnosis. If the mutation is unknown, linkage analysis may be performed to identify inherited mutations. In pregnancies at risk of having a craniofacial syndrome with known mutations, such as Crouzon, Saethre–Chotzen or Muenke, a genetic prenatal diagnosis may be reached by invasive testing. However, the highly variable expressivity of these conditions renders prognostic predictions difficult. Serial sonographic imaging can then be used to assess the actual dysmorphology.

Future development

The rapid expansion of knowledge in genetics will most likely continue. We can expect a continuing development of improved methods to study gene function and epigenetic mechanisms, and to modify gene expression. In this context the importance of basic research, aiming to elucidate the molecular mechanisms in pathogenesis, cannot be emphasized enough. New curative therapies can only develop through increased understanding of these fundamental mechanisms. In plastic surgery, we should expect molecular therapies to increase the healing rate in complicated wounds as well as to prevent excessive scarring and keloids. Gene therapy may become an adjunct to surgical reconstruction. Delivery of factors that stimulate neovascularization and blood flow may be used to enhance the viability of flaps and skin grafts, allowing for larger tissue transfers. "Biological brachytherapy," i.e., the use of microsurgical flaps for local delivery of therapeutic substances, is an exciting development combining reconstruction with adjuvant cancer treatment.

Disappointment with what has been achieved with gene therapy, or with tissue engineering, is frequently expressed. Indeed, the majority of gene therapy clinical trials are still in phase I or II. Moreover, the construction of entire organs or tissues in the laboratory environment cannot be expected in the foreseeable future. However, there is no doubt that we are just at the beginning of a fascinating era in which the combination of gene therapy with cell therapy and biomaterial scaffolds can be used to create composites for tissue regeneration. We can also expect a further understanding of the molecular basis of congenital anomalies. This will obviously be of great value in diagnosis and counseling. Moreover, a better understanding of the genotype-to-phenotype relation will help to guide surgical decisions. It is of paramount importance that the advancement of knowledge and technology for genetic diagnosis and therapy is tightly coupled with a vivid and open debate on all the ethical issues relevant to the field.

 Bonus images for this chapter can be found online at **http://www.expertconsult.com**

Fig. 11.1 History. Timeline with the main milestones of genetic discovery.

 Access the complete reference list online at **http://www.expertconsult.com**

13. Nie X, Luukko K, Kettunen P. FGF signalling in craniofacial development and developmental disorders. *Oral Dis*. 2006;12:102–111.

14. Nie X, Luukko K, Kettunen P. BMP signalling in craniofacial development. *Int J Dev Biol*. 2006;50:511–521.

15. Bonaventure J, El Ghouzzi V. Molecular and cellular bases of syndromic craniosynostoses. *Expert Rev Mol Med*. 2003;5:1–17.

23. Bleiziffer O, Eriksson E, Yao F, et al. Gene transfer strategies in tissue engineering. *J Cell Mol Med*. 2007;11:206–223.

Gene therapy and tissue engineering may play an important role in regenerative medicine for anatomical losses. This paper reviews different strategies of gene delivery in this context.

37. Yao F, Eriksson E. A novel tetracycline-inducible viral replication switch. *Hum Gene Ther.* 1999;10:419–427.

    Temporal regulation of gene expression is an essential component of any useful gene therapy strategy. This paper describes the basis of one such control mechanism.

90. Fleck LM. Ethical Issues In Molecular Medicine and Gene Therapy. In: Kresina TF, ed. *An Introduction to Molecular and Gene Therapy.* Wiley-Liss, New York; 2001:319–346.

    This chapter begins with a discussion of the ethical issues surrounding somatic cell gene therapy. The focus then shifts to germline genetic engineering.

95. Spranger J, Benirschke K, Hall JG, Lenz W, Lowry RB, Opitz JM, et al. Errors of morphogenesis: concepts and terms. Recommendations of an international working group. *J Pediatr.* 1982;100:160–165.

    This article represents a consensus statement intended to clarify terminology applied to disorders of morphogenesis.

Specifically, the authors aim to facilitate diagnostic classification by offering precise terminology to facilitate discussions in a field whose emphasis is evolving from physical description to an analysis of pathogenesis.

105. Mossey PA, Little J, Munger RG, et al. Cleft lip and palate. *Lancet.* 2009;374:1773–1785.

    This is a review of oral clefting. Topics ranging from embryology to clinical management and prevention are discussed.

110. Sivertsen A, Wilcox AJ, Skjaerven R, Vindenes HA, Abyholm F, Harville E, et al. Familial risk of oral clefts by morphological type and severity: population based cohort study of first degree relatives. *Br Med J.* 2008;336:432–434.

185. Jones MC. Prenatal diagnosis of cleft lip and palate: detection rates, accuracy of ultrasonography, associated anomalies, and strategies for counseling. *Cleft Palate Craniofac J.* 2002;39:169–173.

186. Miller C, Losken HW, Towbin R, et al. Ultrasound diagnosis of craniosynostosis. *Cleft Palate Craniofac J.* 2002;39:73–80.

12

Principles of cancer management

Tomer Avraham, Evan Matros, and Babak J. Mehrara

SYNOPSIS

- There has been a gradual progression from radical to more conservative resections of many cancers.
- Neoadjuvant therapies have facilitated resectability and even down-staging of the disease.
- A better understanding of immunology has led to the development of biologic therapies beyond the standard cytotoxic chemotherapies.
- Tailored immunotherapies are being studied and represent a new paradigm in the treatment of cancer.

Background

The introduction of reconstruction after extirpation was a major advance in cancer management. Plastic surgical techniques have facilitated large-scale resections by enabling immediate closure of surgical defects. Furthermore, development of microsurgical techniques enabled transfer of highly vascularized flaps from distant donor sites, thereby increasing the versatility of the reconstructive techniques and obviating the need for time-consuming surgical delay procedures or waltzing flaps.

Improved understanding of tumor pathobiology and prognostic factors has led to a gradual paradigm shift in cancer treatment from a "one size fits all" approach to tailored oncologic therapy. This chapter provides background for the current rationale behind modern treatment of tumors.

History of cancer treatment

While surgery remains the most successful single-modality treatment for solid tumors, the past century has demonstrated an increased role for multimodality therapy. The goal of current treatment for solid tumors is to minimize the deformity of wide-scale surgical extirpation, with assistance of neoadjuvant and adjuvant chemoradiation, to provide the greatest likelihood for cure.

Neoadjuvant treatment is the term used to describe either chemotherapy and/or radiation that are administered prior to tumor excision. Neoadjuvant therapy is used to shrink unresectable tumors rendering them resectable, or to decrease the magnitude of the ablation necessary to achieve negative margins.[1] Patients may undergo a complete response with total preoperative tumor eradication, or a partial response to neoadjuvant therapy. The response to neoadjuvant chemotherapy is an important predictor of outcome and can determine which chemotherapy is used postoperatively.[2] Clinically neoadjuvant therapy is a common part of treatment algorithms for many solid tumors. For example, randomized trials demonstrate lower recurrence rates for T3 and T4 rectal tumors when chemoradiation is delivered preoperatively as compared to postoperatively.[3] Furthermore, for distal tumors lying near the anus, neoadjuvant therapy facilitates sphincter preservation by converting cases which potentially require abdominoperineal resection to low anterior resections.[4]

Disadvantages of neoadjuvant therapy include the possibility for disease progression prior to surgical resection and increased rates of surgical complications due to side-effects of chemoradiotherapy. For example, in a review of nearly 1200 microsurgical breast reconstructions, Mehrara *et al.* demonstrated that neoadjuvant chemotherapy was an independent risk factor for postoperative complications in breast cancer patients undergoing microvascular breast reconstruction resulting in increased rates of wound complications if surgery was performed less than 6 weeks after completion of chemotherapy.[5]

In the adjuvant or postablative setting, chemotherapy or radiation is implemented to decrease locoregional recurrence or systemic disease by treating microscopic tumor deposits or metastases that are not detectable at the time of surgery. It is important to emphasize, however, that even if radiation or chemotherapy is planned postoperatively, all attempts should be made (if surgically feasible) to obtain microscopically negative tumor margins at the time of surgical resection. This concept is based on the fact that negative tumor margins are an important predictor of local or regional metastases in most solid tumors.[6]

Surgery

The earliest treatment for tumors was fulguration using electrocautery, application of toxic materials, or surgical extirpation. Due to the high local recurrence rates seen after tumor excision, surgical management at the turn of the 20th century developed into a "bigger is better" approach with wide margins. The best-known example is the Halsted radical mastectomy for invasive breast cancer advocating the removal of the pectoralis major muscle, all of the breast tissue and axillary nodes.[7] Similarly, head and neck malignancies were treated with internal jugular vein ligation, sternocleidomastoid muscle resection, and spinal accessory nerve sacrifice. Such aggressive approaches to tumor control have

subsequently been shown to be unnecessary for many cancers. Instead, the efficacy of limited anatomic resections has been proven in studies which: (1) demonstrate equivalency with more radical approaches, or (2) combine surgery with multimodality therapy. For example, margins greater than 2 cm have shown no benefit in the treatment of cutaneous melanoma.[8] Additionally, effective treatment of breast cancer no longer mandates mastectomy if lumpectomy is combined with postoperative radiotherapy.[9] Modern surgical therapy uses insight gained from clinical trials to minimize the scope of resection with an eye on preserving form and function *(Fig. 12.1)*. Radical approaches are reserved for only the most advanced cancers with extensive local invasion.

While the utility of primary tumor excision has been established, the role of surgery in management of metastatic disease is less clear. The majority of patients with metastasis receive palliative treatment with radiation to achieve local control and chemotherapy for disseminated disease. However, if thorough evaluation reveals isolated or a limited number of metastases in a patient with a good prognosis, both cure and extended survival have been achieved with surgical "metastectomies." Patients with extremity sarcomas who undergo pulmonary resections have 5-year survival rates up to 25%.[10] Similarly, hepatic lobectomy for colorectal metastasis is associated with 25–40% 5-year survivorship in selected patients.[11]

Finally, the surgeon may be called upon to obtain tissue for diagnosis of a new mass. Depending on tumor size, either incisional or excisional biopsies are performed as a precursor to definitive resection or to establish a diagnosis for cancers treated nonsurgically. Incisional biopsies should always be oriented in a direction that facilitates future wide surgical excision.

Radiation

Ionizing radiation is defined as energy sufficient to release electron(s) from an atom or molecule. Most radiation agents use either photons or electrons to cause ionization. The quantity of ionization produced in air by a beam of radiation is termed the exposure and is measured in units of roentgens. The more clinically relevant measure is the absorbed dose, which is a calculation of the amount of energy absorbed per unit mass.

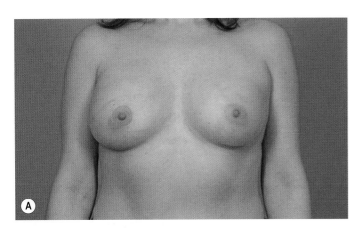
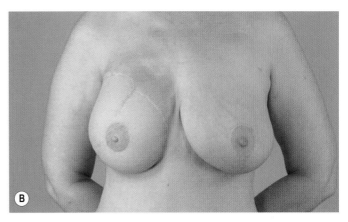

Fig. 12.1 Superiority of lesser resections to radical surgery. **(A)** This patient had less aggressive surgical approach with a nipple-sparing mastectomy followed by immediate autologous tissue reconstruction. **(B)** The second patient had a more aggressive modified radical mastectomy, followed by radiation and delayed reconstruction. Note that while both patients have acceptably cosmetic reconstruction, the outcome of the patient shown in **(B)** is inferior to that of the patient shown in **(A)**. In part due to the extensive nature of her surgery, she has more extensive and noticeable scarring, as well as skin color mismatch.

This is quantified in joules per kilogram, or gray units (Gy). Upon entering tissues, the ionizing agent dose increases, but then degrades exponentially as its distance from the source increases in accordance with the inverse-square law.[12]

The mechanism whereby ionizing radiation achieves tumor cell kill is not completely understood. Ionizing radiation causes cellular damage directly through release of electrons or indirectly by producing free radicals from water. Since oxygen increases the half-life of reactive radical species, radiation is most effective in oxygen-rich environments. When electrons or free radicals come into contact with biologically important molecules, such as DNA, detrimental effects occur. Although cells efficiently repair single-strand DNA breaks, double-strand breaks are less easily handled by cellular machinery. If sufficient DNA damage accumulates prior to the next mitotic cycle the cell is overwhelmed, leading to cell killing. When the interval between successive doses of radiation is increased, greater numbers of cells can repair DNA strand breaks. This principle is termed sublethal damage and provides the rationale for radiation delivery in fractionated daily doses ranging from 1.8 to 2.5 Gy. The success of radiation therapy is predicated on the fact that normal cells have a greater ability to repair sublethal damage between radiation fractions than tumor cells. Radiation therapy is most commonly delivered at a distance from the tumor called external-beam radiotherapy or teletherapy; however, it can also be administered as brachytherapy with high doses given directly into a specified area.[12]

Clinical use of radiation therapy began in the 1940s and 1950s after early pioneers in the field were able to minimize local complications such as radiation burns and secondary skin cancers. Although uncommon, radiation can be used as monotherapy for radiosensitive tumors such as Hodgkin's disease.[13] For other tumor types equivalency between surgical excision and radiation therapy has been demonstrated. For example, treatment of T1/T2 prostate cancer with either radical prostatectomy or external-beam radiotherapy has comparable survivorship, but with different risk profiles for each therapy.[14,15] Choice of treatment is based on patient preference and surgical risk factors as assessed by the treating urologist. Similarly, aerodigestive tumors less than 2 cm respond equally well to either radiation or surgery. In the case of laryngeal neoplasms, radiotherapy is preferred due to its ability for organ preservation.[16]

Surgeons most commonly work with radiation as part of neoadjuvant or adjuvant regimens in combination with extirpation for solid tumors. These two modalities complement each other to improve locoregional control. While surgery fails at tumor margins where cell counts are low or submicroscopic, radiation works best at the periphery where oxygenation levels are highest. Radiation is least effective in the avascular center of necrotic tumor masses where oxygen tension is poor.[17]

The increased role of radiation therapy in cancer management has led to refinements in its delivery. In the past radiation was administered in the neoadjuvant setting with the goal of rendering microscopic tumor deposits, spilled inadvertently at the time of resection, incapable of cell division. However, technical difficulties and increased complication rates, such as wound breakdown and infection associated with this schedule of radiation, have led to its preferred use in the adjuvant setting for many cancers. Although the increased rates of wound-healing complications following surgery in irradiated tissues have been thought to be related to the harmful effects of radiation on the local blood supply, the exact cause(s) of this increased risk remains unknown.[18] In fact, studies have suggested that radiation injury causes depletion of local tissue stem cells and that restitution of these cells with stem cell injections can improve tissue healing.[19]

Chemotherapy

The goals of chemotherapy are similar to those of radiation, namely preferentially kill cancer cells relative to normal tissues while minimizing toxicity. The success of chemotherapy is due to the fact that normal cells have improved ability to repair damaged DNA and survive relative to cancer cells. For chemotherapy to be successful, complete eradication of all tumor cells is essential. Agents that kill 99.99% of 10^9 tumor cells, the approximate number of cells in a 1-cm mass, allow a tumor burden of 10^5 cells to remain. Since agents are unlikely to kill every tumor cell in a single administration, chemotherapies are delivered in several rounds to achieve maximal cell killing. Administration of chemotherapy in fractions takes advantage of the fact that some agents are effective only in certain stages of the cell cycle (termed kinetic resistance) and minimizes toxicity at each time point by allowing decreased dosing.[20] Furthermore, combination chemotherapy using agents with different mechanisms of action and toxicities allows maximal tumor killing while minimizing host side-effects. Recognition of chemotherapy toxicity has led to modifications such as regional administration which allows for increased drug doses with reduced systemic side-effects. Examples of this application include isolated limb perfusion for patients with melanoma in-transit metastases or hepatic artery infusion pumps for colorectal liver metastasis.[21,22]

Chemotherapeutic agents such as nitrogen mustard and methotrexate were first introduced in the 1940s with the intention of avoiding surgery altogether. While effectiveness of chemotherapeutics as single-modality treatment for hematologic malignancies such as leukemia and lymphoma has been demonstrated, their efficacy in primary treatment of solid tumors has not been borne out in most cases. Exceptions include chemotherapy for subtypes of testicular cancer and combined chemoradiotherapy such as the Nigro protocol for anal cancer.[23,24] A common indication for chemotherapy in the management of solid tumors is for palliation of patients with metastatic disease who are ineligible for curative surgery. In such cases chemotherapy is administered with the intent of prolonging survival and improving quality of life.

Surgeons most frequently encounter chemotherapy as part of neoadjuvant or adjuvant treatment in combination with tumor excision. Examples of tumors commonly treated in this manner include breast, colon, and head and neck cancers. Synergy between surgery and chemotherapy is exemplified in the case of extremity sarcomas. Previously patients with osteosarcomas were treated with amputation; however, the introduction of neoadjuvant chemotherapy has increased rates of limb preservation with equivalent long-term survival.[25]

Immunotherapy and biologics

Passive and active immunotherapy are newer forms of cancer treatment which use immune mechanisms to kill tumor cells. In passive immunotherapy the host immune system remains quiescent while therapeutic agents are introduced to eradicate tumor cells. The most common application of this treatment is delivery of monoclonal antibodies against specific tumor antigens (*Fig. 12.2*). Advantages of this approach are the highly specific nature of therapy which theoretically decreases both side-effects and toxicity. A widely used agent is trastuzumab, a monoclonal antibody that binds to the extracellular segment of the HER2/neu receptor, overexpressed in approximately 25% of breast cancers.[26,27]

Adoptive immunotherapy is an alternative form of passive immunotherapy wherein cells with antitumor activity are introduced into the host (*Fig. 12.3*). An

Passive immunity

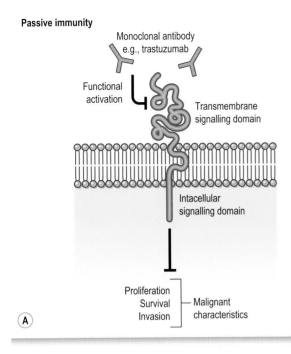

Fig. 12.2 Passive immunotherapy with monoclonal antibodies (mAb). **(A)** Monoclonal antibodies can act by binding a cell surface molecule that acts as a signal transducer. Antibody binding to this molecule inhibits its ability to transduce signals and activate downstream pathways that confer the malignant phenotypes of cell cycle dysregulation, cellular survival, and metastatic potential (e.g., trastuzumab). **(B)** Monoclonal antibodies can contribute to immunotherapy by cytotoxic effects (e.g., rituximab). Antibody binding to tumor-specific antigen can lead to complement fixation and activation, with ultimate formation of the membrane attack complex that punches pores in the tumor cell membrane. Antibody binding may also cause the activation of cytotoxic natural killer cells or phagocytic macrophages. **(C)** Finally, monoclonal antibodies can bind and block the activity of growth factors that are necessary for tumor maintenance. An example of this is bevacizumab, which binds vascular endothelial growth factor (VEGF) and therefore inhibits tumor angiogenesis.

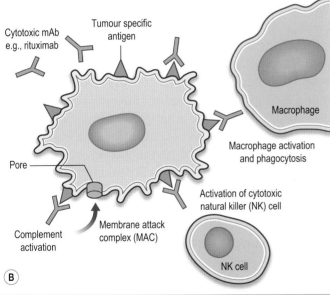

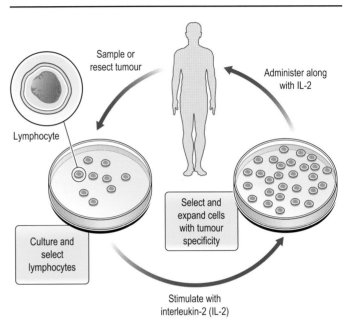

Fig. 12.3 Adoptive transfer of autologous tumor-infiltrating lymphocytes. Lymphocytes are obtained and cultured from tumor specimen. Lymphocyte proliferation is stimulated interleukin-2 (IL-2). Cells with specificity are isolated and expanded. Patient myeloablation is achieved with chemotherapy and radiation. The expanded antitumor lymphocytes are readministered, often along with IL-2.

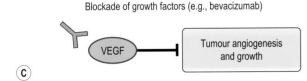

example would be *ex vivo* manipulation of host autologous tumor-infiltrating lymphocytes, which have a naturally occurring reactivity to cancer, in the presence of IL-2 to increase cytolytic potential or tumor antigen recognition.[28] Studies are currently evaluating the utility of this therapy for the treatment of melanoma.[29]

Active immunotherapy describes protocols in which the host immune system is directly stimulated by presentation of antigenic materials. If the antigenic material causes generalized stimulation of the immune system, it is considered nonspecific stimulation *(Fig. 12.4)*. The best-known immunostimulant agent is bacillus Calmette-Guérin (BCG), an attenuated form of bovine

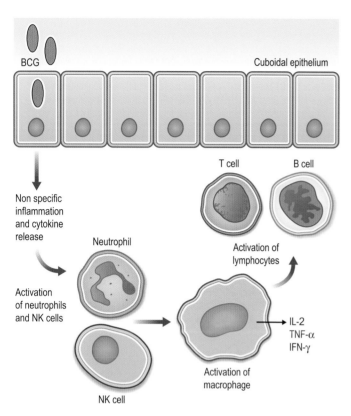

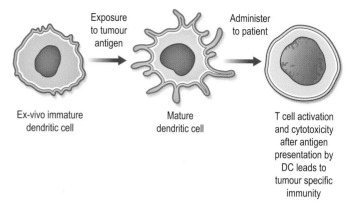

Fig. 12.4 Active immunotherapy with a nonspecific agent such as bacillus Calmette-Guérin (BCG). Administration of the agent causes a nonspecific inflammatory reaction with attendant cytokine release. This results in activation of neutrophils, natural killer (NK) cells, and macrophages. These cells in turn release various cytokines, including interleukin-2 (IL-2), tumor necrosis factor-alpha (TNF-α), and interferon gamma (IFN-γ). These cytokines in turn lead to activation of lymphocytes and resultant tumor cell killing.

Fig. 12.5 Active immunotherapy with tumor vaccination. A variety of approaches to tumor vaccination have been applied, with variable results. An approach that has been advocated recently utilizes *ex vivo* activation of the antigen-presenting dendritic cell (DC). Immature DCs are expanded *ex vivo*. They are then exposed to a tumor-specific antigen and stimulated. The resultant mature DCs are administered to the patient. These cells act as antigen presenters, leading to activation to T cells with specific antitumor activity.

tuberculosis bacillus. Although its mechanism of action is unclear, it has proven benefit in the treatment of superficial bladder cancers, with less promising results as a therapy for melanoma.[30] Infusions with cytokines are another nonspecific form of active immunotherapy. For example, melanoma is a frequent target for agents such as interleukin-2 and interferon-alpha because it is the tumor with the most immunogenic response.[31,32]

Agents which elicit a targeted response to either tumor antigens or effector cells are considered specific *(Fig. 12.5)*. The best example of specific active immunotherapy is development of vaccines derived from antigens expressed on patients' cancer cells. The highly specific nature of this therapeutic approach underscores its limitations. For example, multiple patients' tumors may express different peptide antigens or alternatively different subclonal populations may exist within a single individual.

The latest generation of antineoplastic agents, called biologics, targets molecular pathways identified from basic science tumor biology. In contrast to traditional methods, which develop drugs through trial-and-error testing, drug creation in this manner is referred to as rational design since targets are specified *a priori*. Since many biologics are antibodies, they may be considered as forms of passive immunotherapy. The earliest example, imatinib (Gleevec), was designed to block the abnormal gene product of the Philadelphia chromosome, the constitutively active Bcr-Abl tyrosine kinase.[33] Clinical efficacy with imatinib has led to targeting of other oncogenes such as vascular endothelial growth factor with bevacizumab (Avastin) and CD20 with rituximab (Rituxan). As the newest class of antineoplastic agents, the role of biologics in the chemotherapeutic armamentarium is under investigation. With widespread availability and use, plastic surgeons will increasingly operate on patients who receive them. Few data are available about surgery in this setting, but case reports suggest angiogenesis inhibitors such as bevacizumab contribute to wound breakdown since neovascularization is a key component of normal wound healing.[34]

Photodynamic therapy

Photoradiation uses light within the visible spectrum to produce energy within cells. The most widely known application of photoradiation is lasers. Chemicals called photosensitizers, which are preferentially taken up by cancer cells relative to normal tissues, respond to light by producing free radicals. When light is shone on these cells, accumulation of energy leads to thermal damage and cell killing.[35]

Since photodynamic therapy requires light to be activated, its utility is limited to superficial tumors. Photodynamic therapy is currently being used for the treatment of advanced esophageal and nonsmall cell lung tumors and is under investigation for oral, skin, and other cancers.[36,37]

Pathobiology

Understanding of tumor cell biology provides a foundation for current clinical management of cancers.

Critical mass

Normal cells tend not to overcrowd one another and align themselves in an orderly fashion. In contrast, tumors cells lose this propensity and grow by overlapping each other. Tumor cells grow in a logarithmic fashion, quantified as the doubling time. Each tumor grows at a different rate so doubling times can vary between 2 and 200 days.[38,39] Tumors are generally not detectable until they reach approximately 1 cm in diameter. Depending upon the doubling time, a tumor may be present in a patient for years before it becomes palpable. Understanding this concept affords the oncologic team sufficient time to evaluate newly diagnosed patients properly and thoroughly without rushing therapy. The first step, when technically feasible, is to obtain a biopsy of a tumor mass to establish the cell type and correct diagnosis. Excisional, incisional, or needle biopsies are performed depending on the size and location of the tumor. In some cases, for example, renal cell cancer, needle biopsy or incisional biopsies may be contraindicated as these procedures can cause peritoneal seeding. Tissue diagnosis is usually correlated with imaging studies such as computed tomography scans or magnetic resonance imaging to identify distant and regional tumor spread. Supplied with this information, informed decisions can be made with the patient about the best treatment and timing of adjunctive therapies relative to surgery.

Tumor margins

Variability in the distribution of tumor cells within a given tissue sample can hamper the identification of malignant cells in tissue sections. For example, if 10% of cells in a specimen have a malignant phenotype they are easily visualized using a microscope. However, if the number of malignant cells decreases to 0.1% or 1 in 1000, unless clustered together, identification of these cells can be challenging and may require more sensitive measures such as immunohistochemistry (to label tumor antigens). Even these more sensitive measures may miss small foci of cancer metastases, therefore resulting in false-negative diagnosis. Accurate diagnosis of surgical margins and biopsy specimens is critical since false-negative findings can have a significant effect on diagnosis and treatment.

Clinical findings illustrate this concept. For example, patients with head and neck squamous cell cancers who undergo prophylactic lymphadenectomy have significant rates of local recurrences despite absence of tumor cells on final pathology.[40] A second example can be seen in rectal cancers with negative margins on initial resection. Evaluation of patients with locally recurrent disease shows that 50% occur at the suture line despite negative histology.[41] Tumor recurrence in these scenarios may be attributable to microscopic tumor deposits not detected on pathologic evaluation.

Laboratory studies have also demonstrated the presence of microscopic tumor cells. Examples exist in both head and neck and melanoma specimens where cancer cells cannot be detected in routine histology, but have been successfully grown in vitro.[42,43] More recently, molecular biology techniques such as polymerase chain reaction and immunohistochemistry have been used to perform molecular ultrastaging of histologically node-negative patients for identification of microscopically invisible tumor deposits. Whether such small tumor burdens are clinically significant is the subject of further investigation.[44]

The aforementioned examples provide justification for multimodality treatment of solid tumors managed primarily with surgical extirpation. Although margins are frequently reported as "negative," recurrences often occur. Chemotherapy or, more commonly, radiation is used in these settings to treat potentially viable occult tumor cells. Alternatively, it should be noted that the immune system has the potential to eradicate residual tumor cells remaining after extirpation. Review of patients with positive margins of basal cell cancer demonstrate recurrence rates of only 20–30%, suggesting the body's capacity to destroy small numbers of cancerous cells.[45] Ideally the goal of cancer diagnosis is to identify patients accurately with microscopic spread of tumor to avoid unnecessary delivery of adjuvant agents which have untoward side-effects and toxicities.

Classification

Tumor classification can be based on a number of different factors, including morphology, degree of differentiation, and histologic cell type. Classification schemes differ for each tumor type since factors that determine behavior are variable. Retrospective studies have identified tumor characteristics that may be used to predict the clinical behavior of the tumor type. For example, sarcoma behavior correlates with the number of mitoses identified per high-power field or histologic subtype.[46–48] In contrast, prognosticators for breast cancer include tumor size, lymph node status, and hormone receptor expression.[49–52] The principal goal of classification schemes is to substratify tumors to predict clinical behavior more accurately and guide therapy. Although recent advances have been made in this field, the quest for more accurate diagnosis and prognostication of tumor behavior is a major source of current research. In the future, the goal is to identify tumors based on "genetic signatures" that enable not only more accurate diagnosis, but also targeted treatment.

The oldest classification system is based on clinical findings. Here staging is based on degree of tumor spread, presence of lymph node involvement, and presence of distant metastasis by either radiography or biopsy. The widely used TNM system expounded on clinical classification systems in an attempt to stratify patients further into prognostic groups. In this system, tumor (T) represents the extent of the primary tumor as measured in size, depth of invasion, or degree of anatomic involvement. Node (N) enumerates involvement of lymph nodes, such as the number of affected nodes or node size. Metastasis (M) reflects the involvement of distant organs.

Other classification systems rely on tumor morphology as the basis for prognosis. For example, Lund's classification for basal cell carcinomas is based upon descriptive features of the tumor such as nodular (well-defined margins), ulcerative, morphea and sclerosing patterns (indistinct margins). In this system, the presence of either morphea or sclerosing features is associated with a more aggressive and problematic course.[53] A second example is the morphologic classification established by Clark for melanoma, which includes lentigo maligna, superficial spreading, nodular, acral, and desmoplastic variants.[54]

Histologic classification systems use histologic cell type or category to stratify clinical outcomes. Examples of histologic grading systems include salivary gland tumors, which are separated into mucoepidermoid, adenoid cystic, acinic cell, and squamous cell subtypes.[55] Clark's histologic system categorized melanomas by level of invasion into the papillary and reticular dermis and subcutaneous fat.[54] Using this approach, determination of the depth of invasion was subjective with poor interrater reliability. Subsequently, Breslow's system was developed which more objectively quantitated tumor thickness by measurement with a micrometer attached to the microscope field.[56]

More recently, molecular biology concepts have been applied to tumor classification. Knowledge of the transcriptome and proteasome of tumors has led to identification of unique molecular signatures for each tumor which predict clinical behavior. An example is the reproducible and highly specific molecular signature of the clinically aggressive triple-negative (absent for ER/PR/HER2 receptors) breast tumors.[57] Through use of basic science techniques, investigators aim to subclassify tumors on a molecular level to refine staging schemes and provide tailored therapy.

Management

The oncologist's goal is to apply available treatments options, both surgical and nonsurgical, to minimize morbidity while enabling patient cure. In addition, the relative value of reconstruction in restoration of organ function and cosmesis is not equivalent in all scenarios and may play a role in choosing an oncologic regimen. For example, laryngeal cancer treatment with radiotherapy is strongly preferred over laryngectomy since current methods of voice reconstruction are inadequate.

In contrast, many breast cancers are treated equally well with either lumpectomy and radiotherapy or mastectomy alone. These situations require detailed consultation with a comprehensive oncologic team about the risks and benefits of each therapy with informed decision-making by the patient. Furthermore, the availability of highly effective autologous and implant-based breast reconstruction techniques may further influence the decision to proceed with simple mastectomy. Similarly, limb preservation for osteosarcomas has only become possible through use of neoadjuvant chemotherapy and functional reconstructions with allografts or endoprostheses. These examples highlight a paradigm shift in ablative strategies over the last century from a "Halstead approach" to modern treatment which relies on advances in both multimodality therapy and reconstruction to manage solid tumors.

Beyond primary tumor mass excision, the treatment of draining lymph nodes is an important part of solid tumor management. Since carcinomas drain through regional nodal basins, in contrast to sarcomas which spread hematogenously, removal of regional lymph nodes is crucial for these malignancies. Regional lymphadenectomy is routinely performed as part of staging to determine prognosis and for its potential therapeutic value.[58–62]

For patients with clinically palpable nodes at the time of tumor resection, removal of involved nodes is generally performed to achieve regional control by preventing mass effect and skin breakdown. In cases with no clinical evidence of lymph node involvement either on examination or radiographically, the timing of lymphadenectomy is controversial. Lymph node dissection can be performed either at the time of initial tumor extirpation, termed prophylactic or elective lymph node dissection (ELND), or when the tumor subsequently recurs in a nodal basin (therapeutic lymph node dissection, or TLND). ELND is not routinely recommended for two reasons. First, regional lymphadenectomy leads to increased morbidity such as extremity lymphedema or complications of surgical dissection such as nerve damage. Second, ELND has not clearly demonstrated improved survival compared to TLND for malignancies such as melanoma.[63] Ideally, ELND should be restricted to cases with high probability of occult regional tumor spread such as head and neck cancers with a large primary tumor.[64]

The introduction of the sentinel lymph node concept by Morton et al. has further altered surgical management of clinically negative regional lymph node basins.[65] The sentinel node concept is based on the fact that tissues drain into regional nodes in a reproducible and orderly fashion. After injection of either radioactive colloid or blue dye into the tumor, the first or sentinel node draining the basin is excised to be examined for tumor involvement. The status of the sentinel node is representative of the entire regional nodal chain, suggesting whether or not ELND should be performed. Through careful intraoperative identification of the sentinel node and thorough histologic analysis, false-negative rates for sentinel node biopsy now range from 0 to 11%.[66,67] A subset of patients with negative sentinel nodes on hematoxylin and eosin stain will have micrometastatic disease present on immunohistochemistry. The consequence of such small tumor deposits is unclear since these patients have similar survivorship to controls.[68] An additional benefit of sentinel node mapping is that, since only a single node is harvested, more thorough histologic and pathologic evaluation is performed of the specimen for improved nodal staging accuracy.

Theoretically sentinel node mapping should decrease the number of unnecessary regional lymphadenectomies performed with associated morbidity. Rates of extremity lymphedema with sentinel node mapping have decreased to 5% compared with 35% for complete lymphadenectomies.[69,70] Currently sentinel node mapping is performed for breast cancer and melanoma while reliability of the concept in head and neck, lung, and uterine cancers is under investigation.[71–73]

A second major issue to consider when performing lymphadenectomy is the extent of dissection. Arguments supporting extended or radical lymphadenectomy are that greater node removal more accurately stages disease and failure to remove these nodes leaves residual cancer cells behind. For example, colon cancer guidelines recommend that at least 12 nodes be evaluated histologically to avoid a false-negative nodal status.[74] Arguments against routine use of extended lymphadenectomy include increased morbidity of dissection and lack of a survival benefit compared to limited dissections in randomized trials.

A comprehensive discussion of cancer surveillance is beyond the scope of this chapter, though some points are worth mentioning. Although the premise behind surveillance is to improve outcome through early detection, few protocols demonstrate an actual survival benefit. For example, head and neck patients with asymptomatic recurrences identified through screening methods demonstrate no survival difference compared to patients who presented with symptoms.[75] Concerns have also been raised that reconstruction may obscure recurrence detection, but data do not support this contention. Maxillectomy defects reconstructed with flaps, as opposed to obturators, demonstrate statistically comparable times to recurrence.[76] Similarly, for breast cancer neither implant nor autologous reconstruction has been associated with a delay in diagnosis of recurrent disease.[77,78] Recurrences after transverse rectus abdominis myocutaneous flap reconstruction can be successfully managed with local excision and flap salvage in 80% of cases. Regardless of the type of breast reconstruction performed, recurrent disease is detectable on physical exam, not mammography.

Conclusion

Today, the most common treatment for solid tumors remains surgical excision; however, the last century has demonstrated the advantages of multimodality therapy using chemoradiation. Refined staging and increased knowledge of pathobiology have allowed individualized tumor management with development of targeted treatment regimens. It is incumbent upon plastic surgeons to understand the principles of cancer management in order to perform reconstructions which minimize postsurgical complications, thereby allowing patients to receive adjunctive therapy in a timely manner.

 Access the complete reference list online at **http://www.expertconsult.com**

1. Trimble EL, Ungerleider RS, Abrams JA, et al. Neoadjuvant therapy in cancer treatment. *Cancer*. 1993;72(11 Suppl):3515–3524.

3. Improved survival with preoperative radiotherapy in resectable rectal cancer. Swedish Rectal Cancer Trial. *N Engl J Med*. 1997;336(14):980–987.

   Large trial which unequivocally demonstrated improved outcomes in patients receiving neoadjuvant radiotherapy for rectal cancer. This paradigm is now in use, or being explored in a variety of cancers, including breast and lung. There may be significant implications for reconstructive options.

7. Halsted WS. I. The Results of Operations for the Cure of Cancer of the Breast Performed at the Johns Hopkins Hospital from June, 1889, to January, 1894. *Ann Surg*. 1894;20(5):497–555.

   Seminal manuscript demonstrating the widely held 19th-century belief that wide tumor excision based on anatomic principals provides the greatest chance for cure.

9. Fisher B, Anderson S, Bryant J, et al. Twenty-year follow-up of a randomized trial comparing total mastectomy, lumpectomy, and lumpectomy plus irradiation for the treatment of invasive breast cancer. *N Engl J Med*. 2002;347(16):1233–1241.

   Highly controversial study which demonstrated for the first time that breast-conservative surgery provides similar survival outcomes to modified radical mastectomy. Mastectomy is no longer considered mandatory and is reserved for select patients.

24. Nigro ND, Vaitkevicius VK, Buroker T, et al. Combined therapy for cancer of the anal canal. *Dis Colon Rectum*. 1981;24:73–75.

    Seminal study which demonstrated curative management of a "solid" tumor using chemoradiation alone without the use of surgery. The Nigro protocol now spares many patients from highly morbid abdominoperneal resection (APR).

27. Baselga J, Norton L, Albanell J, et al. Recombinant humanized anti-HER2 antibody (Herceptin) enhances the antitumor activity of paclitaxel and doxorubicin against HER2/neu overexpressing human breast cancer xenografts. *Cancer Res*. 1998;58: 2825–2831.

33. O'Brien SG, Guilhot F, Larson RA, et al. Imatinib compared with interferon and low-dose cytarabine for newly diagnosed chronic-phase chronic myeloid leukemia. *N Engl J Med*. 2003;348:994–1004.

54. Clark Jr WH, From L, Bernadino EA, et al. The histogenesis and biologic behavior of primary human malignant melanomas of the skin. *Cancer Res*. 1969;29:705–727.

56. Breslow A. Thickness, cross-sectional areas and depth of invasion in the prognosis of cutaneous melanoma. *Ann Surg*. 1970;172:902–908.

    Study which demonstrated the biology of melanoma is dictated by lesion thickness. To this day, staging and management of melanoma is guided by a modified version of the Breslow system.

65. Morton DL, Wen DR, Wong JH, et al. Technical details of intraoperative lymphatic mapping for early stage melanoma. *Arch Surg*. 1992;127:392–399.

The sentinal lymph node biopsy was developed for melanoma staging, but has had a significant impact on the management of breast cancer as well. As an alternative to mandatory lymph node disection, this procedure reduces patient morbidity, including lymphedema, and length of stay.

78. Howard MA, Polo K, Pusic AL, et al. Breast cancer local recurrence after mastectomy and TRAM flap reconstruction: incidence and treatment options. *Plast Reconstr Surg*. 2006;117:1381–1386.

13

Stem cells and regenerative medicine

Benjamin Levi, Derrick C. Wan, Victor W. Wong, Geoffrey C. Gurtner, and Michael T. Longaker

SYNOPSIS

- There is a significant biomedical need for tissue reconstruction and regeneration.
- Stem cells are a key building block to any tissue regeneration or engineering strategy.
- Stem cells can be derived from multiple sources and tissues which exist at different stages of differentiation.
- Stem cells can have different *in vitro* and *in vivo* capabilities and are at a different stage in bench and bedside research:
  - embryonic stem cells
  - postnatal and somatic stem cells
  - adipose-derived stromal cells (ASCs)
  - mesenchymal stem cells (MSCs)
  - tissue-specific stem cells
  - induced pluripotent cells.
- Prospective clinical applications for stem cell therapy will likely require multidisciplinary approaches employing tissue engineering and inductive therapies (biomimetic matrices, gene therapy, small molecules, growth factors).

 Access the Historical Perspective section online at
http://www.expertconsult.com

Introduction

- Three characteristics that define a stem cell are:
  1. Self-renewal: stem cells can expand and give rise to a clonal population of cells through cell division, sometimes after long periods of senescence.
  2. Clonality: stem cells are able to give rise to new stem cells.
  3. Differentiation into various cell types: stem cells can differentiate *in vitro* and *in vivo* into multiple cell types and reconstitute a specific tissue type following transplantation.
- Stem cells can come from embryonic or postnatal sources.
- Embryonic stem cells exist in a more pluripotent state than postnatal, somatic, and tissue-specific stem cells.
- MSC differentiation has been elucidated using specific *in vitro* and *in vivo* protocols.
- Adult, or tissue-specific, stem cells are undifferentiated cells which are found in almost all tissues and organs after embryonic development.
- Postnatal stem cells can be reprogrammed into an "embryonic-like" state called induced pluripotent cells.

Discussion of biomedical burden *(Fig. 13.1)*

As the global population continues both to age and expand, so does the associated incidence of diseases, defects, and deficits afflicting patients secondary to a multitude of congenital, postsurgical, posttraumatic, vascular, and degenerative etiologies (arthritis, osteoporosis, chronic wounds, postoncologic resection). In

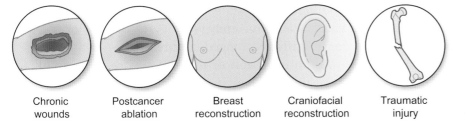

Fig. 13.1 Biomedical burden. Different tissue reconstructive challenges faced by plastic surgeons. From left to right, possible applications of tissue engineering include treatment of chronic wounds, postcancer ablation, breast reconstruction, craniofacial reconstruction, and traumatic injury.

2007, it was estimated that diseases of the musculoskeletal system cost over 26 billion dollars in the US with an average annual growth of 8.5% (second highest growth of all body systems).[1] With regard to cancer reconstructions, the American Society of Plastic Surgery estimates that almost 5.2 million reconstructive procedures were performed by plastic surgeons in 2009, over 3.9 million for cancer reconstruction, and over 86 000 breast reconstructive cases.[2]

Composite tissue reconstruction remains a significant challenge for plastic surgeons treating patients after trauma, oncologic extirpations, and congenital anomalies. Synthetic solutions such as prostheses, plates, and implants to correct soft-tissue defects have greatly improved the lives of millions of patients. Such artificial tissues, however, are plagued by suboptimal durability and infection. Some of these challenges have been mitigated by cadaveric and autogenous grafts; however, these too are limited by durability, availability, and donor site defects.

Thus plastic surgeons struggle due to the inability of current implants and grafts to replicate completely the ability of a dynamic living tissue to remodel and regenerate in response to environmental cues. Ultimately reconstructive strategies must shift from simple tissue repair to tissue regeneration. The fundamental idea behind tissue regeneration is to use a biologically active scaffold seeded with a pluripotent, self-renewing cell type. The synergy of a biomimetic scaffold with a competent cellular element will allow creation of tissues that are able to respond and regenerate in the face of injury. Such cells exist in abundance from embryos to the elderly, namely, stem cells *(Fig. 13.2)*.

Stem cells are defined functionally as a clonogenic population of cells capable of self-renewal and differentiation to committed progenitors and subsequently to differentiated, functional tissues.[3] Traditionally, stem cells have been divided into two categories based on

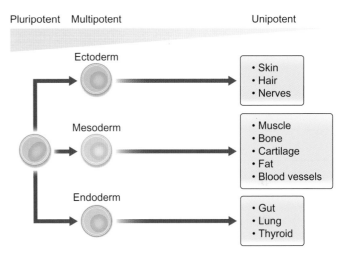

Fig. 13.2 Differentiation of pluripotent stem cells down different multipotent lineages. An embryonic stem cell is a pluripotent stem cell, whereas an adipose-derived mesenchymal cell is a mesodermal multipotent stem cell.

their ability to differentiate. Pluripotent stem cells (embryonic) can differentiate into any cell type in the body, whereas multipotent stem cells (adult) can differentiate into multiple, but not all, cell lineages. In addition to the traditional stem cell classification, a new class of stem cells has recently been described – induced pluripotent stem (iPS) cells – which are derived from genetically reprogrammed adult cells that are believed to have the potential of embryonic stem cells.

Why stem cells and regenerative medicine should be of interest to plastic surgeons

Plastic surgeons stand at the clinical forefront of using ASCs as they have direct access to large quantities of adipose tissue from liposuction as well as body-contouring procedures. The hope of clinicians would be one day to take a patient to the operating room, and in one stage, use a prefabricated biomimetic scaffold construct and seed this with stem cells derived from a small-volume lipoaspirate to address a soft-tissue, skeletal, muscle, cartilage, vascular, or joint defect. Furthermore, as orthopedic surgeons increase their volume in spine surgery and bone morphogenic protein-2 (BMP-2) usage, we foresee plastic surgeons helping with immediate liposuction and ASC harvest in conjunction with growth factors such as BMP-2 for bony regeneration. Recent studies have shown that there may be differences in osteogenic and adipogenic potential in the subcutaneous region from which the cells are harvested and thus surgeons may tailor the region from which they harvest fat to address patient needs best.[4] The potential breakthroughs in the use of human stem and stromal cells have prompted some individuals to store their own tissues in a fee-for-service fashion. The most obvious example is the cryostorage of umbilical cord-derived blood.[5] The process of cell freezing and long-term storage have been applied to human ASCs (hASCs) as well.

Human embryonic stem cells

Definitions

Research in hESCs has been a rapidly developing field, attracting increasing attention over the last decade. The capacity of hESCs to reproduce almost any cell type found in the human body has led to many promising areas of investigation which may yield a deeper understanding of cellular biology and potential cures for many diseases.[37,38] In addition, the ability to repair and regenerate tissues injured by trauma may facilitate the development and implementation of new treatment paradigms employing hESCs to restore areas of organ damage and reverse what was once thought to be permanent functional deficit. Despite recent controversy surrounding political and ethical concerns over the research and clinical use of these cells, studies continue with hESCs and considerable promise still remains for this area of investigation.

The term "embryonic stem cell" was coined by Gail Martin to distinguish them from previously described pluripotent embryonal carcinoma (EC) cells derived from teratocarcinomas.[29] At root, ESCs possess three essential characteristics: (1) derivation from a preimplantation or peri-implantation embryo; (2) the capacity to self-renew and proliferate in a prolonged undifferentiated state; and (3) the ability to form derivates of all three embryonic germ layers – or pluripotency – after prolonged culture.[39]

As an extension of this early work in mice, hESCs were first isolated in 1998.[39] Donated fresh cleavage-stage human embryos produced by in vitro fertilization were obtained by Thomson et al. and cultured to the blastocyst stage, typically reached at 4–5 days postfertilization. From the inner cell mass (which ultimately forms the embryo), five separate hESC lines were established and successfully maintained in culture for 6 months in an undifferentiated state. All five lines also retained the capacity to form teratomas after injection into immunodeficient mice. Histological examination of these teratomas revealed gut epithelium, cartilage, bone, smooth muscle, neural epithelium, ganglia, and stratified squamous epithelium. Similar findings were also described by Reubinoff and colleagues, who derived two additional hESC cell lines and demonstrated expression of the transcription factor Oct-4 in these cells which had previously been shown to be essential for the maintenance of pluripotential capacity in mouse ESCs.[40,41]

With the development of hESCs, enthusiasm flourished surrounding their potential as experimental platforms to study a multitude of disease states. Studies designed to provide insight into human embryogenesis, development of birth defects, and cellular mechanisms of a variety of pathologic states proceeded at a feverish pace. But much of this early scientific fervor was tempered by several significant concerns. In theory, hESC possess the capacity to treat a wide variety of genetic diseases, cancers, diabetes, neurologic degenerative conditions, and spinal cord injuries. Use in such a clinical capacity, however, raises the important issue of graft-versus-host disease associated with allogeneic stem cell transplantation. One solution proffered for this histoincompatibility centers around the development of several hESC cell lines from variegated genetic backgrounds for tailored use in patients to minimize risk of rejection. Other strategies proposed include the use of autologous donor adult stem cells or the more recently described iPS cell.[13,18,42]

While work continues on reduction of donor host rejection, concerns regarding xenogeneic contamination have also been raised. Since their first isolation, hESCs have been traditionally cultured in vitro in the presence of mouse embryonic fibroblast (MEF) feeder layers.[39] In their absence, hESCs have been found to undergo rapid differentiation. A feeder-free culture system was presented by Xu and colleagues employing Matrigel in medium conditioned by MEFs, but in both techniques, hESCs were exposed to murine products to maintain their pluripotency.[43] In 2005, Martin *et al.* reported the presence of a nonhuman sialic acid Neu5Gc on the cell surface of hESCs.[44] As humans are unable to generate this particular sialic acid, this likely represented uptake from media containing animal products and incorporation through the process of glycosylation. When these hESCs and the embryoid bodies they formed were exposed to human serum, rapid binding of immunoglobulin and deposition of complement were noted, ultimately resulting in cellular death.

Circumventing this problem necessitated the creation of a new stem cell line under murine-free conditions. To accomplish this, novel extracellular matrix-coated plates were developed from MEFs and sterilized prior to use.[45] When hESCs were cultured using these plates, undifferentiated proliferation was observed for 6 months and cells maintained the capacity to form all three embryonic germ layers. This system thus eliminated exposure of hESCs to potential contamination from serum and/or live feeder cells and minimized the risk of disease transmission through contact of cells with animal or human pathogenic agents.

Current concepts and research

Scientific investigation with hESCs has begun to reveal the potential of these cells to revamp our contemporary understanding and treatment of disease dramatically *(Fig. 13.3)*. Technologies which may be derived from stem cell research may be used one day to manage spinal cord injuries, degenerative neurologic conditions, and a variety of genetic diseases. While treatment of spinal cord trauma and Parkinson's disease has received more high-profile attention of late, stem cell investigators have also made significant strides in the fields of diabetes, cardiac, and hematopoietic/vascular research.

The ability for ESCs to undergo neuronal differentiation was first demonstrated by Bain and colleagues in 1995.[46] Exposing mouse ESCs to retinoic acid, multiple cellular phenotypes were observed, a large percentage of which produced neuron-like outgrowths. Gene

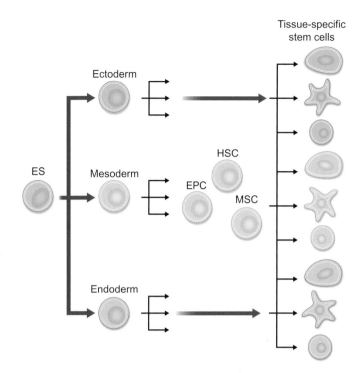

Fig. 13.3 Use of embryonic stem cells. Embryonic stem cells can be used to study genetic changes, screen drugs and design novel therapies.

expression analysis of these cells revealed several neural-associated transcripts including neurofilaments, glutamate receptor subunits, and nerve specific transcription factors. Furthermore, physiologic studies revealed these neuron-like cells could generate action potentials. Paralleling these experiments, Schuldiner *et al.* induced neuronal differentiation from hESCs using both retinoic acid and nerve growth factor (NGF).[47] These neural progenitors were found to be capable of differentiation *in vitro* into astrocytes, oligodendrocytes, and mature neurons.[40,48] When transplanted into the ventricles of newborn mouse brains, these hESC-derived neuronal cells could be observed to distribute widely throughout the brain and integrate in a region-specific manner. These findings therefore reveal the developmental potential of hESCs and their capacity to respond *in vivo* to local environmental cues to differentiate into appropriate neural lineages. While only preliminary, such findings also shed hope for the use of hESCs in the future treatment of neurological disease.

Similar to neural stem cell research, pluripotent hESCs have likewise shown promise in the field of diabetes research. At present, the only therapy considered potentially curative for type 1 diabetes is pancreatic islet cell replacement.[49] Unfortunately, donor shortage has severely limited this modality from becoming a practical therapeutic solution. Furthermore, the risk of potential disease transmission and cellular rejection remains exigent. The discovery of glucose-sensitive insulin-secreting cells derived from mouse ESCs, however, has introduced a new potential source of cells for treatment of type 1 diabetes.[49] Culturing hESCs in suspension and allowing for embryoid body formation also led to the detection of insulin-producing cells after 14 days of differentiation.[50] By immunohistochemical staining, 1–3% of all cells were found to stain positively for insulin and were noted to be interspersed among the mixed population of spontaneously differentiating cells. More recent studies have cast some doubt on the frequency of these cells, though, estimating their true incidence to be less than 1 per 100 000 cells.[51] Continued work must be performed, but these studies nonetheless demonstrate the potential for development of cells capable of β-islet function and insulin release. Such a subset of cells derived from hESCs could theoretically be exploited as a source of cell replacement for treatment of patients with type 1 diabetes.

The study of cardiac tissue development has long been handicapped by the lack of a suitable *in vitro* model. The advent of hESC research, however, has also offered a potential avenue for progress to be made in this field. Kehat and colleagues first noted the presence of spontaneously contracting areas within hESCs cultured in suspension and then plated to form embryoid bodies.[52] Cells from these regions, which comprised approximately 8% of the entire area, stained positively for a variety of cardiac markers, including myosin, desmin, tropinin I, and atrial natriuretic factor. In addition, both positive and negative chronotropic effects were observed with these contracting cells following application of isoproterenol or carbamylcholine, respectively. Differentiation of hESCs into these cells could also be enhanced by the application of 5-aza-2'-deoxycytidine and purified through density centrifugation to obtain a population of cells containing 70% cardiomyocyte progenitors.[53]

In 2003, Mummery *et al.* provided the first demonstration of hESC cardiomyocyte differentiation through co-culture techniques with visceral endoderm-like cells.[54] This approach mitigated the need for spontaneous cardiogenesis and efficiently produced solid aggregates of beating cells consisting of 10–200 cardiomyocytes. Interestingly, these colonies could also be frozen and were observed to resume beating upon thawing. Collectively, the findings presented strongly argue for continued development of hESCs as a model for cardiac research. Their ability to differentiate into cardiomyocytes and potential capability to enrich for these cells naturally lend toward the future development of clinical applications in heart disease.

In concert with work on cardiac differentiation, investigators have also discovered the capacity for hESCs to form vascular endothelial cells. Endothelial cells are critical for tissue repair and regeneration and the potential for hESC-derived vascular cells to participate in treatment of vascular disease is promising.[55] Zambidis *et al.* first described the presence of mesodermal-hematoendothelial cluster colonies within embryoid bodies at days 6–9.[56] These colonies were found to consist of nonadherent cells expressing CD45, which gave rise to hematopoietic lineages, and adherent CD31 cells which expressed markers characteristic for vascular endothelium. Isolation of these hESC-derived endothelial cells was accomplished through flow cytometry using anti-CD31 antibodies.[57] These cells could then be expanded in culture and, when injected into immunocompromised mice, they were shown to form microvascular networks. While their long-term stability is unknown, they represent the first step towards potential treatment of vascular disease and stimulation of ischemic tissue growth using hESCs. They also provide a foundation for future study of the biomolecular mechanisms involved in blood vessel formation.

Clinical correlates

Clinical use of hESCs remains in its early infancy, with several hurdles standing in the way. Obstacles which must be overcome include the risk of tumorigenicity, immunocompatibility, and isolation of desired cell types for therapeutic use. Nonetheless, work continues on what may be the most promising application of hESCs, that being in the field of neuroregeneration. Preliminary work performed in the murine model has been promising and this has led to the first Food and Drug Administration (FDA)-approved clinical trial incorporating hESCs in clinical treatment.

The capacity for regeneration of the central nervous system is limited, making the potential for repair and return of function through hESC therapy compelling. Following trauma, injuries to the brain and spinal cord may result in demyelination secondary to death of local oligodendrocytes.[58] While some axons may be spared, action potential propagation may become disrupted, resulting in irreversible loss of motor function. The ability for hESCs to be differentiated into oligodendrocytes, however, offers some optimism for clinical recovery. As a proof of this concept, Keirstead and colleagues evaluated the ability for hESCs to incorporate, remyelinate, and restore locomotion after spinal cord injury in rats.[59] Spinal cord contusion injuries were induced in Sprague–Dawley rats at the T10 level using a controlled, reproducible force generator capable of delivering a sudden desired impact. Oligodendryocytes derived from hESCs were purified and delivered both above and below the place of contusion 7 days following injury through direct injection into the spinal cord. Histological analysis 8 weeks later revealed significantly greater density of remyelinated axons when compared to control animals. More importantly, however, animals that received hESC-derived oligodendrocytes demonstrated significantly higher locomotor function scores which continued to improve up to 1 month after initial injury. These findings therefore revealed that transplantation of hESCs differentiated into oligodendrocytes may be an effective means of treating acute spinal cord injuries. Of note, no teratomas were observed in this study, suggesting predifferentiation of hESCs prior to clinical use may obviate concerns surrounding this potential complication.[60]

Following these promising data presented in rats for functional recovery, the biotechnology firm Geron petitioned for FDA approval to proceed with human trials in which hESCs would be similarly used to treat patients with spinal cord injuries. A phase I trial for this work was granted in January 2009, allowing for 8–10 patients with severe spinal cord injuries to be treated with hESC-derived oligodendrocytes. However, this trial has been put on hold by the FDA pending further review of preclinical data. While it remains to be seen if the findings described in rats can be clinically replicated, this represents the first step towards future translational therapies designed to incorporate these cells to treat human disease. Though full restoration of function following complete paralysis is not expected at this present time, there is hope that patients with less severe injuries may one day benefit from use of hESCs.[61]

Postnatal and somatic stem cells

Adipose-derived stromal cells

Definitions and harvest

Adipose tissue contains a stromal population that consists of microvascular endothelial cells, smooth-muscle cells, and multipotent cells. ASCs display the capacity to differentiate into adipocytes, osteoblasts, and chondroblasts *in vitro*.[16,18,19,62,63] However, the origin of hASCs has not been clearly defined. Several laboratories have hypothesized that these cells represent pericytes surrounding blood vessels, which may explain their ability to differentiate into endothelial cells; others suspect they are a subpopulation of fibroblasts that reside within adipose tissue *(Fig. 13.4)*.

ASCs, like stem cells from the bone marrow, have an extensive proliferative potential and can self-renew as

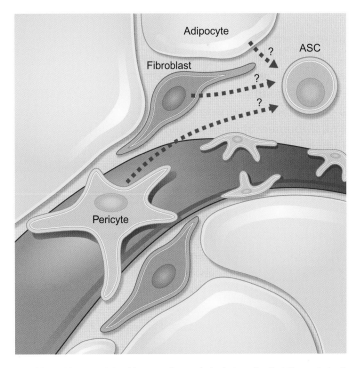

Fig. 13.4 Unknown origin of human adipose-derived stromal cell. Adipose-derived stem cells are thought to be derived from adipocytes or fibroblasts or from perivascular mural cells known as pericytes. ASC, adipose derived stromal cell.

well as undergo osteogenic, chondrogenic, myogenic, and adipogenic differentiation. This population can also be defined by its cell surface markers which have been shown to be positive for CD105, STRO-1, CD29, CD144, and CD166 and negative for CD3, CD4, CD11c, CD14, CD15, CD16, CD19, CD31, CD33, CD38, CD56, CD62p, CD104, and CD144.[24,25]

ASC harvest

Human ASC harvest can be performed on human lipoaspirate or resected adipose tissue. *(Fig. 13.5)*. The benefit of using lipoaspirate is that it removes the step of having to mince the adipose tissue finely. Furthermore, it has been shown that, even following ultrasonic-assisted liposuction, the ASCs retain their ability to undergo osteogenic differentiation.[64] If fat has been harvested from multiple anatomic locations, these specimens should be kept separate and labeled as differences

exist in the differentiative capacity of different subcutaneous depots[4] *(Fig. 13.6)*. Following lipoaspiration, the adipose tissue should be processed as soon as possible in a sterile cell culture environment *(Fig. 13.7)*. Adipose specimens should first be washed in dilute Betadine, followed by two phosphate-buffered saline (PBS) washes of equal volume to each lipoaspiration specimen. Tissues should then be subsequently digested with an equal volume of 0.075% (w/v) type II collagenase in Hank's balanced salt solution at 37°C in a water bath with agitation at 140 rpm for 60 minutes. Every 15 minutes during digestion, the fat should be agitated and vented. Next, the collagenase digest should be

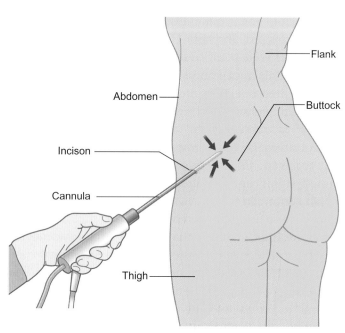

Fig. 13.6 Different locations from which liposuction fat can be harvested. These locations have been shown to demonstrate different osteogenic and adipogenic potentials.

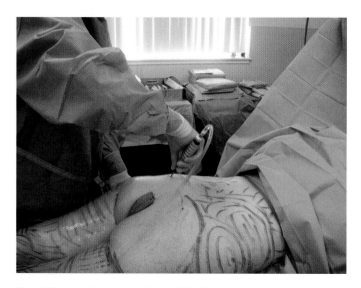

Fig. 13.5 Human liposuction of thigh. ASC, adipose-derived stromal cells.

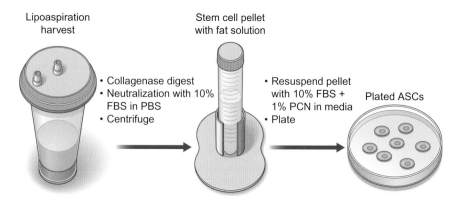

Fig. 13.7 Overview of adipose-derived stromal cell harvest process. Liposuction aspirate (left) is digested, and then centrifuged to pellet the stromal vascular fraction (middle), and then plated in 10-cm dishes for expansion (right). FBS, fetal bovine serum; PBS, phosphate-buffered saline; PCN, penicillin.

inactivated by adding an equal volume of PBS with 10% fetal bovine serum (FBS) and 1% Pen/Strep. The stromal vascular fraction is then pelleted via centrifugation at 1000 rpm for 6 minutes. The supernatant is discarded and the cell pellet resuspended and filtered through a 100-μm cell strainer to remove undigested tissue fragments. The cells are pelleted and resuspended in growth media, and primary culture is established in tissue culture plates incubated at 37°C in an atmosphere of 5% CO_2. Cell counting can be challenging given the large number of erythrocytes in the final cell pellet; however, we do not recommend a red cell lysis step as we believe this decreases the viability of the ASCs. On average, 10 mL of starting adipose tissue will allow the harvest of 1 million hASCs.

Mouse ASC (mASC) harvest is done in a similar manner. The first step involves harvesting the inguinal fat pad bilaterally from at least four mice. Here it is imperative to mince the adipose tissue finely prior to the digestion step. Subsequently, the steps are the same as described above in hASCs, with a digestion step, followed by neutralization, centrifugation, filtration, and plating.

Current concepts and research

Difference between mouse and human ASCs

The study of mASCs is attractive due to the relative ease of cell harvest and the availability of laboratory mice. Moreover, the widespread use of genetic knockout mice makes for potential profitable avenues of investigation. However, there exist important differences between ASCs of mouse and human origin, differences which have not yet been fully investigated. For example, hASCs have been observed to have a significantly more robust *in vitro* osteogenic capacity as compared to mASCs.[65,66] In order to undergo significant *in vitro* osteogenesis, mASCs require an additional osteogenic stimulus such as retinoic acid.[67] Moreover, cytokines such as fibroblast growth factor (FGF)-2 abolish osteogenic differentiation in mASCs, whereas hASC osteogenic differentiation proceeds relatively uninhibited in the presence or absence of FGF-2.[66,68]

In our laboratory, we have observed that ASCs, whether derived from mouse or human origin, contribute to osseous healing of mouse cranial defects.[69,70] For example, a critical-sized mouse calvarial defect shows no healing without ASC engraftment even up to 16 weeks postinjury. Upon hASC engraftment, however, significant bony healing is observed in as little as 4 weeks postinjury.[70]

Enrichment based on cell surface receptors

While substantial progress has been made in the study of ASCs, we are limited by working with a heterogeneous cell population. We believe that a selected, or clonal, subpopulation of cells enriched based on their cell surface markers is necessary to move our investigations forward *(Fig. 13.8)*. By optimizing and selecting for an enriched subpopulation of ASCs that demonstrates a robust ability to differentiate along an osteogenic lineage, we can maximize the outcomes of cell-based therapies for skeletal regeneration. Borrowing an approach used to isolate hematopoietic stem cells (HSCs), ASCs can be enriched based on cell surface markers using fluorescence-activated cell sorting.

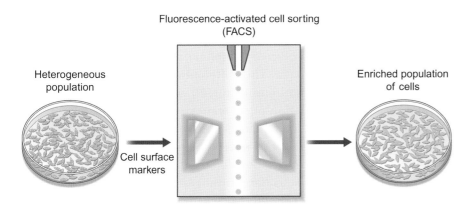

Fluorescence-activated cell sorting
(FACS)

Heterogeneous population

Cell surface markers

Enriched population of cells

Fig. 13.8 Fluorescence-activated cell sorting (FACS) can be used to separate cells based on cell surface receptors. The goal would be to use these surface receptors to identify cells that are more likely to differentiate down a specific lineage. Here, FACS is used on a heterogeneous human adipose-derived stromal cell (ASC) population to isolate an osteoprogenitor population.

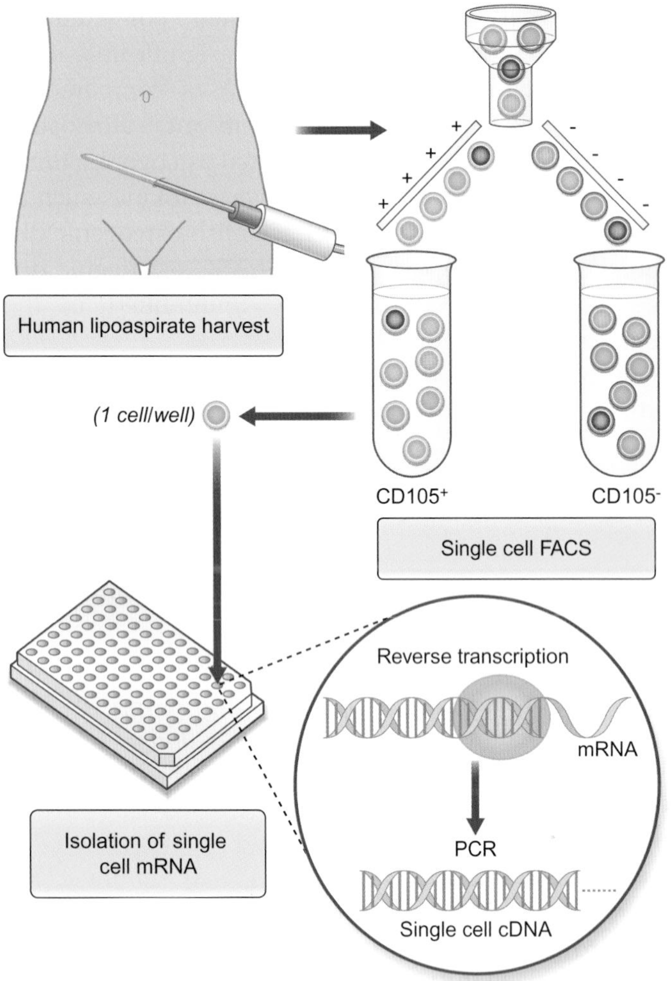

Fig. 13.9 Fluorescence-activated cell sorting (FACS) can be used to isolate cells on a single cell level. Subsequently, human adipose-derived stromal cells can be studied on a single cell level to delineate further the transcriptional properties of each cell. PCR, polymerase chain reaction.

Even within a specific subset of ASCs sorted by a cell surface receptor, heterogeneity persists. While stem cell populations are known to be heterogeneous, the functional consequences of this heterogeneity have not been fully elucidated. The problem of undefined heterogeneity within stem cells must be overcome before they can be used effectively for therapeutic applications. The first step to understand this heterogeneity is to elucidate the gene expression profiles of these complex cells which can be done using single-cell microfluidic technology *(Fig. 13.9)*. This permits precise mixing of nanoliter quantities of quantitative PCR reagents to perform single-cell transcriptional analysis across single cells.

Methods of ASC delivery

Despite accumulating animal research and intriguing case reports, much remains unknown regarding the optimum mode of ASC delivery. A significant and growing number of studies have examined the intravenous (IV) administration of ASCs. Such studies have investigated the natural distribution of ASCs following IV injection. Interestingly, most organs show uptake of ASCs after administration, including bone and bone marrow tissues, and at least some studies show long-term persistence within the host without oncogenic transformation.[71–73] These studies were geared toward disparate interests, but all were rooted in the regenerative capabilities of ASCs. For example, studies have examined IV injection of ASCs for repair of the liver,[72] heart,[74] endothelium,[75] and even olfactory epithelium.[76] An emerging interest as well is in the IV administration of ASCs for autoimmune and inflammatory disorders, such as experimental colitis and abdominal sepsis,[77–79] muscular dystrophy,[80] experimental arthritis,[78] and encephalomyelitis.[81] Two provocative case studies have also been published in humans showing beneficial outcomes of IV-delivered ASCs: the first in rheumatoid arthritis, and the second in chronic autoimmune thrombocytopenia.[82,83] Thus, the use of IV ASCs may be a safe and beneficial future therapeutic modality.

In vitro: protocols on differentiation

Osteogenic differentiation *(Fig. 13.10)*

For osteogenic differentiation, cells should be plated in a six-well plate at a density of 100 000 cells per well, in 12-well plates at a density of 50 000 cells per well, or in a 24-well plate at 25 000 cells per well. After attachment, ASCs are treated with osteogenic differentiation medium (ODM) containing Dulbecco's modified eagle medium (DMEM), 10% FBS, 100 μg/mL ascorbic acid, 10 mM β-glycerophosphate, and 100 IU/mL penicillin/streptomycin. This differentiation media can be enhanced to stimulate increased osteogenesis with the supplementiation of several cytokines, such as insulin-like growth factor, platelet-derived growth factor (PDGF), or BMP-2.[84,85] ODM should be replenished every 3 days.

Early and late osteogenic differentiation have been defined at different time points which differ across species. Whereas mASCs undergo early osteogenesis by

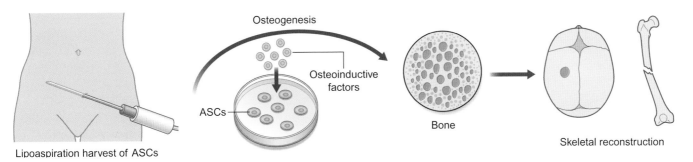

Fig. 13.10 Potential clinical uses for liposuction-acquired fat. Adipose-derived stromal cells (ASCs) are harvested by liposuction (left), cultured *in vitro* with differentiation medium (middle) to bone, and subsequently utilized for reconstructive procedures treating a myriad of diseases (right).

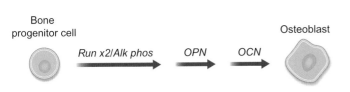

Fig. 13.11 Genes involved in differentiation of a bone progenitor cell to an osteoblast. Lineage-specific differentiation is associated with the ordered sequence expression of various genes. Osteoblast differentiation is associated with expression of runt-related protein-2 (Runx2), osteopontin (OPN), and osteocalcin (OCN), corresponding with early, intermediate, and late osteogenesis.

day 7 and late osteogenesis by day 14, hASCs undergo much more robust osteogenesis and should be analyzed at day 3 for early differentiation and day 7 for late differentiation. To assess osteogenic differentiation, RNA can be analyzed from ASCs. Specific gene markers of osteogenic differentiation include osteocalcin (OCN), osteopontin (OPN), runt-related protein-2 (RUNX-2), collagen Ia (COL1A), and alkaline phosphatase (ALP). ALP staining and quantification can also be performed on day 3 of differentiation to assess for early ostegenic activity *(Fig. 13.11)*. Subsequently, late osteogenic activity can be assessed at day 7 of differentiation by alizarin red staining, which detects extracellular mineralization.

Adipogenic differentiation *(Fig. 13.12)*

To drive ASCs to adipose tissue, cells are seeded in a similar density as described for osteogenic differentiation. Adipogenic differentiation medium contains 10 µg/mL insulin, 1 µM dexamethasone, 0.5 mM methylxanthine, and 200 µM indomethacin. At 3 days, medium should be replaced with 10 µg/mL insulin. Differentiation can be assessed by oil red O staining and quantification or gene analysis. Specific genes expressed by adipose tissue during differentiation that can be analyzed include GCP1, lipoprotein lipase (LPL), and

peroxisome proliferation-activated receptor γ (PPARγ: *Fig. 13.13*).

Chondrogenic differentiation

Chondrogenic differentiation is difficult to perform in monolayer and thus is performed using micromass cell droplets. Each 10 mL droplet contains 100 000 cells which are then seeded in culture dishes and allowed to form cell aggregates and substratum at 37°C for 2 hours. Chondrogenic medium includes DMEM, 1% FBS, 1% penicillin/streptomycin, 37.5 mg/mL ascorbate-2-phosphate, ITS (insulin, human transferrin, and selenous acid) premix, and 10 ng/mL transforming growth factor-β_1 (TGF-β). This medium is carefully added around the cell aggregates. By 24 hours, the aggregates should coalesce and become spherical. Micromasses are fixed with 4% paraformaldehyde/4% sucrose and embedded at day 3 and day 6 for histological analysis. Alcian blue allows for staining of chondrogenic tissues and glycosaminoglycan assays allow for quantification of chondrogenesis. Subsequent gene analysis can be performed using chondrogenic gene analysis such as SOX-9, aggrecan, and collagen II.

In vivo model

Nude athymic mouse 4-mm calvarial defect

To translate *in vitro* findings to the clinical realm, robust *in vivo* data must be obtained to demonstrate the osteogenic capacity of ASCs. *In vivo* models should include large immunocompetent animals such as sheep[86] and dogs,[87,88] as well as smaller immunocompromised animals such as rabbits,[89] rats,[90] or mice.[28] Though several models exist to determine *in vivo* osteogenic healing, we believe the nude mouse model offers a reliable, easily

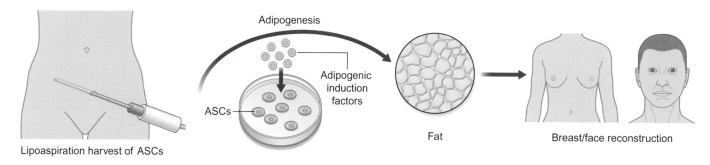

Fig. 13.12 Potential clinical uses for adipocyte differentiation of human adipose-derived stromal cells (ASCs). ASCs are harvested by liposuction (left), cultured *in vitro* with differentiation medium (middle) to fat, and subsequently utilized for reconstructive procedures treating soft-tissue defects (right).

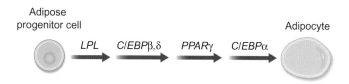

Fig. 13.13 Adipocyte differentiation is associated with expression of lipoprotein lipase (LPL), peroxisome proliferator-activated receptor (PPARγ), and enhancer binding proteins (EbP).

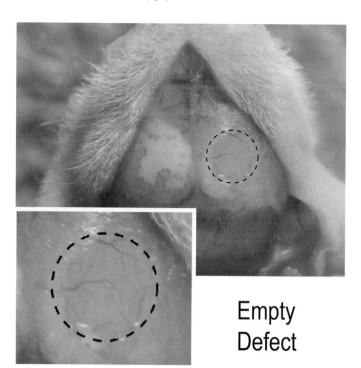

Fig. 13.14 A 4-mm nonhealing critical-sized defect in the right parietal bone of a CD-1 nude athymic mouse.

replicated, and easily followed defect. Immunocompromised animals such as nude athymic mice allow scientists to assess the effect of ASCs on an area while decreasing the innate immune response to xenotransplanted cells which can confound results. Mice are readily available in large quantities and can be studied by most small-animal imaging technologies such as microcomputed tomography (microCT), micropositron emission tomography (micro-PET), and bioluminescent imaging. Mice, however, heal wounds rapidly and effectively and thus scientists must demonstrate that any result is superior to the animal's baseline healing capacity. One way to demonstrate an effect is to create a defect so large that it overwhelms the innate ability to heal the wound. This large defect, that does not heal when followed over time, is referred to as "critical-sized." One such defect we have found to serve as an *in vivo* model is a 4-mm defect in the parietal bone of a nude athymic mouse.[69]

Nonhealing, critical-sized (4-mm) calvarial defects can be created in the right parietal bone of adult (60-day-old) male CD-1 nude mice using a high-speed dental drill. After cleaning the surgical site with Betadine, an incision is made just off the sagittal midline to expose the right parietal bone. The pericranium will be removed using a sterile cotton swab. Using diamond-coated trephine bits and saline irrigation, unilateral full-thickness critical-size calvarial defects are created in the nonsuture-associated right parietal bone. Importantly, the dura mater should be left undisturbed *(Fig. 13.14)*. In preparation for implantation, scaffolds can be seeded with hASCs 24 hours prior to implantation. For scaffold creation, apatite-coated PLGA scaffolds were fabricated from 85/15 poly(lactic-co-glycolic acid) by solvent casting and a particulate leaching process. Briefly, PLGA/chloroform solutions were mixed with 200–300 μm diameter sucrose to obtain 92% porosity (volume fraction), and compressed into thin sheets in a Teflon mold. After freeze-drying overnight, scaffolds were immersed in ddH$_2$O to dissolve the sucrose, and gently removed from the Teflon plate for disinfection and drying.

For apatite coating, simulated body fluid (SBF) solution was prepared by sequentially dissolving $CaCl_2$, $MgCl_2 \cdot 6H_2O$, $NaHCO_3$, and $K_2HPO_4 \cdot 3H_2O$ in ddH_2O. Solution pH was lowered to 6 by adding 1 M hydrochloric acid to increase the solubility. Na_2SO_4, KCl, and NaCl were added and the final pH was adjusted to 6.5 (SBF 1). Mg^{2+} and HCO_3^- free SBF (SBF 2) was prepared by adding $CaCl_2$ and $K_2HPO_4 \cdot 3H_2O$ in ddH_2O and pH was lowered to 6. KCl and NaCl were added and the final pH was adjusted to 6.8. All solutions were sterile-filtered through a 0.22-μm polyethersulfone (PES) membrane (Nalgene, NY). The obtained PLGA scaffolds were incubated in SBF 1 for 12 hours and changed to Mg^{2+} and HCO_3^- free SBF 2 for another 12 hours at 37°C under gentle stirring. Coated scaffolds were washed with ddH_2O to remove excess ions and lyophilized prior to further studies.

We found 150 000 cells/scaffold to be optimal in our laboratory.[70] The hASCs to be seeded on to each scaffold are suspended in 25 μL of growth media, and placed on to the scaffold for 30 minutes. The scaffold will subsequently be submerged in 100 μL of growth media for 12 hours of incubation. Before implantation, cell-seeded scaffolds should be rinsed in sterile PBS to prevent transfer of medium-derived growth factors.

Clinical correlates

Recent case studies have focused on the use of hASCs to replace bone loss.[91] In case reports, defects of the calvaria,[92] maxilla,[93] and mandible[94] have been either healed or enabled to heal faster with the use of hASCs. Such reconstructions eliminate the need for alloplastic materials, and thus reduce the risk of infection, breakdown, or rejection. Despite accumulating translational research, there is a paucity of data defining the mechanisms through which hASCs influence an osseous defect. Do hASCs directly form bone to heal a skeletal defect? In opposition, do engrafted hASCs function as efficient factories to produce potent pro-osteogenic cytokines? In the case of our calvarial defect model, careful examination of calvarial defects engrafted with ASCs yields some profitable insights into the potential derivation of healing. For example, bone is often observed to mineralize from the edges of a cranial defect inwards, which suggests that the host calvarium may contribute to the bony regenerate. Concurrently, small, isolated islands of bone are often observed early

postoperatively, which suggests either contribution from engrafted ASCs or alternatively from host dura mater (another source of significant ostogenic progenitors).[95–97] Finally, uniform and thorough healing of hASC-engrafted defect suggests primary osseous healing derived from the engrafted donor cells themselves. It is likely that all three cell types (donor ASCs, host calvarial osteoblasts, and host dura mater) contribute to bony healing.

Future direction of tissue engineering using ASCs

A significant gap exists between the current knowledge regarding ASC biology and their future translation to clinical use. First, the safety of hASCs must be determined. Oncogenic transformation must be inhibited, such that tumors of mesodermal origin are not produced after cell engraftment.[73] We believe that major breakthroughs in aesthetic and reconstructive surgery using autologous tissue will not come by incremental improvements to technical aspects such as liposuction cannulas or injection syringes. Instead, novel cell-based strategies must be explored to identify and isolate specific fat precursors from hASCs and to coordinate the physiologic induction of adipose tissue differentiation in a biomimetic environment *in vivo* (**Fig. 13.15**). hASC-seeded biomaterial constructs may provide a new direction for autologous fat transfer through the assembly of natural three-dimensional adipose, cartilage, or bone tissues.[98] Our ultimate translational goal is, during the course of a single operative procedure, to harvest subcutaneous adipose tissue, isolate ASC, and implant these cells on an osteoconductive and/or osteoinductive scaffold into the skeletal defect without leaving the operating room (**Fig. 13.16**).

Bone marrow mesenchymal stem cells

Definitions

Bone marrow MSCs are multipotent cells that have been shown to differentiate into a variety of cell types, including adipocytes, chondrocytes, osteocytes, skeletal myocytes, and cardiomyocytes. Following their original identification as cells from bone marrow that could adhere to plastic, numerous studies have documented their plasticity, immunomodulatory properties, and potential for use in tissue-engineering strategies. MSCs

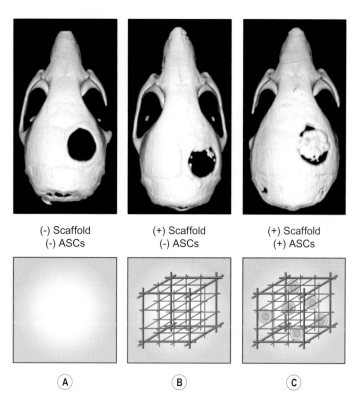

(-) Scaffold	(+) Scaffold	(+) Scaffold
(-) ASCs	(-) ASCs	(+) ASCs
Ⓐ	Ⓑ	Ⓒ

Fig. 13.15 Utilization of adipose-derived stromal cells (ASCs) to heal a skeletal defect. **(A–C)** Microcomputed tomography images of a 4-mm critical-sized mouse parietal bone defect in our P60 nude CD-1 mice. **(A)** Without either a scaffold or ASCs, this defect will not heal by 2 weeks. **(B)** Scaffold only. Wounds treated with scaffold alone also show minimal healing. **(C)** Scaffold with ASCs. Significant remineralization is observed after only 2 weeks postinjury in wounds treated with ASC-seeded scaffolds.

have also been found to be recruited to sites of injury, where they may participate in the body's own natural system of tissue repair. These findings highlight the enormous potential for MSCs in clinical use and therapeutic trials for an increasing range of medical disorders have recently begun. While some debate remains over the true effects MSCs may exert in various disease states, the prospects for use of these cells as an "off-the-shelf" biological therapeutic remains a tangible goal.

The role of MSCs within bone marrow has been debated, with work by Prockop and others helping to elucidate both an intrinsic and extrinsic function to bone itself.[7,99] By infusing genetically marked MSCs into isogenic mice, studies revealed a distribution of these cells to various locations, including cortical and cancellous bone, cartilage, spleen, thymus, lung, and liver.[7] MSCs thus demonstrate the ability to circulate and participate in normal cellular turnover and potentially tissue repair and regeneration.

Current concepts and research

In recent years, the potential use of MSCs in therapeutic modalities for tissue repair has become increasingly promising. As such, a number of studies have focused on phenotypically characterizing these cells both *in vitro* and *in vivo*. The initial isolation of MSCs exploited their ability to adhere to plastic; however, many of the clones isolated by Friedenstein's method proved incapable of osteogenic differentiation.[100,101] This therefore suggested that a considerably heterogeneous population of cells exists within the marrow stroma. Percoll gradients, as employed by Pittenger *et al.*,[13] Caplan,[102] and Haynesworth *et al.*,[103] allowed for a more homogeneous population of MSCs to be harvested, as demonstrated by flow cytometric analysis of cell surface antigens. Alternative methods to obtain higher degrees of homogeneity have also been attempted, including culturing MSCs in low oxygen tension.[104,105] Perhaps the most rigorous means by which to define MSCs, however, has been through the use of cell surface antigens expressed *in vitro*. Numerous antigens have been examined, but the International Society for Cellular Therapy announced specific criteria to define bone marrow MSCs in 2006.[106] Based on these criteria, MSCs are required to be plastic-adherent when maintained in standard culture conditions and express CD73 (ecto 5'-nucleotidase), CD90 (Thy-1), and CD105 (Endoglin) while lacking expression of CD45 (protein tyrosine phosphatase), CD34 (hematopoietic cluster differentiation molecule 34), CD14 (macrophage/neutrophil cluster differentiation molecule 14), CD19 (follicular dendritic cell/B-cell cluster differentiation molecule 19), and human leukocyte antigen (HLA)-DR. Furthermore, MSCs must be capable of differentiation into adipocytes, chondroblasts, and osteoblasts *in vitro*. While these criteria have remained in evolution, they have served as a minimal standard for more recent investigations.

As the *in vitro* characterization of MSCs has progressed, phenotypic delineation of these cells *in vivo* has advanced at a much slower pace and collective data remain far from complete. More recently, investigators have further enriched the STRO-1 fraction through additional positive selection for CD106 (vascular cell adhesion molecule-1: VCAM-1) and CD146 (melanoma cell adhesion molecule), obtaining a purified fraction capable of self-renewal and multipotent

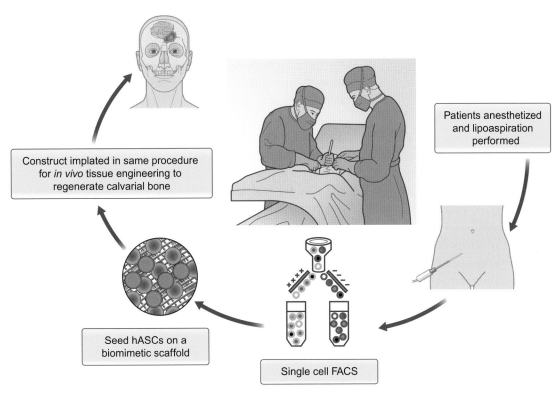

Fig. 13.16 Ultimate clinical translational goal: taking patient to the operating room and harvesting a multipotent, self-renewing cell population such as human adipose-derived stromal cells (ASCs), and then placing them on a scaffold for reconstruction of a tissue defect. FGF-2, fibroblast growth factor-2; BMP-2, bone morphogenetic protein-2.

differentiation.[107] These findings thus lend further support to the notion that MSCs indeed function as an *in vivo* stem cell source for derivation of mesenchymal tissue.

The lineage of MSCs and HSCs has also been carefully evaluated by investigators, looking to determine whether MSCs and HSCs exist as different populations within the bone marrow. Through sex-mismatched HLA-identical bone marrow allografts, researchers have demonstrated marrow-derived stromal cells to be exclusively host-derived while HSC-derived macrophages were found to originate from donors.[108] This finding indicated that MSCs existing within the stromal fraction represent a separate fraction distinct from hematopoietic cells. Contemporary models thus identify at least two types of stem cells within the bone marrow, with HSCs giving rise to hematopoietic cell types and osteoclasts, while MSCs differentiate into a multitude of mesenchymal lineages. Furthermore, it is widely believed that MSCs derive embryologically from mesoderm and that, as these cells stain positive for angiopoietin-1, they likely reside with pericytes located along the walls of sinusoidal blood vessels in bone marrow.[109,110]

Recent investigations have begun to identify an extraordinary property of MSCs with important therapeutic implications. Although still poorly understood, MSCs have been found to possess immunomodulatory properties.[111–116] Baseline expression of MHC class I proteins has been detected in MSCs while MHC class II proteins are entirely absent.[117] This particular profile has been associated with nonimmunogenic conditions, thus potentially allowing for MSC transplantation into allogenic hosts without the requirement of immunosuppressive therapy.[118] Even more surprising, MSCs have been found to be capable of modulating T-cell function.[111,112,114,116] In co-culture conditions, MSCs have been shown to decrease expression levels of proinflammatory cytokines, including tumor necrosis factor-alpha, interferon-gamma, interleukin-4, and interleukin-10 in dendritic cells and helper T cells.[112] MSC secretion of interleukin-1 receptor antagonist has also been reported to contribute to overall MSC-mediated immunosuppression.[119] From a clinical perspective, these properties may one day be exploited for treatment of conditions such as graft-versus-host disease and autoimmune disorders.[118,120]

In vitro: protocols on tissue harvest and differentiation

Contemporary techniques to harvest and culture MSCs are still predicated on the same fundamental property of adherence to plastic employed by Friedenstein *et al.* over 40 years ago.[8] More recently, investigators have incorporated the use of density gradients to eliminate unwanted cell types present in marrow aspirate and increase homogeneity.[13] When working with human MSCs, the iliac crest has been a commonly cited source for bone marrow harvest.[121] Murine MSCs, in contrast, can be harvested from either fibula or tibia by first flushing the marrow contents out with a 27G syringe.[122] Harvested bone marrow is then placed in an aqueous solution of highly branched hydrophilic polysaccharide. By centrifuging for 30 minutes, four layers become visible. Red blood cells may be found on the bottom, above which lies the polysaccharide solution. The third layer contains the majority of mononuclear cells and the top layer contains primarily acellular medium. It is the third layer (mononuclear cells) which is isolated, recentrifuged, and plated on to plastic culture dishes. MSC colonies may often be observed to form after 6–8 days of *in vitro* culture.

Lineage-specific culture conditions to induce differentiation of MSCs into adipocytes, chondrocytes, osteoblasts, and myoblasts have been well described. Adipogenic differentiation can be induced by treatment of MSCs with 1-methyl-3-isobutylxanthine, dexamethasone, insulin, and indomethacin.[13] Fat accumulation can be readily appreciated histologically by the formation of lipid-rich vacuoles within cells. In addition, differentiated MSCs have been shown to express various markers of adipogenic differentiation, including PPARγ2, LPL, and fatty acid-binding protein aP2 *(Fig. 13.13)*. To promote chondrogenic differentiation, MSCs are cultured serum-free in a pelleted "micromass" with TGF-β3.[13] A proteoglycan-rich extracellular matrix can be observed along with expression of type II collagen after 2 weeks, both of which are typically found in articular cartilage. Osteogenic differentiation of MSCs can be

accomplished with the same components as described in the section on ASCs. Finally, culture of MSCs with dexamethasone and hydrocortisone has been shown to induce expression of key regulatory factors for myogenic differentiation, including MyoD1 and myogenin.[123]

Aside from traditional mesenchymal lineages, MSCs have also been found to be capable of *in vitro* transdifferentiation, forming a variety of other tissue types even beyond those derived from mesoderm. Culturing MSCs with 5-azacytidine, Makino and colleagues reported on the formation of spontaneously beating myotube-like structures.[124] These cells were found to express markers consistent with cardiomyocyte differentiation. Neural differentiation has also been reported through treatment of MSCs with β-mercaptoethanol.[125] Under these conditions, cells rapidly assume neuronal morphology and express nestin, neuron-specific enolase, and neuron-specific protein, all proteins associated with early neuronal differentiation. MSCs thus possess a broad differentiation capacity, with plasticity beyond that typically associated with mesoderm-derived mesenchymal tissues. This broad capacity may also provide the future basis for a wide and disparate therapeutic potential.

In vivo models

The ability for MSCs to differentiate along several lineages has made these cells excellent candidates for the repair and regeneration of many tissues. The multipotency of MSCs, along with their ease of isolation and expansion potential, has led to a variety of preclinical studies evaluating their use in cardiovascular disease, central nervous system injury, diabetes, and bone/cartilage regeneration.

Cardiovascular disease remains one of the leading causes of morbidity and mortality worldwide, accounting for nearly 20 million deaths annually.[126] Contemporary approaches to treatment have centered on preservation of myocardium through pharmacologic therapy and revascularization. The ability for MSCs to undergo transdifferentiation along a cardiomyogenic lineage, however, has sparked recent interest in their application for postinfarct myocardial regeneration.[124] Importantly, *in vivo* studies have demonstrated that injected MSCs preferentially migrate to sites of inflammation, thereby allowing for their potential participation in repair of injured cardiac muscle.[127] Myocardial ischemia may promote release of chemoattractive factors, increase vascular permeability, and enhance expression of adhesion proteins to allow for proper homing of MSCs. How these cells truly act at postinfarct sites, however, remains controversial.

Like myocardial infarction, injury to the central nervous system has also contributed to significant death and disability worldwide. As investigators have shown MSCs to be capable of undergoing transdifferentiation into ectoderm-derived neuronal tissue, their use in various animal models of stroke has yielded quite provocative findings.[125] Several studies have demonstrated that injected MSCs can migrate to sites of stroke injury and differentiate into cells expressing neuronal markers.[128–130] Preliminary reports in rats have also shown that MSCs may potentially contribute to restore damaged neurons.[129,130] From a functional perspective, improved sensorimotor function has been shown following injection of MSCs into sites of cortical ischemia.[131]

The treatment of diabetes has been another field where use of MSCs has provided some promising results. Presently, type 1 diabetes may be partially reversed through the replacement of functional pancreatic β cells. Unfortunately, islet cell transplantation has been limited by immune rejection and continued autoimmune-mediated destruction.[132] The scarcity of donor islet cells further lends to the obstacle in treating this disease. The potential ability of MSCs, however, both to modulate the immune system and undergo *in vitro* β-cell transdifferentiation has led to several preclinical investigations employing these cells in animal models of diabetes.[132–135] As with cardiac ischemia and stroke, though, the true role of MSCs in the amelioration of hyperglycemia remains controversial. Introduction of human MSCs into immunocompromised diabetic mice was found to upregulate only mouse insulin production, suggesting that MSCs promote regeneration of endogenous islets rather than undergo transdifferentiation and integration into the host pancreas.[135] Nonetheless, these studies demonstrate that MSCs may one day represent a viable therapeutic option for the treatment of type 1 diabetes.

Of all the work surrounding *in vivo* studies on the preclinical application of MSCs, however, one of the most germane to the field of plastic and reconstructive surgery remains the use of these cells in bone and cartilage regeneration. Bone homeostasis represents a careful balance between bone production by mesenchymal lineage osteoblasts and bone resorption by hematopoietic lineage osteoclasts.[118] MSCs have been found potentially to alter this balance through the modulation of receptor activator of nuclear factor-κB ligand (RANKL) and osteoprotegrin expression.[118] It has also been suggested that a loss of MSC function may contribute to reduced bone regeneration with age.[136] From the perspective of bone repair and regeneration, MSCs have been evaluated as a potential cellular building block for tissue-engineering strategies. Using a canine femoral critical-sized defect model, investigators have shown MSCs to be capable of regenerating bone when loaded on to a hydroxyapatite-tricalcium phosphate cylinder.[88,137,138] By 16 weeks after introduction of MSCs, histological analysis revealed new bone spanning the entire defect.[88] In addition, both autologous and allogeneic MSCs were found to yield equivalent results, with no lymphocytic infiltration or antibody formation noted when leukocyte antigen mismatched allogeneic cells were implanted.[88]

Apart from the appendicular skeleton, investigators have also studied the use of MSCs in promoting bone formation for the spine. Spinal fusion remains the last resort for degenerative disc disease and over 300 000 cases are performed annually in the US.[118] Current research has focused on improvement of spinal fusion through the combination of autologous bone marrow with synthetic scaffolds and cytokine therapy. MSCs implanted on Matrigel and placed into the lumbar fusion bed of rats have been shown to result in a greater rate of successful fusion compared to animals receiving mixed-marrow stromal cells alone.[139] Kai *et al.* reported similar results in rabbits, using a combination of MSCs, calcium phosphate ceramic blocks, and recombinant human BMP-2.[140] These results suggest that MSCs may be a suitable replacement for more traditional methods employing iliac crest bone grafting and may also allow for greater mature osseous tissue formation at earlier time points following spinal fusion.

Repair and regeneration of cartilage remain another challenging problem where MSCs may yield alternative and more compelling strategies than those currently available. The ability to treat damaged cartilage and osteoarthritis is at present quite limited, with prosthetic joint replacement representing the best contemporary solution. Preclinical trials in goats, however, have shown the ability for MSCs to promote cartilage regeneration in knee joints.[141] Following surgical induction of osteoarthritis by excision of the medial meniscus and resection of the anterior cruciate ligament, Murphy and colleagues found that a single injection of MSCs suspended in dilute sodium hyaluronan could result in reduction of articular cartilage degeneration, osteophytic remodeling, and subchondral sclerosis.[141] These findings have also been observed in a mouse model for human rheumatoid arthritis, where allogeneic MSCs introduced intraperitoneally were found to prevent occurrence of severe, irreversible damage to cartilage and bone.[142] Rather than directly providing a cellular contribution to cartilage formation, in this instance MSCs were thought to modulate immune responsiveness and expression of inflammatory cytokines.[142] Future work will undoubtedly need to evaluate whether such an approach may also prove effective in controlling preexisting disease.

Clinical correlates

The last two decades of research with MSCs in both *in vitro* culture and *in vivo* animal models has allowed scientists to begin incorporating these cells into clinical trials for an ever-increasing range of potential medical disorders.[118,120] MSCs have been proposed to treat a wide variety of diseases and patients have already begun enrolling in industry-sponsored studies (Osiris Therapeutics, Waltham, MA) to investigate the use of these cells in graft-versus-host disease, Crohn's disease, and type 1 diabetes. The FDA has also approved the study of autologous MSCs in middle cerebral artery acute stroke treatment. To date, however, the most prominent application of MSCs in clinical trials has been their use in ischemic heart disease.

Following ischemic insult to the myocardium, reperfusion may salvage large regions of viable muscle, but this is often incomplete, resulting in a process of adverse left ventricular remodeling.[143] As previously noted, preclinical trials have shown autologous MSCs to improve cardiac function modestly, whether through transdifferentiation or elaboration of trophic factors capable of stimulating endogenous reparative mechanisms.[144,145]

Similar to ischemic cardiomyopathy, MSCs have also proven to be efficacious in early clinical studies involving skeletal disease. Long-bone distraction osteogenesis has been one emerging field in which researchers have found MSCs to promote improved healing and faster recovery rates.[146] In 17 patients undergoing distraction, injection of MSCs along with platelet-rich plasma into the callus during both lengthening and consolidation phases resulted in accelerated mature bone formation and a reduction in the incidence of complications.[147,148] Horwitz and colleagues have also investigated the use of MSCs in the treatment of osteogenesis imperfecta, a genetic disorder of type I collagen resulting in fragile bones and skeletal deformities.[149–151] While there is no current cure for osteogenesis imperfecta, preliminary reports have shown MSCs to be potentially successful in enhancing bone formation in these patients.[150] Children receiving two infusions of allogeneic MSCs were noted to demonstrate engraftment of these cells in multiple sites, including bone and skin. Importantly, accelerated growth velocity was appreciated during the first 6 months following treatment with no associated complications.[149] These findings thus reveal that MSCs may be safely administered to children, and when injected they can localize to genetically defective tissues.

The breadth of clinical trials involving MSCs is rapidly expanding, as studies have shown these cells to possess a strong propensity to ameliorate a wide range of tissue deficit secondary to injury or disease. While work progresses on their role in ischemic cardiomyopathy and skeletal deficiency, these fields represent only the tip of the iceberg relative to the potential both *in vitro* and preclinical studies have shown for these cells. As studies continue to elucidate how MSCs truly function in disease states, their diverse array of biological mechanisms makes the prospects for the development of a ready-made therapeutic with broad efficacy enticingly close.

Tissue-specific stem cells

Definitions

Adult, or tissue-specific, stem cells are undifferentiated cells which are found in almost all tissues and organs after embryonic development.[152] They fulfill the definition of being a stem cell because of their capacity for both self-renewal and differentiation into specialized cell types of the tissue or organ in which they are found.

Their major function is in maintaining homeostasis and ensuring that various forms of insult or injury are repaired to restore function. It has been hypothesized that defects in adult stem cell function may be responsible for a range of diseases. Further, study of adult stem cell function could reveal important biologic mechanisms that could be exploited for therapeutic purposes.[153]

Although rare, adult stem cells serve a critical function within the hierarchical organization of complex tissues and organs, giving rise to replacement cells to maintain tissue integrity throughout development. A model of coexisting quiescent and active progenitor subpopulations has been proposed to describe adult stem cells with different cell cycle states.[154] It is hypothesized that they exist in tightly regulated zones to ensure that differentiated cells can be rapidly repopulated while keeping a quiescent back-up system to maintain the longevity of adult stem cell pools. Another concept which has been studied in adult stem cells is transdifferentiation, or the ability of lineage-directed stem cells to differentiate into tissues or organs from another embryonic lineage.[155] For example, studies in mice have demonstrated the ability of bone marrow stem cells to differentiate into multiple cell types.

Current concepts and research

Skin

Mammalian skin is a widely available and readily accessible tissue to study adult stem cell function. Gene expression studies have identified critical regulators of epithelial stem cell function, including Wnt/beta-catenin, BMP, notch, and Hedgehog pathways.[156] Further, numerous subtypes of epithelial progenitors have recently been identified and contribute to different skin compartments containing resident epithelial stem cells, such as the hair follicle, sebaceous glands, and the interfollicular epidermis (*Fig. 13.17*).[157] Hair follicle stem cells are located in the bulge region and cycle slowly under normal conditions, but following injury, they become rapidly activated and migrate outwards toward the region of epithelial damage.[158]

These epithelial stem cells are located in discrete skin compartments but have common features which may reveal unifying mechanisms in normal homeostasis.

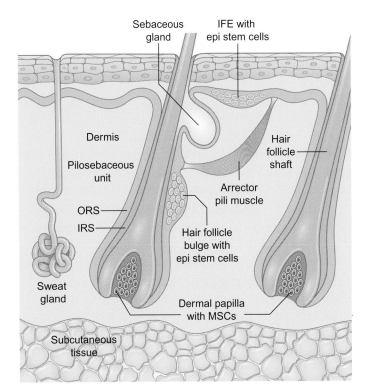

Fig. 13.17 Cells surrounding the hair follicle traffic to the wound site. SG, sebaceous gland; SC, stem cell,

They all express K5, K14, and delta Np63, are adjacent to an underlying basement membrane, and utilize many of the same regulatory signaling pathways.[159] The complex skin environment also houses putative melanocyte stem cells involved in the graying of hair[160] and dermal pericytes which have been implicated as important stem cell regulators of skin regeneration.[161]

Many of the mechanisms underlying skin embryogenesis are recapitulated later in adult life to maintain skin homeostasis.[156] Several models have been proposed to explain the balance of stem cell populations and function. One such model describes asymmetric versus symmetric cell division. Symmetric cell division describes the generation of two daughter cells that eventually acquire the same differentiated fate. Asymmetric division describes the process whereby a stem cell produces one daughter cell with a stem cell fate and another daughter cell destined for differentiation. These models are not mutually exclusive and are both thought to play an important role in the maintenance of skin stem cell populations.[162]

Bone

Osteoblasts are derived from bone marrow MSCs and their differentiation pathways have been well studied. These cells form bone, regulate bone growth and remodeling, and differentiate into mature osteocytes in response to stimuli such as mechanical loading, hormones, and cytokines.[163] A delicate balance is maintained with their osteoclast counterparts, which resorb bone and are derived from monocyte/macrophage precursors. During adult osteogenesis, bone formation proceeds through two different pathways: intramembranous ossification (e.g., skull) or endochondral ossification (e.g., long bones). The former occurs directly from MSC condensation while the latter involves an intermediate MSC-mediated cartilage formation step followed by replacement with bony matrix[164] *(Fig. 13.18).*

Osteoblast differentiation is regulated by several major signaling pathways such as Wnt, BMP, FGF, Hedgehog and transcription factors such as Runx2, Osterix, ATF4, and TAZ.[165] These signals determine the fate of skeletal lineage precursors and can potentially be manipulated to induce bone regeneration. BMPs-2, 4, and 7 have been successfully used to induce osteoblast differentiation and matrix formation *in vivo* and vehicles for BMP gene delivery such as plasmids and viruses have been effectively employed.[166] Combination gene delivery has been successful and is thought to

recapitulate more closely the signaling environment *in vivo*, providing a synergistic stimulus for bone formation. This sensitization effect has been demonstrated with combinations of BMPs, vascular endothelial growth factor (VEGF), RANKL, and Runx2 delivery.[166]

Blood vessels

Regulated blood vessel development in response to tissue injury or ischemia is critical for maintenance of healthy tissues, and dysfunction in this neovascularization process often results in disease.[167] For example, adequate wound healing requires a robust vascular response to deliver immune cells and metabolic substrates necessary for tissue regeneration.[168] In addition, a coordinated pattern of neovascularization signaling and stem cell recruitment is essential for normal organ development during embryogenesis,[169] as well as for tumor growth and metastasis.[170] During embryogenesis, mesoderm-derived angioblasts organize via vasculogenesis to form blood vessels.[171] It was initially believed that all subsequent blood vessel growth occurred through sprouting of pre-existing endothelial cells in a process known as angiogenesis[172] *(Fig. 13.19).* However, it has been discovered that the vascular programming evident during embryonic development is recapitulated in various postnatal states during a process known as adult vasculogenesis[173] *(Fig. 13.19).*

Endothelial precursor cells (EPCs), which are bone marrow-derived progenitor cells that participate in adult vasculogenesis, were first identified by Asahara *et al.*[174] These cells are recruited to the site of ischemia and divide to form syncytial masses which tubularize and canalize to form a patent vascular network.[175] Pericytes, which retain the pluripotency of MSCs,[109] are also intimately involved in vascular morphogenesis. They reside at the interface between endothelial cells and the surrounding tissue and produce proangiogenic signals that regulate endothelial cell differentiation and growth.[176] Through both direct physical interaction and paracrine signaling, endothelial cells and pericytes engage in complex crosstalk that is essential for normal vasculogenesis.[177]

Muscle

Satellite stem cells were first described by Mauro in the 1960s as mononucleated cells situated between muscle fibers and their basement membrane[178] *(Fig. 13.20).*

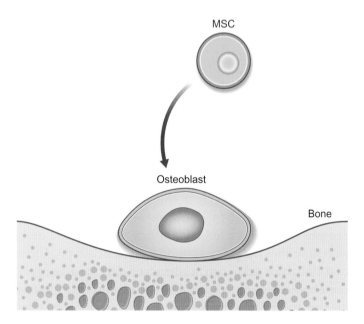

Fig. 13.18 Mesenchymal stem cell (MSC) condensation into an osteoblast as in intramembranous ossificaiton.

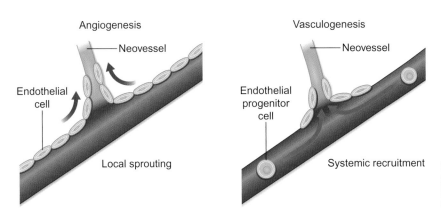

Fig. 13.19 Sprouting of pre-existing endothelial cells in a process known as angiogenesis (left). Formation of new vessel from circulating endothelial progenitor cell known as vasculogenesis (right).

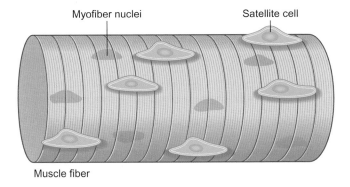

Fig. 13.20 Muscle satellite cells located between muscle fibers and their basement membrane.

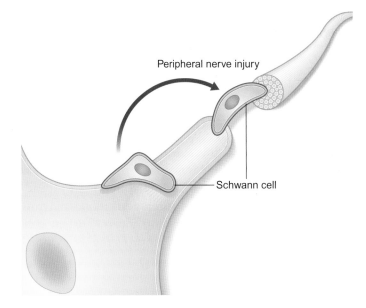

Fig. 13.21 Schwann cell migration to peripheral nerve injury site to assist in repair.

Differential modes of asymmetric cell division have been proposed to regulate satellite cell self-renewal.[179,180] However, symmetric cell division may play a major role in the response to muscle injury whereby large amounts of myogenic cells are needed to replace the missing or dysfunctional muscle mass.[180] Repair mechanisms are also thought to involve recruitment of neighboring satellite cells and circulating myogenic stem cells. Further, satellite cell dysfunction has been proposed to underlie certain muscular diseases such as Duchenne muscular dystrophy, but this hypothesis requires further study.

The major components of the satellite cell niche are the adjacent muscle fiber (including the mechanical, electrical, and biochemical signals which emanate from it), the basal lamina, and the microvasculature. These interrelated components regulate the activity of muscle stem cell populations and include calveolin-1, sphingomyelin, calcitonin receptors, the transmembrane protein Megf10, Notch signaling, and matrix components such as proteoglycans.[180]

Peripheral nerve

Although peripheral nerves have the capacity to regenerate axons following injury, outcomes after repair remain poor due to direct neuronal damage as well as chronic denervation of the distal end.[181] However, when denervated supporting Schwann cells were replaced with healthy ones at the site of injury, nerve regeneration was improved *(Fig. 13.21)*. This suggests that cell-based therapies may have an important role in treating nerve injuries. Guenard *et al.* demonstrated that syngeneic Schwann cells could effectively improve nerve regeneration in rat sciatic nerve injuries.[182] Murakami *et al.* transplanted neural stem cells obtained from the hippocampus of rat embryos into sciatic nerve defects and demonstrated nerve regeneration after 8 weeks.[183] Mean number of myelinated fibers and fiber size were increased compared to controls.

Neurotrophic growth factors have also played an important role in experimental models of nerve repair. These include NGF, brain-derived neutrophic factor (BDNF), neurotrophin-3 (NT-3), NT-4/5, FGF, and PDGF, amongst others.[184] These have been delivered through matrix/conduit release or mini-pump systems but bioavailability throughout the necessary regenerative time scales remains an issue.

Clinical correlates

Skin

Cell-based therapies have been used for decades in the treatment of burn injury and autologous epidermal sheets have been grown *ex vivo* and subsequently reimplanted with varying degrees of success.[185] Bone marrow and fat-derived MSC therapies have proven useful for chronic wounds in the clinical setting, although these are mostly case reports.[186] Dash *et al.* reported a randomized clinical trial using autologous bone marrow MSCs to treat chronic nonhealing ulcers.[187] Stem cell-treated patients demonstrated improvements in pain-free walking and reductions in ulcer size up to 12 weeks posttreatment.

Transplantation of HSCs from peripheral blood and bone marrow has also demonstrated engraftment of cells into skin.[188] Histological evaluation of skin specimens from sex-mismatched transplants showed that up to 7% of cells were XY-positive, indicating that circulating stem cells could differentiate into mature epithelium. However, another study with a similar sex-mismatched transplant design failed to show donor stem cell contribution to keratinocyte populations.[189] Badiavas and Falanga reported on 3 patients with chronic lower extremity wounds refractory to standard therapy who were treated with autologous bone marrow stem cells.[190] Complete wound closure was observed in all 3 patients and there was less wound fibrosis compared to pretreatment wound specimens. It appears that numerous adult stem cell populations can contribute to skin regeneration but the optimal combination of cells and signals remains unknown.

Bone

As previously mentioned, allogeneic bone marrow-derived stem cells were shown to improve osteogenesis in three children with osteogenesis imperfecta with around 2% donor cell engraftment.[150] Three months after treatment, all patients had increased total bone mineral content, growth velocity, and reduced frequency of bone fracture.

Blood vessels

Studies have demonstrated a strong correlation between clinical risk factors for cardiovascular disease and EPC function and quantities. Disease states such as diabetes, coronary artery disease, smoking, and hypercholesterolemia are known to affect EPCs adversely, prompting efforts to improve clinical outcomes through EPC augmentation.[191] Direct injection of EPCs as well as growth factors such as granulocyte–macrophage colony-stimulating factor have been used with some success following cardiac ischemia, and a meta-analysis found that intracoronary bone marrow cell infusions are safe and associated with a minor improvement in left ventricular function at 3–6 months following acute myocardial infarction.[192]

Muscle

Satellite cells have generally been incompatible with systemic administration and exhibit poor viability and migration when delivered intramuscularly. Thus, the therapeutic potential of muscle stem cells has focused more on progenitor populations derived from the endothelial lineage. These cells, which include mesoangioblasts, pericytes, and CD133+ cells, have significant myogenic potential and readily cross the endothelium, making intra-arterial delivery possible.[179] In animal models, these muscle progenitors have shown the ability to restore muscle function and to reconstitute the satellite stem cell compartment to varying degrees.[193] Numerous human trials for Duchenne muscular dystrophy demonstrated effective dystrophin production with the use of injected stem cells, but clinical benefits have not been observed.[194] Clinical trials have also been conducted with muscle stem cells for ischemic heart disease and stress urinary incontinence, with mixed improvements in muscle function.[195]

Nervous system

The vast majority of cell transplantation studies in the treatment of spinal cord injury have been in rodents, with several utilizing human bone marrow stem cells.[196] The FDA recently approved a human trial through Geron Corporation (US) for embryonal stem cell-based treatment of acute spinal cord injury, but this study was put on hold in 2009 due to the development of cysts in the injury site in preclinical studies. Although human-based stem cells have been used in preclinical models of peripheral nerve injury, clinical stem cell-based trials have yet to be conducted.

Prospective clinical applications of stem cell therapy

Scaffolds for stem cell delivery

Stem cells exist in tightly controlled environmental niches and alterations in this microenvironment can dramatically modify their behavior and capabilities. Further, they are often utilized in the setting of disease or injury where toxic signals may be prevalent, which further impair their function. Thus, strategies utilizing biomaterial scaffolds can potentially provide a controlled environment which protects implanted cells from harmful stimuli. Biomaterial matrices are also used to deliver genetic material and/or inductive biochemical cues which allow for some degree of developmental control over the delivered stem cells (*Fig. 13.22*). In terms of tissue and organ regeneration, scaffolds provide the structural template on which to build new tissues and thus can be prefabricated based on their ultimate purpose. For example, rigid scaffolds are much better suited for bone engineering whereas soft flexible scaffolds are ideal for skin applications.

Scaffolds can be broadly separated into two categories: native or synthetic. Native scaffolds include those derived from living or cadaveric donors and can be autogenous, allogeneic, or xenogenic. An excellent example is the treatment of massive burns with dermal substitutes which have been used from a wide range of human and nonhuman sources. Native matrices can also be obtained from decellularization of tissues and whole organs which can then be seeded with exogenous cells.[197,198] These techniques include the use of physical/

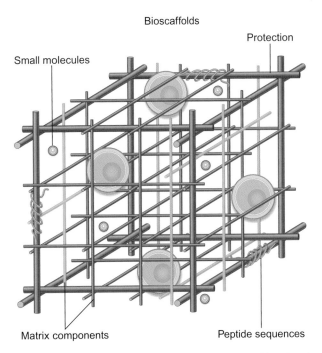

Fig. 13.22 Bioscaffold construct. Bioscaffolds can be tailored based on the stem cell type and small molecule utilized as well the protein type, peptide sequence, and matrix components.

mechanical forces, chemicals, and enzymatic agents to remove cellular material with minimal disruption of the matrix.[199]

Recently, there has been increased focus on so-called "smart" biomaterials.[200] These materials incorporate peptide sequences capable of better mimicking the native cellular environment and can significantly modulate cell differentiation, adhesion, and proliferation.[201] Smart polymers may allow scaffolds to respond to temperature, pH, light, or ionic interactions and these responses include altered mechanical properties, hydrophobicity, and collapse or expansion.[202] The development of these materials reflects the dynamic interactions necessary for successful tissue regeneration.

Numerous studies have demonstrated the benefits of utilizing stem cell–scaffold constructs in regenerative medicine. Scaffolds provide a highly modifiable vehicle for inductive factors as well. Fang *et al.* utilized plasmid DNA loaded on to collagen sponges and demonstrated successful *in vivo* genetic manipulation of fibroblasts to induce bone formation in rats.[203] Poly(lactide-coglycolide) scaffolds loaded with DNA plasmid showed enhanced cell transfection and matrix formation compared to naked plasmid injection alone.[204] Schek *et al.* demonstrated that bone formation was greater with hydrogel delivery of BMP-7-expressing adenovirus in mice compared to nonhydrogel controls.[205] These are just a handful of examples of the benefits of using scaffold-based applications to enhance the regenerative potential of stem cells.

As researchers continue to unravel the complex signals and interactions necessary for stem cell differentiation, it will be increasingly necessary for biomaterial techniques to recapitulate precisely various endogenous stem cell microenvironments.[200]

Genetic induction therapies

Cell-based regenerative strategies are also critically dependent on their biochemical signaling environment. Exogenous administration of specific growth factors and cytokines can induce stem cell differentiation, which provides researchers with a powerful means of manipulating stem cells *in vitro*. They can be coaxed to become numerous types of cells through gene transfer and cytokine therapies *(Fig. 13.23)*. However, before these inductive modalities can be effectively used *in vivo*, they must be delivered in a controlled spatiotemporal manner over the timescales necessary for stem cell repair and tissue regeneration.

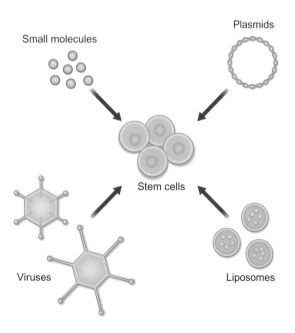

Fig. 13.23 Induction strategies for gene therapy. Small molecules, plasmids, or liposomes can stimulate stem cell differentiation.

Stem cell-directed gene therapy has demonstrated enormous potential following the cure of children with X-linked severe combined immune deficiency and adenosine deaminase deficiency.[206,207] However, two of 10 children treated subsequently developed leukemia, significantly tempering enthusiasm for stem cell gene therapy. Another hurdle has been the lack of relevant *in vitro* and animal models to predict efficacy in humans.[208] Common vector systems employed include Moloney murine leukemia virus, human immunodeficiency virus, and lentivirus, but concerns regarding adverse inflammatory responses are always present.

Gene transfer of growth factors like insulin-like growth factor and FGF has improved wound healing in animal models.[209,210] Recent studies have demonstrated that lentiviral vectors may be preferred for long-term transfection of skin cells whereas adenoviral or adeno-associated viruses may be better suited for short-term skin therapies.[211] Margolis *et al.* used replication-incompetent adenovirus to express PDGF for chronic venous leg ulcers in a phase I clinical trial.[212] Nonviral gene therapies through liposomal gene transfer have also been effectively used for wound regeneration.[213]

Iwaguro *et al.* demonstrated that VEGF gene transfer could be used to augment EPC function for vascular regeneration.[214] They demonstrated improved EPC adhesion, vascular incorporation, and proliferation in a rodent limb ischemia model. EPCs have been transfected to produce anticoagulant proteins in an angioplasty injury model[215] and VEGF-transfected EPCs have been used to fabricate bioengineered vascular grafts.[216] Gene therapy of EPCs has included potential cancer therapy given their avid recruitment to neovascularizing areas.[217]

Stem cell-mediated gene therapy has also been proposed for a wide range of neurologic diseases such as Parkinson's disease, Alzheimer's, amyotrophic lateral sclerosis, and neuropathic pain.[218] Regarding nerve injury, Schwann cells have been transduced to express ciliary neurotrophic factor to augment nerve growth in rats.[219] An adenoviral gene transfer system has also been developed for Schwann cell transfection and peripheral nerve injury.[220] Thus, vector-mediated strategies provide another regenerative tool to control the genetic programming of delivered stem cells with the promise of replacing missing or dysfunctional organs.

iPS Cells

Definitions

Pluripotency is the ability of a cell to differentiate into all cell types of the body and is a property held by blastocyst or inner-cell mass of the early mammalian embryo. As an embryo matures, cells become progressively more specialized and less pluripotent. Though previous studies have made mature cells more pluripotent, in 2007, scientists first described the process of reprogramming or "inducing" pluripotency in a mature cell using a few key transcription factors in the cell for a period of weeks[221] *(Fig. 13.24)*. These cells have been named "induced" pluripotent stem cells as they have stem cell-like properties. The original descriptions of

iPS cells used a set of our transcription factors: Oct4, Sox2, Klf4, and c-Myc *(Fig. 13.25)*. Since these original studies, scientists have been able to reprogram mature cells with only two factors. Dr. Yamanaka, who originally described the iPS cell, used a stochastic model to describe the mechanism behind this type of differentiation. In a stochastic model, most or all differentiated cells have the potential to become iPS cells with the use of four factors. The idea is that a cell represents a "ball rolling down an epigenetic landscape from the totipotent state, going through the pluipotent state and rolling down a lineage committed state." With the development of normal adult cells, pluripotent cells appear briefly and cannot be stopped "on the slope." In contrast, ES cells are blocked by a "bump or roadblock formed by their epigenetic status." Thus, the four

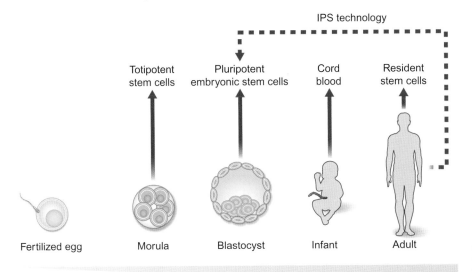

Fig. 13.24 Stem cells can be obtained during the different developmental stages of life. With the development of induced pluripotent stem cell (IPS) technology, adult cells can now be reprogrammed to become embryonic "stem cell-like" cells.

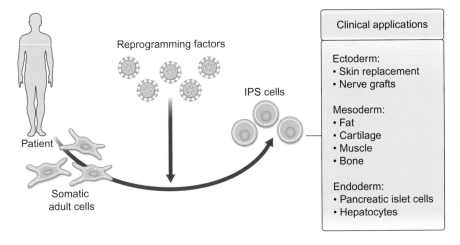

Fig. 13.25 By activation of four transcription factors, adult somatic cells can be reprogrammed into induced pluripotent stem cells, which then can differentiate into all the embryonic lineages: ectoderm, mesoderm, and endoderm.

Yamanaka factors function to reprogram cells back to a pluripotent state.[222]

iPS cells avoid the ethical concerns associated with ES cell derivation as they are derived from adult nonfetal tissues. Furthermore, since these cells are harvested from the same individual that would likely have them reimplanted, they may bypass the immune rejection which limits the use of allogeneic cells. Another advantage of iPS cell derivation is that they can be harvested from several different cell types. Early descriptions of iPS derivation used skin fibroblasts.[223,224] Advantages of this donor site were that a small skin biopsy could be followed by 3–4 weeks of *in vitro* expansion. One major disadvantage of skin fibroblasts, however, is that they have a very low reprogramming efficiency (under 0.01%) when using the four Yamanaka factors and even less without c-Myc. Furthermore, the length of transfection is an additional 3–4 weeks' time for ES cell-like iPS cells to appear.[225]

Based on the epigenetic landscape model, fibroblasts are considered terminally differentiated and thus take a greater amount of time and energy to reprogram.

Keratinocytes from human foreskin biopsies and hair have been used to derive iPS cells.[226] These cells are also easy to access but also require an extended time for *in vitro* expansion. Compared to fibroblasts, these cells, when derived from neonatal/juvenile foreskin, have an approximate 100-fold increase in reprogramming efficiency. This has not, however, been established in adult keratinocytes.

Melanocytes have also been described by Utikal *et al.* after harvest from a skin biopsy.[227] These cells inherently express high levels of Sox2 and thus can be reprogrammed with only three factors (Oct4, Kilf4, and c-Myc). Original studies using all four Yamanaka factors demonstrated a five times higher reprogramming efficiency than fibroblasts. In addition, the melanocytes were able to be reprogrammed in only 10 days.

Umbilical cord blood has recently come in vogue with regard to storage for possible future therapeutic uses. Two laboratories have recently described iPS cell derivation from cord blood cells. One laboratory was able to reprogram these cord blood cells successfully with only Oct4 and Sox2.[228] A benefit of this technique is that cord blood can be stored for over 5 years and still retain the ability to be reprogrammed. Longer cryopreservation, however, should be studied to determine their long-term viability for reprogramming.

A more recent discovery of an even more abundant source of cells for iPS applications is hASCs.[229] Our laboratory has isolated adipose cells from lipoaspirates of adult patients and successfully reprogrammed these using the four Yamanaka factors. Small-volume liposuction, in a minimally invasive outpatient setting, allows for the harvest of millions of cells. It is estimated that 10 mL of fresh lipoaspirate yields 1 million cells after 48 hours of *in vitro* culture. This allows immediate reprogramming without prior *in vitro* expansion. Even in slender patients, as little as 15–50 mL of fat can be used to derive iPS cells. Similarly, due to their rapid expansion, hASCs can be reprogrammed with a 20 times greater efficiency than fibroblasts. Klf4 and c-MYC expression are high in these cells compared to fibroblasts and these cells do not require mouse feeder cells. This ease of harvest and speed of expansion and reprogramming make hASCs an exciting option for scientists exploring translational iPS strategies and will put plastic surgeons at the forefront of tissue harvest.[229]

Despite the excitement generated around iPS cells, methods for their derivation and use need to be further tested and improved. Lentiviruses and retroviruses lead to genomic integration of transgenes which the host cells may not be able to silence completely. Furthermore, both Klf4 and c-MYC are oncogenes. Future directions may involve using small molecules and interfering RNAs, or microRNAs to make iPS cell generation safer. With regard to cell culture, iPS cells still depend on a layer of inactivated MEFs. Though future studies may use fibroblasts derived from the same patient, a Matrigel-coated surface could potentially allow for a feeder-free environment.

Recently laboratories have found ways to circumvent the use of viruses by generating a nonviral minicircle vector to induce iPS formation.[230] Minicircle vectors are nonbacterial supercoiled DNA molecules composed of a eukaryotic expression cassette. Minicircles also offer the advantages of having a higher transfection efficiency and longer ectopic expression due to low activation of exogenous silencing mechanisms. This was successfully done using hASCs from 3 different patients, making it an attractive option if rapid cell expansion and reprogramming are required.[230]

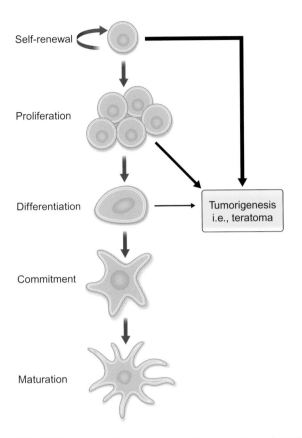

Self-renewal

Proliferation

Differentiation → Tumorigenesis i.e., teratoma

Commitment

Maturation

Fig. 13.26 One potential risk of using a multipotent self-renewing cell is the uncontrolled division of these cells leading to tumor formation. However, usually in tissue engineering a paucity of tissue, rather than excess, is the problem.

Despite the excitement generated behind the use of iPS cells, preclinical studies are still not safe enough for transition into human trials. A human sickle-cell anemia mouse model was successfully treated with iPS cells that were genetically corrected.[231] Although this was a human sickle-cell model, significant safety studies are required to determine the minimal number of undifferentiated iPS cells that can become a teratoma. Second, the oncogenic transgene integration and mutagenesis could induce cancer *(Fig. 13.26)*. Virus-free generated iPS cells offer a potential solution but these also still have not yet undergone rigorous studies. Third, current subcutaneous injection of iPS cells has gone on to differentiate into a teratoma, signifying that these cells will likely need to be differentiated *in situ* prior to implantation to allow for appropriate tissue regeneration *(Fig. 13.27)*. Further, once small-animal models are established, they must be repeated using large-animal models. Lastly, from a commercialization standpoint, it has yet to be determined if a viable business model for

patient-specific iPS treatments is possible given the challenge of their reprogramming and the oncogenic concerns.[225]

In vitro

Culture and Maintenance of iPS cells

IMR90 human fibroblasts or other cell types to be reprogrammed can be maintained with DMEM containing 10% FBS, L-glutamine, 4.5 g/dL glucose, 100 U/mL penicillin, and 100 µg/mL streptomycin. All cells used for reprogramming should be passage two or less. Derived iPS cells can be maintained either on MEF feeder layer or on Matrigel-coated tissue culture dishes (ES qualified; BD Biosciences) with mTESR-1 hES Growth Medium (Stemcell Technology).[229]

Lentivirus production and transduction

293FT cells (Invitrogen) are plated at ≈80% confluence per 100-mm dish and transfected with 12 µg each lentiviral vectors (Oct4, Sox2, Klf4, c-MYC) plus 8 µg packaging plasmids and 4 µg VSVG plasmids using Lipofectamine 2000 (Invitrogen) following the manufacturer's instructions. The resulting supernatant should be collected 48 hours after transfection, filtered through a 0.45-µm pore size cellulose acetate filter (Whatman), and mixed with PEG-it Virus Concentration Solution (System Biosciences) overnight at 4°C. Viruses are precipitated at 1500 g the next day and resuspended with Opti-MEM medium (Invitrogen).

In vitro *differentiation*

iPS cells cultured on Matrigel are treated with collagenase type IV (Invitrogen) and transferred to ultra-low attachment plates (Corning Life Sciences) in suspension culture for 8 days with DMEM/F12 (1:1) containing 20% knockout serum (Invitrogen), 4.5 g/dL glucose, L-glutamine, 1% nonessential amino acids, 0.1 mM 2-mercaptoethanol, 50 U/mL penicillin, and 50 µg/mL streptomycin to allow formation of embryoid bodies (EBs). EBs are then seeded in 0.25% gelatin-coated tissue culture dish for another 3–8 days. Spontaneous differentiation of iPS cells into cells of mesoderm and endoderm lineages can be detected with appropriate markers by immunofluorescence. For osteogenic differentiation,

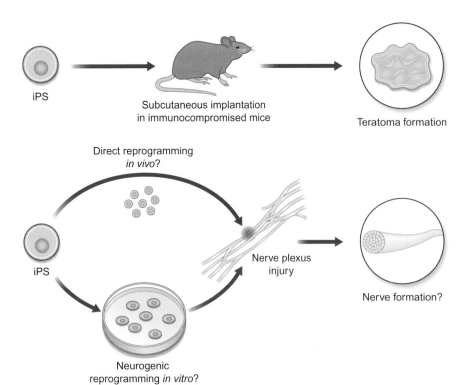

iPS

Subcutaneous implantation
in immunocompromised mice

Teratoma formation

Direct reprogramming
in vivo?

iPS

Nerve plexus
injury

Nerve formation?

Neurogenic
reprogramming *in vitro*?

Fig. 13.27 When induced pluripotent stem cells (IPS) are placed subcutaneously, there is differentiation into all three embryonic lineages, resulting in the formation of a teratoma. The hope is that these cells can be reprogrammed prior to implantation or *in situ* to repair tissues that cannot be repaired with human adipose-derived stromal cells such as neural tissues.

similar osteogenic medium with ascorbic acid, and β-glycerol phosphate have been used along with supplementation of retinoic acid and bone morphogenetic proteins. Furthermore, there remains dispute as to whether the EB formation step is necessary and leads to more efficient osteogenic differentiation or whether omission of this step is possible. Differentiation into dopaminergic neurons can be performed using a co-culture of hASC iPS cells with PA6 cells.

In vivo models and potential clinical correlates

The potential use of iPS technology clinically would revolutionize the field of tissue engineering as it would allow the creation of any of the three germ layers simply from an autologous skin biopsy or lipoaspiration. We believe that the derivation of iPS cells from hASCs holds several advantages compared to other cell types, such as neural stem cells, liver cells, and skin fibroblasts. First, the lipoaspiration procedure for isolating hASCs is relatively simple, fast, and safe. Second, it is easy to obtain a large quantity of hASCs as the starting population for reprogramming after a single lipoaspiration operation. Millions of hASCs can be derived on the same day of lipoaspiration, and the reprogramming can be performed immediately. Up until recently, iPS cells required a layer of mouse fibroblasts to survive in an undifferentiated state, which causes several clinical hurdles as mouse proteins could contaminate these human cells and cause complications in human recipients. Feeder-free derivation of iPS cells from hASCs thus represents a more clinically applicable method for derivation of iPS cells compared to other cell types and should enable more efficient and rapid generation of patient-specific and disease-specific iPS cells.[229] Preclinical testing of iPS cells will require extensive animal modeling. A focal deficit such as those present in spinal cord injuries, Parkinson's disease or type I diabetes might involve direct delivery. More systemic diseases such as muscular dystrophies, however, might require multiple intravenous injections for systemic delivery.[229a] With such models, however, there are several concerns about safety and efficacy that will need to be elucidated prior to use in humans.

Thus three main hurdles exist for iPS utilization to become mainstream:

1. Currently animal proteins are used during the reprogramming of human cells in the form of a mouse fibroblast feeder layer. A potential solution would be to use a feeder-free layer or Matrigel without animal components.

2. Currently viruses used for reprogramming can integrate into the genome and could cause mutations and possible malignancy. What is needed is a nonintegrating viral or robust and efficient nonviral approach such as the minicircle plasmid.

3. *In vivo*, undifferentiated iPS cells form teratomas. What is needed is directly to reprogram an iPS cell to the differentiated cell of interest or to predifferentiate an iPS cell into the desired cell type prior to placing it *in vivo*.

Access the complete reference list online at **http://www.expertconsult.com**

13. Pittenger MF, Mackay AM, Beck SC, et al. Multilineage potential of adult human mesenchymal stem cells. *Science*. 1999;284(5411):143–147.

25. Gronthos S, Graves SE, Ohta S, et al. The STRO-1+ fraction of adult human bone marrow contains the osteogenic precursors. *Blood*. 1994;84(12):4164–4173.

    This paper provides one of the earliest descriptions of the stromal vascular fraction of adipose tissue and characterizes its cell surface markers.

28. Cowan CM, Shi YY, Aalami OO, et al. Adipose-derived adult stromal cells heal critical-size mouse calvarial defects. *Nat Biotechnol*. 2004;22(5):560–567.

    This paper was the first description of using untreated adipose derived mesenchymal cells to heal a calvarial defect. They use novel tissue engineering tecniques and imaging modalities.

35. Moore KA, Lemischka IR. Stem cells and their niches. *Science*. 2006;311(5769):1880–1885.

48. Zhang SC, Wernig M, Duncan ID, et al. In vitro differentiation of transplantable neural precursors from human embryonic stem cells. *Nat Biotechnol*. 2001;19(12):1129–1133.

57. Levenberg S, Golub JS, Amit M, et al. Endothelial cells derived from human embryonic stem cells. *Proc Natl Acad Sci USA*. 2002;26:26.

62. Gimble J, Guilak F. Adipose-derived adult stem cells: isolation, characterization, and differentiation potential. *Cytotherapy*. 2003;5(5):362–369.

92. Lendeckel S, Jodicke A, Christophis P, et al. Autologous stem cells (adipose) and fibrin glue used to treat widespread traumatic calvarial defects: case report. *J Craniomaxillofac Surg*. 2004;32(6):370–373.

    This paper describes one of the first clinical applications of adipose-derived stromal cells to help treat a pediatric patient with an osseous defect. Though a limited patient number, it should set the groundwork for future studies.

222. Yamanaka S. Elite and stochastic models for induced pluripotent stem cell generation. *Nature*. 2009;460(7251):49–52.

    This provides an excellent description of the concept behind iPS derivation. A nice schematic and detailed description of the iPS induction makes a very difficult and ground-breaking discovery appear simple.

225. Sun N, Longaker MT, Wu JC. Human iPS cell-based therapy: Considerations before clinical applications. *Cell Cycle*. 2010;9(5):880–885.

    This provides an excellent review of the different cell types iPS cells can be derived from and the benefits and pitfalls of each cell type. It also concisely and clearly discusses current hurdles to bringing iPS cells to the bedside.

14

Wound healing

Chandan K. Sen and Sashwati Roy

SYNOPSIS

- There are three general techniques of wound treatment: primary intention, secondary intention, and tertiary intention
- The following overlapping phases drive the overall healing response: hemostasis, inflammation, proliferative, and remodeling
- Successful hemostasis or blood coagulation results in prevention of blood loss by plugging the wound within seconds through vasoconstriction and formation of a hemostatic blood clot consisting of platelets and fibrin. The process is divided into initiation and amplification. Initiation is caused by an extrinsic pathway, whereas amplification is executed by an intrinsic pathway
- The inflammatory response during normal healing is characterized by spatially and temporally changing patterns of specific leukocyte subsets. Dysregulated inflammation complicates wound healing. Complete resolution of an acute inflammatory response is the ideal outcome following an insult
- Infection is a common problem in chronic wounds, frequently resulting in nonhealing wounds and significant patient morbidity and mortality. Microorganisms do not always live as pure cultures of dispersed single cells but instead accumulate at interfaces to form polymicrobial aggregates such as films, mats, flocs, sludge, or biofilms
- In an open wound that has undergone contraction, restoration of an intact epidermal barrier is enabled through wound epithelialization, also known as re-epithelialization. During the proliferative phase of wound healing, the granulation tissue is light red or dark pink in color because of perfusion by new capillary loops. It is soft to the touch, moist, and granular in appearance. The granulation tissue serves as a bed for tissue repair
- Wound vascularization may be achieved by angiogenesis or vasculogenesis
- A wound is generally considered chronic if it has not healed in 4 weeks. Chronic wounds can be broadly classified into three major categories: venous and arterial ulcers, diabetic ulcers, and pressure ulcers
- Vascular complications commonly associated with problematic wounds are primarily responsible for wound ischemia. Limitations in the ability of the vasculature to deliver O_2-rich blood to the wound tissue leads to, among other consequences, hypoxia. Three major factors may contribute to wound tissue hypoxia: (1) peripheral vascular diseases garroting O_2 supply; (2) increased O_2 demand of the healing tissue; and (3) generation of reactive oxygen species (ROS) by way of respiratory burst and for redox signaling
- Small RNAs are a new class of regulators of eukaryotic biology. Alongside other small interfering RNAs (siRNAs), miRNAs execute posttranscriptional gene silencing through mRNA destabilization as well as translational repression. miRNAs are emerging as a key regulatory of the overall wound-healing process
- The regenerative potential of injured adult tissue suggests the physiological existence of cells capable of participating in the reparative process. Bone marrow-derived mesenchymal stem cells (BM-MSCs) have been shown to promote the healing of diabetic wounds, implying a profound therapeutic potential for skin defects such as chronic wounds and burns
- Scars (also called cicatrices) are macroscopic fibrous tissue that visibly replaces normal skin after injury. There is a wide spectrum of skin scarring postwounding, including scarless fetal wound healing, fine-line or normal scars, stretched scars, atrophic (depressed) scars, scar contractures, hypertrophic scars, and keloids.

Introduction

Physical trauma represents one of the most primitive challenges that threatened survival. In other words, injury eliminated the unfit. A Sumerian clay tablet (*c.* 2150 BC) described early wound care that included washing the wound in beer and hot water, using poultices from substances such as wine dregs and lizard dung, and bandaging the wound. Ancient scriptures depicting the science of life or *Ayurveda* date from the sixth to seventh century BC, and represent the beginning of planned physical injury with the intent to cure.[1,2] Hippocrates (*c.* 400 BC) detailed the importance of draining pus from the wound, and Galen (*c.* 130–200 AD) described the principle of first- and second-intention healing.[3] Wound healing advanced slowly over the centuries, with major advances in the 19th century in the importance of controlling infection, hemostasis, and necrotic tissue.[4] Today, surgical trauma, taken together with injury caused during accidents and secondary to other clinical conditions, e.g., diabetes, represents a substantial cost to society.[5] Any solution to wound-healing problems will require a multifaceted comprehensive approach. First and foremost, the wound environment will have to be made receptive to therapies. Second, the appropriate therapeutic regimen needs to be identified and provided while managing systemic limitations that could secondarily limit the healing response. This chapter aims to present an overall outline of the cutaneous wound-healing process.

Acute wounds

Any violation of live tissue integrity may be regarded as a wound. Skin is the largest organ of the human body, covering about 3000 square inches (7620 cm^2) in an average adult. The most important role of the skin for terrestrial animals is to protect the water-rich internal organs from the dry external environment. As a primary line of defense against external threats, maintenance of integrity of the skin is a key prerequisite for healthy survival. Thus, healthy skin can regenerate and repair itself under most common conditions. Skin wounds may be open when manifested as a tear, cut, or puncture. Blunt force trauma may cause closed wounds or

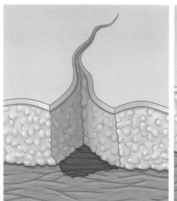 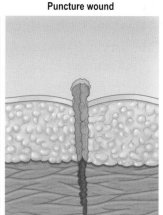

Fig. 14.1 Laceration and puncture wounds.

contusion where the skin appears to be intact but suffers from damage caused to underlying tissues.

Open wounds may be generally categorized as:

- Lacerations – ragged tears and cuts; masses of torn tissue underneath; caused by dull knife, bomb fragments and machinery and may include crushing of tissues; frequently contaminated (*Fig. 14.1*)
- Puncture – e.g., sharp penetrations caused by nails, needles, wire, or bullets (*Fig. 14.1*). These are of great concern in patients with diabetes, as many of these patients have polyneuropathy and have insensate feet, leading to occult injury. Many times these patients will step on thumb tacks, safety pins, or other sharp household objects and not even know it: this, coupled with compromised vascular status, leads to chronic wound infection
- Abrasions – the superficial layer of the skin is removed; skinned knee or elbows and rope burns are examples; an abrasion lends itself to infection
- Avulsions – sections of skin torn off either in part (attached to body) or totally (detached from body); heavy bleeding is common
- Amputations – traumatic amputation results in nonsurgical removal of limb from the body and accompanies heavy bleeding.

There are three general techniques of wound treatment:

1. primary intention, in which all tissues, including the skin, are closed with suture material after completion of the operation

2. secondary intention, in which the wound is left open and closes naturally

3. tertiary intention, in which the wound is left open for a number of days and then closed if it is found to be clean.

The wound-healing process

The entire wound-healing process may be viewed as a cascade that is governed by numerous feedback and feedforward regulatory loops driven by signals from the wound tissue itself, wound microenvironment, as well as interventions under conditions where the wound is subjected to therapy. For simplicity of understanding the several interdigitated biological processes that drive the overall healing response, wound healing is commonly discussed as the following overlapping phases: hemostasis and inflammation, proliferative (granulation, vascularization, and wound closure; closure may be discussed as wound contraction and epithelialization) and remodeling (can continue from weeks to years and encompasses scarring, tensile strength, and turnover of extracellular matrix (ECM) components). These stages, taken as a whole, are also referred to as the wound-healing cascade (*Fig. 14.2*).

Hemostasis

For bleeding wounds, the highest priority is to stop bleeding and this is achieved by hemostasis. Hemostasis is thus a protective physiological response to vascular injury that results in exposure of blood components to the subendothelial layers of the vessel wall. Through successful hemostasis blood loss is prevented by plugging the wound within seconds through vasoconstriction and formation of a hemostatic blood clot consisting of platelets and fibrin. Hemostasis requires both platelets and the blood coagulation system. The process of blood coagulation may be subdivided into initiation and amplification. Initiation is caused by an extrinsic pathway, whereas amplification is executed by an intrinsic pathway. The intrinsic pathway consists of plasma factor XI (FXI), IX, and VIII (*Fig. 14.3*). Tissue factor (TF) generates a "thrombin burst," a process by which

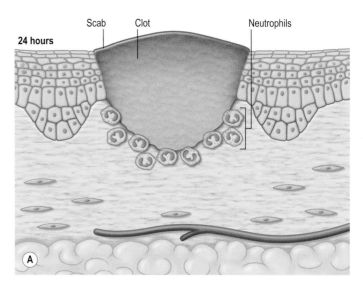

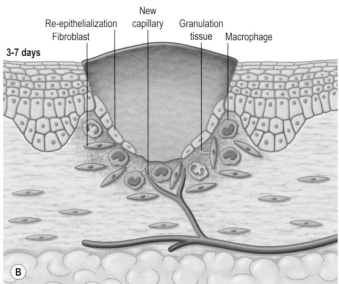

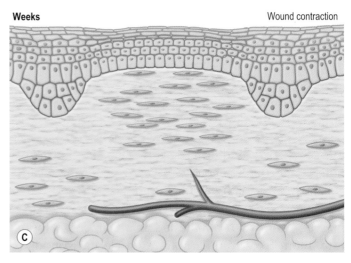

Fig. 14.2 (A–C) Phases of cutaneous wound healing: a simplified representation.

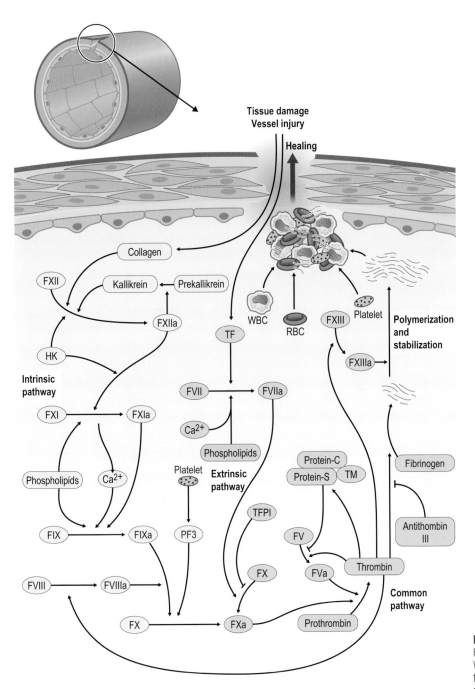

Fig. 14.3 The blood clotting cascade. FXII, factor XII, HK, high-molecular-weight kininogen; TF, tissue factor; WBC, white blood cell; RBC, red blood cell; TM, thrombomodulin; PF3, platelet factor 3; TFPI, tissue factor pathway inhibitor.

thrombin is released instantaneously. Thrombin is a key driver of the overall coagulation cascade.

The extrinsic pathway responsible for the initiation of blood coagulation consists of the transmembrane receptor TF and plasma FVII/VIIa. On the other hand, the intrinsic pathway consists of plasma FXI, FIX, and FVIII.

Under physiological conditions, TF is constitutively expressed by adventitial cells surrounding blood vessels and initiates clotting. Examples of such adventitial cells include vascular smooth-muscle cells, pericytes, and adventitial fibroblasts.[6,7] TF may also contribute to amplification of blood coagulation through its so-called blood-borne form, which is present as cell-derived microparticles as well as through TF expressed within platelets.[6–8]

Levels of FVIIa, a key player of the extrinsic pathway, in the circulating blood are higher than any other activated coagulation factor. Following injury to the blood vessel wall, FVII comes into contact with TF expressed on TF-bearing cells (e.g., white blood cells) and forms an activated complex (TF–FVIIa). TF–FVIIa activates FIX and FX, resulting in FIXa and FXa, respectively. FVII is activated by thrombin, FXIa, FXII, and FXa. The activation of FXa by TF–FVIIa is almost immediately inhibited by the TF pathway inhibitor. FXa and its cofactor FVa form the prothrombinase complex, which activates prothrombin to thrombin. Thrombin is a serine protease that plays a central role in hemostasis after tissue injury by converting soluble plasma fibrinogen into an insoluble fibrin clot and by promoting platelet aggregation. Thrombin activates other components of the coagulation cascade, including FV and FVIII, which in turn activates FXI and cascades to the activation of FIX. Thrombin also activates and releases FVIII from being bound to von Willebrand factor. FVIIIa is the cofactor of FIXa, and together they form the "tenase" complex, which activates FX. In this way the cycle continues. The intrinsic pathway begins with formation of the primary complex on collagen by high-molecular-weight kininogen, prekallikrein, and FXII (Hageman factor). Prekallikrein is converted to kallikrein, and FXII becomes FXIIa. FXIIa converts FXI into FXIa. FXIa activates FIX, which together with its cofactor FVIIIa forms the tenase complex. The tenase complex activates FX to FXa *(Fig. 14.3)*.

The blood clot physically helps plug the wound, minimizing blood loss. It is primarily made up of cross-linked fibrin, cells such as erythrocytes and platelets, as well as other ECM proteins such as fibronectin, vitronectin, and thrombospondin. Current understanding portrays the clot as a dynamic structural matrix containing functionally active proteins and cells. In addition to containment of blood loss, the clot serves as a first aid against microbial invasion. The clot also serves as a provisional matrix for the homing of blood-borne cells, including inflammatory as well as stem or progenitor cells. The provisional matrix is enriched in cytokines and growth factors which then regulate the function of the homing cells.[9,10]

The formation of blood clot is initiated by the proteolytic cleavage of fibrinogen by thrombin. As a result, fibrin is produced and forms cross-links with each other. Cross-linked fibrin entraps platelets, and together they adhere to the subendothelium through adhesion molecules called integrins. Clot fibrin plays a key role in mounting the inflammatory process as well as in facilitating wound angiogenesis and stromal cell proliferation. Fibrin binds to integrin CD11b/CD18 on infiltrating monocytes and neutrophils. It also binds to fibroblast growth factor-2 (FGF-2) and vascular endothelial growth factor (VEGF) that help the wound tissue vascularize. Fibrin also binds to insulin-like growth factor-I and promotes stromal cell proliferation.[11,12]

Blood clot represents the seat of wound chemotaxis. Thrombin, released by platelets at the wound site, is an early mediator of clot development.[13] Thrombin is a serine protease that converts soluble plasma fibrinogen into an insoluble fibrin clot. In addition, it promotes platelet aggregation. Thrombin function may be viewed as an interface between the hemostasis phase of wound healing and the ensuing inflammatory phase as it plays a potent role in mounting wound inflammation. The proinflammatory effects of thrombin include stimulation of vasodilation responsible for plasma extravasation, edema, and an increased expression of endothelial cell adhesion molecules that helps monocytes and others cells extravasate and infiltrate the wound site. Thrombin also induces the release of proinflammatory cytokines like CCL2, interleukin-6 (IL-6), and IL-8 by endothelial cells. These cytokines induce monocyte chemotaxis.[14] Furthermore, thrombin induces the release of inflammatory cytokines by monocytes, including IL-6, interferon-γ, IL-1β, and tumor necrosis factor-α (TNF-α). These early-phase cytokines are typically proinflammatory, which may govern the differentiation of blood-derived monocytes into M1 wound macrophages.[15] Wound chemotaxis is also driven by the degradation of fibrin and subsequent activation of the complement system. As part of this process several chemotactic agents and cytokines are released, which in turn launch the inflammatory phase of wound healing through chemotactic recruitment of blood-borne immune cells.[16] Platelets are one of the earliest sources of cytokines which execute immune cell chemotaxis as well as macrophage activation. Once trapped in the fibrin net, platelets release granules that function as a reservoir for biologically active proteins, such as RANTES (regulated on activation, normal T cell expressed, and secreted or CCL5), thrombin, transforming growth factor-β (TGF-β), platelet-derived growth factor (PDGF), and VEGF. CCL5 is one of the most potent monocyte chemoattractants released by platelets after injury. Other cytokines and chemokines that attract monocytes to the wound bed include monocyte chemoattractant protein-1 (MCP-1) (CCL2), MIP-1α (CCL3), TGF-α, fibronectin, elastin, C5a, C3a, nerve growth factor, and ECM components.[17,18]

Inflammation

Tissue injury triggers an acute-phase inflammation (Latin, *inflammare*, to set on fire) response that is meant to prepare the wound site for subsequent wound closure *(Fig. 14.4)*. Inflammation encompasses a series of responses of vascularized tissues of the body to injury. Local chemical mediators that are biosynthesized during acute inflammation give rise to the macroscopic events characterized by Celsus in the first century, namely, *rubor* (redness), *tumor* (swelling), *calor* (heat), and *dolor* (pain). At cellular and molecular levels, inflammation results from the coordination of manifold systems of receptors and sensors that affect transcriptional and posttranslational programs necessary for host defense and resolution of infection. During normal healing, the inflammatory response is characterized by spatially and temporally changing patterns of specific leukocyte subsets.

Platelets

Formation of the clot or thrombus is dependent on platelet activation. The platelet-rich blood clot also entraps polymorphonuclear leukocytes (neutrophils). This helps amplify blood coagulation and lays the foundation for the subsequent acute-phase inflammatory response. In a matter of hours after injury, large numbers of neutrophils extravasate by transmigrating across the endothelial cell wall of blood capillaries to the wound site. To enable this, local blood vessels are activated by proinflammatory cytokines such as IL-1β, TNF-α, and interferon-γ. These cytokines induce the expression of adhesion molecules necessary for adhesion of

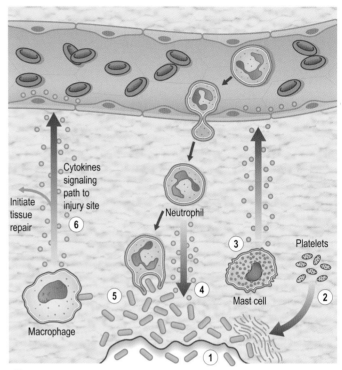

① Bacteria and other pathogens enter wound

② Platelets from blood release blood-clotting proteins at wound site.

③ Mast cells secrete factors that mediate vasodilation and vascular constriction. Delivery of blood, plasma and cells to injured area

④ Neutrophils and macrophages remove pathogens by phagocytosis

⑤ Macrophages secrete hormones called cytokines that attract immune system cells to the site and activate cells involved in tissue repair

⑥ Inflammatory response continues until the foreign material is eliminated and the wound is repaired

Fig. 14.4 The wound inflammatory response.

leukocytes and diapedesis *(Fig. 14.5)*. Adhesion molecules such as integrins as well as P-selectin and E-selectin play a central role in enabling diapedesis of neutrophils *(Fig. 14.6)*. These adhesion molecules bind with integrins expressed on the cell surface of neutrophils, such as CD11a/CD18 (LFA), CD 11b/CD18 (MAC-1), CD11c/CD18 (gp150, 95), and CD11d/CD18. Alongside cytokines, chemokines play a major role in mounting acute-phase inflammation after injury. Chemokines include IL-8, MCP-1, and growth-related oncogene-α. In the case of an infected wound, bacterial products such as lipopolysaccharide and formyl-methionyl peptides can enhance neutrophil recruitment to the wound site *(Fig. 14.7)*.

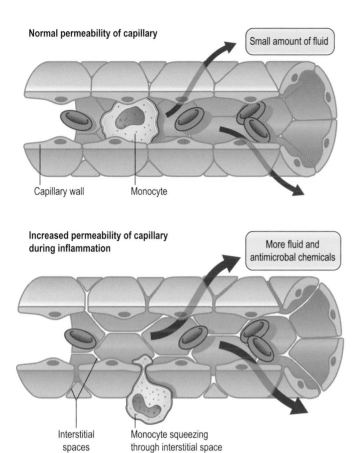

Fig. 14.5 Diapedesis. In healthy permeable capillaries the endothelium lining prevents blood cells from leaving the circulation. In response to injury, blood vessels around the wound site undergo vasodilation, increasing the permeability of capillaries. Such change enables inflammatory cells to extravasate through the capillary wall and migrate to the site of injury. This process includes release of fluid from the vessels to the extracellular space, resulting in the edematous response commonly noted during inflammation. Blood vessels possess a built-in pathway for such diapedesis to occur in response to tissue injury.

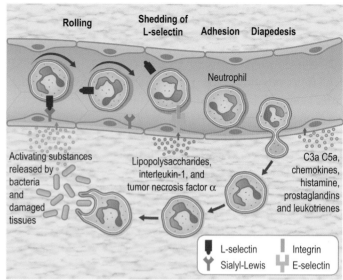

Fig. 14.6 Extravasation of neutrophils in response to tissue injury. Neutrophils move along the capillaries in a rolling motion which is facilitated by the binding and release of L-selectin on the neutrophil surface to sialyl-Lewis, a carbohydrate ligand expressed on the inner wall of capillaries by endothelial cells. Upon injury and/or infection the release of lipopolysaccharides, tumor necrosis factor-alpha, and interleukin-1 results in the shedding of L-selectin by the neutrophils which then strongly adhere to the inner wall of the capillary by the binding of integrin on the neutrophils to E-selectins on endothelial cells. After such adhesion, the process of diapedesis begins, allowing the neutrophils to extravasate to the wound site.

Neutrophils

Neutrophils traverse postcapillary venules at sites of inflammation, degrade pathogens within phagolysosomes, and undergo apoptosis. Neutrophils serve a wide range of functions, ranging from phagocytosis of infectious agents to cleansing of devitalized tissue. When coated with opsonins (generally complement and/or antibody), microorganisms bind to specific receptors on the surface of the phagocyte and invagination of the cell membrane occurs with the incorporation of the microorganism into an intracellular phagosome. There follows a burst of oxygen consumption, and much, if not all, of the extra oxygen consumed is converted to highly reactive oxygen species. This is called

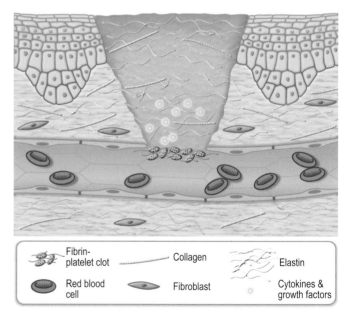

Fig. 14.7 Diapedesis and migration of leukocytes to the wound site.

respiratory burst. In addition, the cytoplasmic granules discharge their contents into the phagosome, and death of the ingested microorganism soon follows. Among the antimicrobial systems formed in the phagosome is one consisting of myeloperoxidase (MPO), released into the phagosome during the degranulation process, hydrogen peroxide (H_2O_2), formed by the respiratory burst and a halide, particularly chloride. The initial product of the MPO-H_2O_2-chloride system is hypochlorous acid, and subsequent formation of chlorine, chloramines, hydroxyl radicals, singlet oxygen, and ozone has been proposed. These same toxic agents can be released to the outside of the cell, where they may attack normal tissue and thus contribute to the pathogenesis of disease.[19] Other products delivered by neutrophils to the wound site include antimicrobials such as cationic peptides and eicosanoids as well as proteases such as elastase, cathepsin G, proteinase 3, and urokinase-type plasminogen activator. As it relates to the overall inflammatory process elicited in response to injury, neutrophils are major players because they can modify macrophage function and therefore regulate innate immune response during wound healing.[20] In the absence of neutrophils, wound site macrophages seem to lack guidance in conducting the healing process.[21]

In a healing wound, neutrophil infiltration ceases after a few days of injury. Expended neutrophils are programmed to die and dying neutrophils are recognized by wound site macrophages and phagocytosed. The wound site contains a small portion of macrophages that are resident. Most macrophages at the wound site are recruited from the peripheral circulation. Extravasation of peripheral blood monocytes is enabled by the interaction between endothelial vascular cell adhesion molecule-1 and monocyte very late antigen-4 ($\alpha4\beta1$ integrin). Factors that guide the extravasated monocyte to the wound site include growth factors, chemotactic proteins, proinflammatory cytokines, and chemokines such as macrophage inflammatory protein 1α, MCP-1, and RANTES. The source of these chemoattractants includes clot-associated platelets, wound edge hyperproliferative keratinocytes, wound tissue fibroblasts and subsets of leukocyte already at the wound site. Once the monocyte leaves the blood vessel to transmigrate into the wound site through the ECM microenvironment, the process of monocyte differentiation to macrophages has started.

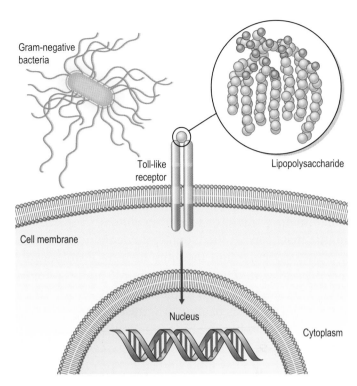

Fig. 14.8 Toll-like receptors: responding to infectious agents and the wound microenvironment.

Mediators present in the microenvironment that the monocyte traverses to reach the wound site interact with receptors on the monocyte cell surface, bringing forth major changes in the transcriptomic as well as proteomic make of the cell. Major examples of such receptors present on the monocyte surface include Toll-like receptors (TLRs: *Fig. 14.8*), complement receptors, and Fc receptors. At the wound site, macrophages function as antigen-presenting cells and phagocytes scavenging dead cells and debris. In addition, they deliver a wide range of growth factors that are known for their abilities to execute the wound-healing process. Such growth factors include TGF-β, TGF-α, basic FGF (bFGF), VEGF, and PDGF. These growth factors enable wound healing by causing cell proliferation and synthesis of ECM and inducing angiogenesis. Macrophages play a crucial role in enabling wound healing. Macrophage depletion is known to impair wound closure markedly.[4,22]

Mast cells

Mast cells are best known for their central role in mediating allergic responses. Beyond that function, it is now known that mast cells are physiologically significant in recognizing pathogens and in regulating immune response.[23] Mast cells may instantly release several proinflammatory mediators from intracellular stores. In addition, they are localized in the host–environment interface. These properties make mast cells key players in finetuning immune responses during infection. Recent studies using mast cell activators as effective vaccine adjuvants show the potential of harnessing these cells to confer protective immunity against microbial pathogens.[24] Mast cell activation helps initiate the inflammatory phase of wound healing. In response to injury, mast cells at the wound site degranulate within a matter of hours and therefore become histologically silent at the wound tissue. After about 48 hours of injury, mast cells are again seen in the wound tissue and their number increases as healing progresses.[25] On one hand, impaired wound healing has been reported in mast cell-deficient mice.[26] On the other hand, mast cells have been implicated in skin wound fibrosis.[27] With the aid of a wide array of newly formed or preformed mediators released by degranulation, the activated mast cell controls the key events of the healing phases: triggering and modulation of the inflammatory stage, proliferation of connective cellular elements, and final remodeling of the newly formed connective tissue matrix. The importance of the mast cell in regulating healing processes is also demonstrated by the fact that a surplus or deficit of degranulated biological mediators causes impaired repair, with the formation of exuberant granulation tissue (e.g., keloids and hypertrophic scars), delayed closure (dehiscence), and chronicity of the inflammatory stage.[28]

Macrophages

Macrophages represent the predominant cell type in a healing wound 3–5 days following injury. The primary acute function of wound macrophages, which arrive at an injury site hours later than neutrophils, is to operate as voracious phagocytes cleansing the wound of all matrix and cell debris, including fibrin and apoptotic neutrophils. Macrophages also produce a range of cytokines, growth and angiogenic factors that drive fibroblast proliferation and angiogenesis.[4,29–32] In a classic study, Leibovich and Ross[33] demonstrated that antimacrophage serum combined with hydrocortisone diminished the accumulation of macrophages in healing skin wounds of adult guinea pigs. Such depletion resulted in impaired disposal of damaged tissue and provisional matrix, compromised fibroblast count, and delayed healing. Today, macrophages have emerged to be a pivotal driver of efficient skin repair.[34,35] Macrophages are plastic and heterogeneous cells broadly categorized into two groups: classically activated or type I macrophages, which are proinflammatory effectors, and alternatively activated or type II macrophages.[36] In the inflamed tissue, it is unclear whether the type II macrophages that appear during the healing phase originate from newly attracted monocytes or from a switch in the activation state of previously proinflammatory macrophages. The macrophage population first taking part in inflammation may change its phenotype and assume the role to resolve inflammation.[37,38] Macrophages from diabetic wounds display dysfunctional inflammatory responses.[39] A persistent inflammatory state of diabetic wound macrophages is caused by impairment in the ability of these cells to phagocytose apoptotic cells at the wound site which in turn prevents the switch from M1 to M2 phenotype.[39]

Resolution of inflammation

Inflammatory responses elicited by injury are only helpful to the healing process if they are timely and transient. Dysregulated inflammation complicates wound healing.[39] Complete resolution of an acute inflammatory response is the ideal outcome following an insult. For resolution to ensue, further leukocyte recruitment must be halted and accompanied by removal of leukocytes from inflammatory sites. Resolution of inflammation is executed by a number of key factors. At the wound site successful phagocytosis of dead neutrophils by macrophages is a key factor. Impairment in macrophage function at the wound site derails the resolution of inflammation.[39] Lipid mediators, such as the lipoxins, resolvins, protectins, and newly identified maresins, have emerged as a novel genus of potent and stereoselective players that counterregulate excessive acute inflammation and stimulate molecular and cellular events that define resolution.[40] Successful resolution paves the path for the healing process to progress towards successful wound closure. Prolonged inflammation may not only compromise wound closure but may also worsen scar outcomes.[41,42]

Infection

Infection is a common problem in chronic wounds, frequently resulting in nonhealing and significant patient morbidity and mortality.[43] Wound infection and the subsequent release of proinflammatory modulators result in pain and delayed healing. The pain, in turn, compromises the immune response to infection.[44] All wounds become contaminated by bacteria from the surrounding skin, the local environment, and autologous patient sources. The local environment is particularly relevant for hospitalized patients. Colonization is defined as the presence of proliferating bacteria without a noticeable host response. Colonization of the wound may enhance or impede wound healing, depending upon the bacterial load. Bacterial loads in excess of 10^5 organisms/gram of tissue are a threat to wound healing, although this threshold may be altered by the status of the host immune system and the number and types of bacterial species present. The concept of critical colonization is controversial and not universally accepted. Critical colonization is characterized by increased bacterial burden or covert infection, and the wound at this stage may enter a nonhealing, chronic inflammatory state. Substantial colonization may not cause the obvious signs of inflammation but will likely affect wound healing with failure to heal or slowing of progression. Signs of critical colonization are atrophy or deterioration of granulation tissue, discoloration of granulation tissue to deep red or gray, increased wound friability, and increased drainage. The transition to infection occurs when bacterial proliferation overcomes the host's immune response and host injury occurs. Several factors determine transition from colonization to infection: the bioburden itself, the virulence of the organisms, the synergistic action of different bacterial species, and the ability of the host to mount an immune response.[43]

During the past decade, there has been rapid progress in the understanding of innate immune recognition of microbial components and its critical role in host defense against infection. The early concept of innate immunity was that it nonspecifically recognized microbes; however, the discovery of TLRs *(Fig. 14.8)* in the mid-1990s showed that pathogen recognition by the innate immune system is instead actually specific, relying on germline-encoded pattern recognition receptors (PRRs) that have evolved to detect components of foreign pathogens, referred to as pathogen-associated molecular patterns (PAMPs).[45] TLRs regulate innate and adaptive immune responses and are important modulators of inflammation during wound-healing responses. The finding that there is activation of TLR signaling during tissue damage in several disease situations in the absence of infection suggests that endogenous molecules serve as TLR agonists, although it is unclear whether this response is biologically important for maintenance of homeostasis, such as tissue repair, or whether this recognition is simply accidental. It is noteworthy that microbial infection triggers the production of modified endogenous molecules (such as high-mobility group protein B1, oxidized phospholipids, β-defensin 2, and nucleic acids) that are recognized by TLRs or other cytosolic PRRs. This may suggest that these endogenous molecules, along with PAMPs, act as adjuvants to activate innate immune programs via TLRs and/or other PRRs, and have key roles in facilitating adaptive immunity against infecting microbes.

Chronic wounds have a complex colonizing flora that changes over time. *Staphylococcus aureus* and coagulase-negative staphylococci are the most commonly isolated organisms. Chronic wounds are colonized by multiple bacterial species and many persist in the wound once they are established. In chronic venous leg ulcers the most common bacteria noted, in order of abundance, were *S. aureus*, *Enterococcus faecalis*, *Pseudomonas aeruginosa*, coagulase-negative staphylococci, *Proteus* spp., and anaerobic bacteria. Resident (colonizing) bacterial species are commonly present in ulcers. The longer an ulcer remains unhealed, the more likely it will acquire multiple aerobic organisms and a significant anaerobic population. Chronic wounds are commonly complicated by underlying ischemia. Thus, they tend to have a low tissue oxygen level. This facilitates the growth of anaerobes in ischemic wounds. Adequate delivery of oxygen to the wound tissue is vital for optimal healing and resistance to infection.[46] Hospitalization, surgical procedures, and prolonged or broad-spectrum antibiotic therapy may predispose patients to colonization or infection, or both, with resistant organisms, including *S. aureus* (methicillin-resistant *S.* – MRSA) or vancomycin-resistant enterococci.[43] Because inflammatory responses to microbial invasion may be diminished in persons with diabetes, clinical signs of infection are often absent in persons with diabetic foot ulcers when infection is limited to localized tissue.[47]

Biofilm

Microorganisms do not always live as pure cultures of dispersed single cells but instead accumulate at interfaces to form polymicrobial aggregates such as films, mats, flocs, sludge, or biofilms. The biofilm state of microorganisms may lead to an increase in virulence and propensity to cause infection. In most biofilms, the microorganisms account for less than 10% of the dry mass, whereas the matrix can account for over 90%. The matrix is the extracellular material, mostly produced by the organisms themselves, in which the biofilm cells are embedded. It consists of a conglomeration of different types of biopolymers – known as extracellular polymeric substances (EPS) – that forms the scaffold for the three-dimensional architecture of the biofilm and is responsible for adhesion to surfaces and for cohesion in the biofilm. The formation of a biofilm allows a lifestyle that is entirely different from the planktonic state. Although the precise and molecular interactions of the various secreted biofilm matrix polymers have not been defined, and the contributions of these components to matrix integrity are poorly understood at a molecular level, several functions of EPS have been determined, demonstrating a wide range of advantages for the biofilm mode of life.

The architecture of biofilms is influenced by many factors, including hydrodynamic conditions, concentration of nutrients, bacterial motility, and intercellular communication, as well as exopolysaccharides and proteins.[48] Chronic wounds offer attractive conditions for biofilm production because proteins (collagen, fibronectin) and damaged tissues are present, which allow attachment. The biofilm impedes healing of chronic wounds. Most of the chronic wound pathogens, such as MRSA and *Pseudomonas* spp., are typical biofilm producers. Compared to bacteria in the unattached free-living planktonic form, bacteria that reside within mature biofilms are highly resistant to traditional antibiotic therapies. Bacteria in biofilms grow more slowly, and slower growth may lead to decreased uptake of the drug and other physiologic changes that could impair drug effectiveness.[43]

Vascularization

Wounds larger than can be closed by diffusion of oxygen from neighboring intact blood vessels or wounds complicated by underlying ischemia largely rely on wound vascularization for their closure. Wound vascularization may be achieved by angiogenesis or vasculogenesis. Angiogenesis represents sprouting of capillaries from existing blood vessels in the wound edge tissue. Vasculogenesis relies on the formation of new blood vessels by mobilization of bone marrow-derived endothelial stem cells.

Wound vascularization is regulated by all phases in wound healing – hemostasis, inflammation, tissue formation, as well as tissue remodeling. The hemostatic plug provides a bed for blood-borne cells to home. Once cells entangle in this plug, the ECM environment modifies cell function towards successful healing. Platelets in the clot serve as a source of growth factors and cytokines which recruit several cell types, including endothelial cells, to the wound site. During the inflammatory phase, leukocytes at the wound site serve as a major source of proangiogenic factors such as VEGF-A and IL-8 that lay the early foundation for successful wound tissue vascularization. As neutrophils are expended and undergo cell death, the number of macrophages at the wound site substantially increases. Macrophage-derived TGF-β, TGF-α, bFGF, PDGF, and VEGF play a key role in driving skin wound angiogenesis. Growing evidence demonstrates that no single angiogenic factor is singularly effective in significantly influencing wound outcomes. Wound vascularization is a sophisticated process requiring dynamic, temporally and spatially regulated interaction between cells, angiogenic factors, and the ECM.

Key processes in tissue vascularization are depicted in *Figure 14.9*. Angiogenic cues are elicited by microenvironmental signals such as hypoxia and are amplified by angiogenic factors such as VEGF expressed by and released from cells at the wound site. VEGF was originally identified as an endothelial cell-specific growth factor-stimulating angiogenesis and vascular permeability. Some family members, VEGF C and D, are

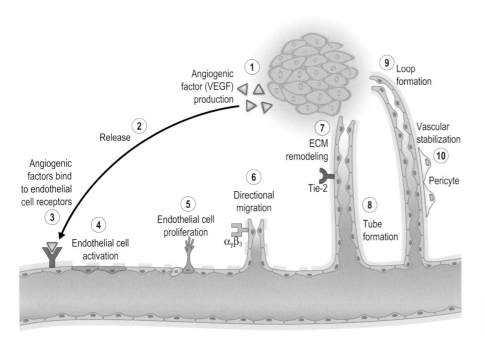

Fig. 14.9 Neoangiogenesis: the formation of new blood vessels. VEGF, vascular endothelial growth factor; ECM, extracellular matrix.

specifically involved in lymphangiogenesis. Ligation of these angiogenic factors with their corresponding receptors elicits a multitude of cell-signaling processes that activate microvascular endothelial cells. For example, VEGF and their endothelial tyrosine kinase receptors are central regulators of tissue vascularization. VEGF signaling through VEGFR-2 is the major angiogenic pathway. VEGFR-3 has also been shown to be important for angiogenesis, acting together with VEGF/VEGFR-2 and Dll4/Notch signaling to control angiogenic sprouting.[49] The biological significance of other angiogenic factors such as EGF and bFGF is mediated by their corresponding receptors, which also belong to the family of tyrosine kinase receptors EGFR, FGFR-1, FGFR-2, FGFR-3, and FGFR-4.

Other tyrosine kinase receptors of outstanding significance in this regard are Tie-1 and Tie-2. Along with the VEGF receptor, these are the only known endothelial cell-specific receptor tyrosine kinases. Tie-2 is induced on the endothelium of neovessels in skin wounds and downregulated as newly formed vessels regress. As an indicator of Tie-2 activation, Tie-2 phosphorylation is detected in skin wounds at all stages of the healing process.[50] Activated microvascular endothelial cells respond by proliferating, which is followed by directional migration of these cells. Migration is a complex process in which cells move in a given direction either in response to changes in the extracellular environment or as a consequence of an intrinsic propensity for directional movement. ECM remodeling by proteases promotes cell migration, a critical event in the formation of new vessels. Temporal and spatial regulation of ECM remodeling events allows for local changes in net matrix deposition or degradation, which in turn contributes to control of cell growth, migration, and differentiation during different stages of angiogenesis. Matrix-bound growth factors released by proteases and/or by angiogenic factors promote angiogenesis by enhancing endothelial migration and growth. Matrix molecules promote endothelial cell growth and morphogenesis, and/or stabilize nascent blood vessels. Hence, ECM molecules and ECM remodeling events play a key role in regulating angiogenesis.[51]

The formation of the capillary-like tubes is specific to endothelial cells and integral to the process of angiogenesis. The basement membrane represents a biologically functional highly specialized ECM on which the basal nonluminal surface of endothelial cells rests. This matrix forms a continuous sleeve around the endothelial cells, and maintains the tube-like structures of the blood vessels. More than 20 years ago Kubota *et al.* observed that endothelial cells plated on a reconstituted basement membrane matrix, rapidly attached, aligned, and formed capillary-like tubules. The cells did not proliferate. The vessels that are thus formed contain a lumen and tight cell–cell contacts. The cells are polarized with the nuclei basally located towards the basement membrane matrix. Furthermore, the capillary-like structures take up acetylated low-density lipoprotein, which is a marker of differentiation for these cells.[52] Angiogenesis not only depends on endothelial cell invasion and proliferation, but also requires pericyte coverage of vascular sprouts for vessel stabilization. These processes are coordinated by VEGF and PDGF through their cognate receptors on endothelial cells and vascular smooth-muscle cells, respectively.[53] Structural support to blood vessels is provided to pericytes and vascular smooth-muscle cells. Normal pericytes are embedded within the basement membrane of capillaries, either as solitary cells or a single-cell layer, where they coordinate intercellular signaling with endothelial cells and other components of the blood vessel wall to prevent leakage. In contrast, vascular smooth-muscle cells form single or multiple layers around arteries and veins to mediate vascular tone and contraction. Pericyte coverage is required for the stabilization of immature endothelial tubes.[54] Pericytes have function beyond angiogenesis that are relevant to wound healing. Skin pericytes may act as mesenchymal stem cells (MSCs), exhibiting the capacity to differentiate into bone, fat, and cartilage lineages. Thus, pericytes represent a potent stem cell population in the skin that is capable of modifying the ECM microenvironment and promoting epidermal tissue renewal from nonstem cells.[55]

Wound closure

Wound contraction and re-epithelialization contribute to closure of wounds that heal by secondary intention. Wound contraction represents an early response to injury that is aimed at juxtaposing the edges of an open wound.[56] This early phase of wound closure appears to be mediated by a contractile "purse-string" force produced by a circumferentially arranged band of fusiform-shaped epidermal cells situated in the wound margin.[57] Fibroblasts at the wound edge tissue are recognized to play a key role in enabling wound contraction.[58] During the inflammatory phase of wound healing, fibroblasts

acquire smooth-muscle cell characteristics and differentiate into contractile myofibroblasts. The first phenotypic transition of wound edge fibroblasts into so-called protomyofibroblasts is characterized by neoformation of contractile β-cytoplasmic actin stress fibers and occurs in response to profibrotic cytokines and to altered properties of the ECM. In the presence of TGF-β1 in a mechanically restrained environment, these cells express α-smooth-muscle actin *de novo*, which significantly increases their contractile activity and is a hallmark of the differentiated myofibroblast.[59] Wound contraction may significantly contribute to wound closure, although this contribution is much larger in loose-skinned rodents than in humans.

In an open wound that has undergone contraction, restoration of an intact epidermal barrier is enabled through wound epithelialization, also known as re-epithelialization.[60,61] A wound that is not epithelialized is not considered "healed," no matter how perfectly restored the underlying dermal structures may be. Thus, wound epithelialization, also called re-epithelialization, is a critical and defining feature of wound repair. Re-epithelialization of the wound can be conceptually viewed as the result of three overlapping keratinocyte functions: migration, proliferation, and differentiation. The sequence of events by which keratinocytes accomplish the task of re-epithelialization is generally believed to begin with dissolution of cell–cell and cell–substratum contacts. This is followed by the polarization and initiation of directional migration in basal and a subset of suprabasilar keratinocytes over the provisional wound matrix. A subset of keratinocytes immediately adjacent to, but not within, the wound bed then undergoes mitosis. Finally, there is multilayering of the newly formed epidermis and induction of differentiation specific gene products to restore the functionality of the epidermis. The most limiting factor in wound re-epithelialization is migration, since defects in this function, but not in proliferation or differentiation, are associated with the clinical phenotype of chronic nonhealing wounds.[62] The process of epithelialization continues until the barrier is re-established and the wound is covered. The process of re-epithelialization is accelerated by a moist environment[63,64] and is facilitated by the enzyme matrix metalloproteinase 1, a collagenase which lessens the affinity of the collagen–integrin contacts.[65]

Proliferative phase

The proliferative phase starts around 2 days after injury and normally lasts up to 3 weeks in a healing cutaneous wound. This phase overlaps with the inflammatory phase and supports re-epithelialization, the formation of new blood vessels, and the influx of fibroblasts and laying down of the ECM. By the time this phase begins, the degradation of the fibrin clot by the macrophages has begun and invading endothelial cells and fibroblasts rapidly fill that space. Migrating fibroblasts produce the cytokines that induce keratinocytes to migrate and proliferate.[66] Activated macrophages produce several cytokines, such as PDGF and TNF-α, which also induce fibroblasts to produce keratinocyte growth factor which in turn induces wound re-epithelialization.[60,61]

Granulation tissue

The fibrin clot formed during hemostasis participates in the early inflammatory phase and is replaced by a perfused, fibrous connective tissue that grows from the base of a wound and is able to fill wounds of almost any size. During the proliferative phase of wound healing, this granulation tissue is light red or dark pink in color because of perfusion by new capillary loops. It is soft to the touch, moist, and granular in appearance. The granulation tissue serves as a bed for tissue repair. The ECM of granulation tissue is created and modified by fibroblasts. Initially, it consists of a network of type III collagen, a weaker form of the structural protein that can be produced rapidly. This is later replaced by the stronger, long-stranded type I collagen, as evidenced in scar tissue. Formation and contraction of the granulation tissue represent integral aspects of the healing wound. In ischemic wounds, contraction of the granulation tissue is impaired because of faulty myofibroblast function, cells responsible for granulation tissue contraction.[67]

Chronic wounds

A wound is generally considered chronic if it has not healed in 4 weeks. Chronic wounds have been also defined as wounds that have not shown a 20–40% reduction in area after 2–4 weeks of optimal therapy. Standard surgical textbooks define chronic wounds as wounds which have not healed in 3 months. Chronic wounds can be broadly classified into three major categories: venous and arterial ulcers, diabetic ulcers, and pressure ulcers.

Venous ulcers

Venous ulcers (stasis ulcer or varicose ulcers) are wounds that are thought to occur due to improper functioning of venous valves, usually of the legs. They are the major cause of chronic wounds, occurring in 50–70% of chronic wound cases.[68] Venous ulcers develop mostly along the medial distal leg, and can be very painful. According to the revised clinical, etiology, anatomy, and pathophysiology (CEAP) classification of chronic venous disease published in 2004, a venous ulcer is defined as a full-thickness defect of skin, most frequently in the ankle region, that fails to heal spontaneously and is sustained by chronic venous disease.[69] Systematically, venous ulcer may be defined as a defect in the skin with surrounding pigmentation and dermatitis, located in the lower leg (usually in the gaiter region) that has been present for greater than 30 days, characterized by persistent venous hypertension and abnormal venous function (result of venous reflux and/or obstruction confirmed by hemodynamic and/or physiologic assessment), without a primary or associated arterial, immunologic, endocrine, or systemic cause. It is recognized that ulcers can be caused purely by venous pathology such as venous reflux or obstruction. When these abnormalities are combined with additional pathologic conditions, they contribute to the causation and perpetuation of the ulcer. The latter situation includes comorbid conditions such as arterial ischemia, swelling and lymphedema, trauma, autoimmune disorders, neurotrophic conditions, and diabetic vascular disease. These ulcers are categorized as of mixed origin, in which the venous component may or may not play a dominant role. Successful treatment of such ulcers includes not only the venous component but also concomitant management of the comorbid condition.

Arterial ulcers

Because both arterial and venous ulcers typically occur on the lower leg, differentiating between them can be challenging for wound care practitioners. However, they have very different pathophysiologies and management pathways. The most common cause of arterial ulcers is atherosclerosis. Risk factors for the development of atherosclerosis include age, smoking, diabetes mellitus, hypertension, dyslipidemia, family history, obesity, and sedentary lifestyle.[70] Ischemia and necrosis are common consequences. Both acute and chronic arterial insufficiency can lead to the formation of lower-extremity ulcers. Arterial insufficiency can occur at any level, from large arteries to arterioles and capillaries. Tissue ischemia that leads to leg ulcers tends to occur more in the setting of large-vessel or mixed disease. Vascular claudication, with exercise, at night, or while one is resting, is often the most distinguishing characteristic of arterial ulcers. Determining the ankle brachial index give an indication of a patient's ability to heal. However, diabetic patients may have falsely elevated ankle brachial index results secondary to vessel calcification. Patients with arterial ulcers must have increased/adequate blood supply to heal and benefit most from revascularization procedures. It should be noted that arterial insufficiency might act in concert with other pathological mechanisms, leading to tissue necrosis and ulceration. Diabetic foot ulcers, for example, may result from the combination of neuropathy, trauma, and arterial insufficiency.

Diabetic ulcers

Diabetic ulcers are the most common foot injuries leading to lower extremity amputation (*Figs 14.10* and *14.11*). In diabetics, the effects of peripheral neuropathy, peripheral vascular disease, and infection often combine to facilitate the development of diabetic ulcers that can lead to gangrene and amputation. Diabetic persons, like people who are not diabetic, may develop atherosclerotic disease of large- and medium-sized arteries, such as aortoiliac and femoropopliteal atherosclerosis. However, significant atherosclerotic disease of the infrapopliteal segments is particularly common in the diabetic population. Underlying digital artery disease, when compounded by an infected ulcer in close proximity, may result in complete loss of digital collaterals and precipitate gangrene. The reason for the prevalence of this form of arterial disease in diabetic persons is thought to result from a number of metabolic abnormalities,

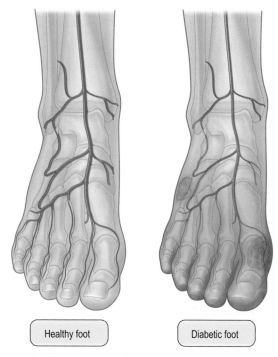

Healthy foot   Diabetic foot

Blood vessel damage in the feet may cause tissue damage such as sores, lesions and poor circulation that can lead to amputation

Fig. 14.10 The ischemic diabetic foot.

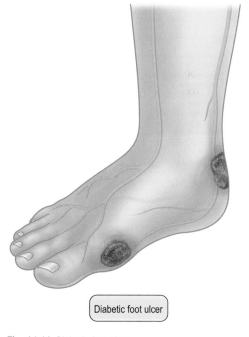

Diabetic foot ulcer

Fig. 14.11 Diabetic foot ulcer.

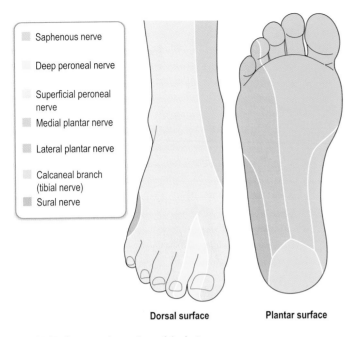

- Saphenous nerve
- Deep peroneal nerve
- Superficial peroneal nerve
- Medial plantar nerve
- Lateral plantar nerve
- Calcaneal branch (tibial nerve)
- Sural nerve

Dorsal surface **Plantar surface**

Fig. 14.12 Cutaneous innervations of the foot.

including high low-density lipoprotein and very-low-density lipoprotein levels, elevated plasma von Willebrand factor, inhibition of prostacyclin synthesis, elevated plasma fibrinogen levels, and increased platelet adhesiveness.[71] When peripheral arterial insufficiency complicates neuropathy there is a 10-fold risk of ulceration progressing to infection, gangrene, and amputation.[72]

Peripheral sensory neuropathy affects 50% of diabetic patients and is attributed to chronic hyperglycemia. It is a major cause of foot ulceration and lower limb amputation. In addition to poor glucose control, traditional cardiovascular risk factors for macrovascular disease are independent-risk factors for incident peripheral neuropathy. In addition, data from the EURODIAB cohort suggest that female sex may be an independent-risk factor. This makes it difficult to identify specific diabetes components of neuropathy.[73] Nerve injuries of the foot can also be caused by penetrating wounds. The sequelae of such injuries depend on the nerve injured and the level of the injury. In the foot and ankle, the main function of the nerves is to provide sensation. Generally, the tibial nerve and its branches (i.e., the medial and lateral plantar nerves) innervate the intrinsic musculature, although the deep peroneal nerve innervates the extensor digitorum brevis and extensor hallucis brevis muscles *(Fig. 14.12)*. Denervation of these

motor nerves can lead to clawing of the toes because of a resulting imbalance of intrinsic and extrinsic muscles. The long-term morbidity of nerve injuries of the foot is predominantly related to sensory nerve injury, except when a tibial nerve injury causes intrinsic muscle function loss. The two main problems associated with injuries to these nerves are the lack of sensation in the distal distribution of the nerve *(Fig. 14.12)* and the formation of a painful neuroma. When the nerve injury occurs in a weight-bearing area of the foot, the presence of a painful neuroma often leads to complex regional pain syndrome type I.[74]

Pressure ulcers

A pressure ulcer is a localized injury to the skin or underlying tissue, usually over a bony prominence, as a result of unrelieved pressure. Pressure ulcers or pressure sores represent a common health problem, particularly among the physically limited or bedridden elderly. Pressure ulcers on the buttocks affect nearly all wheelchair users. Pressure ulcer is a general term covering a number of different tissue injuries, from superficial heel sores to deep pressure sores under the buttocks. Because compressive forces, shearing forces, and/or friction are the major underlying causes some call them decubitus ulcer.[75] Pressure ulcers occur in approximately 5–15% of patients in home care, healthcare facilities, and hospitals. Pressure ulcers are painful, decrease the quality of life, increase susceptibility to infections, risk of death and nursing workload, and create significant costs.[76] Predisposing factors are classified as intrinsic (e.g., limited mobility, poor nutrition, comorbidities, aging skin) or extrinsic (e.g., pressure, friction, shear, moisture). When an ulcer occurs, documentation of each ulcer (i.e., size, location, eschar and granulation tissue, exudate, odor, sinus tracts, undermining, and infection) and appropriate staging (I through IV) are essential to the wound assessment.[77]

While there is little doubt that pressure ulcers are related to the mechanical insult of soft tissue, several hypotheses have been developed pertaining to the link between mechanical loading and tissue necrosis. The two major hypotheses deal with tissue deformation and ischemia.[78] Pressure-induced soft-tissue deformation causes cell necrosis. There is a time/strain relationship, meaning that time does indeed play a role. In other words, external tissue loading for a long time or on a chronic basis results in ulcer formation. Prevention includes identifying at-risk persons and implementing specific prevention measures such as following a patient-repositioning schedule, keeping the head of the bed at the lowest safe elevation to prevent shear, and using pressure-reducing surfaces. Ischemia is a state caused by lack of blood supply to any given tissue. The hypothesis proposes that a mechanical loading of the tissue impinges on the arterial blood vessels, thereby causing local ischemia. Since cells depend on oxygen, heat, and nutrients transported by the blood, they will become hypoxic and subsequently necrotic.

Ischemia and tissue oxygenation

Vascular complications commonly associated with problematic wounds are primarily responsible for wound ischemia. Limitations in the ability of the vasculature to deliver O_2-rich blood to the wound tissue lead to, among other consequences, hypoxia. Hypoxia is a reduction in oxygen delivery below tissue demand, whereas ischemia is a lack of perfusion, characterized not only by hypoxia but also by insufficient nutrient supply.[79] Hypoxia, by definition, is a relative term. It is defined by a lower tissue partial pressure of oxygen (pO_2) compared to the pO_2 to which the specific tissue element in question is adjusted under healthy conditions *in vivo*. Depending on the magnitude, cells confronting hypoxic challenge either induce an adaptive response that includes increasing the rates of glycolysis and conserve energy or undergo cell death. Generally, acute mild to moderate hypoxia supports adaptation and survival. In contrast, chronic extreme hypoxia leads to tissue loss.

While the tumor tissue is metabolically designed to thrive under conditions of hypoxia, hypoxia of the wound primarily caused by vascular limitations is intensified by coincident conditions (e.g., infection, pain, anxiety and hyperthermia) and leads to poor healing outcomes. Oxygen and its reactive derivatives *(Fig. 14.13)* are required for oxidative metabolism-derived energy synthesis, protein synthesis, and the maturation (hydroxylation) of extracellular matrices such as collagen. Molecular oxygen is also required for nitric oxide (NO) synthesis which in turn plays a key

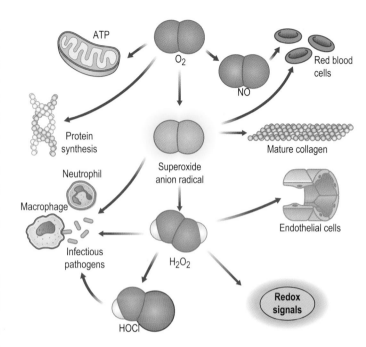

Fig. 14.13 Molecular oxygen and its derivatives in wound healing. ATP, adenosine triphosphate; NO, nitric oxide.

role in the regulation of vascular tone as well as in angiogenesis. In a wound setting, large amounts of molecular oxygen are partially reduced to form reactive oxygen species (ROS). ROS includes oxygen free radicals such as superoxide anion as well as its nonradical derivative, hydrogen peroxide (H_2O_2). Superoxide anion radical is the one-electron reduction product of oxygen. NADPH oxidases represent one major source of superoxide anion radicals at the wound site. NADPH oxidases in phagocytic cells help fight infection. Superoxide anion also drives endothelial cell signaling such as required during angiogenesis. In biological tissues, superoxide anion radical rapidly dismutates to hydrogen peroxide, either spontaneously or facilitated by enzymes called superoxide dismutases. Endogenous hydrogen peroxide drives redox signaling, a molecular network of signal propagation that supports key aspects of wound healing such as cell migration, proliferation, and angiogenesis. Neutrophil-derived hydrogen peroxide may be utilized by MPO to mediate peroxidation of chloride ions, resulting in the formation of hypochlorous acid (HOCl), a potent disinfectant *(Fig. 14.13)*.

Three major factors may contribute to wound tissue hypoxia: (1) peripheral vascular diseases garroting O_2 supply; (2) increased O_2 demand of the healing tissue;

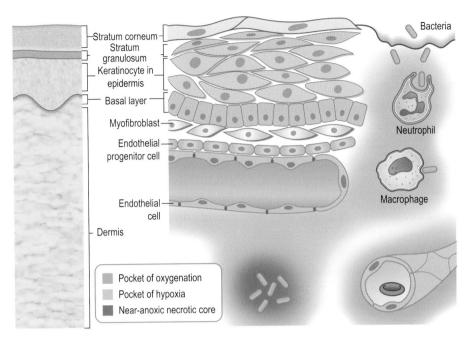

Fig. 14.14 Heterogeneous distribution of oxygen in the wound tissue: pockets of graded levels of hypoxia. Shade of blue represents graded hypoxia. Shade of red or pink represents oxygenated tissue. Tissue around each blood vessel is dark pink in shade, representing regions that are well oxygenated (oxygen-rich pockets). Bacteria and bacterial infection are presented by shades of green on the surface of the open wound.

and (3) generation of ROS by way of respiratory burst and for redox signaling.[80] Other related factors, such as arterial hypoxia (e.g., pulmonary fibrosis or pneumonia, sympathetic response to pain, hypothermia, anemia caused by major blood loss, cyanotic heart disease, high altitude), may contribute to wound hypoxia as well. Depending on factors such as these, it is important to recognize that wound hypoxia may range anywhere from near anoxia to mild to modest hypoxia. In this context it is also important to appreciate that point measurements performed in the wound tissue may not provide a complete picture of the wound tissue biology because it is likely that the magnitude of wound hypoxia is not uniformly distributed throughout the affected tissue, especially in large wounds. This is most likely the case in chronic wounds presented clinically as opposed to experimental wounds which are more controlled and homogeneous in nature. In any single problem wound presented in the clinic, it is likely that there are pockets of near anoxia as well as that of different grades of hypoxia *(Fig. 14.14)*. As the weakest link in the chain, tissue at the near-anoxic pockets will be vulnerable to necrosis which in turn may propagate secondary tissue damage and infection. Pockets of extreme hypoxia may be flooded with hypoxia-inducible angiogenic factors but would fail to vascularize functionally because of insufficient O_2 that is necessary to fuel the repair process. Indeed, uncontrolled expression of VEGF and its receptors leads to insufficient skin angiogenesis.[81] Whether cells in the pockets of extreme hypoxia are O_2-responsive is another concern. Even if such cells may have passed the point of no return in the survival curve, correction of tissue oxygenation is likely to help clean up the dead or dying tissue and replace the void with proliferating neighboring cells. Pockets of moderate or mild hypoxia are likely to be the point of origin of successful angiogenic response as long as other barriers such as infection and epigenetic alterations are kept to a minimum.

Limited supply and high demand: the oxygen imbalance

Peripheral vascular disease can affect the arteries and the veins as well as the lymph vessels. The most common and important type of peripheral vascular disease is peripheral arterial disease, or PAD, which affects about 8 million Americans. The ankle brachial pressure index represents a simple noninvasive method to detect arterial insufficiency within a limb. Arterial diseases, especially those associated with diabetes, represent a major complicating factor in wound healing. PAD is the only identifiable etiology in approximately 10% of leg ulcers. In an ischemic limb, peripheral tissues are deprived of blood supply as PAD progresses, causing tissue loss, ulcers, and gangrene.

Venous insufficiency, on the other hand, is the root cause of most leg ulcers. Chronic venous insufficiency, characterized by the retrograde flow of blood in the lower extremity, is associated with changes in the venous wall and valves generally caused by inflammatory disorders induced by venous hypertension and associated fluid shear stress. Factors causing arterial hypoxemia may also limit O_2 supply to the wound tissue. Compromised pulmonary health, loss of hepatic function, hemodialysis, anemia, altitude hypoxemia, nitroglycerin therapy, nasal packing, critical illness, pain, and hypothermia are examples of conditions associated with arterial hypoxemia. Vasoconstricting drugs may contribute to tissue hypoxia as well.[79]

Increased energy demand of the healing tissue leads to a hypermetabolic state wherein additional energy is generated from oxidative metabolism, increasing the O_2 demand of the healing tissue. Adenosine triphosphate (ATP) thus generated powers tissue repair. At the injury site, extracellular ATP may be contributed by platelets and other disintegrating cells. Extracellular ATP liberated during hypoxia or inflammation can either signal directly to purinergic receptors or, after phosphohydrolytic metabolism, can activate surface adenosine receptors. Purinergic signaling may influence numerous aspects of wound biology, including immune response, inflammation, vascular as well as epithelial biology. ATP may be immunostimulatory or vice versa, depending on extracellular concentrations as well as on expression patterns of purinergic receptors and ectoenzymes. Extracellular ATP induces receptor activation in epithelial cells. ATP, released upon epithelial injury, acts as an early signal to trigger cell responses, including an increase in heparin-binding epidermal growth factor (EGF)-like growth factor shedding, subsequent transactivation of the EGF receptor and its downstream signaling, resulting in wound healing. ATP released from the injured epithelial cells is now known also to turn on NADPH oxidases, the activity of which is critically required to produce the redox signals required for wound healing.[80] Human endothelial cells are rich in purinergic receptors and therefore responsive to extracellular ATP as well. ATP induces endothelium-dependent vasodilation. Both ATP as well as adenosine regulate smooth muscle and endothelial cell proliferation. Recognizing that hypoxia limits ATP synthesis in the ischemic wound tissue, therapeutic ATP delivery systems have been studied for their effect on wound healing. While these approaches may compensate for the deficiency of ATP *per se* in the ischemic wound tissue, they will fail to address the other essential functions of O_2 and its derivatives in wound healing, as discussed below.

Absolute requirements for O_2 arise in several points along the angiogenic sequence. For instance, all vessels require a net or sheath of ECM, mainly collagen and proteoglycans, to guide tube formation and resist the pressures of blood flow. Conditions for collagen deposition and polymerization can be created only if molecular O_2 is available to be incorporated into the structure of nascent collagen by prolyl- and lysyl hydroxylases. Without the obligatory extracellular hydroxylated collagen, new capillary tubes assemble poorly and remain fragile.[82–84] This has a convincing clinical correlate in scurvy, i.e., ascorbate deficiency. Scurvy results from insufficient intake of ascorbate which is required for correct collagen synthesis in humans. Ascorbate is required for the posttranslational hydroxylation of collagen that enables the matured collagen molecules to escape to the extracellular space and provide the necessary tensile strength. In scurvy, the collagenous sheath cannot form because, under ascorbate-deficient conditions, collagen cannot be hydroxylated. Consequently, new vessels fail to mature. Older vessels weaken and break, and wounds fail to heal. Thus, while hypoxia is a proved instigator of molecular signals for angiogenesis, it is also a proven enemy of vessel growth itself in nontumor tissues. Collagen deposition proceeds in direct proportion to pO_2 across the entire physiologic range, from zero to hundreds of mmHg. The K_m for O_2 for this reaction is approximately 25 and the V_{max} is approximately 250 mmHg, suggesting that new vessels cannot even approach their greatest possible rate of growth unless the wound tissue pO_2 is high.[85] Angiogenesis is directly proportional to pO_2 in injured tissues.[83] Hypoxic wounds deposit collagen poorly and become infected easily, both of which are problems of considerable clinical significance.[79]

Redox signaling

Additional high demand for oxygen is placed by a family of enzymes known as NADPH oxidases, which are known to be highly active at the wound site.[86] Recent work has identified that oxygen is not only required to disinfect wounds and fuel healing but that oxygen-dependent redox-sensitive signaling processes represent an integral component of the healing cascade.[80] The widely held notion that biological free radicals are necessarily agents of destruction is now facing serious challenge.[87] Over a decade ago it was proposed that in biological systems oxidants are not necessarily always the triggers for oxidative damage and that oxidants such as H_2O_2 could actually serve as signaling messengers and drive several aspects of cellular signaling.[88] Today, that concept is much more developed and mature. Evidence supporting the role of oxidants such as H_2O_2 as signaling messenger is compelling.[89–99]

Nitric oxide

At the wound site, NO is generated by an oxygen-dependent biosynthetic process. In the late 1970s, research was unfolding that implicated NO involvement in the process of vasodilation. By 1986, research culminated in the identification of NO as the endothelium-derived relaxing factor responsible for the maintenance of vascular tone, thus implicating NO as a potential wound-healing agent.[100] Maximal NO synthase activity is noted early in cutaneous wound healing, with sustained production up to 10 days after wounding. Wound macrophages represent a major source of NO production in the early phase of wound healing.[101] Inhibition of wound NO synthesis lowered wound collagen accumulation and wound-breaking strength, suggesting that NO synthesis is critical to wound collagen accumulation and acquisition of mechanical strength. Later it was demonstrated that wound fibroblasts are phenotypically altered during the healing process to synthesize NO, which, in turn, regulates their collagen synthetic and contractile activities.[102] The blockade of NO synthesis impairs cutaneous wound healing, acting in early and late phases of wound repair.[103] Interestingly, impaired diabetic wound healing is associated with decreased wound NO synthesis.[104]

MicroRNAs

Wound healing is largely dependent on injury-inducible protein-coding genes as they serve as drivers of an inherent tissue repair program that seeks to restore the injured tissue both structurally as well as functionally. There are two key steps that separate a protein-coding gene from its corresponding protein. First, the DNA hosting the gene must transcribe to mRNA. Finally, the mRNA must be translated to protein. Work emerging during recent years demonstrates that both of these critical steps are subject to robust and redundant regulation by microRNAs (miRNAs: 19–22 nucleotides long), which are noncoding RNAs found in all eukaryotic cells. Work during the past decade recognizes small RNAs as a new class of regulators of eukaryotic biology. Alongside other small interfering RNAs (siRNAs), miRNAs execute posttranscriptional gene silencing through mRNA destabilization as well as translational repression. In simple words, whether a gene would code a protein or not is decided upon by miRNAs for which the gene is a target. miRNAs form basepairs with specific sequences in protein-coding mRNAs. Near-perfect pairing induces cleavage of the target mRNA, whereas partial pairing results in translational repression and mRNA decay through deadenylation pathways.[105] According to the miRbase database, the human genome encodes 1048 miRNAs. This count is rapidly growing. These miRNAs may regulate more than a third of all protein-coding genes and virtually all biological processes. Mammalian cells express cell type-specific miRNAs which silence unique subsets of target genes within the cell. While miRNAs are mostly known for being functional in the cytoplasm, nuclear miRNAs may also participate in gene regulation. Initially considered an oddity, miRNA-dependent control of gene expression is now accepted as being integral to the normal function of cells and organisms. miRNAs are emerging as key regulators of the overall wound-healing process.[106]

Inflammation

Disruption of miRNA biogenesis has a major impact on the overall immune system. Emerging studies indicate that miRNAs, especially miR-21, miR-146a/b, and miR-155, play a key role in regulating several hubs that orchestrate the inflammatory process.[107] miRNAs have been directly implicated in the pathogenesis of inflammatory diseases such as osteoarthritis and rheumatoid arthritis. Resolvin-regulated specific miRNAs target genes involved in resolution of inflammation establish a novel resolution circuit involving RvD1 receptor-dependent regulation of specific miRNAs.[108] Furthermore, the brain-specific microRNA-124 can tame inflammation by turning off activated microglial cells and macrophages.[109] Of relevance to tissue repair is also the regulatory loop where cytokines, including those elicited following injury, are regulated by miRNAs as well as regulate miRNA expression.[110,111]

Angiogenesis

In 2005–2008, the first series of observations establishing key significance of miRNAs in the regulation of mammalian vascular biology came from experimental studies involved in arresting miRNA biogenesis to deplete the miRNA pools of vascular tissues and cells.[112] Dicer-dependent biogenesis of miRNA is required for blood vessel development during embryogenesis. Mice with endothelial cell-specific deletion of Dicer, a key enzyme supporting biogenesis of miRNAs, display defective postnatal angiogenesis. NADPH oxidase-derived ROS drive wound angiogenesis. Endothelial NADPH oxidase is subject to control by miRNAs.[113] Hypoxia is widely recognized as a cue that drives angiogenesis as part of an adaptive response to vascularize the oxygen-deficient host tissue. Hypoxia-sensitive miR-200b is involved in such induction of angiogenesis via directly targeting Ets-1.[114] Various aspects of angiogenesis, such as proliferation, migration, and morphogenesis of endothelial cells, can be regulated by specific miRNAs in an endothelial-specific manner. miRNAs known to regulate angiogenesis *in vivo* are referred to as angiomiRs.[115] miRNA-126 is specific to endothelial cells and regulates vascular integrity and developmental angiogenesis. Manipulating angiomiRs in the setting of tissue repair represents a new therapeutic approach that could be effective in promoting wound angiogenesis.

Hypoxia response

Tissue injury is often associated with disruption of vascular supply to the injury site. Thus, the injured tissue often suffers from insufficient oxygen supply or hypoxia. Under conditions of additional underlying ischemia, hypoxia is severe and seriously limits wound healing.[79] Hypoxia induces specific miRNAs, collectively referred to as hypoxamirs.[116] miRNA-210 is a classical

hypoxamir. Expression of hypoxia-inducible factor 1 (HIF-1) is also controlled by specific miRNAs. In turn, HIF-1 controls the expression of hypoxamirs, which are induced in the injured tissue.[117] Hypoxamirs are also induced by HIF-independent pathways. Although hypoxamirs generally favor angiogenesis, their metabolic and cell cycle arrest functions are in conflict with wound healing, especially in an ischemic setting. Silencing specific hypoxamirs may therefore represent a prudent approach to facilitate tissue repair. miRNA-210 represses mitochondrial respiration[116] and exaggerates production of undesired mitochondrial ROS.[118] These outcomes are not compatible with the higher energy demands associated with tissue repair. miR-210 also silences signaling via FGF,[119] a key contributor to wound healing. The injured tissue is highly rich in ROS.[86] In addition, at the site of injury transition metal ions are released from a protein-bound state. Conditions such as these cause DNA damage which opposes tissue repair. DNA repair systems are therefore of key significance in enabling tissue repair. miR-210 antagonizes DNA repair.[120] This is another hypoxamir function that is in conflict with wound healing. Compatible with the common observation that ischemic wounds are refractory to healing response, elevated miRNA-210 in ischemic wounds attenuated keratinocyte proliferation and impaired wound closure.[106,121]

Stem cells

Endogenous miRNA-binding sites have been identified in murine embryonic stem cells (ESCs). miRNAs govern ESCs function by serving as control hubs managing regulatory networks. A central importance of such governance is highlighted by the observation that ESCs lacking miRNAs lose their "stemness." ESCs with deficient miRNA biogenesis systems switch to a mode of ongoing cell division. They do not differentiate on demand because of failure to turn off the pluripotency regulatory program.[122] miRNAs conduct the orchestra of critical gene regulatory networks controlled by pluripotency factors within stem cells. Individual miRNA-dependent pathways that promote the reprogramming of somatic cells into induced pluripotent stem (iPS) cells have been now identified. Manipulation of specific cellular miRNAs helps enhance reprogramming of somatic cells to an ESC-like phenotype, helping to generate iPS cells.[123] Expression of miRNAs is also subject to control by epigenetic factors.[124] Such control influences the balance between proliferation and differentiation of stem cells. In executing such control, the miRNA element of epigenetics cross-talks with changes in chromatin structure as well as with changes in DNA methylation. Collectively, this provides for a mechanism by which the tissue injury microenvironment can influence miRNA-dependent reparative and regenerative processes.

Stem cells

The regenerative potential of injured adult tissue suggests the physiological existence of cells capable of participating in the reparative process. The epithelium of the skin, the epidermis, is in a continuous equilibrium of growth and differentiation and has the remarkable capacity to self-renew completely, which relies on reservoirs of stem cells. In mammals, there are two broad types of stem cells: ESCs that are isolated from the inner cell mass of blastocysts, and adult stem cells that are found in various tissues. In adult organisms, stem cells and progenitor cells act as a repair system for the body, replenished in adult tissues. Stem cells have the property of self-renewal without differentiation and have the potential to differentiate into any type of cell. Totipotent stem cells have the ability to give rise to a whole organism due to their ability to differentiate into embryonic and extraembryonic cells. Pluripotent stem cells are derived from totipotent cells and can differentiate into all cell types but cannot give rise to a new organism *(Fig. 14.15)*. ESCs are derived from the developing embryo, usually from the inner cell mass of a blastocyst or earlier morula stages. Lost or damaged cells can be replaced by differentiation, dedifferentiation, or transdifferentiation *(Fig. 14.16)*. Recent advances have shown that the addition of a group of genes can not only restore pluripotency in a fully differentiated cell state (differentiation) but can also induce the cell to proliferate (dedifferentiation) or even switch to another cell type (transdifferentiation). Dedifferentiation is represented by a terminally differentiated cell reverting back to a less-differentiated stage from within its own lineage. This process allows the cell to proliferate again before redifferentiating, leading to the replacement of those cells that have been

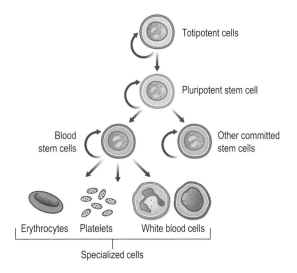

Fig. 14.15 Stem cell renewal.

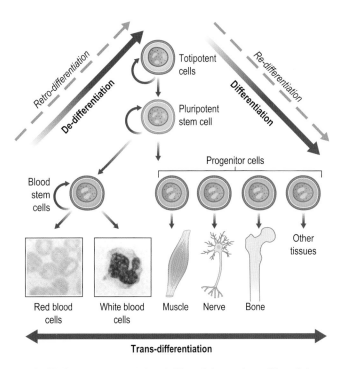

Fig. 14.16 Stem cell differentiation, dedifferentiation, and transdifferentiation.

lost. Transdifferentiation is another naturally occurring mechanism that takes dedifferentiation a step further and sees cells regressing to a point where they can switch lineages, allowing them to differentiate into another cell type. Furthermore, reprogramming aims to revert differentiated cells to pluripotency. From here, they can differentiate into almost any cell type. Although reprogramming occurs naturally during fertilization to produce totipotent cells that can differentiate into any

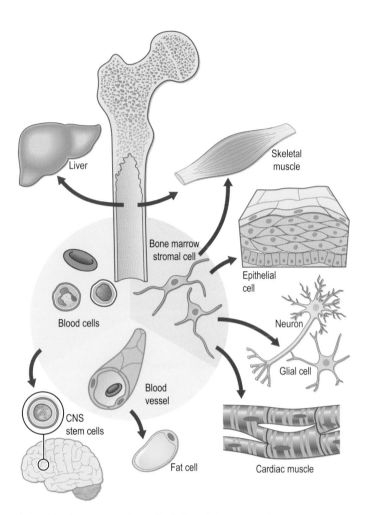

Fig. 14.17 Bone marrow stem cells. CNS, central nervous system.

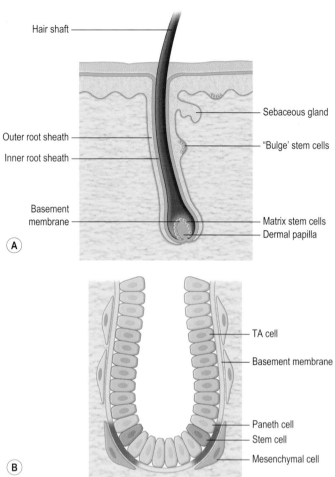

Fig. 14.18 Stem cells in the epidermis. Hair follicles act as reservoirs of stem cells in the skin. (A) Cross-sectional view of a hair follicle. The matrix stem cells differentiate into various parts of the hair while the long-term stem cells are present in the bulge region. The stem cells from the bulge maintain the sebaceous gland and epidermal stem cells. (B) A mammalian gut crypt. Stem cells are located at the basal region with the Paneth cells. The transit amplifying (TA) cells are stem cell progeny which move upwards and differentiate.

cell type, it has not yet formally been shown to be a genuine regenerative response. Furthermore, reprogramming sidesteps the necessity of using embryos for regenerative therapies by using differentiated cells taken from a patient. From a clinical perspective, this comes with the additional bonus of circumventing the immunological problems such as transplant rejection and graft-versus-host disease associated with engraftment.[125]

The bone marrow (*Fig. 14.17*), home of stem and progenitor cells, contributes a significant proportion of cells in the skin. The normal skin has long been known to contain bone marrow-derived cells that are involved in host defense and inflammatory processes, including wound healing. However, recent studies demonstrate that the bone marrow contributes not only inflammatory cells, but also keratinocytes and fibroblast-shaped cells to the skin. Similar to leukocytes in trafficking,

stem/progenitor cells derived from the bone marrow could home to injured tissues and participate in the repair/regeneration. Moreover, culture-expanded bone marrow-derived MSCs have been shown to promote the healing of diabetic wounds, implying a profound therapeutic potential for skin defects such as chronic wounds and burns.[126]

During the inflammatory phase, leukocytes migrating to the wound site are hematopoietic cells derived from the bone marrow. In the skin the bulge of the hair follicle (*Fig. 14.18*) plays a role as a reservoir of stem cells. In mice it has been shown that the bulge region contains hematopoietic cells that are identical to the bone marrow-derived cells and also to those found in fetal circulation.[127] Moreover this region also serves as a reservoir for precursors of mast cells. Discovery of these epidermal stem cells in the hair follicle bulge led to the hypothesis that these cells are necessary for both epidermal renewal as well as wound healing.[128] It was shown that cells from the bulge do not contribute to epidermal regeneration; however upon injury cells from the bulge are recruited into the epidermis and migrate in a linear manner toward the center of the wound.[129] These cells were noted to be transient, living only for a few weeks, thus representing an acute response to injury.

There are two main branches of stem cells in the bone marrow, including hematopoietic stem cells (HSCs) and MSCs. Adult bone marrow-derived HSCs have long been recognized as a precursor to all blood cell lineages, including erythrocytes, platelets, and white blood cells. Additionally, HSCs may also give rise to fibrocytes and endothelial progenitor cells. Circulating endothelial precursor cells play a role in neoangiogenesis which is essential for healing.[130,131] Bone marrow-derived stem cells also contribute to the deposition of collagen III in the wound[132] and differentiate into fibroblasts,[133] keratinocytes,[134] and fibrocytes.[135] Bone marrow-derived MSCs, which are also referred to as bone marrow mesenchymal stromal cells or marrow stromal cells, are self-renewing and expandable stem cells. Although present as a rare cell population in the bone marrow, representing about 0.001–0.01% of the nucleated cells, about 10-fold less abundant than HSCs, MSCs are expandable in culture and multipotent, capable of differentiating into several cell types.

Because of their properties of regeneration and differentiation the use of stem cells to heal problem wounds has long been of interest. Indeed, autologous bone marrow aspirates and cultured cells were helpful in healing chronic wounds.[136] In the case of burn wounds, bone marrow-derived stem cell treatment shows promise as well.[137] Another major source of adult stem cells is adipose tissue.[138] The capability of adipose-derived adult stem cells to differentiate into bone, muscle, fat, or cartilage, or into cells of mesenchymal lineage, makes them a prime target for therapeutic use. It has been shown that adult stem cells enhanced wound healing in a murine model.[139,140]

Hair follicles are an integral part of mammalian skin where they help the epidermis to maintain the body's protective barrier against its external environment. With rare exceptions (such as palms and eyelids), hair follicles are present all over the skin and play an important role in physiological tissue renewal and regeneration after injury. Hair follicles represent an autonomous mini-organ, which provides an excellent model system for studying the biology of adult stem cells.[141] There are obvious differences between human and mouse skin, yet the knowledge gained from lineage-tracing experiments in mice has greatly expanded our understanding of the cellular behavior of the different keratinocyte populations during physiological and injury-induced tissue regeneration. As in most of the body's organs, the skin experiences constant renewal. The upper keratinized layer of the interfollicular epidermis, which consists of terminally differentiated cells, is shed and replaced by cells originating from the actively proliferating layer beneath. In contrast, hair follicles undergo cycles of growth (anagen) and rest (telogen). The potential for proliferation to sustain the lifelong replenishment of normal cell loss and to repair occasional tissue damage lies within the population of epidermal stem cells. The hair follicle bulge harbors stem cells that may help in renewal and repair of the skin. The term "bulge," originally called "der Wulst," was introduced in 1903 by a German morphologist, P. Stöhr, to describe an eminent structure at the site of attachment of the arrector pili muscle in human hair follicles.[141] Similar to many other somatic stem cells, bulge cells are slow-cycling in nature. This feature has permitted their initial identification and isolation as label-retaining cells that can retain a pulse of nucleotide label following a long chase period and is frequently regarded as a defining characteristic of the hair follicle stem cell. In addition, the availability of several immunohistochemical markers, including keratin-15 and CD34, that specifically label murine follicular stem cells has given researchers the ability to examine carefully the signals required for adult stem cell activation and renewal. We now know that the bulge serves as a repository of long-lived multipotent stem cells, imparted with the capacity to differentiate into all cell types that constitute the lower cyclic portion of the hair follicle, as well as the interfollicular epidermis during wound repair.[142,143]

Although research into the use of stem cells for regenerative medicine is on a steep upward slope, clinical success has not been as forthcoming. This has been primarily attributed to a lack of information on the basic biology of stem cells, which remains insufficient to justify clinical studies. Since most clinical protocols use intravenous application of MSCs, it has become important to understand their trafficking in the blood stream. Moreover, since relatively little is known where the transplanted MSCs might locate, a better understanding of involved homing mechanisms will likely shed light on how MSCs exert their therapeutic effects. For instance, it is unclear whether mechanisms used at injured sites are location-specific or whether this recruitment can be modulated for therapeutic purposes. In addition, it has recently been suggested that platelets may play an important role in stem cell recruitment to sites of injury. A better understanding of the mechanisms used by stem cells during tissue homing would allow us to develop strategies to improve recruitment of these rare cells.[144]

Induced pluripotent stem cells

Pluripotent stem cells possess the unique property of differentiating into all other cell types of the human body. The discovery of iPS cells in 2006 has opened up new avenues in clinical medicine.[145,146] Recent breakthrough studies using a combination of four factors to reprogram human somatic cells into pluripotent stem cells without using embryos or eggs have led to an important revolution in stem cell research. It is now possible to convert somatic cells, such as skin fibroblasts and B lymphocytes, into pluripotent stem cells that closely resemble ESCs. Recently, functional neurons, cardiomyocytes, pancreatic islet cells, hepatocytes, and retinal cells have been derived from human iPSCs, thus reconfirming the pluripotency and differentiation capacity of these cells. These findings further open up the possibility of using iPSCs in cell replacement therapy for various disorders, including chronic wounds.

Scar

Scars (also called cicatrices) are macroscopic fibrous tissue that visibly replaces normal skin after injury. There is a wide spectrum of skin scarring postwounding, including scarless fetal wound healing, fine-line (normal) scars, stretched (widespread) scars, atrophic (depressed) scars, scar contractures, hypertrophic scars, and keloids. Postsurgical scar assessment is fundamental for a complete functional evaluation and as an outcome measure. The Vancouver Scar Scale is the most widely used rating scale for scars but the Patient and Observer Scar Assessment Scale is recognized as the most comprehensive tool, taking into account the important aspect of the patient's perspective. Recently, a new scale, called the Stony Brook Scar Evaluation Scale, has been proposed.[147] Although scar remodeling occurs for months to years after the initial injury, complete restoration of the normal ECM architecture is never achieved. Mature scars restore only 70% of the tensile strength of normal skin, and prescar function is never completely recovered.[148]

Scarring is an integral component of the healing process and an outcome of the remodeling stage of wound repair which begins 2–3 weeks after injury and lasts for a year or more.[149] During this stage, all of the processes activated after injury wind down and cease. Most of the endothelial cells, macrophages, and myofibroblasts undergo apoptosis or exit from the wound, leaving a mass that contains few cells and consists mostly of collagen and other ECM proteins.[149,150] Epithelial–mesenchymal interactions probably continuously regulate skin integrity and homeostasis. In addition, over 6–12 months, the acellular matrix is actively remodeled from a mainly type III collagen backbone to one predominantly composed of type I collagen.[151] This process is carried out by matrix metalloproteinases that are secreted by epidermal cells, endothelial cells, fibroblasts, and the macrophages remaining in the scar, and it strengthens the repaired tissue. However, the tissue never regains the properties of uninjured skin.

Fibroblasts at the wound site originating from surrounding tissues as well as supplied in the form of marrow-derived blood-borne cells are recognized as the primary drivers of scar formation. Platelets, macrophages, T lymphocytes, mast cells, Langerhans cells, and keratinocytes are directly and indirectly involved in the activation of fibroblasts, which in turn produce excess ECM. Dermal scarring can result in loss of function, movement restriction, and disfigurement. The mechanism of scar formation involves inflammation, fibroplasia, formation of granulation tissue, and scar maturation. In response to tissue injury, the acute inflammatory response is followed by the proliferation of fibroblasts, which are cells responsible for synthesizing various tissue components, including collagen and fibrin. During the acute inflammatory phase, circulating progenitor cells migrate to injured tissue. Rapid cellular proliferation occurs, which ultimately results in the formation of new blood vessels and epithelium. Fibroblasts then differentiate into myofibroblasts, which are the cells responsible for collagen deposition and wound contraction. Scar formation ultimately results from excess accumulation of an unorganized ECM.[148,152] Sensory nerves, including nonmyelinated C fibers and delta fibers, traverse all cutaneous layers, including the epidermis. These fibers run parallel to capillaries coursing around follicular complexes. A higher density of nerve fiber is associated with scar tissue. Unlike diabetic tissues, hypertrophic scar has excessive neuropeptide activity. In addition, proinflammatory substance P concentration is greater in the hypertrophic scar samples when compared with normal uninjured skin. High substance P and low neutral endopeptidase activity in scar tissue is believed to induce an exuberant neuroinflammatory response contributing to scar formation.[153]

Keloid

Keloid scarring, also known as keloid disease, is a locally aggressive benign fibroproliferative scar that continually grows beyond the confines of the original wound and invades into surrounding healthy skin. Unlike hypertrophic scars which stay within the boundaries of the original wounds and usually regress spontaneously, keloids grow beyond the boundaries of the original wounds and rarely regress. These pathological scars are not only aesthetically displeasing, but can also be both painful and functionally disabling, causing patients both physical and psychological distress. There is a strong genetic predisposition to keloid disease. First, keloids are more common in ethnicities with darker-pigmented skins and have been reported to be 5–15 times more prevalent in blacks than in whites. Familial heritability and prevalence in twins also support the concept of the genetic susceptibility to keloid scarring. The major pathways involved in keloid disease include apoptosis, mitogen-activated protein kinase, TGF-β, IL-6, and plasminogen activator inhibitor-1.[154]

Hypertrophic scar

The pathophysiology of hypertrophic scar formation involves a constitutively active proliferative phase of wound healing.[155] The scar tissue has a unique structural makeup that is highly vascular, with inflammatory cells and fibroblasts contributing to an abundant and disorganized matrix structure. The net result is that the original skin defect is replaced by a nonfunctional mass of tissue. Beyond these observations, investigations into the pathophysiology of the disease have been limited by the absence of a practical animal model and have relied upon the use of human pathological specimens. These studies are problematic in that such specimens represent the terminal stages of the scarring process and may not contain the initiating factors that originally led to the development of the disease. While animal models have provided some insight into the genetics and pathogenesis of cutaneous fibrosis, it is unclear how closely the process of hypertrophic scarring in these models resembles that seen in humans. Specifically, it is unknown whether the same factors that initiate hypertrophic scarring in these species are involved in human disease.[155]

Regenerative fetal healing

In contrast to adult wound healing, early-gestation fetal skin wound healing occurs rapidly, in a regenerative fashion, and without scar formation. The accelerated rate of healing, relative lack of an acute inflammatory response, and an absence of neovascularization distinguish fetal from adult wound healing.[156] Scarless wound healing has been observed in the fetuses of mice, rats, pigs, monkeys, and humans. Fetal skin heals scarlessly before a certain gestational age, after which point typical scar formation occurs. In humans, scarring of wounds begins at approximately 24 weeks of gestation, whereas in mice scarring of wounds begins on embryonic day 18.5 (average gestation period for mice is 20 days). This transition point, however, is modulated by wound size. For example, as wound size increases in fetal lambs, the ability to heal scarlessly is lost earlier during gestation.[148] In response to tissue injury, the fetal dermis has the ability to regenerate a nondisrupted collagen matrix that is identical to that of the original tissue. In addition, dermal structures, such as sebaceous glands and hair follicles, form normally after fetal injury. Although the exact mechanisms of scarless fetal wound healing are still unknown, they are thought to be due to differences between the ECM, inflammatory response, cellular mediators, differential gene expression, and stem cell function in fetal and postnatal wounds.[148]

Acknowledgment

Supported by NIH RO1 grants GM069589, GM077185, NS42617, DK076566, and HL 073087. The authors thank Sabyasachi Biswas PhD, Rashmet Reen PhD, and Viren Patel MD for support in writing this article.

Access the complete references list online at **http://www.expertconsult.com**

30. Martin P. Wound healing – aiming for perfect skin regeneration. *Science.* 1997;276:75–81.

   The healing of an adult skin wound is a complex process requiring the collaborative efforts of many different tissues and cell lineages. This review discusses the key signals and processes that regulate the normal adult cutaneous wound repair.

31. Martin P, Leibovich SJ. Inflammatory cells during wound repair: the good, the bad and the ugly. *Trends Cell Biol.* 2005;15:599–607.

39. Khanna S, Biswas S, Shang Y, et al. Macrophage dysfunction impairs resolution of inflammation in the wounds of diabetic mice. *PLoS One.* 2010;5:e9539.

53. Carmeliet P. Angiogenesis in life, disease and medicine. *Nature.* 2005;438:932–936.

79. Sen CK. Wound healing essentials: let there be oxygen. *Wound Repair Regen.* 2009;17:1–18.

86. Roy S, Khanna S, Nallu K, et al. Dermal wound healing is subject to redox control. *Mol Ther.* 2006;13: 211–220.

   H_2O_2 has been shown to support wound healing by inducing VEGF expression in human keratinocytes. This work presents the first in vivo evidence indicating that strategies to influence the redox environment of the wound site may have a bearing on healing outcomes.

98. Sen CK. The general case for redox control of wound repair. *Wound Repair Regen.* 2003;11:431–438.

   At very low concentrations, reactive oxygen species may regulate cellular signaling pathways by redox-dependent mechanisms. Redox-based strategies may serve as effective adjuncts to jump-start healing of chronic wounds. The review focuses on the understanding of wound site redox biology and novel insights into the fundamental mechanisms that would help to optimize conditions for oxygen therapy.

106. Banerjee J, Chan YC, Sen CK. MicroRNAs in skin and wound healing. *Physiol Genomics.* 2010.

   MicroRNAs (MiRNAs) are small endogenous RNA molecules about 22 nucleotides in length that are capable of posttranscriptional gene regulation by binding to their target messenger RNAs (mRNAs). This review focuses on the role of miRNAs in cutaneous biology, the various methods of microRNA modulation and the therapeutic opportunities in treatment of skin diseases and wound healing.

129. Ito M, Liu Y, Yang Z, et al. Stem cells in the hair follicle bulge contribute to wound repair but not to homeostasis of the epidermis. *Nat Med.* 2005;11: 1351–1354.

   The discovery of long-lived epithelial stem cells in the bulge region of the hair follicle led to the hypothesis that epidermal renewal and epidermal repair after wounding both depend on these cells. This paper discusses the implications of epithelial stem cells for both gene therapy and developing treatments for wounds.

149. Gurtner GC, Werner S, Barrandon Y, et al. Wound repair and regeneration. *Nature.* 2008;453: 314–321.

Skin wound healing: Repair biology, wound, and scar treatment

Ursula Mirastschijski, Andreas Jokuszies, and Peter M. Vogt

SYNOPSIS

- Fast and uneventful wound repair guarantees the integrity of our body and is essential for survival of all living organisms. Overlapping wound healing phases reflect adult repair resulting in a scar in contrast to scar-free fetal skin regeneration.
- Wound healing disorders extend between two extremes: chronic nonhealing ulcers on one side and excessive healing with hypertrophic scarring on the other.
- Multifactorial causes lead to and sustain chronic wounds, while excessive scarring is found predominantly after deep dermal burns. In both cases, biomolecular processes are still not well delineated and focus of intensive research.
- Clinical wound management starts with an assessment of wound type for choosing the appropriate dressing and ends with an interdisciplinary treatment of the wound and accompanying co-morbidities.
- Long-term scar treatment is characterized by physiotherapy, pressure garments and surgical contracture release.
- Innovative therapies for aberrant wound repair are still insufficiently evaluated and mainly experimental. Clinical phase III studies are lacking for proof of efficacy and wide-spread clinical use.

Wound repair biology

A human being has approximately 3000 skin injuries during a lifetime. Small wounds usually heal uneventfully. Questions about normal and pathological processes in the wound-healing scenario only arise when wound repair is disturbed.

Fast and uneventful wound closure restoring the integrity of the outer envelope is a criterion for survival for all living organisms. From prehistoric times up until today's highly developed medicine, the aims of wound repair have not changed: restoring of the outer surface to protect the individual from infection and dehydration. Egyptian papyri document the treatment of wounds and recommend the use of different dressings depending on wound quality.[1] The use of honey as an antiseptic has an astonishing history dating back more than 4000 years and has been rediscovered in recent years for the treatment of chronic wounds.[2] Furthermore, different resins, myrrh, frankincense, and cinnamon were used for wound treatment. South American tribes applied antiseptic resins such as copaiba, Tolu or Peru balm on wounds.[3] The oldest wound suture was detected on an Egyptian mummy dating from the 21st dynasty, around 1100 BC.[1]

Four thousand years later, fast and uneventful repair is still the maxim of skin wound healing, albeit aesthetic issues around tiny and invisible scars play an increasing role. Acute wounds that heal within 3 months are distinguished from chronic nonhealing wounds. The term "acute" comprises burn wounds, traumatic lesions, or surgical incisional wounds.

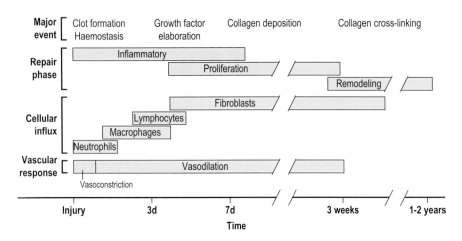

Fig. 15.1 The temporal patterns of repair phase, cellular influx, and vascular response during wound repair. The time points are approximate, and overlap occurs during these repair events.[7]

Adult wound repair

The repair cascade consists of inflammatory, proliferative, and remodeling phases (*Fig. 15.1*). These overlapping phases act in highly coordinated relationships to heal skin defects. During the inflammatory phase, hemostasis occurs and an acute inflammatory infiltrate ensues. The proliferative phase is characterized by fibroplasia, granulation, contraction, and epithelialization. The final phase is remodeling, which is commonly described as scar maturation.

Inflammatory phase

Inflammation is the first stage of wound healing and comprises cellular and vascular responses, including hemostasis. At the injury site, lacerated vessels immediately constrict. Thromboplastic tissue products, predominantly from the subendothelium, are exposed. Platelets adhere, aggregate, and form the initial hemostatic plug.

The coagulation and complement cascades are initiated. The intrinsic and extrinsic coagulation pathways lead to activation of prothrombin to thrombin, which converts fibrinogen to fibrin, subsequently polymerized into a stable clot. As thrombus is formed, hemostasis in the wound is achieved (*Fig. 15.2*). The aggregated platelets degranulate, releasing potent chemoattractants for inflammatory cells, activation factors for local fibroblasts and endothelial cells, and vasoconstrictors. The adhesiveness of platelets is mediated by activated integrin receptors such as GpIIb-IIIa ($\alpha_{IIb}\beta_3$) on their

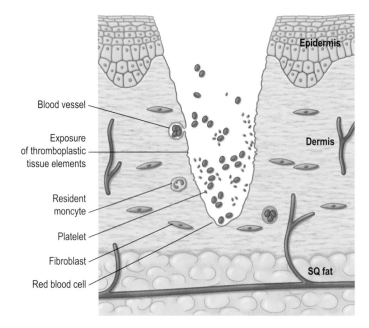

Fig. 15.2 Hemostasis is stimulated by platelet degranulation and exposure of tissue thromboplastic agents immediately after tissue injury.[7] SQ, subcutaneous.

surface.[4,5] Interestingly, under thrombocytopenic conditions, macrophages and T cells at the wound site compensated for lack of platelet-derived growth factors (PDGFs) and initiation of the inflammatory phase.[6]

Immediately, the repair processes are initiated. After hemostasis, local vessels dilate secondary to the effects of the coagulation and complement cascades. Bradykinin is a potent vasodilator and vascular permeability factor that is generated by activation of Hageman factor in the coagulation cascade.[8] The complement cascade

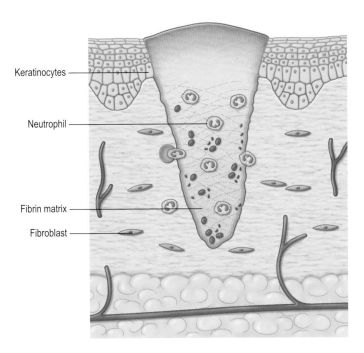

Keratinocytes

Neutrophil

Fibrin matrix

Fibroblast

Fig. 15.3 A neutrophil influx into the wound occurs within 24 hours. The neutrophils scavenge debris and bacteria and secrete cytokines for monocyte and lymphocyte attraction and activation. Keratinocytes begin migration when a provisional matrix is present.[7]

generates the C3a and C5a anaphylatoxins, which directly increase blood vessel permeability and attract neutrophils and monocytes to the wound. These complement components also stimulate the release of histamine and leukotrienes C4 and D4 from mast cells. The local endothelial cells then break cell–cell contact and increase permeability, which enhances the margination of inflammatory cells into the wound site.[8]

The initial influx of white blood cells in the wound is composed of neutrophils *(Fig. 15.3)*. This early neutrophil infiltrate scavenges cellular debris, foreign bodies, and bacteria. Activated complement fragments aid in bacterial killing through opsonization. The neutrophil infiltrate is decreased in clean surgical wounds compared with contaminated or infected wounds.

Within 2–3 days, the inflammatory cell population begins to shift to one of monocyte predominance. Circulating monocytes and mast cells are attracted and infiltrate the wound site.[9,10] These monocytes differentiate into macrophages and, in conjunction with the resident tissue macrophages, orchestrate the repair process. Macrophages not only continue to phagocytose tissue and bacterial debris but also secrete multiple peptide growth factors. These growth factors activate and attract local endothelial cells, fibroblasts, and keratinocytes to begin their respective repair functions. More than 20 different cytokines and growth factors are known to be secreted by macrophages *(Table 15.1)*.[11]

Depletion of monocytes and macrophages in combination with steroid therapy resulted in severe wound-healing deficiency with poor debridement, delayed fibroblast proliferation, and inadequate angiogenesis.[12]

In contradiction to the dogma that inflammation is essential for skin wound healing, mice deficient in the hematopoietic ETS family transcription factor PU.1 showed normal wound repair[13] despite immunoincompetent leukocytes and nonfunctional macrophages.[14] Although the growth factor and cytokine pattern was altered, incisional wounds healed uneventfully and scar-free with phagocytic fibroblasts clearing the wound debris. Obviously, attenuated inflammation is beneficial for wound healing.[9]

Proliferation phase

Extracellular matrix formation

During fibroplasia, fibroblasts synthesize and deposit replacement extracellular matrix (ECM) at the wound site. The proliferative phase begins with degradation of the initial fibrin–platelet provisional matrix. Three major classes of proteases are involved in wound repair. Proteases of the serine, cysteine, and matrix metalloproteinase (MMP) family are secreted to facilitate cellular migration through fibrin clot and provisional matrix. Both tissue and urokinase plasminogen activator are expressed to dissolve the blood clot.[15] MMPs comprise endopeptidases such as collagenases, gelatinases, and stomelysins that can degrade virtually all matrix proteins, activate growth factors, and bind on cell surfaces.[16,17] Cysteine proteases are present in epithelia during wound repair and are involved in signaling and basement membrane protein degradation.[18]

Macrophages, mast cells, and the adjacent ECM release growth factors that stimulate fibroblast activation.[9] Local fibroblasts become activated and increase protein synthesis in preparation for cell division. As fibroblasts proliferate, they become the predominant cell type by 3–5 days in clean, noninfected wounds *(Fig. 15.4)*. After cell division and proliferation, fibroblasts

Table 15.1 A partial list of growth factors present at the wound site*

Growth factor	Cellular source	Target cells	Biologic activity
Activin	Fibroblasts, keratinocytes	Stromal cells	Granulation tissue formation, scarring
TGF-β_1 and TGF-β_2	Macrophages, platelets, fibroblasts, keratinocytes	Inflammatory cells, keratinocytes, fibroblasts	Chemotaxis, proliferation, matrix production (fibrosis)
TGF-β_3	Macrophages	Fibroblasts	Antiscarring?
TGF-α	Macrophages, platelets, keratinocytes	Keratinocytes, fibroblasts, endothelial cells	Proliferation
TNF-α	Neutrophils, mast cells	Macrophages, keratinocytes, fibroblasts	Activation of growth factor expression
PDGF	Macrophages, platelets, keratinocytes, fibroblasts, endothelial cells, vascular smooth-muscle cells	Neutrophils, macrophages, fibroblasts, endothelial cells, vascular smooth-muscle cells	Chemotaxis, proliferation, matrix production
FGF-1, FGF-2, FGF-4	Macrophages, fibroblasts, endothelial cells	Keratinocytes, fibroblasts, endothelial cells, chondrocytes	Angiogenesis, proliferation, chemotaxis
FGF-7 (KGF-1), FGF-10 (KGF-2)	Fibroblasts	Keratinocytes	Proliferation, chemotaxis
EGF	Platelets, macrophages, keratinocytes	Keratinocytes, fibroblasts, endothelial cells	Proliferation, chemotaxis
HB-EGF	Macrophages, keratinocytes	Keratinocytes, fibroblasts	Proliferation, epithelial migration, synergistic with IGF
IGF-1/Sm-C	Fibroblasts, macrophages, platelets	Fibroblasts, endothelial cells	Proliferation, collagen synthesis
IL-1α and IL-1β	Macrophages, neutrophils	Macrophages, fibroblasts, keratinocytes	Proliferation, collagenase synthesis, chemotaxis
CTGF/CCN2	Fibroblasts, endothelial cells	Fibroblasts	Downstream of TGF-β_1
VEGF	Macrophages, keratinocytes, fibroblasts	Endothelial cells	Angiogenesis

*Redundant biologic effects occur through both autocrine and paracrine mechanisms.
TGF-α, transforming growth factor-α; TGF-β, transforming growth factor-β; TNF-α, tumor necrosis factor-α; PDGF, platelet-derived growth factor; FGF, fibroblast growth factor; KGF, keratinocyte growth factor; EGF, epidermal growth factor; HB-EGF, heparin-binding EGF, IGF-1, insulin-like growth factor 1; Sm-C, somatostatin C; IL-1, interleukin-1; CTGF, connective tissue growth factor; VEGF, vascular endothelial cell growth factor.
(Reproduced from Lorenz HP, Longaker MT. Wounds: biology, pathology, and management. New York: Springer-Verlag; 2000.)

begin the synthesis and secretion of ECM products. The initial fibrin matrix is replaced by a provisional matrix of fibronectin and hyaluronan, which facilitates fibroblast migration. The control of ECM deposition by fibroblasts is complex and partially regulated by growth factors and interactions of fibroblast cell membrane receptors with the ECM. Integrins are regulators of cellular function during repair. They are transmembrane receptors with extracellular, membrane, and intracellular protein domains. Integrins are heterodimeric and composed of α and β subunits that interact to form the active protein receptor. Ligands to integrins include growth factors and ECM structural components such as collagen, elastin, and other cells.[19,20] After ligands bind,

phosphorylation occurs in the cytoplasmic domain of the integrin receptor, which starts a signal transduction cascade that ultimately changes gene expression, and new cellular function ensues.

Fibronectin and the glycosaminoglycan hyaluronic acid compose the initial wound matrix.[10] Hyaluronic acid provides a matrix that enhances cell migration because of its large water content. Adhesion glycoproteins, including fibronectin, laminin, and tenascin, are present throughout the early matrix and facilitate cell attachment and migration. Integrin receptors on cell surfaces bind to the matrix glycosaminoglycans and glycoproteins. As fibroblasts enter and populate the wound, they secrete hyaluronidase to digest

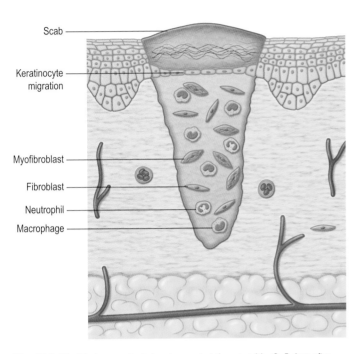

Scab

Keratinocyte
migration

Myofibroblast

Fibroblast

Neutrophil

Macrophage

Fig. 15.4 Fibroblasts are activated and present at the wound by 3–5 days after injury. These cells secrete matrix components and growth factors that continue to stimulate healing. Keratinocytes migrate over the new matrix. Migration starts from the wound edges as well as from epidermal cell nests at sweat glands and hair follicles in the center of the wound.[7]

the provisional hyaluronic acid-rich matrix, and larger, sulfated glycosaminoglycans are subsequently deposited. Concomitantly, new collagen is deposited by fibroblasts on to the fibronectin and glycosaminoglycan scaffold in a disorganized manner, resulting in scar formation. The major fibrillar collagens composing the ECM in skin and scar are collagen types I and III. The ratio of collagen type I to type III is 4:1 in both skin and wound scar. Although type III collagen is initially deposited in relatively greater amounts in wounds, its amount is always less than type I collagen in mature scar.[21]

At least 28 different types of collagen are currently known.[22] Most collagen types of the ECM are synthesized by fibroblasts; however, some types are synthesized by keratinocytes.[23] The collagens share common characteristics: the basic structural unit is a right-handed triple helix. Unique structural properties that distinguish the different collagen types include segments that interrupt the triple helix and fold it into other structures with unique properties.[24]

The major structural component of wound scar is collagen. Fibroblasts synthesize and secrete collagens

through a complex intracellular and extracellular process. Coordinated transcription of genes on different chromosomes (2, 6, 7, 12, 13, 17, and 21) occurs. In addition, several intracellular and extracellular modifications are required to form the new collagen fiber. Collagens contain a high fraction of proline amino acid residues, and this is the basis of its triple helix structure. With regard to collagens I and III, tropocollagen is formed in the ECM.[24] Tropocollagen molecules aggregate laterally and are covalently cross-linked by the enzyme lysyl oxidase to form collagen fibrils.[25] The fibrils interact with other fibril types, which then aggregate into fibers. Fibers then aggregate into bundles and form a collagen-rich scar.

Granulation tissue formation and angiogenesis

Granulation tissue is a dense population of blood vessels, macrophages, and fibroblasts embedded within a loose provisional matrix of fibronectin, hyaluronic acid, and collagen. Granulation tissue is clinically characterized by its beefy-red appearance (i.e., "proud flesh") and is present in open wounds. It is a consequence of the rich bed of new capillary networks (neoangiogenesis) that form by endothelial cell division and migration. The directed growth of vascular endothelial cells is stimulated by tissue hypoxia, and platelet and activated macrophage and fibroblast products.[26] Examples are basic fibroblast and vascular endothelial growth factor (VEGF), which induce migration and proliferation of endothelial cells.[27] A prerequisite for endothelial sprouting is the expression of the integrin $a_v\beta_3$ at the leading capillary tip[28] and the secretion of proteases for matrix degradation. Granulation tissue is a clinical indicator that an open wound is amenable to skin graft treatment. Wounds that benefit from skin grafts are of sufficient size such that the healing time would be decreased after grafting. Because granulation tissue has a high level of vascularity due to the abundance of new capillary formation, it readily accepts and supports skin grafts.

Wound contraction

Contraction is the process in which the surrounding skin is pulled circumferentially toward an open wound *(Fig. 15.5)*. This phenomenon does not occur with closed

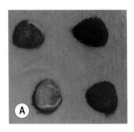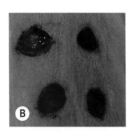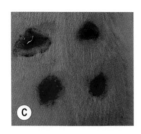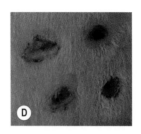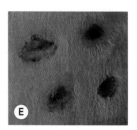

Fig. 15.5 Wound contraction is the process in which the surrounding tissue is pulled radially toward the wound. The wound size is decreased, which shortens the healing time. Full-thickness, rat skin wounds on postoperative days 0 **(A)**, 4 **(B)**, 8 **(C)**, 12 **(D)**, and 14 **(E)** after wounding. Note completely healed wound on postoperative day 14.

surgical incisions. Open wounds after trauma, burns, and previously closed wounds secondarily opened by infection are associated with contraction. Wound contraction decreases the size of the wound dramatically without new tissue formation. This repair process speeds wound closure compared with epithelialization and scar formation alone. In addition, the area of insensate scar is smaller. Animals have a much greater capacity for wound contraction than humans do. Most mammalian animals (e.g., rodents, cats, dogs, sheep, and rabbits) have a panniculus carnosus, which is a myofascial layer between the subcutaneous fat and musculoskeletal layers. This anatomy results in a plane of low resistance between two fascial layers, which allows enhanced skin mobility and therefore contraction. The amount of contraction is related to both the size of the wound and mobility of the skin. In humans, contraction is greatest in the trunk and perineum, least on the extremities, and intermediate on the head and neck. Eighty percent to 90% of wound closure can be due to contraction in the trunk and perineum.[29] These regional differences in contraction are probably due to relative differences in skin laxity.

It has become accepted that myofibroblasts play a key role in wound contraction. After wounding, dermal fibroblasts at wound margins are activated by growth factors released into the wound. Stimulated by mechanical tension and PDGF, they turn into stress fiber-expressing protomyofibroblasts. Protomyofibroblasts are found in early granulation tissue and in normal connective tissue with high mechanical load. Approximately 4 days after wounding, myofibroblasts appear in the wound.[30] Mechanical tension, activated transforming growth factor-β (TGF-β_1)[16] and the splice variant ED-A fibronectin trigger protofibroblast differentiation into alpha-smooth-muscle actin-expressing myofibroblasts.[31] Myofibroblasts exert their contractile

forces by focal adhesion contacts that link the intracellular cytoskeleton to the ECM. Interestingly, intercellular myofibroblast contacts via connexin-containing gap junctions are important for contractility because connexin-43-depleted fibroblasts were incapable to contract collagen matrices.[32] Furthermore, the role of keratinocytes in wound contraction should not be neglected. *In vitro* experiments showed higher contractile forces of keratinocytes compared with fibroblasts.[33] Future research will shed further light on the biology of skin wound contraction.

Wound contraction must be distinguished from contracture. Clinically, contracture is defined as tissue shortening or distortion that causes decreased joint mobility and function. Scar contracture commonly refers to decreased function in the area, whereas scar contraction refers to shortening of the scar length compared with the original wound.

Epithelial resurfacing

Morphologic changes in keratinocytes at the wound margin are evident within hours after injury. Marginal basal cells dissolve intercellular contacts, e.g., desmosomes and adherence junctions, and cell–matrix contacts, e.g., hemidesmosomes. Flattened migratory cells express cytoplasmatic actin filaments, promigratory integrins, e.g., $\alpha_2\beta_1$, $\alpha_5\beta_1$, $\alpha_v\beta_5$, $\alpha_v\beta_6$, and secrete proteases to enable movement.[34] MMP-3 is localized to wound margin keratinocytes and cleaves the intercellular contact protein E-cadherin.[35] MMP-9 cleaves basement proteins, e.g., collagen type IV and VII releasing keratinocytes from their substratum.[36] MMP-1 degrades native collagen type I and III, smoothing the way for newly formed matrix. Furthermore, MMP-1 binds to $\alpha_2\beta_1$ integrin on cell membranes, presumably acting as a migration promoter.[37] Blocking MMP activity with synthetic broad-spectrum inhibitors abolished epithelial migration *in vitro* and *in vivo*.[38,39]

In contrast to keratinocytes are fibroblasts able to adopt an ameboid phenotype and squeeze through the matrix network in the presence of MMP inhibitors.[40] Recently, cysteine proteases, e.g., cathepsin-B, C, K and L, entered the field of skin wound healing, acting as endopeptidases involved in the degradation of ECM proteins.[18]

After the re-establishment of the epithelial layer, keratinocytes and fibroblasts secrete laminin and type IV collagen to form the basement membrane.[41] The keratinocytes become columnar and divide to restore the layering of the epidermis and reform a barrier to further contamination and moisture loss. Keratinocytes can respond to foreign-body stimulation with migration as well. Sutures in skin wounds provide tracks along which these cells can migrate. Fibrotic reactions, cysts, and sterile abscesses centered on the suture can occur. These are treated by removal of the inciting suture and epithelial cell sinus track or cyst.

Remodeling phase

The scaffold that supports cells in both the unwounded and wounded states is the ECM, which is the structural component of skin that must be repaired after injury. The ECM is dynamic and is constantly undergoing remodeling during repair, which can be conceptualized as the balance between synthesis, deposition, and degradation. Lysyl oxidase is the major intermolecular collagen cross-linking enzyme.[25] Collagen cross-linking decreases its degradation and improves wound tensile strength. The balance of collagen deposition and degradation is in part determined by the regulation of MMP activity.[42] MMPs are inactivated by tissue inhibitors of MMPs, α-macroglobulin, and degradation by other proteases.[17,43] Except for reduced wound contraction in MMP-3-deficient mice,[44] other MMP knockout mice have little or no wound-healing disturbances.[36]

Scar formation is the ultimate outcome of wound repair in children and adults. The scar has no epidermal appendages (hair follicles and sebaceous glands), and it has a collagen pattern that is distinctly different from unwounded skin. New collagen fibers secreted by fibroblasts are present as early as 3 days after wounding. As the collagen matrix forms, densely packed fibers fill the wound site. The ultimate pattern of collagen in scar is one of densely packed fibers and not the reticular pattern found in unwounded dermis.

Wound scar remodeling occurs during months to years to form a "mature" scar. The early scar appearance is red due to its dense capillary network induced at the injury site. When closure is complete, capillaries regress until relatively few remain. As the scar redness dissipates during a period of months, the true scar pigmentation becomes evident. Scars are usually hypopigmented after full maturation. However, scars can become hyperpigmented in darker-pigmented patients and in those lighter-pigmented patients whose scars receive excess sun exposure. For this reason, sun protection measures are recommended for patients with early scars on sun-exposed areas such as the scalp, face, and neck. During remodeling, wounds gradually become stronger with time. Wound tensile strength increases rapidly from 1 to 8 weeks after wounding and correlates with collagen cross-linking by lysyl oxidase. However, the tensile strength of wounded skin at best reaches only approximately 80% that of unwounded skin[45] but can be increased by synthetic MMP inhibitors.[46] In addition, scar is brittle and less elastic than normal skin. It is readily visible because of color, contour, and texture differences compared with unwounded skin. Although scars can be hidden well with proper surgical planning and uneventful healing, they may have aesthetically unacceptable appearances in nonelective wounds after trauma and burns and in wounds with healing problems.

Regulation

Growth factors in skin wound healing

Growth factors are the focal regulatory points of the repair process. They are polypeptides that are released by a variety of activated cells at the wound site (*Table 15.1*). They act in either a paracrine or autocrine fashion to stimulate or to inhibit gene expression by their target cells in the wound. In general, they stimulate cellular proliferation and chemoattract new cells to the wound. Myriad growth factors are present in wounds and many have overlapping biologic functions. Most growth factors exist in several isoforms with several receptor types present in wounds, which increases the complexity of growth factor function. In addition to growth factor ligands, their signaling receptors are another locus for regulation of repair. Growth factors do not have an effect on target cells without a functional signaling receptor present on the cell surface. The level of regulation is complex in that the growth factors have multiple different receptor types to which they can bind and induce cell signaling. In recent years, the development of transgenic and knockout mouse models including inducible and cre-lox technologies has generated new knowledge in the function of many growth factors in wound healing. Clinical trials applying various growth factors to chronic nonhealing wounds showed beneficial effects,[47] although treatment efficacy should be confirmed by larger, randomized, double-blinded studies.[48]

Platelet-derived growth factor

PDGF is released from platelet alpha granules immediately after injury. PDGF attracts neutrophils, macrophages, and fibroblasts to the wound and serves as a powerful mitogen. Macrophages, endothelial cells, and fibroblasts also synthesize and secrete PDGF in the wound. PDGF stimulates fibroblasts to synthesize new ECM, predominantly the noncollagenous components such as glycosaminoglycans and adhesion proteins and to contract these matrices.[49] PDGF also increases the amount of collagenase secreted by fibroblasts, indicating a role for this growth factor in tissue remodeling. PDGF strongly induces granulation tissue production and was the first growth factor to be approved for the treatment of diabetic nonhealing wounds.[50]

Transforming growth factor-β

The TGF-β family comprises TGF-β$_{1-3}$, bone morphogenic proteins (BMP), and activins. TGF-β$_1$ predominates in adult wound healing and is a promigratory and profibrotic growth factor that directly stimulates collagen synthesis and decreases ECM degradation by fibroblasts. It is released from all cells at the wound site, including platelets, macrophages, fibroblasts, and keratinocytes. TGF-β acts in an autocrine fashion to stimulate its own synthesis and secretion. TGF-β also chemoattracts fibroblasts and macrophages to the wound, promotes granulation tissue formation,

myofibroblast differentiation, and wound contraction. TGF-β accelerates wound repair when it is applied experimentally to wounds that have no deficiency in repair. However, the increase in repair rate is at the expense of increased fibrosis, which could be a detriment during normal skin healing. In addition, increased TGF-β activity is associated with pathologic fibrosis in multiple different organ systems, including heart, lung, brain, liver, and kidney. TGF-β stimulates ECM synthesis by increasing collagen, elastin, and glycosaminoglycan synthesis. It increases integrin expression, which enhances cell–matrix interactions. TGF-β increases ECM accumulation by decreasing MMP and increasing tissue inhibitor of MMP expression. Through these mechanisms, exogenous TGF-β augments fibrosis at the wound site.[51] Interestingly, studies in mice with a lack of endogenous TGF-β activity demonstrate accelerated healing with an impaired inflammatory response.[52] In chronic wounds, however, significantly reduced TGF-β was found leading to clinical trials with TGF-β treatment that failed showing beneficial effects.[53] Activins and BMP are promigratory proteins secreted by keratinocytes and fibroblasts during wound repair and promote keratinocyte differentiation.[53] These findings underscore the complex effects of TGF-β and other growth factors during the repair process.

Fibroblast growth factors

The fibroblast growth factors (FGFs) are a group of heparin-binding growth factors that are secreted into the ECM, where they remain dormant until activated by tissue injury. They are bound by heparin and the glycosaminoglycan heparan sulfate. They have a broad range of biologic functions, specific to each isoform. FGF-1 (acidic FGF) and FGF-2 (basic FGF) stimulate angiogenesis.[26] Endothelial cells, fibroblasts, and macrophages produce FGF-1 and FGF-2. Basement membrane serves as a storage depot for FGF-2, which is released on degradation of the heparin components of the basement membrane at sites of injury. FGF-1 and FGF-2 stimulate endothelial cells to divide and form new capillaries. They also chemoattract endothelial cells and fibroblasts. FGF-7 (keratinocyte growth factor 1 (KGF-1)), FGF-10 (KGF-2), and epidermal growth factor (EGF) stimulate epithelialization. KGF-1 and KGF-2 are expressed in wound fibroblasts and promote keratinocyte proliferation and migration in a paracrine fashion. Decreased expression of KGF-1 occurs in diabetic and reduced levels of FGF-2 in aged mouse wounds with decreased angiogenic response.[54,55] In an ischemic rabbit wound model, exogenous KGF-2 treatment accelerates epithelialization without an increase in scar formation.[32] Exogenous KGF-2 also increases wound tensile strength, collagen content, and epidermal thickness in animal models of normal healing.[56] Hitherto, only one clinical trial has been conducted using recombinant human KGF-2 for treatment of chronic venous ulcers and showed accelerated wound healing.[57]

Vascular endothelial growth factor

VEGF is also a potent angiogenic stimulus.[58] It acts in a paracrine manner to stimulate vascular permeability and proliferation by endothelial cells after release from platelets, endothelial cells, neutrophils, macrophages, fibroblasts, and keratinocytes.[59–61] Its expression is increased in hypoxic conditions, such as those found at the wound site.[62] Intramuscular gene transfer of VEGF to patients with ischemic ulcers resulted in sprouting of collateral vessels and limb salvage.[63] Despite these promising results, careful use of VEGF is recommended because exogenous VEGF administration yielded vascular leakage and malformation.[64] Placental growth factor (PLGF) is also proangiogenic and acts synergistically to VEGF.[65] PLGF is upregulated in migrating keratinocytes and promotes granulation tissue formation and migration. Unlike VEGF, PLGF does not interfere with lymphatic vessel formation[66] and accelerates wound healing in diabetic mice.[67]

Other growth factors and cytokines

Multiple other growth factors affect wound repair. Epithelialization is also directly stimulated by members of the EGF family, e.g., EGF, heparin-binding EGF (HB-EGF), and TGF-α. These mitogens are released by keratinocytes to act in an autocrine fashion. Insulin-like growth factor 1 (IGF-1) stimulates cell proliferation and collagen synthesis by fibroblasts and interacts synergistically with HB-EGF, PDGF, and FGF-2 to facilitate fibroblast proliferation.[51] Various cytokines comprising interleukins (IL), chemokines, and tumor necrosis factor-α (TNF-α) mediate inflammatory cell functions at the wound site and contribute to tissue remodeling and angiogenesis.[51] IL-6 is crucial for initiation of the wound-healing response[68] whereas overexpression leads to cutaneous scarring. TNF-α and interferon-γ have been shown to downregulate ECM protein synthesis. Granulocyte–macrophage colony-stimulating factor (GM-CSF) is a pleiotropic cytokine stimulating migration and proliferation during wound repair. Experimental treatment of diabetic and chronic wounds showed promising results with faster healing rates.[69,70]

Although further studies are needed to determine the precise growth factor combination that is optimal for specific wound types, therapeutic growth factor application has become a reality. The clinical use of PDGF-BB was approved by the Food and Drug Administration for chronic ulcers. Further promising candidates are VEGF/PLGF, FGF-2, and GM-CSF.

Growth factor interactions with the extracellular matrix

In normal, unwounded conditions, the ECM is a depository of growth factors in latent forms. With injury and matrix destruction, growth factors are released from the ECM in active form and thereby assist in initiating and regulating the repair process. For example, TGF-β is bound in the ECM to the proteoglycan decorin and is inactive when bound. At sites of injury, TGF-β forms complexes with its binding protein, latency-associated protein (LAP), and is released. Under acidic conditions, such as at sites of hypoxia and tissue injury, LAP disassociates and active TGF-β is formed. LAP can also be proteolytically cleaved and released by MMPs and other proteases at the wound site. Active TGF-β immediately binds to its receptors (RI and RII), which are present on fibroblasts, macrophages, and endothelial cells.[71] The TGF-β RI and RII receptors form heterodimeric complexes with each other, and TGF-β biologic activity is initiated in the target cell through the Smad pathway.[72]

The FGFs are another example of growth factors bound by the ECM. PDGF and HB-EGF have also been shown to bind to ECM proteins. Through sequestration of growth factors with their subsequent release during injury, the ECM plays a fundamental role in wound repair by presenting growth factors that regulate the repair processes.

Fetal wound repair biology

The therapeutic solution for the reduction and possible elimination of scar formation may be found in the mechanisms responsible for scarless wound healing in the fetus. The early-gestation fetus can heal skin wounds with regenerative-type repair and without scar formation.[74,75] In scarless fetal wounds, the epidermis and dermis are restored to a normal architecture. The collagen dermal matrix pattern is reticular and unchanged from unwounded dermis. The wound hair follicle and sweat gland patterns are normal as well *(Fig. 15.6)*. The wound is not evident grossly unless a wound edge contour change is present, and this will cast a light shadow under appropriate circumstances.[73] Scarless healing by the fetus does not depend on the fetal environment. Fetal wounds in marsupials[76] or skin graft wounds heal without scar after transplantation to a postnatal environment. Thus, amniotic fluid, the intrauterine environment, and fetal serum factors are not required for scarless healing. Scarless repair appears to be inherent to the fetal tissue and probably depends on factors associated with skin development.[75] Notably, fetal scarless repair in skin is organ-specific with scarring of intestinal wounds at the same gestational age.[77] The fetal environment alone cannot induce scarless healing in adult skin. When adult skin is transplanted on to a fetus and later wounded at a point in gestation when fetal skin heals scarlessly, the adult skin grafts still heal with scar formation.[78] The transformation of adult healing to scarless repair cannot be accomplished simply by perfusion of adult skin with fetal serum or by immersion in amniotic fluid. Thus, induction of scarless healing in adult skin will require more than recreation of the fetal environment. The adult repair processes will likely have to be modified to recapitulate skin development. An understanding of the biology of scarless fetal wound repair will help surgeons develop therapeutic strategies to minimize scar and fibrosis.

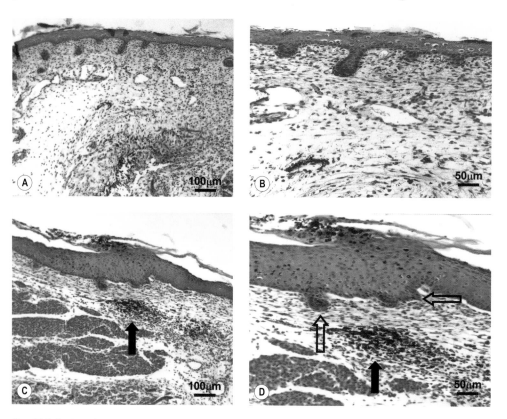

Fig. 15.6 Fetal rat skin wound made at gestational age 16.5 days (term = 21days), stained with hematoxylin and eosin. The hair follicle pattern is normal and there is no dermal collagen scar formation. Black arrows indicate India ink tattoo made at the time of wounding to locate the scarless wound. **(A,C)** Healed wounds harvested at 72 hours (×100). The epidermal appendage (developing hair follicles) pattern shows numerous appendages in the healed wound. **(B,D)** Magnified views of the same wounds show epidermal appendages (open arrows) within the wound site (×200). No inflammatory infiltrate is present. (Modified from Beanes SR, Hu FY, Soo C, *et al.* Confocal microscopic analysis of scarless repair in the fetal rat: defining the transition. Plast Reconstr Surg 2002; 109:160–170.)

Transition from scar-free healing to scar formation

Both gestational age and wound size determine whether the fetus will heal a wound without scar.[79] As gestation progresses, a transition from scarless healing to healing with scar formation occurs before birth. In large-animal models, such as the fetal lamb and monkey *(Fig. 15.7)*, this transition occurs during the early part of the third trimester for incisional, closed wounds. In addition, wound size affects the temporal occurrence of this transition. Open, excisional wounds must be made earlier in gestation than closed, incisional wounds for scarless healing to occur. Also, larger open wounds must be made earlier in gestation than smaller open wounds for scarless healing.[79] The exact reasons underlying these observations remain unknown but probably relate to whether the wound has healed before a certain threshold in development. The shift from scarless healing to scar formation is not abrupt but instead occurs gradually with an intermediate repair outcome that is neither regeneration nor scar: the transition wound. The

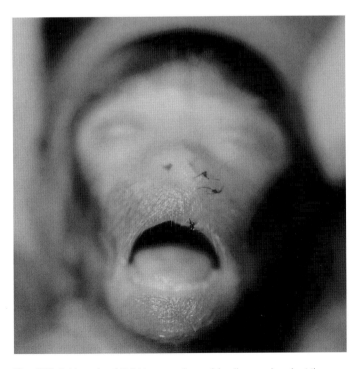

Fig. 15.7 Fetal monkey full-thickness wedge excision lip wound made at the beginning of the third trimester and harvested 2 weeks later. The cutaneous wound is identified by the sutures. No scar was present histologically, and the orbicularis oris muscle reformed across the defect.[73] Interestingly, the naris was deformed compared with the contralateral side.

transition wound has a normal reticular collagen and connective tissue matrix pattern but without restoration of epidermal appendages.[73] Thus, it has features of both scar (no appendages) and scarless (normal ECM) healing.

Differences between fetal and adult repair

Cellular differences

Because fetal fibroblasts deposit matrix in a scar-free pattern, they are crucial for scarless repair. A number of studies have defined the functional differences between fetal and postnatal dermal fibroblasts. First, fetal fibroblasts synthesize more collagen type III and IV with simultaneous proliferation, in contrast to their postnatal counterparts *in vitro*.[80] Fetal fibroblasts failed to respond to TGF-β stimulation with collagen synthesis compared to postnatal fibroblasts *in vitro*.[81] Furthermore, higher gene expression of MMP-1, -2, -3, -9, and -14 is found during fetal wound healing with virtually absent myofibroblasts during early gestation.[82,83] Fetal fibroblasts also migrate at a faster rate than postnatal fibroblasts.[84] Increased migration velocity during repair is likely to affect collagen deposition and crosslinking.

In postnatal wounds, epidermal continuity is restored by proliferating stem cells derived from the epidermal basement membrane and the hair follicle bulge.[85] Because immature fetal skin does not have hair bulges, the stem cell origin is likely to be different to adult wound repair. Indeed, a new stem cell was recently discovered and named dot cell because of its extremely small size.[86] Dot cells are found in basement membranes and in the blood during fetal development and have a strong affinity to wounded tissue. After transplantation of dot cells into adult murine wounds, scarless healing was noted. Despite their small size, these cells seem to have a great future in wound repair.

Differences in wound repair

Several parameters of repair are different in fetal wounds compared with postnatal wounds. The rate of repair for wounds of equal size is faster in the fetus. The collagen synthesis rate is greater in fetal wounds. In addition, the rate of epithelialization is faster in the fetal wound.[80]

Fetal wound repair may be more rapid because there is little or no period of activation for the fetal fibroblast to synthesize ECM at the wound site.

A key difference between fetal and postnatal tissue repair is a reduced inflammatory cellular infiltrate in fetal wound repair.[87] Inflammation plays a prominent role in postnatal repair, but it is not present in significant amounts during scarless fetal healing. This may be due to the immature fetal immune system with decreased platelet degranulation, PDGF and TGF-β production.[87] However a marked inflammatory cellular infiltrate occurs later in gestation after the transition when fetal wounds form scar. The amount of inflammation correlates strongly with the amount of scar formation.

Growth factor expression in fetal wound repair

Few growth factors associated with adult repair have increased expression in scarless fetal wounds. This is likely due to inherent major differences in the regulation between the two repair systems. Growth factors that are upregulated in scarless wounds are increased more rapidly than in postnatal wounds. One example is VEGF, which is expressed rapidly and threefold higher after injury in scarless wounds but is delayed in postnatal wounds.[88] The expression of TGF-β isoforms, receptors, and bioactivity modulators has been analyzed in fetal wounds. Compared with scarring wounds, scarless fetal wounds have more TGF-β_3, receptor type II, and fibromodulin expression.[89] In contrast, increased TGF-β_1, receptor type I, and decorin expression is associated with the transition to scar formation. Thus, the expression profile of isoforms, receptors, and modulators for a growth factor can be different in scarless and scarring wounds. By understanding the scarless repair expression profile for a growth factor, information is obtained that can permit recapitulation of this profile during postnatal repair to reduce scar formation. Exogenous addition of several cytokines to fetal wounds has also been performed and in every case has resulted in accelerated scarring. The cytokines tested include TGF-β_1, TGF-β_2, PDGF, and BMP-2, each of which has increased expression during scar formation in postnatal wounds.[90–92] Thus, growth factors with increased expression in scarring wounds probably modulate scarless

wounds in a similar fashion, and this results in scar formation.

Differences in gene expression

Because fetal skin is growing and differentiating, genes associated with development are likely to have an important role during scarless healing. Their expression may not occur during adult healing because of inactivation at the end of development. Homeobox genes are transcription factors that govern gene expression during embryogenesis. PRX2 is a homeobox gene that has increased expression during scarless fetal wound healing and only weak expression during adult skin healing.[93] New data are available for Wnt proteins involved in skin maturation, fetal and adult wound repair.[94,95] Wnt signaling is increased in postnatal but not in fetal murine wound healing with a TGF-β_1-like profibrotic influence on postnatal but not on fetal fibroblasts.[96] Differential signaling in fetal and adult cells in response to wounding seems to direct the way to either tissue regeneration or scarring.

Differences in matrix composition

Fetal skin and wound matrix are composed of more hyaluronic acid than are postnatal skin and scar. Hyaluronic acid stimulates fibroblast migration and probably affects the ECM deposition pattern.[84] Elastin, present in adult skin, is absent in fetal dermis, although no differences were found in basement membrane proteins or vessel formation.[97] Fetal skin and wound ECM have a relatively greater amount of collagen type III, but how this affects scar formation is not known. The collagen fiber thickness is increased in scarring fetal wounds compared with unwounded fetal skin as measured by confocal microscopy. This distance between collagen fibers is also greater in scarring fetal wounds, but the mechanisms causing these earliest changes in healing associated with scar formation remain to be elucidated.[74] Scarless fetal skin repair is the blueprint for ideal repair. With regard to TGF-β_3, an antiscarring product was developed[98] but failed to prove efficacy in clinical phase III trials. However, the mechanisms responsible for scarless repair still remain to be fully determined and when delineated will likely lead to innovative antiscarring treatment strategies.

Adult wound pathology

Nonhealing wounds

Chronic or nonhealing wounds are open wounds that fail to epithelialize and close in a reasonable amount of time, usually defined as 30 days. These wounds typically are clinically stagnant and unable to form robust granulation tissue. Many factors contribute to inhibit healing in these patients, but no unifying theory can explain the etiopathogenesis of each individual nonhealing wound *(Table 15.2)*. Medical conditions such as diabetes, arterial insufficiency, venous disease, lymphedema, steroid use, connective tissue disease, and radiation injury inhibit wound healing. Nonhealing wounds can also be due to pressure necrosis, infection (especially osteomyelitis), skin cancer, malnutrition, chronic dermatologic disease, and other metabolic conditions. In each case, treatment begins with debridement of any necrotic tissue present.[99] However, despite optimal treatment for each clinical problem, these wounds frequently still do not heal and surgical intervention is required.

Pressure sores

Wounds that develop over a bone prominence, usually in the immobile patient, are termed pressure sores. They are also called decubitus ulcers or bed sores. The sacrum, ischium, and greater trochanter are the most common locations affected.[100] However, the metatarsal heads, ankles, heels, knees, and occiput are susceptible under certain conditions. Another problem is malleolar skin pressure necrosis due to constricting cast placement. The amount of tissue pressure necrosis is determined by both the degree and duration of the pressure. When the tissue pressure is greater than 25–30 mmHg and capillary perfusion pressure is blocked, microcirculation is compromised. Necrosis can occur with as little as 2 hours of sustained pressure at this level.[101] Skin is more resistant to pressure necrosis than are underlying fat and muscle, which explains the common finding of a small area of skin ulceration overlying a large cavitary volume of subcutaneous fat and muscle necrosis. Treatment begins with identification and control of the factors that lead to increased pressure and subsequent wound formation. Paralyzed patients require periodic

rotation and an air mattress or another type of low-pressure bed. Wheelchair seat cushions commonly need to be changed in patients with ischial pressure sore. Behavior, such as prolonged sitting in wheelchairs without equal weight distribution, must frequently be modified. Lower extremity contractures that cause excessive hip, knee, and ankle pressure may need release. Tight casts should be removed and replaced. Improperly fitting lower extremity prostheses can lead to stump wounds and need modification. Other contributing factors, such as malnutrition, infection, and diabetes mellitus, should be identified and treated. Most pressure sores will heal with avoidance of pressure over the involved area. However, they heal with scar, which is less resistant to trauma than is normal skin. Thus, a higher incidence of recurrence exists after spontaneous closure of these wounds than if they are closed surgically with flaps of normal skin and muscle over the bony prominence.[102,103]

Lower extremity wounds

Leg wounds generally arise from either one of two different vascular diseases: arterial or venous insufficiency. Most (80–90%) result from venous valvular disease (venous insufficiency).[104] The role of impaired lymphatic drainage is discussed controversially in being a direct cause of nonhealing wounds or aggravating venous insufficiency.[104a]

Venous

Increased venous pressure in the dependent lower extremity with valvular incompetence leads to localized edema with plasma extravasation. Fibrinogen leakage results in formation of a fibrin layer around the capillaries that impairs oxygen and nutrient diffusion.[105] Leukocytes may be trapped and activated in obstructed capillaries. Oxygen radicals and proteases may then be released, which causes tissue necrosis. Postcapillary obstruction leads to increased perfusion pressure and hypoxia, with further necrosis. Without treatment, the wound size can easily continue to grow.

Arterial

Wounds require adequate oxygen delivery to heal. Ischemic wounds heal poorly and have a much greater risk of infection.[106] Minor trauma, resulting from

Table 15.2 Factors that may impair normal healing and lead to chronic nonhealing wounds

Etiopathology		Examples
Vascular	Arterial	Arteriosclerosis, arterial aneurysm, fat embolism with arterial obstruction, hypertension (Martorell ulcer)
	Lymphatic	Lymphatic edema, lymphangiodysplasia
	Venous	Chronic venous insufficiency, necrotizing thrombophlebitis
	Mixed arteriovenous	Combined arteriosclerosis with venous insufficiency, arteriovenous malformations/dysplasia; steal phenomenon (e.g., arteriovenous shunts, vascular compression/obstruction (due to tumors, enlarged lymphatic nodes, etc.)
	Vasculitis	Wegener granulomatosis, Churg–Strauss vasculitis, Henoch–Schönlein purpura, Sneddon syndrome, systemic lupus erythematosus, rheumatoid arthritis, Felty syndrome, Takayasu arteriitis, polyarteritis nodosa, Kawasaki syndrome, pyoderma gangrenosum, necrobiosis lipoidica diabeticorum, thrombangiitis obliterans (Buerger syndrome), allergic reactions
	Vasculopathic syndromes	Raynaud syndrome, systemic scleroderma, CREST, Klippel–Trenaunay syndrome, proteus syndrome[145,146], CLOVE syndrome,[147] Kasabach–Merritt syndrome
Physical, chemical, and biological causes	Pressure	Immobility, intra- and postoperative bedding, tight shoes and casts, compression therapy
	Trauma	Lacerations, any type of soft-tissue and bone injury, vascular rupture
	Thermal	Burns / frostbite, electrical injury (electrical current/high voltage/lightning)
	Radiation	Radiation therapy
	Chemical-toxic	Extravasation, chemical burns (acids/bases), sclerotherapy
	Infections	Erysipelas, necrotizing fasciitis, septic cutaneous embolism, osteomyelitis, complications after cutaneous infection
		Herpes simplex, cytomegalovirus, human immunodeficiency virus, syphilis, leprosy, tuberculosis
		Tropical ulcers, parasitic and vermicular infections
Neuropathic	Posttraumatic	Spinal lesions with palsy, peripheral nerve injury
	Congenital	Spina bifida, syringomyelia, multiple sclerosis, neurological syndromes
	Systemic neuropathic diseases	Diabetes mellitus, etyltoxic neuropathy, degenerative central and peripheral neuropathies Poliomyelitis, leprosy, tabes dorsalis
Hemopathological	Systemic diseases	Polycythemia vera, sickle-cell anemia, other anemias, thalassemia, thrombocythemia vera, thrombocytopenic purpura, increased blood viscosity (paraneoplastic, paraproteinemia, hyperglobulinemia, leukemia), complication after blood transfusion
	Disturbed hemostasiology	Factor V Leiden syndrome, antiphospholipid syndrome, disturbed fibrinolysis, factor XIII deficiency syndrome, antithrombin III deficiency, protein C/S deficiency, Marcumar necrosis, disseminated intravascular coagulation, necrosis due to vitamin K antagonist therapy
Neoplastic diseases	Cutaneous tumors	Basal and squamous cell carcinoma, melanoma, Bowen syndrome, Marjolin ulcer (scar carcinoma),[148] tumors with cutaneous metastasis or penetration (e.g., Paget syndrome)
Therapeutic modalities		Steroids, vaccination ulcer (BCG), cytostatic drugs, NSAIDs, extravasation of various drugs
Systemic diseases		Hepatic and/or renal insufficiency, immunosuppression, sarcoidosis, homocysteinemia, hemochromatosis
Other causes		Alcoholism, obesity, gout, smoking, advanced age, malnutrition (e.g., vitamin, protein, and micronutrient deficiency, scurvy); psychiatric diseases with self-harming, neglect, intravenous drug abuse; foreign bodies/ projectiles with fistulas

CREST, calcinosis, Raynaud's syndrome; esophageal dysmotility, sclerodactyly, and telangiectasia; CLOVE, congenital lipomatous overgrowth, vascular malformations, and epidermal nevi; BCG, bacillus Calmette-Guérin; NSAIDs, nonsteroidal anti-inflammatory drugs.

scratches and abrasions that would otherwise heal quickly in a well-vascularized extremity, can progress to large wounds in ischemic limbs. Necrotizing infection that is not only limb- but also life-threatening can develop. A reliable clinical sign of adequate arterial inflow for healing is the presence of an arterial pulse. The ankle brachial pressure index (ABPI) represents a simple noninvasive method to detect arterial insufficiency within a limb. ABPI is calculated by dividing the systolic blood pressure measured at the level of the ankle by the systolic blood pressure measured in the brachial artery.[107] Normal ranges of ABPI were defined as being 0.91–1.3, whereas ratios of ≤0.4 imply clinically critical limb ischemia.[108] Transcutaneous oxygen measurement is a noninvasive method with 83% accuracy in predictability of wound closure and 68% in predicting failure in an ischemic extremity.[109,110] To standardize transcutaneous oxygen measurements, tissue hypoxia was defined as <40 mmHg in healthy patients and <30 mmHg in patients with limb ischemia[110] with likely wound-healing disturbances at rates lower than 20 mmHg.[99,111] A nonhealing wound in an ischemic extremity is an indication for revascularization.[112]

Diabetic

Wound healing is impaired in diabetic patients by several mechanisms. Neuropathy is frequently present, which leads to decreased sensation and biomechanical joint instability. Arterial insufficiency is present in 30–60% of cases. Studies have implicated an altered expression profile of growth factors in diabetic wounds.[113] Decreased expression of GM-CSF receptor, PDGFs and their receptors, VEGF and its type II receptor, EGF receptor, IGF-1, and nitric oxide synthase-2 has been demonstrated in human diabetic foot ulcers.[114] Sustained inflammation is marked by an increase in proinflammatory cytokines[115] and cells, e.g., macrophages, B cells, and plasma cells, but decreased number of T cells in the wound margin.[116] MMP production is deregulated with dislocation of proinflammatory MMP-9 to the ulcer bed.[117,118] Advanced glycation end-products and inflammatory mediators commit fibroblasts and vascular cells to apoptosis and impair granulation tissue formation.[119]

Diabetic fibroblasts and keratinocytes have reduced proliferation rates and collagen production.[120] Wound healing is enhanced if glucose levels are well controlled,[121]

which suggests that many of these impairment mechanisms are partially reversible in diabetic wounds.

Radiation injury

External-beam radiation through skin to treat deeper disease has both acute and chronic effects on skin. Acutely, a self-limited erythema may develop that spontaneously resolves. The late effect of radiation is a more significant injury to fibroblasts, keratinocytes, and endothelial cells. DNA damage to these cells propagates and impairs the ability of these cells to divide successfully. Irradiated tissue usually has some degree of residual endothelial cell injury and progressive endarteritis, which results in atrophy, fibrosis, and poor tissue repair.[122] Ultimately, the affected skin may spontaneously break down, but usually after repeated mild trauma.[122] When a surgical incision is placed through irradiated skin on the trunk or extremities, it is not likely to heal. Although improvement in chronic wound repair can be achieved with hyperbaric oxygen therapy,[123] surgical intervention with resection of the wound to normal, nonirradiated tissue and coverage with a vascularized flap are frequently necessary.

Infection

Wound infection is an imbalance between host resistance and bacterial growth.[124] Bacterial infection impairs healing through several mechanisms. At the wound site, acute and chronic inflammatory infiltrates slow fibroblast proliferation and thus slow ECM synthesis and deposition. Although the exact mechanisms are not known, sepsis causes systemic effects that also impede repair. A threshold number of bacteria in the wound is necessary to overcome host resistance and cause clinical wound infection. Bacterial contamination results in clinical infection and delays healing if more than 10^5 organisms per gram of tissue are present in the wound.[125] Skin grafts on open wounds are likely to fail if quantitative culture shows more than 10^5 organisms per gram of tissue, which provides further evidence that bacterial load has an impact on repair.[126] Similarly, well-vascularized muscle flaps heal open wounds successfully if bacterial loads are not greater than 10^5 organisms per gram of tissue.[127] These studies demonstrate that high levels of bacteria inhibit the normal healing processes. Treatment of the closed infected wound depends on whether fluid or necrotic tissue is present. If no fluid is draining or accumulating, the cellulitis can be successfully treated with appropriate antibiotics. The wound should be opened and sutures removed; the wound is irrigated and débrided if pus or necrotic tissue is present. Administration of appropriate antibiotics after wound culture treats surrounding cellulitis. Signs of wound infection include fever, tenderness, erythema, edema, and drainage.

Malnutrition and obesity

Wound healing is an anabolic event that requires additional calorie intake.[128] However, the precise calorie requirements for optimal wound healing have to be calculated for each patient individually.[129] Large injuries such as burns greatly increase metabolic rate and nutritional requirements.[130] Severely malnourished and catabolic patients tend to impaired healing[131] because nutrients such as proteins, vitamins, and minerals that are important for effective wound repair are not substituted. These nutrients are involved in collagen synthesis and cross-linking and re-epithelialisation and promote the inflammatory response in early wound healing. Wound dehiscence risk is increased in humans with hypoproteinemia[132] and in protein-depleted rats, but this can be reversed with protein repletion immediately after wounding.[133]

Vitamin C (ascorbic acid) deficiency results in scurvy. In these patients, wound healing is arrested during fibroplasia. Normal quantities of fibroblasts are present in the wound, but they produce an inadequate amount of collagen.[134] Vitamin C is necessary for hydroxylation of proline and lysine residues,[135] and without hydroxyproline, newly synthesized collagen is not transported out of cells and collagen fibrils are not cross-linked. Both mechanisms decrease wound tensile strength.

Vitamin A (retinoic acid) is involved in multiple facets of repair: fibroplasia, collagen synthesis and cross-linking, and epithelialization.[134] Because vitamin A requirements increase after injury, severely injured patients require supplemental vitamin A to maintain normal serum levels. Animal studies show that vitamin A also reverses the impaired healing that occurs with chronic steroid treatment.[136] Although it is not proved

conclusively in human studies, most surgeons administer vitamin A postoperatively to their patients receiving steroid therapy. Vitamin A is fat-soluble and can be taken in toxic doses, so careful administration is essential. The oral dose is 25 000 IU/day.[134]

Vitamin B_6 (pyridoxine) deficiency impairs collagen cross-linking.[137] Vitamin B_1 (thiamine) and vitamin B_2 (riboflavin) deficiencies cause syndromes associated with poor wound repair. Supplementation with these vitamins does not improve healing unless a pre-existing deficiency is present. Deficiencies of trace metals such as zinc and copper have been implicated in poor wound repair because these divalent cations are cofactors in many important enzymatic reactions.[134] Zinc deficiency is associated with poor epithelialization and chronic, nonhealing wounds.[138] Trace metal deficiency is now extremely rare in both enterally and parenterally fed patients. Excess administration of vitamins and minerals can be detrimental and cause toxic effects, especially by the fat-soluble vitamins. Adequate amounts are present in today's enteral feeding solutions and as supplemental additives to parenteral solutions. Supplemental administration is necessary only in deficiency states and certain unique clinical situations, as described before.

Obesity interferes with repair independently of diabetes.[139] Obese patients with diabetes have impaired wound healing independently of glucose control and insulin therapy. Poor wound perfusion and necrotic adipose tissue probably contribute to impaired healing in both diabetic and nondiabetic obese patients.

Medical treatment

Both topically applied steroids and pharmacologic steroid use impair healing, especially during the first 3 days after wounding.[140] Steroids reduce wound inflammation, collagen synthesis, and contraction.[134] The exact mechanisms by which steroids impair healing are not fully understood. Glucocorticoids decrease PDGF and KGF expression in experimental wounds.[141,142] Steroids stabilize lysosomal membranes and thereby decrease the release of lysosomes at the repair site, which may slow repair processes. Because steroids decrease inflammation, they may decrease host bacterial resistance and thus increase wound infection complications. The entire

Table 15.3 Diagnostic criteria for distinction between hypertrophic scars and keloids[157,182]

	Hypertrophic scar	Keloid
Clinical symptoms	Remain within the boundaries of the wound	Grow beyond the wound borders
	Rarely more than 1 cm in thickness or width	Size variations; growth may be widespread, vertical, or both
	Form scar contractures	No contractures
	Less pruritic and painful	Pruritic and painful
	Occur after injury only: disruption of skin continuity, burns	Spontaneous appearance without skin injury possible
	Generally arise within 4 weeks, grow intensely for several months, then regress often within 1 year	Appear within several months after initial scar, then gradually proliferate indefinitely
	Occur on points with excessive tensile forces: across joint surfaces, sternum, neck, palm, and soles after injury	Occur often on the chest, shoulders, trunk, back of the neck and earlobes, rarely on the palms or soles
	Regress spontaneously	Do not regress spontaneously
Histological features	Fine and thin collagen fibers oriented parallel to the epidermis	Large and thick collagen fibers; closely packed collagen fibrils; increased ratio of type I to type III collagen
	Nodules with increased fibroblast density	Increased fibroblast density in enlarging borders, acellular in keloid center
	Presence of α-smooth-muscle actin-expressing myofibroblasts is typical	Lack of α-smooth-muscle actin-expressing myofibroblasts

repair process is slowed, and risk of dehiscence and infection is increased. Vitamin A administration can reverse this effect.[136,143]

Both radiation and chemotherapeutic agents have their greatest effects on dividing cells. During the proliferative phase of repair, numerous cell types are dividing at the wound site. Antiproliferative chemotherapeutic agents act to slow this process and thus retard healing.[144] After oncologic surgical procedures, in most institutions, chemotherapeutic agents are not administered until at least 5–7 days postoperatively to prevent impairment of the initial healing events.

Excessive healing

Normal wounds have "stop" signals that halt the repair process when the dermal defect is closed and epithelialization is complete. When these signals are absent or ineffective, the repair process may continue unabated and cause excessive scar formation. The underlying molecular mechanisms leading to excessive repair are still a topic of intensive research. Profibrotic cytokine overexpression and reduction of collagenase activity were found in skin tissue of burn patients.[149] In cell co-cultures, keratinocytes from hypertrophic scar tissue or keloids induced increased proliferation and collagen production in dermal fibroblasts.[150,151] A lack of programmed cell death, apoptosis, at the conclusion of repair with the continued presence of activated fibroblasts secreting ECM components has also been implicated.[152] Notwithstanding the molecular regulation of excessive scar formation, there are clinical factors that affect scar formation. To minimize visible scar on skin, elective incisions are least noticeable when they are placed parallel to the natural lines of skin tension (Langer's lines). This placement has two advantages: the scar is parallel or within a natural skin crease, which camouflages the scar, and this location places the least amount of tension on the wound. Wound tension widens the scar. Sharply defined and well-aligned wound edges that are approximated without tension heal with the least amount of scar. Infection or separation of the wound edges with subsequent secondary intention healing also results in more scar formation. Hyperpigmentation and hypopigmentation of the scar increase its contrast with the surrounding skin, making the scar more visible. Sun protection of all wounds is recommended to prevent scar hyperpigmentation.

Hypertrophic scar

Hypertrophic scars and keloids are unique to humans and do not occur in animals for unknown reasons. These pathologic scar types are distinguished on the basis of their clinical characteristics. Hypertrophic scars are defined as scars that have not overgrown the original wound boundaries but are instead raised. They usually form secondary to excessive tensile forces across the wound and are most common in wounds across joint surfaces on the extremities but also commonly occur on the sternum and neck. Physical therapy with range-of-motion exercises is helpful in minimizing hypertrophic scar as well as joint contracture in the extremities. Hypertrophic scar is a self-limited type of overhealing that can regress with time. These scars generally fade as well as flatten to the surrounding skin level. No clear histologic difference between hypertrophic scar and keloid has been demonstrated. Because of similar histologic findings in both hypertrophic scar and keloid,[153] they are more easily differentiated by their clinical characteristics *(Table 15.3)*.[154]

Hypertrophic scars and keloids are both fibroproliferative disorders of wound repair with excess healing.[155] However, because there are no animal models of either condition, there are few biochemical and molecular data that distinguish the two entities in direct comparison. In addition, most studies analyze either one or the other, but not both. In general, both keloid and hypertrophic scar fibroblasts have an upregulation of collagen synthesis, deposition, and accumulation.[154] It may be that keloid fibroblasts respond to a greater degree than do hypertrophic scar fibroblasts to the signals stimulating scar formation. For example, keloid fibroblasts respond to exogenous TGF-β with a much greater increase in collagen production than do hypertrophic scar fibroblasts.[156]

Mast cells and fibrocytes, circulating bone marrow-derived progenitor cells that differentiate into fibroblasts, are proposed to promote tissue fibrosis, especially in burn patients.[157,158] Both cell types are present in hypertrophic scar tissue and secrete profibrotic cytokines. Mast cell histamine enhances collagen production in fibroblasts[159] and is elevated in the plasma of patients developing hypertrophic scar.[160] The keratinocyte's regulatory role in this scenario has gained more interest in the past years. By secreting various factors, keratinocytes stimulate migration, proliferation, and matrix remodeling in a paracrine and autocrine way.[161] Increased collagen production was found in normal fibroblasts co-cultured with hypertrophic scar-derived keratinocytes.[151]

Hypertrophic scar fibroblasts produce more connective tissue growth factor (CTGF/CCN2) after TGF-β stimulation. CTGF stimulates chemotaxis, proliferation, MMP expression and ECM production.[162] The proteoglycan decorin binds TGF-β and regulates collagen fibrillogenesis by downregulating TGF-β production.[163,164] In contrast to normal dermal fibroblasts, hypertrophic scar-derived fibroblasts secrete less decorin and probably contribute thereby to sustained TGF-β activity.[165] A distinct histological difference between keloids and hypertrophic scars is the predominance of myofibroblasts in hypertrophic scar tissue. Controversial findings exist concerning the persistence of fibroblasts after accomplished healing. Programmed cell death is thought to underlie myofibroblast disappearance after wound closure. Whether fibroblast resistance to apoptosis leads to excessive scarring is still unknown.[157]

Keloid

Keloids are scars that overgrow the original wound edges. This clinical characteristic distinguishes keloid from hypertrophic scar. True keloid scar is not common and occurs mainly in darkly pigmented individuals with an incidence of 4.5–16% in African and Asian populations compared to less than 1% in Caucasians.[166,167] Currently, it is proposed that keloids form in areas of high skin tension,[168] although this does not explain why palms or soles are unaffected and why there is a high occurrence rate on tension-free earlobes. Another hypothesis postulates an immune response to the pilosebaceous unit after dermal injury and subsequent cytokine release with fibroblast activation. This is supported by the fact that keloids preferentially occur on anatomical sites with high concentrations of sebaceous glands, such as the chest wall, neck, and pubic area. Patients with keloids have a positive skin reaction to sebum antigen and benefit from desensitization with sebum vaccine.[169] A genetic predisposition is the point of discussion with autosomal-dominant features.[170] Certain syndromes are associated with keloid formation, e.g., Rubinstein–Taybi syndrome,[171] scleroderma,[172] and Touraine–Solente–Golé syndrome.[173] Interestingly, altered TGF-β regulation of the pro-opiomelanocortin (POMC) gene expression in keloid-derived fibroblasts was found.[174] A regulatory role of POMC in keloid formation is conceivable considering the fact that hitherto no human albinos with keloids have been reported.

The keloid scar continues to enlarge past the original wound boundaries and behaves like a benign skin tumor with continued slow growth. However, complete excision with primary closure of the defect results in recurrence in the majority of cases. Keloid patients may have excessive start signals or lack the appropriate stop signals for healing. In the latter instance, the lack of stop signals results in continued and unchecked repair. A possible mechanism of keloid formation may be the presence of persistent signals pushing fibroblasts to keep "healing" the wound site despite complete coverage of the original wound. Studies have looked at apoptosis in normal scar, hypertrophic scar, and keloid. Similar numbers of apoptotic cells at the advancing wound edge in both normal scar and hypertrophic scar have been found.[175] However, proapoptotic gene expression is decreased in keloids, suggesting persistence of activated fibroblasts.[176]

Keloids consist mainly of collagen and are relatively acellular in their central portions with fibroblasts present along their enlarging borders. They do not contain a significant excess number of fibroblasts. Keloid fibroblasts respond differently than normal wound fibroblasts to growth factors found at the repair site.[177] Keloid-derived fibroblasts express increased levels of CTGF,[178] TGF-β,[179] and VEGF[180] compared to normal skin fibroblasts and show increased proliferation and collagen production compared to normal fibroblasts.[181]

Clinical wound management

Management is based on the classification of the wound type. Surgically closed incisions obviously require a different treatment from that of nonhealing open wounds. Hypertrophic scars and keloids with their excessive scarring require other different therapeutic approaches. The treatment options for various wound types are described below.

Incisional wounds

Incisional wounds closed in layers along tissue planes heal with primary intention. Deep sutures are placed in collagen-rich layers such as fascia and dermis. These strength layers can hold sutures under a high degree of tension. Fatty tissue layers, such as subcutaneous fat, do not have significant collagen and cannot hold sutures under tension. For this reason, most surgeons do not close the subcutaneous fat layer, even in morbidly obese patients. Dead space here is better obliterated with a short course of closed suction drainage postoperatively, which can prevent seroma formation and possible infection. The amount of tissue injury and degree of contamination influence the length and quality of healing. Small, clean closed wounds heal quickly with less scar formation, whereas large, open dirty wounds heal slowly with significant scar. To decrease scar formation and risk of infection, meticulous hemostasis should be performed. This limits the amount of hematoma to be cleared and thus decreases the inflammatory phase and probably decreases scar formation. Because hematoma is a culture medium for bacteria, less bleeding also decreases the risk of infection. By limiting the inflammation with sterile technique and tight hemostatic control, repair by activated fibroblasts can begin earlier and shorten the healing period.

Smaller surgical scars are achieved with meticulous approximation of corresponding wound edges, no skin edge trauma, and less resultant inflammation. Forceps crush injury of the epidermis and dermis should be avoided by the use of fine forceps and skin hooks to retract and assist in dermal closure. This decreases the amount of necrotic tissue at the wound edge and thereby reduces inflammation. Because suture material is a foreign body, it generates an immune response and is susceptible to infection. Some surgeons therefore close the epidermis with Steri-Strips. There is no suture to leave a "railroad track" scar or serve as an infection locus in the skin. Fibrin and other biologic glues and sealants are also used especially for superficial wounds in infants without need for anesthesia. Depending on the wound localization, different suture techniques and materials are recommended (*Table 15.4*).[183]

Closed wounds require less care than open wounds. Closed wounds should be kept sterile for 24–48 hours until epithelialization is complete. At this point, water barrier function has been restored and patients can be allowed to shower or wash. This has a psychological benefit during the postoperative recovery period. In addition, gentle cleansing removes old serum and blood, which reduces potential bacterial accumulation and infection risk. Tensile strength of a closed incisional wound is only 20% that of normal skin at 3 weeks when collagen cross-linking is becoming significant. At 6

Table 15.4 Recommended suture materials and techniques for closure of full-thickness skin wounds at various body sites[183]

Wound localization	Suture material	Closure technique	Suture removal (days)*
Scalp	3-0 or 4-0 nonabsorbable, monofilament	Simple, narrow stitches	7–12
Face	4-0 or 5-0 synthetic absorbable or 6-0 nonabsorbable, monofilament	In layers; in case of full-thickness wound: running or single sutures	3–5
Eyelid	5-0 or 6-0 nonabsorbable, monofilament	Single-row stitches or running intracutaneous suture (secured with Steri-Strip for 10 days)	5
Lip, oral cavity	4-0 or 5-0 absorbable for mucosa, muscle, dermis; 6-0 monofilament nonabsorbable for skin	In layer: muscle, mucosa, skin; single stitches	3–5
Neck	4-0 absorbable, 5-0 nonabsorbable, monofilament	Double-layered for better cosmetic result; intracutaneous, running sutures	4–6
Abdomen, back	3-0 or 4-0 absorbable, 3-0 or 4-0 nonabsorbable, monofilament	Single or multilayered sutures; intracutaneous, running sutures	6–12
Limbs	3-0 or 4-0 absorbable,† 3-0 or 4-0 nonabsorbable, monofilament	Single or multilayered stitches (dermis); running intracutaneous sutures; splints for joint-crossing wounds or wounds with high mechanical tension	6–14‡
Hands and feet	4-0 or 5-0 nonabsorbable, monofil	Single layer with simple or Allgöwer / Donati stitches; splints for joint-crossing wounds or wounds with high mechanical tension	7–12
Nail bed	6-0 or 7-0 absorbable	Meticulous approximation with single stitches Use of magnifying glasses is recommended Nail bed splinting with original or artificial nail to avoid adhesions	Resorption

*If nonabsorbable suture material was used.
†Absorbable, monofilament sutures (e.g., polydioxanone) are more suitable for wounds with high mechanical tension, providing higher wound-breaking strength during collagen bundle cross-linking.
‡Nonabsorbable sutures on legs remain for up to 21 days depending on limb perfusion status and skin quality.

weeks, wounds are at 70% of the tensile strength of normal skin, which is nearly the maximal tensile strength achieved by scar (75–80% of normal). Therefore, if absorbable suture is used to close deep structures that are under significant tension, such as abdominal fascia, the suture should retain significant tensile strength for at least 6 weeks before absorption severely weakens the suture. In addition, heavy activity should be limited for a minimum of 6 weeks when healing of abdominal fascial layers is necessary.

Excisional wounds

Open wounds heal with the same basic processes of inflammation, proliferation, and remodeling as do closed wounds. The major difference is that each sequence is much longer, especially the proliferative phase. There is much more granulation tissue formation and contraction. This type of healing process is referred to as secondary intention.

Open wound edges are not approximated but are instead separated, which necessitates epithelial cell migration across a longer distance. Before re-epithelialization can occur, a provisional matrix must be present. Granulation tissue must form. There are variable amounts of bacteria, tissue debris, and inflammation present, depending on wound location and etiology. Infection, with high protein exudative losses and acute and chronic inflammation, can dysregulate repair and transform the healing wound into a clinically nonhealing wound. The exact molecular mechanisms causing this shift from healing to a nonhealing wound with infection remain unknown.

During the proliferative phase of an uncomplicated course of secondary-intention healing, a bed of granulation tissue will be present. If no infection is present and the area is of sufficient size that healing will not be complete for at least 2–3 weeks, placement of a partial- or full-thickness skin graft should be considered. Grafts readily adhere to granulation tissue and will quickly speed the repair process. Partial-thickness skin graft donor sites can heal in as little as 2 weeks, depending on graft thickness. When an open wound heals, which is generally defined as complete epithelialization, the dermal defect has been filled with collagen that is covered by epithelium. This scar has less tensile strength and is more susceptible to trauma than normal skin. Thus, these scars break down more easily from local trauma such as pressure.

Wound treatment

Necrotic material should be removed from open wounds on initial presentation and subsequently as it accumulates. Necrotic tissue serves only as a culture source for bacteria and does not aid healing. The only exception to immediate debridement is a dry, chronic, arterial-insufficiency eschar without evidence of infection. These types of wound may be best treated by revascularization before debridement.

Open wounds heal optimally in a moist, sterile environment. Numerous experimental and clinical studies have demonstrated that a moist environment speeds healing.[184,185] This is thought to occur by preventing desiccation at the base of the wound. Desiccation causes necrosis at the base of the wound until an eschar forms, which may take several days. During this time, the wound is enlarging and initiation of the healing process is delayed. When the wound is kept covered and moist without infection, desiccation necrosis and healing delay are prevented.

Chronic open wounds

A team approach for the treatment of chronic wounds is employed in wound centers. Members include a plastic surgeon, vascular surgeon, orthopedic surgeon, podiatrist, internist, endocrinologist, and specialist in microbiology. The team leader, usually a plastic surgeon, diagnoses the cause of the wound, coordinates appropriate referrals, and directs overall wound care. Prosthetists, physical therapists, enterostomal therapists, and clinical nurse specialists complete the team. Because the etiopathogenesis of chronic wounds is multifactorial, coordinated care by multiple specialists is required for optimal results.

To achieve standardized wound management, the International Wound Bed Preparation Advisory Board and the Canadian Chronic Wound Advisory Board have proposed components relevant for wound bed preparation: tissue debridement, infection/inflammation, and moisture balance. Even when these factors have been corrected, some wounds do not heal and have an abrupt or steep epidermal edge, with no migration of epidermal cells across the wound surface. These four components of wound bed preparation can easily be remembered using the mnemonic TIME – tissue, infection/inflammation, moisture, and edge effect.[99]

Wound bed preparation is the management of a wound in order to accelerate endogenous healing or to facilitate the effectiveness of other therapeutic measures. Treatment begins with debridement of necrotic tissue, which removes a potential source of bacterial infection. Depending on the bacterial load, systemic antimicrobial treatment adjusted to bacterial drug resistance is recommended. To provide optimal healing conditions, wound moisture imbalances should be corrected with adequate dressing and compression therapy.[186] Active medical comorbidities are aggressively treated. The wound characteristics (size, depth, infection, necrotic tissue component, edema, drainage) are documented, and local wound care is initiated. Care is continued until the wound is clean and ready for reconstruction or heals by secondary intention.

Wound dressings

A plethora of wound dressings are available for all types of wounds. High levels of evidence on clinical efficacy could not be demonstrated for any type.[187] However, substantial improvement in both convenience and comfort has been gained compared with saline gauze dressings. A new class of engineered skin replacements that show great promise in chronic wound care has been developed and is changing chronic wound care. The optimal open wound dressing maintains a moist, clean environment that prevents pressure and mechanical trauma, reduces edema, stimulates repair, and is inexpensive. Less frequent dressing changes and prevention of skin irritation are also beneficial.

Different classifications of wound dressings are used depending on their function in the wound (debridement, antibacterial, occlusive, absorbent, adherence), type of material used to produce the dressing (e.g., hydrocolloid, alginate, collagen) and the physical form of the dressing (ointment, film, foam, gel).[48] The latter classifications were used in *Table 15.5* to give an overview of currently available wound dressings.

The films are gas-permeable, maintain a moist environment, and are useful for partial-thickness dermal wounds such as skin graft donor sites. For highly exudative wounds, the absorptive dressings are useful to create a moist environment without excess fluid and proteinaceous material accumulation. Hydrocolloid dressings are useful for locations where adhesion is necessary, such as the extremities and over bone prominences. They are relatively thick and can stay in place for 2–3 days. As their absorptive capacity is reached, they lose adhesiveness, and gentle atraumatic removal is facilitated. Hydrogels are similar to hydrocolloid dressings except that they have little adhesiveness and are especially useful for dressing tendons, ligaments or facial wounds. Alginates can absorb 15–20 times their weight of fluid, making them suitable for highly exuding wounds. However, they should not be used on wounds with little or no exudate as they will adhere to the healing wound surface, causing pain and damaging healthy tissue on removal.[188]

Subatmospheric pressure

A subatmospheric dressing device (VAC, KCI, Texas, US) is available for vacuum-assisted closure. The apparatus consists of a sponge to fill the wound cavity, a vacuum pump, and a transparent film. It can be used in both inpatient and outpatient settings. Vacuum-assisted closure is useful for decreasing the size of large wounds on the extremities and trunk in preparation for reconstruction. The device can aid the healing of pressure sores, skin graft donor sites, and venous stasis ulcers.[189,190] An international expert working group has defined recommendations for the use of vacuum-assisted closure treatment for diabetic foot ulcers, complex leg ulcers, pressure ulcers, dehiscent sternal wounds, open abdominal wounds, and traumatic wounds.[191] Treatment by vacuum-assisted closure has induced granulation tissue formation over exposed bone and tendon. The beneficial mechanism is hypothesized to be due to its reduction of surrounding tissue edema, decrease of bacterial wound colonization, and increase in local blood supply, granulation, and wound cell proliferation. Presumably mechanical transduction, the conversion of mechanical stimuli to biochemical signals, is responsible for the effects seen with vacuum-assisted wound closure.[192] Mechanical forces deform tissues; this leads to cellular deformation, which is followed by stimulation of growth factor pathways, resulting in increased mitosis and production of new tissue.[193]

Recently, the traditional negative-pressure therapy combined with intermittent liquid instillation was introduced for the treatment of problematic acute wounds. Typical instillation solutions include normal saline, antibiotics, antifungals, antiseptics, and local anesthetics to reduce microbial infection or pain, respectively.[194]

Compression therapy

Edema in the lower extremity – whether it is due to venous insufficiency, lymphedema, cardiovascular disease, or metabolic derangement – must be aggressively treated if a wound is present. Elevation and compression therapy must be applied. Four-layer dressing wraps of the lower extremity consisting of gauze, cast padding, Coban, and elastic wraps are commonly used. After a venous stasis wound has healed, 30–40-mmHg pressure stockings must be worn continuously to prevent recurrence, which can be as low as 17% during the next 3 years.[195,196] Caution should be exercised in patients with peripheral neuropathy and arteriosclerosis. Lymph edema associated with chronic leg ulcers that are refractory to conventional compression therapy can be reduced with intermittent pneumatic compression as an adjunct treatment. Through an electrically inflatable boot, compression within a range of 20–120 mmHg at preset intervals is provided, improving venous and lymphatic flow.[196]

Table 15.5 Classes of wound dressings and engineered skin replacements*

Class	Composition	Characteristics and function	Commercial examples
Gauze	Woven cotton fibers	Permeable with desiccation; debridement; painful removal	Curity, Mepilex, Mepitel
Tulles	Open-weave cloth soaked in soft paraffin or chlorhexidine, textiles, or multilayered or perforated plastic films	Low adherent, suitable for flat, shallow wounds with low exudates	Adaptic, Grassolind, Jelonet, Tullegras, Urgotul
Film	Plastic (polyurethane); semipermeable	Allows water vapor permeation; adhesive; impermeable for liquids and bacteria	OpSite, Tegaderm
Foam	Hydrophilic (wound side) and hydrophobic (outer side) polyurethane or silicone foams; semipermeable	Highly absorbent; for necrotic and exudative wounds	Lyofoam, Allevyn, Tielle
Hydrogel	Water (96%) and polymer (polyethylene oxide)	Aqueous environment; requires secondary dressing; no adherence; not recommended if infection is present; semipermeable	Aquaform, Intrasite, Purilon, Vigilon, Aquasorb
Hydrocolloid	Hydrophilic colloidal particles and adhesive	Absorbs fluid; necrotic tissue autolysis; little adherence; occlusive	Comfeel, DuoDERM, IntraSite, Tegasorb
Absorptive powder, paste and fiber	Starch copolymers, hydrocolloid particles	Absorbs exudate; used as a filler; good for deep wounds	Aquacel, Geliperm, GranuGel paste, DuoDERM granules
Alginate	Calcium and sodium salts of alginic acid found in brown seaweed	Absorbs exudate and forms a hydrophilic gel after ion exchange with wound fluid; not suited for dry wounds	Algisite, Algosteril, Kaltostat SeaSorb, Sorbsan, Suprasorb

Antimicrobial dressings	1. Silver (in ionic or nanocrystalline form)
	2. Iodine
	  (a) as povidone-iodine
	  (b) as cadexomer iodine
	3. Metronidazole gel
	4. Octinidine gel
		Suited for colonized or infected wounds:
		1. Absorptive: cadexomer iodine (caution: thyroid diseases)
		2. Control of odor caused by anaerobic bacteria, used for fungating malignant wounds
		3. Used for burns
			1. Acticoat, Actisorb, Silver 200, Aquacel Ag
			2. Iodosorb
			3. Metrotop Gel
			4. Octinidine/Lavanid Gel

Silicone	Silicone sheets	Sheet induces a localized electromagnetic field and increased skin temperature; decreases scar formation?	Sil-K, Mepitel, Mepilex
Subatmospheric pressure	Vacuum pump, sponge, plastic film	Sponge conforms to wound and vacuum removes edema fluid and bacteria; stimulation of granulation, vascularization, and wound cell proliferation	VAC device
Dermal collagen replacement	Fine-mesh fabric (silicone, nylon) with dermal porcine collagens	Nonadherent; semipermeable	Biobrane
Dermal matrix replacement	Acellular matrix	Permeable; increased stimulation of repair?	AlloDerm (human, dermis), SIS (porcine, small-bowel submucosa), Integra (bovine collagen, shark cartilage, and silicone sheet)
Dermal living replacement	Absorbable matrix populated with allogenic human fibroblasts	Permeable; increased stimulation of repair?	Dermagraft (bioabsorbable scaffold), TransCyte (nylon mesh coated with porcine collagen)
Epidermal living replacement	Autologous keratinocytes on murine feeder cells	Permeable; increased stimulation of repair?	Epicel
Skin living replacement	Bovine collagen matrix populated with neonatal human fibroblasts with an outer layer of human keratinocytes	Impermeable; increased stimulation of repair?	Apligraf, OrCel

*Multiple brands within each class are available, and a partial list is given. No particular brands are recommended.
(Modified from Lorenz et al.[7] and Enoch et al.[196])

Pharmacologic treatment

Collagenases, e.g., streptodornase, streptokinase (Varidase), are useful for the treatment of wounds requiring fine debridement of necrotic tissue that is not amenable to surgical debridement. This could be a thin, superficial layer of adherent exudate or small amounts of necrotic tissue remaining after a bedside wound debridement. Theoretically, collagenase would be detrimental to a clean wound in the proliferative phase when ECM synthesis and deposition favor accumulation rather than degradation.

Because of highly sensitizing potential and induction of bacterial resistance, antibiotic wound dressings and ointments have largely been abandoned. Instead, antimicrobial products have become standard therapy for contaminated or infected wounds. In burns, silver sulfadiazine cream has largely been replaced by octinidine gel due to better dressing removal and burn wound assessment qualities of the gel.

Engineered skin replacements

With the biotechnology revolution, several dermal and skin replacements are now available through tissue-engineering technology *(Table 15.5)*. These products have the additional potential benefit of accelerating or augmenting repair because of their biocomponents. Growth factors are present in products with acellular dermal matrices. Some products contain living fibroblast and keratinocyte layers that secrete matrix components, proteases, and active growth factors. These products are typically placed on open wounds similarly to autologous skin grafts under sterile conditions with bolster support.[197] Their major advantages are the lack of a donor site wound and scar and placement in an office setting. Disadvantages are limited shelf-life and high cost, especially if they are applied repeatedly to the same wound, yet models predict that they can be less expensive than nonsurgical therapy.[198] The bilayered human keratinocyte–fibroblast construct on a bovine collagen matrix, Apligraf™, has been shown to improve healing of venous stasis, diabetic, and arterial-insufficiency wounds.[199] However, these studies compare its use against local wound care. No comparison has been made against autogenous skin graft treatment. *In vitro*, reduced keratinocyte migration on a de-epidermized substratum compared to adult split thickness skin.[200] Presumably, artificial skin products accelerate wound healing by growth factor delivery and paracrine stimulation of endogenous wound margin keratinocytes.[201]

Although the unique biology of engineered skin replacement dressings can aid in the treatment of impaired wounds, their efficacy compared with autogenous skin grafts has not been determined. For many biological products, no randomized controlled trials exist and current evidence is based on nonrandomized studies, reviews, and case reports. Products of human origin expose the patient to the danger of disease transmission and bovine, porcine, or human constituents can cause immunological side-effects or have religious and ethical implications.

Cultured epidermal autografts (Epicel) are used for second- and third-degree burns and require a culture time of 2–3 weeks until application to the wound. The patient's keratinocytes are harvested and cultured on irradiated murine feeder keratinocytes. Apart from a long culture time, these products are difficult to handle and lead to blistering, resulting in contractures and scarring.[202]

Excessive scar treatment

Scar classification

Before antiscarring therapy is instituted, an accurate description and classification of the scar type are useful. This assists with assessment of the outcome after late follow-up. A clinically based scar classification scheme has been proposed by the International Advisory Panel on Scar Management, which is composed of plastic surgeons, burn surgeons, and dermatologists *(Table 15.6)*.[203] Consistent and accurate diagnosis of scar types is essential for optimal management and useful literature interpretation.

Therapies

Many treatment modalities have been developed for the prevention and management of hypertrophic scarring and keloids. Many of the techniques have well-documented and time-proven clinical use, but few have been supported by randomized, prospective studies.

Table 15.6 Clinical classification of scars[203]

Scar type	Characteristics
Mature scar	A light-colored, flat scar
Immature scar	A red, sometimes itchy or painful, and slightly elevated scar in the process of remodeling. Many of these will mature normally over time, become flat, and assume a pigmentation that is similar to the surrounding skin, although they can be paler or slightly darker
Linear hypertrophic (e.g., surgical or traumatic) scar	A red, raised, sometimes itchy scar confined to the border of the original surgical incision. This usually occurs within weeks of surgery. These scars may increase in size rapidly for 3–6 months and then, after a static phase, begin to regress. They generally mature to have an elevated, slightly rope-like appearance with increased width, which is variable. The full maturation process may take up to 2 years
Widespread hypertrophic (e.g., burn) scar	A widespread red, raised, sometimes itchy scar confined to the border of the burn injury
Minor keloid	A focally raised, itchy scar extending over normal tissue. This may develop up to 1 year after injury and does not regress on its own. Simple surgical excision is often followed by recurrence. There may be a genetic abnormality involved in keloid scarring. Typical sites include earlobes
Major keloid	A large, raised (>0.5 cm) scar, possibly painful or pruritic and extending over normal tissue. This often results after minor trauma and can continue to spread for years

This inherent problem makes choosing the best treatment modality difficult on the basis of objective scientific evidence. Therefore, most modalities are applied on the basis of the treating physician's personal biases and experiences. Scar therapies, with their respective advantages and disadvantages, are listed in *Table 15.7*.

Prevention

The first step toward treatment of excessive scarring is early recognition and institution of therapy after surgery or trauma. Meticulous tissue handling, suturing, and wound management with efforts to prevent infection are mandatory.[203] Sun protection to reduce scar hyperpigmentation is essential. Patients who are at increased risk of excessive scarring benefit from preventive techniques, which include silicone gel sheeting or ointments, hypoallergenic microporous tape, and concurrent intralesional steroid injection.[203]

Silicone gel sheeting is widely used for hypertrophic scar and keloid treatment. Silicone gel sheeting has a 20-plus-year history with several randomized, controlled trials that support its safe and effective use.[204,205] It is painless and thus useful for children. Proposed mechanisms of action for scar reduction include improved hydration and occlusion,[206] increased temperature elevation of $1°C$ (or less) that can affect collagenase kinetics, and change in the adhesion molecule expression of the lymphocytic infiltrate.[207] When treatment with silicone gel sheeting is not feasible (e.g., scar location on the face, scalp, or neck), silicone oil-based creams are an alternative.[208] For example, silicone-based creams are frequently used on cleft lip repair scars, hypertrophic scars after burns, or hand injury without allergic or other untoward reaction to date.

Microporous hypoallergenic tape can relieve tension across wounds and minimize the excessive scar risk from shearing. Although there are no prospective, controlled studies to support its use, tape is routinely used and recommended by many authors.[203] The tape is applied for a few weeks after surgery. In patients who are at extremely high risk, such as after excision of keloid or hypertrophic scar, concurrent intralesional steroid injections can be given prophylactically, followed by monthly injections as necessary. Success rates, measured by no recurrence, are reported up to 92% for keloids and 95% for hypertrophic scars at a mean follow-up of 30.5 months.[209]

Treatment algorithm

Immature hypertrophic scars (red)

Once excessive scarring is identified, the International Advisory Panel on Scar Management consensus initial management is silicone gel sheeting, steroid injection, and localized pressure therapy *(Fig. 15.8)*.[203] It can be difficult to predict whether immature hypertrophic scars (red, slightly raised) will regress or progress. When erythema persists for more than 1 month, the risk of

Table 15.7 Scar prevention and reduction therapies[203]

Therapy	Advantages	Disadvantages
Surgical excision	Excess scar removed	High recurrence without adjuvant therapy, cost
Surgical lengthening (Z-plasty, W-plasty)	Increased mobility and range of motion	Some excess scar persists, occasionally worse cosmesis
Steroid intralesional injection	Cost, ease	Multiple treatments; telangiectasia, hypopigmentation
Silicone gel sheeting	Cost, ease of use, noninvasive	Difficult application on head, neck, across joints
Pressure therapy	Noninvasive, some proven efficacy	Cumbersome garment, cost high if custom-made, constant use for months to years
Radiation after surgery	Some proven efficacy	Risk of carcinogenesis, cost
Laser	Pulsed-dye 585- or 595-nm laser best for decreasing red color; carbon dioxide, Nd:YAG, pulsed Erb:YAG lasers with some efficacy; selective photothermolysis by erbium-doped fiber lasers (1550 nm)	Costs, multiple treatments Dye laser: reduced efficacy in darker-skinned patients and thick (>1 cm) hypertrophic scars 50% recurrence rate with carbon dioxide laser
Cryotherapy	Some proven efficacy in keloid reduction	Hypopigmentation, pain, skin atrophy
Microporous tape	Ease, low cost	No proven benefit, except uncontrolled reports
Popular treatments (vitamin E, onion extracts, and other plant creams)	Ease, low cost	No proven benefit
Physical therapy treatments: ultrasound, pulsed electrical stimulation, hydrotherapy, massage	Patient participation; increased joint range of motion; can decrease scar pain, pruritus	No quantitative proven efficacy, cost
Recombinant human TGF-β_3 (avotermin), rh Il-10 (ilodecakin), TGF-β_1 inhibitors	Clinical-phase trials	Experimental, high costs, lack of efficacy
Anti-inflammatory/proliferative medication injections (5-fluorouracil, interferons, retinoids, histamine antagonists)	Fluorouracil: repeated application necessary, no systemic effects Retinoids: still experimental, reduce scar tissue and sebum production	Fluorouracil: single administration with recurrence Interferon: high recurrence rate, adverse systemic effects Retinoids: adverse effects with photosensitivity and skin irritation
Calcium channel blockers (verapamil)	Clinical trials ongoing, good efficacy	Still experimental
Experimental therapies (bleomycin, imiquimod, cyclosporine)	Experimental, some efficacy	No proven benefit, systemic side-effects?
Medical needling	Clinical phase trials using the Medical Roll-CIT, low cost, ease	Pretreatment with retinoids, general anesthesia needed for treatment of larger surfaces, short follow-up, recurrence

progression to linear hypertrophic scar increases, and appropriate therapy should be started.

Linear hypertrophic scars (red, slightly raised)

Treatment options include the application of pressure garments or topical silicone sheets, 585-nm pulsed-dye laser therapy, and re-excision. The last option is most useful in cases of excess scar due to wound infection or dehiscence. If the original wound was closed following the basic tenets described and healed otherwise uneventfully, re-excision with primary closure is not likely to result in an improved scar. Recurrence of hypertrophic scar is high in these circumstances, and therefore most plastic surgeons do not treat hypertrophic scar with excision and primary closure unless they plan adjuvant therapy. Silicone gel has proven benefit from randomized, controlled trials and is a recommended first-line

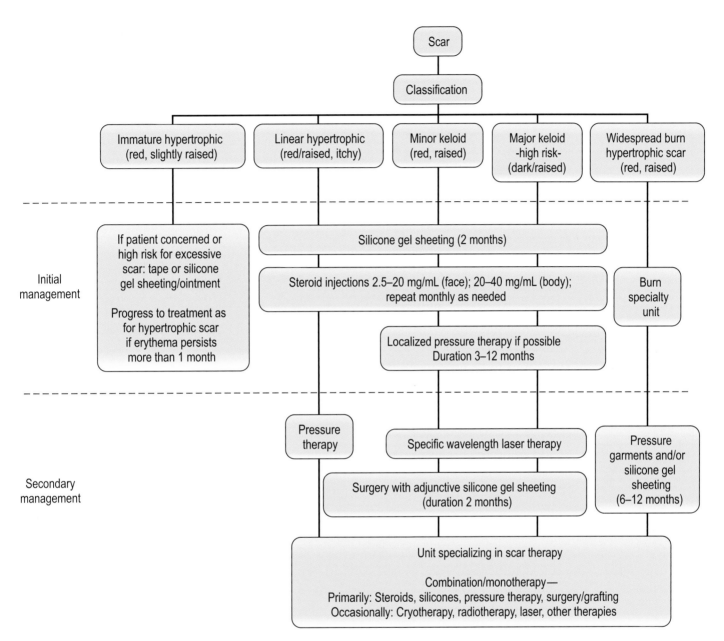

Fig. 15.8 Scar management algorithm. (Reproduced from Mustoe TA, Cooter RD, Gold MH, *et al.* International clinical recommendations on scar management. Plast Reconstr Surg 2002; 110: 560–571, with permission.)

therapy.[203] Concurrent steroid injections are helpful for pruritic or resistant scars. Pressure therapy can be added when feasible. Pulsed-dye laser (585 and 595 nm) treatment of hypertrophic scars is another alternative. Light energy from the pulsed-dye laser is absorbed by intravasal hemoglobin leading to coagulation, vessel obstruction, and tissue hypoxia with necrosis. As a consequence, new collagen synthesis, collagen fiber realignment, and remodeling are the molecular bases for the effects seen after pulsed-dye laser treatment.[210]

Widespread burn hypertrophic scars (red, raised)

Extensive surface-area burn hypertrophic scars may best be treated at burn centers when feasible. Multimodality therapies are generally used; these include silicone gel sheeting, custom-fitted pressure garments, and physical therapy alone or with massage, electrical stimulation, or ultrasound. Steroid injection of especially difficult areas is sometimes necessary. Laser treatment can be useful.[211] Surgical treatment with

Z-plasty, excision and grafting, and flap reconstruction is frequently required.[203]

Minor keloids (red, raised)

No uniformly successful treatment for keloid scar exists. Excision and primary closure invariably result in recurrence. Therefore, additional therapy is necessary, and its efficacy depends on the timing of the patient's presentation. Steroid injection directly into the keloid has the most benefit early in the keloid course.[212] Steroid has been shown to decrease collagen gene expression.[213] Mixed with 2% plain lidocaine in a 50:50 ratio, triamcinolone acetonide 10 mg/mL is commonly used initially; if no response occurs, 40 mg/mL concentration is attempted. Silicone gel sheeting should be used concurrently. Patients presenting with mature keloid lesions of months to years in duration that are slowly changing respond poorly to steroid injection and silicone sheeting. Surgical excision with adjuvant therapy including intralesional steroids, silicone sheeting, and pressure therapy is a reasonable treatment alternative.[210] Careful follow-up is necessary to prevent recurrence. A short course of low-dose radiation therapy to the keloid excision site immediately after excision has been shown to reduce the rate of recurrence.[214]

Major keloids (dark, raised)

Major keloids are difficult to treat effectively, and many are resistant to any treatment. Surgical therapy with all adjunctive therapies described before may still fail and result in recurrence. Radiation therapy is generally used in this group, provided the patient is not young and accepts the possible risk of late cancer formation. Before surgery is performed with postoperative adjuvant therapy, patients should be counseled about the high rate of recurrence with the risk that the next keloid will be larger and more difficult to control. As recommended by the International Advisory Panel on Scar Management, these patients may best be treated by clinicians with a special interest in keloid treatment.[203]

Impact of scar on plastic surgery

Besides hypertrophic scarring and keloid formation in the skin, scar affects every aspect of plastic surgery. Scar and fibrosis are the outcome after tissue repair and,

when excessive, lead to clinical disease. For example, fibrosis of joint capsules leads to contracture, which can be debilitating. Anastomotic fibrosis of free jejunal flaps to the esophagus or pharynx leads to lumen obstruction. Breast implant capsules are the normal fibrotic response to injury, which can be excessive and develop into capsular contracture. Nerve repair sites with excess fibrosis commonly develop neuromas and functional repair failure. Scarring at tendon repair sites restricts motion. Dupuytren disease is a fibroproliferative disorder that involves the palmar fascia and the deep dermis. Each of these excessive scarring conditions leads to morbidity of the patient, which can require further surgical treatment.

Emerging scar therapies

A great deal of research is focused on the development of treatment strategies to reduce or prevent scarring. Prompted by fetal wound-healing observations, investigators initially analyzed the antiscarring effect of anti-TGF-β strategies. Treatment with neutralizing antibody to TGF-β decreased the inflammatory response and reduced scar formation in experimental postnatal rodent wounds.[215] More evidence that TGF-β-related strategies may be successful is provided by a study showing that exogenous addition to wounds of fibromodulin, a TGF-β modulator, reduces scar.[89] Clearly, more studies are needed, and because of the redundancy of action among growth factors, TGF-β is likely not to be the only growth factor targeted to reduce human scar and fibrosis.

Newer treatment modalities, such as intralesional injection of bleomycin, 5-fluorouracil, and, imiquimod may be useful in the future. These act by decreasing inflammation and collagen synthesis; however, their mechanisms of action remain under investigation. Interferon therapy was left because of adverse side-effects and high recurrence rates.[210,216] Other novel strategies include the application of antifibrotic human recombinant growth factors and cytokines (e.g., rh IL-10), anti-inflammatory substances, protease inhibitors, and molecules that interfere with profibrotic cytokine function (e.g., TGF-β) and collagen synthesis at the wound site.[217]

Clinical trials are currently performed using two different novel techniques for scar reduction. Selective photothermolysis is induced by erbium-doped fiber lasers operating at a wavelength of 1550 nm, targeting water as a chromophore. This creates dermal microlesions with controlled width, depth, and densities followed by neocollagenesis.[218] These lasers are used for the treatment of hyperpigmentation and acne scars as well as surgical and traumatic scars. Percutaneous collagen induction therapy is currently used in our department for reduction of hypertrophic scars, striae distensae, wrinkles, and skin laxity. After pretreatment with vitamin A and C cream, patients are treated under anesthesia. Needles of the Medical Roll-CIT create dermal microwounds and separate collagen structures connecting the scar with the upper dermis. Through the following inflammatory reaction, collagen remodeling is induced with consequent scar flattening.[219]

Future perspectives

Growth factor and protease-scavenging therapy

The best-studied growth factors with the most promise to improve healing are PDGF, TGF-β, and members of the FGF family *(Table 15.1)*. However, before widespread use, several obstacles must be overcome, including efficacious application, vehicle development, and cost. For example, nonhealing human wound fluid and tissue have increased protease activity, which probably degrades rapidly exogenously applied peptide growth factors.[118,220] Products targeting excessive activity could be protease-scavenging matrices (e.g., Promogran),[196] selective inhibitors,[221] or specific antibodies.

Experimental and clinical trials have reported some efficacy of growth factors for treatment of chronic or burn wounds. VEGF gene transfer was effective in ischemic leg ulcers with formation of collateral vessels.[222] Topical recombinant bovine FGF, human KGF (repifermin), and GM-CSF increased healing of chronic pressure and venous leg ulcers, respectively. Topical recombinant human EGF had a positive effect on healing of second-degree burn wounds whereas topical recombinant human PDGF-BB (becaplermin), TGF-β$_2$ and granulocyte colony-stimulating factor were effective on diabetic foot ulcers. However, for chronic wound therapy, so far only PDGF-BB has been licensed for commercial use in the US and Europe.[196,223]

Gene therapy

Gene therapy to enhance wound repair through introduction of a growth factor gene, or other therapeutic gene, into repair cells is actively undergoing investigation. With this approach, the gene must be delivered to the target cell and its expression sustained at a therapeutic level; the level and timing of its expression must be reversibly controlled so that it can be stopped when it is no longer needed.[224] Several delivery vehicles are being developed, each with unique advantages and disadvantages. Replication-deficient adenovirus, herpes simplex virus type 1, and retrovirus vectors have been successfully used to transfect epidermal and dermal cells and tissues.[224,225] Other delivery approaches eliminate the virus and its possible risk of untoward side-effects due to antigenicity, potential recombination with wild-type viruses, and cellular damage from persistent viral exposure. Nonviral methods are categorized into chemical and physical methods of gene transfer. Liposome-mediated gene transfer is a chemical method in which the gene is bound to a synthetic liposome vesicle and carried into the target cell by endocytosis. FGF,[226] IGF-1,[224] KGF,[227] and VEGF[228] genes have been successfully transferred into experimental wounds. Particle-mediated gene transfer (gene gun) directly injects DNA into the cells and has been used for TGF-β$_1$,[229] EGF,[230] and PDGF[231] gene transfer in experimental wounds. Gene therapy is likely to become an increasingly important tool for the treatment of nonhealing wounds as its methods advance. In a phase I clinical trial the safety, feasibility, and biologic plausibility of adenovirus-mediated rhPDGF-BB gene therapy to treat venous leg ulcer disease were demonstrated.[232]

Extreme redundancy exists in the function of growth factors at the wound site. In addition, multiple simultaneous processes are occurring during repair. Thus, it is likely that multiple growth factors may need to be added on impaired and even otherwise normal wounds to effect a clinically significant improvement in repair quality and rate. Different growth factor combinations may be needed to treat impaired wounds due to different underlying diseases, such as diabetes versus arterial insufficiency. To complicate matters further, neutralization of certain growth factors may be necessary as well as augmentation of other factors in the same wound.

Stem cell therapy

Multipotent adult stem cells have come into focus as cellular replacement and growth factor delivery source for skin tissue defects and nonhealing wounds because of abundance and easy accessibility in each patient. Furthermore, autologous grafting avoids the risk of rejection and ethical or moral considerations concerning allogenic or embryonic material. Two major types of adult stem cells are available: epidermal and mesenchymal stem cells (MSCs). Epidermal stem cells are located to the basal layer and hair follicles, and contribute to re-epithelialization after wounding.[233] Takahashi et al. reported another promising access to epidermal cells by reprogramming dermal fibroblasts into pluripotent epidermal stem cells.[234]

MSCs are found in various mesoderm-derived tissues. MSCs have the potential either to transdifferentiate into tissues of mesodermal origin, e.g., skeletal muscle, bone, tendons, cartilage, and fat, or to "cross-differentiate" into nonmesodermal cells under appropriate conditions.[235] Promising results were reported treating chronic wounds with bone marrow-derived MSC.[236] Because of easier accessibility and tissue abundance, adipose tissue is an important source of mesenchymal stem cells. Harvesting and labeling techniques have been refined and automatized for better clinical availability.[237,238] Pilot studies using multipotent adipose tissue-derived stem cells (adMSC) for soft-tissue replacement and coverage of nonhealing wounds are currently ongoing in our department.

Our understanding of the biomolecular regulation of repair and handling of autologous cells and tissues is rapidly expanding while modern biotechnology keeps pace with scientific progress. Pilot studies will prove whether it is worthwhile continuing these futuristic approaches with controlled clinical trials.

 Access the complete reference list online at **http://www.expertconsult.com**

10. Singer AJ, Clark RA. Cutaneous wound healing. *N Engl J Med*. 1999;341:738–746.

17. Sternlicht MD, Werb Z. How matrix metalloproteinases regulate cell behavior. *Annu Rev Cell Dev Biol*. 2001;17:463–516.

26. Risau W. Mechanisms of angiogenesis. *Nature*. 1997; 386:671–674.

30. Tomasek JJ, Gabbiani G, Hinz B, et al. Myofibroblasts and mechano-regulation of connective tissue remodelling. *Nat Rev Mol Cell Biol*. 2002;3: 349–363.

42. Toriseva M, Kahari VM. Proteinases in cutaneous wound healing. *Cell Mol Life Sci*. 2009;66: 203–224.

51. Werner S, Grose R. Regulation of wound healing by growth factors and cytokines. *Physiol Rev*. 2003;83: 835–870.

75. Buchanan EP, Longaker MT, Lorenz HP. Fetal skin wound healing. *Adv Clin Chem*. 2009;48:137–161.

86. Kong W, Li S, Longaker MT, et al. Blood-derived small Dot cells reduce scar in wound healing. *Exp Cell Res*. 2008;314:1529–1539.

138. Lansdown AB, Mirastschijski U, Stubbs N, et al. Zinc in wound healing: theoretical, experimental, and clinical aspects. *Wound Repair Regen*. 2007;15:2–16.

161. Werner S, Krieg T, Smola H. Keratinocyte-fibroblast interactions in wound healing. *J Invest Dermatol*. 2007;127:998–1008.

16

Scar prevention, treatment, and revision

Peter Lorenz and A. Sina Bari

SYNOPSIS

- From our most precise aesthetic work to our most challenging reconstructive cases, preventing and treating problem scars are key to patient satisfaction and good surgical outcomes. Understanding scarring determines our surgical planning, our approach, and our technique. In follow-up care, minimizing scarring can lead to both improved form and function. Even long after recovery, patients with pathologic or abnormal scarring may seek the expertise of a plastic surgeon for scar revision. And the most senior of surgeons can attest to the challenges of managing scarred tissue in reoperative surgery.

- To begin to tackle these obstacles, plastic surgeons have created an arsenal of tools based on the central tenets of our discipline. Published in 1957 by Gillies and Millard, *The Principles and Art of Plastic Surgery* defined the fundamental doctrines of plastic surgery and has formed the foundation of our field.[1] Operative scar treatment and revision rely on these principles. Ideas such as diagnosing before treating, making a plan, marking landmarks, "borrowing" tissue from areas that have it to give, and restoring the beautiful normal frame our approach to managing scars. Rather than having a single operation for each defect, the plastic surgeon is charged with crafting these principles to the individual patient.

- To our surgical armamentarium we've added our growing understanding of scar biology. Fetal models have shed light on the complex factors which determine scarring versus scarless wound healing. In addition, we have deepened our understanding of the mechanisms that lead to pathological hypertrophic and keloid scar formation. Advances in cell and tissue biology have revealed many new therapeutic targets currently under active investigation.

- Despite our tools and advances, each treatment, nevertheless, begins with the patient. A good treatment outcome is rarely achieved without first understanding the patient's antecedent experience, current complaints, and future expectations. Herein we will describe important aspects in approaching a scarred patient, assessing a scar and understanding scar biology. We will then focus on strategies in preventing, treating, and revising scars. These strategies increasingly reflect both modern advancements in medicine as well as time-proven principles of surgery.

Personal and social significance of scars

Scars are often deeply emotional. For physicians, scars represent an endpoint in tissue healing. For our patients, however, scars often have deeper, more personal meanings. Deformities from disease, violent trauma, or aberrations of development can result in lifelong physical and psychological burdens. Treating scars requires an understanding of the psychological and social distress a patient may experience.

Scars may arise from both culturally sanctioned and prohibited practices. Ritual scarring, or cicatrization, was an important part of identifying tribal belonging in parts of Africa and Australia.[2] In tribal communities in Sudan and Papa New Guinea, the prevalence of keloid formation in certain racial groups has been exploited for spiritual and cultural markings. Likewise, the Japanese art of tattoo, or *irezumi*, carried sufficient cultural weight as to be banned until 1945, when occupational forces again legalized its practice. Today tattooing and, to a lesser degree, branding and scarification, continues to be a popular form of self-expression. While accepted to some degree within society, the psychology of these scars may overlap with that of the more pathologic, but no less intentional, scars of self-injury and self-mutilation.[3]

In western culture, scars often carry a sinister or menacing connotation. Gender clearly plays a role in the effect of scars. A recent study suggests that some facial scars in men signal risk-taking and bravery, being perceived as more attractive.[4] This effect was not found when observers were shown similarly scarred women. Nevertheless, many scars clearly carry negative social implications for both genders. Studies of quality of life measures in burn patients reveal significant interference with physical comfort as well as social and work life.[5] Depression and posttraumatic stress disorder (PTSD) have been identified as potential long-term sequelae. Rates for PTSD in burn patients range from 23% to 45% at 1 year following injury.[6] Risk factors include avoidant coping strategies and pre-existing psychiatric history as well as hand and face involvement and burn severity.[7] Understanding what specific aspects of the patient's life are most hampered can help direct both medical and nonmedical therapy.

Psychologist Thomas F Cash described the importance in reconciling a patient's "view from the outside" and "view from the inside" in coping with deformity.[8] Understanding the social context and patient's emotional relationship to scars is, therefore, vital to treatment. A potentially useful tool in understanding and assessing these variables is *Psychological Aspects of Reconstructive and Cosmetic Plastic Surgery: Clinical, Empirical, and Ethical Perspectives.*[9] Published in 2006, this title reflects a multidisciplinary effort of leading psychologists, psychiatrists, and surgeons in determining and delivering care to patients with real or perceived deformities.

History and physical examination

As with all forms of treatment, the first step in evaluating a patient with a scar is obtaining a focused history and performing a physical examination *(Box 16.1)*. The etiology of the scar must be determined as well as relevant influencing factors such as prior dissatisfactory surgery, violent crime, or infection. The treating

---

> **Box 16.1 Key points**
>
> **History**
> Etiology
> History of infection
> Associated symptoms (pain, itching)
> Radiation and steroid exposure
> **Physical exam**
> Size, color, texture
> Relationship to normal structures
> Tethering and contracture
> Changes with movement

physician must be careful to empathize with the patient without laying or refuting blame on prior treating physicians. Often this can be accomplished by focusing on the problem and appropriate next steps instead of past mistakes. Little can be gained from implicating other physicians who may earnestly seek your expertise with managing difficult scars.

Physical exam includes assessment of the scar as well as the surrounding tissue. With facial scars, attention must be made to normal folds and features as determined by the aesthetic subunits. Examination of other scars on the patient to determine predisposition to poor scarring is useful. Evaluation of the scar should include written and photographic documentation of size, color, and texture. The relationship of the scar to surrounding structures in motion and repose should be carefully assessed to determine tethering and contracture.

Scars may result in functional, aesthetic, or emotional problems. Most often, patients incur hardship through a complex and changing relationship between all three dimensions. Before initiating treatment, the physician must take the time to understand and diagnose each element. The extent of scar must be considered along with the patient's intent in getting treatment. Arriving at realistic goals and expectations may take multiple visits or a combination of surgery and counseling. Frequently, scheduling a second or third visit to ensure the patient understands with realistic expectations the planned treatment is in the surgeon's best interest.

Assessing scars

Clinical evaluation of a scar is necessary in determining the best course of treatment and, once initiated, the

Table 16.1 The Vancouver Scar Scale	
Pigmentation	
0	Normal: color that closely resembles the color of the rest of the body
1	Hypopigmentation
2	Hyperpigmentation
Vascularity	
0	Normal: color that closely resembles the color of the rest of the body
1	Pink
2	Red
3	Purple
Pliability	
0	Normal
1	Supple: flexible with minimal resistance
2	Yielding: giving way to pressure
3	Firm: inflexible, not easily moved, resistant to manual pressure
4	Banding: rope-like tissue that blanches with extension of the scar
5	Contracture: permanent shortening of the scar, producing deformity or distortion
Height	
0	Normal: flat
1	<2 mm
2	<5 mm
3	>5 mm

(Reproduced from Sullivan T, Smith J, Kermode J, *et al.* Rating the burn scar. *J Burn Care Rehabil.* 1990;11:256–260.)

effectiveness of therapy. Multiple objective and subjective assessment tools have been devised to characterize scars. The ideal scale must demonstrate validity, interobserver reliability, and clinical applicability. While there is yet no universal consensus on scar grading, the most frequently used measure is the Burn Scar Index, also known as the Vancouver Scar Scale (VSS) *(Table 16.1)*.[10] Originally published in 1990, the VSS was designed to assess changes in burn scars with maturity and in response to treatment. Scars are assessed for pigmentation, vascularity, pliability, and height. Scores are then assigned across these four variables based on the

degree of variance from normal skin. When applied, the scale can be a useful tool in prognosis and treatment evaluation. In 1995, Baryza and Baryza[11] found that adding a low-cost instrument could improve interobserver reliability. Their tool combined a ruler, a transparent piece of plastic, and a scoring "cheat sheet" with which to aid in measuring, blanching, and determining the score, respectively.

While perhaps the most commonly used assessment tool, the VSS is limited by its historical focus on burn scars. Other evaluation measures, such as the Visual Analog Scale (VAS), the Patient and Observer Scar Assessment Scale (POSAS), the Stony Brook Scar Evaluation Scale (SBSES), and the MCFONTZL classification system have varying levels of validation and adoption.[12] The large variety of different scales reflects the relative weakness of each system.

The VAS assesses parameters such as color, contour, and texture to correlate intraobserver as well as photographic and histologic findings.[13] The scale can be applied to both burn and surgical scars. Similarly, the POSAS was developed in 2004 for burns and has since been validated for linear scars. This scale has the benefit of incorporating patient opinion and can better assess symptoms such as pain, itchiness, and thickness.[14,15] A third scale, the SBSES, was initially developed as a tool for emergency medicine physicians to evaluate wounds at the time of suture removal.[16] The SBSES has since been adapted for long-term evaluation of scars and has been used as an outcome measure in Food and Drug Administration-mandated clinical trials.[17] Lastly, the MCFONTZL classification system was developed specifically for facial trauma *(Table 16.2)*.[18] This system incorporates billing and uses a mnemonic to divide the face into the maxilla, chin, forehead, orbits, nose, temple, zygoma, and lip. These scales have been useful in comparing outcomes from conventional versus minimally invasive surgery, use of wound closure adhesives, and new therapeutic agents for scar treatment.

A number of instruments have also been used as tools to assess scars objectively. Blood flow has been analyzed by laser Doppler, while depth and color have been studied by ultrasound and spectrometery.[19] Skin elasticity meters, commercialized for evaluation of scleroderma, have also been used to evaluate scars.[20] These instruments have largely been used in research rather than clinical settings.

Table 16.2 MCFONTZL assessment system

A Area	MCFONTZL aesthetic unit designation
S Side	
T Thickness	Depth of penetration
E Extension	Branching
R Relaxed skin tension line conformality	Directionality (relaxed skin tension lines)
I Index laceration	Laceration with maximum continuous skin interruption
S Soft-tissue defect	
K Coding	Current procedural terminology code

(Reproduced from Lee RH, Gamble WB, Robertson B, *et al*. The MCFONTZL classification system for soft-tissue injuries to the face. *Plast Reconstr Surg.* 1999;103:1150–1157.)

Scar biology

Scars form as the body's natural response to injured tissue. The process of scar formation reflects our body's attempt to restore tissue strength and integrity. The imperfect nature of this process, resulting in the morphologic differences between scarred and normal tissue, likely demonstrates a trade-off of organization for debridement and sterilization. The gross differences between scarred and normal tissue reflect histologic differences that define scar. A mature scar, the final product of normal wound healing, is characterized by its disorganized array of collagen and loss of dermal appendages. Rather than a static entity, however, scar represents a broad area in the evolution of a healing wound.

The process of scar formation proceeds temporally from the initial injury through the phases of wound healing into a mature scar, and at times into scar pathology *(Fig. 16.1)*. Wound repair is initiated following injury from trauma, surgery, or disease. The first stage of repair is inflammation, which is characterized by a platelet and white blood cell infiltrate that typically maximizes at 2–3 days. Mediated by the clotting and complement cascades, this initial cellular response is aimed at the establishment of hemostasis and phagocytosis of injured cells. In a noninfected wound, inflammatory cells are then replaced by fibroblasts in the proliferative stage of wound healing. This phase is characterized by synthesis and secretion of the extracellular matrix (ECM).

The ECM is formed by a complex, highly regulated process of synthesis, deposition, and degradation. The initial wound environment is largely composed of fibrin and the glycoaminoglycan hyaluronic acid. As fibroblasts populate the wound, enzymes degrade the matrix and collagen is deposited. Cross-linking and organization of the collagen ultimately create tensile strength across the wound. The process of collagen deposition and degradation is in part determined by the regulation of matrix metalloproteinases (MMPs), which in turn, are inactivated by proteins called tissue inhibitors of metalloproteinases (TIMPs). The balance of MMP-TIMP function is an active area of research in wound healing and scar biology.[21]

At the cellular level, scars are characterized by a lack of connective tissue organization compared to surrounding normal tissue architecture. Grossly, the early or immature scar is red because of its dense capillary network. Over a period of months, the capillaries regress until relatively few remain and the red color fades. The scar remodels slowly over months to years to form a "mature" scar. Mature scars are usually hypopigmented and appear lighter than the surrounding skin after full maturation. Scars can, however, be hyperpigmented and darker than the surrounding skin. Hyperpigmentation is more common in darkly pigmented patients or those lighter-pigmented patients whose scars receive excess sun exposure. For this reason, surgeons recommend sun protection for patients with early scars on sun-exposed areas such as the scalp, face, and neck.

During remodeling, wounds gradually become stronger with time. Wound tensile strength increases rapidly from 1 to 8 weeks postwounding. Thereafter, tensile strength increases at a slower pace and has been documented to increase up to 1 year after wounding in animal studies *(Fig. 16.2)*. Nevertheless, the tensile strength of wounded skin at best only reaches approximately 80% that of unwounded skin. A mature scar, the final result of tissue repair, is brittle, inelastic, and without skin appendages such as hair follicles or sweat glands. The costs of these imperfections are balanced by the benefits of rapid re-establishment of tissue integrity, debridement, and sterilization of contaminated wounds.

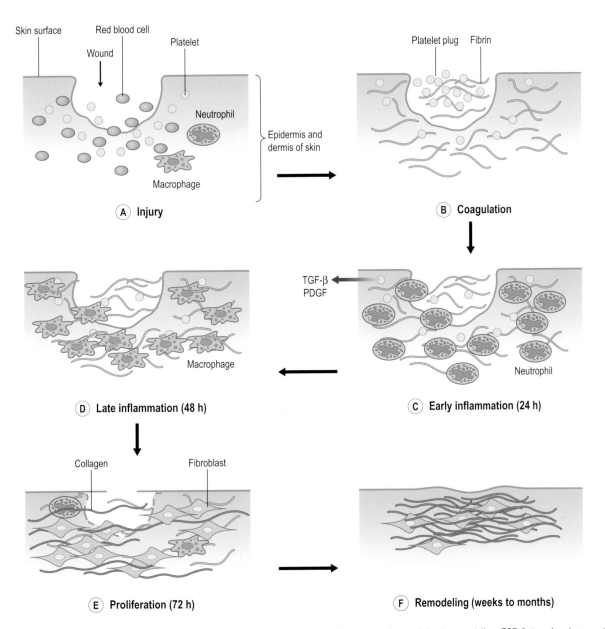

Fig. 16.1 (A–F) Phases of wound healing. Wounds progress through inflammation, proliferation, and finally remodeling. TGF-β, transforming growth factor-β; PDGF, platelet-derived growth factor.

Conditions of excessive scarring

Wound healing is a highly regulated process involving cell–cell signaling and environmental cues. In normal wounds, the repair process slows when the dermal defect is closed and epithelialization is complete. When these signals are absent or ineffective, the repair process may continue unabated and result in conditions of excessive scar. Hypertrophic scars and keloids are both fibroproliferative disorders of wound repair reflecting this excess healing.

In general, both keloid and hypertrophic scar fibroblasts have an upregulation of collagen synthesis, deposition, and accumulation. The underlying regulatory mechanisms leading to excessive repair are not yet known. Profibrotic cytokines such as transforming growth factor-β1 (TGF-β1) have been implicated.[22]

Evidence also suggests a lack of programmed cell death, or apoptosis, of activated fibroblasts secreting ECM components.[23] Hypertrophic scars and keloids are unique to humans and do not naturally occur in other animals for unknown reasons.

Normotrophic, hypertrophic, and keloid scar vary little histologically.[24] Pathological scar types are, therefore, distinguished based on clinical characteristics. Hypertrophic scars continue to thicken and rise instead of flattening and shrinking as mature scars but stay within the original scar boundary; keloid scars continue to grow beyond the boundaries of the initial wound *(Table 16.3)*. Because the time line from immature scar to mature scar to hypertrophic and keloid scar can vary due to a number of factors, diagnosis is not always clear. Important differences, however, do exist and are relevant to treatment.

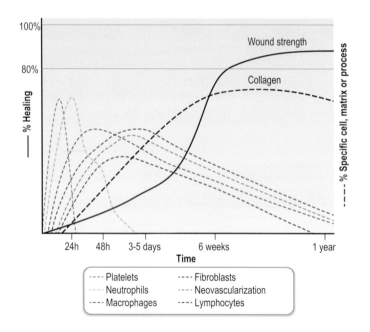

Fig. 16.2 Wound tensile strength with time. Wounds reach approximately 80% of their preinjury tensile strength at 6 weeks. Further gains occur slowly over time and never achieve 100% preinjury strength.

Clinical monitoring of scar evolution with frequent serial examinations is the most important strategy for diagnosing and treating the problem scar. Early application of treatment modalities, discussed in depth later in this chapter, can often prevent further progression and even reverse scar pathology.

Hypertrophic scar

Hypertrophic scars are defined as pathologic scars that have not overgrown the original wound boundaries, but are instead raised *(Fig. 16.3)*. Hypertrophic scar is often painful and pruritic, due to a process that may be mediated by higher levels of the neuropeptide substance P.[25] These scars usually form secondary to excessive tensile forces across the wound and are most common in wounds across flexion surfaces, the extremities, breasts, sternum, and neck.

Hypertrophic scar is a self-limited process after tissue injury, and usually regresses with time. These scars will eventually fade in color as well as flatten to the surrounding skin level, though the unaided process may take years. No clear histological differences between hypertrophic scar and keloid exist. Early studies found that keloids contained bundles of collagen around focal nodules of proliferation.[26] Later studies, however, refuted this distinction. More recently, a study using confocal laser scanning microscopy suggested keloids can be distinguished by the presence of thicker collagen fibers.[24] Advances in animal models of hypertrophic scar, including the rabbit ear, red Duroc pig, and mouse will likely be the key to future understanding of hypertrophic scar biology.[23,27,28]

Keloid

Scars that overgrow the original wound edges are called keloids *(Fig. 16.4)*. This clinical characteristic

Table 16.3 **Types of scar**			
	Appearance	**Growth pattern**	**Cause**
Normal mature scar	Hypo- or hyperpigmented, flat	Contracts slowly over time	Normal tissue repair
Immature scar	Red, slightly elevated, sometimes itchy	Turns into mature scar	Normal tissue repair
Hypertrophic	Raised, itchy, painful, confined to its borders	Self-limited, but may take years	Excess mechanical stress
Keloid	Raised, itchy, extending into normal tissue	Continued growth; recurs	Genetic predisposition, can result from minor trauma

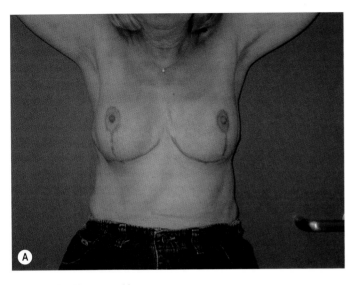
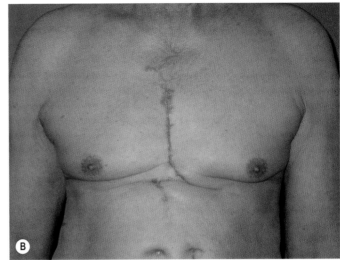

Fig. 16.3 (A, B) Hypertrophic scars.

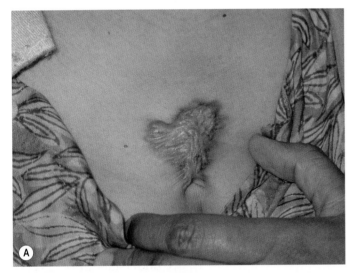
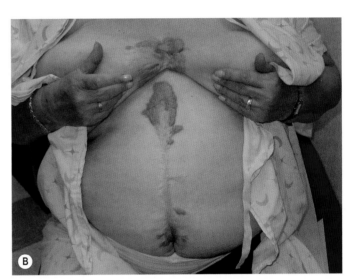

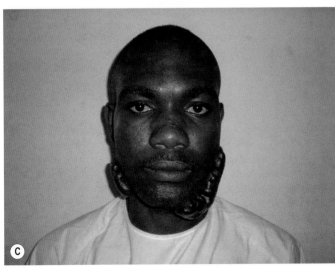
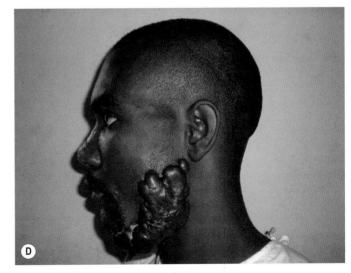

Fig. 16.4 (A–D) Keloids. (With permission from Dr. Shelly Noland.)

distinguishes keloids from hypertrophic scars. True keloid scar is not common and occurs predominantly in darkly pigmented individuals, with an incidence of 6–16% in African populations. It has a genetic predisposition with autosomal-dominant features. The keloid scar continues to enlarge past the original wound boundaries and behaves like a benign skin tumor with continued slow growth. Complete excision and primary closure of the defect, however, result in recurrence in the majority of cases.

Keloids consist mainly of collagen. They are relatively acellular in their central portions with fibroblasts present along their enlarging borders. Keloids do not, however, contain a significant excess number of fibroblasts. Collagen scar deposition outpaces degradation, and the lesion continues to enlarge.

Keloid formation may be the result of excessive stimulation or an inappropriate response to stimulation. *In vitro* studies find that keloid keratinocytes and fibroblasts respond differently than normal wound cells to growth factors found at the repair site. TGF-ß treatment, for example, causes a greater degree of collagen gene expression in keloid compared to normal wound fibroblasts.[29] In addition, a greater degree of profibrotic growth factor expression occurs in keloids compared to normal wounds.[30] These and other studies suggest that keloid formation occurs because of increased expression and activity of proliferative growth factors at the wound site.

Alternatively, a defect affecting the repair process may result in the absence of appropriate "stop" signals for healing. In this proposed mechanism, a lack of stop signals in the wound results in continued and unchecked repair. Studies of apoptotic cell numbers have found similar amounts of apoptotic cells at the advancing wound edge in both normal wound scar and hypertrophic scar. In keloid scar, however, expression of apoptotic genes was decreased.[31] The biology of keloids continues to raise important questions about what factors govern normal and pathologic healing.

Prevention

Surgical technique

Notwithstanding the molecular regulation of scar formation, meticulous surgical technique continues to be

---

> Box 16.2 **Surgical technique**
>
> Atraumatic technique
> Minimizing tension
> Skin eversion
> Perfect apposition
> Use of natural skin tension

the cornerstone of successful scar minimization for the plastic surgeon *(Box 16.2)*. To begin, the plastic surgical craft utilizes fine instruments and atraumatic technique to minimize trauma to tissue. Hooks for retraction and avoidance of double grasping with forceps, for instance, help prevent crush injury to delicate tissue.

Obtaining a fine pencil line scar also relies on relieving tension on the apposed epidermal edges *(Fig. 16.5)*. Undue tension clearly plays a role in widened and hypertrophic scars. Wound tension causes edge separation and scar widening with time. Wound edges that are defined sharply and aligned without tension heal with the least amount of scar. This is accomplished by approximating tissue with deep buried subdermal stitches, relieving tension of overlying tissue, before final apposition. The Gillies near-far pulley can be used to aid approximation of higher tension tissue. Skin eversion is simply the exaggerated application of the principle of tension-free closure. Horizontal mattress and "flask-shaped" simple sutures achieve adequate eversion; however, care must be taken not to strangulate tissue with overly tight stitches.

To prevent Burow's triangles ("dog ears"), sutures should be placed at the wound periphery so that redundancy can be worked towards the middle. Apposition should be performed so as to align the epidermis of the two wound edges. When tissues of differing thicknesses are closed, care should be taken to capture a deeper bite of the thinner tissue and a more superficial bite of the thicker tissue for proper alignment. Likewise, when tissues are at differing heights, taking a deeper bite of the lower tissue can help bring that tissue level.

Final closure can be achieved through fine interrupted and mattress stitches if care is taken for prompt suture removal. Removing sutures on the face should be performed no later than 3–5 days and can be reinforced with adhesive tape strips. Failure to remove stitches in a timely fashion can result in a disfiguring railroad scar pattern from stitch marks. This, no doubt, may serve as an unwelcome calling card of your work.

Alternatively, subcuticular stitches or adhesive tissue glue can be used for final skin apposition. Permanent sutures such as polypropylene (e.g., Prolene, Ethicon) or nylon benefit from inciting less of an inflammatory reaction than absorbable biodegradable sutures. Both permanent and absorbable subcuticular stitches can be left untied with the ends secured by tape to avoid granuloma formation around knots. Removal of permanent subcuticular suture can be aided by interval

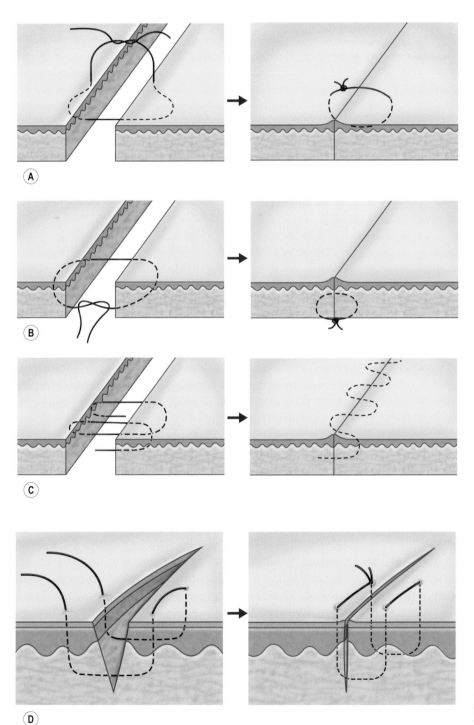

Fig. 16.5 (A–E) Skin eversion technique. Application of deep stitches approximates the dermis and relieves tension on the epidermis, contributing to less scar widening.

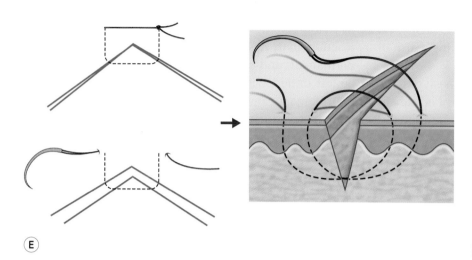

(E)

Fig. 16.5, cont'd

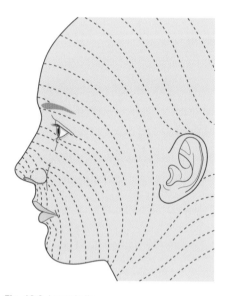

Fig. 16.6 Langer's lines.

externalization of the stitch so as not to have to pull the entire stitch through the wound.

To minimize visible scar, elective incisions are least noticeable when placed parallel to the natural lines of skin tension (Langer's lines) *(Fig. 16.6)*. This placement location has two advantages: the scar is parallel or within a natural skin crease, which camouflages the scar, and the location places the least amount of tension on the wound.

Patient-specific factors

Factors that contribute to poor wound healing may also contribute to poor scarring. Poor nutrition, diabetes, obesity, and radiation exposure may impair healing, leading to an increased risk of infection. Patients with these comorbidities should be considered at higher risk for wound complications and poor scarring. Medications such as corticosteroids and isotretinoin can also negatively affect tissue healing. Lastly, genetics plays a role in scarring, seen most dramatically in keloid formation, though the exact mechanism has yet to be determined.

Wound infections and foreign-body reactions

Wound infections and foreign-body reactions can lead to wound dehiscence and poor scarring. Increased proinflammatory cytokines may trigger abnormal fibroblast responses.[32] Leaving the initial dressing on for 48–72 hours, the time needed for epidermal closure, is a frequently used strategy to maintain wound sterility. Efforts to prevent wound infection, including debridement of any devitalized tissue and perioperative antibiotics when indicated, should be a priority.

Adjunct therapy

Taping and, more recently, coaptive films have been used as adjunctive therapy to prevent abnormal scarring.[33,34] Silicone gel sheeting, discussed in more detail later, should also be considered first-line prophylaxis. Treatment should begin shortly after wound epithelialization, be worn 12–24 hours per day and continued for at least 1 month. Breast and abdominal binders work as external splints to decrease skin tension further. As with internal sutures, care should be taken not to constrict adequate blood flow to the wound edge. Current recommendations encourage the prophylactic use of these measures in patients who have previously developed abnormal scarring or with wounds in high-risk areas such as the breast and thorax.[35]

Studies of over-the-counter remedies such as vitamin E and onion extract have failed to provide good evidence in support of their use.[36–38] These studies have been criticized, however, for their small sample size.[39] Modalities such as massage, hydrotherapy, and ultrasound need additional investigation before their role can be completely elucidated.

Lastly camouflage techniques can be a useful adjunct to address the psychosocial dimension of scar management. These strategies can be incorporated as a nurse-led aspect of a practice and may positively affect patient quality of life.[40,41] A new spray-on, computer color-matched camouflage, Microskin, has been shown to improve psychosocial measures in pediatric burn patients.[42] The product is purported to be water- and sweat-proof, requiring reapplication every 4–5 days.

Treatment

Plastic surgeons today must apply surgical, nonsurgical, and multimodal strategies in treating disfiguring and pathologic scars. Treatment should, again, be guided by diagnoses. Proper diagnosis requires addressing the patient's complaint, assessing the characteristics of the scar, and understanding the state of the scar with respect to scar biology. The approach to a 17-year-old male, for instance, emotionally burdened by mature acne scars involving multiple facial subunits, may require a combination of counseling and nonsurgical modalities. Alternatively, the functional impairment experienced by a 45-year-old woman with hypertrophic scar limiting elbow range of motion may require more invasive intervention. In general, however, noninvasive strategies, described below, offer a good starting point in the treatment algorithm.

Treatment of hypertrophic scar

Treatment options for hypertrophic scars include the application of pressure garments, silicone sheets, corticosteroids, laser therapy, and re-excision with primary closure. The latter option is most useful in cases of excess scar caused by infection or dehiscence. If the original wound was closed following the basic tenets described above, then re-excision with primary closure is not likely to result in an improved scar compared to the initial procedure. Recurrence of hypertrophic scar is quite high in these circumstances. Most surgeons, therefore, do not treat hypertrophic scar with excision and primary closure unless adjuvant therapy is also planned.

Silicone gel sheeting can both prevent hypertrophic scar formation and accelerate their involution. Though a 2006 Cochrane review found only weak evidence to support silicone sheeting, multiple randomized control trials (RCTs) have since reconfirmed its value.[43] Silicone gel sheeting has demonstrated the ability to dramatically hasten hypertrophic scar maturation and decrease associated symptoms of pain, rigidity, and pruritus.[44,45] Studies of polyurethane- and glycerin-based occlusive dressing are mixed, with some studies demonstrating effectiveness equal to silicone.[46,47] Silicone-containing oils and creams have also exhibited mixed efficacy.

Argument exists over silicone's mechanism of action.[48] One line of evidence points to increased hydration from occlusion leading to a decrease in inflammatory cytokines.[49,50] Alternative suggested mechanisms include a direct effect by silicone particles and an increase in static electrical fields.[51,52]

Since adoption in the 1970s, the use of compression garments has been a mainstay of burn scar management. Evidence in the literature, however, has been less resolute. A prospective RCT of 122 burn patients by Chang et al., for instance, failed to show significant improvement in time to scar maturation.[53] A subsequent, more precise RCT in 2005 by van den Kerckhove et al. using both subjective and objective measures found improved scar thickness when garment pressure was above 15 mmHg.[54] Perhaps most discouraging, however, was a 2009 meta-analysis of six RCTs, including those above, which found only marginal improvements of questionable clinical significance in scar thickness.[55]

Intralesional corticosteroid injections offer a second line of therapy for hypertrophic scars refractory to silicone gel sheeting. The exact mechanism is unknown but likely reflects focal suppression of inflammatory cytokines and inhibition of fibroblast proliferation.[56] Despite widespread consensus of its efficacy, few studies have objectively evaluated intralesional steroid treatment. The few studies that do exist suggest response rates well over 50%; however these studies are limited by small sample sizes and unclear evaluation criteria.[57,58] In one such study, multimodality therapy combining steroid injections with surgery improved response rates to 95% with no recurrence.[59] Local side-effects from steroid injection include pain, skin atrophy, telangiectasias, and dyspigmentation, demanding careful application.

Pulsed-dye laser and other wavelength-specific lasers have also been investigated for the treatment of scars. The mechanism of action is unknown; however absorption by hemoglobin with capillary ablation and reduced perfusion has been suggested.[60] Definitive conclusions have been hampered by small sample size, short-term follow-up, and lack of adequate controls in most studies. Review of the dermatologic literature suggests some efficacy when used as a monotherapy, especially in symptomatic relief of pruritic and erythematous lesions.[61] Ablative CO_2 and argon lasers have fallen out of favor in treating proliferative scars due to high recurrence rates. Newer high-energy pulsed CO_2 and Er-YAG lasers, however, are under investigation and may have promise in the treatment of atrophic scars.[62] Larger-scale studies with long-term results are needed to define the role of laser therapy in scar management.

Topical treatments for hypertrophic scars offer the advantage of convenience and, potentially, cost. Unfortunately, an effective salve has yet to be developed. Over-the-counter remedies, including vitamin A, vitamin E, and onion extract, have failed to show conclusive evidence in treating or preventing hypertrophic scarring. Prescription topical immune modular, imiquimod 5%, has also been investigated for scar treatment and prevention. While early results suggested improved cosmesis in postsurgical scars, subsequent studies have failed to reproduce the effects.[63,64] Lastly, skin-lightening agents containing hydroquinone or retinol can aid in the treatment of hyperpigmented scars.[65] Their use, however, carries risk of significant side-effects and should prompt caution. In 2006, concern over the carcinogenic risk of hydroquinone prompted a ban of over-the-counter preparations over 2% in the US and a comprehensive ban in Europe.

Treatment of keloid scar

There exists no uniformly successful treatment of keloid scar. Therefore critical discussion of the risk of recurrence with potential patients prior to embarking on therapy is essential. Nevertheless, the disfiguring physical and psychological burden of keloid scars frequently mandates intervention. Symptoms of pain and burning are common. In such cases, best practice guidelines currently emphasize the importance of multimodal therapy. Even so, appropriate goals must be set and the patient must be aware that lesions may redevelop and may even worsen on recurrence. The only viable treatment options for mature keloids are to monitor and do nothing or to excise and administer adjuvant therapy. Excision and primary closure alone invariably result in recurrence.

Adjuvant therapies include steroid injection, radiation, cryotherapy, laser, and antitumor or immunosuppressive agents. Intralesional corticosteroid injection therapy is the first line in keloid treatment. Additionally, steroid therapy has shown synergistic benefit of other modalities, including laser, radiotherapy, and cryotherapy. Triamcinolone acetonide at 10 mg/mL is generally tried initially, and if no response occurs, then a 40 mg/mL concentration is attempted. The triamcinolone is mixed with 2% plain lidocaine in a 50:50 ratio. Injection into the dense scar is often painful and poses infiltration risk to the surrounding normal tissue. Early, rapidly proliferating lesions respond best to steroid injection while slowly growing, mature keloids respond poorly. Intraoperative and postoperative intralesional steroid therapy following excision has been shown to reduce recurrence to below 50%.[58,66]

A short course of low-dose (20 Gy) radiotherapy to the keloid excision wound immediately after excision has been shown in numerous retrospective studies to reduce the rate of recurrence.[67–69] A more recent prospective study, however, found recurrence rates of 72% at 1 year following excision and radiotherapy, calling into question the efficacy of this approach.[70] The immediate and long-term risks of radiation therapy, including the potential for malignant transformation, implore the need for further study. Nonetheless, radiation therapy may reasonably be considered in adults with lesions refractory to other modalities.

Cryotherapy is a low-cost and effective method of treating selected keloid scar. In multiple retrospective series, complete flattening or greater than 80% volume reduction occurred in 73–85% of lesions treated with liquid nitrogen.[71–73] Early lesions of less than 1–2 years' duration appeared to have more favorable responses. A subsequent prospective study examining cryotherapy of both hypertrophic and keloid scar found an even greater response in hypertrophic scars.[74] In this study, a good to excellent response was found in 78.9% of hypertrophic scars versus only 50.9% of keloids. Interpretation, however, is limited by vague evaluative criteria. Though the mechanism is unknown, the effects of cryotherapy appear to be synergistic with steroid injection.[75,76] Despite its potential efficacy, cryotherapy has been limited to treatment of small lesions due to potential side-effects. These include pain, blistering, lengthy wound healing, skin atrophy, and near-universal dyspigmentation.

As with other modalities in scar treatment, critical evaluation of lasers in keloid treatment has been complicated by small studies with vague diagnostic criteria and inconsistent evaluative measures. These studies are often of low levels of evidence and long-term follow-up is lacking. Additionally, the multitude of laser types and treatment algorithms further complicates direct comparative study. A 1995 study in *The Lancet*, for instance, found decreased pruritus and scar height with pulsed-dye laser treatment but did not distinguish keloid from hypertrophic scar and had follow-up limited to 6 months.[77] Though a significant amount of experience exists from a nearly 20-year history of laser scar treatment, prudent use is best advised pending further study. Our experience has been favorable when combining pulsed-dye laser with intralesional steroid injection for keloids.

In summary, while there is yet no single modality completely effective in keloid management, multimodality approaches offer some promise in management. Current treatment algorithms promote the use of corticosteroids, silicone sheeting, and compression garments as first-line therapy, especially in early, small keloids.[35] Large, recalcitrant keloids can carry significant morbidity and are very challenging to treat. Optimal management may include surgery, steroids, radiation, or other modalities and may best be performed by a surgeon or center with a focus on keloid treatment.

Emerging treatments

Local delivery of antitumor and immunomodulatory drugs presents a new area under intense investigation in the treatment of keloid and hypertrophic scar. Agents such as TGF-β modulators, interferons (IFNs), 5-fluorouracil (5-FU), and bleomycin exploit our growing understanding of scar biology to offer new solutions to age-old problems. While the body of data is still small, early evidence suggests many of these agents may hold promise for safe and effective future treatments.

The TGF-βs are profibrotic growth factors that, among other functions, attract and stimulate fibroblasts to increase collagen synthesis and decrease ECM breakdown. Changes in TGF-β activity have been linked to fibrotic diseases of the kidney, lung, and heart. A robust body of literature implicates the TGF-β family as a major determinant of scar morphology in skin.[78,79] Our deepening knowledge of signaling pathways and TGF-β isomers is now translating into new therapeutic avenues for exploration. Initial phase I/II trials of prophylactically injecting recombinant TGF-β3, for instance, show promise in improving the appearance of scars.[80]

Alternatively, IFNs are antifibrotic cytokines found to suppress the formation of collagen.[81] These findings led to trials of intralesional injections of IFN-α2b and later IFN-γ as monotherapy and postsurgical adjuvant therapy. Promising results from an early study found keloid recurrence rates of 18.7% with adjuvant IFN-α2b injection versus 51.2% with surgery alone at 7-month follow-up.[82] Subsequent studies, however, have been mixed, with some trials showing early recurrence when used as monotherapy and others showing benefits with combined therapy.[83,84] Targeted therapy with IFN, nevertheless, continues to be alluring from a biochemical standpoint, mandating further investigation.

Antineoplastic agents, 5-FU and bleomycin, are promising new pharmacologic treatments for pathologic scarring. Small RCTs have built on the experience of large clinical series to lend impressive preliminary evidence for the efficacy of 5-FU in keloid treatment.[85-87] In one study, side-by-side application of 5-FU and steroid injections on median sternotomy keloids suggested equal efficacy for 5-FU without the side-effects of skin atrophy, hypopigmentation, or telangiectasia.[88] Though far from fully elaborated, 5-FU's effects may in part be mediated via interference of the TGF-β signaling pathway.[89] Bleomycin, on the other hand, is thought to act through binding of DNA to prevent mitosis.[90] The exact mechanism in relation to keloid and hypertrophic scar is yet undetermined, though initial clinical studies from Europe suggest efficacy without systemic toxicity.[91,92] While results have thus far been impressive for both these agents, larger-scale studies are needed to validate the findings of early small studies.

Scar revision

Introduction

Plastic surgery education and techniques allow practitioners to offer surgical, nonsurgical, and combined treatment modalities to patients with scars. Treatment can therefore be dictated by a studied understanding of the pathology rather than limited to a certain tool or device. For the most disfiguring and debilitating scars, surgery is often a necessary component of therapy, if not the only effective therapy. After careful analysis of a scar's characteristics (morphology, maturity, distortion of tissues) and appropriate application of noninvasive measures, the plastic surgeon can then turn to an array of surgical tools to try to transform a difficult scar into a less perceptible one.

Indications

Patients seek scar revision for multiple reasons. As discussed earlier, scars carry both physical and psychologic implications. Understanding what role these factors play in a patient's desire for treatment is important in setting and reaching patient expectations.

Scars eliciting physical symptoms should be examined carefully. Patients will often report discomfort and tightness as a result of scar contraction. An exquisitely painful scar should be examined for a Tinel's sign which may suggest entrapment of a cutaneous nerve. Excision or repair of a neuroma is often an important part of scar revision. Scar contractures across joints, such as occur in burn patients, can result in limitations in range of motion. In such cases, treatment should be directed at restoration of function and be carried out in conjunction with aggressive physical therapy to prevent recurrence.

Scars causing disfigurement can carry powerful personal and social burdens. The surgeon should be sympathetic and nonjudgmental as these scars may be reminders of past trauma. Administering care alongside a mental health professional can help distinguish and address complicating psychological issues. For the surgeon, extra care must be taken in these circumstances to confirm realistic expectations and reinforce the goals of care.

Timing

Timing of scar revision should reflect an assessment of scar maturity and an understanding of the underlying biology. A soft supple mature scar is the ideal starting point from which to consider revision. Immature scars contain the fragile blood vessels of neovascularization, which may bleed excessively during surgery. In addition, the tissue in and surrounding immature scars is more edematous and less mobile, making local tissue rearrangement more difficult. Tissue primed for scar revision should be maximally mobile and soft.

Surgical timing should therefore be based on clinical exam, though some suggest delay for at least 18 months. Interval exams should be used to monitor a scar until one can be certain of maturity. Any uncertainty in scar maturity should prompt the physician to wait longer. This can often be difficult in patients who are eager for a solution. Nonoperative management such as massage and silicone sheeting should be stressed during this period as crucial to the best ultimate outcome. A patient's compliance with nonoperative measures during this period can help assess his or her motivations and expectations. This period can also be a time to build a relationship of trust between patient and physician. Those eager to proceed may not have realistic expectations and should be viewed cautiously. Patients should be advised that early revision will increase the risk of complications and will reset the clock on wound healing and scar maturity.

Hypertrophic scar can be thought of as a chronic inflammatory condition. Early surgery is all the more plagued by immobility and bleeding. Unless planning to excise the whole scar, surgery should be deferred until scar maturity is achieved. This can often take longer than normotrophic scars and should again be dictated by clinical exam. Dr. Millard's principle "When in doubt, don't!" bears stressing.[1]

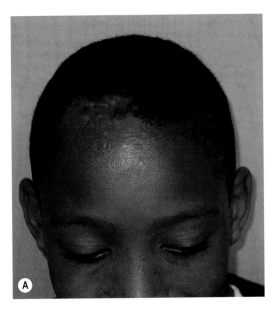 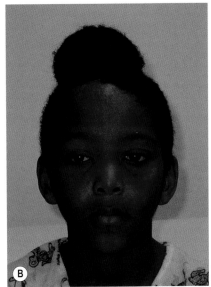 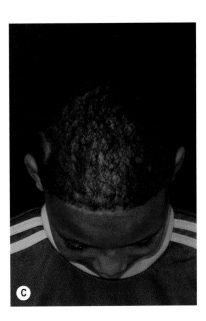

Fig. 16.7 (A–C) Serial excision.

Planning

In addition to timing, several others factors are important to consider when planning for surgical scar revision. For complex reconstructions involving multiple areas, management is best directed from larger to finer areas. Burn scars involving the head and neck, for instance, should start with resurfacing of the cervicofacial region before addressing ectropion.

Surgeons must also determine if each scar is best treated by single or multistaged revision. Single-staged operations include both simple direct excisions and more complex soft-tissue rearrangements. Unless an initial wound was widened due to infection and dehiscence, direct excision alone is rarely effective. When applicable, however, preoperative suturing and on-table tissue expansion can be used to decrease tension on a wound after direct excision. Undermining and advancement of skin edges similarly allow for reapproximation of skin edges without tension. This can be performed asymmetrically to change the degree of tension and deformity in neighboring tissue.

Serial excision and tissue expansion are staged strategies for scar revision. While seemingly simplistic, staged serial excisions of scars may provide the best results *(Fig. 16.7)*. Two or three serial excisions of large scar may accomplish what is hazardous or even impossible in a single stage. Serial excision is accomplished by circumferentially excising the margin of a scar, then undermining and advancing bordering normal tissue. The pliability of the normal tissue should be assessed before making the incision. This will dictate how much scar is safe to excise and timing of subsequent stages. Tissue expansion provides another alternative for staged scar revision. This has been especially valuable in scalp reconstruction of patients with burn alopecia, though it does carry the additional risk of infection associated with implant placement and requires two procedures for insertion and subsequent removal.

Scar release

Scarring is a three-dimensional process that often extends from superficial to deep tissue. Scar contracture in deep layers can result in puckering and tethering of the overlying tissue. This can happen even in the absence of superficial injury. Fat necrosis following blunt tissue trauma, for instance, can result in a concave skin defect without laceration. Treatment of tethered scar requires release from the underlying tissue and sometimes interposition of muscle or fascia. Soft-tissue fillers, fat autograft, and acellular dermis have all been used successfully to fill depressed scars, although long-term data are lacking.[93–95]

Acne scarring poses special considerations for the treatment of the tethered scar. The multiple pitted scars of "icepick" acne can be disfiguring and result in considerable psychological stress for the patient. Mild to moderate acne scars may benefit from resurfacing procedures such as with the CO_2 laser or chemical peels to even out contour deformities.[96] Most serious acne scars, however, require formal excision to achieve adequate depth. Focal excision with release of tethered tissue can be extremely effective but should first be applied to one or two test lesions to assess patient-specific results.

Principles of tissue rearrangement

The surgical approach to scar revision should begin with the principles outlined for scar prevention. These include atraumatic technique, tensionless closure, and proper skin eversion. Scar revision that involves tissue rearrangement, discussed further below, also requires consideration of anatomic landmarks and lines of tension. Restoration of anatomic landmarks such as the vermillion border, eyelid position, or alar base should take primacy over scar characteristics.[1] The use of local flaps in the face to prevent distortion of anatomic landmarks demonstrates this principle. Herein, a larger scar of a flap may be preferred when local tissue recruitment with a shorter scar would result in deformity of these landmarks. The first step in scar revision should similarly be restoring anatomic structures to their correct location.

Scars should be hidden in the resting lines of skin tension. Presented originally in 1861, Karl Langer's eponymous "lines" resulted from examination of the vertical wounds left by circular stab marks into a cadaver.[97] Reorientation of a scar to these lines allows for the least tension across a wound.[98] This is achieved in scar revision surgery with tissue rearrangement techniques such as Z-plasty. The lines of resting tension form the basis for the aesthetic units and subunits that dictate facial surgery.[98,99] The face, however, is dynamic and patients should be cautioned that scars may be more apparent with changes in expression.

Scar elongation and irregularization are other principles that reflect consideration of tension lines caused by scars themselves. Myofibroblasts within a mature scar cause scar contracture in the axis of the scar. A long, straight scar will result in uniform contracture in one axis, resulting in greater deformity in the surrounding tissue and greater depression of the scar. The resultant tight scar can cause limitations in movement while the change in contour can be aesthetically displeasing. In addition to reorienting a scar, local tissue rearrangement techniques break up the length of the original scar by incorporating neighboring tissue. A longer scar relaxes the pull on each end of the scar towards the center of the scar. Contractile forces are displaced into the axis perpendicular to the length of the scar. Multiple applications of this technique result in an irregular scar, wherein contractile forces are dispersed into multiple axes. This, in turn, results in less tissue deformation and an easier ability to camouflage.

Scar revision techniques

Techniques of local tissue rearrangement require an understanding of tissue properties, careful planning, and meticulous technique. When applied successfully, these simple but fundamental techniques embody the art of plastic surgery. These techniques accomplish the goals of scar reorientation, elongation, and irregularization necessary to treat difficult scars.

Though some argument exists, Z-plasty can be dated at least as far back as Horner in 1837 and Denonvilliers in 1854.[100] Their procedure for transposing triangular flaps to relieve cicatricial ectropion has evolved into the modern Z-plasty. In current nomenclature, Z-plasty refers to transposition of two triangular flaps, usually of equal size and equal angle, into each other's defect.

Planning and performing Z-plasty requires an understanding of geometric principles. The first published mathematical analysis came from Limberg in 1929.[101] Through the pythagorean theorem he revealed the theoretical gains in length achievable with changes in the angle of the lateral limbs (*Table 16.4*).[102] In practical application, however, the elasticity of skin and rigidity

Table 16.4 Z-plasty gains in length	
Angle of lateral limb of Z-plasty	Theoretical gain in length of central limb (%)
30	25
45	50
60	75
75	100
90	120

of scar create unequal deformation of the central and lateral limbs.[103] This deformation results in lower gains in length *in vivo* than would be expected in theory. Deformational forces are magnified with smaller flaps and with serial Z-plasties. Nevertheless, proper execution of a Z-plasty is essential to accomplishing what has been described as four fundamental functions: to lengthen a scar, to break up a line, to move tissue, and to obliterate or create a web or cleft *(Box 16.3).*[104]

Z-plasties have been further characterized as simple, planimetric, skew, and multiple. The simple or stereometric Z-plasty has two flaps of equal angle and length *(Fig. 16.8).* Traditionally, these flaps are raised at 60° as this angle offers the best balance between elongation in the axis of the scar and the creation of tension forces pulling perpendicular to the scar. Last-minute flap revisions can be avoided by incising and

---

Box 16.3 The four fundamental functions of Z-plasty

1. To lengthen a scar
2. To break up a straight line
3. To move tissues from one area to another
4. To obliterate or create a web or cleft

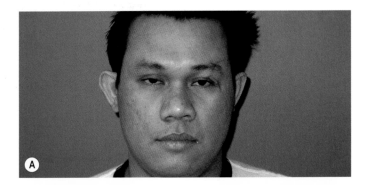

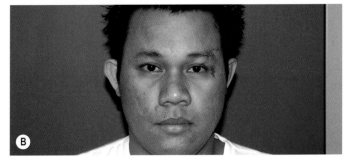

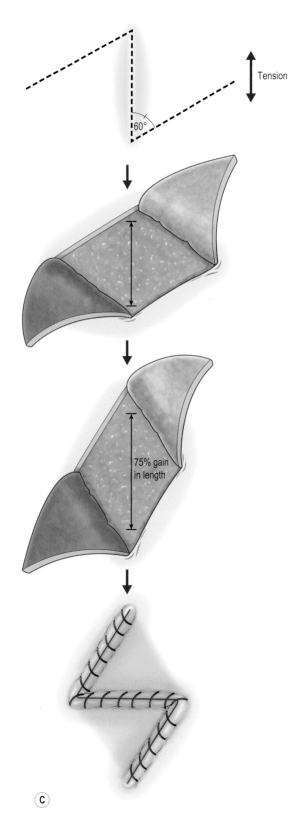

Fig. 16.8 (A–C) Simple Z-plasty.

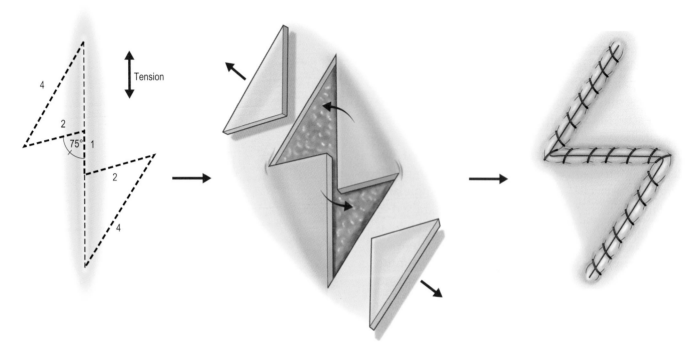

Fig. 16.9 Planimetric Z-plasty.

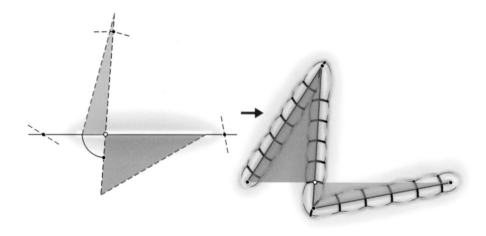

Fig. 16.10 Skew Z-plasty. (Reproduced from Furnas DW. Transposition of the screw z-plasty. Br J Plast Surg 1966;19:88-89.)

transposing one flap to determine excursion accurately *in vivo* before cutting your second flap.

The planimetric Z-plasty is a variation of the classic Z-plasty that maintains the flaps in the same plane *(Fig. 16.9)*.[105] By minimizing the amount of rotation and excising redundant tissue, this flap design avoids the contours and depressions created by simple Z-plasty. Flaps may theoretically be designed with lateral limb angles ranging from 60° to 90°, though most often they are planned at 75° angles. The planimetric Z-plasty is ideal for scar releases on flat surfaces where lengthening is the primary objective and contour deformities would be suboptimal.

Skew Z-plasties have lateral limbs departing at different angles from one another *(Fig. 16.10)*. This flap has been suggested when anatomic landmarks mandate asymmetric movement of one flap. Furnas and Fischer's topographic study in dogs revealed that the narrow flap

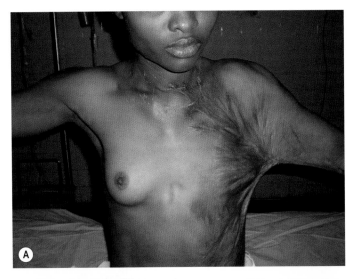

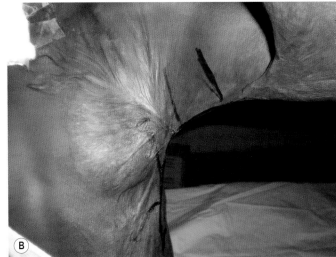

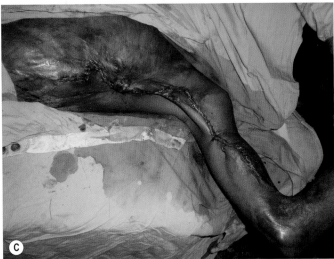

Fig. 16.11 **(A–C)** Multiple Z-plasties. (With permission from Dr. Shelly Noland.)

transposed easily but was likely to form a "dog ear," while the wider flap was difficult to transpose and caused more stretch at its base.[103] This is counterintuitive to some degree as the narrow flap has to travel through a larger arc of rotation to traverse the wide flap. For this reason, deformational forces created by skew Z-plasty flaps can be difficult to predict and its use should be avoided.

Multiple-flap Z-plasty refers to multiple Z-plasties along a scar length as well as Z-plasties designed with more than two flaps *(Fig. 16.11)*. When performing multiple Z-plasties in series, the previous Z-plasty exerts deformational forces on the tissue of the next Z-plasty, further limiting the actual gain in length. A single large Z-plasty a specific angle will therefore create more length than multiple small Z-plasties at that same angle. A large Z-plasty, however, is not always in keeping with the aesthetic and functional goals of a scar revision. Numerous Z-plasties utilizing multiple flaps have been devised. Among them, the Limberg's four-flap and Mustarde's "jumping man" five-flap Z-plasties are frequently used for release of first-webspace contractures *(Fig. 16.12)*.[101,106]

Regardless of design, care must be taken to widen the tip of flaps to avoid tip necrosis.[107] The thickness of flaps is dictated by the quality and location of the tissue. Scars often have distorted and unreliable blood supply, therefore thicker flaps are necessary. In unscarred tissue, care must be taken to elevate the subdermal vascular plexus to include the cutaneous microvasculature in your flap.

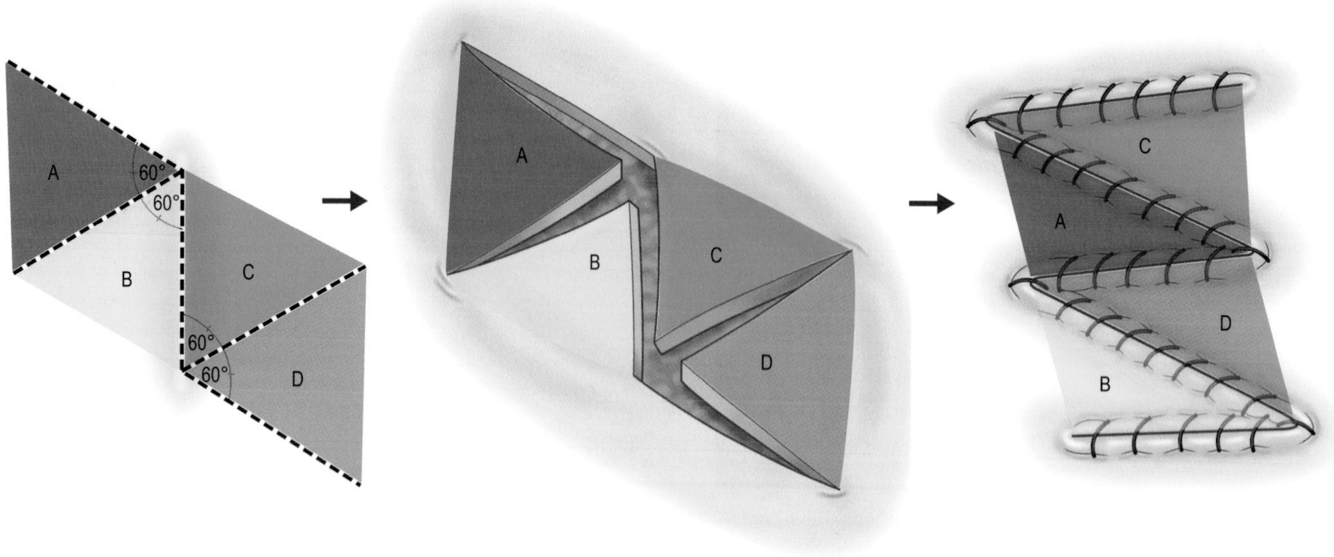

Fig. 16.12 Four-flap Z-plasty.

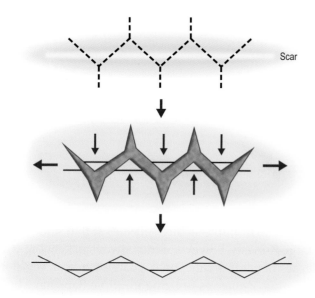

Fig. 16.13 V-Y and Y-V advancement flaps.

V-Y and Y-V advancement flaps allow for the incorporation of adjacent tissue without the threat to vasculature necessary for Z-plasty *(Fig. 16.13)*. These flaps are not transposed and therefore they do not require undermining. Like Z-plasties, these flaps can be carried out in tandem through careful flap design.

W-plasty and geometric broken line are techniques for scar irregularization *(Figs 16.14, 16.15)*.[108] W-plasty uses a zigzag pattern excision of the scar followed by reapproximation of small interdigitated limbs. There is no elongation of the scar and tissue is removed, therefore a net increase in tension is produced in the axis perpendicular to the scar. In contrast, Z-plasty trades relaxation in the axis of scar for tension perpendicular to the scar, resulting in no change in overall tension. Master artisan, Albert F Borges of Church Falls, Virginia, suggested w-plasty as a good revision technique in facial scars not in the resting lines of skin tension and without excessive tension across them.

Lastly, geometric broken line is a refined technique wherein 5–6 mm randomly distributed triangles, squares, trapezoids, and semicircles are incised at the wound edge with reciprocating shapes planned opposite them. The technique is challenging and labor-intensive; however, it may have some utility in further camouflaging facial scars that cross aesthetic subunits.

Postoperative care and follow-up

Initial postoperative care should be directed towards optimal wound healing, including adequate nutrition,

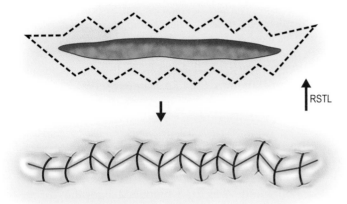

Fig. 16.14 W-plasty. RSTL, relaxed skin tension lines.

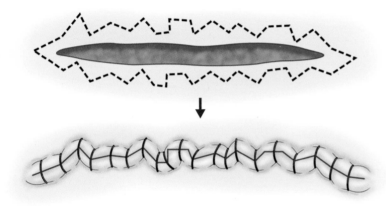

Fig. 16.15 Geometric broken line.

blood sugar control, smoking cessation, and activity precautions. Long-term scar implements techniques aimed at prevention and treatment. Following a revision, risk of recurrence should be minimized through aggressive use of taping, silicone sheeting, compression, and scar massage. Specific follow-up care should be dictated by patient-specific factors. Regardless of complexity, however, both the patient and physician benefit from long-term follow-up to evaluate personally the efficacy of any treatment strategies.

 Access the complete references list online at **http://www.expertconsult.com**

1. Gillies HD, Millard DR. *The Principles and art of plastic surgery*. Boston: Little, Brown, and Company; 1957.

   Gillies and Millard initially published 16 principles of plastic surgery in The Principles and Art of Plastic Surgery. These were later extended to 33 in The Principilization of Plastic Surgery. Millard ultimately condensed these ideas into the plastic surgeon's creed: Know the ideal beautiful normal.

9. Sarwer DB, Pruzinsky T. *Psychological aspects of reconstructive and cosmetic plastic surgery: clinical, empirical, and ethical perspectives*. Philadelphia, PA: JB Lippincott; 2006:xiii, 338.

10. Sullivan T, Smith J, Kermode J, et al. Rating the burn scar. *J Burn Care Rehabil*. 1990;11:256–260.

35. Mustoe TA, Cooter RD, Gold MH, et al. International clinical recommendations on scar management. *Plast Reconstr Surg*. 2002;110:560–571.

In 2002, The International Advisory Panel on Scar Management brought together world leaders in plastic surgery, burn management, and dermatology to evaluate critically the literature on scar therapy and set evidence-based treatment guidelines.

48. Stavrou D, Weissman O, Winkler E, et al. Silicone-based scar therapy: a review of the literature. *Aesthetic Plast Surg.* 2010;34:646–645.

55. Anzarut A, Olson J, Singh P, et al. The effectiveness of pressure garment therapy for the prevention of abnormal scarring after burn injury: a meta-analysis. *J Plast Reconstr Aesthet Surg.* 2009;62:77–84.

77. Alster TS, Williams CM. Treatment of keloid sternotomy scars with 585 nm flashlamp-pumped pulsed-dye laser. *Lancet.* 1995;345:1198–1200.

78. Lin RY, Sullivan KM, Argenta PA, et al. Exogenous transforming growth factor-beta amplifies its own expression and induces scar formation in a model of human fetal skin repair. *Ann Surg.* 1995;222: 146–154.

Landmark studies from the laboratories of pediatric surgeons, Michael R. Harrison and N. Scott Adzick, explored the molecular underpinnings of fetal development. This work enriched and corroborated the development of the field of in utero fetal surgery.

98. Borges AF. Relaxed skin tension lines (RSTL) versus other skin lines. *Plast Reconstr Surg.* 1984;73:144–150.

Cuban-born plastic surgeon Alberto F. Borges (1919–90) extolled the importance of reorienting wounds to the relaxed lines of skin tension. Though himself a master craftsman, his work in examining the principles of scar revision beyond simple technique places him among historic artisans who have helped translate craft into science.

102. Rohrich RJ, Zbar RI. A simplified algorithm for the use of Z-plasty. *Plast Reconstr Surg.* 1999;103:1513–1517; quiz 1518.

Rohrich and Zbar's review of the history and technique of Z-plasty highlights key points in flap design including flap thickness, angle, and location. Facile application of Z-plasty is necessary for all plastic surgeons to master.

17

Skin graft

Saja S. Scherer-Pietramaggiori, Giorgio Pietramaggiori, and Dennis P. Orgill

SYNOPSIS

- History of skin grafting mirrors many of the important advances of plastic surgery.
- There are complex biologic mechanisms that allow skin grafts to take.
- There are a variety of types of skin grafts that can be selected based on clinical application.
- Technique should be adjusted to avoid most complications.
- There are exciting areas of research that will help minimize donor sights and improve function and appearance of skin grafts.

 Access the Historical Perspective section online at
http://www.expertconsult.com

Skin grafting is a technique for the transfer of cutaneous tissue from one site of the body to another, often to cover large defects. Depending on the thickness of the dermis of graft that is harvested, skin grafts are defined as full-thickness or split-thickness.

Anatomy and physiology

The skin represents approximately 8% of our total body weight, with a surface area of 1.2–2.2 m². The skin is 0.5–4.0 mm thick and covers the entire external surface of the body, including the walls of the external acoustic meatus and the lateral tympanic membrane. The main function of skin is to protect body contents from the environment, including pathogens, temperature, and excessive water loss. Insulation, temperature regulation, sensation, immune function, and the synthesis of vitamin D are all critical functions of the skin. Skin loses regenerative capacity when lesioned down to the lower dermis and results in scar tissue when injured.

Epidermis

Skin has a complex three-dimensional structure characterized by two overlapping layers, the epidermis and the dermis. The epidermis, as the nervous system, derives after gastrulation from the neuroectoderm. Epidermis is the outer or upper layer of skin, which is a thin, semitransparent, water-impermeable tissue, consisting primarily of keratinocytes. These cells form a multilayered keratinized epithelium, similar to a wall of bricks. The basement membrane separates the epidermis from the dermal tissue and consists of a protein structure produced by basal keratinocytes. Basal keratinocytes are partially differentiated stem cells of the epidermis that provide the proliferative and regenerative capacity of the skin epithelium. The epithelium is metabolically active and continuously self-renews to maintain an efficient barrier function. Cellular homeostatic regulation is, as a consequence, very important: too little proliferation would bring a loss of barrier and excessive activity to hyperproliferative disorders, such as psoriasis. Homeostasis is granted by the basal epidermal cells, which periodically cycle, executing their program of terminal differentiation, a process that takes approximately 28 days. The differentiation of the keratinocytes is characterized by the progressive production of alpha-keratin, with migration towards the surface until the cells lose their intercellular connections (desmosomes), die, and become corneal lamina.

During this process, called cornification, basal keratinocytes produce tonofilaments (precursor of keratin) and then transform into the stratum spinosum as the desmosomes stretch the cells into spikes visible with a microscope. In the plasmalemma, the tonofilaments are connected to the desmosomes. Cells next start to produce keratohyalin, which aggregates in dense and basophilic granules, giving the name to the stratum granulosum. In these granules a histidine-rich protein, profilaggrin, becomes progressively filaggrin, which ultimately acts as a glue to keep keratin filaments together once the cells die and the cell membrane degrades.

As the cells divide and move up through the epidermis they eventually transform into the stratum corneum, a layer of dead cells, which ultimately is highly mechanically and chemically resistant due to chemical bonds between lipids and proteins. It is thought that cells die as the increasing proteins in their cytoplasm start to activate lysosomes. The stratum corneum provides an extremely effective barrier layer to keep water in and microorganisms out.

Also contained within the epidermis are melanocytes, Langerhans cells, Merkel cells, and sensitive nerves. Around 10% of the epidermal cells are represented by melanocytes, which derive from the neural crest. These complex dendritic cells produce melanin granules (contained in the melanosomes) that are then transported through dendrites into keratinocytes, providing color to the skin and protecting basal epithelial nuclei from ultraviolet damage. Melanocytes are anchored to the basal lamina by hemidesmosomes, but do not have desmosomic connections with other cells.

Langerhans cells are the immune cells of the epidermis and are important in generating a response to foreign agents, playing an important role in allograft rejection and contact dermatitis. These cells are situated in the stratum spinosum and, with long dendrites, slide between epithelial cells, without desmosomic connections to them. Langerhans cells share several features with macrophages of connective tissues.

Merkel cells are commonly found in the epidermis of palms, soles, nail beds, oral and genital areas. Merkel cells act as mechanoreceptors and thus are responsible for neurosensory transmission. These cells reside in the basal layer of the epidermis, often protruding into the dermal layer like nails. Merkel cells are connected by desmosomes to the neighboring cells.

Skin adnexal structures are epidermal derivatives that invaginate into the dermis with a lining of epithelial cells. They include hair follicles, sweat and sebaceous glands. These structures provide the basis for re-epithelialization following the harvest of an STSG.

Sensitive nerve supply to the skin is rich and extends through the basement membrane into the epidermis. Nerve fibers also go to skin adnexal organs that allow hair to become erect and sweat glands to secrete.

Dermis

The dermis is a tough fibrous layer that provides the mechanical features of the skin. It is composed primarily of collagens, glycosaminoglycans, and elastins. Skin grafts without the dermis result in a closed but often unstable skin. Grafting a part of the dermis is therefore very important to consider in terms of functionality of the future skin.

The upper part of the dermis has a particular architectural organization that is called papillar and contains blood vessels and nerve fibers. The papillar layer of dermis consists of fine collagenous fibers that form an undulating interface with the overlying basement membrane and epidermis. This structure increases the contact area between dermis and epidermis, allowing for maximal mechanical stability of the two layers and exchange surface for diffusion. Deeper, we find the reticular dermis, with increasingly thicker collagenous fibers (mainly of type I) as we move toward the subcutaneous tissue. The reticular dermis has larger collagenous fibers with substantial strength. The mechanical properties of the dermis are critical to allow movement while providing stability and protection from mechanical trauma. The dermis is remarkably self-healing, mainly due to the presence and activation of myofibroblasts following injury.

Blood vessel supply of the skin

Dermal vascularisation is particularly important, as blood vessels are not directly present in the relatively more metabolically active epidermal layer, glands, and hair follicles. Blood vessels set up a rich superficial plexus just underneath the basement membrane in the papillary dermis, facilitating nutrient transport to the epidermis. The blood vessels in the papillary dermis are arranged in the papillary plexus, with a rich network of capillaries in the papillae, which come in close contact with the epidermis. Deeper in the dermis is the reticular plexus from which small vessels distribute to the subcutaneous and deep dermal tissues to vascularize adnexal organs, including the hair follicle bulb. Arterial capillaries generate venous plexi, which have the same distribution of arterial vasculature. In the deep layers of dermis it is possible to find several arteriovenous anastomoses, particularly at the extremities (hands, feet, ears), where they exhibit strong muscular sphincters. The function of these structures is mainly under the control of the visceral nervous system, with the main function of thermoregulation and intravascular volume redistribution.

Blind-ended lymphatic structures are present in the dermis from where they connect to the reticular plexus and to larger vessels in the subcutaneous tissue. In this region, lymphatic vessels are larger, with valves, and drain in deeper lymphatic vessels called regional collectors. In the skin the lymphatic drainage is very active with multiple interconnections enabling lymphatic exchange. Circular skin and subcutaneous damage can therefore lead to problematic lymphatic stasis in extremities or in the genital area.

Stem cells and regeneration of skin

Basal epithelial keratinocytes are the committed stem cells of the epidermis. Constant self-renewal provides a new protective layer at the skin surface.[7–12] Hair follicles contain multipotent stem cells that are activated upon the start of a new hair cycle and upon wounding to provide cells for hair follicle and epidermal regeneration. In the hair follicle stem cells reside in the bulge area. Bulge cells are relatively quiescent compared with other cells within the follicle.[9,10] However, during the

hair cycle, bulge cells are stimulated to exit the stem cell niche, proliferate,[13] and differentiate to form the various cell types of the hair follicle.[14] In addition, bulge cells can be recruited during wound healing to support re-epithelialization.[15,16]

The relative importance and exact contribution of bulge cells to wound healing are currently unknown as areas of the body such as the palms and soles that lack hair follicles still exhibit normal healing.

Hair follicles

Hair differentiates in a craniocaudal direction, 9 weeks after gestation, as mesenchymal cells populate the skin to form the dermis. Specialized cells in the dermal layer stimulate epithelial cells to proliferate and migrate downward into the epidermis, forming hair canals. The complete developed hair follicle contains an ectoderm-derived matrix and an underlying mesoderm-derived follicular papilla. There are three bulges that attach to the hair bulk. At the base the erector muscle develops, the middle part gives raise to the sebaceous gland, and the superficial bulge develops into an apocrine unit (*Fig. 17.1*).

Histological structures of the hair follicle can be divided as follows. The part that reaches from the entrance of the hair follicle into the skin to the apocrine gland is the infundibulum. The zone between the apocrine gland and the sebaceous gland is referred to as isthmus. The stem of the hair follicle is located between the sebaceous gland and the base of the erector muscle. The bulb is the deepest part of the hair follicle and contains the follicular matrix and papilla. This part is growing and regenerates the hair after injury. If the bulb is lesioned the hair will not recover from injury.

Follicles can be found in different phases: anagen (proliferating phase), catagen (regression phase), and telogen (resting phase).

Although no new hair follicles are made postnatally, the lower portion of the hair follicle regenerates in order to produce new hair. Some of this capacity has been linked to the presence of multipotent epithelial stem cells. These cells can be found in the lowest permanent portion of the hair follicle – the bulge.[13] Bulge stem cells are activated during the transition from telogen to anagen, to restart hair growth.

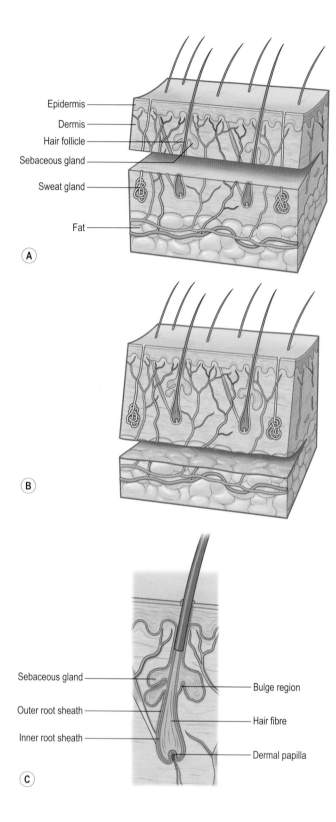

Epidermis
Dermis
Hair follicle
Sebaceous gland
Sweat gland
Fat

(A)

(B)

Sebaceous gland
Outer root sheath
Inner root sheath

Bulge region
Hair fibre
Dermal papilla

(C)

Fig. 17.1 Skin grafts. **(A)** Split-thickness skin grafts (STSGs) are the preferred approach for the treatment of large superficial skin defects such as dermal burns. STSGs consist of the partial-thickness dermis and the epidermis. Depending on the thickness, STSGs are referred to as thin or thick STSGs. In thick STSGs superficial hair follicles can be included into the graft and restore hair growth and functional sweat glands in the future skin.
(B) Full-thickness skin grafts are limited in availability and are used in the reconstruction of aesthetic (face) or functional (hand) body areas. The graft is usually taken from behind the ear, or the inguinal or elbow fold. The graft consists of the complete dermal and epidermal layer, including hair follicles and glandular structures.
(C) Hair follicle: histological structures of the hair follicle. The presence of epidermal cells as far as the bulb explains the fast re-epithelialization after STSG harvest at the donor site. The infundibulum reaches from the entrance of the hair follicle into the skin to the apocrine gland. The zone between the apocrine gland and the sebaceous gland is referred to as the isthmus. The stem of the hair follicle is located between the sebaceous gland and the base of the erector muscle. The bulb is the deepest part of the hair follicle and contains the follicular matrix and papilla. This part grows and regenerates the hair after injury. If the bulb is lesioned the hair will not recover from injury. (Revised from Orgill, D. P. Excision and skin grafting of thermal burns. *N Engl J Med* 360: 893–901, 2009.[62])

Glandular structures

Sabaceous glands are small saccular structures residing throughout the dermis, but are more common in thicker areas. These glands produce lipid-rich sebum on the surface of the skin and around the hair shaft. The function of sebum is still partially unknown but probably is linked to protection of the hair and contributes to the impermeabilization of the skin, giving protection from stings, parasites, and smell. Sebaceous glands are particularly large on the face, trunk, shoulders, and genital and perianal regions. When excessive quantities of sebum are produced – such as during puberty – the duct can be obstructed and ultimately bemay become infected or form cysts.

Sweat glands are divided into eccrine and apocrine glands. There are numerous eccrine glands in every region of the body except the tympanic membranes, lips, nail bed, nipples and clitoris. Their body has a glomerular structure and they excrete a clear odorless, hypotonic liquid. The secretion is stimulated mainly by an increase in body temperature, with the exception of some regions, such as palms, face, and axilla, where the main stimulus is emotional.

Apocrine glands are found exclusively in the axillar, perianal, periumbilical, areolar, preputial, scrotal, pubic and vulvar areas. While their structure is similar to that of the eccrine glands, these glands differ as regards the quality of their excretions, which are characterized by a thick milky, protein-rich fluid, which has a striking odor after bacterial colonization.

Science

Mechanisms of skin graft take

Skin grafting is the transfer of autologous skin cells left in anatomic order but without an intact blood supply. Therefore time and the recipient surrounding conditions limit the vitality. The operative procedure allows for nearly immediate coverage of large wound areas. Meshed grafts allow further expansion of skin but leave multiple small wounds that are re-epithelialized, mainly from the mesh within a few days. Skin can also be expanded through multiple small skin island grafts (as in Reverdin's technique) that stimulate granulation tissue, probably by excreting growth factors. In STSGs, keratinocytes on the basal layer show high proliferation rates, which may ultimately stimulate growth factor excretion.[17]

Three phases of skin graft take are commonly described: (1) serum imbibition; (2) revascularization; and (3) maturation (*Fig. 17.2*).

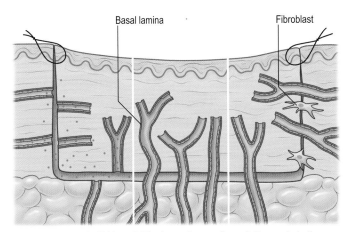

Basal lamina   Fibroblast

1. Plasma imbibition   2. Blood vessel connection   3. Revascularisation

Fig. 17.2 The concept of revascularization of the graft. Skin graft take is characterized by three main phases: (1) Plasma imbibition: The graft is initially nourished by the plasma circulation from the wound side. (2) Blood vessel connection: three different theories of how the skin graft revascularizes on the wound bed are described: (**a**) graft vessels regress and leave a basal lamina infrastructure followed by ingrowth of host epithelial cell ingrowth; (**b**) the reconnection of graft and host open ends; and (**c**) the ingrowth of endothelial cells from the host into the graft. (3) Revascularization of the skin graft. (Revised from Capla, J. M., Ceradini, D. J., Tepper, O. M., *et al.* Skin graft vascularization involves precisely regulated regression and replacement of endothelial cells through both angiogenesis and vasculogenesis. Plast Reconstr Surg 117: 836–844, 2006.)

Serum imbibition

In the first days, before the graft revascularizes, oxygen and nutrients diffusing through the plasma between the graft and the wound bed will nourish the skin graft. Huebscher in 1888[18] and Goldmann in 1894[19] theorized that skin grafts might be nourished by host fluid before vascularization of the graft occurs. They referred to this as "plasmatic circulation."[18,19] Later, Converse *et al.*[20] altered the term to "serum imbibition," as fibrinogen changes into fibrin that fixes the skin graft on to the wound bed in the absence of real plasmatic flow. Converse's studies show that skin grafts gain up to 40% of their initial weight within the first 24 hours after grafting and then this gain is reduced to 5% at 1 week postgrafting.[20] In the first hours, passive absorption of serum from the wound bed causes edema, which resolves when the revascularization is functional (*Fig. 17.2*).

Revascularization

Revascularization is critical for long-term skin graft survival. Early studies in the 19th century[21–24] suggested a connection between the wound bed and graft vessels, referred to as inosculation,[18,19,25,26] but the mechanism of revascularization remained unclear for many years.

Three hypotheses of revascularization are supported by the literature, each of them probably contributing to the process: anastomosis, neovascularization, and endothelial cell ingrowth. Anastomosis is the process of reconnection between the blood vessels in the recipient site wound bed and the graft.[21,23,24,27–29] Neovascularization is characterized by new vessel ingrowth from the recipient site into the skin graft. The last mechanism describes endothelial cell proliferation and sliding from the recipient site, utilizing pre-existing vascular basal lamina as a structure, while in the graft endothelial cells gradually degenerate.[22,24,30–32]

The process of revascularization begins as early as 24–48 hours after grafting.[33,34] Many authors describe vessel ingrowth mainly from the wound bed and less so from the wound margins, since no significant increase in blood vessels was seen in graft margins after skin grafting.[21,24,33–36] Studies supporting vessel ingrowth from the host as the main mechanism of skin graft revascularization have been controversial with respect to time course and the mechanism of host–graft vessel interactions.[23,37] Some early studies demonstrated by intravenous injection with radioisotopes that blood flow in the graft was established 4 days after grafting.[38] Similarly, studies using India ink showed graft vessel stain as early as 2 days postgrafting.[23] More recently, it was demonstrated, using a transgenic tie2/pacZ mouse model, that vessel ingrowth appears in the periphery of the graft (following blood vessel regression in the graft) from day 3 until day 21.[39] Zarem et al.[22] suggested that the process of vascularization of full-thickness skin grafts in the mouse is dominated by vascular ingrowth from the recipient using a modified transparent skin chamber. Henry and Friedman[37] proposed the theory that endothelial cells of superficial graft vessels degenerate and that host vessels profit from the basement membrane-covered infrastructure for new vessel ingrowth. In 1967, other investigators confirmed this theory using the graft hamster cheek pouch and showed a similar vessel pattern before and after grafting.[40] Converse and Ballantyne further investigated endothelial cell ingrowth into the graft using diaphorase, a marker of viable vascular endothelium. They found increased diaphorase levels in the graft bed 4 days after grafting, supporting the theory of vascular ingrowth from the host. As very few functional anastomoses were present, the authors concluded that both mechanisms, inosculation and vascular ingrowth, were important in the process of revascularization.[32] Vessel regression was also supported by NADH diaphorase activity loss during the first 4 days after grafting that was probably taken up by new vessel ingrowth.[30,39,40] The conclusion that endothelial cells utilize preformed tunnels of basal lamina was triggered by the observation that initially empty graft vessels subsequently became infiltrated with leukocytes and that ingrowing vessels used the white blood cell-filled channel as a conduit.[22] Later studies showed a central refilling of the graft vasculature as early as 48 hours, leading to the conclusion that early ansastomosis between host and graft vessels may play a major role in graft revascularization, as vessel growth takes about 5 μm/hour and angiogenesis would take at least 5 days to reach the 600-μm-thick murine dermis.[22,41] In 1987 Demarchez et al.[42] supported this hypothesis by grafting athymic mice with human STSGs. Double labeling of cross-reacting antifactor VIII and a human specific antitype IV collagen antibody showed initial anastomosis between graft and host vessels. Murine host cells gradually replaced vascular structure and the extracellular matrix of the skin graft. Later studies confirmed this hypothesis by observing a similar blood vessel network of the skin graft at the donor site and after revascularization of the graft between 96 and 120 hours after grafting.[33]

Capla et al. further showed that about 20% of blood vessels supporting the microcirculation on day 7 after grafting occurred by bone marrow-derived endothelial progenitor cell-derived vasculogenesis.[39] Recent studies measured increased levels of growth factors related to hypoxia-induced angiogenesis (hypoxia-inducible factor-1 and vascular endothelial growth factor) 24–240 hours after grafting, a process that may also contribute to host vessel ingrowth *(Fig. 17.2)*.[33]

Maturation

Once the skin graft is completely integrated, the same graft and surrounding tissues remodel and contract, similar to the last phase of wound healing after re-epithelialization is complete. Skin grafts take at least 1 year to complete maturation, with the extension of this process continuing for several years in burn victims and children. Scars from skin grafts can continue to improve for a number of years, often making prolonged conservative therapy worth considering.

Skin graft vascularization contributes to prevent underlying tissue contraction. Fibroblasts from surrounding tissues and from blood circulation become activated and repopulate the wound at the interface between the graft and the recipient site. As collagen is deposited, cross-linking allows the extracellular matrix to resist mechanical insults. Fibroblasts develop fibers called alpha-smooth-muscle actin (alpha-SMA) that exert contractile forces on the extracellular matrix. The development of alpha-SMA coincides with the differentiation of fibroblasts into myofibroblasts and wound contraction. During wound maturation, the epithelium from the edges of the wound produces a basal lamina on the open surface while sliding across and progressively covering the immature granulation tissue.

During the remodeling phase, all immature blood vessels necessary to support the initial phases regress and eventually disappear. The remodeling phase of wound healing is the longest, lasting from several months up to years.

Skin appendages and functional structures

Hair follicles, sweat glands, and dermal nerves can often be transferred within thick, STSGs and full-thickness skin grafts *(Fig. 17.1)*. Thin STSGs will not allow the transfer of hair or other adnexal glands, as the regenerating bulb is not harvested. Hair regrowth can occur in STSGs but, due to the shallow depth of harvest, is rather unlikely. Full-thickness and composite grafts will show hair regrowth 2–3 months after grafting.

It is still unclear how nerves regrow into the skin graft. Studies demonstrated that recipient nerves use the basal lamina infrastructure of degenerated blood vessels and Schwann cells of donor nerves to grow. Although histological images reveal similar neural structures between healthy skin and integrated skin grafts, patients report abnormal sensation, including hypersensitivity and pain, up to 1 year. Usually patients regain sensitivity of the grafted area after 1 year, but the result is not completely normal.

Neural reconnection to sweat glands will reactivate their function up to 3 months after grafting. For this reason, moisturizing of the skin graft is advised for at least 3 months to avoid dryness.

Full-thickness skin grafts include skin appendages that can survive and be functional at the recipient side, while STSGs do not contain the deep structure skin appendages and remain without glandular function or hair growth.

Clinical application

Skin wounds that extend into the deep dermis heal through the mechanisms of scarring and wound contraction. For large wounds this process leaves the body at risk of infection and when it occurs around joints, this can lead to significant scar contractures that affect functionality. For example, in anterior neck wounds, the contractile processes can be so strong that, over time, the chin can be fixed to the chest, often with a thick scar. Also, wounds that are left open for months to years can degenerate into skin cancer (Marjolin's ulcer). For these reasons, methods that rapidly facilitate wound coverage or resurfacing are desired.

Skin grafting is still the gold standard to cover large areas of skin loss. The concept is to take skin from an area where the donor site will heal with minimal

Table 17.1 Definition of origin of the skin graft

Graft type	Graft origin: donor and recipient of:
Autograft	Same subject
Homograft Isograft	Same species Different subject Same genetic background
Allograft	Different subjects Same species
Hetero- or xenograft	Different subjects but same species

(Revised from Andreassi A, Bilenchi B, Biagioli M, et al. Classification and pathophysiology of skin grafts. Clin Dermatol 2005, 23.)

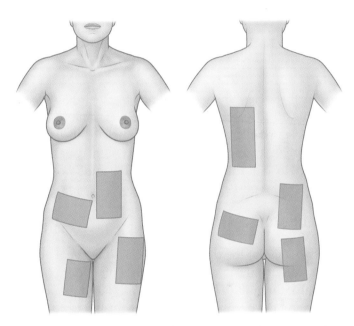

Fig. 17.3 Split-thickness donor sites. Split-thickness donor sites are commonly chosen from the anterior thigh or abdomen. Color-matched and aesthetically less evident areas can only be chosen if healthy skin is available. In burn patients with only limited availability of nonaffected skin, skin will be taken from any part of the body. Face and hands are preferentially spared from skin harvest. (Revised from Knipper, P: Mission: Plastic surgery under challenging conditions. Maîtrice Orthopédique, 2002:118 and 2003:112.)

scarring and transplant it to an area of need. As skin grafting always leaves some sort of scar, donor site considerations are important when balancing the needs of the recipient site for a given skin graft.

Skin grafts can be of different origin *(Table 17.1)*, from different anatomical sites *(Fig. 17.3)*, and can be harvested in different thicknesses *(Table 17.2)*. Depending on the histological level of the graft the skin graft type is classified by thin and thick STSGs, full-thickness skin grafts, and composite grafts *(Fig. 17.1)*. Skin grafts

Table 17.2 Indications, advantages, and disadvantages of thin split-thickness skin graft (STSG), thick STSG, and full-thickness skin graft (FTSG)

	Indications	Advantages	Disadvantages
Thin STSG	Debrided burn wounds Chronic wounds with less vascularized wound beds Exposed flap areas Acute well-vascularized wounds	Fast donor site re-epithelialization Multiple possibilities to reharvest the same area Good graft take	Contraction of the skin graft Graft quality limited because of minimal dermal thickness
Thick STSG	Same indications as thin STSG	Less secondary graft contraction compared to thin STSG Graft more stable because of thicker dermal layer Good graft take	Slower donor site re-epithelialization
FTSG	Reconstruction of functional areas such as in the face or hand Noninfected, well-vascularized wound beds	Minimal to no secondary graft contraction Excellent skin quality, stability Hair regrowth and skin appendage function	Limited availability Nontake risk is higher in a less vascularized wound bed

are further classified according to their thickness into thin (0.15–0.3 mm, Thiersch–Ollier), intermediate (0.3–0.45 mm, Blair–Brown), and thick (0.45–0.6 mm, Padgett). Skin grafts thicker than 0.6 mm usually correspond to full-thickness skin grafts and are called Wolfe–Krause grafts.[43–45]

Split-thickness skin graft

The thickness of the dermal layer classifies the STSG as either thin or thick. An STSG consists of epidermis and a variable amount of superficial to profound (papillary) dermis. As the dermis is responsible for the viscoelastic property of the skin, it is crucial for stability of the future skin. The amount of dermis grafted is key to the outcome: body areas with high mechanical friction are ideally grafted with thicker dermal layers. If donor sites do not allow this, skin quality can be improved with a combination of skin and dermal substitute grafts.

Thin STSGs include the epidermis and a thin layer of the dermis (*Fig. 17.1*). STSGs are commonly taken from the lateral thighs and trunk (*Fig. 17.3*). They do not include the full length of appendages and are therefore unlikely to grow hair or to develop full sweat gland function. The main advantage of thin STSGs is the reduced morbidity of the donor site and the possibility of performing multiple harvests from the same donor area about 2 weeks after the previous harvest. Although thinner grafts allow for more frequent reharvest, they result in additional wound contraction. The clinician

must weigh the advantages and disadvantages of these conflicting goals when deciding the thickness of the graft.

Thick STSGs include more dermis with a greater number of full hair follicles and glandular structures (*Fig. 17.1*). These grafts will likely develop some hair growth and sweat gland function about 2–3 months after grafting. Thick STSGs are commonly selected to cover areas of high mechanical friction, such as joints, plantar soles, and the palm. Since hair regrowth is common in thick STSGs, the donor site should be carefully chosen to avoid unpleasant hair growth. The sensitivity and function of sweat glands are often better in thick than in thin STSGs. Because of decreased nutrient diffusion, thick grafts require a better recipient wound than thin grafts during the revascularization process. Therefore, thick grafts should be avoided in unhealthy wound beds such as in chronic ulcers. The donor site usually heals with more obvious scarring and discoloration but less graft contraction.

Technique

To reduce bleeding during skin harvest some surgeons prefer to infiltrate the donor site area primarily with epinephrine diluted in saline subcutaneously (diluted technique: *Fig. 17.4*). If small to medium-sized areas of skin are needed and a dermatome is not available, surgeons can skillfully take skin grafts with a surgical knife or with the oscillating Gulian knife (*Fig. 17.5*). The

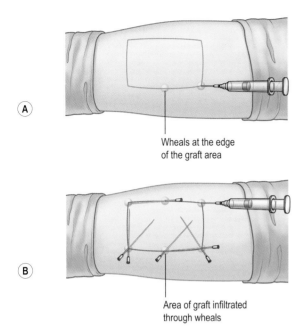

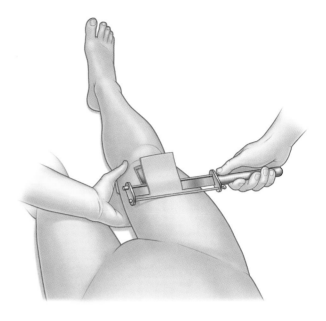

Fig. 17.4 Donor site preparation. Bleeding is one of the most important complications of excision and grafting. To reduce the severity of bleeding during excision, the fatty tissue under the graft can be infiltrated with a solution of epinephrine diluted in saline ("tumescent technique"). (Modified from King M, Bewes P. Skin grafts and flaps: The general method for split skin grafting. In Primary Surgery, Vol. 2. Trauma. Oxford: Oxford University Press, 2009. By permission of Oxford University Press Inc.)

Fig. 17.5 Split-thickness harvest with a manual knife. Alternatively, if no electrically driven dermatome is available, skin grafts can be carefully harvested with a manual knife. This procedure requires experience and harvest of even thickness is difficult. (Revised from Knipper, P. Mission: Plastic surgery under challenging conditions. Maîtrise Orthopédique, 2002:118 and 2003:112.)

disadvantage of skin grafts taken manually is the difficulty of achieving uniform depth that can result in aesthetically unpleasant donor and recipient site skin pattern. To increase the uniformity and expedite the harvest of skin grafts, a number of electrical or air-powered dermatomes have been designed to take uniform small to large skin grafts. Powered dermatomes have adjustable guards to set the graft thickness. There is a fair amount of variability in thickness depending on how hard the operator pushes on the dermatome. Drum dermatomes are precision instruments that can take large graft areas reliably *(Fig. 17.6)*. They require placement of adhesive on the skin and an oscillatory movement by the operator.

When possible, harvesting the skin graft first and covering the donor site will avoid contamination from the wound. When the excisional preparation of the recipient site needs to be performed first, a separate instrument set-up for the donor site can be considered. The size of the graft needed should be accurately measured prior to harvest. The graft thickness can be adjusted by a lever near the end of the dermatome between 0.1

and 1.0 mm. The surgeon presses the dermatome in 45° to the skin surface on to the tissue and moves the device from distal to proximal with uniform pressure and speed *(Fig. 17.6)*. A second assistant can pick up the skin graft with two anatomical forceps during the harvest process to avoid damage of the graft. If the desired length is taken, the dermatome will cut the edge when elevating it while running the motor. Keeping the graft moist with saline-impregnated gauze is of vital importance if not immediately grafted.

Larger skin grafts should be incised with an 11 knife multiple times to allow wound fluid drainage and prevent collections between the skin graft and the wound bed.

Meshed skin graft

STSGs can be enlarged up to six times their original size. Enlargement of the graft can vary from just a few manually applied perforations with an 11 blade to a systematic enlargement with a hand-powered meshing device (mesher) that applies multiple slits at regular intervals *(Fig. 17.6)*. Meshed grafts are often used following large burns when the wound area exceeds available healthy

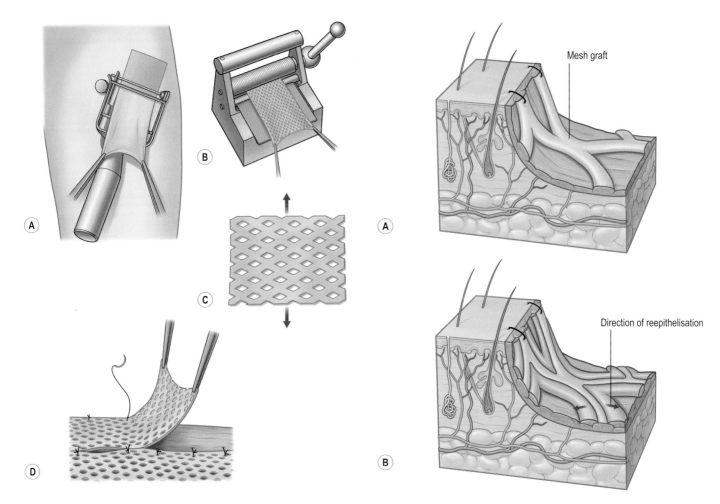

Fig. 17.6 Split-thickness harvest and grafting. **(A)** Split-thickness skin graft (STSG) harvest with an electrically driven dermatome at the anterior thigh. **(B)** The skin graft should be positioned flat on the mesh template: this can be perforated by multiple slits to **(C)** expand the graft up to six times its original size. **(D)** Meshed STSGs are ideal to cover large and uneven wounds. Stapler fixation is a time-saving method to fix large grafts. (Revised from Orgill D. P. Excision and skin grafting of thermal burns. *N Engl J Med* 360: 893–901, 2009.)

Fig. 17.7 Meshed split-thickness skin graft (STSG) and re-epithelialization. The pattern of the meshed STSG is evident even after completely healed skin and is more evident with the enlargement ratio used. Therefore, surgeons possibly prefer to expand with 1 : 1.5–1 : 2 ratios as maximum. **(A)** The meshed skin graft can be fixed with staplers or sutures. **(B)** Open surfaces will be gradually re-epithelialized from the skin stripes. In largely expanded grafts the stimulation of the wound bed from the engrafting cells leads to hypergranulation, resulting in an unpleasant aesthetic pattern. (Revised from Orgill, D. P. Excision and skin grafting of thermal burns. *N Engl J Med* 360: 893–901, 2009.)

donor sites. Meshed skin grafts are also very helpful to cover irregular geometric surfaces such as around joints as they minimize folds in the graft. Development of contractures should be taken into consideration in functional areas. If meshing is not necessary, the graft should be perforated multiple times to allow fluid removal under the graft (pie-crusting) that can minimize the risk of hematoma, seroma, or infection under the graft. Using different mesh templates, from 1:1 to 1:9, can regulate the extent of the enlargement of meshed grafts. The most commonly used mesh ratio is 1:1.5 in smaller wounds, while a mesh ratio of 1:3 and 1:6 is often needed to cover large burns.

Meshing devices are manual and come with different plastic templates where the skin graft is placed on upside down. The graft should be taken with anatomical forceps to avoid mechanical damage. The mesh gaps will be subsequently filled by keratinocytes from the skin stripes *(Fig. 17.7)*. This process takes longer with higher mesh expansion ratios. Since grafted cells excrete growth factors, underlying granulation tissue will be stimulated until full re-epithelialization occurs. Aesthetically unpleasant hypergranulation in the open areas of the mesh are therefore more often seen in large mesh ratios. Meshed skin grafts leave unsightly long-term results that

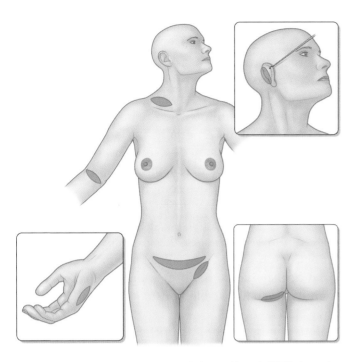

Fig. 17.8 Full-thickness donor sites. Full-thickness skin graft (FTSG) donor sites are limited and require primary wound closure or split-thickness skin grafting after harvest. FTSG are indicated in the reconstruction of smaller lesions in aesthetic (face) or functional areas (hand). Larger FTSG can be taken from the buttock fold and the infra-abdominal fold. Ideal for reconstruction of the hand is the hypothenar area and the anterior wrist fold. The main axis of the elliptically shaped hypothenar graft should be positioned slightly dorsal to the glabrous–skin border to avoid a hypersensitive scar. For face reconstruction, FTSG are taken from the retroauricular or, often used in children, the superior eyebrow regions for optimal color match. The inguinal fold is frequently used because of good aesthetic outcome at the donor site. Other areas are the subclavicular, the infra-abdominal, and the elbow fold as well as the inner upper arm. (Revised from Knipper, P: Mission: Plastic surgery under challenging conditions. Maîtrise Orthopédique, 2002:118 and 2003:112.)

need to be considered when selecting this technique. Very thin meshed skin grafts used in combination with dermal substitutes or keratinocyte cultures are other strategies to mitigate the result *(Fig. 17.7)*.

Full-thickness skin graft

Full-thickness skin and composite grafts are limited in availability but show excellent function and sensitivity after engraftment. Full-thickness grafts should be considered in the reconstruction of aesthetically dominant (face) or functionally important areas (hand). Full-thickness grafts from the retroauricular region and above the eyebrows are an excellent choice to maintain tissue quality and color of the surrounding skin in the face *(Fig. 17.8)*. If needed, foreskin can also be used and in adults retroauricular skin is helpful in face

reconstruction. Also, excess skin from the upper eyelid and submental area can be taken into consideration for full-thickness reconstruction if the patient is comfortable with an aesthetic-like intervention.

In hand reconstruction, elbow crease and wrist fold grafts have been described but should be avoided in cultures where these donor site scars may result in stigmatization of the patient as they can be associated with suicide. Hypothenar skin is useful for glabrous reconstruction but can leave a painful scar that can cause an unpleasant sensation if the hand is positioned on a table in a relaxed position. Therefore, full-thickness skin graft from the hypothenar area should be harvested elliptical with the main axis and slightly more dorsal in relation to the glabrous–skin border *(Fig. 17.8)*.

Full-thickness skin grafts are taken in an area where loose surrounding skin is available to achieve primary closure. Skin grafts can be designed elliptical and excised with a knife. Harvesting should be carried out trying not to elevate the underlying tissue. Most of the full-thickness grafts need defatting and this can be easily performed by spreading the graft over the index finger and trimming the fat tissue tangentially to the skin. Defatting of the graft will encourage graft take *(Fig. 17.9)*.

Composite graft

Composite grafts include a layer of subcutaneous fat tissue under the dermal and epidermal layer. The donor sites are principally the same as the full-thickness donor sites. Since fat tissue is less vascularized and more vulnerable to ischemia, optimal revascularization is needed in order to achieve graft survival. Composite grafts can be used in children as they show a remarkable capacity to revascularize thicker grafts. Some surgeons use composite grafts to reconstruct the nasal tip, the alar, and the columella in cleft lip patients.[46]

Over time, the appearance of skin grafts tends to improve in both color and texture. Nevertheless, skin grafts rarely have the aesthetic appearance of normal skin and patients should be advised about the likely final appearance of the graft.

Skin fixation and dressing

Once the autologous skin is grafted on to the wound site the revascularization depends on multiple factors. One

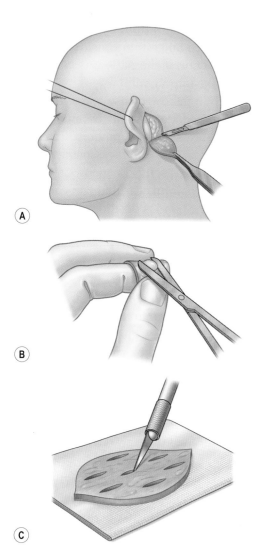

Fig. 17.9 Full-thickness skin graft (FTSG) harvest and preparation. FTSGs should be designed elliptically to achieve primary wound closure without deforming surrounding tissues. This fact is usually given if a length: width ratio of 1:3 is followed. **(A)** After sharp excision of the graft the surgeon should elevate the graft if possible without fat tissue and protect the graft by handling it with a skin hook or anatomical forceps. **(B)** Defatting is an important process to avoid fat necrosis after grafting and to facilitate direct revascularization of the wound bed. The graft can be easily defatted with scissors by stretching the graft upside down over the index finger. **(C)** To allow fluid exit from the wound bed, FTSG should be incised with a sharp knife in multiple sites. (Revised from Knipper, P: Mission: Plastic surgery under challenging conditions. Maîtrise Orthopédique, 2002:118 and 2003:112.)

of the most important factors to achieve stable taking is the immobility of the graft during the revascularization process. An open technique requires labor-intensive monitoring on the graft and any fluid that is formed beneath the graft is rolled out with a cotton-tipped applicator. More often, skin grafts are fixed through a series of sutures and overlying compressive dressing

materials (bolster: *Fig. 17.10*). Scattered sutures through the graft on to the wound bed can additionally immobilize larger skin grafts. If large and multiple skin grafts are placed as frequently needed in burn victims, fixation can be performed with staplers to shorten operation time. Staples are painful when removed and may be overgrown by skin, especially in large skin grafts. Vacuum-assisted pressure devices can be used with a protective interface of petroleum gauze or a silicone sheet to permit continuous compression on to the graft and fluid removal. The suction dressing is especially useful if fast mobilization is desired in patients with wounds in joint regions or the lower extremities *(Fig. 17.10)*. Compression to stabilize the graft on to the wound bed should be performed until 5–10 days when the graft is usually stable and wound areas are completely closed.

Splints can be used as adjuncts if the risk of wound contraction is high, such as in chin scar release or in joint and web space release of the hand. These splints or casts should be worn up to several months after grafting, in the beginning 24 hours per day, later during the night, to avoid the loss of mobility. Physiotherapy and scar massage are also important elements for obtaining better results with skin grafts.

Negative-pressure wound-healing devices also make very effective bolsters, especially on largely grafted surfaces and chronic ulcers.[47–49]

Sealants

Fibrin glue can also be helpful to assist skin graft fixation. In this case, some surgeons spray fibrin glue on to the skin graft dermis just before placing it on to the wound site. The fibrin network may even act as a provisory extracellular matrix under the graft.[50]

First dressing change

The first dressing change should occur once the skin graft is revascularized and has a stable physical connection to the wound bed. Early dressing change around the third day after grafting may allow predicting the "take rate" of the graft but risks secondary graft loss through shear forces that disturb nascent vessel connections. More commonly the dressings are taken off for the first time 5–10 days after grafting.

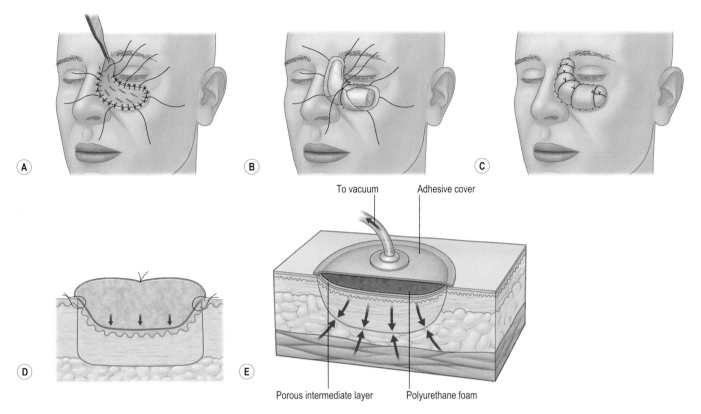

Fig. 17.10 Fixation of a skin graft. Skin grafts require precise contact with the wound surface and fluid collections and micromovements are to be avoided. A bolster dressing is an excellent method to press and stabilize smaller skin grafts on to the wound, particularly in the face or hand areas. **(A)** The graft is placed and sutured on to the wound and sutures are left intentionally long. (Revised from Knipper, P: Mission: Plastic surgery under challenging conditions. Maîtrise Orthopédique, 2002:118 and 2003:112.) **(B)** A first layer of nonadhesive fat dressing is placed on the graft and covered with a bolster of cotton or gauze that is sutured face to face over the second layer. (Revised from Chase RA, Atlas of Hand Surgery. Philadelphia, WB Saunders, 1974.) **(C)** The second layer will subject mild pressure on to the graft that stabilizes the graft and allows fluid exit into the bolster dressing. (Revised from Knipper, P: Mission: Plastic surgery under challenging conditions. Maîtrise Orthopédique, 2002:118 and 2003:112.) **(D)** The bolster dressing will precisely adapt the skin graft on to the wound bed to optimize the conditions for the revascularization process. **(E)** Vacuum-assisted closure dressing to fix skin grafts: The fixation of the skin graft is an elegant method, especially if larger and uneven areas that cover joints are grafted. Continuous suction and compression on to the wound bed ensure fluid removal and stabilization of the graft. The skin graft will be fixated as usual and the first dressing should be either a nonadhesive perforated silicone dressing or a petroleum gauze to avoid maceration of the graft by the open polyurethane foam. Some surgeons use the moist white foam without interface to fix the graft.

Recipient site considerations

Before planning a skin graft, several factors have to be taken into consideration to achieve optimal tissue cover at the wound site. The wound bed quality has to be optimized for a successful "take" of the graft and the skin color, thickness, and mechanical resistance of the donor site area should ideally match the recipient site skin quality. Wound conditions often found in chronic or insufficiently debrided burn wounds and characterized by low wound bed vascularization or high bacterial loads will not allow skin grafts to be taken.

Wound bed preparation

The successful engraftment of skin grafts highly depends on the quality of the wound bed. Revascularization particularly depends on a vital recipient wound bed. A good quantity of blood vessels near the surface is critical in order to support graft viability. Irradiated, ischemic and scar tissue, bone, and tendon do not ordinarily have sufficient blood supply to allow the skin graft to take. If highly vascularized peritendon and periosteum are still intact, skin grafts can be performed. In chronic wounds re-epithelialization occurs at the wound margins that can grow into the tissue and may inhibit the lateral reconnections of the graft. Therefore, wound margins should be sharply excised with a blade before grafting.

Experimental data suggest that the bacterial level must be brought down below the critical level of 10^5 bacteria per gram of tissue to allow a skin graft to take. The practical problem with quantitative bacterial cultures is that it takes about 48 hours to obtain the result, long after the decision to graft is typically made. As a result, this methodology seems most commonly applied to research studies. Surgeons often take a fairly aggressive approach to making sure all necrotic tissue has been debrided and that the wound is clinically "clean" prior to grafting.

Wound debris or necrotic tissue physically inhibits and chemically slows ingrowth of blood vessels into the skin graft. Wounds that were left open for several days contain high bacterial loads and therefore need to be extensively debrided before skin grafting. Preparation of the recipient site commonly occurs by sharp excision, but can also be performed using a variety of other debridement techniques, including laser, water jet, and ultrasound as well as standard dressing changes. Surgeons have learned over time that a "granulating" wound has a high likelihood of taking a skin graft. Active bleeding of the wound bed will likely lead to blood collection between the graft and the wound bed, inhibiting graft take. Accurate homeostasis can be performed with bipolar cautery and larger blood vessels can be ligated with fine resorbable sutures.

If tendons or bones are exposed without peritendon or periosteum, the surrounding soft tissue can often be adapted to cover critical structures before skin grafting. Small areas of tendons and bones can either be prepared by vacuum-assisted closure therapy to grow granulation tissue from the sides or dermal substitutes can be used to cover functional structures.

Functional consideration

Skin grafts can often provide functional and aesthetic skin reconstruction. Consideration needs to be given to the size of graft needed, the degree of wound contraction expected, the color and texture of the skin required, and the need for adnexal glands. The amount of wound contraction expected is inversely related to the amount of dermis in the skin graft.

Full-thickness grafts, those that take the entire epidermis and dermis, maximally restrain contractile forces and give excellent cosmetic results. Full-thickness skin grafts are frequently used for nipple–areola reconstruction, syndactyly release, or ectropion release. Full-thickness grafts are in short supply and can be augmented by tissue expansion prior to harvesting full-thickness skin grafts.

Very thin grafts such as epidermal grafts result in a donor site that heals quickly with minimal contraction but provide little constraint to wound contraction. The surgeon can use this as an advantage if wound contraction is desired. For example, on large scalp wounds or abdominal wounds, wound contraction may be desired to keep the skin graft as small as possible while pulling the wound edges together over time. Secondary excision of the contracted skin graft and primary wound closure can be performed in a second stage to achieve best functional and aesthetic results.

As the skin thickness varies throughout the body, a variety of skin thicknesses are available for use. For example, full-thickness upper eyelid skin is very thin but provides good resistance to wound contraction. Thicker skin is available in the trunk and leg region, where thick STSGs can be taken, leaving enough adnexal structures and dermal thickness to minimize donor site scarring.

Aesthetic considerations

Skin color is determined by a complicated integration of skin texture, melanin pigmentation, and blood flow. In general, replacement of tissue from a similar or adjacent site will give the best color match. In the face, this is often the most critical aesthetic area and choosing donor sites such as supraclavicular, posterior auricular, upper eyelid or scalp skin grafts can often lead to an excellent color match. For darker areas of the skin, such as the nipple–areola complex, grafts from the contralateral areola or genitalia have been used. More commonly today, skin grafts in this area can be tattooed with vegetable dyes to give an excellent color match.

Skin texture is most commonly an issue when dealing with glabrous skin (palms and soles of feet). In this case, placing a nonglabrous skin graft to cover these areas can result in a very unnatural look, often with significant color match differences. Glabrous skin grafts are obviously in short supply but can be harvested from the hypothenar eminence. Skin adnexal glands are difficult to replace but can sometimes be successfully transferred with full-thickness grafts.

Donor site considerations

The obligatory scarring or discoloration associated with donor sites must be considered when taking a skin graft. For large surface area burns, the surgeon must use whatever donor site is available to close the wound; in contrast, for smaller grafts, a thorough discussion of the donor site possibilities with the potential risks and benefits allows for the best skin match with the least iatrogenic damages.

Common donor sites include the thigh, trunk, and buttocks, regions frequently covered by clothing (see *Fig. 17.3*).

When defects of the face need to be covered, full-thickness skin grafts are often preferred. The donor area for a graft on the face should be preferably chosen among scalp, neck, and supraclavicular area to obtain the best color match. Important aspects are the thickness, color, and texture of the graft, which should closely match those of the recipient site.

Eyelid skin, which is thin with a few glandular structures, is generally best replaced by eyelid skin. Thick, highly glandular nasal skin can be replaced by skin from the nasolabial folds, supraclavicular area, or anterior auricular area.

In trauma, avulsed (degloved) skin can often be prepared by extensive defatting and regrafted primarily[51] or stored and used later.

Full-thickness donor sites in the head and neck are pre- and postauricular regions (the first is generally thicker), nasolabial crease, supraclavicular region, eyelids, and neck.

Other common regions include the inguinal crease that is often used to cover large defects. In this case it is important to harvest laterally and away from potentially hair-bearing regions of the pubis. This area generally heals well and is hidden *(Fig. 17.8)*.

In nipple–areola reconstruction after mastectomy, a full-thickness graft from the contralateral region is often taken in combination with a full-thickness graft from the groin.

Donor sites from full-thickness skin grafts are generally closed primarily. Particular attention should be taken when supraclavicular donor sites are used, as this region is prone to develop hypertrophic scars. Sometimes large donor sites that cannot heal primarily are used for covering extensive defects, for example, in the face or joints. In this case, an STSG can be used to cover the donor site.

Donor site dressing

Topical gauze soaked with diluted epinephrine solution is useful to stop bleeding at the donor site and can be left until the operation is ended, adding an analgesic effect. The donor site of an STSG generally heals (re-epithelializes) in 7–21 days depending on the size and depth of the graft taken and the age of the patient. A myriad of donor site dressings are available with multiple studies on a variety of products. Traditionally, fine-meshed gauze, often impregnated with a petroleum-based product, is placed over the wound and fixed in place. Cotton gauze is placed over this and removed a day or two after the operation. The wound heals under this dressing and the dressing spontaneously comes off when healed. The advantages of this type of dressing system are its simplicity, low cost, and minimal wound care requirement. The work of Winters in the early 1960s[52] showed that a moist wound heals faster. As a consequence many have advocated a simple semiocclusive adhesive, semipermeable polyurethane dressing, although it promotes serum accumulation between the wound and the dressing that should be evacuated by a drain or a syringe. This process can be labor-intensive for a busy inpatient service or difficult to manage on an outpatient basis. In addition, when an infection develops, it can rapidly spread to the entire donor site area with this dressing.

A large number of other dressings, including silver-based, absorptive, and biological, have been studied. In most of the cases the donor site heals spontaneously, thus simple impregnated gauze is still the gold standard. When some complications occur, the harvest site can deepen and become a full-thickness defect, mainly due to infections in the elderly, infants, or critically ill patients. As a consequence, excision and grafting of the donor site may be required.

Skin graft storage

Skin grafts can be stored on a moist gauze at 4°C for up to 2 weeks, although the viability decreases over time. Experimentally, storage can be extended using cell culture media. For degloving injuries, the skin can be defatted acutely and reapplied as a full-thickness graft.

Complications

Hematoma

Any liquid between the wound and skin graft can impair skin graft take. Since bleeding represents one of the most important complications after excision and grafting with up to 100–200 mL of blood, every 1% of body surface area that is excised, particularly from the scalp.[53] The surgeon must be certain that bleeding has stopped prior to dressing the wound. Suture ligation or cautery can be used to control larger bleeding vessels; oozing can be controlled with pressure and/or pharmacological methods such as topical thrombin, epinephrine, or fibrin glue. To reduce bleeding during excision the area can be primarily injected with epinephrine diluted in saline (tumescent technique: *Fig. 17.4*).[54] As discussed above, incisions of the graft should be done to allow fluid evacuation through a compressive or suction dressing.

Seroma

Serum imbibition is essential for early skin graft survival. Excessive serum, such as a seroma, will prevent or delay skin graft take. Seromas are better tolerated than hematomas, and adequate fenestrations (pie crusting) can prevent this problem.

Infection

When skin graft infections occur, pus often accumulates beneath the skin graft and can rapidly spread. If an infection is found early, prompt incision and drainage of the fluid beneath the graft can often salvage some or all of the skin graft. A large number of dressings have been developed that carry a variety of topical antimicrobial agents. Silver nitrate, mafenide acetate, and silver ion dressings are commonly used. Bacteria seem not to develop resistance easily to silver products, making these products desirable.

A contaminated wound will not heal and reject a graft. Some microorganisms, such as *Pseudomonas*, can contaminate the wound and cause nonpurulent infections. Even systemic or nonskin-localized infections have been proven to delay or prevent skin graft taking.

Nontake

Unfavorable conditions such as malnutrition, vasculitis, malignant diseases, steroids, and chemotherapeutic medications have all been shown to cause or accelerate nontake of the graft.

Wound contraction

Wounds covered with skin grafts can still undergo wound contraction leading to a scar contracture. After the acute inflammation phase the contraction starts. Fibroblasts from surrounding tissues and from blood circulation start to be activated and repopulate the wound between the graft and the wound bed. Cells at the interface need to build new collagen-rich tissue to replace fibrin and anchor the graft to the wound bed. While fibrin is crucial for early cell migration in the wound bed, collagen deposition allows wound maturation. As collagen is deposited, cross-linking occurs so that the extracellular matrix becomes mechanically resistant. This increase in mechanical resistance allows mechanical interaction with fibroblasts that develop fibers called alpha-SMA. The development of alpha-SMA coincides with the differentiation of fibroblasts into myofibroblasts that induce wound contraction.

Instability

Shear forces are a major cause of skin graft failure that can disrupt the nascent fragile blood vessel connections. Later, thin skin grafts have less collagen content and are prone to delamination due to shear forces.

Cosmetic issues

Unpleasant net-like patterns of meshed STSGs are much more prominent than nonmeshed or full-thickness grafts. Color differences are a common problem if donor sites could not be optimally chosen. If excess skin surrounds the grafted area, the skin graft can be excised in multiple steps until primary closure can be reached.

Donor site

Infection at donor sites can occur from bacterial contamination during the operation or in the postoperative period. These infections are treated with topical antimicrobial agents, including silver dressings. The delay in healing of donor sites due to infection can lead to hypertrophic scar formation. Hypertrophic scar or keloid formation can also result from deep donor sites or in patients with a propensity for scarring. Itching is a common reaction to donor sites as well as hypersensitivity to changes in temperature.

Future

Dermal substitutes

Burke *et al.* first described a collagen–glycosaminoglycan scaffold to treat dermal defects in the early 1980s.[55] Dermal substitutes *(Table 17.3)* are widely used in large burn injuries, when skin lesions are so extensive and unaffected donor skin areas are often limited. Cadaver skin (allograft) or dermal substitutes can be used initially to cover large defects. Dermal substitutes can also

be used to improve functional and aesthetic outcome. Dermal regeneration is very limited in our skin and full-thickness skin defects heal by secondary intention with scar tissue formation. The difference of scar tissue and healthy skin besides the aesthetic appearance is the viscoelasticity and therefore stability. Scar tissue shows histological parallel-oriented collagen fibers, while healthy dermis consists of randomly oriented collagen fibers. In some patients and for restricted donor sites keratinocyte cultures or very thin STSGs can be attempted to close full-thickness defects. The resulting skin is usually fragile and dry, leading to reopening and ulcers through normal mechanical friction. This poses a particular problem if functional structures underlie the new thin skin. The introduction of the first commercially available skin substitute, Integra, is a bovine-derived collagen type 1 cross-linked matrix with glycosaminoglycans that is similar to the dermal structure and covered by a silicone sheet to recreate temporarily the function of the epidermis. Integra can be applied to a vascularized wound bed followed by blood vessels and cell growth into the collagen matrix to create a vascularized neodermis after 2–3 weeks. During the avascular period, the dermal graft is very sensitive to infection, one of the main disadvantages of the two-step strategy.

Once revascularization is accomplished, the silicone layer can be removed and the epidermal replacement can be granted by either keratinocyte cultures or a thin STSG *(Fig. 17.11)*. To improve dermal graft integration,

Table 17.3 Permanent and temporary dermal and epidermal skin substitutes

Origin	Dermal	Epidermal	Mixed
Permanent			
Autograft	Fibroblast culture	Keratinocyte culture Skin graft	
Allograft	Human cadaver dermis (Alloderm)		
Synthetic	Integra Matriderm		
Temporary			
Mixed	Dermagraf (polyglactin mesh + human fibroblasts)		Apligraft (bovine collagen matrix + neonatal human fibroblasts and keratinocytes)
Temporary			
Xenograft	Xenoderm (porcine-derived acellular dermis) Mediskin (porcine-derived acellular dermis) Strattice (porcine-derived acellular dermis)		

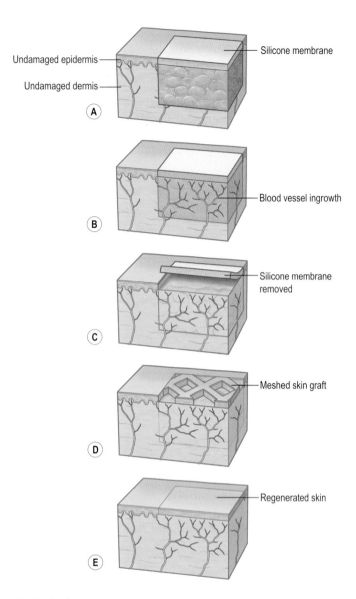

Undamaged epidermis — Silicone membrane
Undamaged dermis —
(A)

Blood vessel ingrowth
(B)

Silicone membrane removed
(C)

Meshed skin graft
(D)

Regenerated skin
(E)

Fig. 17.11 Skin regeneration with dermal substitutes. If large, deep skin defects have to be covered with thin split-thickness skin grafts, dermal substitutes can be used to augment the dermal layer and therefore the aesthetic and functional outcome. (Revised from www.integra-ls.com.)

surgeons have successfully seeded dermal substitutes with keratinocytes.[23] Newer clinical studies show that small areas of exposed tendon or bone without remaining peritendineum or periosteum can be successfully grafted with Integra.

After the invention of Integra, a number of other human- and animal-derived dermal substitutes are now commercially available. Another synthetically engineered dermal substitute is Matriderm (Dr. Suwelack Skin and Health Care), a bovine-derived collagen matrix with noncross-linked collagen fibers of types I, III, and V matrix coated with elastin fibers. Synthetically dermal substitutes such as Integra and Matriderm are permanent dermal regenerative templates that will be ultimately covered by an epidermal autologous graft. For temporal coverage of large wounds there are available dermal allografts (human, Alloderm, Lifecell) or xenografts such as porcine-derived lyophilized split-thickness Xenoderm (Asclepios Medical Techics, www.ascelpios.de), porcine-derived acellular dermis, Permacol (Tissue Science Laboratories, Hampshire, UK), and Strattice (Lifecell, KCI) or a frozen irradiated porcine xenograft with a dermal and epidermal layer, Mediskin (Brennen Medical, www.brennenmedical.com). Allografts and xenografts will be rejected by the recipient and may adhere in patients with large burn injuries for several weeks because of the posttraumatic immunosuppressed stage. After 2–3 weeks dermal dressings will be removed and a well-vascularized wound bed is found underneath that is ready for final skin reconstruction by autologous grafts. Infection of the acellular dermis demands careful wound dressing and infection control. Another drawback for human- and porcine-derived dermis is possible viral infection transmission.[56]

Cell cultures

Epithelial cell culture autografts were first introduced by Rheinwald and Green in 1975 and pose a milestone in skin regeneration.[57] In patients with extensive burns, donor sites are often limited. Cultured epithelial autografts (CEA) are keratinocytes harvested from a small biopsy of the same patient that are then expanded manifold in the laboratory *(Fig. 17.12)*.

The time needed to expand keratinocyte cultures *in vitro* for clinical use is dependent upon the delivery method. In order to obtain sheets of confluent keratinocytes as in normal epidermis, it may take up to 5 weeks. This time can be shortened to less than 2 weeks[58] by expanding the cultures on bioscaffolds that allow cell attachment and proliferation prior transplantation. Hyaluronan or collagen scaffolds have been demonstrated to be very useful in delivering cell-seeded sheets with approximately 80% confluence up to even multilayered epithelial tissue constructs. Cell suspensions have the advantage of being delivered faster, reducing

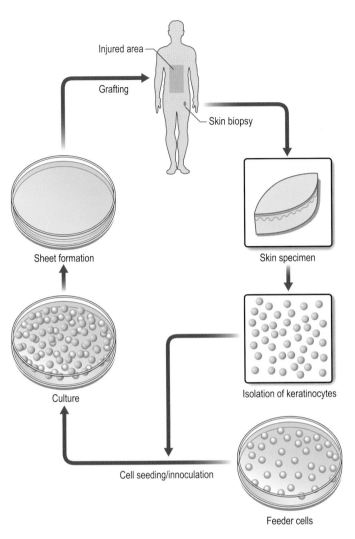

Fig. 17.12 Keratinocyte cultures. Epidermal cells can be harvested from a small biopsy from the patient and expanded manifold *in vitro*. Once the expansion is achieved the autologous keratinocytes can be delivered back to the patient. (Revised from Autologous Cultured Epidermis, www.jpte.co.jp.)

the *in vitro* time to only 5–7 days. Recently, Recell, invented by Fiona Wood *et al.*, introduced an even faster method, applying noncultured keratinocytes in a one-step procedure.[59] Since in deep wounds time is a critical issue, this strategy, offering accelerated delivery, is promising, although still poorly characterized. One major concern is whether cells directly sprayed on the wound surface are able to find attachment sites to engraft and survive.

The introduction of CEA in clinical practice dates back more than 20 years, but the best delivery method as well as efficacy and indications has not been

identified yet. Published studies have reported taking rates of CEA on biomaterials varying from 0 to 80%, raising many questions about their effectiveness. Boyce *et al.*[60] described bilayered autologous skin constructs with keratinocytes and fibroblasts on collagen–glycosaminoglycan matrixes that showed promising results in burn treatment. Direct comparison of autologous bilayered skin constructs versus STSGs showed higher initial nontake rates and regraftment after treatment with the skin construct, while STSG-treated areas healed spontaneously. Once wound closure occurred, the outcomes showed similar results in skin quality at longer time points. The variability may be explained by heterogeneous wound cohorts, inconsistencies in the time at which wounds were analyzed, treatment techniques, and measuring systems.

Bioengineered cultured allogenic bilayered constructs

Cell-seeded skin constructs were first described in the early 1980s, when autologous keratinocytes and fibroblasts were seeded into collagen glycosaminoglycan matrixes by centrifugation.[61] Further research found neonatal skin cells to be very efficient in accelerating wound healing. Neonatal foreskin keratinocytes and fibroblasts were than used in combination with biological or synthetically engineered scaffolds to stimulate wound healing in topically applied allogenic skin constructs. Other than autologous cells, which seem to integrate into wound tissues, allogenic constructs rather stimulate healing by growth factor release and initial production of extracellular matrix proteins, but are rejected eventually. Apligraf (Organogenesis, Canton, MA, US and Novartis Pharmaceuticals, East Hanover, NJ, US) is a bilayered living skin-equivalent composed of type I bovine collagen and allogenic keratinocytes and fibroblasts obtained from neonatal foreskin. Fibroblasts are cultured in the collagen matrix where they proliferate and augment the extracellular matrix with all kinds of proteins. Keratinocytes are then added and build up the epidermal layer. The living skin construct supports skin graft take in difficult wounds, such as burn wounds, or accelerates healing in chronic wounds. With a shelf-life of 5 days at room temperature Apligraf has to be applied fresh either as a temporary dressing or over meshed STSGs.

Dermagraft (Advanced Tissue Sciences, La Jolla, CA, US) does not contain keratinocytes and is described as a living dermal skin construct consistent with a cryopreserved bioabsorbable polyglactin mesh seeded with allogenic neonatal fibroblasts. Fibroblasts were shown to proliferate and produce dermal collagen, growth factors, glycosaminoglycans, and fibronectin while the mesh material is gradually absorbed. Dermagraft can be used as a temporary or permanent covering of meshed STSGs in combination with allografts to support their take.

Future products that are less immunogenic might be useful for improving skin regeneration.

Access the complete reference list online at **http://www.expertconsult.com**

6. Tanner Jr JC, Vandeput J, Olley JF. The Mesh Skin Graft. *Plast Reconstr Surg.* 1964;34:287–292.

12. Blanpain C, Fuchs E. Epidermal stem cells of the skin. *Annu Rev Cell Dev Biol.* 2006;22:339–373.

   Review of the current knowledge of epidermal stem cells of the adult skin.

14. Fuchs E. Scratching the surface of skin development. *Nature.* 2007;445:834–842.

   Review article giving insight into recent developments that have focused on epidermal stem cell population to maintain hair follicle regeneration and re-epithlialization in response to wound healing.

30. Converse JM, Smahel J, Ballantyne Jr DL, et al. Inosculation of vessels of skin graft and host bed: a fortuitous encounter. *Br J Plast Surg.* 1975;28:274–282.

34. O'Ceallaigh S, Herrick SE, Bennett WR, et al. Perivascular cells in a skin graft are rapidly repopulated by host cells. *J Plast Reconstr Aesthet Surg.* 2007;60:864–875.

39. Capla JM, Ceradini DJ, Tepper OM, et al. Skin graft vascularization involves precisely regulated regression and replacement of endothelial cells through both angiogenesis and vasculogenesis. *Plast Reconstr Surg.* 2006;117:836–844.

57. Rheinwald JG, Green H. Serial cultivation of strains of human epidermal keratinocytes: the formation of keratinizing colonies from single cells. *Cell.* 1975;6:331–343.

   A milestone article in skin regeneration, introducing the cultivation of keratinocytes for autologous cell treatmeant.

60. Boyce ST, Goretsky MJ, Greenhalgh DG, et al. Comparative assessment of cultured skin substitutes and native skin autograft for treatment of full-thickness burns. *Ann Surg.* 1995;222:743–752.

   Clinical study comparing an autologous bilayered skin construct based on keratinocytes, fibroblasts, and a collagen matrix versus the gold standart therapy: autologous skin graft in burn patients.

62. Orgill DP. Excision and skin grafting of thermal burns. *N Engl J Med* 2009;360:893–901.

   Review article on current guidelines of the treatment of thermal burns.

18

Tissue graft, tissue repair, and regeneration

Wei Liu and Yilin Cao

SYNOPSIS

- Tissue grafting is an important technique for tissue repair in reconstructive plastic surgery.
- More importantly, with the advancement of scientific research and newly developed biotechnologies as well as their applications in plastic surgery, the conventional tissue-grafting approach is likely to be switched to a tissue regeneration strategy using stem cell therapy and tissue engineering, and thus to avoid undesired appearance or functional disturbance at the graft donor site.
- This chapter introduces the history and surgical techniques for tissue harvesting and repair of dermal graft, fat graft, fascial graft, tendon graft, and skeletal muscle graft as well as composite graft.
- Also included are recent developments in tissue graft research and their clinical applications, such as adipose-derived stem cells, acellular tissue graft, and engineered tissue graft fabrication.

 Access the Historical Perspective sections online at
http://www.expertconsult.com

Introduction

Plastic surgery is defined as a specialized branch of surgery concerned with the repair of deformities and the correction of functional deficits.[1] In this specialty, preparation and transfer of tissue graft for tissue reconstruction and repair are among the most important surgical techniques to achieve the goal of deformity repair and deficit correction. The surgical technique to create a tissue graft such as skin tube or forehead pedicle flap can be traced back to as early as 1597 and 1794.[1] In

today's practice, many conventional tissue grafts are still used as clinical routine procedures for tissue repair and reconstruction, for example, dermal, fat, fascial and tendon grafts or muscle flap or composite graft consisting of more than two types of tissues. In modern plastic surgery practice over the past 200 years, an obvious drawback of tissue grafts, i.e., tissue damage on donor site, has been a problem troubling both physicians and patients and has yet to be overcome. Fortunately, the rapid development of biotechnology in the past 20 years has also shed light on this puzzle. In particular, the development of tissue engineering and stem cell biology makes it possible to generate autologous tissue graft without causing donor site tissue damage.[2]

The purpose of this chapter is to provide a general introduction of conventional tissue grafts, but also introduce recent scientific developments on how to generate related autologous grafts with tissue-engineering techniques for tissue repair and regeneration.

Dermal graft and repair

Dermal graft is defined as a graft that contains a deep layer of the papillary dermis and the entire reticular layer of the dermis along with a minimal amount of adherent subcutaneous fat and indigenous subepidermal extensions of the epithelial appendage *(Fig. 18.1)*.[3]

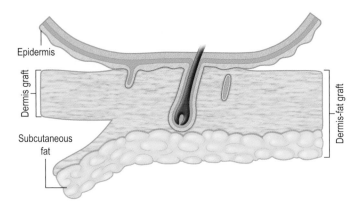

Fig. 18.1 A dermal graft contains the deep layer of the papillary dermis and the entire reticular layer of the dermis, along with a minimal amount of adherent subcutaneous fat and indigenous subepidermal extensions of the epithelial appendages. (Reproduced from Chiu DWT, Bradford WE. Repair and grafting of dermis, fat and fascia. In: McCarthy JC, ed. Plastic surgery. Philadelphia: WB Saunders; 1990:509–526.)

Surgical technique[3]

The general requirements for creating a dermal graft and successful application include selection of an inconspicuous donor site, good preparation of a recipient bed to insure it is free of infection and scar tissue, meticulous hemostasis, and adequate immobilization. The dermal graft can be harvested from the groin, gluteal fold, lateral gluteal region, submammary region in females, or lower abdomen. Due to natural contraction, a 25% excess in surface area should be considered when harvesting the graft and an ellipse shape is desired in order to close the wound in a linear fashion. Conventionally, the epidermis is removed by Reese dermatome.[3] The epidermis can also be removed by Dispase treatment to maintain the whole structure of the dermis.[4]

The fate of implanted dermal graft

According to histological study, dermal graft along with skin appendage can survive well in subcutaneous environment but the appendage structure may disintegrate after 5 years. However, these structures tend to form dilated excretory duct and epidermoid cyst, eventually resulting in considerable fibrosis around them *(Fig. 18.2).*[3]

Clinical application for tissue repair and recent development

As a conventional technique, autologous dermal graft remains widely used in clinical treatments. Lemma *et al.* reported the repair of hernia of abdominal wall with autologous dermal graft.[5] Maguina *et al.* reported its use in breast reconstruction and treatment of breast implant malposition.[6] Karacaoglu reported the application in augmentation mastopexy in 21 patients with 20.6-month follow-up and the procedure was found to be cost-effective and could improve breast appearance.[7] It has also been applied to repair parotid surgery wound, which can limit the common complication of depression deformity or neck scarring.[8] Samson *et al.* have applied autologous dermal graft to the repair of large infected abdominal wall hernias in obese patients with success.[9]

The disadvantage of this traditional technique is the need to harvest a full-thickness skin graft, which is limited by the availability of the donor site skin and can cause scarring. In addition, buried skin appendage can also lead to cyst formation, as illustrated in *Figure 18.2.* One of the approaches to overcome this problem is the development of allogenic acellular dermal graft, and thus there will be no limitation in the graft supply. Additionally, the allogenic acellular graft will not cause immune response due to the elimination of immunogenic cells.

Alloderm is the first commercially available product of acellular dermis developed by LifeCell Corporation from human cadaveric allograft skin. During the process, the entire epidermis and all dermal cells are removed by detergent treatment or a freeze-drying process, which results in an undamaged cell-free dermis that contains an intact basement membrane structure, collagen, and other native extracellular matrices.

One important application of Alloderm is for abdominal wall reconstruction, which has been tested for its efficacy in both experimental study and clinical trials with success,[10–19] including the repair of ventral hernia or contaminated and high-risk abdominal wall defect. It has been observed that implanted Alloderm could be fast revascularized and gradually remodeled into autologous tissue. In 2005, Butler *et al.* reported the multiple applications of Alloderm for pelvic, chest, and abdominal wall reconstruction, demonstrating its great potential in tissue repair.[17] The other applications include

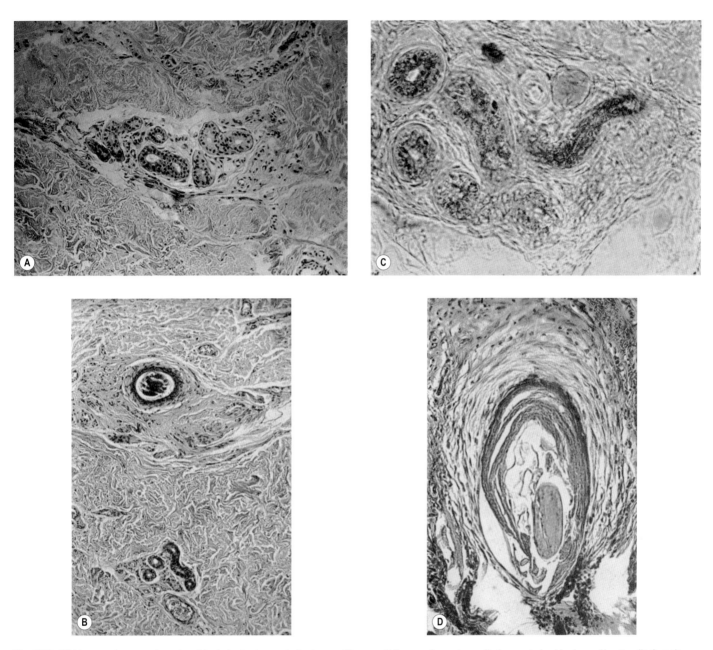

Fig. 18.2 **(A)** Human autogenous dermal graft buried subcutaneously for 4 years. The essentially normal secretory coil of a sweat gland is shown. Hematoxylin & eosin (H&E), ×120. **(B)** From the same section as **(A)**. The greatly dilated excretory duct containing a secretion cast in its lumen (above) is shown with its associated sweat gland (below). H&E, ×75. **(C)** The dark granules represent sites of succinic dehydrogenase activity inside the cells of a surviving sweat gland. Succinic dehydrogenase, an enzyme in the Krebs citric acid cycle, is essential for the vital processes of mammalian cells. Neotetrazolium method ×300. **(D)** Human autogenous dermal graft buried subcutaneously for 5 months. An epidermoid cyst derived from a hair follicle is shown at an intermediate stage of disintegration. The epithelial lining is becoming thinned after the accumulation of keratohyaline debris inside the cyst. There is considerable surrounding reactive fibrosis. H&E, ×210. ((C,D) Reprinted from Chiu DWT, Bradford WE. Repair and grafting of dermis, fat and fascia. In: McCarthy JC, ed. Plastic surgery. Philadelphia: WB Saunders; 1990:509–526.)

gingival augmentation,[20] facial soft-tissue reconstruction,[21] and burn treatment.[22]

Future

One direction will be the use of xenogenic acellular dermal matrix (ADM) as a replacement when concerning the source of donated human skin. Mirzabeigi *et al.* reported the use of porcine ADM (Permacol) to repair chest wall defects resulting from desmoid tumor resection *(Fig. 18.3)*.[23] However, an apparent immunogenic response was observed in xenogenic ADM compared to allogenic ADM during a clinical trial in burn treatment.[24] It has been found that amino-terminal propeptide is the most immunogenic part of type I procollagen.[25] In the future, transgenic pigs that are genetically modified to produce human type I procollagen might be an ideal source for generating less immunogenic ADM given the fact that such a genetic technique is already available for expressing some human molecule in pigs,[26] and given the available technique that can provide pathogen-free animals.

Fat graft and repair

Fat graft is defined as a graft containing fat cells along with stromal tissues. Fat graft can be transplanted by the means of free fat transfer, or transfer with dermal

tissue in the form of dermis fat graft or microvascular transfer of fat graft using microsurgery.[3] FIG **18.4** APPEARS ONLINE ONLY

Clinical application for tissue repair and recent developments

The use of fat injection as a way of transplanting free fat graft was established soon after the introduction of liposuction. Free fat graft has been widely used for various types of tissue repair.[27] Breast cosmetic surgery or reconstruction is the most important application. The indications include treatment of micromastia, correction of postaugmentation deformity (with and without removal of implant), treatment of tuberous breasts and Poland's syndrome, surgical repair of postlumpectomy deformity and postmastectomy deformity, treatment of deficits or tissue damage caused by conservative or surgical reconstruction, and nipple reconstruction.[28–34] Facial augmentation and correction of defects are also important indications, including rhinoplasty with lipoinjection,[35] facial contouring,[36,37] and facial tissue augmentation.[38] Guyuron and Majzoub developed a core fat graft technique for lip augmentation and correction of malar and buccal deficiency.[39] *Figures 18.5–18.7* demonstrate the procedure and the results for lip and buccal augmentation with fat transfer.[39] In addition, free fat transplantation has been applied to gluteal augmentation and repair of contour deformities,[40,41] hand rejuvenation,[42] and penile enlargement and aesthetic improvement.[43,44]

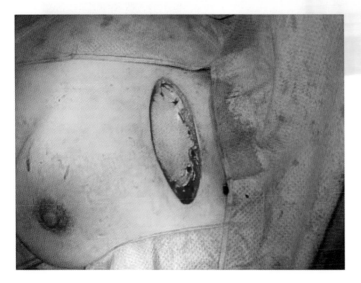

Fig. 18.3 Permacol sewn into place with 1-0 polydiaxanone (PDS): periosteal drilling was utilized to anchor the suture material. (Reprinted from Mirzabeigi MN, Moore JH Jr, Tuma GA. The use of Permacol for chest wall reconstruction in a case of desmoid tumour resection. J Plast Reconstr Aesthet Surg. 2011;64:406–408.)

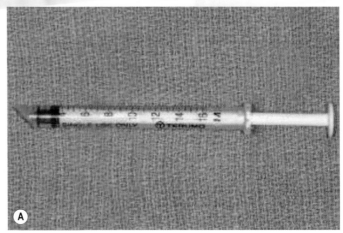

Fig. 18.5 Procedures for harvesting fat graft. **(A)** The tip of a conventional syringe is cut obliquely and is thin-walled to harvest fat and deliver it to the tissue bed.

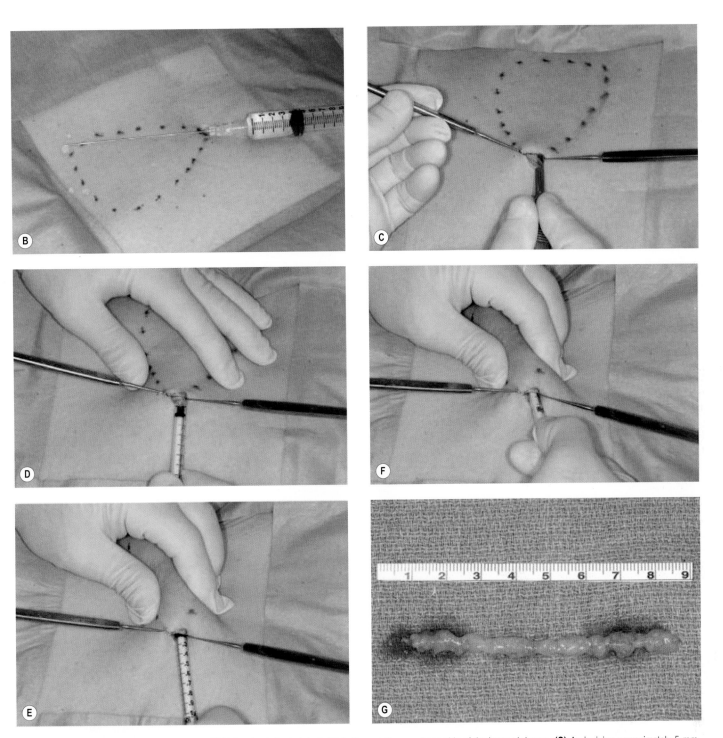

Fig. 18.5, cont'd **(B)** Xylocaine containing 1:100 000 epinephrine is injected into the umbilicus and one side of the lower abdomen. **(C)** An incision approximately 5 mm long is made in the inner portion of the umbilicus. **(D)** The beveled syringe is inserted in the deep subcutaneous plane, and the incision margins are stabilized using skin hooks. **(E)** As the beveled syringe is advanced, it is rotated and the plunger is retracted enough to accommodate the cored-out fat. No vacuum is created. **(F)** While the syringe is being advanced, the fat is pushed into it. **(G)** A sample of extracted fat using "core" fat grafting technique. The fat graft has an intact structure. (Reprinted and modified from Guyuron B, Majzoub RK. Facial augmentation with core fat graft: a preliminary report. Plast Reconstr Surg. 2007;120:295–302.)

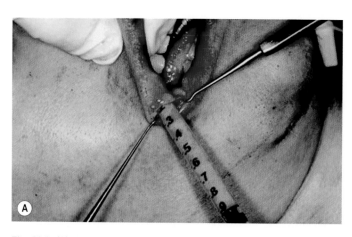

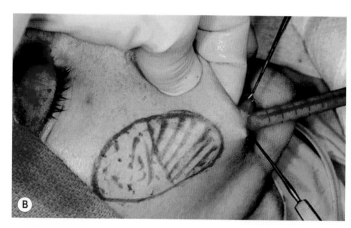

Fig. 18.6 **(A)** Upper lip augmentation with core fat graft. The syringe delivers an *en bloc* graft to the upper lip as the syringe is withdrawn and the piston is pushed forward. **(B)** Correction of malar and buccal deficiency with core fat graft technique through an oral commissure incision. (Reprinted and modified from Guyuron B, Majzoub RK. Facial augmentation with core fat graft: a preliminary report. Plast Reconstr Surg. 2007;120:295–302.)

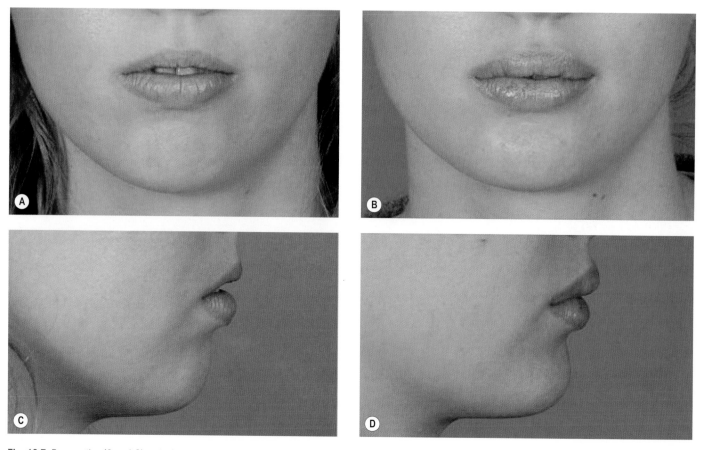

Fig. 18.7 Preoperative **(A and C)** and 16-month postoperative **(B and D)** frontal and profile views of a patient after lip augmentation with core fat graft.

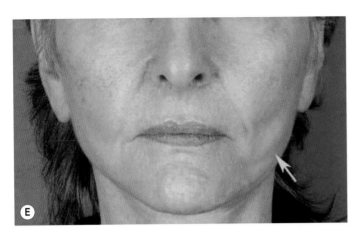
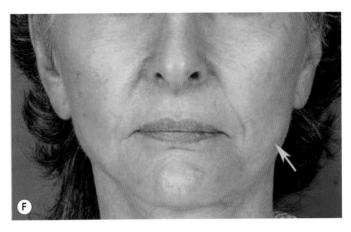

Fig. 18.7, cont'd Frontal views of a patient before **(E)** and 8 months after **(F)** core graft to the buccal area. (Reprinted and modified from Guyuron B, Majzoub RK. Facial augmentation with core fat graft: a preliminary report. Plast Reconstr Surg. 2007;120:295–302.)

To harvest free fat graft, minimal invasiveness and high tissue viability are the general principle. It is thus suggested to use 3–4-mm blunt cannula or similar needle and utilize minimal amounts of suction force to avoid mechanical damage. In addition, cell damage caused by centrifugation force and air exposure should be avoided.[27] In regard to complications, in addition to infection, seroma, hematoma formation, graft volume loss via reabsorption and necrosis are the primary causes of poor results.[27] Tissue or cell damage during harvest is also one of the reasons. The other factor is poor vascularization of implanted fat graft.[45]

There are several reports on improving vascularization and survival of transplanted fat by incorporating vascular endothelial growth factor (VEGF) gene-transfected adipose stem cells.[46] Potentially, other angiogenic growth factors like basic fibroblast growth factor (bFGF) and platelet-derived growth factor can be integrated into the fat grafts to support their survival by enhancing *in vivo* angiogenesis at the transplantation site.[47] Circulating endothelial progenitor cells (EPC) are considered an important factor for promoting tissue vascularization, which can be recruited to an ischemic region by locally released factors.[48] Therefore, mixing EPCs with fat graft will also potentially enhance vascularization and tissue survival.

Although the translation of experimental discovery to clinical application remains at an early stage, Yoshimura *et al.* reported a practical approach for cosmetic breast augmentation called cell-assisted lipotransfer (CAL), which has benefited from the basic research

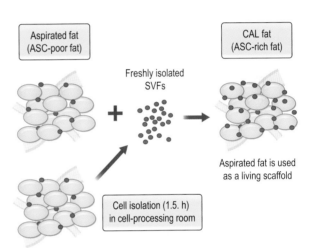

Fig. 18.8 Scheme of cell-assisted lipotransfer (CAL). Relatively adipose-derived stem/stromal cell (ASC)-poor aspirated fat is converted to ASC-rich fat by supplementing ASCs isolated from the other half of the aspirated fat. The ASCs are attached to the aspirated fat, which is used as a scaffold in this strategy. SVF, stromal vascular fraction. (Reprinted from Yoshimura K, Sato K, Aoi N, et al. Cell-assisted lipotransfer for cosmetic breast augmentation: supportive use of adipose-derived stem/stromal cells. Aesthet Plast Surg. 2008;32:48–55.)

of stem cell biology.[28] In the reported study, adipose-derived stem/stromal cells (ASCs) were isolated from stromal vascular fraction and then mixed with lipoaspirated fat to form ASC-rich fat (*Fig. 18.8*). Because ASCs are much more angiogenic and potent than mature adipocytes and lipoaspirated fat can serve as the scaffold to support the growth and function of seeded ASCs, such an ASC-rich fat graft will have a better survival rate than a regular free fat graft due to better angiogenesis after implantation. The result of clinical application demonstrated good tissue survival (*Fig. 18.9*) with soft

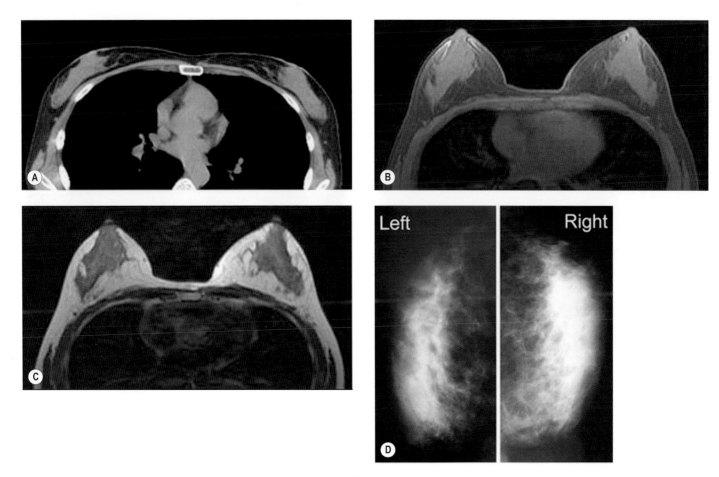

Fig. 18.9 Radiologic evaluation of augmented breast by cell-assisted lipotransfer. **(A)** A preoperative computed tomography (CT) image in the horizontal plane at the level of the nipples. **(B and C)** Horizontal images by magnetic resonance imaging (MRI) 12 months after surgery: **(B)** T1 image; **(C)** T2 image. The adipose tissue is augmented around and under the mammary glands. A small cyst (<10 mm) appears in the fatty layer under the right mammary gland. **(D)** Mammograms at 12 months show no abnormal signs such as calcifications. (Reprinted from Yoshimura K, Sato K, Aoi N, *et al.* Cell-assisted lipotransfer for cosmetic breast augmentation: supportive use of adipose-derived stem/stromal cells. Aesthet Plast Surg. 2008;32:48–55.)

breast and natural contour and breast volume could be stabilized 2–3 months after transplantation. More importantly, a 4–8-cm increase in breast circumference was observed in this CAL, trial, in contrast to only 2–3-cm increase in conventional procedure *(Fig. 18.10)*.[28] The potential mechanisms of CAL method may include ASCs differentiating into adipocytes and endothelial cells, promoting angiogenesis and graft survival, releasing angiogenic growth factors in response to hypoxia and other conditions, and contributing to the turnover of implanted adipose tissue.[28]

In addition to free fat graft, dermis fat graft and microvascular fat graft are also the methods for fat tissue transplantation. Many applications have been reported for this type of grafting, including facial reconstruction and correction of forehead depression scar,[49,50]

orbital reconstruction,[51] and nerve or tendon covering.[52] However, volume loss remains a concern for this type of graft, as revealed either by experimental study[53] or by the study of transplanted human dermis fat graft.[54] One of the approaches to overcome volume loss is microvascular transfer of fat graft such as free omental fat flap or de-epithelialized dermis fat graft for various tissue repairs, which will be described in other chapters.

Future

Application of ASCs and fat tissue engineering are apparently important directions towards fat tissue repair and regeneration. As shown in *Figure 18.11*, ASCs are located at the stromal vascular fraction and

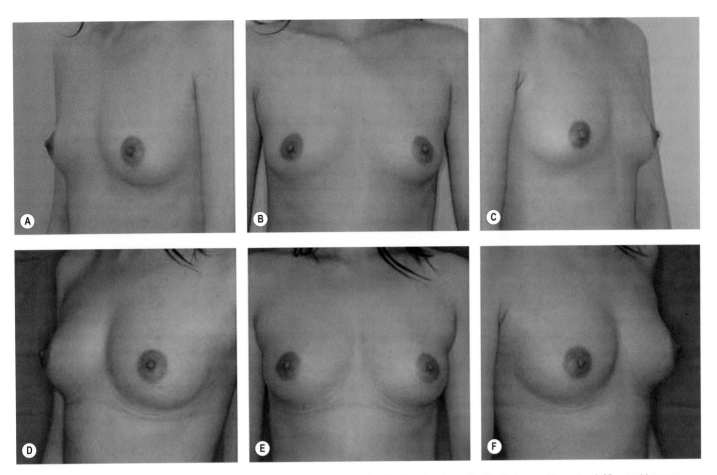

Fig. 18.10 Clinical views of breast augmentation by cell-assisted lipotransfer. Preoperative **(A–C)** and postoperative **(D–F)** views at 12 months. A 32-year-old woman underwent breast augmentation with cell-assisted lipotransfer (CAL) (280 mL in each breast). Her breast circumference difference increased from 9 cm (baseline) to 14.5 cm (at 12 months). The breast mounds are soft and natural-appearing with no visible injection scars. (Reprinted from Yoshimura K, Sato K, Aoi N, *et al.* Cell-assisted lipotransfer for cosmetic breast augmentation: supportive use of adipose-derived stem/stromal cells. Aesthet Plast Surg. 2008;32:48–55.)

can be concentrated by centrifugation.[55] As previously described, mixing isolated ASCs with lipoaspirated fat graft can better maintain tissue survival via several mechanisms.[27] To master this process, Cytori Therapeutics developed a special facility called Celution system, which allows for separating and collecting ASCs from freshly harvested fat tissue in about 1 hour in the operating room and enables surgeons to mix ASCs with fat tissue for breast augmentation or other soft-tissue repair (information derived from Cytori website: www.cytori.com). Therefore, the concept of ASC-assisted fat tissue transplantation proved by experimental study and clinical trials is likely to be translated into a therapeutic procedure.[56]

Another important approach, adipose tissue engineering, may represent a more suitable alternative for adipose tissue regeneration via *de novo* adipogenesis. In particular, to correct a large adipose defect, adult stem cells like ASCs or adipose progenitor cells can be seeded on a three-dimensional scaffold and implanted *in vivo* for adipogenesis. The advantage of this approach is the possibility of incorporating angiogenic growth factors like VEGF or bFGF into the scaffold or mixing EPCs or endothelial cells along with ASCs. In addition, implantation of adult stem cells is likely to be induced for angiogenesis and/or vascularization during the *de novo* adipogenic process, and eventually develop a fully vascularized fat tissue to ensure correct tissue volume and function. In contrast to mature adipocytes, implanted ASCs or adipose progenitor cells also provide a means of self-repair or regeneration via their self-renewal function.[57]

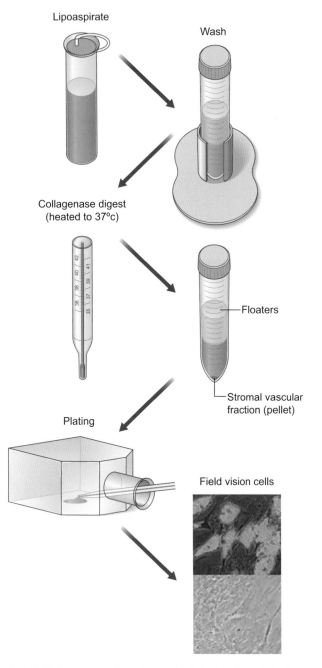

Lipoaspirate

Wash

Collagenase digest
(heated to 37°c)

Floaters

Stromal vascular
fraction (pellet)

Plating

Field vision cells

Fig. 18.11 Processing of lipoaspirate and isolation of adipose-derived stem cells. (Reprinted from Gimble JM, Katz AJ, Bunnell BA. Adipose-derived stem cells for regenerative medicine. Circ Res. 2007;100:1249–1260.)

Fascial graft and repair

Fascial graft is defined as a graft of broad dense fibrous tissue, which can be transferred with or without a vascular supply.

Surgical technique and tissue repair application

Fascia is characterized by its unique dense collagen structure, which can provide great mechanical strength. As an example, the average tensile strength of fascia latae is approximately 7000 lb per square inch or 10.73 lb per quarter-inch strip.[3,58,59] Because of this unique character, fascial graft is usually employed to repair a defective tissue that requires mechanical strength to carry out its normal function. These indications include repair of facial palsy,[60] paralytic lagophthalmos,[61] congenital unilateral lower lip palsy,[62] reconstruction of ruptured Achilles tendon,[63] promoting watertight dural closure to prevent cerebrospinal fluid leakage postsurgery,[64] assisting closure of abdominal wall after multiple organ transplantation,[65] and reconstruction of the palatal aponeurosis.[66]

Fascia latae is the most common donor site for nonvascularized fascia. Generally, a strip 10–15 mm wide can be harvested; removing a further wider fascia strip is likely to make muscle herniate through the fascia defect. *Figure 18.12* demonstrates the procedure of harvesting a strip of fascia latae by a refined version of a fascia tripper developed by Wilson and Castroviejo.[3] For vascularized fascial graft, the temporoparietal fascial flap is the common type of fascia free flap; it is ultrathin and leaves a minimal donor site defect.[3] In recent years, the endoscope has been used to harvest temporoparietal fascial flap with fascular pedicle. This fascial flap can either be used in local repair or in distant areas as a free flap. *Figure 18.13* demonstrates the process of harvesting a temporoparietal fascial flap and its application in auricular reconstruction.[67]

Future

It remains difficult to find a biological tissue to replace fascia graft fully due to fascia's unique tissue structure and its great mechanical strength. One potential approach is the fabrication and application of tissue-engineered fascia. Hung *et al.* reported the formation of tissue-engineered neofascia in an animal study which may potentially be applied for reconstructive pelvic surgery.[68] Fann *et al.* reported a model of tissue-engineered ventral hernia repair employing novel aligned collagen tube and autologous skeletal muscle

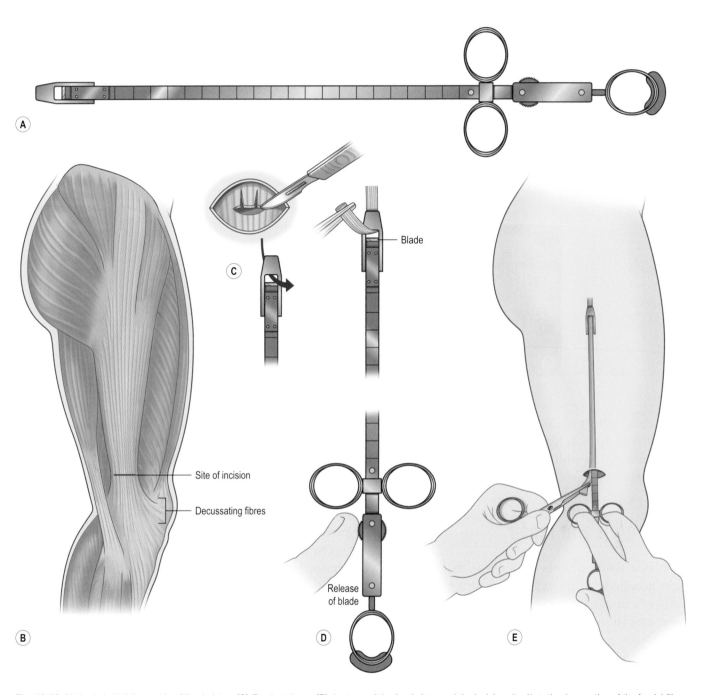

Fig. 18.12 Method of obtaining a strip of fascia latae. **(A)** Fascia stripper. **(B)** Anatomy of the fascia latae and the incision site. Note the decussation of the fascial fibers. **(C)** A flap of fascia is raised parallel to the direction of the fibers. **(D)** The flap of fascia is introduced into the stripper and held by a heavy clamp. **(E)** The stripper is advanced while downward traction is maintained on the clamp. The knee should be flexed, thus maintaining the fascia latae under tension. When a fascia strip of sufficient length is obtained, the upper end of the strip is severed by means of the guillotine. (Reprinted from Chiu DWT, Bradford WE. Repair and grafting of dermis, fat and fascia. In: McCarthy JC, ed. Plastic surgery. Philadelphia: WB Saunders; 1990:509–526.)

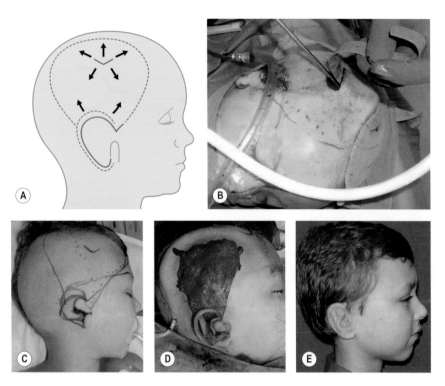

Fig. 18.13 Endoscope-assisted temporoparietal fascia harvest for auricular reconstruction. **(A)** Schematic illustration of the flap harvest. Red marks indicate incisions; red dots mark the limit of flap dissection; black arrows show directions of dissection, and periauricular dotted lines denote planned ear position. Note that medial dissection is performed initially at the posterior base of the flap and not the lateral access incision. **(B)** The scalp is elevated with an insulated malleable retractor (superficial to the temporoparietal fascia), beginning with the endoscopic portion of the lateral access cavity dissection. Endoscopic brow lift sheath is used later as needed at the periphery of the dissection. **(C)** Flap area is outlined. **(D)** Flap is delivered. **(E)** Final outcome of its application in auricular reconstruction. (Reprinted and modified from Helling ER, Okoro S, Kim G 2nd, *et al.* Endoscope-assisted temporoparietal fascia harvest for auricular reconstruction. Plast Reconstr Surg. 2008;121: 1598–1605.)

satellite cells, which could form a "living repair," and the established approach may potentially be applied for clinical therapy.[69] In addition, decellularized fascia may be a potential strategy.

Tendon graft and repair

Tendon is a white fibrous cord tissue that connects a muscle to a bone to transmit the contracting force for the movement of extremities. It may lie in a paratenon, a loose areolar tissue surrounding tendon, or it may pass through a tendon sheath, a tube of condensed fibrous tissue surrounding tendon. The anatomy of tendon as well as its related structures is shown in *Figure 18.14*.[70]

Surgical technique and tissue repair application

The characteristics of an ideal donor tendon include: easy access, consistent in all its dimensions, sufficient length and mechanical strength for defect repair, and thin enough for adequate revascularization. The commonly used tendon grafts include the palmaris longus;

the plantaris; the extensor digitorum longus tendons to the second, third, and fourth toes; a flexor digitorum superficialis tendon; or an undamaged tendon in an amputated digit. None of these graft candidates meets all the requirements, but each candidate has some of these characters.[70] *Figures 18.15–18.17* demonstrate the procedure of harvesting several common tendon grafts.[70]

The healing of tendon grafts may include three phases[70]: (1) cellular phase: the space between the graft and host tissue is filled with blood clot, inflammatory cells, and granulation tissue. Epitenon cells may proliferate and invade to participate in the repair; (2) collagen synthesis phase, beginning at the first week and lasting for several weeks with extracellular matrix production along with ongoing revascularization process; (3) remodeling phase: during this phase, transplanted graft gains strength and peritendinous adhesions become loose and filmy and lose their strength, allowing the graft to glide. However, it may need 9 months to remodel the collagen fibers to a relatively normal pattern. In addition, intrinsic and extrinsic healings are both possibly involved in the repair. The former employs cells within the tendon (tenocytes or endotenon) to heal the wound, whereas the latter uses the cells on the surface of tendon (epitenon) or cells in the surrounding tissue

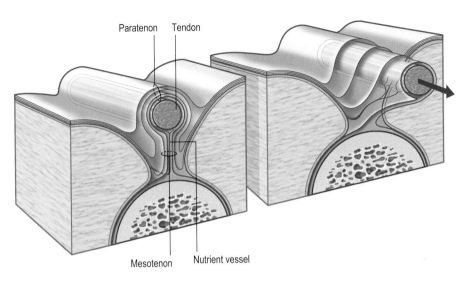

Paratenon Tendon

Mesotenon Nutrient vessel

Fig. 18.14 The multilayered paratenon forms a barrier between the tendon and the surrounding structure and serves as a source of nutrition via the vincular vessels. The mesotenon is the part of the paratenon draped over the nutrient vessels functioning as an umbilicus. Its pliability and length allow the tendon to glide and yet maintain continuous perfusion. (Reproduced from Chiu DWT, Bradford WE. Repair and grafting of tendon. In: McCarthy JC, ed. Plastic surgery. Philadelphia: WB Saunders; 1990:527–545.)

(fibroblasts) to repair the wound. Generally, intrinsic healing is the preferred type because of better functional restoration, whereas the extrinsic pattern is likely to cause fibrotic adhesion between repaired tendon and the surrounding tissue.[70,77]

Tendon graft may primarily be used in hand surgery to repair flexor profundus injury,[78,79] extensor pollicis longus tendon rupture,[80] or for reconstruction of extensor hood deficits with subluxation.[81] Importantly, when there is an unsuitable bed for tendon grafting, a two-stage tendon grafting procedure is necessary. This technique was first described by Carroll and Bassett[3,82] and Hunter.[3,83] In the first stage, a good recipient bed is prepared, including contracture release, skin cover, nerve repair, scar removal, and implantation of a silicone rod to create a space for tendon graft; in the second stage, tendon graft is transplanted to a well-prepared bed.[84] In addition, a bone tendon graft has also been applied for Achilles tendon defect repair[85] and patellar tendon grafts have been reported for posterior cruciate ligament reconstruction[86] and lateral ankle ligament reconstruction.[87]

Tendon substitute and engineered tendon

As described above, none of the available autologous tendon grafts is able to meet all the requirements of an ideal tendon graft.[70] In particular, it is almost not possible completely to avoid functional disturbance to the donor area where a tendon graft is harvested. This becomes a major concern when large quantities of autologous tendon grafts are needed to repair severe tendon injury and defect. Therefore it has been a challenge in plastic surgery for long time. To address this concern, several strategies have been proposed and developed.

Tendon allograft is one of them. After experimental studies, Liu reported the use of refrigerated flexor tendon graft for second-stage tendon graft and the results showed 63% had good flexion, 21% fair, and 16% poor; and 8% had good total active motion, 71% fair, and 21% poor. It was concluded that allograft could be applied for tendon repair but was inferior to autograft.[88] Peacock and Madden reported the transplantation of composite allograft of complete flexor apparatus which was stored for a few days at 4°C, and the result showed seven of 10 patients achieved satisfactory functional result.[89] According to the literature, there are few reports on the application of allograft for tendon repair in the hand. In contrast, there are relatively more reports on using allografts for cruciate ligament reconstruction,[90,91] suggesting that knee joint, a relatively immune-privileged environment, may be a more suitable recipient site for allograft transplantation than the hand. Tendon xenograft remains at an experimental stage[92] and a clinical trial reported the failure of this application,[93] possibly due to the antigenicity of xenocollagen.

Artificial tendon is also one of the strategies which employed nondegraded materials to substitute tendon tissue. This is not a new area and much work has already been done, as reviewed by Murray and Semple in 1979.[94]

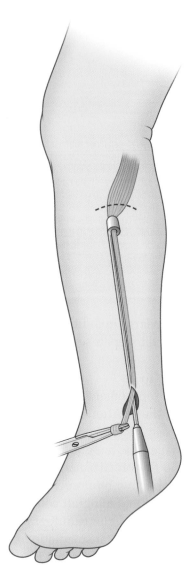

Fig. 18.15 Securing the distal stump of the plantaris tendon with a hemostat avoids the embarrassment of losing the tendon graft when advancing the tendon stripper. The maneuver also allows fine adjustments of tension when advancing the tendon stripper. (Reproduced from Chiu DWT, Bradford WE. Repair and grafting of tendon. In: McCarthy JC, ed. Plastic surgery. Philadelphia: WB Saunders; 1990:527–545.)

The difficulty in healing between host tissue and artificial tendon, fibrotic tissue formation, and the fatigue of implanted materials remain the challenges to functional repair. In recent studies, cells have been incorporated into the material to promote healing and integration.[95] In addition, attempts have been made to develop a biological interface between the prosthesis and the host tissue.[96]

The most promising strategy might be tissue engineering because it is able to generate autologous graft without causing donor site morbidity.[97] The two key factors in tendon engineering are scaffold materials and seed cells.

Tendons are the connective tissue that links muscles to bones, so that the tensile force created by muscles can be transmitted to bone for body movement. The main tendon extracellular matrix is type I collagen, which is highly organized in a hierarchy of bundles that are aligned in a parallel fashion. This unique structure provides the unique biomechanical properties of tendon tissues. Therefore, the parallel alignment structure and strong mechanical property should be considered for tendon scaffold design. It was proposed that an ideal tendon scaffold should fulfill the following requirements[98]:

1. Biodegradability with adjustable degradation rate

2. Biocompatibility before, during, and after degradation

3. Superior mechanical properties and maintenance of mechanical strength during the tissue regeneration process

4. Biofunctionality: the ability to support cell proliferation and differentiation, extracellular matrix secretion, and tissue formation

5. Processability: the ability to be processed to form desired constructs of complicated structures and shapes, such as woven or knitted scaffolds.

Based on the literature search, the major categories of scaffold materials for tendon engineering include: poly (α-hydroxy acids), collagen derivatives, acellular tendon, xenogenic acellular extracelluar matrix, silk derivatives, and polysaccharides.

Regarding seed cells, tenocytes,[99–101] dermal fibroblasts,[102,103] and bone marrow stem cells (BMSC)[104] have become the candidates for tendon engineering. As early as 1994, Cao *et al.* performed a pioneer research of tendon engineering using polyglycolic acid (PGA) fibers as the scaffold and calf tenocytes as the cell source for *in vivo* tendon engineering in a nude mouse model.[99] First, unwoven PGA fibers were arranged in a parallel fashion, then tenocytes isolated from calf tendons were expanded *in vitro* and seeded on the scaffold, followed by *in vivo* implantation in the subcutaneous tissue of nude mice. After 12 weeks of implantation, tendon-like

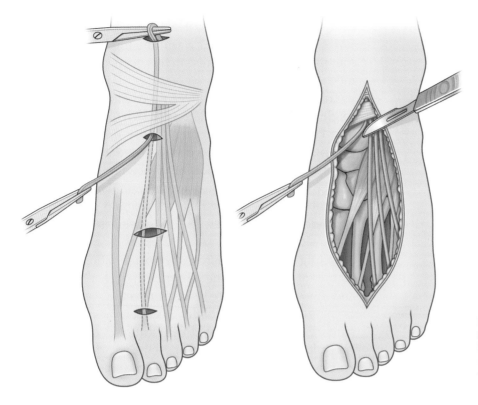

Fig. 18.16 The anatomic relationship between the long and short toe extensors and the "closed" and "open" methods of tendon removal. (Reproduced from Chiu DWT, Bradford WE. Repair and grafting of tendon. In: McCarthy JC, ed. Plastic surgery. Philadelphia: WB Saunders; 1990:527–545.)

tissue formed and revealed longitudinally aligned collagen fibers.[99]

To test further the possibility of engineering tendon in immunocompetent animal models, Cao *et al.* reported *in vivo* tendon engineering using hen claw as a model for tendon regeneration and repair inside a tendon sheath.[100] Similarly, unwoven PGA fibers served as a scaffold and were arranged into a cord-like shape. Autologous tendon tissues were harvested and tenocytes were isolated by enzyme digestion. After *in vitro* expansion, cultured tenocytes were seeded on to the scaffold PGA fibers and the cell–scaffold construct was cultured *in vitro* for 1 week before *in vivo* implantation. For *in vivo* tendon repair inside a tendon sheath, two small transections were made at a distance of 3–4 cm apart *(Fig. 18.18A)*, and a 2.5-cm-long fragment was removed from the second digital flexor profundus tendon *(Fig. 18.18B)*, resulting in a 3–4-cm tendon defect, then a cell–scaffold construct was inserted into the tendon sheath to bridge the tendon defect *(Fig. 18.18C)*. At 12 and 14 weeks postrepair, mature tendon tissue

was formed when observed grossly *(Fig. 18.19)*. Histologically, longitudinally aligned collagen fibers with a curving pattern could be observed with proper cell–collagen ratio and ideal interface healing between engineered and host tendons *(Fig. 18.20)*. Importantly, engineered tendon reached 83% of native tendon's tensile strength, suggesting the possibility of functional repair by engineered tendon.[100]

For practical applications, an alternative cell source must be considered because no autologous tendon will be available to extract tenocytes after tendon injury and defect formation. BMSCs are the first cell type that was used to replace tenocytes for tendon engineering. Awad *et al.*[105] and Young *et al.*[106] initially used BMSCs as seed cells for tendon engineering. They mixed BMSCs with a collagen gel to repair the defects of patellar and Achilles tendons respectively in a rabbit model. Although the biomechanical properties were improved when compared with the control tissue formed by the scaffold that was implanted without cell seeding, the engineered tissues failed to display a histological

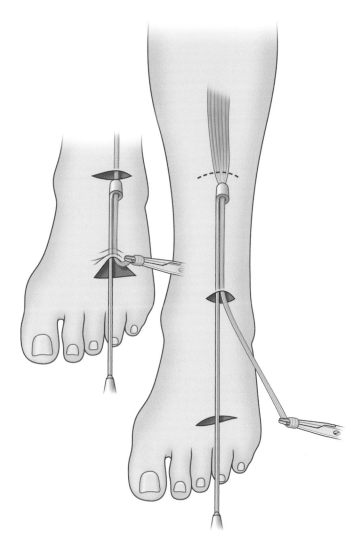

Fig. 18.17 To obtain a single long-toe extensor, serial transverse incisions are made over the course of the tendon. The authors recommend using a fine small tendon stripper, which may obviate the need to incise the extensor retinaculum. (Reproduced from Chiu DWT, Bradford WE. Repair and grafting of tendon. In: McCarthy JC, ed. Plastic surgery. Philadelphia: WB Saunders; 1990:527–545.)

structure similar to that of a normal tendon. Ouyang et al.[104] reported successful engineering of a rabbit Achilles' tendon using allogeneic BMSCs. The experiment showed that knitted poly-lactide-co-glycolide scaffolds seeded with BMSCs could generate a tendon tissue with a histological structure similar to that of a normal tendon. However, it remains unclear which factors should be used to induce tenogenic differentiation of BMSCs, and proper tenogenic marker molecules need to be determined to characterize tenogenically differentiated cells. Additionally, committed tenogenic differentiation of implanted BMSCs is certainly an

important issue. Harris *et al.* reported the formation of ectopic bone at the site of a tendon defect where a BMSC–collagen construct was implanted,[107] suggesting that more fundamental research is needed to define the mechanism.

Transdifferentiation between two similar cell types might also be an appropriate approach to find a replaceable cell source. Considering similar origin, cell morphology, and function, we have tried to use dermal fibroblasts to replace tenocytes as seed cells to engineer tendon and repair tendon defects. As similarly described, dermal fibroblasts were first isolated and cultured and expanded *in vitro*, then the cells were seeded on to unwoven PGA fibers for 1 week of *in vitro* culture. Scanning electron microscope examination revealed abundant matrix production by both dermal fibroblasts and tenocytes that were seeded on to the scaffold, indicating good cell compatibility between the cells and the scaffold. The prefabricated cell–scaffold construct was transplanted *in vivo* to repair a 3-cm-long defect created on flexor digitorum superficialis tendon. When examined at 26 weeks postrepair, mature tendon tissue was formed, which was similar to the tendon tissue engineered by autologous tenocytes in a gross view. Histologically, similar tissue structure was observed among dermal fibroblast and tenocyte-engineered tendons and native tendon tissues. Interestingly, with long-term *in vivo* tissue remodeling under mechanical loading, dermal fibroblast-engineered tendon produced predominant type I collagen similar to tenocyte-engineered tendon, suggesting cell phenotype shift *(Fig. 18.21)*. Importantly, strong mechanical property was also achieved in engineered tendons. All these factors indicate that dermal fibroblasts are a possible cell source for tendon engineering.[102]

Although the studies mentioned above proved that engineered tendon repair is possible via an *in vivo* approach using different types of cells, a greater challenge would be to provide surgeon-engineered autologous tendon graft for immediate repair and thus to achieve early functional recovery, instead of implanting a cell–scaffold which involves a more complicated *in vivo* tissue formation process and takes a relatively long time. Our center has explored the possibility of *in vitro* tendon engineering.

Cao *et al.* reported a preliminary study on tendon engineering *in vitro* using hen tenocytes and unwoven

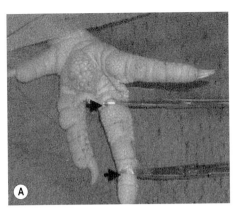
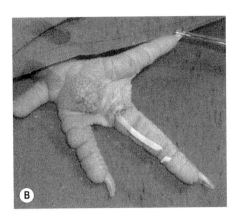
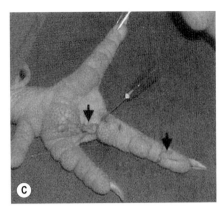

Fig. 18.18 *In vivo* model for engineered tendon repair. **(A)** Two transections (arrows) were made 3–4 cm apart. **(B)** A 2.5-cm-long fragment was removed from the second digital flexor profundus tendon, resulting in a 3–4-cm tendon defect. **(C)** A cell–scaffold construct (arrows) was inserted into the tendon sheath to bridge the tendon defect. (Reprinted from Cao Y, Liu Y, Liu W, *et al.* Bridging tendon defects using autologous tenocyte engineered tendon in a hen model. Plast Reconstr Surg. 2002;110:1280–1289.)

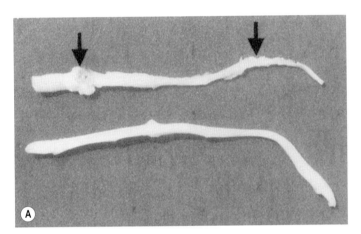
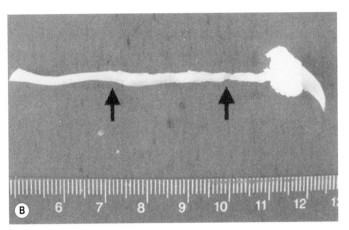

Fig. 18.19 Gross views of engineered tendons at **(A)** 12 weeks and **(B)** 14 weeks. **(A)** Engineered tendons (above, between arrows) resembled normal tendon (below) in color, texture, and thickness. An interface between the normal and engineered tendons (above, left arrow) was noticed. **(B)** The engineered tendons at 14 weeks (between arrows) matched the structure of the normal tendons (left side of left arrow). Ideal interface healing (left arrow) was observed between the normal and engineered tendons. Tendons at both 12 and 14 weeks were uniform in diameter throughout the length. (Reprinted from Cao Y, Liu Y, Liu W, *et al.* Bridging tendon defects using autologous tenocyte engineered tendon in a hen model. Plast Reconstr Surg. 2002;110:1280–1289.)

PGA fibers.[101] First, unwoven PGA fibers were arranged into a cord-like construct and fixed on a U-ring with static tension. Next, tenocytes were extracted from hen tendon tissue by collagenase digestion and expanded *in vitro* and then seeded on to the PGA scaffold. After culture of the cell–scaffolds for 6 or 10 weeks *in vitro*, a neotendon tissue was formed when examined grossly *(Fig. 18.22)*. Histologically, collagen fibers with longitudinal alignment were observed in the tissue section. Interestingly, PGA fibers were mostly degraded through *in vitro* culture. Apparently, the engineered neotendon became more mature in the group with static loading comparing to that with no tension *(Fig. 18.23)*.[101]

Furthermore, we recently also tested the feasibility of using human dermal fibroblast to engineer neotendon *in vitro*. In this study, both human dermis and tendon were harvested from an amputated extremity and both fibroblasts and tenocytes were extracted from respective tissue with enzyme digestion. After *in vitro* expansion, cells were loaded on to PGA unwoven long fibers that were secured on a U-shaped spring which is able to provide a static mechanical loading. As shown in *Figure 18.24*, with extended culture time, neotendon became relatively more mature than neotissue of early time points. More importantly, both fibroblast- and tenocyte-engineered neotendons exhibited similar gross views

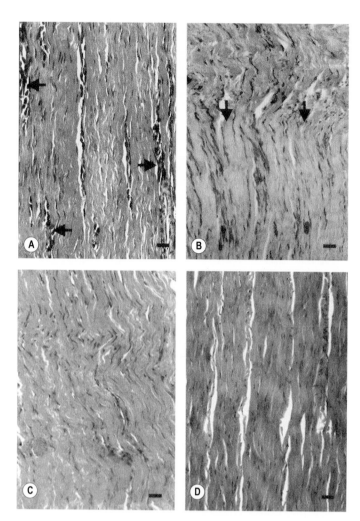

Fig. 18.20 Histologic findings of the engineered tendons. **(A)** Hematoxylin and eosin (H&E) staining of an engineered tendon of 12 weeks and arrows shows undegraded polyglycolic acid fibers. **(B)** Trichrome staining demonstrates the interface healing between engineered tendon (lower portion) and normal tendon (upper portion), as indicated with arrows. **(C)** H&E staining of engineered tendons of 14 weeks. **(D)** H&E staining of a native hen tendon. (Original magnification, ×100; bar represents 15 µm.) (Reprinted and modified from Cao Y, Liu Y, Liu W, et al. Bridging tendon defects using autologous tenocyte engineered tendon in a hen model. Plast Reconstr Surg. 2002;110:1280–1289.)

and histologic structures when observed at 9 weeks of *in vitro* culture. Furthermore, they also exhibited similar tensile strength and collagen fibril diameter.[103] These preliminary results indicate that dermal fibroblasts are a possible cell source for generating engineered tendon graft *in vitro*.

The drawback of these reported studies is the weakness of *in vitro*-engineered tendons and the tensile strength is usually less than 5 N. This is probably due to the lack of proper mechanical loading that is applied to native tendon tissue in daily life. In a recent study

performed in our center, we developed a bioreactor to provide dynamic mechanical loading to the *in vitro*-engineered tendon at a certain frequency and the results showed that tissue quality as well as the mechanical strength of loaded engineered tendon were significantly improved after 10–12 weeks of *in vitro* culture (data not shown). This probably represents the future direction of this area.

In addition to linear tendon engineering, our center has performed a pioneering study of engineering extensor tendon complex by an *ex vivo* approach.[108] In this study, PGA long fibers and human fetal extensor tenocytes (isolated from a 3-month-old aborted fetus donated by the patients for research only) were used to engineer extensor tendon complex equivalent. The PGA long fibers were arranged to mimic the extensor tendon complex-like structure *(Fig. 18.25)* followed by cell seeding on to the scaffold. After *in vitro* culture for 6 weeks, the cell–scaffold constructs were further divided into three groups: (1) *in vitro* culture with mechanical loading; (2) *in vivo* implantation without mechanical loading; (3) *in vivo* implantation with mechanical loading by suturing the construct to fascia, and thus mouse movement can provide a natural dynamic loading. The results showed that human fetal tenocytes could form an extensor tendon complex structure *in vitro* and become further matured *in vivo* by mechanical stimulation *(Fig. 18.25C)*. In contrast to *in vitro* loaded and *in vivo* nonloaded tendons, *in vivo* loaded tendons exhibited bigger tissue volume, better-aligned collagen fibers, more mature collagen fibril structure with D-band periodicity, and stronger mechanical properties *(Fig. 18.26)*. These results indicate that *in vivo* mechanical loading via an *ex vivo* approach might be an optimal approach for engineering functional tendon tissue. Therefore, a reasonable strategy for engineered functional repair of tendon defect might be to generate a neotendon tissue first *in vitro* and then to implant *in vivo* for its further maturation and carrying out its functions.

In plastic surgery practice, the most important task of tendon repair might be the flexor tendon repair in the zone 2 area where tendons are surrounded by a tendon sheath. In hand injury, tendon injury often comes with tendon sheath injury or defect. Tendon sheath is a membrane-like structure surrounding the tendon, which separates the tendon from surrounding tissue and allows

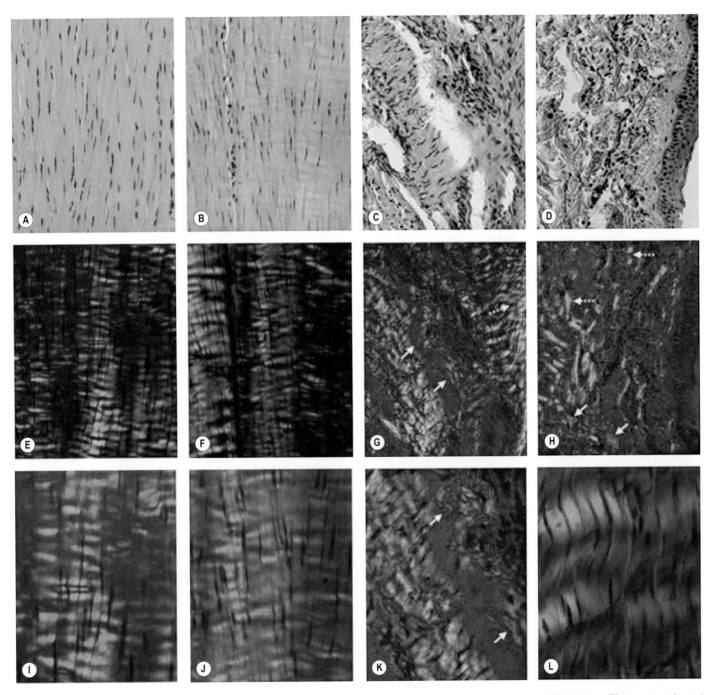

Fig. 18.21 Histological finding of formed tissue at 26 weeks. Hematoxylin and eosin (H&E) staining shows histological structures of **(A)** fibroblast, **(B)** tenocyte-engineered tendons, **(C)** a control tissue in control group 2, and **(D)** normal pig skin. Collagen III (delicate collagen fibers with a light-green color) is detected only in the polarized images of control tissues **(G and K)** and in normal pig skin **(H)**, as indicated by white arrows. In addition, collagen I (golden color, indicated by white dotted arrows) is also detected in these tissues. In the polarized images of fibroblast **(E and I)** and tenocyte **(F and J)** engineered tendons and natural tendons **(L)**, collagen I (golden color) is the predominant collagen type. (Original magnification ×400 (I–K); ×200, all others.) (Reprinted from Liu W, Chen B, Deng D, *et al.* Repair of tendon defect with dermal fibroblast engineered tendon in a porcine model. Tissue Eng. 2006;12:775–788.)

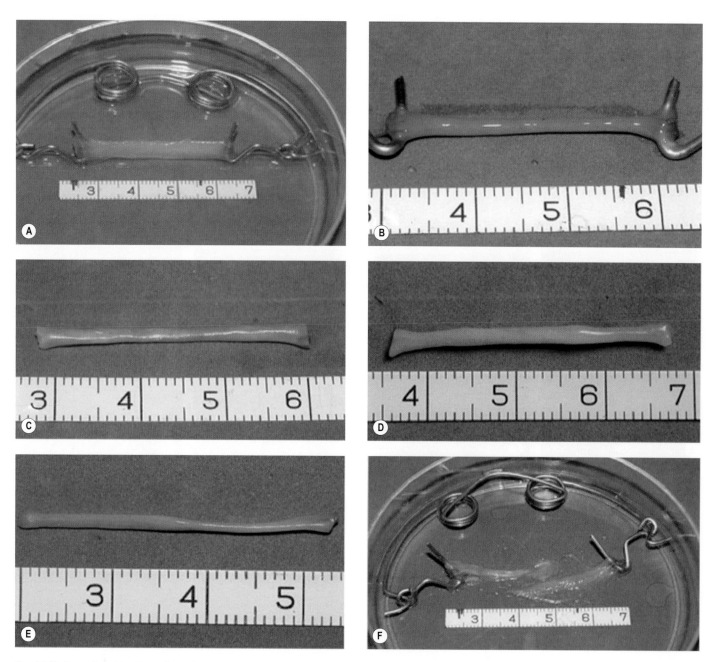

Fig. 18.22 Gross view of *in vitro*-engineered tendons and cell-free constructs cultured for different time periods. **(A)** Tenocyte polyglycolic acid (PGA) construct cultured without tension for 1 week. **(B)** *In vitro*-cultured tenocyte PGA construct without tension at 4 weeks. **(C and D)** Engineered tendons cultured without tension for 6 and 10 weeks, respectively. **(E)** Engineered tendons cultured with tension for 6 weeks. **(F)** Partially degraded PGA fibers of the cell-free scaffold after 4 weeks of incubation. (Reprinted from Cao D, Liu W, Wei X, *et al. In vitro* tendon engineering with avian tenocytes and polyglycolic acids: a preliminary report. Tissue Eng. 2006;12:1369–1377.)

tendon to glide smoothly inside the sheath. Additionally, the synovial sheath itself is a good biological barrier that prevents invasion of peripheral fibrous tissue and inhibits exogenous healing of the tendon. Also, the sheath is the source of synovial fluid, which provides nutrition to the tendon and serves as a lubricant to maintain normal tendon gliding. Although methods like hyaluronic acid membrane[109] or vein graft[110] have been tried for repairing the sheath defect, the long-term results were less satisfactory because they cannot replace native sheath tissue for the function of synovial fluid production. To search for a better functional repair method, our center has recently reported the engineering of a functional tendon sheath in a hen model.[111]

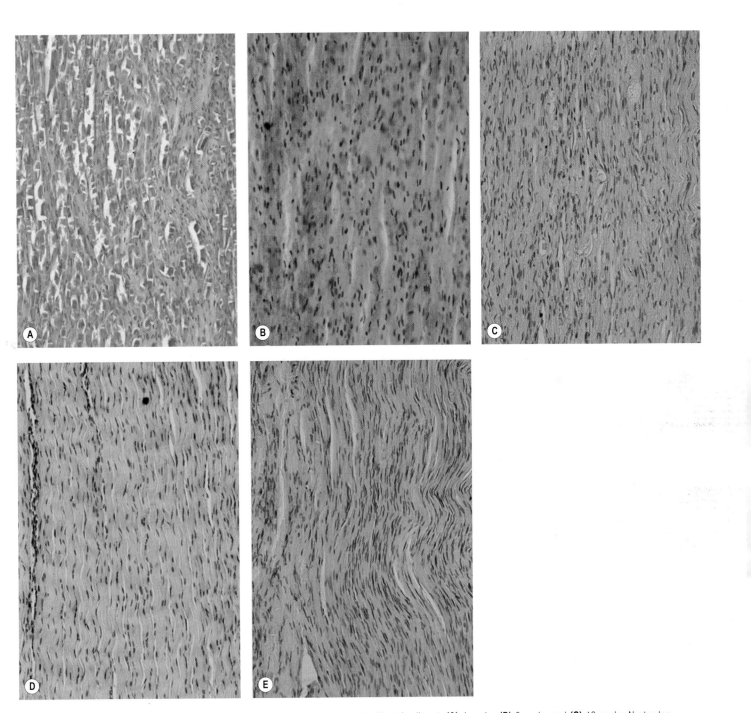

Fig. 18.23 Histological findings of *in vitro*-engineered tendons. Neotendon engineered without loading at: **(A)** 4 weeks; **(B)** 6 weeks; and **(C)** 10 weeks. Neotendon engineered with static mechanical loading at 6 weeks **(E)** and histology of native tendon **(D)**. (Original magnification × 100.) (Reprinted from Cao D, Liu W, Wei X, *et al. In vitro* tendon engineering with avian tenocytes and polyglycolic acids: a preliminary report. Tissue Eng. 2006;12:1369–1377.)

In this study, autologous tendon sheath tissues were first harvested and tendon sheath cells (containing both synoviocytes and subintimal fibroblasts) were extracted with enzyme digestion. After *in vitro* expansion, cells were seeded on the PGA unwoven fibers, and then a 1-cm defect was created by separating the sheath from the tendon and segmental removal. Afterwards, the sheet of cell–PGA construct was inserted at the defect site and wrapped around the tendon without suturing to repair the defect in the experimental group, or repair with PGA only in the scaffold control or unrepair in the blank control group.

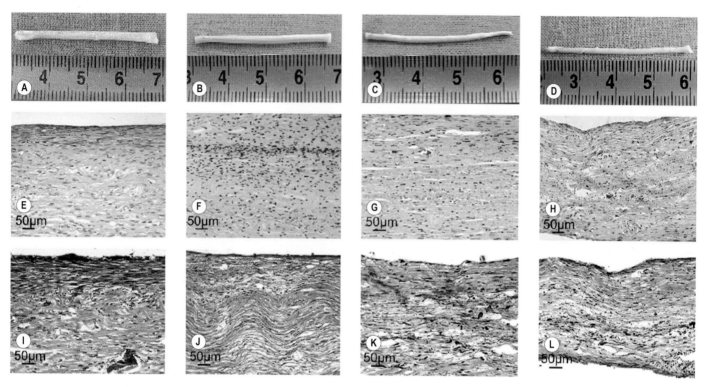

Fig. 18.24 Gross view **(A–D)**, histology **(E–H,** bar, 50 μm) and Masson's trichrome staining **(I–L,** bar, 50 μm) of *in vitro*-engineered neotendon under static tension by human dermal fibroblasts at 5 weeks **(A, E, I)**, 9 weeks **(B, F, J)** and 14 weeks **(D, H, L)**, or by human tenocytes at 9 weeks **(C, G, K)**. (Reproduced from Deng D, Liu W, Xu F, *et al.* Engineering human neo-tendon tissue *in vitro* with human dermal fibroblasts under static mechanical strain. Biomaterials. 2009;30:6724–6730.)

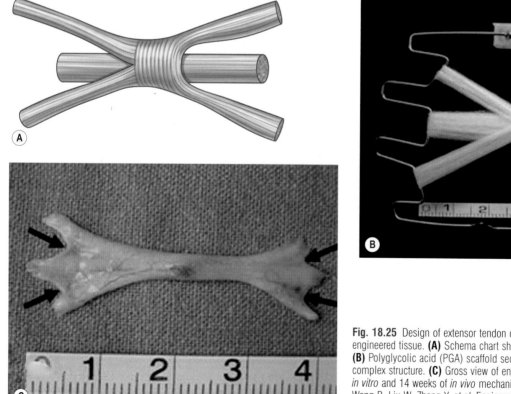

Fig. 18.25 Design of extensor tendon complex scaffold and gross view of engineered tissue. **(A)** Schema chart showing the central slip and two lateral bands. **(B)** Polyglycolic acid (PGA) scaffold secured on a custom-made spring to mimic the complex structure. **(C)** Gross view of engineered tendon complex after 6 weeks of *in vitro* and 14 weeks of *in vivo* mechanical loading. (Reprinted and modified from Wang B, Liu W, Zhang Y, *et al.* Engineering of extensor tendon complex by an *ex vivo* approach. Biomaterials. 2008;29:2954–2961.)

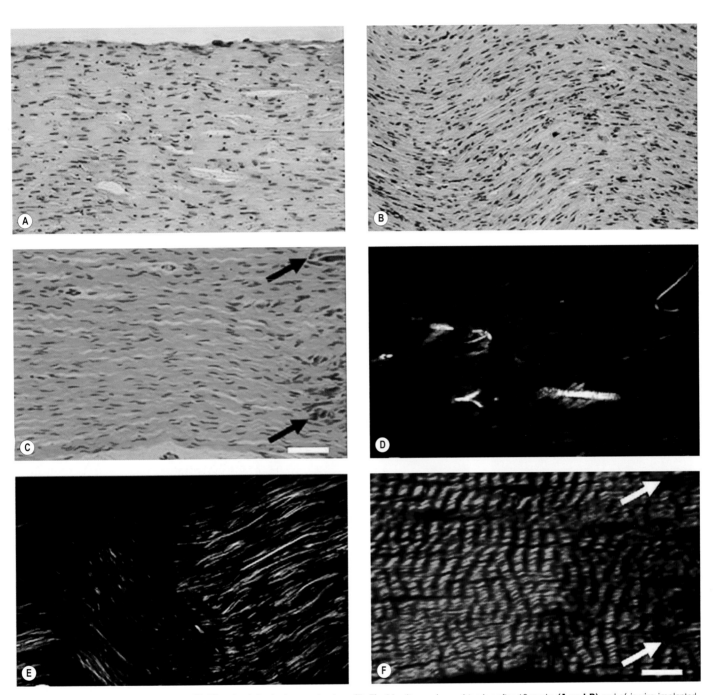

Fig. 18.26 Hematoxylin and eosin staining **(A–C)** and polarized microscopic views **(D–F)** of *in vitro*-engineered tendon after 12 weeks **(A and D)** and of *in vivo* implanted tendons for 14 weeks without **(B and E)** and with **(C and F)** loading. Arrows represents relatively immature collagen fibers. (Original magnifications: ×200; bar represents 50 μm for all.) (Reprinted from Wang B, Liu W, Zhang Y, *et al*. Engineering of extensor tendon complex by an *ex vivo* approach. Biomaterials. 2008;29:2954–2961.)

The results showed that tendon sheath cells seeded on a PGA scaffold were able to produce hyaluronic acid. At 12 weeks postrepair, a well-developed tendon sheath structure was observed, which could be easily separated from the tendon tissue with a smooth inner surface and no fibrotic adhesion. In contrast, there was severe fibrotic adhesion between tendon and surrounding tissue in two control groups, which severely limited the sliding of the tendon tissue *(Fig. 18.27)*. Electronic scanning microscopic examination also confirms the smooth

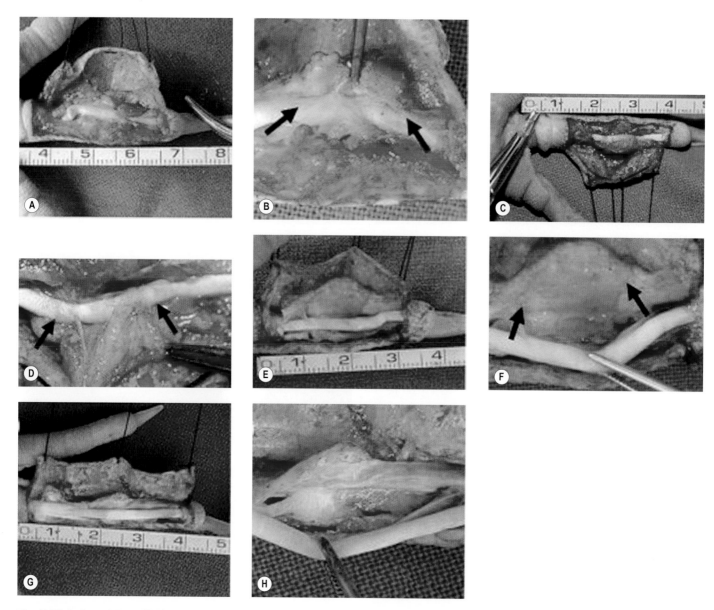

Fig. 18.27 Engineered sheath **(E, F)** revealed a smooth surface with good healing to adjacent native sheaths **(F,** repaired area between arrows) and there was no obvious adhesion between the tendon and the sheath, similar to a native sheath **(G, H)**. The untreated defect **(A, B)** healed with fibrotic tissue formation surrounding the tendon and on the tendon surface with severe adhesion **(B,** repaired area between arrows). Similarly, defect repaired with scaffold alone **(C, D)** also formed fibrotic tissue with severe adhesion **(D,** repaired area between arrows). **B, D, F,** and **H** are amplified pictures of **A, C, E,** and **G** respectively. (Reprinted from Xu L, Cao D, Liu W, *et al. In vivo* engineering of a functional tendon sheath in a hen model. Biomaterials. 2010;31:3894–3902.)

surface superstructure of the experimental group, which is similar to that of the native tissue.

To reveal the process of engineered sheath repair, engineered tissues were harvested at 2, 5, and 12 weeks postrepair for hematoxylin and eosin staining to observe the structural relationship between the tendon and the newly formed tissue. As shown in *Figure 18.28*, the engineered sheath structure in the experimental group started to form at the second week postimplantation and became more mature at the 12th week, which was mostly equivalent to that of native sheath. A clear space was also observed between the engineered sheath and the tendon. In contrast, there was no sheath formation in the other two control groups and fibrotic tissue was observed to fill in the space between the tendon and the surrounding tissues. More importantly,

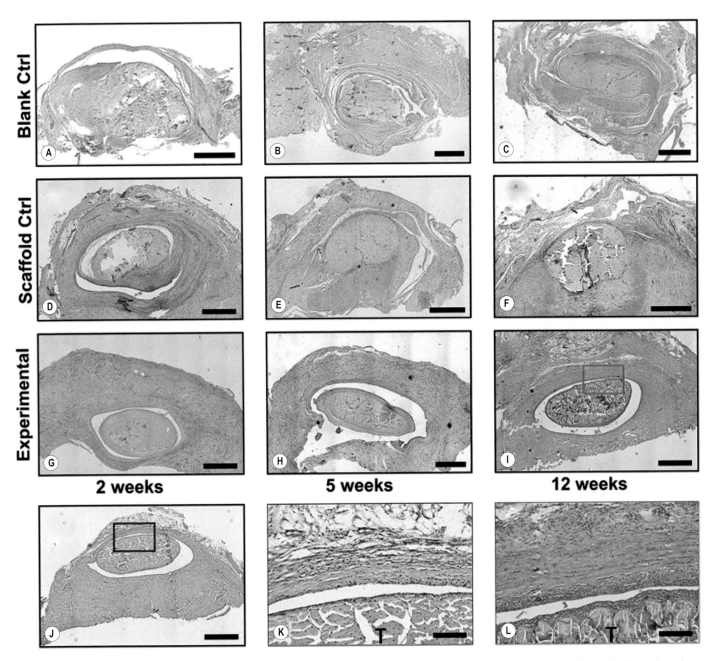

Fig. 18.28 Hematoxylin and eosin staining of scar-repaired surrounding tissues of blank control group (**A–C**) or scaffold control group (**D–F**) and of *in vivo*-engineered tendon sheath (**G–I, L**) or native tendon sheath (**J, K**) at postsurgery weeks 2 (**A, D, G**), 5 (**B, E, H**), and 12 (**C, F, I, L**). Engineered sheaths formed a tendon sheath complex structure (**I, L**) similar to that of a native sheath (**J, K**) with a clear space between the engineered sheath and its surrounded tendon. Fibrous tissue formation and disturbance of normal tendon sheath complex structure were observed in both control groups (**C and F**). The bar represents 100 μm for K and L, and represents 1 mm for the rest. (Reprinted from Xu L, Cao D, Liu W, *et al. In vivo* engineering of a functional tendon sheath in a hen model. Biomaterials. 2010;31:3894–3902.)

the result of work of flexion assay indicated that much less energy was needed to make tendon slide in the engineered group than in the other two control groups. The results of this preliminary study indicate that a tissue-engineered approach is possible to generate autologous tendon sheath for potential functional repair of tendon sheath defect.

Future

Functional repair of massive tendon tissue defect remains a challenge in plastic surgery not because of surgical technique, but rather due to the lack of autologous tendon graft. As reported in the literature, current experiments demonstrate the possibility of generating autologous tendon graft via a tissue-engineering approach. One future direction is to employ a proper bioreactor system with dynamic mechanical loading to generate engineered autologous tendon graft and therefore to enhance matrix production and maturation of *in vitro*-engineered tendon tissues. In addition, design of a proper scaffold material with enhanced mechanical strength would also help to provide an engineered tendon graft that is strong enough for functional requirements after *in vivo* implantation. The other potential direction is to employ acellular allogenic/xenogenic tendon tissue to reconstitute tendon graft given that new methods can be applied to facilitate cell penetration.[112,113]

Skeletal muscle graft and repair

Striated muscle is the organ system which makes up 30–40% of body weight and its function is to contract and to move extremities or body parts. Although variable in different muscles, most muscles shorten about 40% of their length during full contraction.[114] As such, defect of important muscle type can lead to functional disability. A muscle graft by definition is a muscle completely removed from its origin, insertion, and nerve and blood supply, and replaced into the original bed (orthotopic) or another anatomic location (heterotopic).[114] Generally, muscle graft types include free muscle transfer (without nerve/vascular anastomosis) or microneurovascular muscle transfer.

Surgical technique and tissue repair application

In the clinic, microneurovascular transfer of muscle graft is essential in order to preserve muscle contraction function. In order to maximize reinnervation potential, the general technical aspects of the procedure can be summarized as: (1) selection of a donor muscle with a single artery and nerve that can be removed with little residual functional disability; (2) reduction of the length of ischemia time; (3) proximal neural repair; (4) the donor muscle should have functional characteristics that closely parallel the specific anatomic deficit.[114,117–119]

Examples of clinical applications include: (1) treatment of facial paralysis with microneurovascular transfer of free gracilis muscle[120,121] and pectoralis minor flap[119]; (2) treatment of forearm muscle avulsion[122]; (3) treatment of traumatic loss of long flexor musculature by microvascular transfer of gracilis and pectoralis major muscle[118]; (4) closure of large myelomeningocele defects with latissimus dorsi muscle flap[123]; and (5) breast reconstruction with latissimus dorsi muscle flap.[124] Details of surgical repair of tissue defects with various muscle flaps will be described in related chapters.

Future

Like other tissue types, a tissue-engineering approach may potentially generate an autologous muscle graft without causing donor site defect. Conconi *et al.* reported an interesting study of engineered muscle repair of abdominal defect in a rat model. They isolated myoblasts and seeded on an acellular muscle matrix after *in vitro* expansion, and the cell-seeded patches were implanted between obliqui abdominis muscles. The results demonstrated that, after 2 months of *in vivo* implantation, the patches displayed abundant blood vessels and myoblasts, and electromyography evidenced in them single motor unit potentials, sometimes grouped into arrhythmic discharges *(Fig. 18.29)*, suggesting the potential of engineering functional muscle *in vivo* using acellular muscle matrix as a scaffold.[125] Another example is the reconstitution of a "beating heart" by perfusion of decellularized heart matrix with cardiac and endothelial cells, which further supports the potential of muscle engineering.[126] In

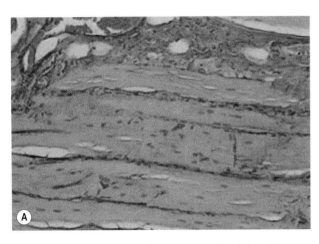
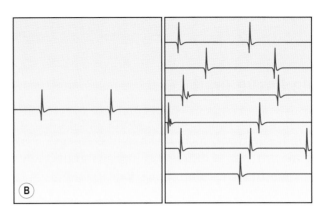

Fig. 18.29 Vertical section of implant composed of acellular matrix seeded with autologous myoblasts 60 days after surgery **(A)** (×100), and corresponding electromyographic record **(B)**. (Reprinted from Conconi MT, De Coppi P, Bellini S, *et al.* Homologous muscle acellular matrix seeded with autologous myoblasts as a tissue-engineering approach to abdominal wall-defect repair. Biomaterials. 2005;26:2567–2574.)

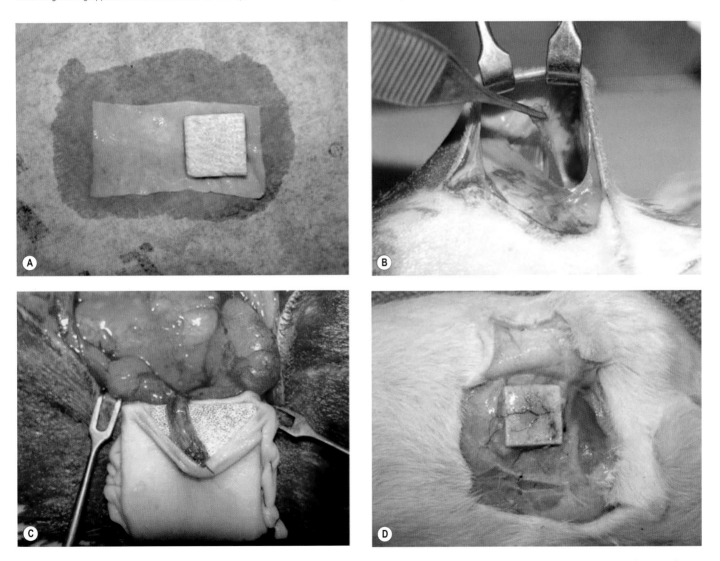

Fig. 18.30 Creation of vascularized composite graft. **(A)** Sheets of AlloDerm are enveloped around square wafers of hydroxyapatite to create composite grafts measuring 2 × 2 cm. **(B)** The superficial epigastric arteriovenous unit is dissected and ligated and then **(C)** placed between the hydroxyapatite and acellular dermal matrix within the midportion of the construct, establishing the experimental specimen. Control specimens were placed on the opposite side without attachment to vascular structures. **(D)** Photograph suggestive of superficial vessel formation at the time of graft harvest. (Reprinted from Woo AS, Jang JL, Liberman RF, *et al.* Creation of a vascularized composite graft with acellular dermal matrix and hydroxyapatite. Plast Reconstr Surg. 2010;125:1661–1669.)

addition, stem cell-based cell therapy may also be a potential approach for muscle regeneration and repair.[127]

Composite tissue graft

The definition of a composite graft is a graft composed of two or more tissue types, such as skin and cartilage. There can be many types of different composite grafts, for example, myocutaneous flap, bone flap, fingertip graft, and full-thickness ear segment tissue. The details of their applications in tissue repair can be found in respective chapters.

As with other types of tissue, the shortage of proper composite grafts or donor site morbidity resulting from tissue harvest remains a major concern in plastic surgery. Engineered composite graft may represent a potential approach in the future. As an example, Woo *et al.* reported an experimental trial of generating vascularized bone composite graft, as shown in *Figure 18.30*.[128]

Access the complete references list online at **http://www.expertconsult.com**

3. Chiu DWT, Bradford WE. Repair and grafting of dermis, fat and fascia. In: McCarthy JC, ed. *Plastic Surgery*. Philadelphia: WB Saunders; 1990:509–526.

17. Butler CE, Langstein HN, Kronowitz SJ. Pelvic, abdominal, and chest wall reconstruction with AlloDerm in patients at increased risk for mesh-related complications. *Plast Reconstr Surg*. 2005;116:1263–1275.

28. Yoshimura K, Sato K, Aoi N, et al. Cell-assisted lipotransfer for cosmetic breast augmentation: supportive use of adipose-derived stem/stromal cells. *Aesthetic Plast Surg*. 2008;32:48–55.

    The authors evaluate a technique in which fat grafts for breast augmentation are enriched with adipose-derived stem cells. They report consistent augmentation after 2 months of follow-up.

39. Guyuron B, Majzoub RK. Facial augmentation with core fat graft: a preliminary report. *Plast Reconstr Surg*. 2007;120:295–302.

    A cylindrical fat-grafting technique is described to allow for less traumatic en bloc harvest and implantation. Predictable results were achieved with shorter operative and recovery times.

50. Lapiere JC, Aasi S, Cook B, et al. Successful correction of depressed scars of the forehead secondary to trauma and morphea en coup de sabre by en bloc autologous dermal fat grafts. *Dermatol Surg*. 2000;26:793–797.

83. Hunter JM. Artificial tendons. Early development and application. *Am J Surg*. 1965;109:325–328.

84. Alnot JY, Masmejean EH. The two-stage flexor tendon graft. *Tech Hand Up Extrem Surg*. 2001;5:49–56.

    This review of two-stage flexor tendon repair begins with a historical perspective and discusses the procedure's indications, technical steps, and complementary procedures. Possible complications are also addressed.

100. Cao Y, Liu Y, Liu W, et al. Bridging tendon defects using autologous tenocyte engineered tendon in a hen model. *Plast Reconstr Surg*. 2002;110:1280–1289.

103. Deng D, Liu W, Xu F, et al. Engineering human neo-tendon tissue *in vitro* with human dermal fibroblasts under static mechanical strain. *Biomaterials*. 2009;30:6724–6730.

    The authors report a method for the successful differentiation of dermal fibroblasts to neotendon tissue. A critical role is identified for static strain in this process.

111. Xu L, Cao D, Liu W, et al. *In vivo* engineering of a functional tendon sheath in a hen model. *Biomaterials*. 2010;31:3894–3902.

    This study describes in vivo generation of tendon sheaths from sheath cells seeded on PGA scaffolds. Histological and biomechanical results indicated formation of functionally useful constructs.

19

Tissue engineering

Andrea J. O'Connor and Wayne A. Morrison

SYNOPSIS

- Tissue engineering, i.e., a growth of three-dimensional (3D) tissues using cells, scaffolds, and blood supply, calls on the skills and expertise of cell biologists, engineers, and clinical surgeons.

- It aims to replicate the embryological process of tissue regeneration rather than adult healing and, given the complexity of the process, much of our efforts to date may seem simplistic.

- Nevertheless, much progress has been made across the full spectrum of the research field. This chapter outlines the historical beginnings of tissue engineering and discusses the current status, addressing the three structural components of tissue: cells, matrix, and vascular supply.

- Biomaterials science and applications are discussed under matrix.

- Much of the work in tissue engineering has been performed *ex vivo* and unfortunately many of these experiments do not predict the fate of cells and matrices *in vivo*.

- Models of *in vivo* tissue engineering are discussed along with the progress in specific fields.

- Very few clinical trials have been undertaken, controls or placebo groups are difficult to incorporate in trial design, and tracking the fate of implanted cells is difficult in humans.

- All this needs to be viewed with the perspective that, to date, very few truly tissue-engineered products have come to market despite huge expectations and investments.

 Access the Historical Perspective section including Fig. 19.2 online at **http://www.expertconsult.com**

Introduction

Traditional reconstructive plastic surgery techniques "rob Peter to pay Paul." The long-held hope for the ultimate reconstruction has been allotransplantation but to date drug morbidity makes the risk–benefit ratio unfavorable for nonvital organs except in rare circumstances. Tissue engineering has emerged as a possible new direction where ideally our own body is stimulated to generate its own replacement tissue.

Definition of tissue engineering

The definition of tissue engineering quoted by most authors is that it is "an interdisciplinary field that applies the principles of engineering and the life sciences toward the development of biological substitutes that restore, maintain, or improve tissue function."[1] It stressed the key roles of engineering techniques, material science, biochemical expertise, and cell biology. What it did not stress was the role that blood supply would play if and when such engineered tissues were to be transplanted into the body. It is to this piece of the tissue-engineering puzzle that plastic surgeons may hold the key and why the clinical application of tissue engineering will become the province of the plastic surgeon.

Regenerative medicine

While tissue engineering has predominantly surgical roots with research directed by cell biologists and engineers, regenerative medicine, a modernized branding for cellular therapy, was the province of physicians and cell biologists. It was a natural progression from bone marrow transplantation and initially focused on hematological stem cells. It has since expanded to target organ regeneration and includes pancreatic islets, liver, cardiac, brain, and spinal cord stem cells and others. There is now considerable crosstalk between the disciplines: tissue engineers are borrowing regenerative medicine's applications of stem precursor cells and regenerative medicine the tissue engineer's scaffold technology for implantable device delivery. For the purpose of this chapter, we distinguish tissue engineering as the pursuit of 3D structural tissue generation and regenerative medicine primarily as a cell-based injection therapy. Although there is obvious overlap only tissue engineering directed towards producing 3D structures is discussed further in this chapter.

The classical paradigm of tissue engineering followed Jack Burke's artificial dermis skin model of seeding cells on to a biodegradable matrix scaffold and implanting it into a vascularized bed.[2] This would rapidly nourish the graft and, by a combination of survival of implanted cells and substitution, the "new skin" would become functional. Clinical needs for bone and cartilage determined early research directions and this gave preeminence to the engineering materials side of the tissue-engineering pendulum as structural load, stability and ideally biodegradability were clearly essential. The spectacular image of the "human ear" in the mouse (see *Fig. 20.22*) galvanized scientists and the public alike as to the potential offered by tissue engineering and reinforced the dogma of expanding cells in culture, seeding them *ex vivo* into scaffold matrix and implanting the composite into the body.[3] The journal *Tissue Engineering* was established in 1996 and many publications focused on novel synthetic biomaterials attempting to replicate pore size and connectivity of nature's extracellular matrix (ECM) using sophisticated machinery and mathematical modeling. Toxicity, structural integrity, biodegradability, surface modifications, cell survival, adherence, migration, and proliferation could all be tested in *ex vivo* models. Bioreactors could greatly expand cell numbers and mimic *in vivo* physical environments to allow more sophisticated *ex vivo* experimentation.

The *ex vivo* paradigm stumbled when attempts were made to translate advances into the living animal. Biomaterials proved toxic to cells in some cases and acted as foreign bodies.[4] Their dynamic structural behavior was very different to *ex vivo* testing and cells found life hostile in the new world. Despite the obvious need for multidisciplinary cooperation, most early research was directed in isolation and this has led to delayed progress in tissue engineering. The engineer's mind set is focused on scaffold structure, tensile strength, biocompatibility, and surface modification while the cell biologist's is on cell identification, expansion, and differentiation. Scaffold modeling was based on sophisticated replication of human ECMs with respect to pore size, but evaluation was largely done *in vitro*. Both teams are laboratory-based, observing cell responses outside the living animal, and had limited access to a practicing clinician's observations, especially plastic surgeons, with respect to the behavior of foreign bodies *in vivo*. Furthermore, surgeons know from bitter experience with skin grafting that cells seeded on to an implanted scaffold *ex vivo* and then implanted are unlikely to connect to a blood supply in sufficient time to avoid ischemic death. Vascularization is vital to cell survival and is a key to any successful multidisciplinary partnership towards clinical translation of tissue engineering. Unfortunately, early tissue engineers were beguiled by selecting tissues that were very thin, such as skin, which could rapidly connect to a blood supply or tissue that did not need a blood supply, namely cartilage. Once 3D soft tissues were attempted such as adipose, muscle, or organs, it became evident that cell survival was poor and that blood supply was paramount.[5–7]

Embryology

Tissue engineering at its core is an attempt to replicate embryology or fetal healing. Here, new tissues form in response to certain signals, both biochemical and biomechanical.[8] The tissues are determined or patterned according to a genetically guided time sequence where growth factors and their chemical gradients as well as changing physical forces in the matrix attract, guide, and differentiate primitive cells into functional clusters. In this process, cells will link with a capillary bed, lay down their own matrix, and create an environment appropriate to their expansion and development. This relatively new concept of "self-assembly" is important to appreciate when translating embryogenesis into a model for tissue engineering. As cells change their phenotype, for example, from precursor to differentiated or from motile and proliferative to resting and clustered, their ECM requirements alter accordingly. Many cells secrete their own matrix suitable to their needs. This constant change cannot easily be replicated in the laboratory and it is simplistic to believe we can seed cells on to one specific matrix and assume this will be appropriate for the cells' needs throughout their development *in vivo*, nor is it easily conceivable that "smart surfaces" can be imprinted on synthetic matrices in layers programmed to be released according to the changing cells' needs when at this point we do not know what these needs are.

Examples from nature

Nature has given us many examples of spontaneous tissue regeneration or engineering which give clues to how this might be modeled artificially. The liver has been known since ancient times to self-regenerate and is captured in the legend of Prometheus, a Titan, who stole fire from Zeus and gave it to mortals. As punishment, he was bound to a rock while a great eagle ate his liver each day, only to have it grow back to be eaten again.

A salamander regrows its legs, the fetus repairs wounds with minimal scarring, and humans have the capacity to gain and lose adiposity rapidly. Ruptured tendons can regenerate across gaps when their ends are retained within their synovial sheath where their matrix and cellular environment are maintained and axial mechanical force signals are transduced into biochemical stimulation *(Fig. 19.1)*. Muscles also will regenerate across gaps in the same way. FIG **19.2** APPEARS ONLINE ONLY

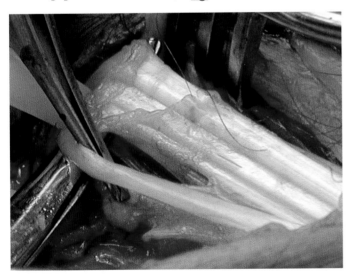

Fig. 19.1 Spontaneous regeneration of ruptured extensor digiti minimi tendon at the wrist (lower tendon held with forceps).

Components of tissue engineering

Simplistically, our tissues can be viewed as a composite of: (1) cells; (2) matrix; and (3) blood vessels.

Each must be considered in the context of tissue engineering. Cell maintenance and behavior including growth and regeneration are influenced by biochemical (growth factors/cytokines) and biomechanical interplay. Each of these components is the purview of the tissue engineer.

Cells

Cell sources

Cells used for tissue engineering may be autologous, heterologous, or xenogenic and each type may be mature differentiated or in precursor stem cell form. Embryonic stem (ES) cells are totipotent, infinitely proliferative, and can be differentiated into all tissue types but they are unstable and form teratomas. Adult stem cells are multipotent and limited in their proliferation capacity and differentiation. Originally found in bone marrow, two distinct adult stem cell types were recognized: (1) hemopoietic (HSC), which differentiated into the white blood cell population; and (2) mesenchymal (MSC), the progenitors of bone, cartilage, fat, and muscle.[14,15] Endothelial precursor cells (EPCs), also known as angioblasts, are thought to derive from hemoblasts, a common ancestor for HSCs. MSCs and EPCs are now known to be present not only in bone marrow but also in fat tissue associated with the microvasculature,[16] where they are known as adipose-derived stem cells (ASCs). Skin, muscle, cord blood, and amnion are also sources of MSCs. Tissue-specific stem cells have now been isolated from almost every organ as well as mesenchyme and they include cardiac, liver, lung, kidney, brain, breast, and others.

Ideally, cells for tissue engineering should be our own cells, and endogenously mobilized to participate in the regenerative process, thereby avoiding issues of rejection and *ex vivo* cell processing or manipulation. This is in essence wound healing, where key cells, both local and distant, are mobilized in response to biochemical gradients and biomechanical forces. A parallel in regenerative medicine is the mobilization and expansion of white blood cells with granulocyte–macrophage colony-stimulating factor (GMCSF), where bone marrow hemopoietic precursors are signaled and released to migrate to their target site. Unlike adult wound healing, which involves deliberate sloughing of damaged tissue and repair by rapid wound closure, scar, and contracture, tissue engineering tries to achieve a more scarless regeneration from stem cells, matrix, and growth factors delivered according to a sequence and type learned from embryology. In the traditional *ex vivo* model of tissue engineering, mature differentiated cells are expanded *in vitro* culture and seeded on to scaffolds prior to *in vivo* implantation. Cartilage, bone, Schwann cells for nerves, and fibroblasts for ligament and tendon engineering are highly proliferative in culture and were early candidates. All these cells have significant proliferative potential *in vitro* but, once implanted, assuming they survive, are not expected to expand further. Other differentiated cells such as adult cardiomyocytes, hepatocytes, and adipocytes are notoriously difficult to culture and expand *in vitro*. MSCs have therefore become more favored sources of cells for mesenchymal tissues which are the main building blocks employed for plastic and orthopedic reconstruction.

On activation, stem cells divide into a daughter cell committed to a particular lineage pathway given the appropriate differentiation stimulus and another which retains the stem properties. Most of our understanding of the properties of these cells comes from studies of bone marrow MSCs, but because of their ease of harvest by liposuction and their abundance, ASCs are now the preferred source. For the most part, they have the same properties but are more abundant, more easily cultured, grow more rapidly, and can be cultured for longer periods than bone marrow stem cells before senescence. A 100-mL sample of lipoaspirate can yield as many as 2 $\times$ 10^8 ASCs (estimated to range from 1/100 to 1/1500 cells).[17] ASCs from different subcutaneous sites display differences in their density, differentiation potential, and adipose function.[18–20] Their potential also varies with age.

Lipoaspirate is washed to lyse red blood cells, collagenase-digested, filtered, and centrifuged to produce a pellet of cells called stromovascular fraction (SVF). This fraction contains ASCs which can be isolated by their adherence to tissue culture plates. Other cells in SVF include EPCs, pericytes, fibroblasts, endothelial cells, anti-inflammatory M2 cells, and hemopoietic cells. Isolation of ASCs using surface markers has been elusive and there is no specific marker currently that specifies these cells. With progressive culturing of ASCs, the hemopoietic markers (CD34) are lost along with their angiogenic potential. They do not express markers of differentiated vascular origin (CD31 or hemopoietic CD45, nor human leukocyte antigen (HLA)-major histocompatibility complex (MHC) class II origin) and cannot be compared with primary isolated SVF cells. They regularly express CD29, CD44, CD90, and CD146. Rodeheffer *et al.* reported that CD24 was a key marker of ASCs.[21] For tissue-engineering and fat injection purposes, it is clear that obsessive attempts to isolate the "pure ASC" may be counterproductive as the other cells of the SVF, especially the EPCs, may also contribute to the apparent functional effects of stem cell application.

For tissue-engineering purposes the ideal would be to have a stem cell that could be predifferentiated *in vitro* and then delivered *in vivo* where it would expand and become a particular tissue type. It is becoming clear that many of the initial claims for stem cell survival, differentiation, and their replacement of damaged tissue could not be substantiated. More commonly, increased angiogenesis or other beneficial anti-inflammatory paracrine effects are observed consistent with their known growth factor and cytokine capacities, including SDF-1, which allows them to home in to injured tissue.[22–26]

MSCs do not express MHC class II markers and several studies suggest they are relatively immune-privileged and may be used as allografts. This is a potentially attractive concept where cells could be sourced from stem cell banks for tissue engineering.[27,28]

Some researchers have persisted with ES cell research based on their allure of totipotency, their infinite capacity for proliferation, and the potential to study diseases at a genetic level. Successful differentiation protocols have been found to induce ES cells along specific lineage pathways from all germ layers towards many specific tissues and organs, including adipocytes.[29] These cells are probably immunogenic and ethical issues will persist. There are many regulatory and organizational issues which will make pathways into the clinic difficult for elective procedures such as tissue engineering, especially proving that they will not form cancer.

Takahashi *et al.*[30] described a method of converting somatic fully differentiated skin cells, mostly fibroblasts, to an embryonic-like state using four transcription factors. Unlike ES cells, they are derived from the patient and present no issues of allogenicity or ethics. They can be induced back through all germ layers to differentiated tissue types, potentially for repair of the donor. They are termed induced pluripotent stem (iPS) cells and they offer an unlimited supply of cells of specific donor identity. Disease models based on these adult-induced cells will also become powerful tools for investigations into genetically based diseases. Rather than using viral transfection to upregulate the induction genes, the proteins they produce can now be used for induction, eliminating issues of viral contamination and reducing the risks of cancer formation. Mice have been cloned from their own iPS cells by implantation into an enucleated ovum. These animals have reproduced and no cancers have been detected.[31]

Biochemical signaling

Metalloproteins, growth factors, and chemokines play vital roles locally and systemically in repair and tissue development, especially via macrophages. Inflammatory cytokines and local angiogenic growth factors stimulate endothelial cell migration, proliferation, and mitogenesis. Systemically, growth factor cytokines signal distant precursor cells, including EPCs.[32,33] Embryogenesis is critically dependent on growth factor cascades released sequentially according to a genetic code and time clock. Gradient concentrations and specific time release of growth factors can theoretically be programmed into materials by incorporating them between layers with a controlled degradation profile to be released according to an orchestrated script but it is a tall order to imagine that anything but the simplest of growth factor combinations could be incorporated into bioengineered materials, so-called "smart surfaces," so as to instruct cell behavior *in vivo*.

Growth factors are expensive, have short half-lives and angiogenic growth factors particularly risk reactivating dormant cancer when used for postcancer resection reconstruction.

Biomechanical signaling and 2D and 3D culture

Cells change behavior in response to both their chemical and physical environments. When cultured on two-dimensional (2D) tissue culture plastic, the equivalent of cells being firmly stretched in clinical situations, their surface receptors sense the rigidity and adhere. They then move, migrate, and proliferate until they reach confluence. The same cells when placed in a soft 3D culture gel environment sense a modulus that encourages the cells to cluster together into spheroids *(Fig. 19.3)*. Integrin-mediated adhesion between cells and the

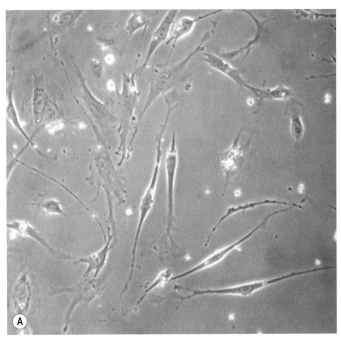

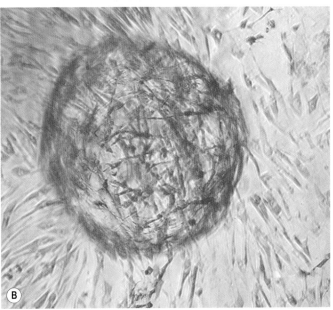

Fig. 19.3 (A) Preadipocytes growing on two-dimensional tissue culture plastic; **(B)** the same cells growing in three-dimensional gel culture form spheroids. (Reproduced with permission from Stillaert et al. Plastic and Reconstructive Surgery Intrinsics and Dynamics of Fat Grafts: An In Vitro Study. Plast Reconstruct. Surg. 2010.)

ECM modulates critical cellular events such as gene expression, embryonic development, cell movement, and differentiation. When the cells pull on the soft matrix they pull it into a ball, stop dividing, and many apoptose. If they are stem cells the environment promotes differentiation.[34–36] By manipulating the ECM modulus cell behavior can be changed accordingly. Physiologically stiff substrates signal stimulation of tyrosine kinase or inhibition of tyrosine phosphatase which stabilizes focal adhesions. The cell measures the flexibility of its substrate cytoskeleton myosin push/pull on the focal adhesion. The response then leads to changes in tyrosine phosphorylation to signal transduction to the nucleus. The mechanical properties of the cell's surrounding substrate environment could be modulated by synthesis/degradation of ECM proteins, movement of cells, or fluid shear from blood flow. These events continually occur during embryonic development and wound healing.[37]

Thus responses to culture in 3D can differ significantly from those on 2D surfaces.[38–43] Culture on traditional hard 2D surfaces such as tissue culture plastic does not replicate the 3D architecture or physical cues of the natural cellular microenvironment in the ECM and it has been shown that a 3D culture environment is important to physiological function of cells *in vitro*. Chondrocytes, for example, change morphology and lose their chondrogenic capacity in 2D monolayer culture but can maintain these features in 3D culture.[44]

Distraction osteogenesis exploits these phenomena. Periods of stretch promote proliferation and migration while relaxation incites cells to cluster together and terminally differentiate into bone. GTR similarly works by presenting the cells with a hard surface which stimulates them to divide and to migrate. Stem cell mechanobiology is attracting increased attention as understanding develops of the influence of substrate mechanics and architecture on differentiation.[45] Cells may be cultured in 3D on biomaterial supports such as porous scaffolds, hydrogels, or microspheres under conditions designed for the desired cell attachment, migration, proliferation, and differentiation.[46] The design of such biomaterial constructs is discussed further later. Bioreactors which magnify cell proliferation or differentiation in culture are based on the same principles of manipulating mechanical forces, such as fluid flow and substrate flexibility.

Co-culture

Tissues cultured *ex vivo* generally are of one cell type and following implantation into an animal rely on recruitment of supporting cellular structures and matrix to evolve into a stable, functional tissue. Co-culturing cells with other types prior to implantation can facilitate their survival and function, such as endothelial cells for vasculature[47] or MSCs for paracrine effects, or for their ability to incorporate into developing tissues *in vivo* such as blood vessels.[16] *In vitro* co-culturing beating cardiomyocytes with ASCs to initiate differentiation into cardiac lineage is a further application.[48]

Bioreactors

Cell culture in 3D constructs presents challenges in delivery and removal of nutrients and waste products in the absence of a blood supply.[49] The delivery of oxygen is challenging due to its relatively low solubility in cell culture media and the time required for diffusion to occur into human-scale 3D constructs. Delivery of macromolecules such as growth factors also presents challenges due to their large size and thus relatively slow diffusion. In addition, mechanical forces and hydrodynamic conditions can significantly affect cellular processes and tissue development. Therefore, bioreactors may be used to provide fluid flow around or through the construct to enhance mass transport and suit the hydrodynamic requirements of the tissue.

It is challenging to obtain uniform conditions throughout a bioreactor due to the difficulty of seeding cells uniformly, mass transport limitations, and variations in fluid shear rates, and this can lead to nonuniform tissue development. Bioreactors which apply additional mechanical forces on the developing tissue construct are also used, particularly for tissues which experience significant forces *in vivo*, like tendons and ligaments. The significant effects of physical forces were demonstrated in engineered cartilage constructs grown in rotating bioreactors in microgravity in comparison to controls grown on Earth *(Fig. 19.4)*.[50] The constructs grown in microgravity for 4 out of the 7 months' culture time showed markedly lower aggregate modulus and glycosaminoglycan content than constructs grown for 7 months on Earth, which showed comparable values to natural cartilage.

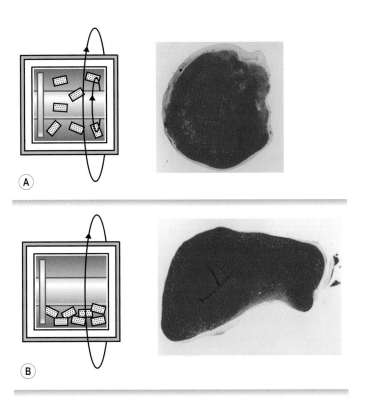

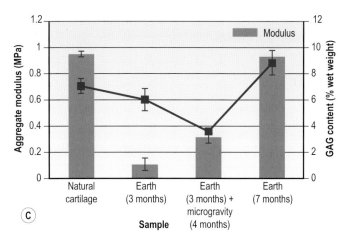

Fig. 19.4 Effects of physical forces on tissue engineering: cartilage grown *in vitro* in microgravity and in Earth's gravity. **(A)** Tissue constructs obtained from growth in rotating bioreactors on Earth for 3 months and in microgravity for 4 months; and **(B)** on Earth only for 7 months (tissues are stained with safranin-O to show glycosaminoglycan in red); **(C)** graph of tissue construct aggregate moduli and glycosaminoglycan (GAG) content. (Based on data from Freed LE, Langer R, Martin I, *et al.* Tissue engineering of cartilage in space. Proc Natl Acad Sci USA 1997;94:13885–13890. © 1997 National Academy of Sciences USA.)

The challenges and approaches developed for cell culture for tissue engineering of a range of specific tissue types have been reviewed in the text edited by Vunjak-Novakovic and Freshney.[51]

Applications for stem cells and tissue engineering

Specific tissues grown using stem cells with traditional tissue-engineering techniques are discussed later. Initial reports of injecting MSCs into tissues for various indications, including cardiac, peripheral vascular disease, and irradiation injury in humans as well as a large experience in the horse-racing industry, boasted survival, differentiation, and function. Few studies were controlled and tracking of cells was absent or difficult to assess. With the exception of brain, almost no cases could confirm that the MSCs survived in significant numbers or that these survivors differentiated into the injured tissue type. Most studies now concede that the paracrine-growth factor-hormonal-cytokine immune-modulatory effects probably account for the benefits seen with these stem cells. Ischemia increases homing of these cells to the injured site where MSCs release high levels of vascular endothelial growth factor (VEGF) to modulate the

repair of capillaries. MSCs injected intravenously in cardiac infarct models do not implant in the heart nor become heart tissue but lodge in the lung, where they are activated to secrete the anti-inflammatory protein TSG-6,[23] and it is probably the anti-inflammatory factor that induces the beneficial effects. Partially purified ASCs which still retain CD34 and CD90 markers grown into spheroid clusters in gel culture differentiate into endothelial cells and capillary structures in methyl cellulose and these produce high levels of VEGF. They also rapidly differentiate into adipocytes in adipogenic media, making them potentially suitable for adipose tissue engineering.[52] Nonexpanded SVF has shown efficacy after injection into Crohn's tissue and in equine studies due to its anti-inflammatory effects.[53] More recently, MSCs have been used as intravenous infusions for the treatment of multiple sclerosis, with promising results. It is felt that the response was anti-inflammatory in nature due to the release of high numbers of M2 anti-inflammatory macrophages.[54] Other growth factors released from ASCs include macrophage colony-stimulating factor, GMCSF, VEGF, antiapoptotic factors, hepatocyte growth factor, and transforming growth factor-β (TGF-β_1). In hypoxia, the VEGF levels are significantly increased, leading to angiogenesis and decreased apoptosis.

Matrix

Biomaterials

An increasing variety of synthetic and naturally derived biomaterials have been considered for application in tissue engineering. Early tissue-engineering attempts tended to utilize materials which had already been used in other clinical applications, such as the polymers used in degradable sutures. Natural materials such as porous coral and hydrogels like alginate or collagen were also trialed. More recently, numerous alternatives have been formulated for particular tissue targets as researchers aim to develop multifunctional biomimetic biomaterials with superior performance characteristics to suit the specific demands of tissue engineering, which can differ significantly from those of other biomaterial applications. Newly developed materials require extensive testing *in vitro* and *in vivo* before clinical acceptance, with very high costs and relatively low rates of translation from the laboratory to the clinic to date.[55] Despite this, a range of such materials are in this testing pipeline.

The role of biomaterials in tissue engineering depends on the application. Biomaterials may be used to provide mechanical support and space for cell and tissue growth; they may affect cellular behavior via adhesion or other interactions; and they may release bioactive factors over time.

Criteria for biomaterials to be suitable for tissue engineering applications include:

- biocompatibility, i.e., eliciting a suitable host response in the specific application
- suitable mechanical properties for target tissue and implantation site
- biodegradability over desired timeframe with suitable mechanical properties and nonharmful degradation products
- not containing harmful impurities
- a host response *in vivo* that does not prevent desired tissue development; i.e., inflammation and foreign-body response are not excessive
- ability to be fabricated into desired structures

- cost-effective
- ability to be sterilized without harmful changes to their chemical or physical properties
- adequate stability and shelf-life
- ability to promote desired cellular responses, e.g., proliferation, differentiation, gene expression.

Biomaterials currently available for use in tissue-engineering approaches do not generally ideally satisfy all of these criteria and development of better biomaterials for tissue engineering is an area of active research worldwide. Whilst it may be feasible to produce complex biomimetic materials to influence cell fate *ex vivo*, simplicity is also desirable to facilitate regulatory approval and translation of new materials into clinical application.[56] Selection of biomaterials will depend on the specific requirements of the tissue being targeted.

Degradation of biomaterials may result in relatively sudden changes in their properties, such as their mechanical strength before the biomaterial is completely removed. The rate of degradation can vary widely so the mechanical integrity may be retained for as little as days or weeks, or as long as a year or more. The rate of degradation and loss of integrity will depend on the type of biomaterial, the site of implantation, properties of the biomaterial construct such as surface area to volume ratio, size, and surface chemistry. *Figure 19.5* shows examples of the loss of mechanical strength of biodegradable polymers tested *in vitro*. As well as the loss of physical integrity, rapid degradation may lead to excessive concentrations of the degradation products of a biomaterial which can cause adverse tissue reactions. This is well known for the polylactides and polyglycolides which can undergo autocatalytic degradation with decreasing pH inside a thick-walled construct and "acid burst" leading to reduced local pH and tissue necrosis. For this reason, it is important to consider degradation rates and mechanisms in designing the composition and architecture of tissue-engineering constructs using biomaterials.

Biomaterials for tissue engineering may be naturally occurring in the human body or derived from other natural or synthetic sources. They may be ceramics, polymers, hydrogels, or composites of these. Decellularized tissues are also used as biomaterials to support tissue growth, wherein cells are removed from allografts or xenografts to reduce immunogenicity but some of the

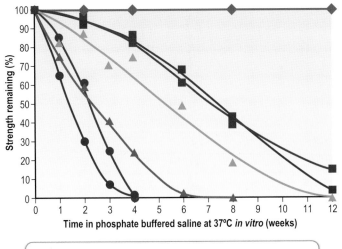

PGA (polyglycolide)

MONOCRYL (Glycolide-ε-caprolactone copolymer)

BIOSYN (glycolide-p-dioxanone-trimethylenecarbonate copolymer)

MAXON (glycolide-trimethylenecarbonate copolymer)

P(LA/CL) (L-lactide-ε-caprolactone copolymer) 75/25

PDS (poly-p-dioxanone)

PLLA (poly-L-lactide)

Fig. 19.5 Changes in tensile strength of biodegradable polymers during degradation *in vitro*. (Reproduced from Suzuki M, Ikada Y. Biodegradable polymers in medicine. In: Reis RL, Román JS (eds) Biodegradable systems in tissue engineering and regenerative medicine. Boca Raton: CRC Press, 2005.)

complex composition and architecture of the ECM may be retained. The physical form of biomaterials for tissue-engineering applications can also vary to suit the application – solid materials, porous scaffolds, microspheres, hydrogels, injectable materials which may cross-link *in situ*, or other configurations can be fabricated.

Natural biomaterials

Natural biomaterials may have the benefits of being chemically similar or identical to molecules in the body, readily degraded *in vivo*, and able to interact with cells on a molecular level. However, they can be difficult to obtain and purify, vary in properties between batches, may be difficult to sterilize, alter their properties during storage, and they may elicit significant immunogenic responses. Naturally derived biomaterials investigated for tissue engineering include proteins (e.g., collagen, gelatin, silk), polysaccharides (e.g., chitosan, hyaluronic acid), polynucleotides and extracts of ECM components.[57] These materials may be modified to tailor their properties, such as via chemical cross-linking to slow degradation and increase mechanical strength.

Synthetic biomaterials

Numerous synthetic polymers are used in medicine and some of these are biodegradable (or bioresorbable) *in vivo*. *Figure 19.6* shows examples of the chemical structures of biodegradable polymers that could be used in tissue engineering. Among these, the polyesters poly(glycolic acid), poly(lactic acid) and poly(ε-caprolactone) (PCL) and their copolymers such as poly(lactide-co-glycolide) (PLGA) have been widely used in tissue-engineering approaches.[58,59] The mechanical strength and degradation rate of these polymers can be tuned over a wide range by changing the polymer properties (molecular weight, composition, crystallinity).[60] As can be seen from the chemical structures, many biodegradable synthetic polymers are quite hydrophobic, unlike the ECM. Exposure of such surfaces *in vivo* can lead to nonspecific adsorption of proteins of mixed orientation and states of denaturation, potentially resulting in a foreign-body reaction (FBR) to the material.[61]

Ceramic biomaterials

Ceramic biomaterials are primarily utilized in tissue engineering of hard tissues. Calcium phosphates, such as hydroxyapatite, and bioactive glasses have been developed as bioceramics for bone tissue engineering. Bioceramics are brittle but have high compressive strength, can bond strongly to bone, and can be osteoinductive.

Hydrogels

Hydrogels are water-swollen cross-linked polymer networks which can absorb up to thousands of times their dry weight of water, which gives them the advantage of being more like most natural tissues and allowing mass transport to and from cells.[49,62] They also allow relatively easy incorporation of cell-binding ligands or ECM molecules to facilitate cell interactions. They may be formed by physical (hydrogen bonds, ionic interactions, molecular entanglements, hydrophobic interactions) or chemical interactions (covalent bonds) and this will affect their stability and degradation rates. The mechanical strength of hydrogels is limited and their degradation tends to be faster than for other biomaterials. Hydrogels may be naturally derived (e.g., collagen, gelatin, hyaluronic acid, alginate) or synthetic (e.g., poly(ethylene glycol) (PEG)-based polymers).[63]

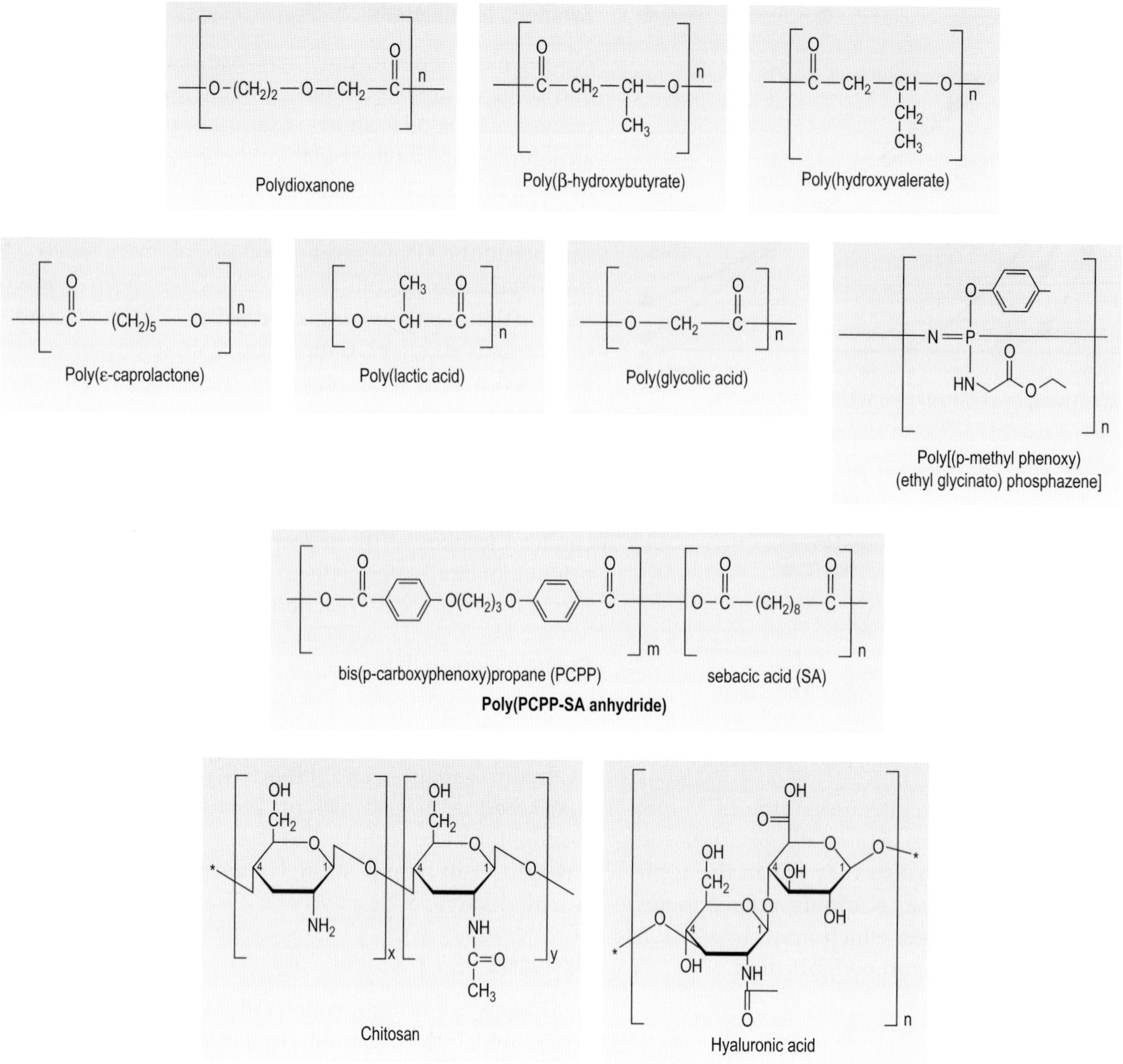

Fig. 19.6 Chemical structures of selected biodegradable polymers of potential interest in tissue engineering. (Reproduced from Kohn J, Abramson S, Langer R. Bioresorbable and Bioerodible Materials. In: Ratner BD, Hoffman AS, Schoen FJ, *et al.* (eds) Biomaterials Science. Amsterdam: Elsevier, 2004, pp. 115–217. Chitosan reproduced from Guibal E, Vincent T, Blondet FP. Biopolymers as supports for heterogeneous catalysis: Focus on chitosan, a promising aminopolysaccharide, in Ion Exchange and Solvent Extraction: A Series of Advances A. SenGupta, Ed. 2007, Taylor & Francis: Boca Raton. 151–292. Hyaluronic acid reproduced from Yannas, IV, Natural Materials, in Biomaterials Science – An Introduction to Materials in Medicine, B.D. Ratner, et al., Eds. 2004, Elsevier: Amsterdam.)

Gelation or changes in molecular conformation may be caused by environmental changes, resulting in so-called smart polymers, as shown in *Figure 19.7*. These types of change can be used to encapsulate and release payloads of cells or drugs, to form gels upon injection *in vivo*, or for cell sheet engineering.[61,64,65]

Research efforts to improve biomaterials for tissue engineering include efforts to create cell-responsive materials, which degrade in response to cellular processes (e.g., secretion of matrix metalloproteinase) during tissue development such that the biomaterial degradation rate adapts to the tissue growth rate.[66] Another key challenge is the FBR seen *in vivo* with almost all synthetic biomaterials used clinically, be they polymers, ceramics, or hydrogels.

Approaches to reduce the FBR to biomaterials *in vivo* may use physical properties, such as by creating spatial features which lead to reduced fibrosis (e.g., porous

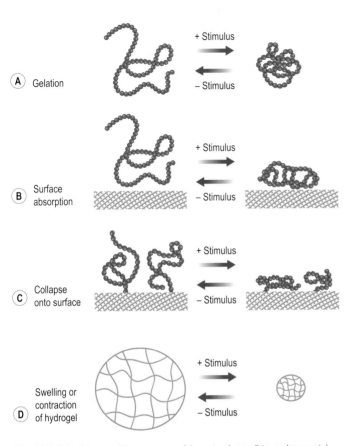

Fig. 19.7 Potential reversible responses of "smart polymers" to environmental stimuli. **(A)** Gelation; **(B)** surface adsorption; **(C)** collapse on to surface; **(D)** swelling or contraction of hydrogel. (From Hoffman AS. Applications of "smart polymers" as biomaterials. In: Ratner BD, Hoffman AS, Schoen FJ, *et al.* (eds) Biomaterials Science. Amsterdam: Elsevier, 2004, pp. 107–115.)

polymers with pores of around 30 μm[67] or small-diameter fibers[68]). Surface chemical properties can also be used to reduce the FBR to biomaterials, such as via attachment of oriented cell adhesion ligands (e.g., oriented osteopontin on a polymer surface[69]), or by modifications to minimize nonspecific adsorption of host proteins, which can be denatured and lead to an immune reaction (e.g., by layer-by-layer assembly of polyelectrolytes ending with a nonadhesive outer layer,[70] or attachment of PEG[71]). However, many strategies which show promise *in vitro* suffer from enzymatic attack and changes to the biomaterial surface *in vivo* during the acute inflammatory stages of the wound-healing response, and so their *in vivo* performance may be disappointing.[72]

Tissue-engineering construct fabrication

Biomaterial constructs for tissue engineering can be fabricated into structures such as porous scaffolds and hydrogels, meshes, or microspheres using a variety of techniques, such as the solid free-form fabrication and rapid prototyping methods illustrated in *Figure 19.8*. In addition to these methods, polymer phase separation, particle or foam templating, and electrospinning have been widely investigated to produce 3D constructs for tissue engineering.[39,73–75] The techniques for tissue-engineering scaffold fabrication have been recently reviewed.[55,76–78]

The design of biomaterial constructs for tissue engineering is complex and varies significantly depending on the tissue target. Even for specific tissue types, various design criteria may be considered and the definition of ideal designs is not yet well established. Some of the key parameters are:

- biomaterial composition (chemical composition, molecular weight, polydispersity)
- internal 3D porous architecture
- surface chemistry and roughness
- degradation properties and products
- mechanical properties (initially and during degradation)
- effects on cellular processes (adhesion, migration, proliferation, and differentiation)
- ability to be fabricated reproducibly and economically
- ability to be sterilized without unacceptable property changes.

The interaction of cells with a biomaterial surface alters depending on whether the surface has binding sites of suitable orientation and conformation to enable attachment of the cells, and the density of such sites. This in turn can affect cell morphology and migration rates, as shown in *Figure 19.9*.

Scaffolds of various internal architectures can be produced, as shown in *Figure 19.10*. The porosity must be interconnected and of sufficient size for molecular transport, cell migration, and vascularization. The size required may be larger than the minimum size required to fit cells or blood capillaries. Cao *et al.* found that pores of at least 300 μm were needed for tissue survival in PLGA scaffolds where a significant FBR occurred inside

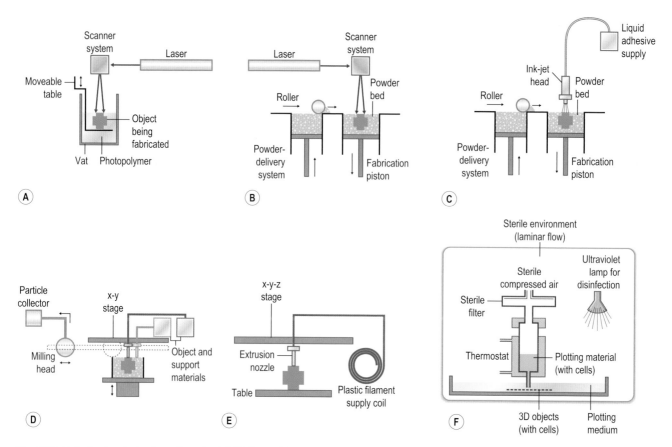

Fig. 19.8 Methods of producing three-dimensional (3D) biomaterial constructs via solid freeform fabrication. **(A)** Stereolithography; **(B)** selective laser sintering; **(C)** 3D printing; **(D)** wax printing; **(E)** fused deposition modeling; **(F)** bioplotter. ((A–E) The Worldwide Guide to Rapid Prototyping website © Copyright Castle Island Co. All rights reserved; (F) From Hollister SJ. Porous scaffold design for tissue engineering. Nat Mater. 2005;4:518.)

Intracellular contraction forces / Substratum adhesive strength	Large	Intermediate	Small
Typical cell morphology			
Migration speed	Negligible	Significant	Negligible

Fig. 19.9 Effects of cell–substrate interactions on cell migration speed. (Reproduced from Palsson BO, Bhatia SN. Tissue Engineering. Upper Saddle River, NJ: Pearson Education, 2004.)

the scaffolds.[79] Scaffolds may have up to 90% porosity or more and the extent and architecture of the porosity can be used to control the scaffold strength, as shown in *Figure 19.11*. Ideally the mechanical strength of tissue-engineering constructs would be designed to match that of the tissue targeted to favor the desired cellular behavior, as discussed above, and avoid stress shielding, which can lead to osteolysis in the case of bone implants.[80]

The mechanical properties of tissues and their components vary widely (*Table 19.1* and *Fig. 19.12A*) and so the physical microenvironment of particular cells *in vivo* also varies significantly. Engler *et al.*[36,45] have shown that MSC lineage specification can be altered *in vitro* when cells are cultured on substrates of different stiffness (*Fig. 19.12*). Soft hydrogels of similar elastic modulus to brain tissue were found to be neurogenic, stiffer hydrogels of similar modulus to muscle were

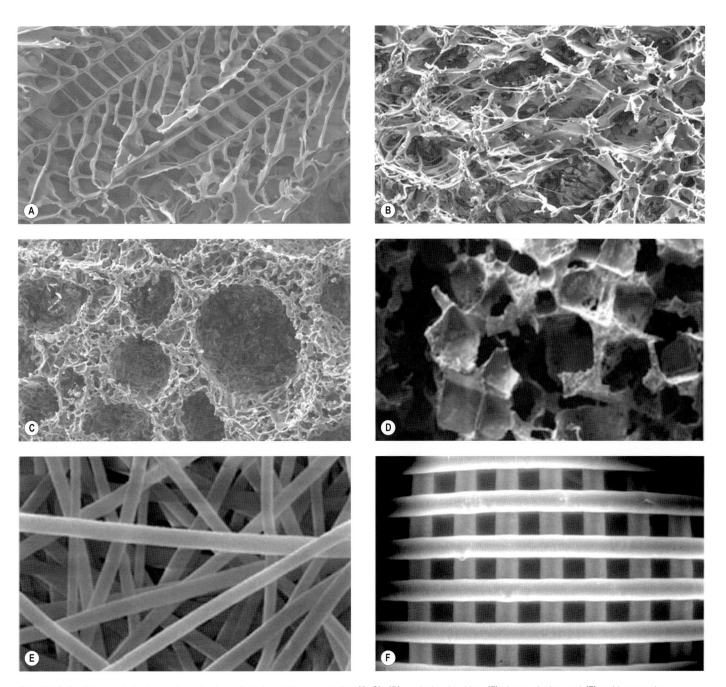

Fig. 19.10 Scaffold morphologies produced by thermally induced phase separation **(A–C)**; **(D)** particulate leaching; **(E)** electrospinning; and **(F)** rapid prototyping. (**A–C,** Reproduced from Cao Y, Croll T, Cooper-White JJ, O'Connor AJ, Stevens GW. Production and Surface Modification of Polylactide-Based Polymeric Scaffolds for Soft Tissue Engineering. In: Hollander AP, Hatton PV, editors. Biopolymer Methods in Tissue Engineering. Totowa, NJ: Humana Press; 2004. p. 87–112; **(D–E)** reproduced from Kretlow JD, Mikos AG. From material to tissue: biomaterial development, scaffold fabrication, and tissue engineering. Aiche J 2008;54:3048–3067; **(F)** reproduced from Shor L, Guceri S, Chang R, Gordon J, Kang Q, Hartsock L, *et al*. Precision extruding deposition (PED) fabrication of polycaprolactone (PCL) scaffolds for bone tissue engineering. Biofabrication. 2009;1:1–10.)

myogenic, and hydrogels of modulus similar to collagenous bone were osteogenic. Cellular morphology, gene expression, migration, and proliferation are also modulated by the mechanical properties of their microenvironment.[35,38,43,66]

An alternative approach to the use of biomaterial constructs in tissue engineering is to fabricate scaffold-free constructs, which can be achieved using emerging rapid prototyping methods.[81,82] Forgacs and coworkers have demonstrated this concept using multicellular

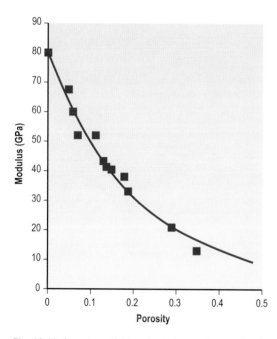

Fig. 19.11 Ceramic scaffold mechanical properties as a function of porosity. (From Boccaccini AR. Ceramics. In: Hench JRJ (ed.) Biomaterials, artificial organs and tissue engineering. Cambridge, UK: Woodhead, 2005.)

Table 19.1 Typical mechanical properties of selected tissues and tissue components

Material	Elastic modulus	Yield stress	Maximum strain
Elastin	100 kPa	300 kPa	300%
Cartilage	10 MPa	8–20 MPa	70–200%
Skin	35 MPa	15 MPa	100%
Muscle fascia	350 MPa	15 MPa	170%
Tendon	700 MPa	60 MPa	10%
Cortical bone	17.4 GPa	160 MPa	1.8%

(Adapted from Palsson BO, Bhatia SN. Tissue Engineering. Upper Saddle River, NJ: Pearson Education; 2004; and Cowin SC. The mechanical properties of cortical bone tissue. In: Cowin SC (ed.) Bone Mechanics. Boca Raton, FL: CRC Press, 1989.)

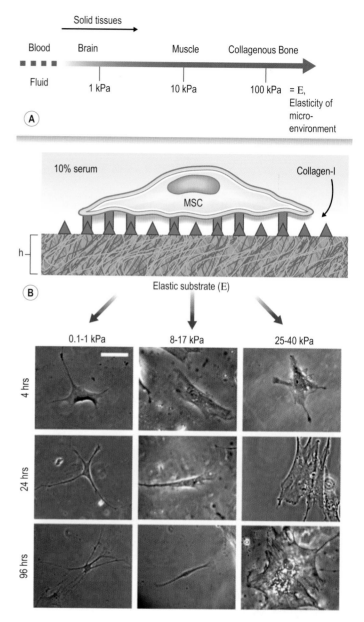

Fig. 19.12 Effects of substrate mechanical properties on differentiation. **(A)** Range of microenvironment elasticity for various solid tissues; **(B)** mesenchymal stem cells (MSCs) grown on collagen I-coated hydrogels of various elastic moduli differentiate to phenotypes corresponding to tissues of the same elasticity as the hydrogels. (From Engler AJ, Sen S, Sweeney HL, *et al*. Matrix elasticity directs stem cell lineage specification. Cell 2006;126:677–689.)

aggregates to create a "bio-ink" which was printed in layers to produce 3D tubular structures, which fused over several days in culture.[81,83]

Tailored delivery systems

Bioactive molecules play a critical role in natural tissue morphogenesis and control of their delivery both spatially and temporally to growing tissue may significantly enhance tissue-engineering outcomes.

Molecules such as growth factors, anti-inflammatory peptides, and drugs may be incorporated into biomaterial delivery vehicles for release at the desired time during tissue development. The release systems may be designed for continuous or pulsatile delivery; the latter may be programmed or triggered by some change in the local environment.[84] Delivery systems can be fabricated

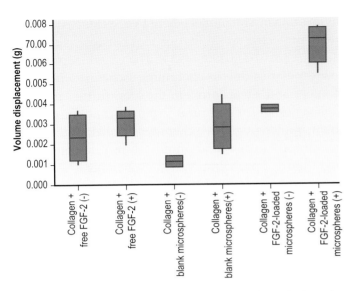

Fig. 19.13 Effect of controlled release of a growth factor on tissue development *in vivo*. Cross-linked gelatin microspheres suspended in collagen were used to deliver fibroblast growth factor-2 (FGF-2) in a tubular mouse tissue-engineering chamber enclosing superficial epigastric vessels in the groin of mice, with (+) or without (−) an autologous fat graft. (From Vashi AV, Abberton KM, Thomas GP, *et al.* Adipose tissue engineering based on the controlled release of fibroblast growth factor-2(FGF-2) in a collagen matrix. Tissue Engineering. 2006;12:3035–3043.)

from biodegradable polymers in the form of micro- or nanoparticles or capsules, or incorporated into other biomaterial constructs such as within the walls or on the surfaces of scaffolds or hydrogels.[43] It is critical to the design of an effective delivery system that the payload of bioactive molecules retains its conformation and bioactivity throughout the loading and release processes. An additional challenge is the prediction of release rates *in vivo*, which generally differ significantly from those *in vitro*.

Growth factors regulate numerous cellular fate processes, including adhesion, proliferation, differentiation, migration, and gene expression. Controlled delivery of these molecules is desirable as they have short half-lives *in vivo*, are relatively slow to diffuse due to their size, and may have undesired effects if delivered systemically.[38] The potential benefits of growth factor delivery on adipose tissue engineering were demonstrated *in vivo* using gelatin microspheres to deliver fibroblast growth factor-2 (FGF-2) over an extended time in a mouse tissue-engineering chamber.[85] Chambers containing an autologous fat graft and the gelatin microspheres loaded with FGF-2 grew significantly more tissue than controls with free FGF-2 or blank microspheres *(Fig. 19.13)*.

Similar approaches are also being investigated for cell delivery, wherein cells may be loaded on to degradable microspheres *in vitro*, allowed to attach, migrate, and proliferate on or within the spheres and then delivered to a target site for tissue growth. This significantly increases the surface area available for attachment of adherent cells and using biodegradable beads that can be delivered *in vivo* avoids the need to detach the cells from the culture surface for delivery.[86] It has been shown that ASCs loaded into chitosan microspheres were viable and maintained their multipotency after *in vitro* culture.[87]

Blood vessels: vascularization – nutrition

Cartilage is nourished predominantly via diffusion and blood supply is not critical for survival. Tendons and ligaments are relatively acellular and they too can be nourished by tissue fluids but other 3D tissues require an intimate connection with capillary vasculature. Generally, cells do not survive beyond 150 µm from a capillary,[6,88] but certain cells and tissues vary in their oxygen needs. Brain, muscle, and kidney cells are particularly sensitive to anoxia while stem cells and fetal tissues live happily in an environment of low oxygen tension. This issue of vascularization is one of the major hurdles in translating laboratory-based tissue-engineering products into human practice.

Extrinsic vascularization model of tissue engineering

To date, most *ex vivo* products are avascular and once implanted rely on diffusion until vascularization invades the construct from the periphery through into its core. This model of "extrinsic tissue engineering" has been the traditional prototype for 3D tissue engineering from its inception. Certain modifications have been trialed to facilitate rapid vascularization on implantation, including angiogenic growth factors, endothelial cells and MSC co-culturing for their angiogenic and paracrine effects, patterning of synthetic matrices with artificial vascular channels,[89–91] bioactive scaffolds containing growth factors for controlled release,[92–95] or decellularized whole-organ tissues that retain a skeletonized vascular tree[96] which may be seeded with endothelial cells *ex vivo* or spontaneously endothelialized *in vivo*. Alternatively, cells may be subjected to ischemic preconditioning prior to seeding *in vivo* to tolerate the new environment better.[5,97,98]

Inosculation, where existing vessels in a graft directly link with those in a recipient bed, has been proposed as a potential way of rapidly reconstituting a functional circulation to implanted tissue-engineered constructs that have their own internal vasculature. Laschke *et al.*[99] implanted PLGA scaffold disks into rats and, 20 days later, after vascular invasion, transplanted them into the back of syngeneic rats. Using intravital fluorescence microscopy, the authors observed that after 6 days the existing vessels in the graft reperfused, demonstrating that they had directly connected to the new host vasculature. Previous studies of inosculation have favored a progressive replacement of the graft vasculature with invading host vessels, using the graft as a scaffold conduit.[100,101] No matter by which method the vasculature connects, it is clear that 6 days is too long to expect anything but very thin tissues as were used in this model would survive the transplantation anoxia.

It is mostly conceded that reliance on a 3D prefabricated structure to survive implantation by the random invasion of capillaries from the implantation bed is unlikely to be a viable concept, especially for tissues sizeable enough to be clinically useful.

Intrinsic vascularization models and *in vivo* bioreactors

Prefabrication of flaps, where a blood vessel pedicle is implanted into living tissues to vascularize a dedicated territory such as skin,[102,103] or prelamination, where several tissues are grafted around the pedicle so that they can be subsequently transferred as a composite tissue graft,[104] has given tissue engineers insights into the importance of blood supply and how such vascularization might be incorporated into tissue-engineered products grown in the body. This process involves the establishment of an intrinsic vascularization that grows in tandem with the tissue-engineered product and nourishes it progressively. When a vascular pedicle or loop is tunneled into a tissue plane, the surgical trauma, inflammation, and hypoxia stimulate release of proangiogenic growth factors and promote angiogenic sprouting, which links to the pre-existing vasculature *(Fig. 19.14)*. We have exploited this concept for tissue

engineering in a rat model where a vessel loop is directed into a protected space that cannot collapse, such as a chamber box[105] *(Fig. 19.15–19.18)*. The vessel loop sprouts new capillaries due to continuing ischemia within the chamber and shear forces in the loop further promote angiogenesis. The "wound" cannot contract or shut down, prolonging the ischemic stimulus, and altered mechanical forces and fluid shifts influence cell migration and proliferation within chamber. The inflammatory environment of the chamber attracts neighboring and distant cells to participate in this frustrated repair process in an attempt to close the dead space which is progressively replaced with new vascularized predominantly fibroblastic tissue *(Fig. 19.18)*. As the tissue grows the angiogenic front moves centripetally and corresponds to the retreating zone of ischemia.[106] Tissue growth is enhanced when collagen matrix is included in the chamber and the angiogenic tissue will readily accept a skin graft, thereby creating a vascularized flap. The angiogenic stimulus continues for at least 20 weeks but is maximal between 7 and 10 days[107] *(Fig. 19.19)*. Simcock *et al.*[33] injected human angioblasts intravenously into rats with an arteriovenous loop chamber and observed that they could home to the chamber site. This was enhanced by SDF-1 delivery directly into the chamber and implies that vasculogenesis plays a role in the vascularization process *(Fig. 19.20)*. The contribution of vasculogenesis to skin graft and flap healing has been elegantly investigated by Capla *et al.*[108] If fibroblasts are added to the chamber at the time of creation of the loop they survive and can proliferate.[109]

We have developed a similar model of tissue engineering in the mouse using a "flowthrough" epigastric artery and vein in the groin surrounded by sealed silicone tube, which includes Matrigel matrix, a mouse sarcoma extract composed largely of laminin and FGF,[110] which has also been described by Walton *et al.*[111] *(Figs 19.21 and 19.22)*. We have studied the mechanism of angiogenic invasion into Matrigel, as has been done also by Tigges *et al.* in mice.[112] This highlights the pre-eminent role of bone marrow-derived macrophages and pericytes. Macrophages burrow into the matrix, creating channels which are lined initially by pericytes. Only later do endothelial cells follow and line the hollow tubes. Vessel-like networks form initially without any endothelial cell contribution but these cannot form without macrophages. This elegant exposé of the process

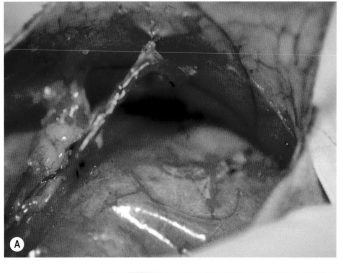

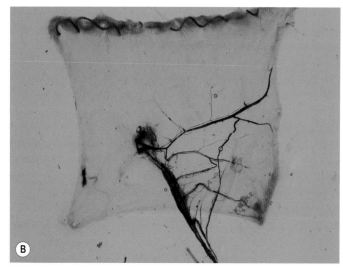

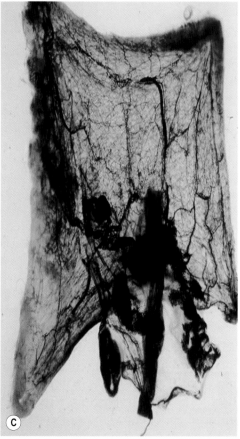

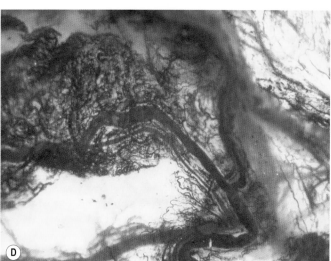

Fig. 19.14 Prefabricated flap in a rabbit thigh. **(A)** Implantation of a vascular pedicle into the subcutaneous layer of the rabbit thigh; **(B)** injection study at 1 week; **(C)** injection study at 3 weeks; **(D)** close-up capillary budding. (Courtesy of M Hickey, O'Brien Institute.)

of vascularization was specific to Matrigel and may not necessarily reflect the vascularization process of wounds comprising other matrices.

This intrinsic system of vascularization can support seeded cells and the histological pattern of their survival clearly demonstrates the intimate role of the neovasculature in nourishing the cells. Fibroblasts,[109] as well as specialized cells including neonatal cardiomyocytes[113] *(Fig. 19.23)*, islet cells,[114] and myoblasts[5] survived in the chambers but quantification of survival is difficult and almost certainly many cells apoptose. Delayed seeding of cells into a

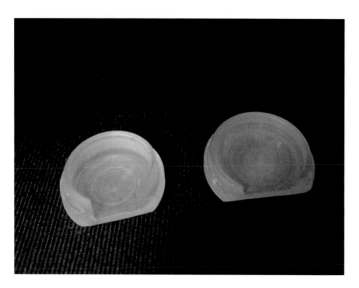

Fig. 19.15 Polycarbonate chamber (top) comprising a base plate and a lid (below).

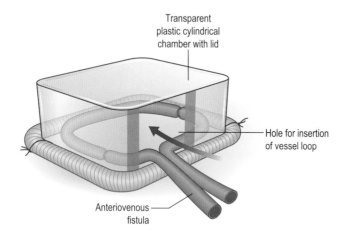

Transparent
plastic cylindrical
chamber with lid

Hole for insertion
of vessel loop

Anteriovenous
fistula

Fig. 19.16 Chamber box with arteriovenous loop.

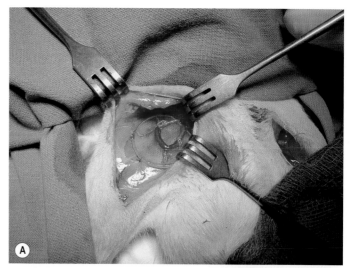

Ⓐ

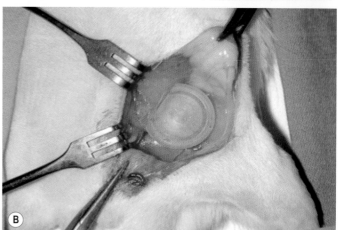

Ⓑ

Fig. 19.17 Chamber implanted **(A)** in rat groin, where **(B)** it is closed and buried.

prevascularized chamber enhances cell survival in the rat[5] and mouse chambers.[114]

When ASCs were implanted into the mouse chamber model in Matrigel and traced by sex mismatching or human to animal stains, new fat tissue formed but the stem cells were found to contribute only to new blood vessel formation. New fat was of host origin, indicating that the stem cells did not differentiate into fat but were inductive for endogenous fat formation. It is well recognized that MSCs have paracrine effects, including angiogenesis, cell recruitment, homing, anti-inflammatory, and antiapoptotic effects.[115] We have compared survival of liver precursor cells cultured on 2D plastic delivered as cell suspensions with 3D gel-cultured spheroids. In the spheroid form greater numbers of cells implant and survive in the chamber, suggesting that survival is related to other factors such as cell–cell microenvironment apart from pure vascularization. When solid tissue pieces such as muscle were implanted into the chamber they did not survive but regularly the dead tissue induced endogenous fat replacement.[116]

Khouri et al.[117] designed a tissue-engineering chamber (BRAVA) to induce fat growth for breast tissue replacement. It consists of a suction device applied to the external surface of the breast which, when worn regularly for prolonged periods, pulls the tissue away from the chest wall, creating tissue injury, inflammation, and a potential space. These are the key elements of our tissue-engineering chamber where inflammatory cytokines

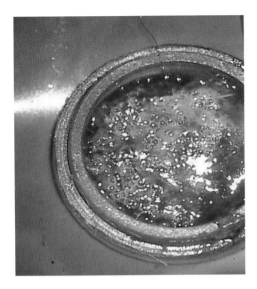

Fig. 19.18 Chamber opened after 6 weeks showing tissue formation.

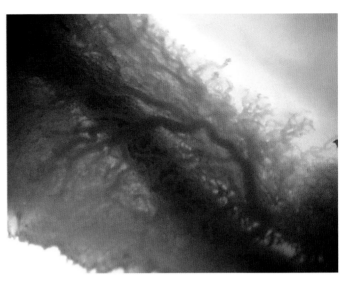

Fig. 19.19 Angiogenic sprouting from the vessel loop at 10 days. (Courtesy of Dr. Z Lokmic.)

Fig. 19.20 Human angioblast, DiI-labeled, homing to the rat chamber after intravenous injection. (Courtesy of J Simpcock and G Mitchell, O'Brien Institute.)

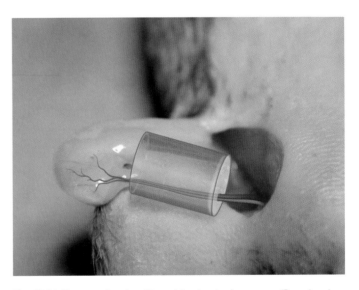

Fig. 19.21 Tissue-engineering silicone tube chamber in a mouse. (Reproduced from Cronin KJ, Messina A, Knight KR, *et al*. New murine model of spontaneous autologous tissue engineering, combining an arteriovenous pedicle with matrix materials. Plast Reconstruct Surg 2004;113:260–269.)

stimulate angiogenesis and attract stem cells while the vacuum creates the space. Biomechanical forces including fluid shifts also influence cell behavior. More recently Khouri has included fat injection. This modification is akin to our model of seeding cells into a preconditioned prevascularized chamber.

In another original concept of intrinsic vascularization for tissue engineering using "autologous microcirculatory beds," Chang *et al.*[118] devised an *ex vivo* perfusion chamber where an explanted flap of tissue which is in essence a preformed vascular bed can be continuously perfused with oxygen carrying nutrient fluids for periods of up to 24 hours through its vascular pedicle. During this time, the flap was infused with cells intravascularly, including stem cells which egressed from the microcirculation into the tissues to form cell clusters. The flap was then reimplanted by microvascular anastomosis into the animal. This model points to a

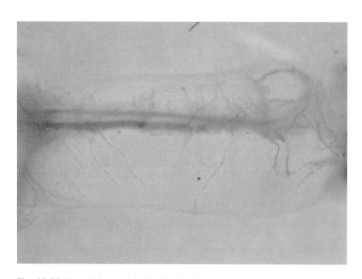

Fig. 19.22 Vascularization into the Matrigel in a mouse chamber at 4 weeks.

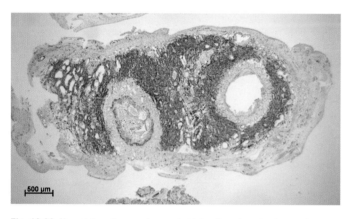

Fig. 19.23 Neonatal cardiomyocytes seeded into rat camber showing maximum survival around the vessel loop. (Courtesy of A Morritt, O'Brien Institute.)

new direction in organ regeneration or cell transfection to deliver deficient proteins.

In a different model of intrinsic 3D tissue engineering, a vascularized flap of fat tissue when implanted into an empty chamber space will expand and attempt to fill the space. We initially observed in our mouse Matrigel model that if a fat pad was used to plug one end of the chamber tube and wax the other, fat gradually replaced the Matrigel by direct extension from the pad.[110] When we placed an isolated fat pad on a vascular pedicle into the chamber in a rat even without matrix, the fat tissue expanded. When perforations were included in the chamber shell the space completely filled with tissue, approximately 40% of which was new fat.[119] This result was repeated in a pig model which grew over 50 mL of new fat *(Fig. 19.24)*.[119a] Although surgical trauma, ischemia, and inflammation play a role through

biochemical signaling in this new tissue growth, it is likely that the tissue flap finding itself in an empty space reacts to the changed biomechanical environment through focal adhesion transmembrane pathways as discussed earlier,[37] stimulating cell migration and growth. Quantification of this effect is difficult *in vivo* and the precise process remains unclear.

Testing and characterization of tissue-engineering approaches

Characterization of new or modified biomaterials, cells, and methods for tissue engineering is critical to their potential pathway to clinical trials and ultimately to clinical and commercial success. Systematic testing is not only a requirement of regulatory and ethical approval during the development process, but also crucial to developing understanding and thus being able to improve tissue-engineering methods further. Testing should aim to allow prediction of the long-term safety and efficacy of the tissue-engineering approach under consideration. Ideally, *in vitro* testing would be used to screen tissue-engineering constructs and methods in order to minimize animal testing for ethical reasons. However, it remains a significant challenge to predict *in vivo* responses from *in vitro* tests and so significant animal testing is normally required before initial clinical trials can be designed.

Standardized testing methods are highly desirable so that objective comparisons can be made between different approaches and construct components across different laboratories. Testing should be undertaken under conditions simulating the targeted tissue-engineering application, rather than relying on test results for the same material in different applications.[63] For example, the requirements for biomaterials in tissue engineering may differ significantly from those in other applications of the same materials, such as in degradable sutures which are used in low volumes and degrade relatively quickly.

Mathematical modeling may assist in design of tissue-engineering constructs and methods, helping to minimize the requirements for testing many alternatives. For example, different cell-seeding patterns and timing can be investigated using a mathematical model of a tissue-engineering scaffold during vascularization *in*

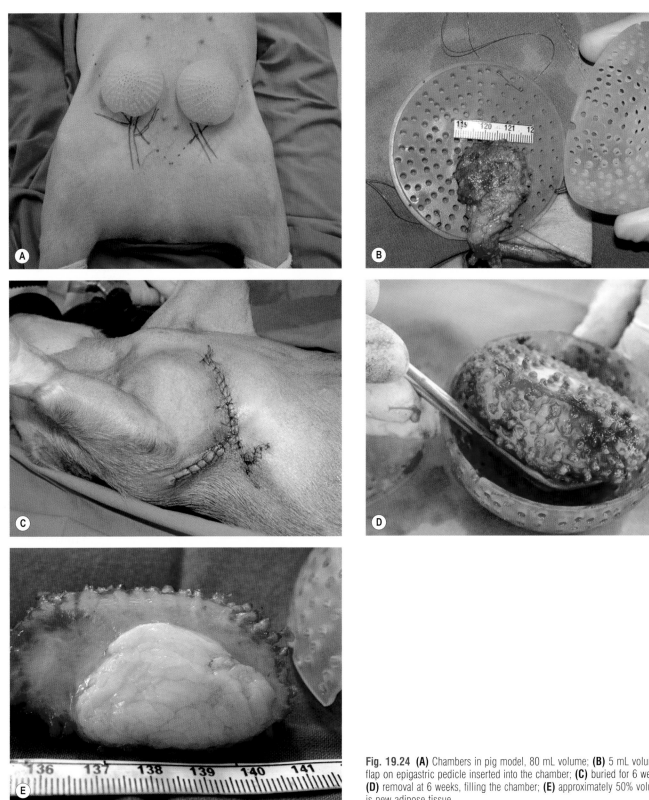

Fig. 19.24 (A) Chambers in pig model, 80 mL volume; **(B)** 5 mL volume fat flap on epigastric pedicle inserted into the chamber; **(C)** buried for 6 weeks; **(D)** removal at 6 weeks, filling the chamber; **(E)** approximately 50% volume is new adipose tissue.

vivo to provide insights into the optimal arrangement and governing parameters.[120,121]

Physicochemical characterization of biomaterials and constructs made from biomaterials should be undertaken to ensure the targeted composition, absence of significant residues or impurities, and desired morphology, are achieved. Materials which are nominally the same may perform differently in tissue-engineering applications due to differences such as the presence of impurities, differences in molecular weight or polydispersity in polymers, or variations in surface properties.

Risk management, regulation, and ethics

Risk management is a critical consideration in clinical and commercial tissue-engineering efforts. A number of potential products developed early this century suffered from problems with regulatory trials and product launches, along with challenging investment conditions internationally, contributing to a downturn in the commercial aspect of the tissue-engineering field.[122] Tissue-engineering approaches have significant potential benefits to patients and the health system but also involve risks, which may include human error (e.g., mix-ups of autologous cells), biomaterial performance variations from predictions (e.g., changes in degradation rates *in vivo*), quality control problems (e.g., microbiological contamination), and variations in patient-specific responses. Most of these can be minimized by rigorous management and scientific processes, whilst patient-specific responses will only be fully assessed once sufficient clinical trial data have been collected. Many of the commercial successes in the field of tissue engineering to date have avoided the risks involved in delivering biological materials, rather using acellular products.[122]

The ethical considerations related to tissue engineering have been reviewed in the literature.[123,124] Many of these apply to other fields of medicine and biomaterials and are not unique to tissue engineering. The sources of biological material to be used, particularly the potential use of ES cells, are, unsurprisingly, prime considerations. The extent of animal testing is a further issue of concern, which may be partly addressed by effective *in vitro*

testing and well-designed experimental approaches, as discussed above. Animal trials should be designed to simulate the final clinical application as closely as possible to avoid incremental approaches to the final design with numerous animal trials at every stage.

The regulatory approvals required for tissue-engineered products depend on the jurisdiction involved and have evolved significantly over the last decade around the world. In the case of the US Food and Drug Administration (FDA), products may be characterized as tissues, biological products, medical devices, or combination products and numerous standards and guides have been developed for particular categories of products.[125]

Case studies and status of tissue engineering for specific tissues

Skin tissue engineering

Skin tissue engineering has focused on generating a dermal component to the long-established keratinocyte laboratory expansion sheet technology. While the skin banks have been instrumental in saving burns patients' lives, graft durability and functionality are poor. Commercially, the target for tissue-engineered skin substitutes is for the treatment of chronic wounds, skin disease modeling, especially vitiligo and psoriasis, and drug design.

The principles of skin tissue engineering follow the same concept as other tissues and involve cells, scaffold, and vascularization. Cell sources include fibroblasts to promote collagen structural integrity but also to address the fundamental problem of biofilm that protects bacteria from attack by neutrophils and renders local fibroblasts senescent. Live fibroblasts can be incorporated into the implant to attract and activate neutrophils,[126,127] epidermal-derived stem cells,[128] and MSCs, especially for wound healing.[129] Bulge cells from hair follicles and co-cultures, especially with neonatal dermal fibroblasts, offer some hope of regeneration of functional skin elements, including hair follicle and sebaceous glands.[130]

Scaffold plays a key role in engineered skin. Substitutes initially served as passive matrices for ingrowth from the wound bed full of blood vessels and dermal elements, but more recently more complex structures comprising biomimetic proteins and material, 3D culture techniques, and altered surface chemistry and topography to influence cell adhesion, growth and differentiation, durotaxis, spatial cueing, and mechanoregulation.[131,132]

Current products suffer from poor integration to the wound bed as a result of inadequate vascularization and impact on the survival of implanted cells. Stem cells secrete angiogenic growth factors, especially following ischemic preconditioning, and submandibular and pancreatic-derived stem cells also have been shown to promote angiogenesis via growth factor release in *in vivo* studies when seeded into dermal regeneration scaffolds.[133]

Adipose tissue engineering

Adipose tissue engineering holds great interests to plastic surgeons for reconstruction of deformities such as Poland syndrome, Romberg syndromes, aging, breast postmastectomy and traumatic deformities, burns, and postirradiation defect.

Adipocytes are fragile, prone to ischemic death,[134] very difficult to grow in cell culture, and do not proliferate *in vivo*. Consequently, precursor populations derived from bone marrow or fat SVF and sorted by adherent cell culture or fluorescence-activated cell sorting (FACS) are the preferred cell source for the traditional loaded-scaffold paradigm of tissue engineering. This direction has been singularly unsuccessful for fat, no matter what scaffold is chosen, and most clinically focused research is returning to modifications of fat injection, possibly with matrix material as a more likely route to clinic.

Attempts to understand the fate of fat-grafting dates back almost a century when Marchand[135] grafted fat on to the brain of animals and identified two cell types at exploration: (1) fat, which he interpreted as having survived a graft; and (2) histiocytes which had come from the hosts and appeared to be turning into fat. This, he labeled replacement. The debate continues as to whether fat cells survived or signal endogenous fat productions. When we inserted human fat grafts into our mouse chamber tissue-engineering model containing Matrigel and FGF-2, new fat formed but it was of mouse origin *(Fig. 19.25)*. Similarly, when FACS-sorted or SVF-derived human ASCs or bone marrow stem cells were implanted, endogenous fat formed.[136] If the fat graft or stem cells are substituted by an inflammagen such as yeast particle zymosan, fat also forms in Matrigel. This, together with the early appearance of the macrophages in the chamber, suggests that the signaling mechanism by which fat grafts stimulate fat growth is an inflammatory one. This is consistent with the emerging concepts that MSCs largely function through their paracrine effects especially to promote angiogenesis and cell signaling. The growth factor profile of the mouse chamber contents clearly shows inflammatory angiogenesis predominating for the first 7 days, at which time it changes

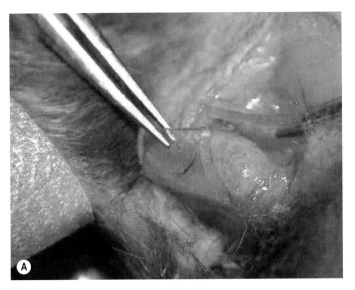
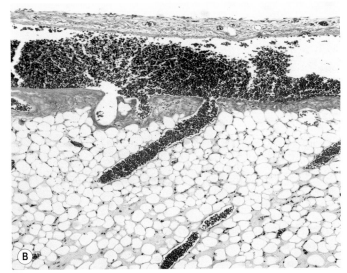

Fig. 19.25 (A) Spontaneous endogenous fat formation in Matrigel in a mouse model of tissue engineering after insertion of a small nonvascularized fat allograft; **(B)** normal fat tissue grown in the chamber. Note the extensive vascularization sprouting from the vascular pedicle. (Courtesy of F Stillaert, O'Brien Institute.)

to adipogenesis with the appearance of peroxisome proliferation-activated receptor-γ and other markers. Whether this event sequence is peculiar to Matrigel matrix is not yet clear and it seems from recent human clinical reports of clearly successful fat grafting that at least some injected fat does survive based on the observation that the volume is maintained from the time of injection rather than initially diminishing and then refilling, which would be expected if a final product is endogenous in origin. In animal studies, endogenously produced fat first appears at 4 weeks and is maximum by 8 weeks. This timeframe may still be consistent with injected fat not having resorbed before 8 weeks, by which time endogenous fat has replaced it. The recent reports by Yoshimura *et al.*[137] and by Cytori (http://www.cytori.com/) of increased graft efficiency by the concurrent injection of a bedside-processed lipoaspirate concentrated from the SVF add to the confusion. Are these injected stem cells surviving and turning into fat or are they merely a concentrated dose of inflammatory paracrine factors which induce endogenous fat production? It is probably safest to sit on the fence at present and assume that both fat survival and replacement mechanisms account for the results observed.

Mechanical forces influence cell behavior, including differentiation, and we believe that this is critical to the growth seen in the chamber space, particularly in those models where there was no matrix or seeded cells such as the adipose tissue growth seen in the pig model *(Fig. 19.24)*.

Matrix plays a key role in adipogenesis, as does angiogenesis. Multiple synthetic and natural scaffolds have been trialed *in vitro* and *in vivo* with and without FGF and/or seeded cells. Matrigel is both angiogenic and adipogenic[138] and several Matrigel substitutes are under study, including derivatives of muscle (myogel)[57] and adipose ECMs.[139] Most need growth factor additives[140] and this limits their clinical application because of cost and regulation hurdles. The ultimate clinical product would be an adipogenic injectable matrix gel with or without processed lipoaspirates.

Muscle tissue engineering

Tissue engineering of skeletal muscle has potential *in vivo* applications for the treatment of muscular dystrophy, muscle loss from injury and post tumor resection, chronic denervation, and targeted delivery of proteins and drugs by gene transfection of muscle cells. *Ex vivo* applications could include models for the study of exercise physiology or muscle diseases or drug screening. It could also in theory find a commercial use for tissue-engineered meat production from animal stem cell sources.[141]

Muscle is unique functionally with its densely packed parallel-aligned multinucleated muscle fibers which contract axially through calcium-sensitive actin and myosin filaments. This in turn involves neural connections functionally linked through acetylcholine release and its receptors.

Cells for tissue engineering can be sourced from satellite cells, a stem cell type that resides below the basal lamina of myofibers. They represent 1–5% of the cell population and are capable of self-assembly into new myotubes following injury and stimulation.[142,143]

As with other tissues, the standard tissue-engineering design model is to seed scaffolds with cells *ex vivo* followed by *in vivo* implantation with the expectation of vascularization cell survival and function. Myoblasts from skeletal muscle can be cultivated and expanded *in vitro*,[144,145] but differentiation in 2D culture after extended passaging is difficult. ECM composition plays a key role in myoblast alignment and differentiation. 3D culture techniques using collagen or Matrigel[115,146] more closely mimic the *in vivo* ECM environment and allow cell expansion, differentiation and fusion in a mold.[115,146] (ref Matsuda 18L; Van Den Berg 19L) By co-culturing the myoblasts with fibroblasts on Seran wrap or laminin-coated plates stretched out between pins, myoblasts oriented themselves axially and on differentiation they separated from the wrap and assembled into a cylindrical core of contractile muscle using the pins as tendon-like anchors. These were termed myoids.[147–149] Modifications included fibrin gel to replace fibroblasts and laminin,[150] which also had the advantage of shorter culture periods and stronger muscle contraction, although this was still miniscule by comparison with functional muscle. Electrical stimulation of myoblasts in 3D collagen gel culture mimics nerve stimulation and promotes differentiation to myotubes, which has been shown to be due to increased nox expression.[151] VEGF is also upregulated and this may have potential for *in vivo* applications.[152] Mechanical stretch or force organizes myoblasts into functionally aligned myotubes and favorably influences fiber diameter and cell number[153,154] by myofilament gene regulation and protein expression.[155,156] *In vitro* preconditioning of myoblasts by cyclic strain in a bioreactor improved the contractile forces generated after implantation.[157] Co-culture with neural tissue in a 3D matrix enhanced *in vitro* muscle function,[158] as well as generating neuromuscular junctions with functioning acetylcholine receptors.[159]

ECM compositions play a key role in the alignment and differentiation of myoblasts. Various synthetic matrices, including PLGA mesh,[160] PCL,[161] chitosan,[162] glass fibers,[163] micropatterned nanofibers,[164,165] and wavy silicone surfaces,[166] influence regulation of cell alignment differentiation and proliferation but the elasticity, toxicity, and biodegradability are critical to *in vivo* application. Myoblasts seeded into decellularized biological scaffolds including skeletal muscle itself are attractive because they are nonimmunogenic, have a preformed shape, and may retain biologically active cytokines and growth factors and functional cues. *In vivo* implantation of such homologous myoblast seeded acellular muscle matrix pieces into the rat abdominal wall defects showed survival (Y chromosome) integration with host muscle and good vascularization.[167,168]

Vascularization of thick *in vitro*-formed tissues remains a large hurdle to clinical applications. This has been addressed using 3D multiculture systems *in vitro* combining myoblasts with embryonic fibroblasts and endothelial cells on polymer scaffolds.[150,169,170] This resulted in endothelial cell networks in *in vitro* models which when implanted *in vivo* integrated with host vasculature forming chimeric vessels. This model was also associated with increased muscle survival. It is likely however that repeated implantation of small numbers of cultured myoblasts with or without co-culture will achieve greater *in vivo* survival than attempting large 3D implantation. We have seeded rat myoblasts into an *in vivo* chamber containing an arteriovenous vessel loop and observed that the cells survive and spontaneously differentiate into highly vascularized confluent myotubes by 4 weeks. However, by 6 weeks, these cells had all but disappeared, presumably due to the absence of neural stimulation. Others have reported the formation of functional neuromuscular junctions *in vitro* by co-culture of myoblasts with neural tissue in 3D fibrin matrix. These could be electrically stimulated, causing contraction of the 3D muscle. Furthermore,

acetylcholine receptors were identified.[158,159] To date, the dream of muscle replacement therapy for reversal of muscle dystrophy remains elusive[171] and the alternative of using gene-transfected myoblasts for targeted delivery of deficient growth factors such as insulin-like growth factor, erythropoietin, and vasculogenic factors may prove more beneficial.

Tissue engineering of nerves

Nerves in different locations have distinct microenvironments and thus the optimal tissue-engineering strategies for each will differ. Tissue-engineering strategies may be used for guided nerve regeneration using, for example, degradable biomaterial tubes or scaffolds. Hollow tubes can function effectively as nerve guides for gaps of up to 10 mm in the peripheral nervous system under a range of clinical situations; these are often made from nondegradable polymers but may also be made from degradable materials. For example, tubular collagen nerve guides (Neuragen from Integra Life Sciences) are being used clinically to treat peripheral nerve injuries.[172] The critical gap length that may be successfully treated using nerve guides can be longer than 10 mm in primates and can be further increased by addition of cells and cell supports such as biomaterial fibers or hydrogels.[172] It has been shown that use of oriented hydrogel matrices (e.g., fibrin or collagen) within nerve guides results in a larger critical gap length than use of the same matrices without alignment. Fibers can also be used to guide nerve regeneration, depending on their diameter, alignment, and spacing.[39,172,173] Schwann cell grafts and the addition of controlled-release vehicles containing drugs or neurotrophic factors can also increase the success of tissue-engineering strategies for nerves.[173,174]

The environment and cellular responses to injury in the central nervous system tend to inhibit regeneration. A range of tissue-engineering investigations for the spinal cord have been reported, involving acellular scaffolds or cellular substrates containing spinal and/or stem cells. Stem cells have shown some regenerative responses in trials, although the mechanisms of how they may repair the spinal cord are not well understood.[172] It may be desirable to use stem cell-derived precursor cells for tissue-engineering strategies in the central nervous system, as stem cells may not differentiate as desired at an injury site *in vivo*. Scaffolds or hydrogels with oriented pores may also improve cellular regeneration in the spinal cord; neurites and cells have been shown to penetrate into oriented porous scaffolds.[172] Strategies for nerve tissue engineering that combine cells, biomaterials, and biomolecule delivery over the relevant time scales are subject to ongoing research which may lead to more clinical treatments in the future.

Tissue engineering of blood vessels

A number of strategies to tissue engineer blood vessels *in vitro* or *in vivo* as an alternative to autografts, allografts, or nondegradable polymer prostheses have been developed and tested in animal models and in the clinic with promising results.[175] Biodegradable scaffolds made from natural or synthetic materials, or a combination of these, have been developed and seeded with endothelial cells to tissue engineer blood vessels. Incorporation of angiogenic growth factors within scaffolds has been shown to increase microvascular growth.[176] Collagen-based scaffolds containing a polyester mesh have been tested extensively and are now available commercially (Omniflow II from Bio Nova International) and are used clinically for blood vessel tissue engineering.[177] In a contrasting approach, cell sheet engineering has been used to create autologous-engineered blood vessels *in vitro* without exogenous scaffold materials, by rolling sheets of cultured dermal fibroblasts and their surrounding ECM into tubes which are then seeded with the patient's endothelial cells.[178] This approach has progressed to clinical trials as the Lifeline tissue-engineered blood vessel.[178,179] In another alternate strategy, Campbell *et al.* have grown tubular vessels in the peritoneal cavity *in vivo* to create tissue-engineered blood vessels comprising autologous cells. These vessels have been successfully grafted into the circulatory system of the host animal where they were shown to remodel in response to the new environment and remain patent for up to 16 months in rabbits.[180,181]

Tissue-engineering strategies to create vascular networks have also been developed. Networks of capillary-like vessels have been assembled *in vitro* by culture of endothelial cells, EPCs, or human umbilical vein endothelial cells on a range of substrates, including plastic, hydrogels, and decellularized human skin.[176]

Biomaterial constructs have also been engineered with microchannels to encourage development of a vascular network in 3D constructs *in vitro*.[182] Recent research has proposed the use of bioprinting of preformed multicellular aggregates to create 3D tubular structures and organ constructs with vascular networks which can be perfused *in vitro* and could be connected to the patient's circulatory system *in vivo*.[81,82]

However successful *in vitro* development of vascular networks may be, the challenge of transplanting and connecting them to the patient's blood supply is significant. This has been achieved in some animal model studies, with newly developed blood vessels connecting to the host blood supply and surviving in severe combined immunodeficiency mice.[176] Problems may arise though, due to immunorejection and delays in inosculation between the vessels in the implanted construct and the host's circulatory system. Thus, intrinsic vascularization *in vivo* may prove to be a more successful strategy in some cases, as discussed above.

Bone tissue engineering

Significant research efforts have been made to tissue engineer both load-bearing and nonload-bearing bone to meet the demands for alternatives to autografts or allografts which have their inherent disadvantages and supply limitations. However, limited translation to clinical application has occurred to date.[78] Progress and challenges in this area have been recently reviewed in the literature.[4,78,80,183] Bone tissue-engineering strategies generally involve a biomaterial scaffold of suitable mechanical strength with or without added cells and/or biomolecules to encourage bone growth.

Tissue-engineered constructs for bone should be osteoconductive to allow bone cells to adhere, proliferate, and migrate. A range of ceramics (e.g., β-tricalcium phosphate and hydroxyapatite) and polymers have been reported to meet this requirement and a number have been used as bone substitutes clinically. Slowly degrading polymers, such as poly(L-lactic acid) and PCL, have been widely investigated to produce tough porous scaffolds for bone tissue engineering. PCL-based scaffolds produced by fused deposition modeling have been developed for bone tissue engineering by a team based at the National University of Singapore and commercialized (Osteopore International). These have been approved by the FDA and used clinically as burr plugs and sheets for orbital floor reconstruction in more than 200 patients.[183]

Scaffolds which are osteoinductive have also been produced and shown to enhance bone growth. Among these, bioactive glasses composed of silica-containing calcium, sodium and phosphorous oxides, have been termed "bioactive" because they can form strong bonds to hard and soft tissues *in vivo*.[80] These materials have been marketed commercially as Bioglass and used clinically, primarily in nonload-bearing applications.

Porosity is required in bone tissue-engineering scaffolds for cell and nutrient transport as well as vascularization (pores >300 μm have been recommended).[79,183] It is also important to match the mechanical properties of an implanted tissue-engineering construct to that of the target tissue to ensure the construct will not collapse under the forces applied *in vivo* but will also not cause stress shielding to the surrounding bone, which can lead to bone resorption. The construct should maintain its strength during tissue development until the newly formed tissue can withstand the mechanical forces at play.[184] Scaffold mechanics can be varied by adjusting the scaffold material, porosity, grain size (for ceramics) and using composites such as nanoparticles of hydroxyapatite in a polymer matrix of poly(L-lactic acid).[62] Whilst porosity is critical for transport and vascularization, it reduces the mechanical strength of scaffolds; purely ceramic scaffolds with the porosity desired for effective vascularization may therefore not have sufficient strength for load-bearing bone tissue engineering and this limits their current clinical application.[183]

Composite materials are attractive as they can overcome the brittleness of ceramics. This strategy mimics the composite structure of bone, being an inorganic–organic composite structure. Coral has been used in bone tissue engineering as it is a naturally occurring composite material with suitable mechanical properties and porous architecture for some bone tissue-engineering applications.[183] Suspensions or pastes of ceramic or composite materials may also be used in surgical repair or via injection to encourage bone growth for small-volume repairs.

In addition to the influence of the scaffold, the osteoinductive growth factors, bone morphogenic proteins (BMPs), may be used to enhance bone tissue growth. Other growth factors (e.g., TGF-β_1, FGF-2, platelet-derived growth factor) may also enhance bone formation, as summarized by van Gaalen *et al*.[80] Tissue engineering utilizing BMPs has progressed to a number of clinical trials, primarily in spinal surgery, showing some promising results.[80,184] One disadvantage of incorporation of growth factors remains their high cost. Bone progenitor cells, such as bone marrow-derived stromal cells, may also be added to a tissue-engineering construct *in vitro* and cultured for some time prior to implantation into the patient. This allows cells to migrate into the scaffold, adhere, proliferate, differentiate, and begin to lay down ECM within the construct, provided the construct is not too large to allow sufficient diffusion of oxygen and other molecules to and from the cells. Scaling this approach up to human-sized implants is therefore presents challenges which are yet to be resolved. Further complexity arises in designing bone tissue-engineering strategies incorporating cells, as it is often not clear whether new bone growth originates from transplanted cells.[80]

Cartilage tissue engineering

Tissue engineering of cartilage is relatively well developed as the problem is simplified by not requiring vascularization within the developing tissue. Several cell and tissue-engineering treatments for cartilage repair have been established clinically. However, clinical use is not widespread as yet due to limitations in efficacy, consistency, and applicability.[185] Autologous chondrocyte implantation for articular cartilage repair has been approved by the FDA and implemented clinically (Carticel, Genzyme Biosurgery, US).[78] Although this procedure has shown good clinical outcomes, it is labor-intensive in the cell expansion in the surgery and limited in the defect size that can be treated.[186,187]

Biomaterial support structures may be used to treat larger cartilage defects, deliver cells, and provide critical mechanical support until the tissue is sufficiently developed. A possible timeline for cartilage repair using a biomaterial implant is shown in the idealized schematic shown in *Figure 19.26*. The 3D arrangement of chondrocytes is important to their function and the ECM synthesis required for tissue development and this may be encouraged by suitable biomaterial scaffold design.[86,188] Native articular cartilage is not isotropic but contains zones of different ECM and cell organization and

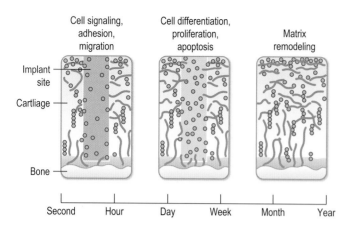

Fig. 19.26 A timeline for cartilage tissue engineering from *in vivo* implantation to formation of the final tissue. (From Palsson BO, Bhatia SN. Tissue Engineering. Upper Saddle River, NJ: Pearson Education, 2004.)

function. Current research aims to develop biomaterial scaffolds which mimic this feature of cartilage more effectively to achieve engineered tissues with the normal zonal organization.[185]

A range of biodegradable polymers, including PLGA, PCL, hyaluronan, gelatin, and collagen, have been used to produce scaffolds and microspheres to support chondrogenesis.[39,86,186,188] Hyalograft (a form of the biomaterial product Hyaff-11 from FIDIA Advanced Biopolymers, Italy) is a hyaluronic acid-based 3D scaffold product for cartilage tissue engineering which is available commercially and has been used clinically.[44,186]

Biomaterial scaffolds for cartilage tissue engineering may be seeded with cells and cultured *in vitro* or simply implanted into the defect site, where host cells may migrate into the scaffold. The physical microenvironment of the cells is again important to tissue development. For *in vitro* culture, forces such as gravity and hydrodynamic forces from the fluid motion affect the quality and size of cartilage tissue formed *(Fig. 19.4)*.[50,188] A number of bioreactor designs have been devised to provide favorable *in vitro* growth conditions for chondrocytes, among other cell types.[86,185]

Tissue engineering of other organs

Organ regeneration is the grail of tissue engineering. Early reports suggested that systemically injected MSCs could home to injured tissues such as the heart, survive, and differentiate into functional cardiac tissues. Apart from in the brain, it is now largely accepted that most of these cells do not survive or at least are undetectable except in the microvasculature and their main efficacy is via paracrine hormonal effects. To engineer specific organs, stem cells are generally needed and, although many have been identified in adult organ tissue, because of their scarcity, their differentiation from embryonal stem cell sources has received intensive research. Differentiation protocols have been defined for several tissues but ethical issues and cancer risks are ongoing barriers. iPS cells derived from adult fibroblasts offer a new direction for personalized organ repair.

In vitro cell-seeded scaffolds face the same hurdles of vascularization as other tissues following implantation. Perhaps for this reason, few studies have attempted 3D organogenesis *in vivo*. We have had success in animal *in vivo* models with cardiac tissue using cultured neonatal rat cardiomyocytes inside an arteriovenous loop chamber model in the rat. By 4 weeks a beating syncytium of well-vascularized cardiac muscle was regularly grown which responded to chemical and electrical pacing.[113] In order to resolve the problem of cardiac cell source in this model, human ASCs were able to be differentiated into beating cardiomyocytes expressing cardiac markers by co-culturing them with rat neonatal cardiomyocytes.[48] This opens the way for a customized nonimmunogenic cell source from an individual's own fat tissue. We have also engineered tissue capable of secreting growth hormone after implantation of mouse pituitary stem cells into a vascularized chamber in mice[189] and restored thymus function in athymic rats after implantation of human thymic tissue in vascularized chambers as evidenced by the postoperative appearance of processed T cells in the blood and by the rejection of skin allografts.[190] Most recently, small-animal models of decellularized heart,[96] liver,[191] and lungs[192] have been seeded with organ-specific fetal or neonatal cells *in vitro* and some function has been demonstrated. More exciting still is the demonstration that the vascular tree is essentially preserved and that it can be seeded with endothelial cells and allow short-term function when transplanted *in vivo*.

Notably, research by Atala *et al.* into tissue engineering of the urological system has progressed from animal studies to clinical trials.[193–195] Acellular collagen matrices obtained from human bladder tissue have been used successfully for onlay urethral repairs clinically in over 200 patients. However, attempted tubular

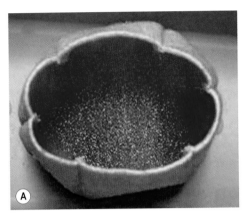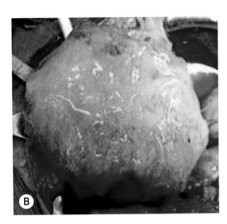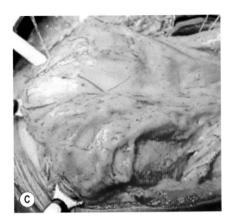

Fig. 19.27 Tissue engineering of the bladder: **(A)** a biodegradable scaffold was seeded with autologous cells, **(B)** anastomosed to the patient's native bladder, and **(C)** covered with fibrin glue and omentum. (From Atala A, Bauer SB, Soker S, *et al*. Tissue-engineered autologous bladders for patients needing cystoplasty. Lancet 2006;367:1241–1246. Copyright Elsevier 2006.)

reconstructions using small-intestinal submucosa did not show adequate tissue regeneration clinically.[193] A significant milestone in organ tissue engineering was the report that engineered bladder tissue showed promising outcomes in a clinical trial for cystoplasty reconstruction.[194,196] Autologous cells from a bladder biopsy were seeded on to biodegradable scaffolds and grown *in vitro* prior to transplantation *(Fig. 19.27)*. The bladder function was shown to improve and this was sustained for several years. In 2009, it was reported that FDA phase II studies on this technique had been completed but further studies are required before it could be disseminated broadly.[193]

 Bonus images for this chapter can be found online at
http://www.expertconsult.com

Fig. 19.2 (A) Thumb stump with distraction device; **(B)** X-ray of bone distraction; **(C)** new bone filling the gap.

Access the complete reference list online at **http://www.expertconsult.com**

3. Cao Y, Vacanti J, Paige K, et al. Transplantation of chondrocytes utilizing a polymer-cell construct to produce tissue-engineered cartilage in the shape of a human ear. *Plast Reconstr Surg*. 1997;100(2):297–302.

58. Dijkhuizen-Radersma Rv, Moroni L, Apeldoorn Av, et al. Degradable polymers for tissue engineering. In: van Blitterswijk C, Thomsen P, Lindahl A, et al., eds. *Tissue Engineering*. Amsterdam: Elsevier; 2008. pp. 193–221.

   A textbook on tissue engineering which addresses the field in detail, with chapters written by experts in individual aspects that include grounding in the biological basis for tissue engineering of different tissues.

79. Cao Y, Mitchell G, Messina A, et al. The Influence of Architecture on Degradation and Vascularisation of Three Dimensional Poly(lactic-co-glycolic) Scaffolds *in vitro* and *in vivo*. *Biomaterials*. 2006;27(14):2854–2864.

99. Laschke MW, Vollmar B, Menger MD. Inosculation: Connecting the Life-Sustaining Pipelines. *Tissue Engineering Part B: Reviews*. 2009;15(4):455–465.

105. Tanaka Y, Tsutsumi A, Crowe DM, et al. Generation of an autologous tissue (matrix) flap by combining an arteriovenous shunt loop with artificial skin in rats: preliminary report. *British Journal of Plastic Surgery*. 2000 Jan;53(1):51–57.

   This paper describes the first realization that the "tissue" that grows into a space is not only vascular tissue.

107. Lokmic Z, Stillaert F, Morrison WA, et al. An arteriovenous loop in a protected space generates a permanent, highly vascular, tissue-engineered construct. *FASEB J*. 2007 February 1, 2007;21(2): 511–522.

   This paper provides a detailed analysis of angiogenesis from a vascular loop in a dedicated space.

113. Morritt AN, Bortolotto SK, Dilley RJ, et al. Cardiac Tissue Engineering in an In vivo Vascularized Chamber. *Circulation*. 2007 January 23, 2007;115(3): 353–360.

   Captures the imagination and potential of tissue engineering; significant because of the spectacular image of beating tissue grown in a chamber in vivo.

122. Lysaght MJ, Jaklenec A, Deweerd E. Great Expectations: Private Sector Activity in Tissue

Engineering, Regenerative Medicine, and Stem Cell Therapeutics. *Tissue Engineering, Part A.* 2008;14(2): 305–315.

Outlines the commercial activity in the tissue engineering field, with discussion of the reasons for numerous early failures and insights about risk management and practicably achievable outcomes.

137. Yoshimura K, Suga H, Eto H. Adipose-derived stem/ progenitor cells: roles in adipose tissue remodeling and potential use for soft tissue augmentation. *Regen Med.* 2009 Mar;4(2):265–273.

192. Petersen TH, Calle EA, Zhao L, et al. Tissue-Engineered Lungs for *in vivo* Implantation. *Science.* 2010;329:538–541.

20

Repair, grafting, and engineering of cartilage

Wei Liu and Yilin Cao

SYNOPSIS

- Cartilage is one of the most important tissue grafts in plastic surgery and is widely used in auricular reconstruction, rhinoplasty, and facial countoring.
- This chapter introd uces the background knowledge and surgical skills required for harvesting cartialge graft and managing donor site tissues.
- Additionally, recent development in engineered cartilage fabrication and their potential application in plastic surgery are described.

Introduction

Cartilage is a kind of connective tissue which is mainly composed of chondrocytes and their extracellular matrices (ECM) of type II collagen fibers, proteoglycans, and elastic fibers. According to its composition, cartilage can be classified into three types[1]: (1) hyaline cartilage; (2) fibrocartilage; and (3) elastic cartilage. *Figure 20.1* shows the histology of the three types of cartilages.

Hyaline cartilage is the most common type of cartilage and can be found in costal, articular, tracheal, and nasal cartilage. With the exception of articular cartilage, the free surface of most hyaline cartilage is covered with perichondrium. In addition to collagen II, hyaline cartilage is rich in glycosaminoglycans and is thus characterized by its stiffness, that permits sustained compressional loading.

Fibrocartilage is composed of bundles of thick collagen fibers along with intervening unicellular islands of cartilage arranged in small chains. Because of this unique structure, fibrocartilage can provide high tensile strength and supporting function and is thus present in areas that are most subject to frequent stress, such as meniscus, intervertebral discs, symphyseal joints, and the joint portion of bone and tendons/ligaments. In contrast to other cartilage, fibrocartilage also contains type I collagen. In addition, it has moderate amounts of proteoglycan but little glycosaminoglycans.

Elastic cartilage is characterized by its extremely high elasticity because of the presence of abundant amounts of elastic fibers. It is histologically similar to hyaline cartilage but contains many elastic fibers which form an elastic fiber network along with collagen fibers. This unique feature provides great flexibility so that elastic cartilage can withstand repeated bending. It is mainly found in the outer ear structure, and also in the larynx and epiglottis. It is also surrounded with perichondrium.

The perichondrium is a layer of dense irregular connective tissue that consists of two separate layers, an outer fibrous layer and an inner chondrogenic layer. Collagen fibers and fibroblasts constitute the fibrous layer. In contrast, the chondrogenic layer remains partially undifferentiated and is likely to contain mesenchymal stem cells and chondrogenic progenitor cells,[2,3] which can play a role in cartilage repair and regeneration.

Cartilage is a unique tissue with low metabolic rate due to the sparsity of its cell population and its

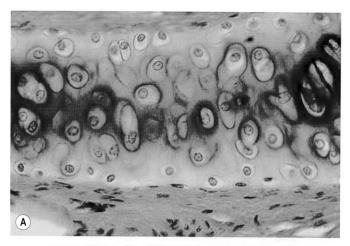

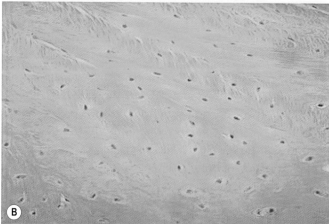

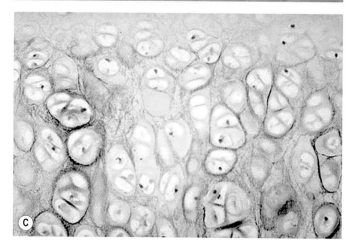

Fig. 20.1 Histology of **(A)** hyaline cartilage, **(B)** fibrocartilage, and **(C)** elastic cartilage (silver staining). (Courtesy of Dr. Roger C. Wagner Prof. Emeritus of Biological Sciences at University of Delaware and Prof. Fred E. Hossler, East Tennessee State University.)

avascular structure. The glycolytic activity and oxygen consumption of cartilage approaches anaerobic condition and the tissue is nourished by tissue fluid diffusion. Because of this unique feature, cartilage graft is relatively easy to survive when being implanted. In term of cartilage grafting, Sushruta Samhita in India probably is the first person to perform cartilage grafting in the form of a composite graft.[4,5] Cartilage graft is widely used for repairing nasal or auricular defects as well as for reconstructing other tissues either as a pure cartilage graft or as a composite graft. According to surgical procedures, cartilage can be transferred either as a free graft or as a microvascular composite graft. Generally, autologous cartilage graft will not have metaplastic changes even being transferred to a different locations.[6] In addition, grafting of free perichondrial tissue is also a common procedure for cartilage reconstruction because it has been observed long time ago that perichondrium possesses the ability to regenerate cartilage.[7]

Autologous cartilage grafts and applications[6]

Although cartilage is considered as "immunologically privileged," and allogeneic cartilage may serve as a potential graft, autologous cartilage grafting remains the most applicable cartilage graft. Generally, common donor sites for harvesting autologous cartilage grafts include auricular, nasal, and rib cartilage.

Auricular cartilage graft

As an elastic cartilage, auricular cartilage is an ideal graft for transplantation and perhaps is the most versatile of all cartilage grafts because it can be easily fashioned and contoured into different shapes for various uses. Auricular cartilage can be harvested easily under local anesthesia and a significant portion of the concha can be removed without causing donor site deformity.[6]

However, in practice, harvesting of the entire conchal cartilage is likely to cause collapsed conchal bowl, cymba concha, and a horizontally short ear. To overcome this problem, Han *et al.* proposed the surgical procedure that involves: (1) using a postauricular incision to minimize visible scars; (2) harvesting the entire cymba concha and cavum concha separately, with at least 5 mm

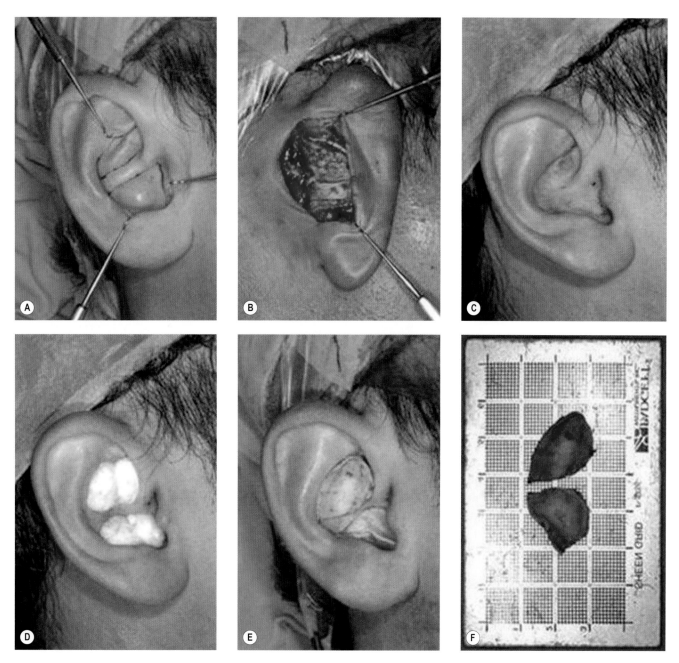

Fig. 20.2 The surgical technique for harvesting the maximal amount of conchal cartilage graft. **(A)** Markings. It was necessary to leave at least 2 mm of the superior outer rim along the conchal wall in order not to cause a noticeable change in the conchal bowl of the donor ear. Note the helical crus with its lateral extension between the cymba concha and cavum concha. **(B)** The entire unit of the cymba concha and cavum concha was removed separately, leaving at least 5 mm of the crus helicis with an extension to prevent collapsing. **(C)** There is almost no external evidence that the large conchal cartilage graft had been removed. **(D)** Two peanut cotton balls were placed into the interstices of the ear and sutured in place with through-and-through 4-0 nylon sutures, which were removed 5 days later. **(E)** The harvested cymba and cavum conchae were placed *in situ* to demonstrate their relationship with the intact helical crus and its lateral extension. **(F)** The surface area was 224.0 mm² at the cymba concha and 247.0 mm² at the cavum concha. (Reproduced from Han K, Kim J, Son D, *et al*. How to harvest the maximal amount of conchal cartilage grafts. J Plast Reconstr Aesthet Surg 2008;61:1465–1471.)

of the helical crus, leaving a lateral extension as a strut between them, as well as a 2-mm outer rim along the conchal wall; and (3) by using a tie-over bolster dressing that can serve as a mold for the conchal bowl. *Figure 20.2* presents the technique to avoid contour irregularity

or deformity after harvesting the maximal amount of conchal cartilage graft.[8]

Auricular cartilage graft is often used as a framework for ear reconstruction or auricular deformity correction, as reported by Brent,[9] Ono *et al.*,[10] Firmin *et al.*,[11] and

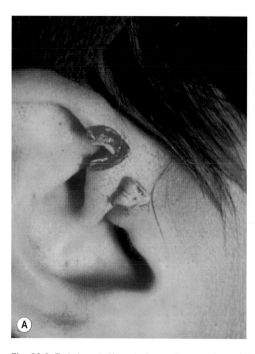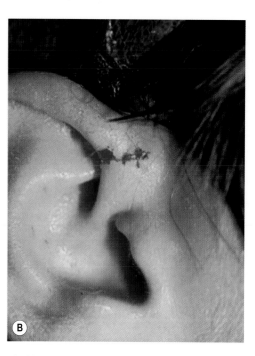

Fig. 20.3 Technique 1: Harvest of a small composite graft (<1 cm) with primary closure by running the dog ear anteriorly into the hairline. This closure preserves contour of the ear. (Reproduced from Singh DJ, Bartlett SP. Aesthetic management of the ear as a donor site. Plast Reconstr Surg 2007;120:899–908.)

others. In addition, conchal cartilage can be used as a single-layered graft for nasal, tarsal, and nipple reconstruction.[6]

The other important application of auricular cartilage is to transfer as a composite chondrocutaneous graft for nasal reconstruction. How to manage the donor site of auricular composite graft aesthetically is important for its successful application. Singh and Bartlett have summarized several techniques to deal with the donor site of free auricular composite grafts according to different applications[12]:

1. Technique 1: A composite graft that is less than 1 cm can be harvested from the root of the helix and the dog ear is run anteriorly toward the hairline with primary closure of the defect *(Fig. 20.3)*.

2. Technique 2: This is designed to close the donor site wound of the composite graft with cartilaginous base of 1–1.5 cm, which is usually needed to repair a wider defect of the alar rim *(Fig. 20.4)*.

3. Technique 3: To repair a nasal defect with short vertical dimension (height), the composite graft can be harvested from the anterior aspect of the helical root and the dog ear must be run superiorly and inferiorly. As shown in *Figure 20.5*, this technique can provide adequate tissue for nasal reconstruction and an aesthetic closure without disturbing the size of the ear.

4. Technique 4: For harvesting grafts with width of 1–1.2 cm from the base of the helix, the defect may be closed primarily by advancing the helical rim forward. The possible resulting overprojection of the ear might be addressed with a postauricular incision and a scaphomastoid suture to match the prominence with the contralateral ear *(Fig. 20.6)*.

5. Technique 5: After harvesting composite graft wider than 1.5 cm from the base of helix, the closure of such a wound became more intricate. A simple helical advancement would result in significant distortion and overprojection *(Fig. 20.7)*. To overcome this, a V-shaped wedge of skin is harvested, but a "half-star" pattern of cartilage at the apex of the V is taken *(Fig. 20.8B–E)*. In addition, a postauricular incision with a scaphomastoid suture is needed. With these procedures, this technique can prevent cupping of the ear with closure *(Fig. 20.8F)*.

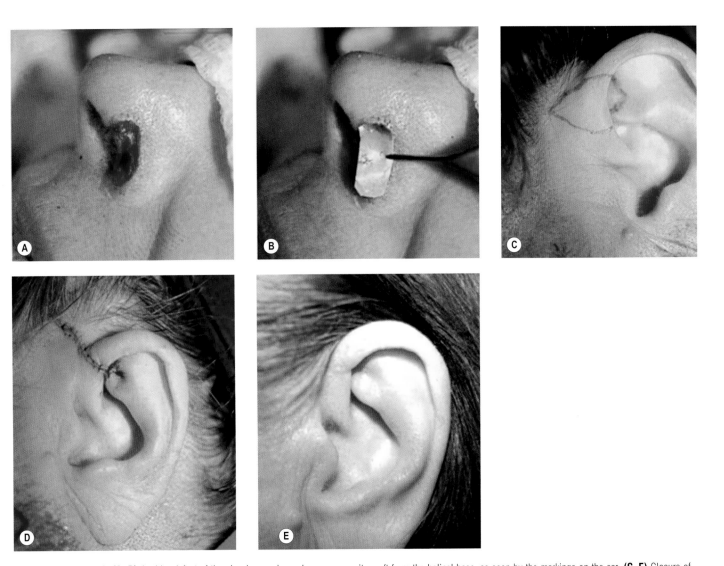

Fig. 20.4 Technique 2: **(A, B)** A wider defect of the alar rim requires a larger composite graft from the helical base, as seen by the markings on the ear. **(C–E)** Closure of the defect is accomplished by running the dog ear anteriorly into the hair line and posteriorly into the triangular fossa. A full-thickness wedge of cartilage must be removed from the triangular fossa to prevent buckling of the ear. (Reproduced from Singh DJ, Bartlett SP. Aesthetic management of the ear as a donor site. Plast Reconstr Surg 2007;120:899–908.)

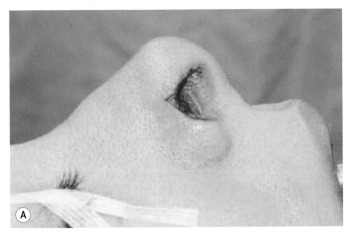

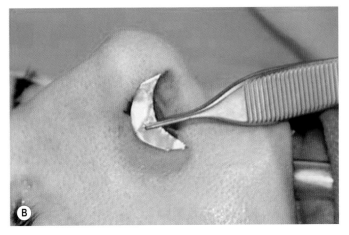

Fig. 20.5 Technique 3: **(A, B)** The nasal defect is wide but short in its vertical dimension. This allows harvest from the anteroinferior helical rim.

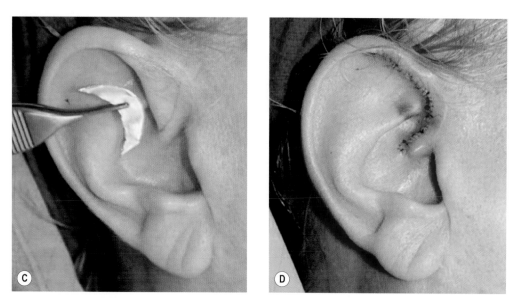

Fig. 20.5, cont'd (C, D) Primary closure is achieved by running the dog ear superiorly and inferiorly. (Reproduced from Singh DJ, Bartlett SP. Aesthetic management of the ear as a donor site. Plast Reconstr Surg 2007;120:899–908.)

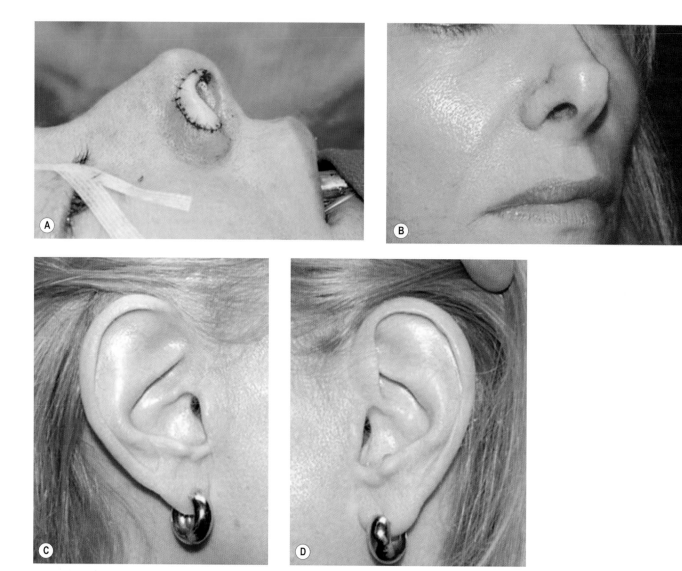

Fig. 20.6 Technique 4: **(A, B)** Inset of graft and aesthetic outcomes of nasal reconstruction and **(C)** the auricular donor site in comparison with **(D)** the contralateral ear. (Reproduced from Singh DJ, Bartlett SP. Aesthetic management of the ear as a donor site. Plast Reconstr Surg 2007;120:899–908.)

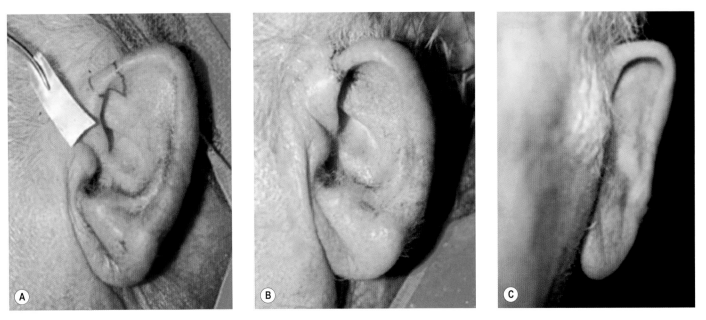

Fig. 20.7 (A–C) With harvest of a small (1–1.2 cm) composite graft, closure can be achieved by helical rim advancement. However, overprojection of the ear may result, as seen in this series of photographs. (Reproduced from Singh DJ, Bartlett SP. Aesthetic management of the ear as a donor site. Plast Reconstr Surg. 2007;120:899–908.)

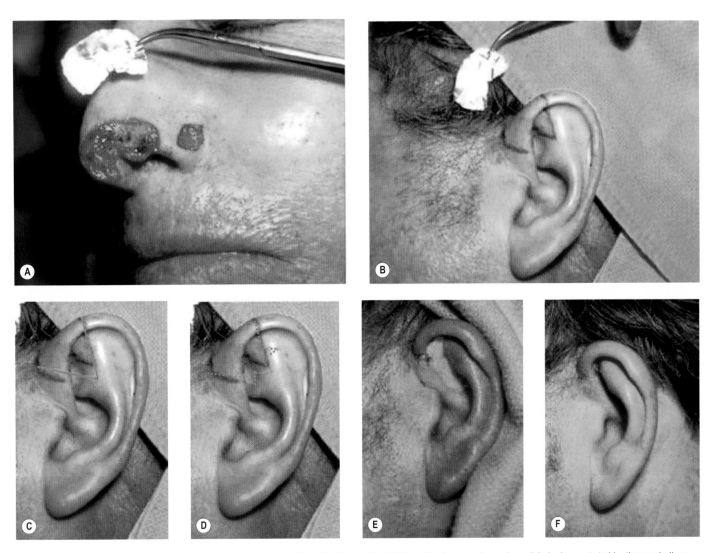

Fig. 20.8 Technique 5: **(A)** This nasal defect requires a larger composite graft with a width of 1.8 cm. The harvest site on the auricle is demonstrated by the purple lines. **(B–E)** To overcome distortion and overprojection resulting from tissue harvest, closure for this size auricular defect involves a V-shaped wedge of skin and a half-star pattern of cartilage excision at the apex of the V. The solid lines indicate skin incision and the dotted star pattern demonstrates cartilaginous incisions. In addition, a postauricular incision with a scaphomastoid suture is performed. **(F)** This technique of wound closure prevents the cupping of the ear and relatively normal shape and projection of the ear are maintained after the closure. (Modified from Singh DJ, Bartlett SP. Aesthetic management of the ear as a donor site. Plast Reconstr Surg 2007;120:899–908.)

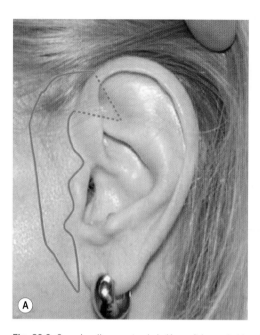 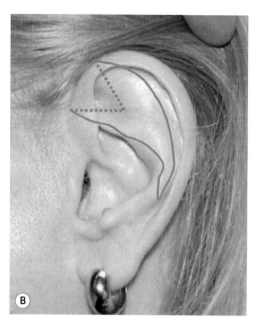

Fig. 20.9 Occasionally, an extended skin graft is needed in addition to the composite graft for reconstruction of nasal defects. **(A)** The solid lines indicate skin incisions and the dotted line indicates a cartilaginous incision. **(B)** The solid lines represent the harvest of a postauricular full-thickness skin graft. (Reproduced from Singh DJ, Bartlett SP. Aesthetic management of the ear as a donor site. Plast Reconstr Surg 2007;120:899–908.)

6. When an extended skin graft component is needed with the composite graft, the composite tissues can be taken either preauricularly or postauricularly, as demonstrated by the markings on *Figure 20.9*.

The techniques described above provide simple methods to close the wounds of auricular chondrocutaneous composite grafts primarily with appreciable aesthetic outcome.[12] Other methods of rotational flap or skin graft have also been described in the literature.[13,14] Importantly, the functional and aesthetic aspects should be well balanced for both the repair site and donor site when a physician decides to harvest an auricular composite chondrocutaneous graft of a particular size and shape.

One concern for the clinical application of free auricular composite grafts is their limited size due to the lack of immediate blood supply after transplantation. In contrast, microvascularly transferred auricular composite grafts can overcome this limit and are particularly useful when repairing large nasal defects. Zhang *et al.* have recently reviewed their experiences of surgical treatment of large nasal defects with vascularized preauricular and helical rim flaps based on the superficial temporal vessels in 63 clinical cases. The repaired deformities include unilateral alar defect, alar and side wall defects, tip and columellar defects, entire lower third of the nose missing, and composite defects involving cheek and maxilla. The total flap survival rate reached 97%. The results demonstrate that such an approach, using vascularized preauricular and helical rim flaps, is a reliable method for reconstructing nasal defects.[15] *Figure 20.10* demonstrates the surgical technique for repairing an alar lobule defect with vascularized helical rim composite tissue and preauricular skin.[15]

Nasal cartilage graft

Although limited in its available amount, nasal cartilage has been employed as a composite chondromucosal graft for eyelid reconstruction. Septal cartilage is an important source of nasal cartilage graft. As reported by Murrell, the septal cartilage can be accessed via a hemitransfixion incision with dissection around the caudal margin of the quadrangular cartilage. After both sides of mucoperichondrium are raised, the septal cartilage can be harvested.[16] Importantly, as shown in *Figure 20.11*, an L-shaped septal strut should be preserved to give nasal support and avoid nasal collapse.[6,16] Nevertheless, the amount of L-shaped strut cartilage necessary to provide good support can vary greatly depending on the strength, thickness, and dimensions of the nasal septum and other nasal tissues (i.e., upper lateral cartilages, lower lateral cartilages, nasal bones).[16]

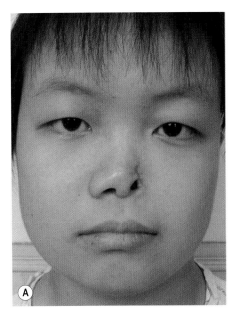 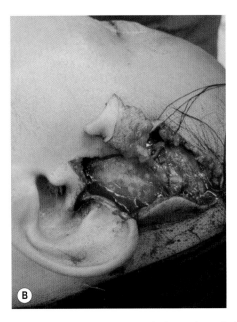 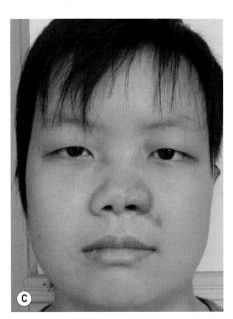

Fig. 20.10 A 17-year-old female with a deformity of the left alar lobule after laser treatment of a hemangioma. An ipsilateral reverse-flow flap consisting of both the helical rim and the preauricular skin (2.2 × 1.8 cm) was used. The anastomosis was made to the proximal end of the superficial temporal vessels by means of 11-cm vascular grafts from the descending branch of the lateral circumflex vessels. **(A)** Preoperative and **(B)** intraoperative views of the harvest of a reverse-flow flap based on the distal superficial temporal vessels. **(C)** Postoperative view at 3-month follow-up. (Reproduced from Zhang YX, Yang J, Wang D, *et al.* Extended applications of vascularized preauricular and helical rim flaps in reconstruction of nasal defects. Plast Reconstr Surg 2008;121:1589–1597.)

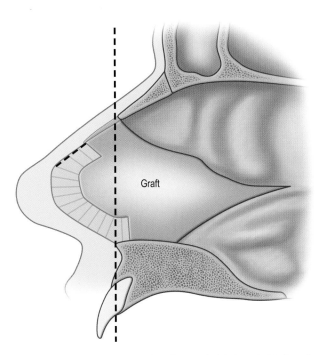

Fig. 20.11 Harvest of nasal septal cartilage graft. It is important to keep the L-shaped strut cartilage (shown in stripes) to provide nasal support. The area of septum that attaches to the upper lateral cartilages should also be preserved. Generally, nonsupportive quadrangular cartilage, which is pictured posterior to the dashed vertical line, can be harvested freely. (Reproduced from Murrell GL. Dorsal augmentation with septal cartilage. Semin Plast Surg 2008;22:124–135.)

As early as 1962, Millard published his work of repairing eyelid defect with a chondromucosal graft harvested from nasal septum. Later, Mustardé also described the technique in the book *Repair and Reconstruction in the Orbital Region.*[6]

The other region available for harvesting nasal chondromucosal graft is the upper lateral nasal cartilage, as reported by Tessier in 1979.[6] In clinical practice, repairing a large defect of the upper eyelid is always a challenge. Scuderi and colleagues have developed a surgical technique to address such a concern. In their report, a pedicled nasal chondromucosal flap was designed along the lateral nasal wall based on the terminal branch of the dorsal nasal artery. The flap includes the subcutaneous tissues down to the periosteum and the cranial portion of the upper lateral cartilage. It can be harvested either unilaterally or contralaterally and a skin graft is applied for cutaneous coverage. In their reported 15 patients, the flap was viable in every patient and satisfactory functional recover was achieved, indicating that this one-stage procedure can reconstruct a thin and mobile eyelid.[17] *Figure 20.12* demonstrates its design and surgical procedure as well as its clinical outcome.[17] In addition to eyelid repair, septal cartilage graft has

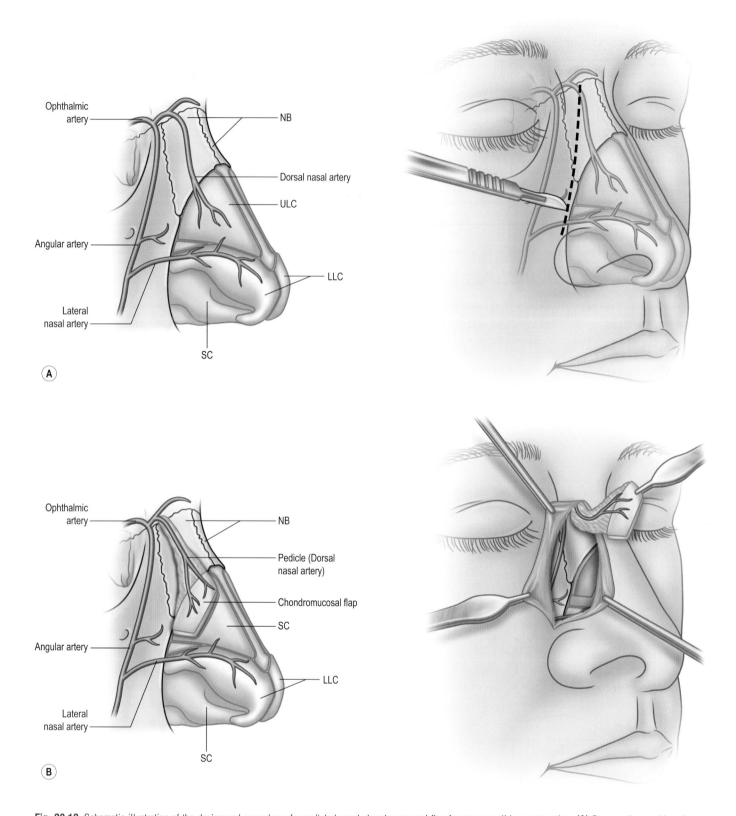

Fig. 20.12 Schematic illustration of the design and procedure of a pedicled nasal chondromucosal flap for upper eyelid reconstruction. **(A)** Preoperative markings for harvest of the upper lateral cartilage in the nasal chondromucosal flap, which is based on the lateral terminal branch of the dorsal nasal artery. **(B)** After skin incision and undermining, the flap is raised after a portion of the upper lateral cartilage (ULC) is harvested. NB, nasal bone; LLC, lower lateral cartilage; SC, septal cartilage. (Modified from Scuderi N, Ribuffo D, Chiummariello S. Total and subtotal upper eyelid reconstruction with the nasal chondromucosal flap: a 10-year experience. Plast Reconstr Surg 2005;115:1259–1265.)

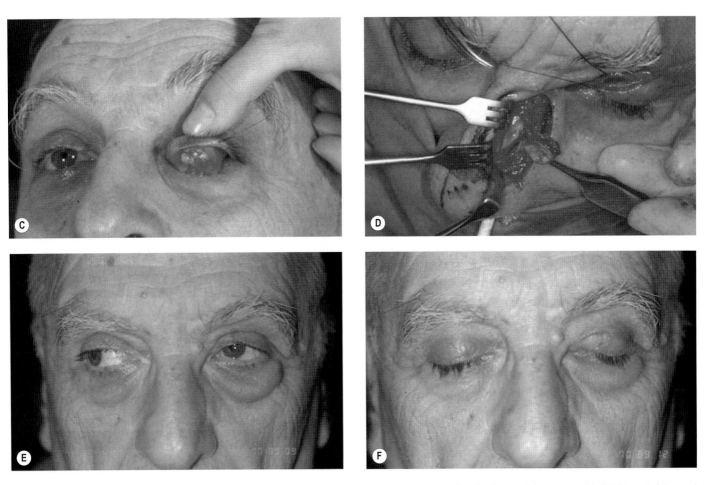

Fig. 20.12, cont'd (C) Clinical outcome of upper eyelid defect repaired with pedicled nasal chondromucosal flap. Carcinoma of the upper eyelid. **(D)** Harvest of the nasal chondromucosal flap. **(E,F)** One-year postoperative result after reconstruction with the nasal chondromucosal flap. (Reproduced from Scuderi N, Ribuffo D, Chiummariello S. Total and subtotal upper eyelid reconstruction with the nasal chondromucosal flap: a 10-year experience. Plast Reconstr Surg 2005;115:1259–1265.)

been used for dorsal augmentation,[16] tracheal repair,[18] and extended septal graft for controlling the projection shape of nose tip.[19]

Rib cartilage graft

Costal cartilage may serve as the best donor site for cartilage graft in terms of available tissue amount and mechanical strength. The autologous rib cartilage can be virtually contoured into any desired shape and it can retain form and bulk after implantation if basic surgical principles are followed.[6] The costal cartilage graft is often used as a cartilage framework for total ear reconstruction. Tanzer,[20] Thomson et al.,[21] and Brent[22] have respectively described the technique to harvest costal cartilage to construct auricular framework. In the procedure, the synchondrosis of the sixth and seventh cartilages as well as the eighth costal cartilage is harvested, usually along with the perichondrium.[20–23] In contrast, Nagata's method for total auricular reconstruction requires the harvest of four costal cartilages in the first-stage operation and one or two costal cartilages for the second-stage operation.[24–28] *Figure 20.13* is a schematic illustration of the harvest of rib cartilage designed for ear reconstruction or chin contouring.[29]

In clinical practice, harvest of costal cartilage can be associated with donor site morbidity. Uppal et al. have reported their investigation on morbidity associated with the harvest of costal cartilage in 42 patients who underwent ear reconstruction. The commonest complaints included pain and clicking of the chest wall, which usually peaked in the first week postsurgery and gradually diminished over 3 months. The other problems were scar and chest wall deformity.[30] Among them,

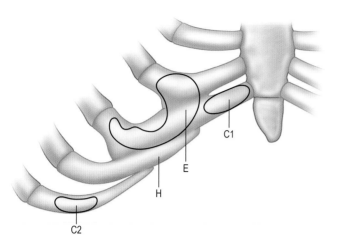

Fig. 20.13 Donor site for costal cartilage grafts in auricular framework and chin graft construction. E, ear base block; H, helix; C1, chin graft, first layer; C2, chin graft, second layer. (Reproduced from Brent B. Repair and grafting of cartilage and perichondrium. In: McCarthy JC (ed.) Plastic surgery. Philadelphia: WB Saunders; 1990, pp. 559–582.)

the most challenging problems are pneumothorax during the surgical procedure and resulting abnormal chest wall contour. This is particularly true for Nagata's method, which requires more and extra cartilage grafts for auricular reconstruction.[24–28]

To address this concern, Kawanabe and Nagata developed a new method for harvesting rib cartilage to avoid intraoperative and postoperative complications and problems. In this modified procedure, the costal cartilages were harvested *en bloc* with the perichondrium left completely intact at the donor site. In addition, after the fabrication of the auricular cartilage frame, the remaining costal cartilage was cut into small blocks that acted as spacers to fill the dead space formed in the perichondrial pocket. The retained perichondrium not only helps to avoid the injury of pleura, but may also promote cartilage regeneration because of the presence of chondrogenic stem cells.[2,3] In an investigation of 270 cases of total auricular reconstruction performed using Nagata's method and the new method of rib cartilage harvesting, the incidence of infection and pneumothorax was reduced to less than 1%. More importantly, there were no postoperative chest wall deformities when costal cartilage was harvested with this new technique.[31] Interestingly, a follow-up study revealed that returned hyaline cartilages were mixed with fibrocartilage with visible margins at 6 months postsurgery. Twelve months after the first-stage operation, homogeneous

hyaline cartilage was observed histologically, and the regenerated cartilages were similar to native costal cartilages in their hardness, which enabled the second harvest.[32] *Figure 20.14* gives a schematic illustration of harvesting costal cartilage with the new method of retaining perichondrium and returning the remaining costal cartilage to the donor site.[31]

Modification of previously established methods of making auricular framework is also considered as an alternative option to avoid harvesting extra cartilage and thus help to prevent chest wall deformity. As an example, Chin *et al.* recently reported several modifications of auricular framework and these methods required less cartilage graft and meanwhile could also generate individualized and harmonious ear frameworks to meet the need for satisfactory three-dimensional (3D) outline of a reconstructed auricle.[33] The framework may consist of the helix, the base frame, the Y-shaped antihelical complex, and the tragus attached with an additional cartilaginous cube depending on individualized need *(Fig. 20.15)*. In addition, bone cement is used as the support material during the ear elevation stage, and therefore extracostal cartilage harvesting became unnecessary.[34] *Figure 20.16* demonstrates the clinical outcome of reconstructed ear with modified frameworks based on the individualized 3D auricle structures.[33]

In addition to auricular reconstruction, rib cartilage graft also has other applications, including reconstruction of significant saddle-nose deformity,[35] treatment of maxillonasal dysplasia (Binder's syndrome),[36] nipple reconstruction,[37] for septorhinoplasty,[38] and in tracheal reconstruction.[39]

Autologous perichondrial graft

In 1959, Lester first reported the potential of neocartilage formation by transplanted perichondrium.[40] This phenomenon has also been observed by others.[41–44] Despite the enthusiasm and optimism derived from the pioneering observations, the clinical application of perichondrial grafts for cartilage regeneration remains limited to certain conditions, such as the reconstruction of degenerated knee joint cartilages. The potential causes of limiting the application include the technique of harvest, the oxygenation of the recipient bed, and the

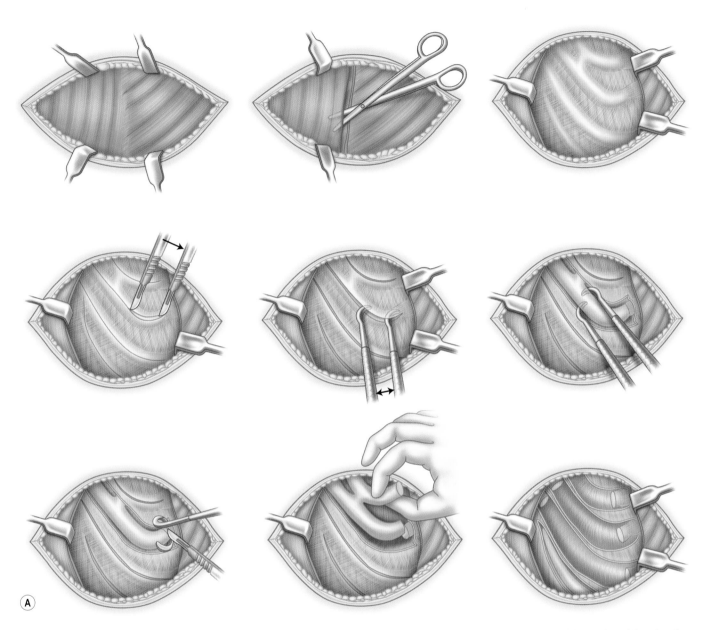

Fig. 20.14 (A) Schematic illustration of the new method of costal cartilage harvest. (Above, left) The muscular fascia of the rectus abdominis muscle and the external oblique muscle are exposed. (Above, center) A longitudinal incision is made between the rectus abdominis muscle and the external oblique muscle with delicate dissecting scissors. (Above, right) The perichondrium is completely exposed. (Center, left) The line of incision is marked in the center of the costal cartilage, and, taking special care not to injure or damage the cartilage, the incision is made with a scalpel. (Center, center) The anterior surface of the perichondrium is first undermined with an elevator. (Center, right) The undermining of the posterior surface of the perichondrium requires extreme precaution because the risk of pneumothorax exists; therefore, the tip of the elevator is placed on the cartilage or must face the cartilage to avoid accidental puncture of the thoracic wall. The approximately 1 cm of periosteum at the costochondral junction is undermined for easier harvest of the costal cartilage. (Below, left) A Doyen rib raspatory is placed (inserted) underneath the undermined costal cartilage between the cartilage and the perichondrium at the costochondral junction. The costal cartilage is excised with a scalpel and the costochondral junction is to be left behind at the donor site. (Below, center) Harvesting of the costal cartilages is easier if the sixth and seventh costal cartilages are harvested from the side of the costochondral junction instead of the sternal side. (Below, right) The appearance of the donor site immediately after the harvest of the costal cartilages. The perichondrium is left completely intact at the donor site. (Reproduced from Kawanabe Y, Nagata S. A new method of costal cartilage harvest for total auricular reconstruction: part I. Avoidance and prevention of intraoperative and postoperative complications and problems. Plast Reconstr Surg 2006;117:2011–2018.)

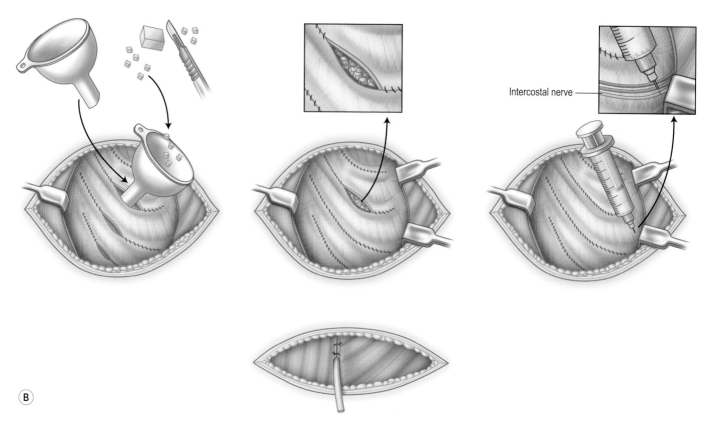

Fig. 20.14, cont'd (B) (Above, left) The perichondrium is sutured with 4-0 nylon at 5-mm intervals with the exception of one area for the return of the remaining costal cartilage after fabrication of the three-dimensional costal cartilage framework, which is cut into 2–3-mm blocks. A small funnel is placed in the unsutured opening of the perichondrium for returning the cut cartilage blocks. (Above, center) The appearance after the return of cut cartilage blocks. The cartilage blocks are visible at the opening of the perichondrium. (Above, right) Intercostal nerve block is performed for reducing postoperative pain with 0.25% Marcaine under direct vision. A total of 5 mL is administered per each rib. (Below) The muscle and muscular fascia are sutured with 4-0 nylon and a Penrose drain is placed under the muscular layer. (Reproduced from Kawanabe Y, Nagata S. A new method of costal cartilage harvest for total auricular reconstruction: part I. Avoidance and prevention of intraoperative and postoperative complications and problems. Plast Reconstr Surg 2006;117:2011–2018.)

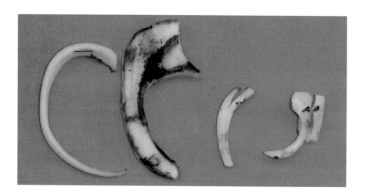

Fig. 20.15 The modified rib cartilage framework may contain these parts to provide prominent structures. From left to right, the helix, the base frame, the Y-shaped antihelical complex, and the tragus attached with an additional cartilaginous cube. (Reproduced from Chin W, Zhang R, Zhang Q, et al. Modifications of three-dimensional costal cartilage framework grafting in auricular reconstruction for microtia. Plast Reconstr Surg 2009;124:1940–1946.)

presence of chondroprogenitors at the recipient site, which can all have an influence on the composition of the new tissue.[45] With proper microenvironments, perichondrium-mediated cartilage regeneration remains possible, as revealed by experimental studies. For example, Sari et al. reported neocartilage formation in a folded-ear perichondrium at 6 weeks postimplantation under the abdominal muscle in rabbit.[45]

One of the major clinical applications is for joint repair. As early as 1975, Engkvist et al. reported a pilot experimental study of regenerating articular cartilage of cavitas glenoidalis by transplanting ear perichondrium in a rabbit model. Further, clinical trials were formed in 5 cases of arthritis patients. After removal of the degenerated cartilage, rib perichondrium was grafted and

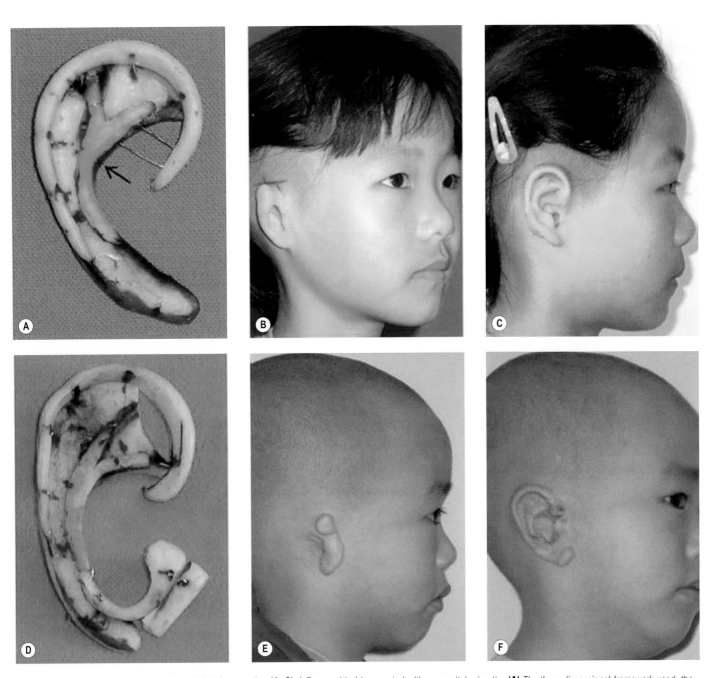

Fig. 20.16 Auricular reconstruction with modified frameworks. **(A–C)** A 7-year-old girl presented with congenital microtia. **(A)** The three-dimensional framework used: the arrow indicates the Y-shaped antihelical complex attached on the base frame. **(B)** Preoperative oblique view of conchal-type microtia. **(C)** Close-up appearance of the reconstructed auricle 8 months after grafting of the framework. **(D–F)** A 6-year-old boy presented with congenital microtia. **(D)** The completed costal framework with Y-shaped antihelical complex and the tragus attached with an additional cartilaginous cube. **(E)** Preoperative lateral view of sausage-type microtia. **(F)** Postoperative oblique view, 3 months after grafting of the framework. (Modified from Chin W, Zhang R, Zhang Q, et al. Modifications of three-dimensional costal cartilage framework grafting in auricular reconstruction for microtia. Plast Reconstr Surg 2009;124:1940–1946.)

articular cartilage regeneration took place.[46] Following the initial trials, there were some reports of the application of perichondrium graft for clinical repair of human knee joint articular cartilage,[47,48] but there were few on repairing articular cartilage of human digits.[49] Instead, transplantation of costal osteochondral grafts became the major tissue graft for functional restoration of injured digital articular cartilage.[50,51]

The other important clinical application might be nasal reconstruction either as a perichondium graft or

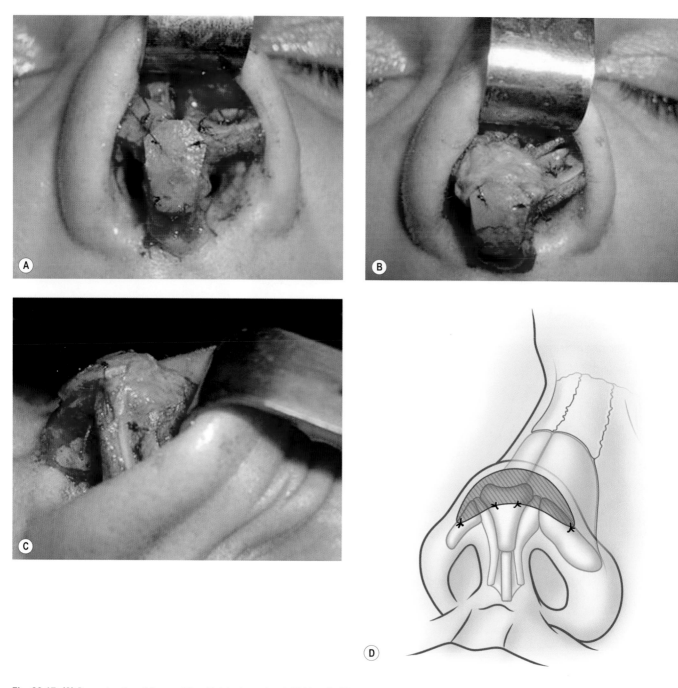

Fig. 20.17 **(A)** Reconstruction of the nasal tip with lateral crural and shield grafts (Sheen-type) harvested from the cartilage of the auricular concha. **(B)** Graft of the perichondrium stretched over and secured to cartilaginous grafts to make the contours smooth and disguise tip grafts. **(C)** Lateral view of the same graft. **(D)** Schematic illustration of the perichondrium graft positioning and fixation. The presence of numerous grafts inevitably leads to sharp ridges and irregularities in the cartilaginous contour that can be eliminated by means of the perichondrium graft. (Modified from Boccieri A, Marianetti TM. Perichondrium graft: harvesting and indications in nasal surgery. J Craniofac Surg 2010;21:40–44.)

as a perichondrocutaneous graft. Recently, Boccieri and Marianetti reported the application of perichondrium graft for nasal surgery. Because of its thinness and malleability, perichondrium is particularly suitable for covering every part of the cartilaginous graft, and is easy to fold into various layers if greater thickness is required in filling certain areas and therefore is commonly used in secondary rhinoplasty.[52,53] *Figure 20.17* demonstrates the surgical procedure of nasal tip reconstruction with auricular perichondrium.[52]

In addition, perichondrocutaneous graft is a common graft type. Brent and Ott reported the graft and proposed its application in reconstructive facial surgery in 1978.[54] The donor source for the graft should be restricted to concha in order to prevent deformity.[6] This graft has wide applications. It has been reported to be used for facial reconstruction,[55,56] for reconstruction of nasal defect,[57,58] for auricular defect repair,[59] and repairing ectropion.[60] Overall, although both perichondrium and perichondrocutaneous grafts have been widely used for clinical repair of tissue defect, there remains no solid clinical evidence to support the theory that transplanted perichondrium is able to regenerate a significant amount of cartilage tissue.

Cartilage engineering

Introduction and basic principle

Cartilage probably is one of the most commonly used tissue grafts in plastic surgery and has been employed in auricular reconstruction, rhinoplasty, and other surgical procedures, as described above. However, autologous cartilage graft is limited in its available amount and tissue harvest may cause donor site morbidity.

Tissue engineering is a new biotechnology developed from the late 1980s and early 1990s, which aims to repair and regenerate human tissue via an engineering approach to produce autologous tissue. Actually, cartilage is closely related to the development of tissue engineering because it was used as a tissue target to prove the basic principle.[61,62] Interestingly, the success in the engineering of human ear shape cartilage in a nude mouse model vividly revealed that this tissue-engineering technique has great potential in plastic surgery for tissue repair and reconstruction.[63]

As outlined by Stock and Vacanti,[64] the basic concept of tissue engineering includes a scaffold that provides an architecture on which seeded cells can organize and develop into the desired organ or tissue prior to implantation. The scaffold provides an initial biomechanical profile for the replacement tissue until the cells produce an adequate ECM. During the formation, deposition, and organization of the newly generated matrix, the scaffold is either degraded or metabolized, eventually leading to a vital organ or tissue that restores, maintains, or improves tissue function.

Generally, the tissue-engineering process involves three major components: (1) seed cells: the component for matrix production, deposition, and tissue formation; (2) scaffold: the substance that provides a 3D place for cells to reside, proliferate, and produce matrix; (3) tissue formation environment: after being seeded on the scaffold, cells start to grow and produce and deposit ECMs on the scaffold. In a proper environment, with gradual degradation of the scaffold, cell proliferation, matrix production, and proper tissue remodeling, an engineered tissue gradually forms and becomes mature.

In the past 20 years, tremendous progress has been made in basic and applied research of cartilage engineering, including the search for different biomaterials as scaffolds, seeking different cell sources and chondrogenic induction of stem cells as well as advances in the techniques of cartilage tissue formation, such as *in vitro* reconstruction of cartilage tissue. Among them, some have already revealed the great potential in plastic surgery, for example, auricular reconstruction, rhinoplasty, and facial contouring. The following gives a few examples of the techniques for generating and the results of engineered cartilages that may potentially be used for cartilage repair and reconstruction.

Engineering of auricular cartilage

An important achievement in cartilage engineering research is the development of the technique that enables generation of a human ear-shaped cartilage, because it vividly reveals the application potential in plastic surgery. The procedure is described below to provide an example of translational research of cartilage engineering.[63]

To generate a human ear-shaped cartilage, selection of seed cell, scaffold materials, and an animal model should be determined according to the principle. In this study, chondrocytes derived from calf cartilage, polyglycolic acid (PGA), unwoven fibers, and a nude mouse model served as the basic components to construct the cartilage.

To isolate the cells, cartilage fragments were first harvested from the articular surface of glenohumeral and humeroulnar joints and then subjected to collagenase digestion (3 mg/mL) in culture medium at 37°C for

12–18 hours. The resulting tissue digestion solution was filtered and centrifuged to collect the chondrocytes and the cells were expanded *in vitro*.

To prepare the scaffold for the human ear shape, the ear of a 3-year-old child was cast using alginate as the impression material, and then a final cast of plaster was fashioned from the alginate impression. Using the plaster cast as a mold, PGA nonwoven mesh in about 100 μm thickness was coated with 1% (w/v) solution of polylactic acid (PLA) in methylene chloride. Following immersion, the fabric was removed and shaped into the form of a human ear using the plaster prosthetic mold.

To prepare a cell–scaffold construct, the ear-shaped scaffold was placed in a culture dish and seeded with 3 mL of chondrocyte suspension (1.5×10^8 cells) and placed in an incubator for 4 hours to allow seeded cells to attach on the scaffold and then culture medium (Hamm's F-12 supplemented with 10% fetal calf serum, 5 μg/mL ascorbic acid, 292 μg/mL L-glutamine, 100 U/mL penicillin, and 100 μg/mL streptomycin) was added, and the construct was incubated *in vitro* at 37°C in 5% CO_2 for 1 week. As shown, the cell–seeded construct could maintain a good ear shape *(Fig. 20.18A)* and scanning electron microscope revealed good cell attachment on the scaffold and matrix production *(Fig. 20.18B)*.

After 1 week of *in vitro* culture, the cell–scaffold construct was implanted into the subcutaneous tissue of a nude mouse with the support of an external stent outside the skin to keep the shape *(Fig. 20.19)*. As shown in *Figure 20.20*, an ear cartilage structure is formed with the 3D shape that is almost identical to that of a human ear after 12 weeks of *in vivo* implantation. To verify the formation of engineered ear cartilage, tissues were harvested and subcutaneous tissues were stripped and the resulting gross view and histology confirmed a well-formed ear shape cartilage *(Fig. 20.21)*. Through this pioneering study, the result provides an example of how to translate cartilage engineering research to plastic surgery application, particularly for engineered auricular reconstruction.[63]

To explore the possibility of translating this technique to clinical application, a technique of *in vitro* engineering human ear shape cartilage was developed with the assistance of computer-aided design (CAD) and computer-aided manufacture (CAM) technologies.[65]

To proceed, computed tomography was employed to scan a patient's normal ear to collect the geometric data;

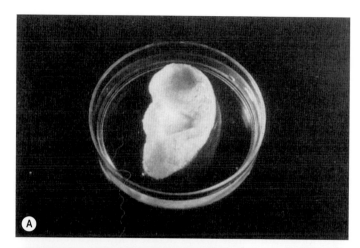

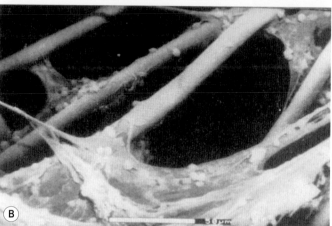

Fig. 20.18 Chondrocytes seeded on to the polymer ear mold *in vitro*. **(A)** Gross appearance of the ear polymer mold seeded with chondrocytes (1.5×10^8). **(B)** Scanning electron micrograph showing adherence of chondrocytes to polyglycolic acid device before implantation. (Reproduced from Cao Y, Vacanti JP, Paige KT, *et al*. Transplantation of chondrocytes utilizing a polymer–cell construct to produce tissue-engineered cartilage in the shape of a human ear. Plast Reconstr Surg 1997;100:297–302.)

the information was then processed by a CAD system to generate both positive and negative image data of the normal ear. The resultant data were then input into a CAM system to print a mold with 3D structure of a normal ear in half size. Then, PGA unwoven fibers were inserted into the mold and coated with 0.3% PLA solution, thus generating a relatively solid ear shape scaffold material. The resulting scaffold was laser-scanned to generate a 3D image, which could be digitally compared with the original ear 3D image to analyze the similarity in 3D structure. As revealed in *Figure 20.22*, the resulting ear-shaped scaffold achieved a similarity level of above 97% compared to the positive mold of original ear shape, indicating that the mold fabricated by CAD/

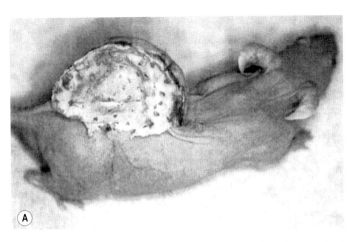
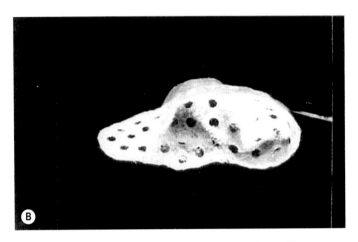

Fig. 20.19 An external stent was fixed on the outside skin of the polymer ear implant to maintain polymer mold shape **(A)** and the view of an external stent **(B)**. (Reproduced from Cao Y, Vacanti JP, Paige KT, et al. Transplantation of chondrocytes utilizing a polymer-cell construct to produce tissue-engineered cartilage in the shape of a human ear. Plast Reconstr Surg 1997;100:297–302.)

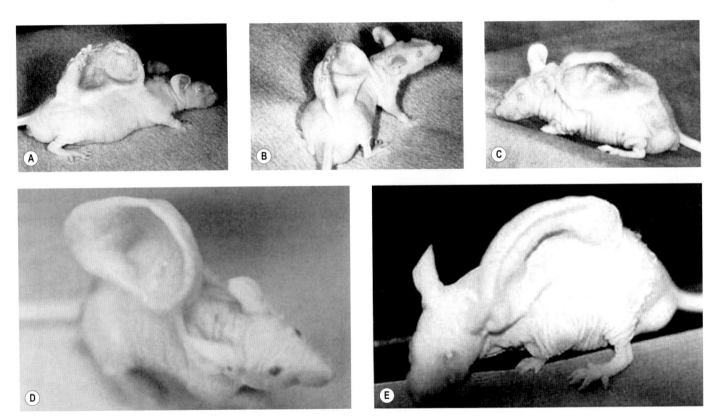

Fig. 20.20 (A–E) Gross appearance of the constructs 12 weeks after subcutaneous implantation into nude mice. Note the three-dimensional shape that is almost identical to that of a human ear. (Reproduced from Cao Y, Vacanti JP, Paige KT, et al. Transplantation of chondrocytes utilizing a polymer-cell construct to produce tissue-engineered cartilage in the shape of a human ear. Plast Reconstr Surg 1997;100:297–302.)

CAM can fabricate a scaffold accurately into an ear shape that is mirror-symmetrical to the normal ear.

Afterwards, a total of 50×10^6 cells in 1 mL volume were evenly seeded on to the ear-shaped scaffold and cultured *in vitro* with medium change at regular time intervals. Interestingly, a human ear cartilage could be generated *in vitro* after 12 weeks of culture with good elasticity *(Fig. 20.23)*. The engineered cartilage also revealed relatively mature histological structure of cartilage with lacuna structure formation and strong

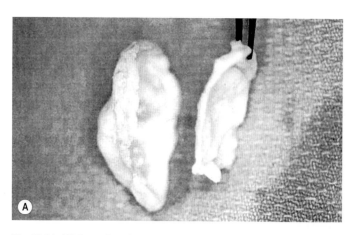
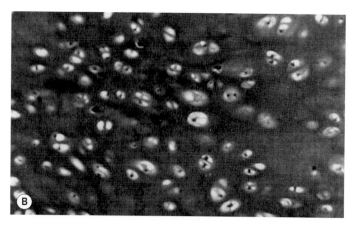

Fig. 20.21 (A) Gross view of engineered ear shape cartilage with (left) or without (right) external stent fixation. Note: fine contour of the new cartilaginous ear is maintained in the group with stent application. **(B)** Histology of engineered ear shape cartilage (hematoxylin and eosin, ×320). (Modified from Cao Y, Vacanti JP, Paige KT, *et al.* Transplantation of chondrocytes utilizing a polymer-cell construct to produce tissue-engineered cartilage in the shape of a human ear. Plast Reconstr Surg 1997;100:297–302.)

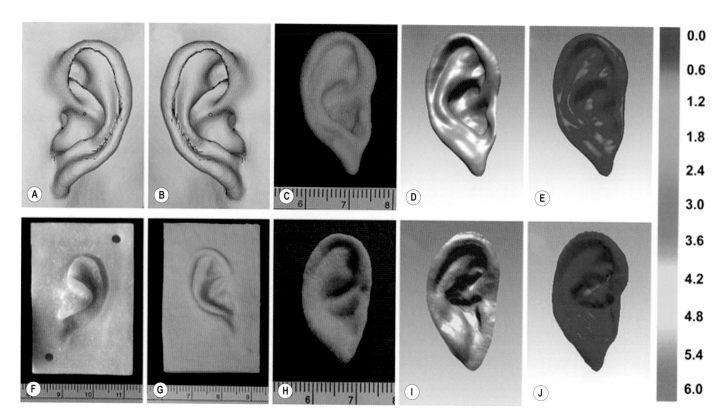

Fig. 20.22 Preparation and shape analysis of the ear-shaped scaffolds. **(A)** Three-dimensional (3D) image of the normal ear; **(B)** the mirror image of A; **(C)** the half-sized resin-positive mold; **(D)** laser scan image of C; **(E)** color map of D; **(F)** inner part of the resin-negative mold fabricated by 3D printing; **(G)** outer part of the negative mold cast from F with silicone rubber; **(H)** the ear-shaped polylactic acid/polyglycolic acid scaffold; **(I)** laser scan image of H; **(J)** color map of I compared to D. Color bar at the right side represents similarity from highest (top, blue) to lowest (bottom, red). (Reproduced from Liu Y, Zhang L, Zhou G, *et al. In vitro* engineering of human ear-shaped cartilage assisted with CAD/CAM technology. Biomaterials 2010;31:2176–2183.)

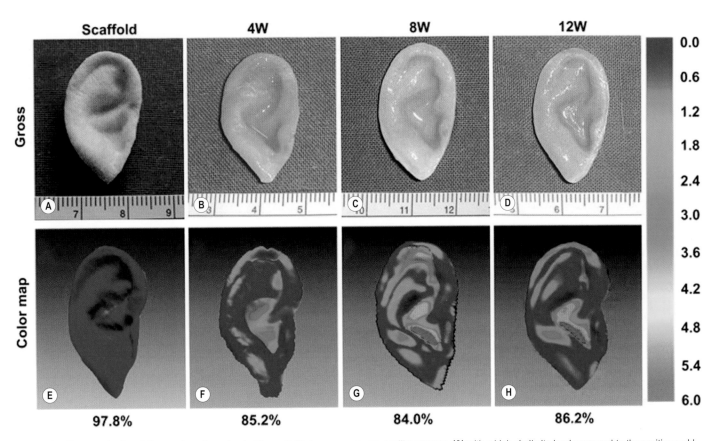

Fig. 20.23 Shape evaluation of the ear-shaped constructs. The scaffold shows an accurate ear-like structure **(A)** with a high similarity level compared to the positive mold **(E)**. All the cell scaffold constructs largely maintain their original ear-like structures at 4 weeks **(B)**, 8 weeks **(C)**, and 12 weeks **(D)**. Quantitative analysis shows over 84% shape similarity in all the samples **(F–H)** compared to the positive mold. (Reproduced from Liu Y, Zhang L, Zhou G, et al. *In vitro* engineering of human ear-shaped cartilage assisted with CAD/CAM technology. Biomaterials 2010;31:2176–2183.)

staining for Safranin-O and collagen II, as shown in *Figure 20.24*. More importantly, the human ear-shaped cartilage formed *in vitro* could reach a morphological similarity of 82.6% to the positive ear mold, indicating that this technique not only can generate cartilage tissue *in vitro* but is also able to maintain a designed 3D tissue structure *(Fig. 20.23)*.[65] Currently, continuous effort is being made in our center to study the fate of the *in vitro*-engineered ear-shaped cartilage after *in vivo* implantation and the progress in this area is expected to pave the way for the eventual clinical application of engineered human ear-shaped cartilage.

One of the unique properties of human ear cartilage is its excellent elasticity and flexibility that allow for torsion and bending without causing a fracture. Mimicking such mechanical properties of the native tissue should also be an important consideration for engineering ear-shaped cartilage and its application. In 2005, Xu *et al.* reported a new method of generating

flexible auricular cartilage.[66] In their study, auricular chondrocytes were isolated from swine ear cartilage by enzyme digestion and fibrin polymer was used as the scaffold. In addition, auricular perichondrium was harvested and lyophilized. During the engineering process, equal volumes of both the chondrocyte fibrinogen suspension and the thrombin solution were mixed together to give rise to a chondrocyte–fibrin polymer suspension. The suspension was then placed into an ear-shaped well made from bone wax to allow for polymerization. To produce a flexible cartilage, the polymerized chondrocyte–fibrin construct was sandwiched between two layers of lyophilized swine perichondrium to form a trilayer, ear-shaped construct and then implanted into athymic mice subcutaneously. As a control, chondrocyte–fibrin construct without perichondrium was implanted as well. At 12 weeks of implantation, engineered cartilaginous tissue was formed in both the experimental and control groups.

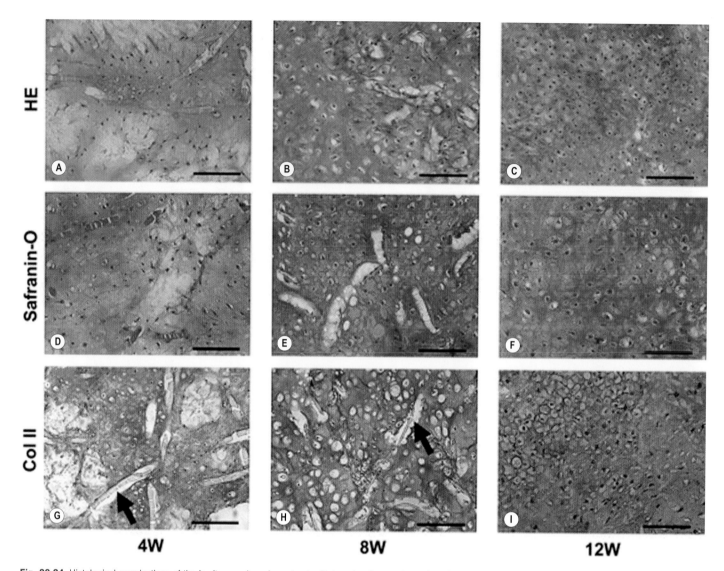

HE

Safranin-O

Col II

4W   **8W**   **12W**

Fig. 20.24 Histological examinations of the *in vitro* ear-shaped constructs. At 4 weeks, the constructs form heterogeneous cartilage-like tissue along with undegraded polyglycolic acid fibers **(A, D, G)**. With prolonged culture time, the histological structure of the constructs gradually becomes compact, accompanied by increased numbers of lacuna structures at 8 weeks **(B, E, H)**. Homogeneous cartilage with abundant extracellular matrix and mature lacunae is observed at 12 weeks **(C, F, I)** with no visible scaffold residuals in the constructs. The black arrows indicate the undegraded polyglycolic acid fibers. Scale bar = 100 μm. (Reproduced from Liu Y, Zhang L, Zhou G, *et al. In vitro* engineering of human ear-shaped cartilage assisted with CAD/CAM technology. Biomaterials 2010;31:2176–2183.)

Importantly, engineered cartilage laminated with perichondrium exhibited mechanical properties similar to those of the native swine ear, and could tolerate severe torsion and bending without fracture, although the 3D structure remains to be improved. Histology also revealed good integration between the engineered cartilage and lyophilized perichondrium *(Fig. 20.25)*. In contrast, the engineered cartilage of control group became fractured after the test of torsion and bending. The result of this study indicates that lamination with lyophilized perichondrium is a reliable method of conferring elastic-like flexibility to an engineered ear

cartilage. In the future, selection of a proper solid scaffold may help to control the precise and detailed structure better in order to generate flexible auricular cartilage with better 3D structure.[66]

In addition to the experimental studies that employed animal chondrocytes, human chondrocytes have also been investigated for their ability to form engineered cartilage. Kamil *et al.* reported a comparative study of normal chondrocytes and microtia chondrocytes from patients and the results showed their similar abilities in cell proliferation and cartilage tissue formation, indicating that cartilage derived from microtia patients may

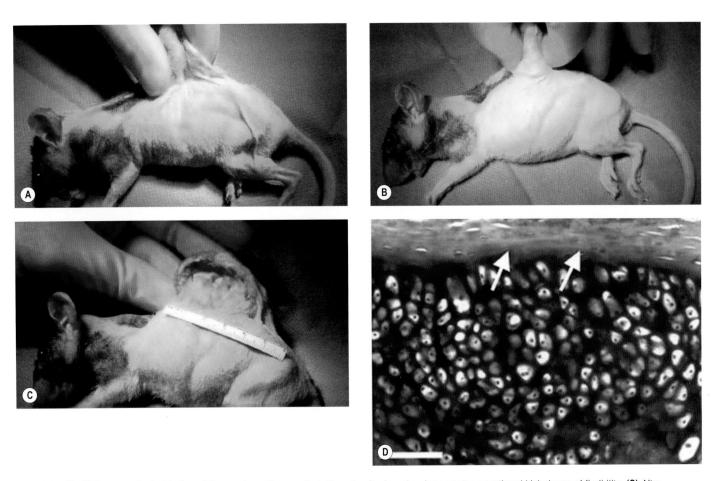

Fig. 20.25 (A, B) Gross mechanical testing of the ear-shaped framework at 12 weeks after insertion demonstrates a continued high degree of flexibility. **(C)** After mechanical testing, the framework easily recovers its initial shape. **(D)** Hematoxylin and eosin staining of flexible tissue-engineered cartilage (original magnification ×100; bar = 100 μm), demonstrating the tight adherence at the interface between neocartilage and the lyophilized swine perichondrium laminate (arrows indicate interface). (Modified from Xu JW, Johnson TS, Motarjem PM, *et al.* Tissue-engineered flexible ear-shaped cartilage. Plast Reconstr Surg 2005;115:1633–1641.)

potentially serve as the cell source to engineer human auricular cartilage.[67]

Interestingly, Yanaga *et al.* reported a clinical trial of auricular reconstruction with fabricated human cartilage. In this trial, chondrocytes isolated from the cartilage remnant of microtia patients were cultured *in vitro* using a multilayer culture method, then the expanded cells along with their produced gelatinous chondroid matrices were collected into a syringe in the cell density of $0.5-1 \times 10^7$ cells per mL. Afterwards, 40–73 mL of cells/gelatinous matrices was injected into a subcutaneous pocket on the fascia of a patient's lower abdomen using a 16-gauge indwelling needle in order to generate an engineered cartilage block which could be sculptured to an auricular framework *(Fig. 20.26)*. The results showed that a large piece of elastic cartilage was formed at the abdominal environment at 6 months

postimplantation, which was also verified by histology examination. Importantly, this engineered cartilage block provides sufficient cartilage to create an ear framework. Furthermore, the framework could well support the reconstructed auricle without obvious absorption after being implanted for several years *(Fig. 20.26)*. This preliminary study provides important supporting evidence for the future clinical application of engineered auricular reconstruction.[68]

Engineered cartilage for rhinoplasty and facial contouring

In addition to auricular reconstruction, rhinoplasty is another area where tissue-engineered cartilage may potentially be applied clinically. In contrast to auricular

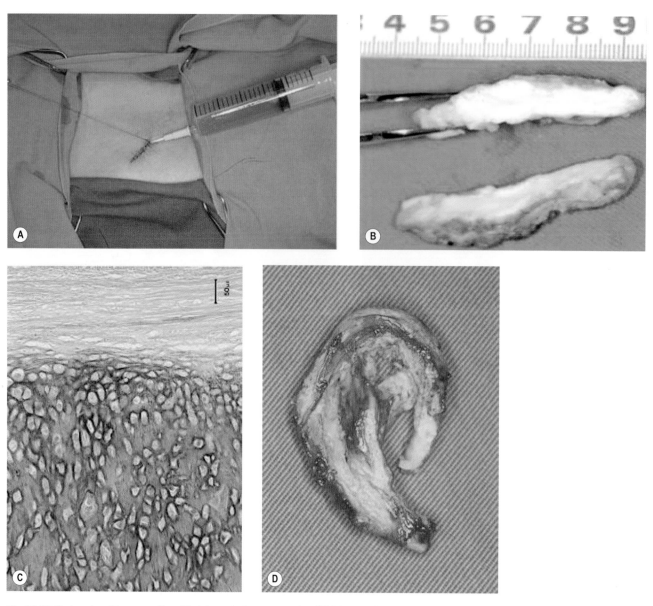

Fig. 20.26 Engineering of human cartilage block for auricular reconstruction. **(A)** Injection of cultured chondrocytes subcutaneously; **(B)** formation of engineered cartilage block with good elasticity; **(C)** histological verification of engineered elastic cartilage; **(D)** an ear framework, sculptured from the engineered neocartilage block;

reconstruction, injectable cartilage is an important physical form for transplanting engineered cartilage.

In the early stage of tissue engineering research, injectable cartilage was employed to explore the feasibility of cartilage engineering using slowly polymerizing calcium alginate gels[69] or Pluronic gel,[70] amongst others. In recently published studies, human chondrocytes have also been confirmed to be able to form injectable cartilage using different injectable scaffolds.[71,72]

Although most engineered injectable cartilage research remains at the experimental stage using either animal cells or an animal model, there are a few reports of the clinical application of injectable cartilage.[73,74] Yanaga et al. reported a clinical trial of injecting cultured autologous chondrocytes for nasal augmentation. First, a piece of cartilage was harvested from auricular concha to extract chondrocytes and the cells were expanded in vitro into a gel-type cell-containing mass. Then, a subperiosteal skin pocket was created on the nasal dorsum of the patients and the chondrocytes were transplanted within a gel mass and the wound was closed. The implantation site was fixed with splint and

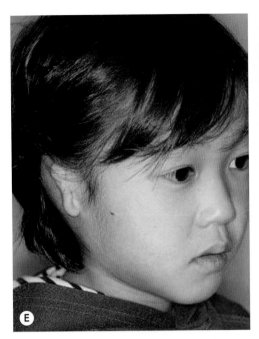
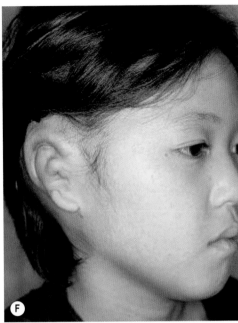

Fig. 20.26, cont'd (E) a 9-year-old boy with microtia before operation; **(F)** 2 years after auricular reconstruction with engineered framework. (Modified from Yanaga H, Imai K, Fujimoto T, *et al.* Generating ears from cultured autologous auricular chondrocytes by using two-stage implantation in treatment of microtia. Plast Reconstr Surg 2009;124:817–825.)

tape for 3 weeks. Biopsy of injected tissue confirmed the formation of engineered cartilage after 1 month of implantation.

The procedure was applied in 8 patients for primary nasal augmentation or to correct a deformity resulting from silicone implant exposure or deviation. The patients were followed up for 6 months to 2 years and injected cartilage could maintain its shape without resorption.[73] Later the same group further reported clinical trials in 32 patients for both nasal augmentation and facial contouring, with excellent clinical evaluation results and patient satisfaction in most cases.[74] *Figure 20.27* demonstrates the clinical outcome of injected cartilage for nasal augmentation. Additionally, the authors used injected autologous chondrocytes for chin augmentation and to correct temporal and forehead depressed deformity.[73,74]

In addition to injectable cartilage, *in vivo*-engineered cartilage may potentially be used for nasal reconstruction. For example, Farhadi *et al.* reported the engineering of human nasal cartilage. In the study, chondrocytes were isolated from nasal septum and seeded on to nonwoven meshes of esterified hyaluronan (Hyaff-11). The cell–scaffold construct was cultured *in vitro* for 2 or 4 weeks and then implanted into nude mouse. The results

showed that the cartilage was well formed after 2 weeks of *in vivo* implantation and the engineered cartilage exhibited good mechanical property.[75] Similar results were also reported in another study.[76] With enhanced mechanical strength, these *in vivo*-engineered cartilages may provide the autologous cartilage grafts potentially for septum or nasal alar reconstruction or nasal augmentation. *In vitro* engineering of cartilage with a nasal tip has been reported many years ago to aim for nasal reconstruction with specifically shape-designed cartilage,[77] but its relatively weak mechanical strength might prohibit *in vitro*-engineered cartilage from immediate transplantation in nasal reconstruction.

Engineered cartilage for joint cartilage repair and reconstruction

Engineered cartilage may also serve as a composite graft to repair or reconstruct articular cartilage. There are two potential targets: temporomandibular joint (TMJ) and digital joints. In 2001, Weng *et al.* reported a preliminary study of mandible condylar reconstruction with tissue-engineered composites of bone and cartilage. In the study, scaffold of PLA-coated PGA was molded into the shape of human mandible condyle and respectively

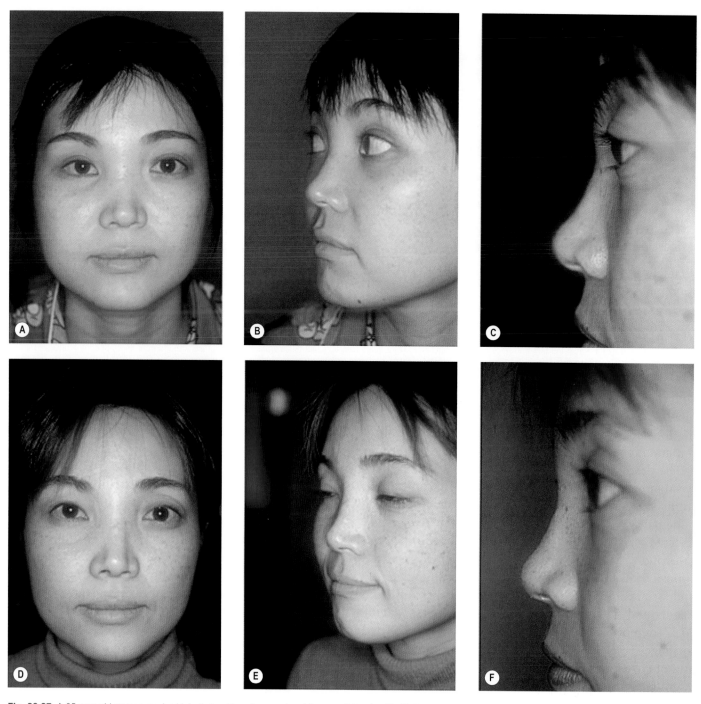

Fig. 20.27 A 35-year-old woman received injected cartilage to correct saddle-nose deformity. **(A–C)** Preoperative views. The autologous cultured auricular chondrocytes were grafted to the nasal dorsum. **(D–F)** Postoperative views after 34 months. The projection radix is higher than before grafting. The shape and contours of the nasal dorsum have aesthetically improved. Good contours have been maintained, and there has been no absorption of the grafted chondrocytes. (Reproduced from Yanaga H, Yanaga K, Imai K, *et al.* Clinical application of cultured autologous human auricular chondrocytes with autologous serum for craniofacial or nasal augmentation and repair. Plast Reconstr Surg 2006;117:2019–2030.)

seeded with osteoblasts and chondrocytes followed by *in vivo* implantation in nude mouse. After 12 weeks, a condyle-shaped bone tissue was well formed with articular cartilage on the surface and histology confirmed the formation of trabecular bone and hyaline cartilage, suggesting a potential approach for clinical TMJ reconstruction.[78] In addition, engineered cartilage was proposed for TMJ disc reconstruction to potentially restore TMJ function.[79]

Cartilage presents as the major tissue component in interphalangeal joints or metacarpophalangeal joints and plays an important functional role. As early as 1999, Isogai *et al.* reported a preliminary study on constructing small phalanges and the whole joints using a tissue-engineering approach.[80] The approach included the use of PLA or PGA as the scaffold and fresh bovine periosteum was harvested to wrap around the scaffold for bone engineering. Additionally, chondrocytes and tenocytes were seeded on the scaffold to form articular cartilage and associated tendon tissue. The results showed that a preliminary composite tissue formed with the shape and dimensions of human phalanges as well as the joints.[80] A study with much larger sample size was also performed to engineer composite tissue of human phalanges and a small joint, with successful results.[81] Although these studies were preliminary, the results revealed the promise of the future application of engineered cartilage in joint reconstruction.

Future directions

Despite a few preliminary clinical trials of engineered cartilages in auricular and nasal reconstruction, there remains much to do in both basic and applied research prior to true translation of cartilage research to clinical application. To fulfill the goal, the following areas may represent future directions.

Stem cell-based cartilage engineering

Although both auricular and nasal cartilages have been used as the sources to extract chondrocytes, the available tissue amounts are limited. Although more tissue volume can be harvested from rib cartilage, the amount of cells that can be harvested is limited due to low cellular density. Stem cells, particularly adult stem cells, have become an alternative cell source because of their multidifferentiation potential (including chondrogenic) and strong proliferation capability.

The adult mesenchymal stem cells derived from bone marrow and adipose tissue are the most feasible cell source for cartilage engineering.[82] Chondrogenic differentiation can be achieved with growth factor induction[83] or co-culture with chondrocytes[84] or with chondrogenic matrices.[85] In recent years, mimicking native histoarchitecture and the molecular signaling of cartilage microenvironment in scaffold design have been considered important to facilitate stem cell chondrogenic differentiation and cartilage formation.[86] Therefore, optimization of chondrogenic induction regime by proper combination of paracrine factors, chondrogenic matrices, and suitable topographical structure of scaffold is likely to enhance chondrogenic differentiation of stem cells, and improve the structure and function of stem cell-engineered cartilage.

In vitro engineering of cartilage with enhanced mechanical strength

As described above, the application of plastic surgery requires immediately available cartilage graft to generate an auricular or a nasal frame for reconstructive surgical procedures. *In vivo* engineering cartilage, first using the human body as a bioreactor and then reshaping the *in vivo*-engineered cartilage block into a desired frame, would require at least two-stage operations.[68] Furthermore, patients may undergo unnecessary suffering if the first stage of *in vivo* engineering fails. Therefore, *in vitro* cartilage engineering can not only avoid two-stage operations, but also reduce the risk of failure because more back-up engineered cartilages can be made simultaneously *in vitro* without causing patient suffering.

Today, *in vitro* cartilage engineering has already been proven feasible by experimental studies using either chondrocytes[65] or mesenchymal stem cells.[87] Nevertheless, the mechanical strength of *in vitro*-engineered cartilage remains relatively weak compared to that of *in vivo*-engineered cartilage.[88] This is likely caused by the differences between *in vitro* and *in vivo* microenvironments, and the latter can promote the maturation of engineered cartilage and thus lead to differential expression of key matrix molecules such as collagen IX and pyridinoline, and enhanced mechanical strength.[88] Although it remains difficult to define the environmental mechanism, partially mimicking *in vivo* microenvironmental factors may help to enhance the mechanical property of *in vitro*-engineered cartilage. For example, when an articular cartilage was engineered in a bioreactor with dynamic loading, it was found that continuous dynamic loading could significantly increase Young's modulus of the engineered cartilage. In addition, the loaded cartilage increased the production of cartilage oligomeric matrix protein and collagens II and IX.[89] In the future, mechanical loading as well as other factors that are able to facilitate collagen maturation may represent one of the future directions for *in vitro* cartilage engineering.

Design and precise control of engineered cartilage 3D structure

For engineered cartilage application in auricular and nasal reconstruction, precise control of 3D structure is necessary to achieve the goal. As previously described, a CAD/CAM system is essential to collect the 3D information and to fabricate the scaffold with a specific 3D structure that matches a patient's own auricular or nasal structure. In addition, the fabrication of a suitable scaffold that is able to maintain the precise 3D structure during cartilage formation may be an important consideration. Furthermore, an inner core stent with slow degradation rate may help to maintain the 3D structure if the inner core starts to degrade after mature cartilage formation.

 Access the complete references list online at **http://www.expertconsult.com**

6. Brent B. Repair and grafting of cartilage and perichondrium. In: McCarthy JC, ed. *Plastic Surgery*. Philadelphia: WB Saunders; 1990:559–582.

8. Han K, Kim J, Son D, et al. How to harvest the maximal amount of conchal cartilage grafts. *J Plast Reconstr Aesthet Surg*. 2008;61:1465–1471.

12. Singh DJ, Bartlett SP. Aesthetic management of the ear as a donor site. *Plast Reconstr Surg*. 2007;120:899–908.

   The ear is a popular donor site for chondrocutaneous grafts in nasal reconstruction. The authors review their experience with these procedures to offer insights in maximizing aesthetic donor site outcomes.

17. Scuderi N, Ribuffo D, Chiummariello S. Total and subtotal upper eyelid reconstruction with the nasal chondromucosal flap: a 10-year experience. *Plast Reconstr Surg*. 2005;115:1259–1265.

   A technique for upper eyelid reconstruction with a nasal chondromucosal flap is presented. Excellent flap viability and an average of 13-mm levator excursion is reported.

23. Brent B. Auricular repair with autogenous rib cartilage grafts: two decades of experience with 600 cases. *Plast Reconstr Surg*. 1992;90:355–374.

30. Uppal RS, Sabbagh W, Chana J, et al. Donor-site morbidity after autologous costal cartilage harvest in ear reconstruction and approaches to reducing donor-site contour deformity. *Plast Reconstr Surg*. 2008;121:1949–1955.

31. Kawanabe Y, Nagata S. A new method of costal cartilage harvest for total auricular reconstruction: part I. Avoidance and prevention of intraoperative and postoperative complications and problems. *Plast Reconstr Surg*. 2006;117:2011–2018.

63. Cao Y, Vacanti JP, Paige KT, et al. Transplantation of chondrocytes utilizing a polymer-cell construct to produce tissue-engineered cartilage in the shape of a human ear. *Plast Reconstr Surg*. 1997;100:297–302.

   This paper describes a strategy to tissue engineer cartilage in the shape of a human ear on the dorsum of athymic mice. Histological and morphometric outcomes are assessed.

65. Liu Y, Zhang L, Zhou G, et al. *In vitro* engineering of human ear-shaped cartilage assisted with CAD/CAM technology. *Biomaterials*. 2010;31:2176–2183.

   The authors report their efforts in tissue engineering CAD/CAM-designed tissue engineered auricles on PLA/PGA scaffolds in vitro.

68. Yanaga H, Imai K, Fujimoto T, et al. Generating ears from cultured autologous auricular chondrocytes by using two-stage implantation in treatment of microtia. *Plast Reconstr Surg*. 2009;124:817–825.

   A technique for in vivo chondrogenesis in a heterotopic abdominal pocket is reported. Cartilaginous frameworks for auricular reconstruction were successfully modeled and implanted from this neocartilage in four patients, with promising reconstructive outcomes.

21

Repair and grafting of bone

Iris A. Seitz, Chad M. Teven, and Russell R. Reid

SYNOPSIS

- This chapter will concentrate on the principles and concepts of bone repair, grafting, and reconstruction.
- The embryology, physiology, microanatomy, and histochemistry of bone will be reviewed.
- Principles of mechanotransduction and cellular mechanisms of bone turnover will also be discussed.
- Pathophysiology of traumatic injury to bone (fractures, segmental loss, defects) will be categorized and reviewed.
- Bone-remodeling mechanisms (osteoconduction, osteoinduction, osteointegration) will be described.
- After a brief history of autogenous bone grafting, the clinical application of bone transfer and transplantation will be captured by a brief atlas of harvest of each subtype.
- The reader will also be provided with a brief overview of bone substitutes.

Microanatomy and histochemistry

Bone is a complex structure that serves many important roles within the human body. It is crucial for maintaining mineral homeostasis, and providing both protection to delicate internal organs and structural support for locomotion and stature. Bone undergoes constant remodeling, during which old bone is degraded and subsequently replaced by newly formed bone. Most other organs in the adult human, rather than regeneration, undergo repair with scar tissue. This and many other attributes makes bone a unique organ system.

The formation of bone occurs by two distinct mechanisms: intramembranous ossification and endochondral ossification. Direct condensations of mesenchymal stem cells (MSCs) initiate the process of intramembranous ossification to create the flat bones of the craniofacial skeleton. During intramembranous ossification, osteoblasts that line the surfaces of the skeleton deposit new bone upon previously laid bone in a process called apposition. Alternatively, endochondral ossification occurs when MSCs form a hyaline cartilage template that is subsequently replaced by bone. Endochondral ossification is responsible for the development for the tubular long bones of the appendicular skeleton as well as the bones of the vertebral column and pelvis.[1-4]

Bone is characterized by the presence of osteocytes located within open cavities within bone, called lacunae. Osteocytes project radiating processes that travel through microscopic canals called canaliculi that adjoin neighboring lacunae. Osteocytic cytoplasmic processes are linked to one another via gap junctions,[5] through which osteocytes are thought to communicate.[6]

Cortical versus cancellous bone

The entire skeleton is comprised of two types of bone: cortical bone and cancellous bone (*Fig. 21.1*). Cortical or compact bone comprises the outer layer of the skeleton and accounts for 80% of all bony tissue. It is characteristically dense, strong, and stiff, and serves to support

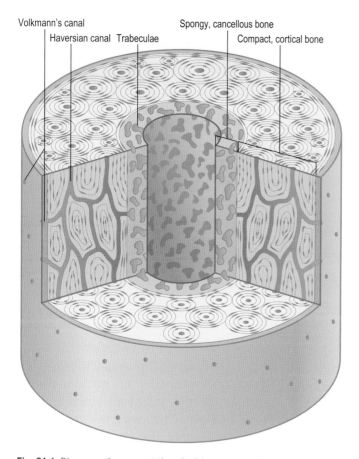

Fig. 21.1 Diagrammatic representation of axial compact cortical bone microarchitecture.

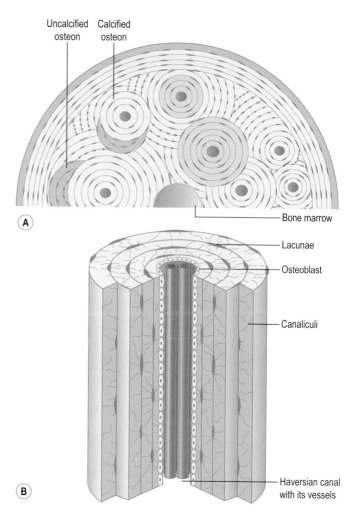

Fig. 21.2 (A) Cross-section of compact bone as seen by microradiography. Note that the osteons are oriented in the longitudinal axis of long bone. The dark masses represent recent decalcified osteons. The light masses represent older calcified osteons. **(B)** A single osteon of the haversian system.

the body and protect the internal organs. A two-layered cellular membrane known as the periosteum covers cortical bone. The outer layer is composed of a dense fibrous membrane that contains flat fibroblast-like cells and serves as an attachment for muscles and tendons. Large plump cells line the inner periosteal layer (cambium layer) and can differentiate into osteoblasts when induced. In addition, bone contains a thin layer of vascular connective tissue that lines the medullary cavity, known as the endosteum.

The primary functional unit of cortical bone is the osteon, or haversian system *(Fig. 21.2)*. Each osteon consists of concentric layers of cortical bone tissue (lamellae) that surround a central canal (haversian canal). The haversian canal contains nervous tissue and blood vessels that innervate and supply bone. Nutrient vessels within haversian canals anastomose to blood vessels within the bone marrow and periosteum. Volkmann's canals run perpendicular to haversian canals and are responsible for the aforementioned interconnection

between the haversian efferent vessels and those in the bone marrow and periosteum.

Cancellous (trabecular) bone, which comprises approximately 20% of the human skeleton, is characteristically porous compared to cortical bone. Cancellous bone is located deep to cortical bone within the medullary cavity, typically at the ends of long bones. It consists of bony trabeculae that are oriented along the lines of stress. Cancellous bone is identical in chemical composition to cortical bone; however, because of its greater surface area for remodeling, cancellous bone has increased metabolic activity. Cancellous bone provides internal support for both bone marrow elements and cortical bone.

The chemical composition of bone

Inorganic phase

Bone is a calcified tissue composed of 60% inorganic matter, 30% organic matter, and 10% water.[7–9] The inorganic component of bone is responsible for approximately 40% of bone volume, while the organic component and water comprise 35% and 25%, respectively.[7–10] The inorganic phase primarily consists of calcium phosphate (hydroxyapatite), which has the following chemical formula: $Ca_{10}(PO_4)_6(OH)_2$. Hydroxyapatite is a mineral crystal that measures 20–25 nm in length, 15 nm in width, and 2–5 nm in thickness.[7] It is the hydroxyl endmember of the apatite group; however, impurities arise when hydroxyl groups are replaced by potassium, magnesium, or sodium, or phosphate groups are replaced by carbonate.[7,10–14] By storing a mixture of minerals in the form of impure hydroxyapatite, bone serves as an important reservoir of such minerals within the human body.

Organic phase

The organic component of bone, know as demineralized organic bone matrix or osteoid, is deposited by osteoblasts during bone formation. Osteoid primarily consists of type I collagen, but also includes nearly 30 noncollagenous proteins.[9] Collagen is a trilaminar protein composed of two α1 chains and one α2 chain that interact to form a unique right-handed helical structure. Within the rough endoplasmic reticulum of osteoblasts, procollagen undergoes hydroxylation and glycosylation before subsequent transfer to the Golgi apparatus, where it is packaged and secreted. Outside the cellular membrane, procollagen peptides are cleaved into tropocollagen. Lysyl oxidase, an important copper-dependent enzyme, mediates covalent cross-linking within and between tropocollagen molecules to create mature collagen fibers. The strength of bone is primarily derived from interactions between collagen fibers and inorganic minerals.

The cellular composition of bone

Three cell types are predominantly found in bone: osteoblasts, osteocytes, and osteoclasts *(Table 21.1)*. Osteoblasts are responsible for the formation of bone matrix. Osteocytes are the terminal differentiation product of osteoblasts. Both cell types are derived from a common MSC precursor. Osteoclasts, which are responsible for bone resorption, are derived from hematopoietic stem cells.

Table 21.1 Bone cells

Cell type	Morphology	Location	Function	Source	Precursor cell	Differentiation product
Osteoblast	Rounded, basophilic cells Stain strongly for alkaline phosphatase	External surfaces of bone in areas of active remodeling and bone formation Bone surfaces in fractures	Produce bone matrix	Periosteum Endosteum Bone marrow ? Others	Preosteoblast ? Bone-lining cells	Osteocyte
Osteocyte	Stellate cells with thin cytoplasmic processes	Embedded in lacunae	Exact function unknown Potential functions: Mechanosensory Mineral homeostasis Bone resorption	Osteoblasts that become embedded in osteoid	Osteoblasts	Terminally differentiated cell
Osteoclast	Large, multinuclear cells with ruffled border Stain positive for tartrate-resistant acid phosphatase	Endosteal and periosteal surfaces of bone in areas of active remodeling On fractured bone surfaces	Bone resorption	Bone marrow Spleen ? Lung, peritoneum, peripheral blood	Hematopoietic stem cell	None

Osteoblasts

Histology and function

Osteoblasts are derived from pluripotential MSCs that have the capacity to differentiate into several connective tissue cell types.[15] Within the appropriate osteogenic environment, MSCs first differentiate into osteoprogenitor cells and become committed to an osteoblastic lineage. Though they may continue to proliferate, osteoprogenitor cells eventually become preosteoblasts, prior to their maturation into osteoblasts. Osteoprogenitor cells are seemingly ubiquitous in bone, located within Volkmann's and haversian canals, the cambium layer of periosteum, the endosteum, and within the perivascular tissue adjacent to bone.[16]

Osteoblasts are plump, basophilic cuboidal or columnar cells located on the external surfaces of bone at sites of active bone formation during bone development and fracture repair. Ultrastructurally, osteoblasts have a vast endoplasmic reticulum capable of abundant collagen production. Osteoblasts also contain many mitochondria and a large Golgi apparatus, both necessary to package and secrete large amounts of procollagen. Osteoblasts are chiefly responsible for the production of the organic component bone matrix. They also play a role in the mineralization of osteoid by aiding the process of hydroxyapatite deposition and also by the liberation of matrix vesicles.[16–18] Osteoblasts may eventually surround themselves with bony matrix, at which time that may terminally differentiate into osteocytes.

The phenotypic characteristics of an osteoblast depend upon its stage in maturation. As an osteoprogenitor cell matures into a preosteoblast, it will begin to express enzymes and markers characteristic of the osteoblastic lineage. For example, preosteoblasts, which are typically located near but not at bone-forming surfaces, express low levels of alkaline phosphatase (ALP), a well-described marker of early osteogenesis.[4,19,20] Preosteoblasts also produce bone matrix proteins, though not to the extent of mature osteoblasts.

As osteoblasts mature, they begin to take their characteristic basophilic appearance, stain strongly for ALP, and lose the ability to proliferate. In addition to osteoid, osteoblasts secrete numerous noncollagenous proteins, including bone sialoprotein (BSP), osteonectin, osteopontin, and osteocalcin. Osteoblasts also secrete colony-stimulating factors, which play an important role in myelopoiesis.[16,21]

Mature osteoblasts express receptors for hormones that have important roles in both bone metabolism and mineral homeostasis, including parathyroid hormone receptor (PTH-R) and 1,25-dihydroxyvitamin D receptor (1,25-$(OH)_2D_3$-R). Mature osteoblasts also secrete a number of cytokines with many pleiotropic functions, including transforming growth factor-beta (TGF-β), bone morphogenetic proteins (BMPs), insulin-like growth factors (IGFs), and platelet-derived growth factors (PDGFs). Eventually, most osteoblasts undergo apoptosis or become bone-lining cells; nearly 20%, however, differentiate to osteocytes (see below).[22]

Regulation of osteoblast differentiation

Major signaling pathways

Under the control of multiple signaling pathways, preosteoblasts differentiate into mature osteoblasts. The Wnt pathway,[23–26] the TGF-β/BMP superfamily[19,27–29] (see below), notch signaling,[30–32] hedgehog proteins,[33–36] and fibroblast growth factors[37–40] (FGFs: see below) have all been implicated in the molecular signaling of osteogenesis. Although the exact mechanisms of osteogenesis are complex and only partially elucidated, advances have been made regarding the initiation and molecular control of this process. Wnt/β-catenin signaling has been shown to control the differentiation of both osteoblasts and osteoclasts, which may be important in postnatal bone acquisition.[41] Wnt/β-catenin signaling is also important during skeletogenesis in the fetus, and is considered to be partially responsible for both osteoblast and chondrocyte differentiation.[42,43] Notch signaling is a highly conserved signaling system involving cell–cell communication. In addition to cell fate division and homeostatic maintenance, the notch pathway is believed to be important in osteogenesis because of notch1–BMP-2 interactions that promote osteogenic differentiation.[44] Additionally, Engin *et al.*[45] showed with osteoblast-specific gain of Notch function studies that Notch not only stimulates terminal osteoblast differentiation, but that it also plays a role in the proliferation of immature osteoblasts. In addition, loss of notch signaling is associated with the expression of an osteoporotic phenotype.[45]

Hedgehog signaling plays a role in many embryonic processes and also is involved with the maintenance of stem cells in adults. There are three mammalian Hedgehog orthologs: Desert, Sonic, and Indian. Sonic Hedgehog and Indian Hedgehog both have important roles in osteogenesis.[33,34,46–49] Specifically, Indian Hedgehog is critical for endochondral bone formation,[50] whereas Sonic Hedgehog appears to be important for skeletal patterning.[51]

Transcriptional regulation

In addition to numerous signaling pathways, many transcription factors play a significant role in osteogenesis. Runt-related transcription factor 2/core-binding factor alpha 1 (Runx2/cbfα-1) and osterix have many important effects on osteoblast differentiation.[52–57] Runx2 is the mammalian homologue of the *Drosophila* transcription factor Runt and is believed to be evolutionarily conserved in humans to serve a critical role throughout the many steps of osteoblastogenesis, including osteoblast induction, proliferation, and maturation. Homozygous deletions of the Runx2 gene are uniformly lethal in mice due to a complete lack of mineralized bone matrix.[53] Runx2 haploinsufficiency causes cleidocranial dysplasia, an autosomal-dominant disease in humans characterized by hypoplastic clavicles, dental deformities, shortened stature, brachycephaly, hypertelorism, and other skeletal defects.[58] While the exact mechanisms that control the regulation of Runx2 have not been fully decoded, studies have shown that various histone acetyltransferases are important Runx2 cofactors.[59,60] Additionally, microRNAs appear to regulate Runx2 protein expression.[61] MicroRNAs play critical roles in stem cell function,[62,63] and thus may have important clinical implications for diseases due to dysfunctional MSC/Runx2 interactions. Many other regulators also play an important role in Runx2 function[64–70]; however, their exact roles are currently under study.

The zinc finger-containing protein osterix (Osx) is also a key transcription factor to bone formation.[55,71] Osx-null mice form neither cortical nor cancellous bone. Unlike Runx2-null mice, however, osx-null mice still produce normal cartilage.[72] As a result of the findings that Osx expression is absent in Runx2 knock out mice, whereas Runx2 expression is normal in Osx-null mice, the Osx gene is thought to be downstream to Runx2.[55] Nishio *et al.*[73] confirmed this using overexpression experiments to show that Runx2 transactivates the Osx gene promoter significantly, indicating that there is a Runx2-binding element within the promoter region.

The signaling pathways and transcription factors responsible for osteoblastogenesis are exquisitely detailed and only a brief review has been described. For the reader interested in further study, excellent review articles have been published.[74,75]

Osteocytes
Histology and function

Osteocytes are terminally differentiated cells of the osteoblast lineage and comprise 90–95% of all bone cells. Despite being the most abundant cell in bone, osteocytes are the least well characterized. Osteocytes are located within lacunae. Multiple cytoplasmic processes radiate from osteocyte somas and travel through canaliculi between lacunae. Gap junction connections between adjacent cytoplasmic processes enable osteocytes to communicate with one another. Osteocytes communicate with osteoblasts by way of this canalicular network as well. Processes also must extend to the haversian canals so that osteocytes can rid themselves of waste products and receive nutrients necessary for survival. Compared with osteoblasts, osteocytes have qualitatively similar cellular organelles, but the organelles are smaller in both size and number.[76]

Osteocyte functions

Bone is a dynamic substance that maintains its viability by constantly adapting to the environment in which it lives. Victim to mechanical loading and various traumas, bone must have a way to recognize such stressors. It is believed that osteocytes are mechanosensory cells that translate (via mechanotransduction) physical stress into chemical and/or electrical signals that stimulate bone remodeling.[77–79] This hypothesis has been derived from various lines of evidence. Anatomically, osteocytes form a syncytium with surrounding cells via their cellular processes. These connections may provide communication between mechanical stimuli and effector cells (osteoblasts and osteoclasts). Recent evidence has shown that osteocyte processes also attach to ECM proteins and may mediate mechanotransduction by the amplification of shear stress experienced at the ECM.[80] In addition, mechanical loading alters osteocyte gene expression. Osteocytes rapidly produce increased levels of *c-fos*,

IGF-1, prostaglandin (PG), and nitrous oxide (NO) when mechanically stimulated.[81-83] These and many other molecules (see below) have numerous effects on bone turnover. Molecular studies have implicated the activation of the Wnt/β-catenin pathway in response to loading.[84,85] The osteocytic Wnt/β-catenin pathway appears to be triggered by crosstalk with various signaling pathways when the osteocyte senses a load strain, thereby decreasing negative regulators of the Wnt/β-catenin pathway,[82] an important regulator of bone mass. Finally, Tatsumi *et al.*[86] have shown that targeted ablation of osteocytes induces osteoporosis with defective mechanotransduction.

One potential function of the osteocyte, termed periosteocytic osteolysis, has remained elusive. Osteocytes may fulfill an osteoclast-like activity by resorbing varying amounts of calcified bone matrix surrounding their lacunae. Evidence for periosteocytic osteolysis comes from studies that have shown a larger than expected size of lacunae in conditions characterized by increased bone resorption.[87-89] However, criticisms for these studies were raised regarding the methodology used to determine the size of lacunae. More recently, the administration of parathyroid and thyroid hormone has been shown to induce microradiographic enlargement of lacunae, thought to be the result of the hormones' actions on osteocytes.[90,91]

Osteoclasts

Histology and function

Osteoclasts are multinucleated cells primarily responsible for bone resorption, a process necessary for bone growth, tooth eruption, fracture repair, and calcium homeostasis. Osteoclasts typically have between three and 25 nuclei per cell and are approximately 40 μm in diameter. Histologically, osteoclast cytoplasm has a characteristic homogeneous, "foamy" appearance due to a high concentration of vesicles and vacuoles. Osteoclasts are derived from hematopoietic progenitor cells and are related to the monocyte/macrophage lineage. Osteoclasts are found on the endosteal and periosteal surfaces of bone in areas of active remodeling.

Bone resorption is a complex process by which crystalline hydroxyapatite is dissolved and organic bone matrix is degraded. *In vitro* bone resorption models using primary osteoclast isolates provided the basis for the resorption cycle.[92,93] The cycle is a complex series of actions which includes osteoclast migration to the resorption site and attachment to bone, membrane polarization, dissolution of hydroxyapatite followed by degradation of organic bone matrix, removal of degradation products, and osteoclast inactivation or apoptosis.[94] Clinically, bone resorption is an extremely important process, as evidenced by pathologic conditions characterized by dysfunctional resorption. For example, increased osteoclastic function leads to excess bone resorption, thereby causing osteoporosis. In contrast, osteoclast underactivity decreases bone resorption, which causes osteopetrosis.

Bone resorption is key for both bone remodeling at sites of injury and also as a mechanism of calcium homeostasis. Osteoclasts are stimulated to resorb bone by growth factors and cytokines secreted by local osteoblasts.[95] Once osteoclasts localize to the area in need of resorption they form a tight seal that separates the area of bone to be resorbed from the extracellular environment. Evidence has pointed to integrins (in particular integrin $\alpha v \beta_3$) and cadherins as playing a prominent role in the attachment of this sealing zone.[96-98] Myosin and actin-binding proteins are also important for such attachments.[99,100] After sealing zone attachments are completed, osteocytes polarize such that the area adjacent to the resorbing bone surface becomes ruffled. The ruffled border is a specialized membrane domain formed by the fusion of intracellular acidic vesicles and functions as the osteocyte's resorbing organelle.[101,102] Finger-like projections from the ruffled border increase the effective surface area of resorption. Before proteolytic cleavage of the organic matrix occurs, osteoclasts dissolve hydroxyapatite crystals by targeted secretion of hydrochloric acid through the ruffled border toward the resorption pit (Howship's lacuna).[94] After the dissolution of inorganic matter, many proteolytic enzymes, including matrix metalloproteinase-9 and cathepsin K, are secreted into the resorption lacuna to degrade the organic components of bones.[103,104] Both phases of bone are subsequently removed from the resorption lacuna via transcytosis through the ruffled border and sent to the secretory domain of the osteoclast, which then expels these degradation products into the extracellular space outside the osteoclast.[105-107] The osteocytic marker tartrate-resistant acid protease (TRAP) has been localized to transcytotic vesicles of resorbing osteoclasts, and is believed to generate reactive oxygen species that degrade matrix degradation products within these vesicles.[108]

Osteoclast differentiation

The mechanisms surrounding osteoclast differentiation are complex and have been the subject of intense study. Depending on local stimuli, hematopoietic stem cells may differentiate into osteoclasts, macrophages, or dendritic cells. Macrophage colony-stimulating factor (M-CSF) and receptor activator for nuclear factor κ B (RANK) and RANK ligand (RANKL) are early mediators that signal osteoclastogenesis.[109–114] In murine studies, M-CSF is functionally lacking in *op/op* mice, which express an osteopetrotic phenotype.[115,116] In addition, in order for osteoclastogenesis to commence, RANKL (found on the cellular membrane of osteoblasts) must interact with RANK, a receptor found on osteoclast precursors.[117–119] RANK–RANKL interaction must occur in order for osteoclast precursor cells to begin expressing phenotypic markers (e.g., TRAP) that characterize osteoclasts. Similar to *op/op* mice with functionally absent M-CSF, RANK and RANKL knockout mice also express an osteopetrotic phenotype.[112,114,120]

Osteoprotegerin (OPG), a TNF-related soluble protein secreted by osteoblasts, is also an important regulator of osteoclastogenesis. OPG has effects on bone density and bone mass[117,121] by acting as a decoy receptor for RANK, thereby blocking RANK–RANKL interaction. Transgenic mice that overexpress OPG suffer from an osteopetrotic phenotype,[121] while OPG knockout mice display an osteoporotic phenotype.[122,123]

The RANK molecule lacks enzymatic activity, and thus must recruit adaptor proteins when stimulated by RANKL to promote differentiation.[124–126] TNF receptor-associated factor (TRAF) family members appear to be important adaptor proteins, with TRAF6 serving the most critical role.[127–129] TRAF6 knockout mice develop severe osteopetrosis as a result of either the dysfunction or total absence of osteoclasts.[130,131] Moreover, TRAF6 activates NF-κB, another essential modulator of osteoclast differentiation.[132,133] NF-κB enters the nucleus of osteoclasts stimulated with RANKL, and regulates transcription of target genes critical for osteoclastogenesis.[134]

Extracellular matrix

The extracellular matrix (ECM) is a complex scaffolding from which bone derives much of its strength and characteristic architecture. Most molecules found within the ECM are produced by osteoblasts. The ECM contains nearly 30 types of collagen, as well as noncollagenous phospho- and glycoproteins. Type I collagen is the predominant form found within the ECM, making up approximately 90% of bone matrix. The significance of type I collagen is highlighted by patients with osteogenesis imperfecta (OI), a disease characterized by bone fragility and repeated fracture. OI often occurs in patients with pro-α1 or pro-α2-chain gene mutations, or from a mutation in one of the enzymes responsible for posttranslational hydroxylation of collagen.[135] In addition, bone mineralization takes place within the ECM. Bone mineralization is a well-orchestrated process during which hydroxyapatite crystals are laid down within the organic matrix of bone and calcify proteins that are secreted by osteoblasts.

In addition to type I collagen, many noncollagenous proteins are found within the ECM *(Table 21.2)*. Osteopontin is a ubiquitous phosphoprotein that exists in multiple forms. It has been localized to most cells within bone, including osteoblasts, osteocytes, osteoclasts, and bone precursor cells.[136–138] Osteopontin plays a role in the nucleation of hydroxyapatite crystals during matrix mineralization and also in osteoclast adhesion during bone remodeling.[139–144]

Osteonectin is a glycoprotein that binds to calcium and type I collagen and also initiates and regulates bone mineralization.[145,146] BSP is another important noncollagenous protein that, in contrast to osteopontin and osteonectin (both of which are expressed by many tissues throughout the body), is mainly expressed by cells within the skeleton.[147] BSP is an acidic phosphoprotein that binds to collagen and also promotes hydroxyapatite nucleation.[148] BSP-null mice express a phenotype characterized by small and undermineralized bones.[149]

Osteocalcin (bone Gla protein) is a vitamin K-dependent γ-carboxyglutamic acid-containing protein, similar to factors II, VII, IX, and X of the coagulation cascade. The most abundant noncollagenous protein in bone, osteocalcin is secreted by osteoblasts and odontoblasts and is an important marker of increased bone turnover.[150] Osteocalcin plays a role in bone

Table 21.2 Extracellular matrix molecules in bone

Molecule	Protein structure	Cell source	Present in nonosseous tissues	Function	Phenotype of knockout animals or deficiency in humans
Collagen type I	Trilaminar protein consisting of 2 α1 chains and 1 α2 chain	Many Mature and immature osteoblasts in bone	Yes	Primary scaffold of bone 90% of matrix	Osteogenesis imperfecta in humans
Alkaline phosphatase	Metalloenzyme	Mature and immature osteoblasts Different isoforms expressed by cardiac and hepatic cells	Yes	Enzyme Regulator of extracellular matrix mineralization Regulator of cellular migration, adhesion, and differentiation	Hypophosphatemia and defects in skeletal mineralization in knockout mice
Osteopontin	Phosphorylated glycoprotein	Osteoblasts/ osteoclasts Tumor cells (e.g., breast)	Yes	Osteoclast activation and extracellular matrix mineralization Anchor osteoclasts to mineralized matrix	Alterations in extracellular matrix remodeling in knockout mice
Osteonectin	Glycoprotein	Osteoblasts Endothelial cells, megakaryocytes	Yes	Binds calcium and collagen type I Regulator of mineralization	Unknown
Bone sialoprotein	Phosphorylated glycoprotein	Almost exclusively produced by skeletal cells (osteoblasts, osteocytes, hypertrophic chondrocytes)	No	Exact function unknown Regulator of cellular adhesion	Unknown
Osteocalcin	Vitamin K-dependent γ-carboxyglutamic acid-containing protein	Osteoblasts Odontoblasts Hypertrophic chondrocytes	No	Regulator of bone turnover Regulator if osteoclast migration Binds hydroxyapatite	Osteopetrosis in knockout mice
Biglycan	Proteoglycan	Mature and immature osteoblasts Nonosseous cells	Yes	Exact function unknown Regulates function apatite formation	Osteoporosis and small, thin, short limbs in knockout mice

turnover,[151,152] osteoclast differentiation,[153] and energy metabolism.[154,155]

Osteoblasts also produce proteoglycans, the most abundant of which is biglycan (BGN). BGN, a leucine-rich noncollagenous protein, is believed to play a role in the mineralization of bone given that *bgn*-deficient mice express an osteoporotic phenotype.[156] However, BGN seems to play an important role outside the skeleton as well, as *bgn*-knockout mice manifest spontaneous aortic rupture and dissection,[157] dental and muscular abnormalities, thinning of skin, and osteoarthritis.[158]

A variety of enzymes produced by bone cells also function within the ECM. The most prominent is ALP.

Like osteocalcin, ALP is often used as a marker of bone turnover.[159] While the exact function of ALP is unknown, it is believed to be important for bone mineralization, during which it regulates apatite formation.

Principles of bone homeostasis and turnover

Unique to bone is its ability to undergo regeneration rather than repair with scar formation, as is typified by most other tissues within the body. As described previously, bone is subject to constant remodeling, a process mediated by osteoclasts and osteoblasts. Physiologically, bone homeostasis is maintained by the counterbalancing of bone resorption with formation, and vice versa. When one of these two processes becomes dysfunctional, patients often manifest a distinct pathology. Excessive bone resorption resulting in an excessive loss of bone is the fundamental pathogenesis underlying osteoporosis.[160] Conversely, decreased bone resorption due to decreased osteoclast activity leads to an osteopetrotic phenotype.[161] Decreased bone resorption due to increased osteoblast activity, however, will produce an osteosclerotic phenotype.

The structure of bone is a function of its material composition as well as the genetic blueprint of an individual. In addition, various loads to which bone is subjected define its structure. This process of functional adaptation mediates repair of damaged bone and also facilitates prevention of damage before it may occur. Bone exhibiting suppressed remodeling and resorption suffers increased microdamage and fracture accumulation.[162,163] It has been demonstrated that sites of microcracks are subsequently associated with new bone remodeling more often than expected by chance,[164–166] which has led to the belief that bone remodeling and repair are often targeted to specific locations.[167]

Wolff's law and mechanotransduction

Wolff (1892) derived a mathematical formula to describe how changes in the form and function of bone could lead to a change in its internal architecture and external structure.[168] Wolff believed that, during the functional adaptation of bone to new loads that occur during one's life (e.g., as a result of trauma), the trabeculae within bone would reorient to align with the new principal stress trajectories of these environmental loads. While various authors have criticized Wolff's beliefs because he did not take into account that bones are subject to dynamic applied loads,[169] the overarching importance of his contributions to our understanding of bone adaptation cannot be denied.

Since Wolff's time, ongoing research has examined the initial events that stimulate bone adaptation. It is believed that the stimulus for bone remodeling is strain (the physical deformation of bone tissue).[170] Osteocytes, the mediators of mechanotransduction,[171] respond molecularly to mechanical loads. Osteocytes undergo direct deformation by bending and also are deformed by the electrical potential induced by the flow of surrounding interstitial fluid.[172,173] In addition, osteocytes are subjected to shear stress by the physical flow of interstitial fluid around their cellular membranes.[174–178]

When strained, osteocytes convert the mechanical stimulus into chemical or electrical activity in a process thought to require various signaling molecules, including NO and PGs.[171] Interestingly, NO synthase, a calcium/calmodulin-dependent enzyme, becomes activated under conditions of increased intracellular calcium; intracellular calcium concentrations appear to increase in response to fluid flow.[179,180] Not surprisingly, Klein-Nulend and colleagues[181] demonstrated that a pulsating fluid flow model led to the release of NO from osteocytes. Taken together, these studies indicate that NO may be important in osteocyte mechanotransduction.[182] Additional studies have showed that pulsating fluid flow treatment also stimulates osteocytes to synthesize increased levels of PGE_2 and PGI_2,[183,184] as well as increased levels of cyclooxygenase-2 (COX-2) mRNA.[185] COX-2 production is also stimulated by mechanical loading.[186,187] Thus, COX-2 induction and the production of PGs are thought to be important mediators in the conversion of mechanical shear forces into signals that trigger bone turnover.

Bone regeneration: the role of the stem cell

In the last decade, the field of regenerative medicine has exploded with the discovery of new techniques to isolate cells capable of differentiating into many different tissues. In particular, the MSC (*Fig. 21.3)* has considerable therapeutic potential for fracture repair and other bone pathologies. For concordance, Dominici and colleagues[188] have proposed that MSCs meet the following criteria: (1) isolated MSCs must adhere to plastic in culture; (2) MSCs should express the CD105, CD73, and CD90 surface antigens as well as not express the CD34, CD45, CD14 or CD11B, CD79A or CD19 and human leukocyte antigen-DR (HLA-DR) surface antigens; and (3) MSCs must have the capacity to differentiate into osteoblasts, adipocytes, and chondroblasts. MSCs and MSC-like are derived from bone marrow, but can also be expanded from skeletal muscle,[189] adipose tissue,[190] dental pulp,[191] the circulatory system,[192] synovium,[193]

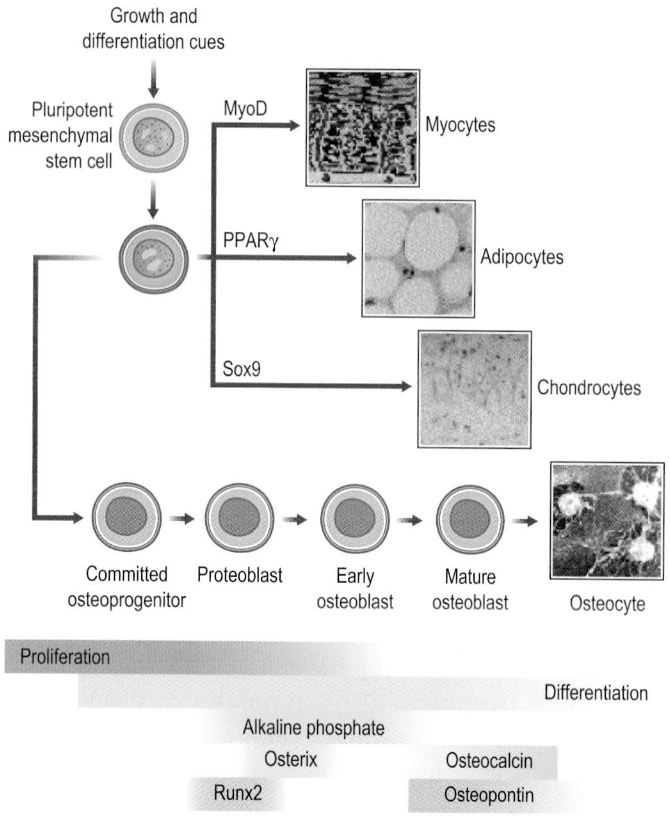

Fig. 21.3 Schematic representation of mesenchymal stem cell (MSC) differentiation pathways. MSCs are pluripotential stem cells that are capable of differentiating into several lineages with distinct growth and differentiation cues. These lineages include osteogenic, chondrogenic, adipogenic, and myogenic lineages. Lineage-specific differentiation is a well-coordinated process that is regulated by master regulators, such as MyoD for myogenesis, peroxisome proliferator-accepted receptor (PPAR)-γ for adipogenesis, Sox9 for chondrogenesis, and Runx2 and Osterix for osteogenesis. Osteogenic differentiation can be staged by measuring alkaline phosphatase (early marker) and osteopontin and osteonectin (late markers). (From Tang N, Song W-X, Luo J, et al. Osteosarcoma development and stem cell differentiation. Clin Orthop Relat Res. 2008;466:2114–2130.)

amniotic fluid,[194] the umbilical cord,[195] and fetal tissues.[196,197]

The capability of MSCs to differentiate into and assist with the restoration and repair of bone has been extensively studied.[198,199] MSCs are also used clinically in patients with various bone disorders.[200] In a clinical trial[200] that examined MSC administration to children with OI, bone mineral density, growth velocity, and ambulation all improved after MSC administration. However, the concentration of MSCs detected in bone, skin, and other tissues was less than 1%. These data and evidence from additional studies[201,202] have led authors to postulate that MSCs may actually secrete soluble factors that alter tissue microenvironment, which may be an important mechanism by which MSCs repair tissue.[203,204]

Molecular mechanisms of bone regeneration

Bone regeneration consists of a complex interplay of molecular processes that promote MSC migration, proliferation, and differentiation. Recently, there has been a great deal of research aimed at the identification of these molecular processes, and advances in our understanding of the molecular mechanisms of bone regeneration have been made. Many have been able to identify important signaling molecules as well as transcriptional regulators of bone regeneration (*Table 21.3*).

Bone morphogenetic protein

In the 1960s, Urist[205] discovered the function of BMP from their work with demineralized bone matrix (DBM). To date, approximately 20 BMP isoforms have been characterized. BMPs are pleiotropic members of the TGF-β superfamily. BMPs, while important for brain and bone formation *in utero*,[206–208] have generated much of their recognition from their osteoinductive properties.

BMPs are synthesized as large precursor molecules that consist of characteristic subsections. A series of seven cysteine residues are located at the carboxyl termini of BMPs, and is important for proper protein folding. BMPs also contain a signal peptide, a prodomain, and a mature peptide.[209] BMPs are thought to be secreted from cells in their active form.

BMPs are natural ligands for type I and type II serine/threonine kinase transmembrane cellular surface receptors. There are three type I and three type II receptors that are capable of binding BMPs.[208] Upon ligand (BMP) binding, a heterotetrameric complex is formed, after which type II receptor kinase domains phosphorylate Gly-Ser domains in the type I receptor kinases. This process activates type I receptors to recruit and phosphorylate intracytoplasmic Smad proteins (Smads 1, 5, and 8). Following Smad phosphorylation, Smad 1, 5, or 8 will bind to Smad 4, and this Smad4-phosphorylated Smad 1, 5, or 8 complex will relocate to the cell nucleus. Transcription factor activation occurs, leading to the transcription of bone morphogenetic target genes.[210]

Table 21.3 Growth factors and fracture repair

Molecule	Ectopic bone formation	Segmental defect healing	Effect on fractures	Combination with other growth factors	Effective in lower vertebrates	Effective in primates	Potential clinical use
BMP	Yes	Endochondral ++++ Membranous ++++	Increase callus volume Increase mechanical strength ? Increase rate of healing	Synergistic with TGF-β	Yes	Yes	Spinal fusion Alveolar bone deficiency Segmental defects Augment bone graft healing Dental implants
TGF-β	No	Endochondral ++ Membranous ++	Increases callus size Increases mechanical strength	Synergistic with BMP Increases FGF-2 expression Increases VEGF expression	Yes	No (limited study)	Role alone unclear
FGFs	No	Endochondral+/− Membranous+/−	Increase callus and bone volume Increase mechanical strength	Increase VEGF expression ? Synergistic TGF-β	Yes	Yes (limited study)	Potential for augmenting angiogenesis in compromised wounds
PDGF	No	Endochondral − Membranous −	Increases callus volume Increases mechanical strength	Increases VEGF Synergistic TGF-β for chemotaxis	Yes	No	Unknown

++++, very active; +/−, minimally active; −, no activity
BMPs, bone morphogenetic proteins; TGF-β, transforming growth factor beta; FGFs, fibroblast growth factors; VEGF, vascular endothelial growth factor; PDGF, platelet-derived growth factor.

Bone morphogenetic protein function

BMP exerts pleiotropic effects throughout the lifespan of an organism. In the early stages of human development, BMP plays a key role in skeletogenesis.[207] Also during this time period, BMP signals epidermal induction,[211] directs the development of neural crest cells,[212] and induces a sympathetic adrenergic phenotype.[213] BMP-2-null mice typically die between 7 and 10 days of gestation due to cardiac defects, even before the formation of bone begins.

BMP is the only signaling molecule capable of singly inducing de novo bone formation. It has been hypothesized that BMP-2, -6, and -9, and to a lesser extent, -4, and -7, various BMP isoforms, have the greatest osteogenic capacity.[19,209] Luu and colleagues[19] infected HEK293, C2C12, and C3H10T1/2 cells with adenoviral vectors containing various BMP isoforms (AdBMP). The authors measured the expression of early (ALP) and late (osteocalcin) osteogenic markers *in vitro*. They also assessed *in vivo* induction of heterotopic ossification by implanting AdBMPs into nude mice and evaluating radiographic and histologic results at 3 and 5 weeks. BMP-2, -4, -6, and -7 were shown to induce increased ALP elevation compared to other BMPs. In addition, BMP-2, -4-, -6, -7, and -9 stimulated increased osteocalcin expression compared to others. The authors also found that BMP-2, -6, -7, and -9 induced the greatest degree of osteogenesis *in vivo*. The authors concluded that BMP-2, -6, and -9 have the greatest osteogenic potential, and that BMP-4, and -7 also have a significant degree of osteogenic potential.

BMP-2 promotes osteoblast differentiation by stimulating Runx2 in a process mediated by Smad proteins.[214] In addition, BMP-2 affects osteoblast differentiation via activation of the β-catenin signaling pathway.[215] Interestingly, endogenous activation of β-catenin induces ALP mRNA expression; however, BMP-2 must be present for β-catenin signaling to induce osteocalcin expression as well.[216] Thus, β-catenin-dependent differentiation processes likely require BMP-2 to promote the later stages of osteoblast differentiation. Recently, it has been demonstrated that BMP-2-mediated osteoblast differentiation is also dependent upon Akt2 selective signaling.[217] IGFs are important for osteoblast differentiation and normal bone growth,[218–221] and Akt2 is a key molecule within the insulin signaling pathway. Mukherjee et al.[217] showed that, although BMP-2 signaling is normal, osteoblast differentiation does not occur in Akt2-knockout mice. Delivery of Runx2 to Akt2-deficient mice restores osteoblast differentiation; thus, Akt likely serves a specific role in osteoblast differentiation through its regulation of Runx2 gene expression.

Furthermore, BMP-2 appears to improve bone healing in large osseous defects. Many studies have evaluated recombinant human BMP-2 (rhBMP-2) in *in vivo* animal models. In rabbits, rats, dogs, and nonhuman primates, rhBMP-2 has been shown to augment bone growth successfully and also close critical-sized osseous defects.[222–226] Both retrospective and prospective studies have assessed the efficacy of rhBMP-2 in humans as well.[227–236] Slosar *et al.*[237] demonstrated that anterior lumbar allografts filled with rhBMP-2 experienced higher fusion rates than lumbar allografts without rhBMP-2 in patients who underwent lumbar fusion. The authors demonstrated that at 6 months and at 2 years, allografts with rhBMP-2 shortened the timeframe for expected improvement, and also improved patients' Oswestry Disability Index scores. Thus, it has been concluded allografts with rhBMP-2 can offer reliable and clinically significant benefits.

At the present time, rhBMP-2 (INFUSE, Medtronic, Inc.) is one of only two rhBMPs that are approved by the Food and Drug Administration (FDA) for human application. The other is rhBMP-7 (rhOP-1). As described, rhBMP-2 is often used in spinal fusion, as well as orthopedic trauma and dental procedures. rhBMP-7 has shown clinical benefits in spinal fusion and in tibia repair.[238,239] Interestingly, although BMP-2 may be more osteoinductive than BMP-7 based on in vitro analyses,[29] there has been relatively little *in vivo* data comparing the two. Barr and colleagues[240] have found that rhBMP-7 promotes similar bone quality but greater bone volume induction than rhBMP-2 in murine muscle pouch assays analyzed by microscopic computed tomography and histology. However, other studies have found different results.[28,241] Conflicting results among these studies may be due to differences in experimental design.

Transforming growth factor-β

TGF-β also has protean effects on cellular processes within the human body. TGF-β has been implicated in cell cycle regulation, angiogenesis, wound healing, and skeletogenesis. TGF-β also appears to have significant roles in human disease.[242] There are three distinct human TGF-β isoforms (TGF-β1, -β2, and-β3). Though they exhibit differences, each isoform shares similar functions with one another, including roles pertaining to the regulation osteogenesis and osseous repair.

TGF-β, like BMP, contains a cluster of conserved cysteine residues.[243] In addition, each isoform is produced as a precursor molecule consisting of TGF-β and a propeptide region. In contrast to BMPs, however, TGF-β is secreted as an inactive molecule and stored in its latent form within the ECM. TGF-β becomes active after the noncovalent disulfide bond linking TGF-β and its propeptide region is broken.

TGF-β signal transduction has been the subject of much study.[243–245] There are four TGF-β receptors identified to date: types I, II, and III, and endoglin. TGF-β-initiated signaling, like BMP-mediated signaling, uses Smad protein intermediates. Active TGF-β binds to either type III or type II receptors, both of which promote the phosphorylation of type I receptors. Phosphorylation of Smad2 or Smad3 follows, which in turn leads to the binding of Smad4 to the phosphorylated Smad2 or Smad3 proteins. This complex translocates to the cellular nucleus, where transcription factors activate specific target gene transcription, thereby mediating the effects of TGF-β at the cellular level.

Evidence that TGF-β may play a role in osteogenesis has come from experiments demonstrating that TGF-β stimulates the production of collagen and osteopontin, as well as studies demonstrating that TGF-β is produced by osteoblasts.[246–250] In addition, many *in vivo* studies have demonstrated an osteoinductive effect of TGF-β.[251–253] TGF-β1, in particular, has been the subject of a considerable body of literature with respect to its osteogenic potential, in part because it is the dominant TGF-β isoform expressed by bone cells.[254] *In vitro* analyses have demonstrated that TGF-β1, by recruiting and stimulating the proliferation of osteoblast progenitors, increases bone formation.[255] Interestingly, TGF-β1 seems to have a differential effect on osteoblast differentiation. Early phases of differentiation appear to be promoted by TGF-β1, while later phases are blocked.[256]

In addition, TGF-β1 modulates the processes of osteoclastogenesis and bone resorption. At high TGF-β1 concentrations (0.1–10 ng/mL), osteoclastogenesis appears to be downregulated.[255] TGF-β1 binds to its receptor on osteoblasts and augments the expression of OPG while also decreasing RANKL expression. A lower RANKL:OPG ratio results in maximal RANKL occupation by OPG, thus decreasing maturation of osteoclasts. TGF-β1 appears to serve a bifunctional role, however, as low concentrations are associated with high levels of both RANKL and RANK, and subsequent osteoclastogenesis.

TGF-β1 may also be important for the coupling of bone resorption and formation, as is found at bone resorption sites. Along these lines, Tang and colleagues[257] injected green fluorescent protein (GFP)-labeled osteogenic bone marrow stromal cells (BMSCs) into the femur cavity of *Tgfb1*[+/+] *and Tgfb1*[−/−] immunodeficient mice. Using anti-GFP antibodies, injected BMSCs were detected at both 1 and 4 weeks. After 1 week, BMSCs were localized to the bone surfaces in *Tgfb1*[+/+] mice; BMSCs were widely dispersed in the bone marrow (i.e., not at bone surfaces) of *Tgfb1*[−/−] mice. After 4 weeks, BMSCs were embedded in trabecular bone in *Tgfb1*[+/+]mice but not in *Tgfb1*[−/−] mice. The authors concluded that TGF-β1 plays an essential role in the coupling of bone resorption to bone formation by their induction of osteogenic BMSCs to sites of resorption.

In addition, TGF-β expression is elevated during fracture repair.[258] Given its apparent role in many physiologic bone processes, TGF-β has been considered for exogenous use to augment bone growth and repair. Studies support that TGF-β isoforms, both alone and in conjunction with other cytokines, can significantly induce the formation of endochondral bone at extracranial sites in rapid fashion.[259,260] However, studies observing the effects of TGF-β on calvarial defects revealed little osteoinductive potential.[261,262]

Fibroblast growth factor

FGF consists of a family of structurally related cytokines that mediate processes such as cellular proliferation, migration, and differentiation, as well as mitogenesis, angiogenesis, embryonic development, and wound healing. There are at least 23 known members of the FGF family, all possessing a characteristically high affinity for heparin. Most FGF isoforms share a similar internal core region that has important FGF receptor (FGFR)-binding properties.[263] Mutations in FGFs or FGFRs are thought to play an important role in the development of various skeletal dysplasias, including achondroplasia and craniosynostosis.[38,264,265]

There are four known FGFRs (FGFR-1, -2, -3, -4). Following FGF ligand binding, receptor dimerization occurs, which promotes the transphosphorylation of each receptor monomer by an intrinsic tyrosine kinase domain. Phosphorylated tyrosine residues on FGFRs become docking sites for adaptor proteins necessary for downstream signaling.[266] Human gene studies have identified many associations between diseases of bone and the skeleton and FGFRs. Specifically, Pfeiffer syndrome has been linked to FGFR1 gene mutations,[267] Crouzon syndrome to FGFR2 gene mutations,[268] and achondroplasia to FGFR3 gene mutations.[269]

FGF has been implicated in a variety of osteogenic mechanisms. FGF-2, in particular, is thought to play an important role in endochondral bone growth. Coffin *et al.*[270] have found that increased concentrations of FGF-2 are found at the epiphyseal growth plate, specifically within the proliferation and hypertrophic zones. FGF-2 also appears to accelerate fracture repair as well as closure of critical-sized defects in endochondral bone.[271] In addition, FGF-2 appears to affect cell function during intramembranous bone growth.[265] There appears to be a differential effect of FGF-2 treatment with respect to its method of delivery. Although continuous FGF-2 treatment stimulates osteoblast proliferation, it decreases levels of differentiation markers (e.g., ALP) and augments osteoclast formation, thus resulting in net bone resorption. Oppositely, intermittent FGF-2 treatment enhances both *in vitro* and *in vivo* bone formation.

The effects of FGF-2 in combination with other growth factors on osteoblast differentiation have also been studied. Maegawa and colleagues[272] examined MSCs deposited in osteogenic media supplemented with BMP-2, FGF-2, or both. MSCs supplemented by both FGF-2 and BMP-2 concurrently expressed the highest levels of ALP, osteocalcin mRNA, and bone matrix formation. In addition, Sabbieti *et al.*[273] investigated whether FGF-2 modulates the anabolic response of bone to PTH. Primary calvarial osteoblasts were isolated from

FGF-2$^{+/+}$ (wild type) and FGF-2$^{-/-}$ mice. By immunocytochemistry, FGF-2-null osteoblasts expressed decreased Runx2 protein synthesis as well as significantly less Runx2 expression within perinuclear and nuclear spaces than wild-type variants when exposed to PTH. Given the importance of Runx2 on osteogenesis (see earlier), it was concluded that FGF-2 expression is required for PTH to promote an anabolic response by bone.

Platelet-derived growth factor

PDGF plays an important role in a number of biological processes, including embryological development, inflammatory reactions, angiogenesis, organogenesis, and wound healing. Four unique isoforms of PDGF have been characterized (PDGF-A, -B, -C, -D), which are inactive in their monomeric forms, and thus must dimerize to become active. Five dimeric PDGF compounds have been indentified (PDGF-AA, -BB, -CC, -DD, and -AB).[274] All PDGF molecules share a highly conserved PDGF/vascular endothelial growth factor (VEGF) homology domain, a motif that is also found in VEGF.[275] PDGFs interact with two receptor tyrosine kinases, termed PDGF receptor-α (PDGFR-α) and PDGFR-β. PDGFRs as well must dimerize in order to activate.[276] Receptor dimerization results in autophosphorylation at a specific tyrosine residue on a PDGFR, a necessary step for signal transduction to proceed. Although it has been shown in tissue culture-based systems that PDGF can promote similar responses by interacting with PDGFR-α or PDGFR-β, it is thought that these two receptor types in fact mediate distinct events during organism development because of their unique temporospatial expressions *in vivo*.[277]

PDGF is a potent mitogen and chemotactic agent for cells and tissues of mesenchymal origin and is crucial in bone homeostasis and repair. At sites of bone fracture, platelets congregate and release PDGF. PDGF attracts many other cell types important for tissue repair and the formation of granulation tissue. PDGF has also been shown specifically to attract osteogenic cells derived from calvaria, periosteum of long bones, trabecular bone, and BMSCs.[278] In addition, angiogenesis is crucial for bony healing (to be discussed later) and PDGF, in addition to its direct mitogenic effect on osteoblasts, indirectly enhances bone regeneration by stimulating angiogenic factors such as VEGF.[279,280]

PDGF also appears to stimulate bone healing indirectly via interactions with other growth factors. Levi et al.[281] studied the ability of IGF-1, PDGF-A, and a mixture of the two to induce osteogenic differentiation. IGF-1 promoted differentiation of human adipose-derived stromal cells down an osteogenic lineage, whereas PDGF-A did not. IGF-1 and PDGF-A in combination, however, enhanced osteogenesis more than IGF-1 alone. This finding may be the result of enhanced IGF-1 transcription in the presence of PDGF-A. In contrast, PDGF-BB may decrease IGF-2 mRNA expression by osteoblasts.[282]

Clinical studies of the effects of PDGF on osseous repair have been performed mainly within the disciplines of periodontology and orthopedics. For example, a randomized controlled trial was performed assessing the effectiveness and safety of the administration of 300 μg/mL of recombinant human PDGF-BB (rhPDGF-BB) with beta-tricalcium phosphate (β-TCP) for the treatment of advanced periodontal osseous defects.[283] Compared to β-TCP alone, β-TCP plus rhPDGF-BB treatment promoted significantly greater linear bone gain as well as percent defect fill at 6 months. Patients who received rhPDGF-BB were also found to have a significant gain of clinical attachment level compared to patients who did not receive treatment with rhPDGF-BB at 3 months. Moreover, the efficacy of rhPDGF-BB in a β-TCP matrix as a bone graft material was evaluated in a pilot study of 20 adult patients with ankle or hindfoot fusion.[284,285] Patients were randomly assigned to receive either a β-TCP matrix enhanced with rhPDGF-BB or an autologous bone graft. At 12 weeks postsurgery, computed tomography scan results showed that in 7 of 11 (64%) patients who received the β-TCP matrix with rhPDGF-BB, there was greater than 50% osseous bridging across the fusion site. Greater than 50% osseous bridging across the fusion site was found in only 3 of 6 (50%) patients who underwent bone graft with autologous tissue. These preliminary results have paved the way for a larger study of approximately 400 patients for which the results have not yet been published.[278]

Healing of fractures

Bone repair is the physiologic process by which the body facilitates the healing of fractures. In many ways,

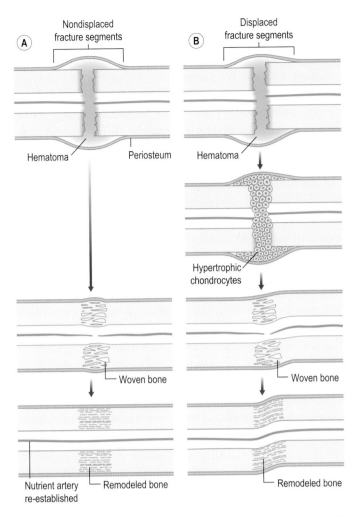

Fig. 21.4 Schematic representation of primary and secondary (callus) bone repair. **(A)** Primary bone repair: nondisplaced bone fragments heal without cartilaginous intermediate. **(B)** Secondary (callus) bone repair: displaced (or unstable) bone segments heal with cartilaginous intermediate. (Modified from Mehrara BJ, McCarthy JG. Repair and grafting of bone. In: Mathes SJ, ed. Plastic surgery. vol. 2. Philadelphia: WB Saunders; 2005:639–718.)

fracture repair recapitulates the events that occur during skeletogenesis. Successful fracture healing is dependent upon many factors. The mechanism of disruption, the fracture pattern, and the method and timing of fixation will all affect the outcome of bone repair. For example, fractures that create more than two fragments of the same bone (comminuted fractures) require swift surgical intervention to heal successfully. In addition, the biologic milieu surrounding a fractured bone may play a role in the fate of the fracture.

Originally distinguished based on their histology, two types of bone repair have been described *(Fig. 21.4)*. Primary bone repair refers to direct cortical healing of

two fracture ends without a cartilaginous intermediate. During secondary (callus) bone repair, a cartilaginous intermediate is formed by mechanisms that occur within the periosteum, soft tissues, and bone marrow. Most fracture repair is by secondary bone healing.

Primary bone repair

Primary bone repair involves the direct deposition of woven bone by osteoblasts to re-establish mechanical continuity between fracture fragments. Similar to intramembranous ossification, the periosteum provides osteoprogenitor cells and undifferentiated MSCs during primary bone repair. In order for primary bone repair to occur, the fracture fragments must be reduced to anatomic position.[286] This is usually accomplished through rigid internal fixation. The interfragmentary strain must also be at a minimum for direct bone healing to occur.[286] In addition, bone healing occurs under axial compression and fails under tension *(Fig. 21.5)*.

During primary bone repair, new bone is synthesized in parallel to the long axis of the bone by osteoprogenitor cells. This process is initiated by the formation of cutting cones at the junction of live and necrotic skeletal segments. A cutting cone is a system of cells, mainly composed of active osteoclasts. It burrows its way through cortical bone across the fractured bone segments, thereby allowing the ingrowth of blood vessels and undifferentiated MSCs. MSCs then differentiate into bone-producing osteoblasts. New haversian systems are created and provide pathways for blood vessel penetration. Initially, bone is laid down in a woven-matrix configuration. Within a few weeks, the woven bone becomes more lamellar-like in its orientation. As the proportion of lamellar bone increases over the course of months, complete fracture repair occurs. The benefits of rigid plate osteosynthesis include increased stability, decreased incidence of non- and malunion, and decreased incidence of infection.[287] Orthopedic surgeons, as well as cardiac surgeons, commonly perform rigid internal fixation.[288]

Secondary (callus) bone repair

Fractures left untreated or those that are treated with external or intramedullary fixation or by sling or cast immobilization heal by secondary bone repair without

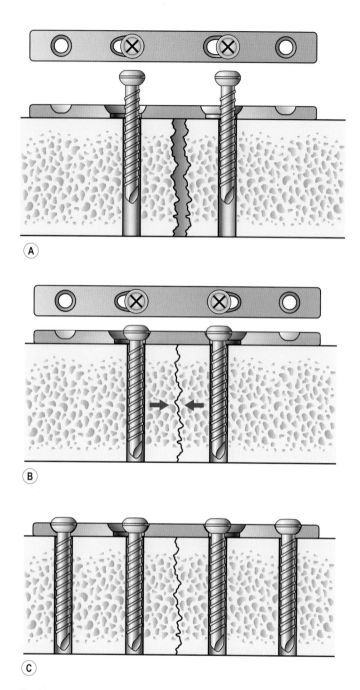

Fig. 21.5 The compression mode of miniplate fixation. **(A)** A four-hole plate. Note that the inner holes are eccentrically shaped so that, as the screws are tightened, the head falls into the wider portion and compresses the bone margins **(B)**. **(C)** Completed view of the skeletal fixation.

inflammatory phase, reparative phase, and remodeling phase *(Fig. 21.6)*. However, at least five distinct stages of healing have been described.[289]

When a bone fractures, the disruption of osseous tissue, surrounding soft tissue, and blood vessels initiate the inflammatory phase of secondary bone repair. This phase peaks at approximately 48 hours and typically lasts 7 days. The inflammatory phase supports immobilization at the fracture site by promoting pain and swelling.[290] A hematoma forms at the site of fracture, which also serves to immobilize the area (via a fibrin network). In addition, the hematoma provides a source of signaling molecules that initiate cellular events necessary for fracture repair.[291] Platelets within the hematoma release PDGF and TGF-β, which promote MSC proliferation and differentiation into an osteoblastic lineage. Moreover, neutrophils, lymphocytes, blood monocytes, and tissue macrophages are recruited to remove necrotic debris and stimulate angiogenesis at the fracture site.

Approximately 3–4 days postfracture – before the inflammatory phase subsides – the reparative phase commences. This phase lasts several weeks to months and is characterized by the development of a fracture callus that will stabilize and unite fracture segments before being replaced by bone. The callus is chiefly composed of cartilage, but also contains woven bone, osteoid, fibrous connective tissue, and blood vessels. MSCs from the surrounding periosteum and marrow migrate to the injured site and mature into many cell types, including osteoblasts, chondrocytes, and fibroblasts, which form the callus.

The fracture callus undergoes both intramembranous and endochondral ossification.[289] Endochondral ossification occurs during the second week of fracture repair, when abundant cartilage overlying the fracture site (formed by chondrogenesis of the callus) undergoes calcification. Blood vessels grow into this calcified cartilaginous callus, bringing with them osteoblast progenitor cells. As the calcified cartilage is resorbed by chondroclasts, osteoblasts begin to lay woven bone. Intramembranous ossification, on the other hand, occurs adjacent to the fracture site.

The remodeling phase of fracture repair is characterized by the replacement of woven bone with lamellar bone and may remain active for several years. Osteoclasts resorb poorly located trabeculae and new bone is formed

rigid fixation. During secondary or callus bone repair, undifferentiated MSCs proliferate and differentiate into cartilage prior to bone formation at the fracture site. This involves a combination of both intramembranous and endochondral ossification. There are the three overlapping phases of secondary bone repair: the

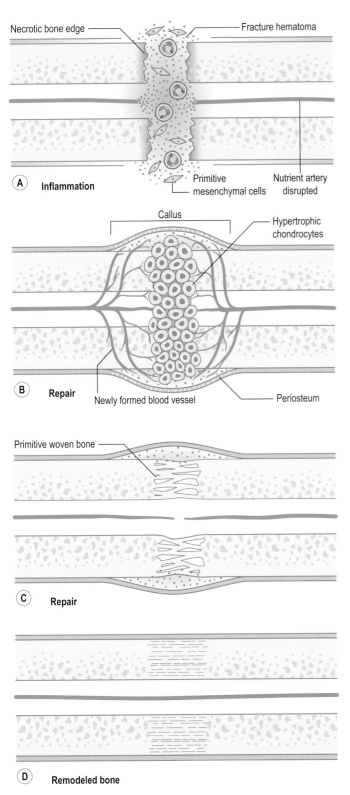

Fig. 21.6 Schematic diagram of callus fracture repair in endochondral bone. **(A)** Early stages of fracture repair characterized by hematoma formation, inflammatory cell migration and differentiation (polymorphonuclear neutrophils), and scattered primitive mesenchymal cells. **(B)** As healing progresses, a callus is formed between the bone edges, and hypertrophic chondrocytes can be seen. In addition, newly formed blood vessels sprout from the nutrient artery and local blood vessels. **(C)** Primitive woven bone has bridged the fractured bone segment. **(D)** Woven bone is remodeled into lamellar bone.

along the lines of stress. In response to varying mechanical loads, bone will gradually modify at the fracture region until optimum regeneration is achieved. During remodeling, pain subsides and the normal activities can be resumed.

Variables influencing bone repair

Blood supply

Blood flow to bone represents approximately 10–20% of total cardiac output. The pattern of vascularization to the majority of the appendicular skeleton is similar in organization to the vascular pattern of a typical long bone.[292] A tubular long bone in the adult human receives blood by three distinct arterial systems that anastomose with one another extensively *(Fig. 21.7)*. The primary supply of blood to the inner two-thirds of the cortex and the medullary cavity is derived from the diaphyseal nutrient artery. As the nutrient artery traverses the cortex, it passes through to the medullary cavity, where it divides into ascending and descending medullary branches. Metaphyseal and epiphyseal arteries represent the second significant source of blood flow. These vessels, which arise from arteries supplying adjacent joints, deliver blood to cancellous bone found at the end of long bones. The third principal blood flow source stems from periosteal arteries, which carry blood to the outer one-third of bone cortex.

As blood moves through bone, from endosteum to periosteum, it flows through sinusoids and arterioles within the haversian system. Exchange vessels (i.e., vessels connecting the arterial and venous systems) within osteons lie in parallel to the axis of the bone. Collecting sinuses and veins with similar names to their arterial counterparts receive deoxygenated blood from exchange vessels. A high intramedullary pressure is likely responsible for the centrifugal flow of blood through bone.[293]

Angiogenesis is critical for bone growth maturation, and repair.[294] Although the mechanisms that regulate angiogenesis during fracture repair have not been fully elucidated, many important angiogenic cytokines have been described *(Table 21.4)*. The prototypical molecule thought to play a pivotal role in angiogenesis within developing and healing bone is VEGF. Molecules described previously (BMP, TGF-β, FGF-2, and PDGF)

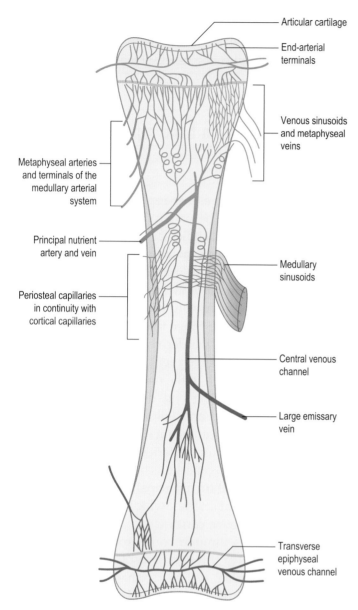

Articular cartilage

End-arterial terminals

Venous sinusoids and metaphyseal veins

Metaphyseal arteries and terminals of the medullary arterial system

Principal nutrient artery and vein

Medullary sinusoids

Periosteal capillaries in continuity with cortical capillaries

Central venous channel

Large emissary vein

Transverse epiphyseal venous channel

Fig. 21.7 The three sources of bloody supply to the long bone. The nutrient artery provides the principal source of blood supply to the marrow cavity and the inner cortex. The diaphyseal periosteal vessels supply the outer cortex of the diaphysis. The metaphyseal epiphyseal periosteal vessels penetrate the cortex of the bone in the adult and anastomose with the nutrient artery, providing adequate supply to the marrow cavity and inner cortex in cases of disruption of the nutrient artery.

have also been implicated in angiogenic processes necessary for osteogenesis. VEGF and FGF-2 are the only two directly acting regulators of angiogenesis; other growth factors serve indirect roles. In addition, the hypoxia-inducible factor-1α (HIF-1α) pathway is crucial to the coupling of angiogenesis with osteogenesis.[295,296] Discoveries associated with this pathway have led

some authors to hypothesize that skeletal angiogenesis and osteogenic–angiogenic interactions are rate-limiting processes in bone growth.[294] Not surprisingly, the HIF-1α pathway is intimately linked to VEGF expression.[297]

A potent regulator of both vasculogenesis and angiogenesis, VEGF mediates many important functions during the embryologic stage of development, and throughout the lifetime of organisms. Deletion of even a single VEGF allele is associated with lethality *in utero* in a mouse model.[298,299] VEGF, which is structurally related to PDGF, is expressed by many different of cell types, typically in especially high concentrations within highly vascularized tissues. VEGF mediates its effects on cells through its interactions with two receptor tyrosine kinases (VEGF-1 and VEGF-2).

The hypothesis that VEGF plays an essential role in skeletogenesis mainly comes from studies examining endochondral bone formation. At the epiphyseal growth plates of long bones, hypertrophic chondrocytes have been shown to express high levels of VEGF.[300,301] In addition, injection of an anti-VEGF monoclonal antibody results in inhibition of vascular invasion of the non-human primate growth plate, thereby hampering longitudinal bone growth.[302] Moreover, mice treated with a VEGF inhibitor manifest significantly decreased bone capillary invasion and trabecular bone formation.[301] Cessation of anti-VEGF treatment is associated with capillary invasion and restoration of bone growth.

The therapeutic utilization of VEGF and other angiogenic cytokines is a subject of great promise in the treatment of patients with both complicated and uncomplicated fractures.

Fracture fixation

Critical to the success of fracture repair in long bones is the extent of movement at the fracture site after fixation.[303] Delayed union and nonunion are both associated with excess motion; however, some movement, known as micromotion, can enhance bone healing. The mechanism by which absolute immobilization hampers fracture repair may be related to increased resorption in a stress-protected environment. In addition, the degree of mechanical strain endured at the site of a fixed fracture has differential effects on chondrogenesis and osteogenesis.[304]

Table 21.4 Growth factors and angiogenesis

Growth factor	Structure	Angiogenesis	Function	Role in fracture healing	Regulation of expression	Receptor
BMP	Single large propeptide molecule Cleavage enables dimerization Member of the TGF-β superfamily Conserved series of seven cysteine residues at carboxyl terminal At least 15 known isoforms	Indirect regulator of angiogenesis	Mitogen and chemoattractant for osteoblasts and mesenchymal cells Apoptosis Patterning	Expressed by mesenchymal cells early in fracture repair Also expressed by osteoblasts and osteoclasts Exogenous BMPs can heal critical-sized defects Ectopic bone formation ? Accelarate fracture repair ? Actions synergistic with TGF-β	Patterning genes and transcription factors (e.g., Cbfa1)	Serine-theronine kinase receptors
TGF-β	Propeptide Cleavage necessary for activation At least three different isoforms	Indirect regulator of angiogenesis	Chemoattractant and mitogen for osteoblast precursors and osteoblasts Inhibits osteoblast differentiation Regulates expression of other growth factors important in angiogenesis and osteogenesis Increases matrix synthesis	Produced for osteoblasts, mesenchymal cells, osteoclasts Increases callus formation and volume Subperiosteal injection promotes both chondrogenesis and membranous ossification Exogenous TGF-β may heal some critical-sized defects	Patterning genes and transcription factors Mechanical strain	Serine-theronine kinase receptors
FGF-2	Heparin-binding glycoprotein At least nine different isoforms	Direct regulator of angiogenesis	Angiogenesis Regulator of bone development and skeletal patterning Can regulate osteoblast differentiation and proliferation (actual effect is dose-dependent)	Increases angiogenesis in fracture site Increases expression during fracture repair Exogenous FGF-2 can increase mechanical strength of fractures ? Accelerates fracture repair or promotes healing of critical-sized defects	Inflammatory cells and acute inflammation Patterning genes and transcription factors	Tyrosine kinase receptors
VEGF	Dimeric glycoprotein	Direct regulator of angiogenesis	Increases vascular permeability Increases vascular sprouting Increases endothelial cell migration, proliferation adhesion	Increased expression during fracture repair Expressed by osteoblasts, osteoclasts, and mesenchymal cells Increases blood vessels in growth during fracture repair	Microenvironment (e.g., pH, hypoxia, lactic acid concentration) Growth factors (e.g., TGF-β, FGF, BMP, IGF), inflammatory cytokines (e.g., PGE_2)	Tyrosine kinase receptors

Table 21.4 Continued

Growth factor	Structure	Angiogenesis	Function	Role in fracture healing	Regulation of expression	Receptor
PDGF	Dimeric, disulfide-bonded polypeptide chain α and β subunits determine isoform (AA, AB)	Indirect regulator of angiogenesis	Promotes chemotaxis of osteoblasts and inflammatory mediators Decreases cellular differentiation Increases collagen synthesis Increases collagen degradation and turnover May promote osteoblast proliferation	Released by degranulating platelets and acts to increase osteoblast chemotaxis, and possibly proliferation Expressed by osteoblasts, macrophages, and mature/immature chondrocytes during fracture repair Promotes synthesis of angiogenic molecules (e.g., VEGF) Promotes matrix deposition and turnover	Inflammation and injury Mechanical strain TGF-β (decreased expression)	Tyrosine kinase receptors

BMP, bone morphogenetic protein; TGF-β, transforming growth factor-beta; FGF-2, fibroblast growth factor; PDGF, platelet-derived growth factor; VEGF, vascular endothelial growth factor; IGF, insulin-like growth factor; PGE$_2$, prostaglandin E$_2$.

Age

Increasing age causes characteristic changes in bone. Pediatric fractures tend to heal at an accelerated rate compared to adult fractures.[305,306] The reasons for this are multifactorial. Age appears to affect angiogenesis,[307] and angiogenesis affects fracture healing (see earlier). With this in mind, Lu and colleagues[308] designed a study to examine the effect that age has on vascularization during fracture healing. Tibial fractures were created in 4-week-old, 6-month-old, and 18-month-old (juvenile, middle-aged, elderly, respectively) rats. At 7 days postfracture, there was a higher surface density of blood vessels in juvenile fracture calluses compared to those of middle-aged and elderly rats. In addition, juvenile rats expressed increased levels of HIF-1α and VEGF at 3 days postfracture versus older rats. Although these results do not provide definitive data that a younger age augments osteogenesis via vasculature-mediated mechanisms, they do offer insight into the fact that angiogenic potential during fracture healing does change throughout the lifespan of rats. Age may also influence fracture repair via its effects on periosteal structure and cell population[309] and chondrogenic potential,[310] stem cell function,[311] and biologic signaling.[312]

Bone remodeling

Osteoinduction

Albrektsson and Johansson[313] have written that osteoinduction is the process by which undifferentiated pluripotent cells are stimulated to become cells within the osteoblast lineage. This phenomenon occurs naturally during skeletogenesis and fracture repair.

Although osteoinduction is an intrinsic biologic process, it can also be manipulated exogenously. For example, purified and recombinant human isoforms of BMP are commonly used in experimental settings to induce bony formation. Various biomaterials have also been used for the same purpose. Bioglass and other osteoinductive materials have shown promise when used for craniomaxillofacial applications.[314] After bioactive glass is mixed with saline or blood, an apatite surface layer is formed at the biomaterial–bone interface, which incorporates collagen and proteins from surrounding native bone. In addition to producing a chemical bone at the interface, the apatite layer stimulates the production of osteogenic cytokines from surrounding osteoprogenitor cells, and this results in new bone formation.[315]

The use of osteoinductive effector cells such as MSCs and osteoprogenitor cells is currently an area of large focus. This is because the use of exogenous or autologous stem cells capable of differentiating into bone, in addition to osteoinductive cytokines, appears to have clear benefits. Adipose tissue may provide an ideal source of MSCs capable of undergoing osteoinduction as they have been shown to have the ability to differentiate into osteogenic cells.[316] In addition, Caballero et al.[317] examined whether and to what extent MSCs from the umbilical cord of neonates and palatal periosteum of older infants could undergo osteoinduction. After isolation and subsequent MSC incubation within osteogenic media, it was found that umbilical cord- and palatal periosteum-derived MSCs both stained positive for calcium deposition and also expressed increased levels of BMP-2, ALP, and osteocalcin. Given that MSCs from both sources appear to be capable of undergoing osteoinduction, they may be of benefit for children with critical osseous defects (defects that cannot ossify on their own without intervention).

Osteoconduction

Osteoconduction refers to the ability of a material to serve as a scaffold on to which bone can attach and grow. During primary bone repair, opposing fragments at the fracture site mediate osteoconduction. In secondary bone repair, callus ECM acts as a scaffold on to which new bone can attach and grow. In the field of regenerative medicine, many implanted materials serve an osteoconductive role. It is believed that an osteoconductive substrate must be porous to allow for the ingrowth of bone and fibrovascular tissue during osteoinduction.[318] Currently, there are many osteoconductive materials that are used in an effort to improve bone healing in clinical practice. Surgeons can choose from allografts (processed human bone), autogenous bone grafts, purified collagen, calcium phosphate (CaP) substitutes, and synthetic polymers. Different osteoconductive materials have differing innate osteoinductive potentials as well. Native bone, for example, will mediate both osteoconduction and osteoinduction, whereas CaP substrates are purely osteoconductive. CaP, however, can express osteoinductive properties if enhanced with osteoinductive substances such as BMPs.[319]

Osseointegration

There are varying definitions of ossoeintegration,[312,320] but many authors would agree that the phenomenon implies a stable anchorage between bone and implant that results in a structural and functional connection between the two. Osseointegration has been compared to primary fracture healing because, during osseointegration, native bone and an implant unite without a cartilaginous intermediate (similar to fragment ends in primary fracture repair). A key difference between primary fracture repair and osseointegration, however, is that during the latter, unification occurs between native bone and a foreign body. As such, implant structure and composition play a vital role in this process.

In order for osseointegration to occur, certain prerequisites must be met.[321] The material that composes the foreign body (i.e., implant) must be either bioinert or bioactive. A bioinert material is one that does not stimulate an adverse reaction from the native tissue into which it is placed. Commercially pure titanium is an example of a bioinert material that is extensively used in dental, craniofacial, and orthopedic procedures. A bioactive material is one that promotes a favorable tissue reaction, typically by stimulating bone production or chemical bond formation between implant and native tissue. Bioactive agents are typically applied as a coating to implants with an otherwise unfavorable mechanical quality. In addition, the degree and strength of bone–implant contact depend on the surface properties of an implant. The extent of bone–implant interface has been shown to be positively correlated to implant surface roughness.[322] This may be related to the fact that roughness of an implant increases resistance against shear stress, whereas smooth implants display little resistance. In addition, Butz and colleagues[323] assessed the intrinsic biomechanical properties (hardness and elastic modulus) of bone tissue integrated to titanium implants with varying degrees of surface roughness. The authors found that bone deposited around acid-etched titanium implants displayed enhanced biomechanical properties compared to bone deposited around implants with smoother, machined surface topography. Similarly, compared with machined surfaces, implant surfaces subjected to anodization exhibit increased bone-to-implant contact.[324]

Distraction osteogenesis

Distraction osteogenesis, the formation of new bone from the gradual separation of osteotomized fronts, was pioneered by the work of Codvilla at the turn of the 20th century and expanded by Ilizarov in orthopedic surgery.[325-327] Through a set of rigorous experimentation, Ilizarov[327] was the first to establish the hypothesis that gradual controlled separation of osteotomized bone results in a "tension stress effect" leading to angiogenesis and new bone formation. These initial observations and classic experiments were based upon the axial skeleton. It was not until the early 1970s that the concept of craniofacial distraction was introduced, first in a canine model,[328] in which the authors demonstrated correction of an iatrogenic crossbite by an external distraction device (1 mm/day for 2 weeks). The application of distraction to the human craniofacial skeleton was finally introduced by McCarthy *et al.* in the early 1990s.[329-331] Since its inception in the human mandible, the indications of distraction osteogenesis have expanded from congenital cases to cases of craniofacial skeletal deficiency with tumor-, trauma-, or iatrogenic-related etiologies.

Distraction osteogenesis requires three main stages for successful augmentation of bone formation: latency, activation, and consolidation. The first stage, latency, occurs immediately after osteotomy and refers to the period during which bone healing is initiated at the bony gap, periosteal integrity is restored, and callus formation begins. Latency typically ranges between 1 and 7 days, and is typically gauged according to the patient's age; the younger the patient, the shorter the latency period. During the second stage, activation (distraction), osteogenesis is induced with the generation of immature bone. Distraction occurs by the turning of an axial screw at a predetermined rate for a certain number of days until target bone augmentation is achieved. The third and final stage, consolidation, refers to the phase during which immature bone remodels into mature bone. In practical terms, consolidation is the period from the end of distraction to the removal of the device. The parameters for these stages are established by the craniofacial surgeon in response to specific patient profiles and the region of the skeleton undergoing distraction.

Histology

Successful distraction osteogenesis results from membranous ossification in the absence of a cartilaginous intermediate.[333-337] In the early phases of regenerate formation, distraction angiogenesis is a more accurate term to describe the cellular response to ischemia and traction. This phase is characterized by the appearance of multipotent precursor cells and type I collagen matrix expression in the distraction zone. Recently, Cetrulo and colleagues were able to demonstrate the honing of MSCs to the distraction zone in rat mandibles after intra-arterial transfer,[338] an indication that paracrine factors expressed in ischemia (e.g., HIF-1α) are chemoattractants and eventual agents of osteoinduction. Specifically, endothelial precursor cells are enriched at midactivation through 1–2 weeks into the consolidation period, when distracted rats were compared to controls.[338] CD31, CD34, and Flk-1, markers of neovascularization, stem cells, and endothelial precursors, respectively, have all been demonstrated by immunohistochemistry. Further in the activation period, dense collagen fibrils are formed and organized in the direction of distraction as a template for mineralization.[335,339-341]

It has been recognized that bone precursor cells respond to mechanical cues in order to differentiate. Distraction appears to be no exception to this tenet. In a rat model, Rhee and colleagues demonstrated increased intranuclear expression of signal transduction factors ERK1/ERK2 early in the distraction phase.[342] This expression paralleled upregulation of BMP2/BMP4, two relatively potent osteoinduction agents. Mineralization by active mature osteoblasts starts 10–14 days after the onset of distraction, and begins at the osteotomy fronts, proceeding centrally towards the relatively avascular fibrous interzone[327,335,339,343] *(Fig. 21.8)*. This leads to the formation of the primary mineralization front. Thin-walled vascular channels and bony spicules are slowly converted to normal lamellar bone and marrow. Interestingly, during the latter phase of activation, the infantile regenerate is still malleable and can remodel according to external forces. One can therefore take advantage of the gradual process and judiciously manipulate the distracted bone clinically in order to obtain a more precise occlusion, for example. This clinical principle, which is based on the gradual histomorphogenesis of the distraction zone, is termed molding

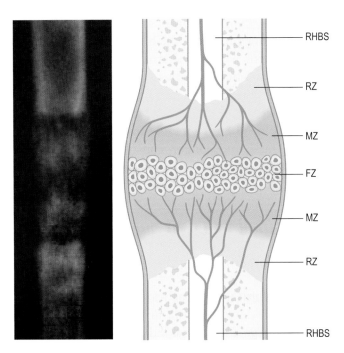

Fig. 21.8 Schematic drawing of bone formation during distraction osteogenesis. After approximately 10 days of distraction and during the distraction period, the regenerated tissue can be divided into three zones: **(1)** an avascular fibrous interzone (FZ); **(2)** two mineralization zones (MZ) or fronts; **(3)** and two regenerate zones (RZ). Regenerate zones are adjacent to residual host bone segments (RHBS). (From Samchukov ML, Cope JB, Cherkashin AM. Craniofacial distraction osteogenesis. St. Louis: Mosby; 2001.)

the regenerate.[344,345] Several studies have confirmed that molding the distraction bone, clinically by use of an orthopedic appliance, does not lead to disturbance of the regenerate or fibrous nonunion.[344,345]

Variables affecting osteogenesis

To understand the variables that have a negative or positive impact on osteogenesis in the context of distraction, one must understand the factors that promote successful regenerate formation and bony union. These tenets are aptly described by Ilizarov[346]: (1) device stability; (2) a latency period; (3) a gradual distraction (activation) period; and (4) a sufficient consolidation period. First, osteocyte viability reflects osteoblastic activity and thus the selection of a strong area of bone for osteotomy and distractor placement is critical. A stable device placed in stably healing bone results in the formation of strong cortical bone within the regenerate and minimizes the chance of fibrous nonunion. It follows that any thermal or mechanical injury to the bone can

damage the blood supply to the bone, resulting in ischemic fibrogenesis. Fibrogenic damage leads to irregular and disorganized collagen formation from arterial insufficiency or cystic degeneration from venous outflow obstruction. Previous concerns of periosteal damage resulting in poor osteogenesis have recently diminished as increasing experience among craniofacial surgeons has demonstrated that, even with complete osteotomy, the periosteum is sufficiently osteogenic for strong bone production.

Inappropriate timing of the distraction stages can result in osteogenic failure. In terms of the latency period, this translates into either too short a period (immediate distraction) or a prolonged period (delayed distraction). Important for primordial callus and ultimately regenerate volume, latency periods range between 0 and 7 days, depending upon patient variables, such as age, osteotomy site, blood supply, and other factors that may affect regenerate formation (see below). The majority of experimental evidence points to an optimal latency period of 5–7 days. Theoretically, immediate distraction may prevent adequate hematoma and primordial callus generation, culminating in a regenerate of suboptimal volume/mechanical strength, and, in extreme circumstances, fibrous nonunion. It follows that disruption of initial fracture hematomas, which simulates an abbreviated latency period, results in a 26% decrease in callus cross-sectional area, and a significant impairment in the mechanical strength of the newly formed bone.[347] On the other hand, deferment of the distraction period >14 days results in premature consolidation of the distraction site and device failure.[333,339,348,349]

Overall, latency periods have been a source of debate among craniofacial surgeons and their significance held in question ever since the inception of the technique. To this end, studies comparing latency periods of 7, 14, and 21 days have failed to underscore any difference in protocols in terms of osteogenesis.[332,350] Clinically, Hollier and colleagues demonstrate a low complication rate with the elimination of the latency period and implementation of a rapid distraction rate (2 mm/day) in their pediatric population.[351] It is important to note that the nonunion rate in this series was 4.5% and was attributed to the only distracted bone graft in the study. It is generally accepted that reduced latency periods and faster distraction rates formulate an acceptable protocol in children, due to improved blood supply and osteogenic potential. Flexibility in the timing and rate of distraction needs to be inherent in any successful protocol, with respect to patient profile (see below).

Patient factors

Age

It has been well recognized that increasing age contributes negatively to the overall outcome of distraction osteogenesis, presumably secondary to limited ability of older subjects to recruit osteoprogenitor cells to the site of injury. In support of this concept, studies have demonstrated that the rate of bone formation and bone mineral deposition in pediatric distraction patients (385 mm/day) is far more superior than adults (213 mm/day).[332] This age-related difference in osteogenic potential, however, is not a contraindication to distraction osteogenesis, as older individuals can undergo surgery successfully. In this context, latency and consolidation periods may be extended to allow for protracted regenerate formation in the older patient.

Blood supply

Several studies have demonstrated that, on a molecular level, the establishment of neovascularization is critical to the formation and eventual mineralization of the regenerate. Accordingly, factors that impair vascularization of the distracted field may result in failed bone formation. Osteocyte survival depends on the proximity of less than 0.1 mm to nutrient vessels.[352] The factors critical in osteogenesis of the axial skeleton (e.g., periosteal preservation) appear to be less important for osteogenesis in the craniofacial skeleton.[326,333,343,347,349,353,354] There are however, factors that unify both regions.

Radiation

Radiotherapy, by compromising vascularity, cellularity, and local oxygen supply, has been known to impair osteogenesis.[355–357] Limited clinical[355–357] and animal studies[358–361] have been performed in this regard; these studies have had mixed results. In the experimental realm, animals exposed to 36 Gy of radiation prior to the distraction process show a definitive decrease in bone mineralization microdensitometric analysis.[362]

These authors therefore propose finding an optimal radiation dosing protocol which would make distraction osteogenesis a viable alternative in the head and neck cancer patient. Regardless of the optimal conditions for radiation delivery and in consideration of the reduced vascularity within the irradiated field, such patients may need an extended latency period, slower distraction rate, and longer consolidation period to achieve similar outcomes in osteogenesis to the nonirradiated patient.

Clinical application of bone transfers

Indication for bone transfers

A variety of clinical approaches are currently used to repair skeletal defects in plastic surgery. In order to provide an optimal outcome, a detailed analysis of the bony defect and the mechanical requirements of the reconstructed part is needed. Reconstruction of bony deficiencies can be performed using autografts (obtained from the patient), allografts (obtained from another individual), xenografts (obtained from another species), bone substitutes, or implants. The standard of care is to use autologous bone grafting if possible, and the type of bone graft has to be chosen based on the clinical scenario; medical condition of the patient; previous radiation, infection, or severe scarring of the recipient site; bone graft donor site availability; and the patient's and surgeon's preference.

Typical indications for the use of bone grafts are bone gaps as a result of trauma or comminuted fractures, delayed or nonunion of fractures, bony defects after benign or malignant lesion resection, and reconstruction of functional and contour deficits in the craniofacial skeleton. Other indications include arthrodeses, limb-lengthening procedures, and spinal fusion. The structure and biomechanical properties of the graft determine the clinical application.

Bone graft healing and graft survival

Bone graft incorporation and fracture healing go through similar stages (see above). Graft incorporation is the process of graft resorption and replacement of necrotic bone by vascular ingrowths and new bone formation, also known as creeping substitution.[363] The incorporation of the bone grafts depends on various factors: the type of graft (i.e., autogenous versus allogeneic and vascularized versus nonvascularized), the quality of transplanted bone and recipient site, the mechanical properties of the graft, and systemic and local disease. The molecular and mechanical environment of the graft site, the contact between the graft and recipient bed, and the osteoinductive, osteoconductive, and osseointegrative capability of the graft influence bone graft healing.

Bone formation during remodeling is stimulated by compression, which leads to periosteal and endosteal apposition; traction, in contrast, promotes periosteal resorption and intracortical osteolysis.[364] Successful grafting requires a well-vascularized bed and adequate graft fixation.[365] Mechanical stability of the healing defect allows for revascularization of the graft.[366] Mechanical stress on a rigidly fixated graft prevents graft resorption,[367–369] and an intact periosteum also improves graft survival.[367]

Cancellous versus cortical grafts

Cancellous and cortical bone grafts have different applications in skeletal reconstruction. Compared to cortical bone, cancellous bone has little immediate strength or structural support but has higher osteogenic, osteoinductive, and osteoconductive properties. It is more quickly incorporated and revascularized than cortical bone, usually within 2 weeks. In the transplanted cancellous bone graft, the viable cells are composed of osteoblasts and endosteal cells lining the graft surface. Cancellous bone grafts serve as an osteoconductive substrate to support creeping.[370–373] They are indicated to bridge gaps less then 5–6 cm in nonstress-bearing areas. Typical sources of cancellous bone grafts are the iliac crest, the cranial diploe, the upper tibial epiphysis, and the distal radius.

Cortical bone has limited osteogenic properties as it is less osteoconductive and less osteoinductive than cancellous bone.[374] Creeping substitution is the main mechanism of cortical bone graft incorporation, and the graft largely relies on plasmatic imbibition from the recipient bed to keep the outer layer of osteocytes alive after transplantation.[371] The incorporation and revascularization of cortical grafts are slower than cancellous grafts, usually taking 1–2 months.[375–377] However, cortical grafts provide immediate structural support and are able to bridge defects up to 12 cm in length. Cortical grafts should be tailored to fit exactly into the defect and, usually, rigid fixation is needed to prevent fracture of the healing graft.[378] Pure cortical grafts are often used for onlay augmentation of contour deficits. Typical grafts sites arise from the fibula, the rib, and the iliac crest.

Clinical considerations

To optimize the chances of bone graft survival, the bone graft should be handled as follows[379]:

1. Graft exposure time to air at room temperature should be minimized (ideally to less than 1 hour to maintain cell viability).[380] However, longer periods of ischemia can be tolerated by bone cells if the medullary nutrient blood supply is later reconstituted, as in vascularized bone.[381]

2. To enhance bone viability by 4–6 hours, a graft should be covered in a blood-soaked sponge with a moist saline gauze on top. If longer periods of graft exposure are required, cell viability can be maintained if the graft is stored in 10% human serum albumin and a 90% balanced salt solution at 3°C in Collins–Terasaki solution.[381]

3. Grafts should be kept cool, as temperatures over 42°C may cause cell death.

4. Antibiotic washes are not only bactericidal but are also cellucidal and therefore should be used with caution.

5. Dead space around the graft should be avoided.

6. The cancellous portion of the graft should be placed in contact with the cancellous bone in the bed.

7. Ideally, the graft should be placed in a previously prepared vascularized bed to increase graft survival.

Techniques of harvest: autologous bone grafts

Ilium

The ilium has become the most commonly used site for corticocancellous bone grafts (*Figs 21.9, 21.10*). The

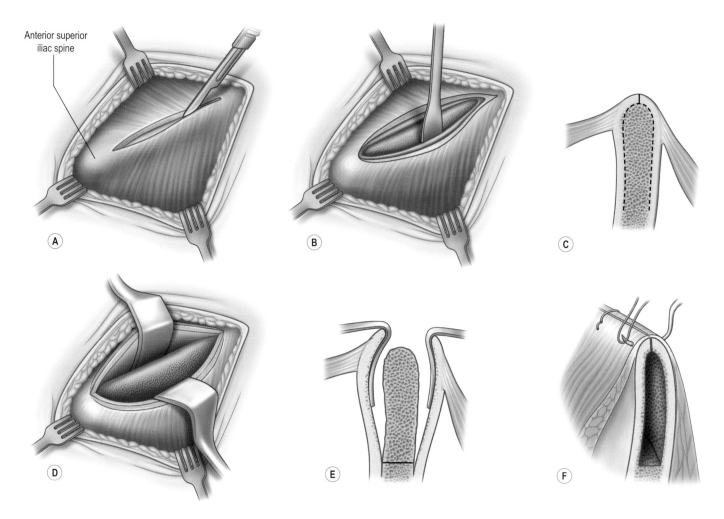

Anterior superior
iliac spine

(A) (B) (C)

(D) (E) (F)

Fig. 21.9 A technique for removal of cancellous bone from the ilium. **(A)** Incision of the periosteum after exposure of the crest. **(B)** Separation of the cortex with an osteotome. **(C)** Cross-section showing lines of separation of the inner and outer cortex from the cancellous bone. **(D)** Exposure of cancellous bone. **(E)** Cross-section showing exposure. **(F)** Reunion of the inner and outer cortex by stainless steel wire suture. ((A-F) From Cutting CB, McCarthy JG, Knize DM: Repair and grafting of bone. In McCarthy JG, Plastic Surgery Vol 1, Elsevier 1990; (F) After Tessier P, Kawamoto H, Matthews D, et al. Taking bone grafts from the anterior and posterior ilium – tools and techniques: a 6800-case experience in maxillofacial and craniofacial surgery. Plast Reconstr Surg. 2005;116(Suppl):25S–37S; see also Wolfe SA, Kawamoto HK. Taking the iliac-bone graft. J Bone Joint Surg Am. 1978;60:411.)

clinical indications are wide due to the versatility of the ilium, the large amount of cortical and cancellous bone, and the possibility to transfer it as a vascularized flap. The iliac crest is relatively easily accessible and has limited morbidity if the proper technique is used. Commonly reported complications include chronic harvest site pain, sensory changes, and gait abnormalities.[382]

Principally, the harvest technique should preserve the shape of the iliac crest by careful and proper splitting. Correct handling of the iliac wing permits its regeneration and allows for further or repeat harvest. Additionally, wiring the split iliac crest back together can decrease

postoperative pain. Furthermore, care must be taken to avoid stretching the lateral femoral cutaneous nerve by unnecessary superior dissection, to avoid tearing the gluteal muscles, and to avoid removing the iliac crest itself.

Also, preservation of the insertion of the abdominal and the gluteal muscles on the iliac crest is important. Dependent upon the amount of graft taken, the outer, inner, or both cortical plates of the iliac wing need to be preserved. The amount of cancellous bone that can be harvested from the ilium is quite large – down to the cotyloid ridge above the glenoid fossa. A large subcrest corticocancellous graft up to 11 cm, a 6 × 10 cm

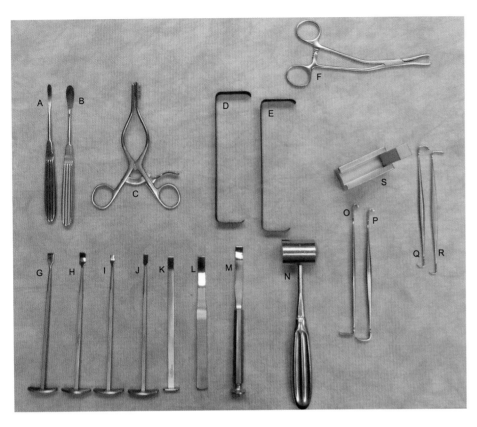

Fig. 21.10 Instruments for ilium harvest.
(A) Obwegeser periosteal elevator, 6 mm.
(B) Obwegeser periosteal elevator, 12 mm.
(C) Wheatlander retractor. **(D, E)** Farabeuf retractors.
(F) Digman bone-holding forceps. **(B–M)** Osteotomes,
4–12 mm, straight and curved. **(N)** Mallet. **(O, P)** Senn
retractors. **(Q, R)** Ragnel retractors. **(S)** Cottle crusher.

corticocancellous inner plate, and an approximately 5 × 8 cm corticocancellous outer plate can also be harvested. Harvest of the anterior iliac crest *(Fig. 21.9)* is more convenient due to the supine position of the patient. However, the posterior iliac crest provides a larger amount of graft material and avoids aberrant entry into the abdomen. In order to prevent avulsion fractures of the anterior superior iliac spine (ASIS), the anterior approach should stop 2–3 cm posterior to the ASIS. The posterior approach should stop 4 cm anterior to the posterior superior iliac spine to prevent injury to the sacroiliac joint.[374]

The anterior approach can be performed in supine position or with a roll underneath the patient's hip to raise it. The following landmarks are drawn: ASIS and the tubercle of the iliac crest. The incision is placed over the iliac crest and is 6–10 cm in length. By pulling the skin medially, the incision actually lies 3–5 cm below and lateral to the iliac crest. No subcutaneous dissection is necessary; the abdominal soft tissue is retracted medially and the crest, tuberosity, and anterior spine are palpated. A cartilaginous cap is frequently encountered

overlying the bone and this must be split to access the cortical plate. The next step is to split the iliac crest; the split is extended just behind the anterior spine. The medial leaf of the split crest is created and moved medially as a single piece with the attachments of the abdominal muscles. The same maneuver is performed for the lateral leaf with attention to the convexity of the lateral crest. The grafts are extracted according to defect size and shape.[383] Excessive retraction can potentially cause injury to the lateral femoral cutaneous nerve, which travels retroperitoneal on the deep surface of the iliac muscle, down to the inguinal ligament near the ASIS. This can result in postoperative paresthesias.

Closure is performed after obtaining hemostasis, using electrocautery and bone wax, specifically if bleeding occurs from the central artery of the iliac bone.

Gelfoam can be placed in the periosteal pocket, and the iliac leafs are wired back together. Muscles, subcutaneous tissue, and skin are closed in a layered fashion over a suction drain. A pain pump catheter delivering local anesthetics can be inserted in the wound for better postoperative pain control.[384] In similar fashion, the posterior iliac crest can be harvested from the supine or prone position. When harvesting this region of the crest in the prone position, one must take care to avoid injury to the cluneal nerves.[384] Also, in order to prevent injury to the sacroiliac joint, the most posterior mark with the osteotome is made 4 cm anterior to the posterior iliac spine.[374]

Complications are rare if proper technique is used, as shown in a summary of 5600 patients with a resultant complication rate of 0.5 % (hematoma, hernia, paresthesia of the lateral femoral cutaneous nerve, broken wires with bursa formation, and late sponge removal).[383]

Tibia and fibula

The tibia was mainly used as a source of corticocancellous bone graft during World Wars I and II. Its use has decreased in popularity due to donor site morbidity and pathologic fractures. The tibia remains a favorable donor site in various centers in Scandinavia and the UK when only small amounts of cancellous bone are needed (e.g., alveolar bone grafting).[385,386] A detailed description of technical aspects of tibial harvest has been given *(Fig. 21.11)*.[387]

The use of fibula grafts has decreased with the availability of allograft. Currently, the fibula is mainly used as a vascularized transfer for mandible reconstruction, as well as midface and extremity reconstruction.

Greater trochanter and olecranon

The greater trochanter and the olecranon are potential sites of cancellous bone harvest, specifically when small amounts are needed. The harvest technique is similar to a bone biopsy. A small incision is made overlying the area of interest, dissection is carried down to the bone, and the periosteum is removed from the desired area. An osteotome can be used to transect the cortex or a small drill bit can be used to create perforations in an elliptical pattern, which then can be connected with an osteotome. Through this opening, cancellous bone can then be harvested with a curet. After completion of the harvest, the cortical bone piece can be reinserted, or if need be, can be used as part of the graft. Hemostasis is achieved using gelfoam and thrombin. A layered closure is performed and a compression dressing applied.[382]

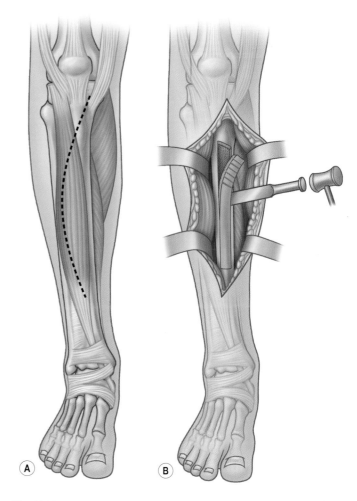

Fig. 21.11 Tibial bone grafts. **(A)** Incision for removal of the graft. **(B)** Removal of the graft with an osteotome.

Rib

Rib is another source of bone for use as a graft or as a vascularized transfer. The advantages of rib grafts are the flexibility of the bone, which allows for easy bending and wire fixation. Also, rib integrates easily to the host bone. Disadvantages include the fact that ribs are fragile and do not allow for stable screw fixation. Furthermore, the amount of cancellous bone is minimal and a second harvest is implausible as a result of poorly regenerated rib.

When harvesting rib, short skin incisions should be used and one rib should be skipped to preserve contour and stability of the thoracic wall *(Figs 21.12, 21.13)*. If possible, the surgeon should avoid subcutaneous dissection and transection of the rectus muscle. Also, one must be cognizant of bleeding from the intercostal vessels as well as air leaks. The harvest can be performed with the patient in the supine or lateral position. The skin incision should be located over the rib that is to be harvested or over the skipped rib if two ribs are required. Dissection is carried down to the rib, and the periosteum is incised longitudinally on the lateral aspect of the rib. Subperiosteal elevation should then be performed up to the costochondral junction. The length of the rib to be harvested is determined based on the amount needed: a long segment from one rib is preferred over a short segment from two ribs. If cartilage is needed, it can be included in the harvest.

After harvest, the wound should be irrigated and examined for an air leak and then closed in a layered fashion. This takes place by suturing the edges of the periosteum and performing a layered closure of the muscles, subcutaneous tissue, and skin. A suction drain and local pain pump can be added if the surgeon desires.

The associated donor site morbidities and risks include pneumothorax, which can easily be prevented if careful and proper technique is used. In addition, the chest wall might become deformed if consecutive ribs

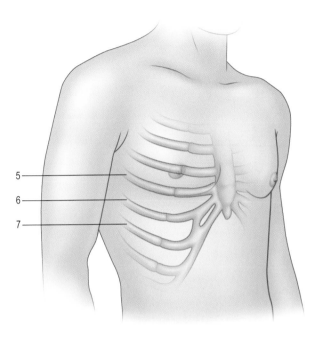

Fig. 21.12 Ribs 5–7 are the most commonly used donor ribs. (From Tessier P, Kawamoto H, Matthews D, *et al.* Taking long rib grafts for facial reconstruction – tools and techniques: III. A 2900-case experience in maxillofacial and craniofacial surgery. Plast Reconstr Surg. 2005;116:38S.)

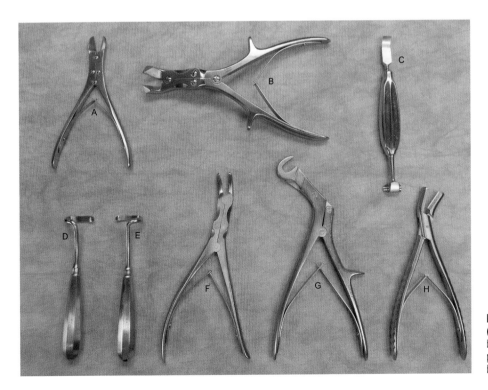

Fig. 21.13 Instruments for rib harvest. **(A)** Bone-cutting forceps. **(B)** Stille–Listor angled bone-cutting forceps. **(C)** Alexander–Farabeuf periosteotome. **(D, E)** Doyen elevators. **(F)** Frykholm bone rongeur. **(G)** Rib shears. **(H)** Tessier bone bender.

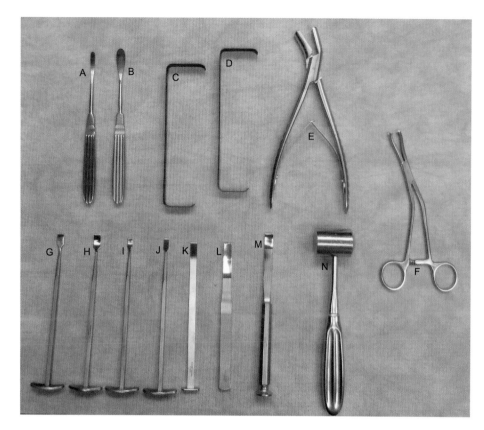

Fig. 21.14 Instruments for calvarial harvest.
(A) Obwegeser periosteal elevator, 6 mm.
(B) Obwegeser periosteal elevator, 12 mm.
(C, D) Farabeuf retractors. **(E)** Tessier bone bender.
(F) Digman bone-holding forceps. **(G–K)** Dautry-Munro osteotomes, straight and curved. **(L)** Straight osteotome. **(M)** Stille osteotome, 15 mm. **(N)** Mallet.

are harvested. Postoperative breathing difficulties secondary to pain can affect postoperative recovery time. Overall the complication rate is low but varies within the literature. Complications may include pain, intraoperative bleeding and air leaks, secondary bleeding, and rarely, chest wall deformities or scoliosis.[388]

Calvarium

Calvarial bone grafts are of ectomesenchymal nature, with a rich diploic vascular system that allows for rapid revascularization of the haversian systems. This allows for osteocyte survival and thereby leads to less resorption as well as increased maintenance of their structure.[389] Calvarial bone grafts are ideal for calvarial, midfacial, nasal, and orbital reconstruction.[390] Calvarial grafts can be obtained as split- or full-thickness grafts. In young children, however, a split graft may not be possible because the calvarium may be too thin. Harvest can occur via *in situ* splitting of the outer table or full-thickness harvest and on-the-table splitting to increase the surface area of graft available.[391] It is important to

use the correct instruments and to make certain they are in good condition *(Fig. 21.14)*. The surgeon must also be aware of the location of the sagittal and coronal sutures, as the corticotomy should not occur less than 1 cm from the coronal suture or less than 1.5 cm from the sagittal suture. It is additionally important to locate the perforating vessel posteriorly near the sagittal suture.

The technique of calvarial bone graft harvest includes a coronal incision that is made through scalp and galea. The pericranium is then incised and elevated. Bone wax and/or gelfoam can be used to halt bone bleeding. The landmarks include the coronal suture, the sagittal suture (with its posterior perforating vessels), the anterior temporal crest, and the intraosseous lateral vein. When taking a split *in situ* outer-table graft, the design can be outlined and traced with an oscillating saw followed by burring until diploe is seen. The alternating straight and curved osteotomes are used to split the calvarium. After the splitting of the outer table, further strips of diploe can be harvested until the inner table is encountered specifically at the thicker, posterior border near the lambdoid suture. If during this process the dura becomes exposed, it can be covered with bone chips. The pericranium can be closed over Surgicel and the scalp should be closed in layers over suction drains.

There are several factors that make an intracranial approach for calvarial bone graft harvest a better option. Specifically, an intracranial approach should be undertaken in children with a thin calvarium, when a large graft is needed, in a patient with an irregular skull shape, or if, for graft design purposes, the inner table is more feasible. Availability of a neurosurgeon is recommended for this approach. Once the full-thickness piece is obtained, it can be split on the back table. One should not use a saw but rather an osteotome to reduce the waste of bony substance and to reduce heat damage to the graft. It is important to make sure that no cerebrospinal fluid leak is present and that hemostasis is achieved. One split segment is returned to the donor site; the other is used for reconstruction.

Overall, complications are rare (0.25%). Intraoperative incidents such as bone bleeding, dural bleeding, and dural laceration are usually controlled during surgery. Postoperative complications include minimal pain and occasional paresthesia, subscalp hematoma and calvarial irregularities, infection, and rare brain injury with transient neurological sequelae.[392]

Vascularized bone flaps

Vascularized bone flaps avert the reparative phase of nonvascularized grafts and do not depend on recipient bed vascularity. Specifically in circumstances of prior irradiation, extensive trauma, or chronic scarring, vascularized bone flaps are superior to nonvascularized bone grafts.[393–396] The survival of osteocytes in vascularized bone grafts leads to a decrease in the remodeling process during revascularization as well as the maintenance of bone mass and strength.[397–400] Other advantages include increased blood flow to compromised recipient sites; utilization of composite tissue flaps, including skin, muscle, and nerves; and the growth potential when including a growth plate in the graft.[401–406] An important indication for the use of vascularized bone flaps is segmental defects of greater than 6–8 cm after traumatic or oncologic bone loss; composite tissue loss; bony nonunion; avascular necrosis; osteomyelitis; or after biologic failure due to infection, scarring, or irradiation.[407–410]

Vascularized iliac transfer

The ilium is not only a great source of bone graft material but also has a rich periosteal blood supply in addition to the nutrient artery. Many studies have been performed to identify and choose the best blood supply to the ilium.[411,412] The superficial circumflex iliac vessels are often utilized in conjunction with a groin fasciocutaneous flap, but the deep circumflex iliac vessels are a better blood supply to the bone (*Fig. 21.15*).[411,412] Furthermore, a piece of vascularized iliac crest can be harvested in conjunction with the anterolateral thigh flap based off the lateral femoral circumflex system, with the ascending branch giving a small vascular pedicle to the anterior superior iliac crest.[413,414] Details of vascularized bone transfer can be found in the clinical chapters of this book.

Vacularized fibula

The free fibula transfer is utilized mainly in mandibular and occasionally in midface reconstruction as well as for long-bone defects or nonunions. The fibula provides a straight cortical piece of bone up to 30 cm in length. The principal blood supply to the fibula is via the nutrient artery, a branch of the peroneal artery with a diameter of 1.5–3 mm (*Fig. 21.16*). The fibula is further supplied by periosteal branches from the peroneal artery before the nutrient vessel and by musculoperiosteal branches more distally. The dissection can be performed through an anterior or posterior approach. Bone can be transferred with adjacent muscles such as soleus, peroneal muscles, or flexor hallucis longus. Fasciocutaneous perforators allow for a skin paddle up to 10 × 20 cm in size.[415] The surgical steps will be described in another chapter. It is important to leave 6 cm distally to maintain stability of the ankle joint. Another important component is rigid fixation of the transferred bone to the recipient site to improve healing. Complications include instability of the ankle joint, persistent pain, neurological compromise, and wound breakdown or delayed skin graft healing over the donor site if a skin paddle was included. Various series have shown a high complication rate, reaching levels between 20% and 50%.[416,417]

Vascularized scapula

The vascularized scapular bone flap can be combined with a variety of possible composite flaps, including

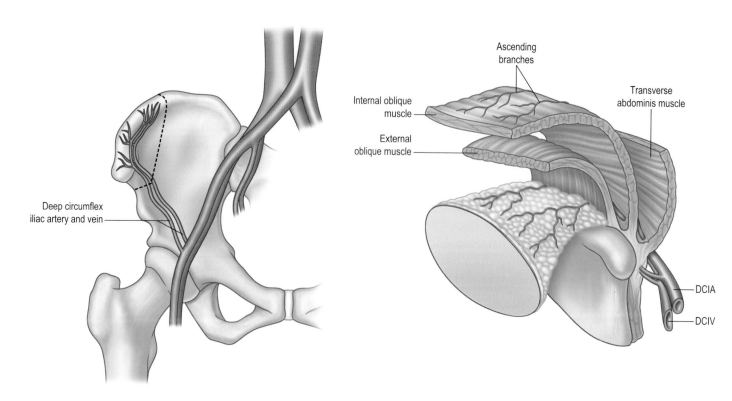

Fig. 21.15 The deep circumflex artery vascularized bone flap. Vascularized bone based on the deep circumflex iliac artery and vein (DCIA/DCIV) is harvested and can be taken with an overlying skin paddle.

various amounts of muscle and skin. The scapula can be transferred as a vascularized bone based on the nutrient artery, which enters inferior to the lateral attachments of the acromion to the scapula plate.

The scapula bone flap can be based on the lateral border (lateral scapular osteocutaneous flap)[418] supplied by the circumflex scapular circulation or on the medial ridge of the scapula[419,420] based on the same pedicle and also on periosteal blood supply *(Fig. 21.17)*. The scapular bone can further be based on an additional branch of the thoracodorsal system called the angular branch, which supplies the wing of the scapula.[421] The mean pedicle length of the circumflex scapular system is 7.5 cm. It can, however, be increased up to 13–15 cm by clipping the circumflex scapula perforators, which allows the bone to be supplied by the angular vessels, thus avoiding the need for vein grafts.[422]

During flap dissection the teres major and minor muscles need to be divided, and this can lead to shoulder impairment. Another potential complication is scapular winging from division of the serratus anterior. Vascularized scapular bone might offer an advantage over fibula or iliac crest in the older patient in whom ambulation is essential for postoperative recovery.[423]

Vascularized rib

The rib provides a curved, malleable piece of bone up to 30 cm long that receives its vascular supply through nutrient vessels and periosteal vessels. The nutrient vessel arises from the posterior intercostal vessels and the periosteal blood supply comes from various surrounding sources (intercostal perforators from the thoracodorsal system, the superior epigastric system, the internal mammary vessels, the lateral thoracic vessels, and the thoracoacromial vessels). The overlying muscle, skin, and fat of each region can be transferred with the flap.[424] A composite flap can be particularly helpful, for example, in the reconstruction of complex three-dimensional cranial defects.[425,426] A dissection that includes the nutrient vessel within the rib flap requires thoracotomy. As such, it adds a level of difficulty and is not without its associated risks and complications.

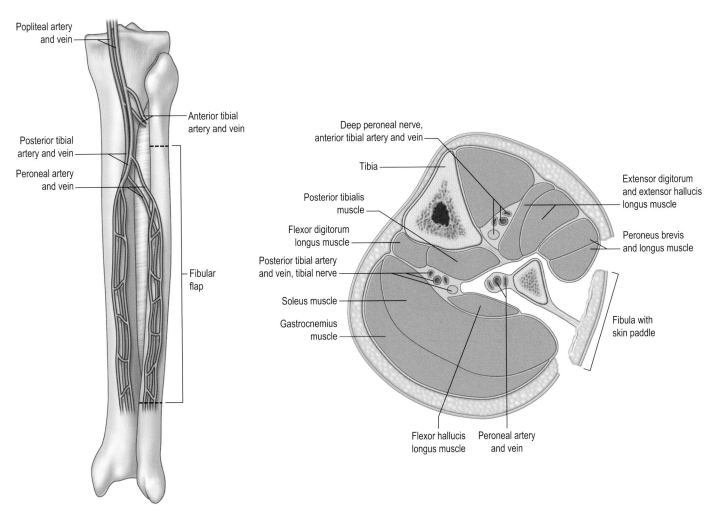

Fig. 21.16 The fibula free flap. Vascularized fibula is based on the peroneal artery and vein pedicle and can be raised with or without an overlying skin paddle.

Therefore, most vascularized rib transfers are based on the periosteal blood supply.

Vacularized calvarium

The vascularized calvarial bone flap is useful for unfavorable recipient sites (irradiated or scarred tissue) as well as in midface reconstruction.[427] An understanding of the anatomy of the temporoparietal region is important to be able to utilize the area for reconstructions with vascularized bone. The calvarial bone is covered with pericranium, overlying temporal muscle, temporal fascia with a deep and superficial layer, subgaleal fascia, superficial temporal (temporoparietal) fascia, subcutaneous tissue, and skin. Different flap types based off the superficial and deep temporal system can be useful to reconstruct facial defects, specifically in the midface.[427]

A temporoparietal fascial flap can be harvested with parietal bone that is vascularized by periosteal vessels from perforators of the superficial temporal system. A vascularized calvarial flap can also be harvested with a fused segment of the deep and superficial temporal fascial flap 2 cm above the orbital rim.[391] This flap is based on the middle temporal artery. A third option is a temporalis myo-osseous flap, which transfers the temporalis muscle and distal periosteum with the underlying bone as one unit. This is based off the deep temporal vessels.[428] The parietal bone can be harvested as partial (outer table) or full-thickness flap while avoiding the sagittal sinus (*Fig. 21.18*).

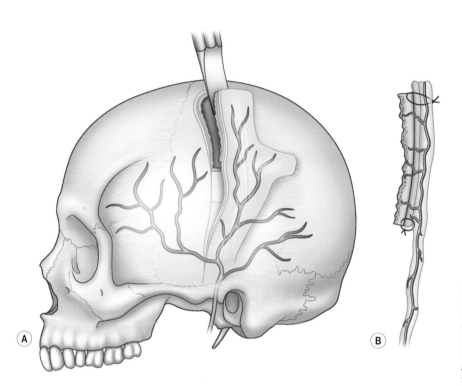

(A)

(B)

Fig. 21.17 (A) The outer table of the parietal bone is harvested with a curved osteotome after a trough is created around the periphery of the bone flap. The blood supply of the bone flap is maintained by preserving the periosteal blood vessels in continuity with the superficial temporal artery system within the galea superficial musculoaponeurotic system and the deep temporal fascia. **(B)** Sutures passed between the overlying galea, periosteum, and calvaria are helpful in keeping the periosteum attached to the bone and preserving the blood supply.

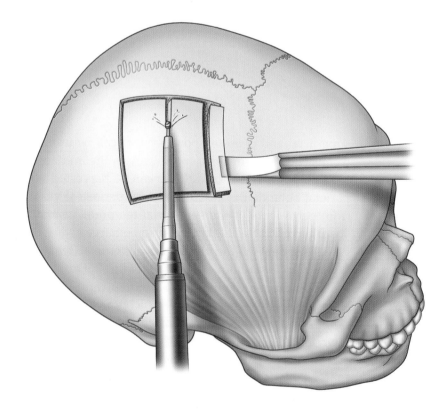

Fig. 21.18 The parietal bone donor site. (From Tessier P, Kawamoto H, Posnick J, *et al.* Taking calvarial grafts, either split *in situ* or splitting of the parietal bone flap *ex vivo* – tools and techniques: V. A 9650-case experience in craniofacial and maxillofacial surgery. Plast Reconstr Surg. 2005;116:55S.)

The surgical steps include a preauricular incision extending into the hairline, the elevation of flaps and dissection down to temporoparietal fascia, and a decision of flap level elevation and flap harvest with the appropriate pedicle, as described above. The pedicle is dissected into the pericranium of the desired calvarial bone. The bone flap design is based on the defect and reconstructive needs of the patient. Multiple strips can be harvested for complex three-dimensional defects. Stable fixation of the cranial bone flap at the recipient site is essential for reliable early bone integration.

Principles of bone transfer

In order to optimize clinical outcomes the principles of bone grafting need to be understood. Knowledge of such principles arises from the accumulation of three components: individual experience, experience of others (literature review), and the knowledge acquired from basic science research.[429] There are general principles and specific doctrines. The general principles include defining one's goals and priorities; taking into consideration the location, size, depth, and etiology of the defect; the quality of the surrounding tissue; presence of history of infection; pre- or postoperative radiation; age and health of the patient; status of disease (control or palliation); and functional and appearance-related considerations.[430] The specific doctrines include the harvesting of bone from areas with which one is familiar, contouring of the bone graft to fit the defect, fixing the bone graft in a tension-free manner, ensuring absolute graft immobilization, differentiating between child and adult grafts, avoiding contaminated sites, proper handling of the graft, ensuring adequate blood supply over the graft, and assessing graft take periodically.[429]

If the recipient site is compromised due to scarring, infection, or irradiation or if greater biomechanical strength is required for segmental defects greater then 6 cm in a load-bearing area, a vascularized bone transfer should be considered. The maintained/re-established vascular supply to the transferred bone leads to rapid healing with less resorption and greater biomechanical strength.[398,399]

Allogeneic bone grafts

Bone allografts are taken from different individuals of the same species. The use of allogeneic bone for reconstruction of large bony defects in the axial and peripheral skeleton has grown in the last decade due to improved methods for bone preservation and sterilization. Nonvascularized bone allografts are free of any viable donor cells after antigen extraction and autolysis. These acellular constructs therefore mainly act as a scaffold for ingrowth of recipient mesenchymal cells which repopulate the donor by creeping substitution. Advantages over autogenous bone grafts include an unlimited supply, a lack of donor site morbidity, and decreased operative time. Disadvantages include the lack of osteogenic properties in prepared allografts as well as the immunologic response of fresh bone allografts. Due to slow union, long-term fixation is required.

Processing and preservation

Allografts cause an immune response in the host and need to be prepared in such a way as to remove all viable cellular components and thereby decrease the host immune reaction. The goal of the processing is to create a sterile, acellular, biocompatible, and osteoconductive product. During the preparation and preservation process in tissue banks, the allograft should lose all osteogenic and osteoinductive properties.

Processing techniques include mechanical debridement, ultrasonic or pulsatile water washes, ethanol washes, antibiotic soaks and terminal sterilization with moderate-dose (<20 kGy) irradiation. Larger doses (>30 kGy) are needed to neutralize significant viral loads, but will weaken the bone significantly.[431] The preservation of allografts can be achieved with deep-freezing (−70°C) and freeze-drying. Freeze-drying appears to cause a larger decrease in bone strength compared to deep-freezing.[432]

Risk of disease transmission

The risk of disease transmission from processed allografts is minimal due to extensive donor screening and testing as well as the acellular nature of the graft.[433,434] The pathogens of main concern are human immunodeficiency virus (HIV), hepatitis B virus, and hepatitis C virus. The transmission risk for HIV is thought to be extremely low (1 in 1.6 million).[434] However, this risk appears to decrease to virtually zero with newer screening techniques as well as by removing blood and blood products from the graft.[428]

Immunogenicity

The immune response caused by allografts varies and depends upon the degree of antigen mismatch between donor and host and upon the degree of graft processing. The immune response to fresh allografts is both humoral and cell-mediated in nature; fresh frozen allografts, however, predominantly activate T lymphocytes but not a humoral response. The cell-mediated immune response is to cell surface major histocompatibility class I and II antigens. Freeze-dried allograft implants only elicit a minimal cellular or humoral immune response.[435] Signs of graft rejection are not as clear as in organ transplantation: the main clinical signs include resorption and mechanical dysfunction. The process of allograft implant remodeling can be disturbed by sequestration of the bone implant in a fibrous capsule as a sign of chronic rejection. The rejection process can be arrested by cyclosporine administration.[436]

Incorporation of allograft bone

The phases of allograft incorporation are similar to fracture repair. They include an initial, limited inflammatory response with increased vascularity, resorption, and bone formation and remodeling. The incorporation of cancellous bone chips occurs more quickly than cortical grafts. The biomechanical strength of allografts after incorporation is lower than that of autografts, and this needs to be taken into consideration when reconstructing weight-bearing bones.

Formulations of allogeneic bone grafts

There are several formulations of allograft bone available: DBM (osteoinductive), morselized cancellous chips (osteoconductive), cortical and corticocancellous grafts, and whole bone segments (structural support). Demineralized bone preparations are not osteogenic, but they are osteoinductive and provide scaffolding upon which new bone can be formed.[437–439]

Xenogeneic bone grafts

Xenografts are taken from a species different than the patient. These grafts undergo a high rate of resorption, and their immunogenicity, specifically due to matrix and serum proteins, limits their clinical utility.

Deproteinated and defatted xenograft preparations show decreased immune response but also show destruction of BMPs and other growth factors and therefore are inferior substitutes for autografts and allografts.[440]

Bone substitutes

Alloplastic cranioplasty is a concept as old as trephination. From the Incan use of precious metals, to the first documented use of a synthetic material to repair a cranial defect (Fallopius, 16th century), to Meekeren's use of canine bone in a human subject, the quest for a suitable nonautologous material has been ever present.[441] The ideal bone substitute has the following characteristics: (1) chemically inert; (2) hypoallergenic or incapable of inducing a foreign-body reaction; (3) easily contoured; (4) stable and durable shape retention; (5) noncarcinogenic; and (6) capable of incorporation into or replacement with living tissue from the recipient. Although this ideal has not been achieved, several products are available and are discussed below. The following discussion is based upon the three broad categories of substitutes used in clinical practice: (1) cement pastes; (2) biomaterials replaced by bone; and (3) prefabricated polymers.

Cement pastes

Calcium phosphates

Resembling the inorganic form of bone, hydroxyapatite and related composites have been available for FDA-approved clinical use since 1994. Calcium phosphate substitutes have supplanted calcium sulfate variants due to their closer resemblance to bone, higher biocompatibility, and tendency to undergo less resorption. Two main forms are available for use: ceramic pastes and cement pastes. Ceramic hydroxyapatite constructs (e.g., Interpore, Interpore International, Irvine, CA), although difficult to mold, demonstrate less resorption and better osteoconduction than their cement counterparts, as demonstrated in a series of animal experimentation.[442] These authors were able to demonstrate that the higher the pore size, the greater degree of osteoconduction and osteoinduction, as substitutes composed of pure ceramic hydroxyapatite, or cement forms of higher TCP (80% TCP/20% hydroxyapatite) exhibited greater replacement by lamellar bone histologically.[442] The latter formulation was osteoinductive by virtue of the relatively high TCP content that yields to resorption and replacement by macropores. The cement form of this material has been quite popular, due to its biocompatibility, malleability, and relative ease of handling. Due to the limited scope of this chapter in this regard, only two major commercially available forms of bone cement will be discussed: BoneSource and Norian.

BoneSource

The first commercially available calcium phosphate cement,[443] BoneSource (Stryker Leibinger, Inc.) is based on a mixture of tetracalcium phosphate and dicalcium phosphate dehydrate and activated with water at a 4:1 ratio prior to use. After an isothermic reaction, the resulting paste can be contoured on the field, setting into pure hydroxyapatite within 20–25 minutes. Final set time is 4–6 hours.[444] A dry operative field is mandatory for this biomaterial to reach its final cured state. In this state, BoneSource achieves a compressive strength of 50 MPa and a diametral strength of 8 MPa.

BoneSource has been used over the years in numerous applications on the craniofacial skeleton. Providing one of the largest series to date, Burstein and colleagues[445] reviewed their experience with this product in 61 patients retrospectively (20-month mean follow-up). Inlay and onlay grafting were performed over a 3-year period. Postoperative complications were present in 11% of patients, mainly seromas. Interestingly, the authors used slow-release antibiotic therapy (1 gram cephalosporin mixed with 10 grams of cement prior to use). In another large trial in cranioplasty patients ($n = 103$),[446] an overall infection rate of 5.8% was achieved.

Norian SRS/CRS

Norian (Synthes, Inc.) is a unique carbonated calcium phosphate that mimics the inorganic phase of bone. Conferring solubility at a low pH, Norian has the theoretical advantage of resorption and replacement by true bone.[447] This calcium phosphate cement is produced intraoperatively by mixing a base powder (monocalcium sulfate, monohydrate, α-TCP, calcium carbonate) and a solvent containing sodium phosphate at room temperature.[448] After a 5-minute interval, the material becomes implantable, and continues to cure for approximately 24 hours to become a microporous polycrystalline apatite with a maximum compressive strength of 50 MPa and tensile strength of 2.1 MPa. For comparison, the compressive and tensile properties of cancellous bone are 1.9 and 2.42 MPa, respectively.[449] The commercial product is available in regular and fast-setting formulations.

FDA-approved since 1998, Norian CRS has now been subject to long-term clinical outcome analysis. Providing the largest series specific to this bone cement in the context of craniofacial surgery, Gilardino and colleagues[450] report a rather substantial complication rate (26% overall) when using this product, regardless of the type of cranioplasty (onlay, full-thickness inlay). The majority of complications were infectious, attributable to the sheer amount of material used, or its use in a contaminated field. Stratifying according to type of cranioplasty (inlay versus onlay), the authors report the following limitations with Norian: (1) increased trending complication rate when >25 cm^2 inlay defects are reconstructed with this bone cement; (2) statistically significant increased complication rate when onlay constructs were placed in areas of high bacterial contamination (paranasal sinuses). Such results indicate that this bone cement, not dissimilar to others, is likely not osteoconductive, as supported by several experimental studies.[451]

Osteoactive materials

Osteoactive materials include bioactive glass (Nova Bone, Porex Surgical Inc.) and DBM. Composed of silica dioxide, sodium dioxide, calcium dioxide and phosphate, bioactive glass confers its osteogenic properties when these components are mixed together to form an apatite surface layer. This layer recruits and stimulates osteoprogenitor cells to produce cytokines that have an autocrine and paracrine effect. Osteoblasts proliferate and differentiate on this surface, leading to new bone formation. In turn, the particulate glass is resorbed via osteoclastic activity.

The formulation that comprises DBM is based upon the landmark work of Urist and Strates[452] and Reddi and Huggins.[453] To date, manufacturers produce this bone substitute with the standard methodology: human cadaver long diaphyses are morselized to 250–600-mm particle sizes, demineralized in 0.6 N hydrochloric acid, and washed with deionized water, ethanol, and ethyl ether. In contrast to bioactive glass, DBM contains trace amounts of BMP, which makes this biomaterial both osteoconductive and osteoinductive. At baseline, however, DBM alone is hard to handle, making it difficult to apply clinically. In order to improve handling characteristics, manufacturers have added various types of carriers to the formulation (e.g., glycerol, gelatin, calcium sulfate). Therefore, not all preparations of DBM are the same. To this end, Acarturk and Hollinger[454] have performed comparative analysis of all the different DBM products. In an athymic rat critical-sized calvarial defect model, they found that there was indeed a differential bone-regenerative effect among the different formulations. One unifying principle was that those formulations that handled better (DBM + glycerol (Grafton, Osteotech, Inc.), DBM + hyaluronan (DBX, Synthes US)) demonstrated statistically significantly higher bone formation than other groups, as assessed by histomorphometry. Overall, however, the bone-regenerative capacity was not as robust as the authors predicted, which could be related to not achieving the threshold quantity of particulate DBM required for complete ossification of the defect.

Prefabricated polymers

Methylmethacrylate

An acrylic-based construct, methylmethacrylate[455–457] forms when a powdered mixture of methyl methacrylate polymer, methyl methacrylate-styrene copolymer, and benzoyl peroxide monomer is combined. The reaction is caustic, leading to an exothermia that approaches 85°C and pungent fumes that are carcinogenic. In fact, the premixing recommendations of this construct recommend use in an approved fume hood. After mixing for 8–10 minutes, the polymerization process yields a rigid, durable material that can be contoured, is radiolucent, and can be fixed rigidly to the cranioplasty site. Advantages of this material include a relatively low cost, possibility of *in situ* contouring, and lack of biodegradation. A prefabricated, customized, modified version of this material (Hard Tissue Replacement, Biomet Corporation, Jacksonville, FL) is composed of polymethylmethacrylate-polyhydroxyethyl methacrylate and available based on preoperative computed tomography data[458] (see below). The major drawback to acrylic-based resins, and in particular methylmethacrylate, is the substantial exothermic reaction involved in curing, which *in situ* can lead to severe thermal tissue injury. The cured, rigid substance has a high bacterial adhesion profile, and thus the high incidence of infected cranioplasties when using this substance.

Medpor

A high-density, porous polyethylene construct (pore size 100–250 mm), Medpor has gained some popularity in the reconstruction of select sites of the craniofacial skeleton. Current applications include nasal/malar augmentation, orbital floor reconstruction, genioplasty, and cranial augmentation. In this last application, Medpor has been found to augment successfully resorptive areas of the craniofacial skeleton (e.g., temporal fossa). Due to its porous nature, this implant permits native tissue ingrowth and therefore may provide some resistance to infection. Other advantages include the ability for intraoperative contouring, and customized prefabrication based on three-dimensional volumetric data (DICOM) from computed tomography. Despite these benefits, there are clear disadvantages to this material (risk of infection, exposure, extrusion) that limit its use to well-vascularized recipient sites. As with all alloplastic cranioplasties, an irradiated field bears a relative contraindication from the use of this implant.

Access the complete references list online at **http://www.expertconsult.com**

74. Deng ZL, Sharff KA, Tang N, et al. Regulation of osteogenic differentiation during skeletal development. *Front Biosci.* 2008;13:2001–2021.

   This paper provides an important review of skeletal development at molecular and genetic levels. Both the major signaling pathways involved with and the transcriptional control of osteogenic differentiation are detailed.

326. Ilizarov G. The tension-stress effect on the genesis and growth of tissues. Part I. The influence of stability of fixation and soft-tissue preservation. *Clin Orthop Relat Res.* 1989;238:249–281.

   This paper describes a pioneer study on distraction osteogenesis. Among other parameters, this study evaluated optimum conditions during limb lengthening as well as examined changes that occur in soft tissues that undergo elongation.

329. McCarthy JG, Schreiber J, Karp N, et al. Lengthening of the human mandible by gradual distraction. *Plast Reconstr Surg.* 1992;89:1–8; discussion 9–10.

   This paper describes a pioneer study on distraction osteogenesis of the craniofacial skeleton. Early evidence on the efficacy of bilateral mandibular distraction is described in the context of clinical experience.

333. Ilizarov G: The tension-stress effect on the genesis and growth of tissues. Part II. The influence of the rate and frequency of distraction. *Clin Orthop Relat Res.* 1989;239:263–285.

364. Chamay A, Tschantz P. Mechanical influences in bone remodeling. Experimental research on Wolff's law. *J Biomech.* 1972;5:173–180.

374. Finkemeier CG. Bone-grafting and bone-graft substitutes. *J Bone Joint Surg Am.* 2002;84-A:454–464.

   This paper reviews the concept of bone grafting and bone graft substitutes. Various options for bone grafting, including autologous bone grafts, allografts, and ceramic composites, are discussed.

378. Tessier P, Kawamoto H, Matthews D, et al. Autogenous bone grafts and bone substitutes – tools and techniques: I. A 20 000-case experience in maxillofacial and craniofacial surgery. *Plast Reconstr Surg.* 2005;116(suppl):6S–24S; discussion 92S–94S.

383. Tessier P, Kawamoto H, Matthews D, et al. Taking bone grafts from the anterior and posterior ilium – tools and techniques: II. A 6800-case experience in maxillofacial and craniofacial surgery. *Plast Reconstr Surg.* 2005;116(suppl):25S–37S; discussion 92S–94S.

   This paper reviews the use of the ilium for bone grafts. Advantages, disadvantages, and techniques regarding iliac graft use are discussed.

400. Weiland AJ, Phillips TW, Randolph MA. Bone grafts: A radiologic, histologic and biomechanical model comparing autografts, allografts and free vascularized bone grafts. *Plast Reconstr Surg.* 1984;74:368–379.

431. Stevenson S. Biology of bone grafts. *Orthop Clin North Am.* 1999;30:543–552.

22

Repair and grafting of peripheral nerve

Renata V. Weber, Kirsty U. Boyd, and Susan E. Mackinnon

SYNOPSIS

- Primary neurorrhaphy is the gold standard by which all other nerve repair techniques are judged.
- Primary repair, delayed primary repair, and secondary repair indicate timing of the repair with respect to the injury.
- Excessive tension will inhibit nerve regeneration; however a small amount of tension to achieve primary coaptation is acceptable.
- Nerve autograft is the gold standard for reconstructing a nerve gap.
- In the event of a nerve gap, options for repair include:
  - mobilization and primary coaptation
  - nerve repair with nerve graft or conduit
  - nerve transfers.
- Factors most affecting nerve recovery include:
  - age of the patient
  - location of injury (proximal versus distal peripheral nerve)
  - type of injury: crush versus avulsion versus transection
  - timing or repair
  - technique or repair (tension, alignment, scarring).

Introduction

Nerve repair and grafting have not significantly changed over the last several decades. The major advancements over the last 20 years have been in our understanding of the internal neural topography and tension at the neurorrhaphy site, advancement in suturing techniques, and the development of nerve transfers. While the future of nerve surgery holds exciting possibilities, the major limitation to peripheral nerve recovery is the time limit of nerve regeneration. This remains true regardless of the technique used for that repair. Without prompt motor nerve input, denervated muscle after a prolonged period of time becomes resistant to nerve regeneration. While we are able to help speed up the regenerative process to some extent, the ultimate success is dependent on several conditions, such as number of neurorrhaphy sites, supply and type of donor nerves, and the condition of the surrounding tissue. At every coaptation site, a percentage of nerve fibers are lost. Excessive tension is harmful to a repair site, and in the case of a large gap, a nerve graft is often used to fill in the deficit. Autologous nerve grafts are limited: the sural nerve is the most common source for autologous nerve graft. Alternatives to standard treatment include vein grafts, commercially available nerve conduits, nerve allografts, and nerve transfers. Schwann cell-lined nerve conduits and tissue-engineered substitutions are still experimental, but may offer the solution to enhanced nerve regeneration in the future.

Types of nerve injury

Nerve injury

A peripheral nerve injury can be classified in several ways. Historically, the first classification system by Sir Herbert Seddon (1943) was based on gross and

Table 22.1 Classification of nerve injury

Seddon	Sunderland	Injury	Recovery
Neurapraxia	Degree I	Conduction block resolves spontaneously	Fast/excellent
Axonotmesis	Degree II	Axonal rupture without interruption of the basal lamina tubes	Slow/excellent
	Degree III	Rupture of both axons and basal lamina tubes, some scar	Slow/incomplete
	Degree IV	Complete scar block	None
Neurotmesis	Degree V	Complete transection	None
	Degree VI (Mackinnon)	Combination of degree I–IV ± normal fascicles	Mixed

histologic anatomical changes rather than mechanism of injury.[1] He described three types of nerve injuries. Firstly, neurapraxia involves a local conduction block at a discrete area along the course of the nerve. Wallerian degeneration does not occur and the recovery is excellent. Secondly, axonotmesis implies direct axonal damage, while thirdly, neurotmesis is the transection of a peripheral nerve. In both axonetmesis and neurotmesis, wallerian degeneration occurs distal to the site of injury; however while the former recovers, the latter does not. Within axonotemesis, Seddon described a degree of injury associated with scarring and less complete recovery. Within neurotmesis he described an "in continuity," total scar, and no recovery injury. However it was Sunderland who expanded upon the earlier Seddon classification and emphasized five degrees of nerve injury.[2] Mackinnon later went on to include a sixth *(Table 22.1)*.[3,4] First-degree (neurapraxia) and second-degree (axonotmesis) injuries recover spontaneously, the latter at the classic rate of 1 inch (2.5 cm)/month or 1–1.5 mm/day.[5] Fourth- and fifth-degree injuries do not recover, while third- and sixth-degree injuries recover partially for different reasons. The difficulty with surgical correction of a sixth-degree injury is limiting the repair to the fascicles affected by fourth- and fifth-degree damage and not damaging fascicles with the potential for spontaneous recovery.

Nerve injuries can also be grouped by mechanism of injury and whether they are open or closed. This clinical classification is useful in evaluating nerve injuries, determining the likelihood for spontaneous recovery, and provides an algorithm for managing these injuries. *Table 22.2* lists the typical nerve injury patterns and their significance with respect to assessment and treatment. For simplicity, nerve injuries can be grouped as:

(1) penetrating injuries; (2) crush and compression injuries; and (3) stretch and avulsion injuries. While generally, avulsion and crush injuries tend to be closed injuries, they may be open. This implies a more severe force, is associated with soft-tissue, vascular, and orthopedic injuries and the extent of muscle and skin damage will ultimately influence the outcome of the nerve repair. More extensive soft-tissue and/or bony injuries raise the complexity as well as the likelihood for a staged reconstruction. Often, the nerve reconstruction is delayed in light of more acute vascular and orthopedic injuries.

Penetrating injuries

Penetrating trauma can be a result of sharp or blunt penetration, and will often have concomitant vascular structures and tendons injured in addition to the nerve. A sharp laceration, such as a hand laceration from a knife or piece of glass, will almost always necessitate exploration if a nerve deficit is present: the likelihood that the nerve is partially or completely transected is high. It is recommended to explore these injuries semielectively within the first week. The further from the time of injury, the less likely the two ends of the nerve can be mobilized enough to coapt primarily and the more likely a nerve graft will be needed to overcome a gap. In our practice, however, acute nerve grafting is frequently performed if there is concern about a degree of injury that would make it difficult to reoperate in the future. In the event of a penetrating trauma with an associated vascular injury, immediate exploration is warranted. Occasionally in proximal injuries with large arterial injuries with or without underlying fractures, the nerve injury is overlooked in the face of more urgent

Table 22.2 Classification of nerve injury by mechanism. The significance of each type of injury in terms of ability to repair and outcome is discussed

Type	May be injured	Significance
Stretch/avulsion injury		
Avulsion	Nerve roots Nerves exiting Foramen, bony fracture	Unable to be repaired primarily Indication for nerve transfer
Stretch	Any nerve	Mixed nerve injury (degree VI)
Crush and compression injury		
Injury		
Complex crush	Skin, subcutaneous Tissue, muscle, nerve, ± bone	Varying degree of depth, loss of function is related to amount of tissue destruction
Chronic compression	Nerve	Slow onset, reversible
Acute compression	Nerve ± muscle	Quick onset, reversible muscle ischemia, variable recovery of both muscle and nerve
Compartment syndrome	Nerve + muscle	Quick onset, reversible muscle ischemia if ischemia less than 6 hours; no or variable recovery of muscle if released after 6 hours
Penetrating injury		
Sharp	Skin, subcutaneous tissue, muscle, nerve ± bone All levels	Needs surgical exploration because of high probability of nerve severance
Blunt	Variable	Injury may extend further than expected
Blast	Variable	Injury pattern depends on ballistic makeup and velocity
Electrical	Variable	Neuropathy is from damage to myelin sheath and ranges from neuropathy to causalgia

vascular and orthopedic injuries. Rather, the deficit is noticed postoperatively, when it is unclear if the nerve injury is from the inciting event, iatrogenic during the repair of the vascular injury, or secondary to edema or hematoma. While a computed tomography scan or magnetic resonance imaging may be helpful to evaluate for the latter, internal scarring of the nerve may not always be clearly determined.

Blunt penetrating and blast injuries are usually treated conservatively, similar to closed crush and stretch injuries, because they are may recover spontaneously. The local-tissue edema often causes a neurapraxia that resolves; however, those that do not recover after 3 months should be evaluated by electrodiagnostic studies and the algorithm for traction or crush injury followed *(Fig. 22.1)*.

Crush injuries

Crush injuries comprise the most common peripheral nerve injuries to the extremity. External compression may be complicated by increased internal pressure from hematomas, fractures, and local tissue edema. When minor, this may cause a temporary neurapraxia, but with greater compression, the likelihood of a permanent injury increases. The most severe consequence of a crush injury is the progression to compartment syndrome, which is a surgical emergency. Often an early sign of impending compartment syndrome is a decrease in vibration sensibility.[6] Compartment syndrome is discussed in greater detail in another chapter.

While nerves are fairly resistant to injury, especially when the surrounding tissue is not significantly

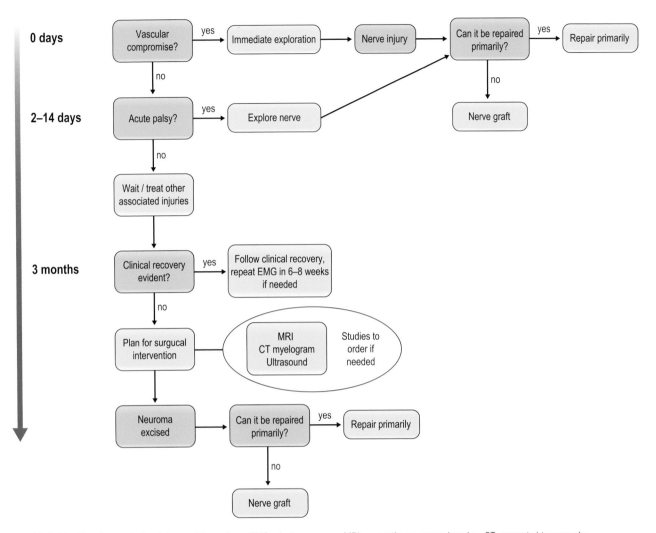

Fig. 22.1 Algorithm for penetrating injury and lacerations. EMG, electromyogram; MRI, magnetic resonance imaging; CT, computed tomography.

damaged, a mixed nerve injury can often occur. A more extensive crush injury can cause local tissue damage that contributes more to the loss of function than the nerve injury. Muscle tissue is the most susceptible to external forces. Even if the injury is not significant enough to cause a compartment syndrome, the local destruction of muscle may lead to muscle death. Tendon and skin are more resistant and can withstand higher compressive forces before irreversible damage to the cells results.

The nerve portion of the injury is usually treated conservatively and exploration is warranted if the nerve recovery does not follow an expected pattern. Along with avulsion injuries, the algorithm is to follow recovery for 3–4 months and intervene if the expected recovery does not appear to be forthcoming *(Fig. 22.2)*.

Stretch and nerve avulsion injuries

Stretch injuries occur because the strain on the nerve exceeds the maximum limit and the internal structure of the nerve becomes injured without any appreciable external evidence of injury.

Nerves that are stretched to the point of avulsing from the proximal end suggest a high-velocity or high-impact injury that is often associated with limb-threatening injuries that take precedence over the nerve injury. The nerves tend to be avulsed around areas of tethering, such as bony foramina and the spinal cord. If the proximal nerve can be accessed, as in injuries of the obturator nerve in the pelvis, a graft can be placed through the orifice and a neurorrhaphy with nerve graft may be performed. For areas such as the cranial nerves

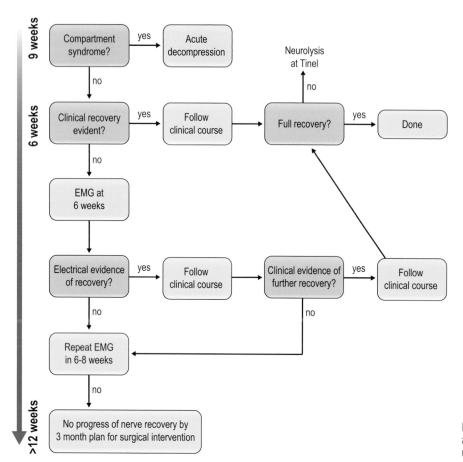

Fig. 22.2 Algorithm for closed traction, stretch, and avulsion injuries. EMG, electromyogram; MUPs or nascent units.

or the spinal roots, where the portion proximal to the avulsion is either central nervous tissue or inaccessible due to skeletal constraints, reconstruction is done via nerve transfers.[7] Our current surgical algorithm focuses on nerve reconstruction first, followed by tendon transfers and associated procedures to augment or complement the nerve reconstruction when warranted *(Fig. 22.2).*[8]

Nerves avulsed at the neuromuscular junction present a different problem, as the distal end is unavailable. In the case of motor nerves that are avulsed from the muscle bellies, implantation of the proximal nerve directly into the muscle is the alternative when no distal end is available. Some studies show as good as M4 motor recovery 1–2 years after direct nerve to muscle neurotization[9]; however, experimental studies do not support these findings; rather, recovery is much less than a nerve coaptation would produce.[10]

Hint: Sharp injuries with acute nerve deficit should be explored early (within 1 week) in order to be able to perform a primary neurorrhaphy. Crush and traction injuries should be treated conservatively with serial exams and electromyograms (EMGs) at 3 months if no clinical evidence of recovery is noted.

Evaluation of nerve injuries

A thorough physical exam remains the most reliable method for determining the neurologic defect. Sensation, or lack thereof, can be tested using Semmes–Weinstein filaments, two-point static and moving discrimination, or the "ten test." The quick and easy ten test sensory exam uses the patient's own subjective perception to moving light touch in order to elicit differences in sensation.[11] For example, to test for a median nerve injury, both the injured and uninjured index fingers of the patient are touched at the same time over corresponding areas of each finger and the patient is asked if the subjective sensation is the same or different. This technique is particularly useful in young children who may not be able to cooperate with a two-point discrimination test.

In patients who present with an acute motor deficit or palsy, determining if the nerve will recover spontaneously or if surgical intervention is needed can often be difficult. The mechanism of the injury can often assist in the preoperative evaluation. Any sharp penetrating injury with no clinical evidence of recovery should be explored. Optimal timing is 0–7 days, as long as the patient is surgically stable and a skilled surgical team is available. Any injury where there is a high index of suspicion of nerve transection should be explored and repaired. The advantage of repair within the first 2 weeks of injury is that at this early time point the nerve ends have not retracted and primary neurorrhaphy is often possible.

Closed traction injuries, partial avulsion, and crush injuries with palsy are more difficult to evaluate. Waiting 3–4 months with serial physical examinations to assess for evidence of spontaneous recovery is recommended. At 3 months, electrodiagnostic testing is advised when no clinical recovery is evident as EMG changes precede clinical recovery. If there is no evidence of reinnervation occurring by 3 months (e.g., motor unit potentials), surgical exploration and reconstruction are warranted.

There are clinical investigations using newer ultrasound machines that can detect digital nerve neuromas; however these studies are still investigational and are highly operator-dependent.

Hints: We prefer to evaluate the patient early and follow the clinical exam, as well as ordering electrodiagnostic testing, in order to minimize delay in recognizing a nerve deficit that will not resolve spontaneously.

Nerve repair

Timing of repair

When there is a high index of suspicion that a nerve transection exists, there is no reason to wait as long as the patient is clinically stable and able to be taken to the operating room for exploration and repair of the nerve. Nerves repaired acutely within the first 2 days are considered repaired primarily. A delayed primary repair occurs between 2 and 7 days. In either case, the proximal and distal ends of the nerve are freshened and an end-to-end coaptation performed. Nerves repaired after the first week are considered repaired secondarily.

Clearly these cut-off days of 2 and 7 are arbitrary numbers. Often even at 2–3 weeks from injury, the nerve can be coapted without need for a graft; however, the longer the time from injury, the less likely that a primary neurorrhaphy can be achieved, even with significant mobilization of the proximal and distal nerve ends.

Tension and nerve repair

Excessive tension across a nerve repair is known to increase the scarring at the coaptation site and impair regeneration. In an uninjured nerve, a 15% strain of the nerve causes a reduction in microvascular flow and, for an hour after relaxation, a delay of peak velocity to 66% of initial value persists.[12] Mild tension, on the other hand, is actually believed to be beneficial to the repair by stimulating neurotropic growth factors.

In clinical practice we do not formally measure the tension across a neurorrhaphy; however we always avoid tension on a repair. The two ends of a nerve are mobilized in order to bring the ends in reasonable approximation. Strain on the nerve decreases the microcirculation and excessive tension will cause the repair to break down. In addition, tricks such as positioning the arm in adduction or placing the wrist and fingers in flexion will significantly decrease the tension across the repair depending on the location of the injury and may increase the total length of available nerve; however, we recommend avoiding postural manipulation in order to force primary repair. Not only can dehiscence occur when the joint near the repair is moved too early, but it may create significant stiffness from prolonged immobilization.[13] An immobilized nerve also results in scarring at the repair site.

Type of repair: epineural versus fascicular

Any repair that withstands gentle range of motion is considered a "tension-free" repair. Giddins et al.[14] showed in a cadaveric study comparing suture size to the strength of an acute repair of the median nerve that 9–0 nylon withstood the greatest distractive forces. At a lower tension 10–0 snapped, and 8–0 sutures pulled out of the nerve tissue. However, in clinical practice, 10–0 and 8–0 sutures are often used based on the size of the nerve, the thickness of the epineurium, and the amount of inflammation.

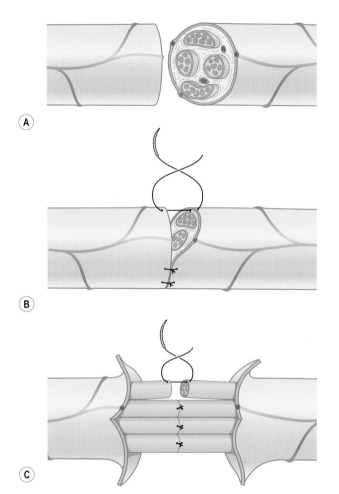

Fig. 22.3 Schematic depicting an epineural **(B)** versus perineural **(C)** repair after transection of the nerve **(A)**. The native artery and the fascicular pattern are used to align the neurorrhaphy properly. The least number of epineural sutures using 8–0, 9–0, or 10–0 nylon is used.

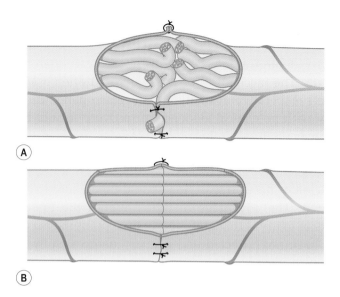

Fig. 22.4 **(A, B)** Alignment of the fascicles is crucial to optimal outcome.

Alternatively some surgeons use fibrin glue, especially when there is no tension in the repair. Laser energy for epineurial coaptation has been investigated experimentally; however it produces heat that damages nerve tissue and results in unacceptably decreased tensile strength at the repair site. The gold standard remains microsuture applied under microscope control.

Epineural repair is the preferred method of repair once the severed ends are freshened surgically. External markers such as a vessel on the surface and matching the fascicular patterns are used to align the fascicles without overlapping *(Fig. 22.3)*. For major peripheral nerves, an argument for perineural repair can be made to improve alignment of the larger fascicular groups individually; however, clinical studies support both techniques as equally effective as long as the fascicles were not overlapped *(Fig. 22.4)*.[15] The disadvantage of a perineural repair is that the extensive dissection and the permanent intraneural stitches can lead to increase fibrosis.[16] In practice, it is often difficult to align the fascicles accurately, as trauma, edema, and scarring can distort the normal topography.

Our preferred method for repair is an epineural repair using the native artery as a guide *(Fig. 22.2)*. The least number of epineural sutures using 8–0, 9–0, or 10–0 nylon to approximate and keep the repair intact through a full range of motion is used.

Type of repair: end-to-end versus end-to-side

Most nerve repairs are performed end-to-end. This is irrespective of primary neurorrhaphy or a nerve graft repair. The controversy of end-to-side repair continues to be debated. Currently, we recommend end-to-end repair for all motor, mixed nerves and sensory nerves in critical distributions. We use sensory end-to-side repair for noncritical sensory nerves, such as the dorsal cutaneous branch of the ulnar nerve. We also use end-to-side to restore sensation to a donor sensory nerve graft territory, such as transferring the distal end of the medial antebrachial cutaneous to the sensory (lateral) side of the median nerve.

When we do sensory end-to-end transfers (for example, the third web space median to ulnar sensory), we do an end-to-side of the distal end of the donor nerve to an adjacent normal sensory nerve. This transfer is conducted to restore sensation in the donor nerve distribution.

With respect to motor end-to-side, we know that motor axons, unlike sensory axons, will not spontaneously collateral sprout; the axons must be injured for "traumatic" sprouting to occur.[17] We therefore rarely use this technique. One setting where this technique is employed is for suprascapular nerve reconstruction, where partial neurectomy and proximal crush of the accessory nerve are performed with an end-to-side nerve transfer. This allows reinnervation of the suprascapular nerve and still preserves some function in the trapezius muscle.

Intraoperative nerve stimulation

For uncomplicated nerve injuries such as a transection or a neuroma in continuity involving the entire cross-section of the nerve in which the surgical plan is to resect the entire scarred tissue and repair or reconstruct, intraoperative nerve stimulation may not be useful; however, in closed traction injuries, especially of the brachial plexus or injuries to larger mixed peripheral nerves in the extremities that have variable recovery, formal intraoperative monitoring or a handheld nerve stimulator may offer guidance in surgical decision-making. If the nerve is injured at several segments along its length, or in the case of a partial brachial plexus injury, we will often use formal intraoperative nerve mapping to assist in the surgical decision-making. In addition, we use formal intraoperative electrical stimulation in cases where the preoperative EMG results were equivocal or that additional recovery may have occurred between the time of the previous study and the operation, since the results may affect the surgical plan.

A handheld nerve stimulator, which provides muscle contraction but no information about sensory recovery, is used when motor nerve transfers are performed. It allows us to pick out grossly redundant motor nerve fascicles, which will be spliced into nonfunctioning motor nerves to restore animation. For routine lacerations that require grafting or primary repair, there is no additional benefit to the use of nerve stimulation, unless it is performed in motor and mixed motor nerves transected and repaired within 72 hours. For a partial nerve injury with neuroma involving only a portion of the nerve's cross-sectional area, a nerve stimulator can help determine which nerve fascicles to preserve while resecting the damaged tissue. In nerves that are purely or mostly sensory fibers, a handheld nerve stimulator is not useful.

Factors affecting outcome

Several factors will affect nerve repair. The age of the patient seems to be the most predominant factor. We know from historical data that nerve repair in children and young adults (sensory and motor) yields better results than in adults. In part, this is due to the fact that children are smaller, thus if nerve regeneration is 1–1.5 mm/day, a child's nerve is expected to recovery sooner than an adult's because of the shorter distance to the target organ, whether it is muscle for a motor nerve or a sensory receptor for a sensory nerve. A child's brain plasticity has an equally important role in the overall outcome, since children's ability to process the reinnervated motor and sensory within the brain cortex is more facile than an adult's.

The degree and type of injury also affect outcome. Proximal injuries are usually mixed nerves containing both motor and sensory fibers. Reconstructing these larger nerves with optimal alignment is more difficult than distal nerves that are more likely to be "pure" sensory or motor. Crush and avulsion injuries are more likely to have associated soft-tissue injuries and thus tend to be worse than a sharp injury occurring at the same level. The internal damage of the nerve is often underestimated acutely and poor recovery is usually a result of repair within the zone of injury when re-explored.

The timing of repair historically revealed that earlier repair led to better prognosis, most likely because a primary neurorrhaphy was possible. Good prognosis is expected if the repair occurs before 6 months, and best results occur if the repair is performed before 3 weeks. In general, functional recovery (FR) is inversely proportional to the time of denervation, and directly proportional to the number of motor axons reaching the target endplate. "Time is muscle."

$$FR \, \alpha \, \frac{\text{Number of motor axons reaching target endplate}}{\text{Time of denervation}}$$

Bridging the gap: current techniques

Prompt primary neurorrhaphy is universally held as the ideal repair, and multiple animal studies support the idea that a single nerve repair results in a better outcome over a nerve repaired with two neurorrhaphy sites.[18] Since at each repair site, a percentage of fibers are lost, fewer neurorrhaphies ensure a greater percentage of proximal nerve axons reaching the target organ. Some investigators believe that as many as 50% of regenerating sensory or motor axons may never reach the correct end organ.[19] However, the key points for a nerve repair are excellent microneurosurgical technique to avoid tension, doing the repair outside the zone of injury, matching accurately sensory/motor topography, and early controlled movement to allow neural gliding.

In the event that a primary neurorrhaphy is not immediately possible, mobilization of the nerve ends may overcome a small (less then 5 mm) gap because of the elastic property of a nerve.[20] If the repair is performed in the face of extreme tension and contamination, unfavorable scarring will occur. In this case, two neurorrhaphy sites under favorable conditions are preferable to a single neurorrhaphy under unfavorable conditions.[13,21] If primary repair by mobilization and elongation cannot be achieved, there are several techniques to address the resultant nerve graft *(Table 22.3)*.[22] The most common technique for repairing defects in peripheral nerves is autologous nerve grafts.

A nerve graft serves as a guide for the axon as it regrows toward the distal stump. The sural nerve is the most commonly used donor nerve, although other suitable donor nerves include the lateral and medial antebrachial cutaneous nerve distal sensory end of the posterior interosseous nerve, and the terminal portion of the anterior interosseous nerve.[23–25] Our favored donor graft for upper extremity reconstruction is the medial antebrachial cutaneous. Experimental studies comparing motor, mixed, and sensory nerve grafts support the idea that motor and mixed nerve grafts achieve better regeneration across the repair.[26,27] However, motor nerve grafts exist in even more limited supply and, in clinical practice, the gracilis muscle nerve and the distal anterior interosseous nerve are the two motor grafts that cause the least morbidity.

Current practices that account for the success of nerve grafts include the use of small thin grafts that are cabled when necessary. Historically, when full-thickness nerve trunks were used as grafts, poor results ensued.[28] For the graft to be successful, it must survive long enough for the nerve to regenerate through it. Small, thin grafts revascularize more easily than larger nerves, and this contributes to the success of functional outcome. No agreement exists on the maximum length that may be bridged by a nerve graft; however, 20 cm and longer nerve grafts have been used with varying degrees of success.[29,30] Free vascularized nerve grafts were introduced in 1976 by Taylor and Ham in order to treat these longer gaps.[31] For smaller defects, a vascularized graft and conventional graft do not appear to differ in clinical outcome; however, Doi *et al.*[32] recommend using free vascularized nerve grafts when the gap distance is greater than 6 cm with associated soft-tissue loss over the repaired area. Currently the indication for a free vascularized nerve graft is for reconstruction of large-diameter nerve grafts, such as the ulnar nerve in brachial plexus avulsion surgery.[33,34]

While nerve grafts are the standard by which gaps are reconstructed, the major disadvantages are the limited number of donor nerves available and the resulting donor site morbidity. This has led to the development of new techniques for bridging the nerve gap, including vein grafts, biological and synthetic conduits, and nerve allograft. Current consensus is that for a sensory deficit less than 3 cm, any of these options is equally reliable.[35]

Nerves repaired with a sutureless technique are usually wrapped at the neurorrhaphy site with a nerve guide or vein wrap and then covered with fibrin glue. This is especially useful if there is a slight mismatch in size, as in the setting of a nerve transfer, or if two smaller nerves are coapted to one larger nerve.

Autologous vein grafts are the oldest conduit and are still used both as a primary conduit and as a wrap.[35] Biological conduits, including bone, artery, collagen,[36] and muscle,[37] have been used but are not as conventionally used as vein or small-intestine submucosa.[38] Biodegradable synthetic conduits such as polyglycolic acid are currently used, while nondegradable nerve guides made from silicone have also fallen out of favor.[39] Their major disadvantage is leaving foreign material

Table 22.3 Options for management of the nerve gap

	Advantages	Disadvantages
Nerve autograft	Gold standard for reconstruction Schwann cells in extra cellular matrix	Second operative site Results in donor sensory loss Potential for neuroma formation/pain Sensory nerve autografts do not support motor regeneration as well as motor or mixed sensorimotor nerves Limited available length
Allograft	Can potentially allow functional recovery equivalent to autograft No donor site morbidity	Requires patient systemic immunosuppression (~18 months) Patients vulnerable to opportunistic infections
Conduits	Circumvents adverse effects of autografts and allografts Guides regenerating nerve to intended target	Length limitation (<3 cm) Only for small-diameter sensory nerves No Schwann cells No matrix Expensive
Acellularized graft	Retains scaffolding matrix of nerve tissue Nonimmunogeneic and inert Biological substrate for nerve regeneration without need for immunosuppression	Length limitation (<5 cm) No Schwann cells Only for small-diameter nerves Very expensive
End-to-side	No length limitation	Poor sensory results Motor requires donor neurectomy
Reverseend-to-side	Augment partial motor/sensory nerve injury	Requires knowledge of topography Requires knowledge of expendable donors May need nerve autograft or acellular graft
Nervetransfer	Earlier motor/sensory target recovery	Requires expendable donor Requires motor (sensory) re-education Requires knowledge of nerve topography

that potentially causes a chronic reaction with excessive scarring.

All of these conduits can be used as primary conduits or as nerve wraps. Nerve conduits may be used in sensory nerve gaps less than 3 cm, and are not recommended for longer gaps or in motor defects. They provide at least protective sensation and, in some cases, good sensory recovery.[40] When using the conduit, at least 5 mm of the nerve should be inserted into the conduit to minimize the risk for pull-out of either end of the nerve *(Fig. 22.5)*. The nerve can either be sutured to the conduit or laid in place and secured with a sealant, such as one of the fibrin glue products available. When using a conduit, we recommend placing a small portion of the proximal nerve into the conduit to provide a source of Schwann cells.

Since the request for nerve wraps has increased many nerve tube companies offer nerve wraps in addition to the conduit. In cases where a primary repair is performed but there is concern that motion may disassociate the repair, a nerve wrap offers the protection of a covering in the event the neurorrhaphy separates but stays within the tube and allows for the possibility that nerve recovery may still occur. The newer nerve wraps are thinner than the standard conduits and are usually pre-cut to allow easier application around the nerve *(Fig. 22.6)*. We have also used Seprafilm adhesion barrier (Genzyme, Cambridge, MA) as a "nerve wrap," placing a small piece above and below the repair.

Because these tubes have no structure, experimental studies have shown that placing morselized nerve into the tube can help to augment nerve growth.[41] Most recently, acellular human processed nerve allografts have been introduced as an alternative to conduits. Initial clinical trials show that the recovery for small sensory gaps is better than conduits and more comparable to autografts.[42] Because this is human tissue, it retains its three-dimensional structure, including

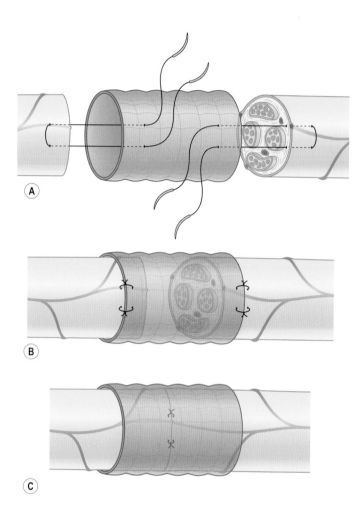

Fig. 22.5 When a neural tube is used to bridge a nerve gap **(A)**, a nerve tube slightly wider than the diameter of the nerve is chosen. A simple or horizontal mattress suture is placed to secure the epineurium to the edge of the neural tube, tucking in the end of the nerve about 2–5 mm within the tube to prevent dislodgement of either end **(B)**. When used to cover a neurorrhaphy site, the tube may be slid over one end of the nerve prior to suturing the nerve, then slid back over the neurorrhaphy site to protect the repair, or it can be cut longitudinally and wrapped around the neurorrhaphy site. A suture may be placed around the outside of the conduit to help keep it in place **(C)**.

epineurium, fascicles, endoneural tubes, and laminin, and it is believed that the scaffold allows for repopulation of the host cells similarly to autologous nerve tissue *(Fig. 22.7)*. The product is expensive at longer lengths but competitive with conduits for the 15 mm lengths. It shortens operative time and eliminates a donor deficit. It handles similarly to autologous nerve, comes in various widths (ranging from 1 to 5 mm) and lengths (ranging from 15 to 50 mm), and may be sutured in place or aligned and secured in place with a sealant such as fibrin glue. In addition, the neurorrhaphy site may also be covered by a nerve wrap such as in the case of autologous nerve repair.

A recent study by Whitlock et al.[43] showed that the acellular allograft with its extracellular matrix was superior to an empty conduit, but inferior to an autograft (which provides not only extracellular matrix but also Schwann cells). We use acellular allografts for short gaps (5–10 mm), small-diameter nerve gaps, noncritical nerve gaps, and nerve gaps in which a conduit could be safely used. Otherwise we prefer nerve autografts.

Nerve transfer: alternative to conduits

A nerve gap easily repaired with a graft or neural tube should be treated in the standard fashion; however, when the nerve injury is more complicated than a gap in nerve tissue, nerve transfers now offer the ability to repair injuries that prior to the 1990s were largely thought to be irreparable. The procedure has a higher learning curve than a standard nerve repair and should be reserved for situations such as those listed in *Box 22.1*.

Motor nerve transfers grew out of the knowledge of tendon transfers, are modeled after their analogous tendon transfers, and thus have some similar principles. Only expendable nerve fascicles are used. Nerves with redundant fascicles or branches make excellent donor nerves. Unlike a tendon transfer, a nerve transfer does not rely on amplitude and excursion of the tendon muscle unit, nor is it limited to the one tendon, one function and the straight line of pull principles. The type of muscle fiber unit and the insertion of the tendon will influence the ultimate effectiveness of that muscle's contraction in its new position.[44,45] The major advantages of a nerve transfer over that of a tendon transfer are that: (1) nerve transfers can restore sensibility in addition to motor function; (2) a nerve that innervates multiple muscle groups can be restored with a single nerve transfer; and (3) the insertion and attachments of the muscle(s) in question are not disrupted, thus the original muscle function and tension are maintained. While a synergistic nerve transfer is ideal, antagonistic nerve transfers can be successfully utilized in some cases such as branches of radial nerve used to restore median nerve function.

A significant advantage of nerve transfers over long nerve grafts is the ability to convert a proximal

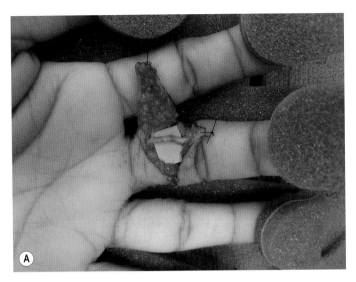

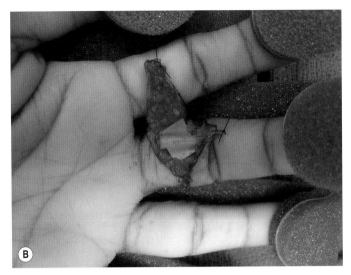

Fig. 22.6 The nerve is repaired primarily **(A)** and the wrap is placed over the repair **(B)** to protect it. The wraps are more translucent than the conduits and the suture of the primary repair is seen through the wrap.

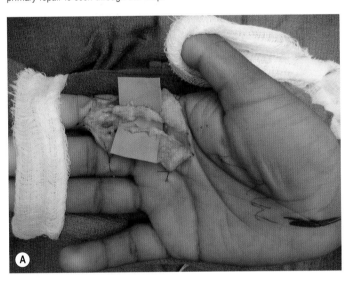

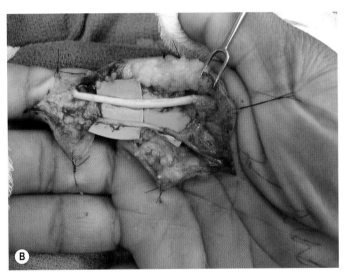

Fig. 22.7 The nerve allograft **(B)** can be chosen to match the width of the injured nerve. Here are two different size grafts that were sutured in place with 9–0 nylon sutures after resection of two digital-nerve neuromas **(A)**.

Box 22.1 Indications for nerve transfers

1. Brachial plexus injury with only very proximal or no nerve available for grafting
2. High proximal injury that requires a long distance for regeneration
3. Scarred areas in critical locations with potential for injury to critical structures
4. Major limb trauma with segmental loss of nerve tissue requiring several grafts
5. Prolonged time from injury to reconstruction as an alternative to nerve grafting
6. Partial nerve injury with a defined functional loss
7. Spinal cord root avulsion injury
8. Idiopathic neuritides, radiation trauma, and nerve injuries where the level of injury is uncertain

high-level nerve injury to a low-level nerve injury. This is especially important in high median nerve and ulnar nerve injuries. The donor nerves close to the injured nerve as well as to the motor end-plate are selected, and nerve grafts are rarely needed in addition to a nerve transfer. An internal neurolysis allows for separation of donor and recipient fascicles from the main nerve so that an end-to-end repair is performed. Nerve transfers will be discussed in greater detail in another chapter.

When choosing donor nerves for transfer, a nerve that innervates a synergistic muscle group is preferable, as it facilitates postoperative re-education. While a nerve supplying a nonsynergistic, or even antagonistic, muscle group may be used, more motor retraining may be necessary to learn to contract the newly reinnervated muscle.

Our preferred method for the neurorrhaphy is an end-to-end repair. As previously discussed, there are increasingly common instances where we do perform a nerve transfer with an end-to-side neurorrhaphy.[7] Our experimental studies show that, while sensory nerves will spontaneously sprout from an epineural or perineural window, a motor nerve requires a partial neurectomy to facilitate end-to-side regeneration.[46] Sensory nerve transfers developed as a natural extension of motor nerve transfers.

Nerve transfers are possible in part because of the redundancy existing in proximal mixed nerve fibers. Knowledge of the internal topography facilitates the separation of fascicle groups even in the proximal extremity. Whereas in the past it was believed that nerve fibers to a distinct fascicular group remained separate proximally and merged distally, closer to the target organ, we now know that these fibers run adjacent to each other even in the proximal limb, albeit following extensive plexus pathways.[47] Motor fibers for specific distal function are grouped together and thus can be electrically identified intraoperatively when being selected for possible nerve transfer.

Bioengineering: the future?

On the horizon is the bioengineering of neural tubes to be populated with Schwann cells and neurotrophic agents in order to facilitate the regenerative process. Trophic (growth-promoting) factors studied include nerve growth factor, brain-derived neurotrophic factor, fibroblastic growth factors, ciliary neurotrophic factor, and interleukin-6, among others.[48,49] The mechanism by which these growth factors stimulate axonal regeneration is not yet clear, nor the timing of their effects, although many of these growth factors and cytokines are released into the surrounding tissues after a nerve injury. In theory, a gap at the nerve repair site should allow budding axons to identify the target end organ correctly; investigations have shown that optimal nerve regeneration requires tightly coapted nerves with

no gap and with accurate alignment.[50] Finally, the ability of certain axon membrane glycoproteins to attract either motor or sensory axons preferentially has been investigated as a method of guiding nerve regeneration.[51]

The ultimate bioengineered nerve conduit will be able to enhance regeneration, block invasion of scar tissue and autodegrade when it is no longer needed. Schwann cells inside a conduit are known to improve nerve regeneration, and early clinical trials of Schwann cell-lined neural tubes are in progress. Growth factors have been studied to determine the usefulness and timing of the doses. Insulin-derived growth factor[52] does not promote nerve regeneration through a nerve guide, while nerve growth factor[53] and fibroblastic growth factor[54] showed enhanced nerve regeneration across the guide. External modalities to enhance nerve regeneration include the use of pulsed electromagnetic fields. The rate of regeneration is not increased; however, the number of motor neurons as well as their ability to reach the target organ are significantly improved.[55] It appears to be driven by an upregulation of brain-derived neurotrophic factor.[56] At present there is no benign modality for increasing the rate at which a nerve regenerates; however, the ability to alter the rate at which the motor end plates resorb has been experimentally possible. Leupeptin, a calpain inhibitor, blocks the calpain protease-mediated absorption of the motor end-plates, and may offer an important advancement in nerve repair and nerve recovery at the peripheral and spinal cord level.[57]

Postoperative management

After simple neurorrhaphy, we immobilize the area for 1–2 weeks, but start gentle protected range of motion at 2–3 days. We believe that early, protected range of motion is critical for neural gliding and an excellent result. At the time of primary nerve repair, we assess the degree of movement tolerated without providing tension at the repair site. This guides our protected range of motion, which begins within 2–3 days. In patients with concomitant tendon or bony injuries, the postoperative protocol is guided by the injury most difficult to rehabilitate. For example, in finger lacerations in which both tendon and nerves are transected, a flexor tendon protocol is followed postoperatively in order to maximize tendon gliding. The nerve repair, while important, is easier to reconstruct if necessary later. In the case of fractures in addition to nerve and soft-tissue injures, the bony fixation takes precedence.

No consensus exists on what length of time for immobilization is necessary. One clinical study suggests that early range of motion may not be as detrimental to the long-term results as previously believed. Patients with isolated digital nerve injuries were compared to patients with patients with combined flexor tendon and digital nerve injuries. The patients with isolated nerve injuries were immobilized for 21 days, while patients with combined injuries were started on protected motion at around 4 days postoperatively. At follow-up, the repaired nerve had less sensibility than the uninjured nerve. There was no significant difference in final two-point discrimination and Semmes–Weinstein testing between the two repaired groups, challenging the long-held belief that nerve repairs should be completely immobilized after surgery.[58]

Most patients complain in the postoperative period of paresthesia and electrical shocks, which extend beyond the area of the injury. Most of these can be controlled with neurotropic medications such as nortriptyline, gabapentin, or pregabalin. In some patients, the recovering nerve pains are so severe, they require significant narcotic and neuroleptic medications and the involvement of a pain specialist becomes paramount to managing the associated chronic pain these patients experience. Physical therapy and occupational therapy continue for an extended rehabilitative period to prevent joint contractures while the nerve recovery is in progress, to fabricate and adjust protective splints, and to assist in motor and sensory re-education as the recovery process is underway.

Summary

Primary neurorrhaphy remains the gold standard for all nerve repair techniques, while an autologous nerve autograft is the gold standard for bridging a nerve defect. Since the first implementation of a nerve allograft in 1870 by Philipeaux and Vulpian, significant contributions regarding suturing technique, neural topography, and the biology of nerve regeneration have transformed the way we approach nerve reconstruction. While primary neurorrhaphy and autografts are the most common methods for repair, several newer options are at our disposal. Nerve transfers have revolutionized our approach for treating from devastating brachial plexus injuries converting them to highly selected upper and lower motor and sensory nerve injuries. Nerve allografts and conduits offer alternatives to autologous nerve grafting when needed. Bioengineering of nerves and conduits, as well as therapies to augment the regenerative properties of the peripheral nerve, is the current issue being investigated in academia and industry. Breaking these barriers of nerve regeneration limitation will push peripheral nerve surgery to the next level.

 Access the complete reference list online at **http://www.expertconsult.com**

14. Giddins GE, Wade PJ, Amis AA. Primary nerve repair: strength of repair with different gauges of nylon suture material. *J Hand Surg Br*. 1989;14:301–302.

15. Cabaud HE, Rodkey WG, McCarroll Jr HR, et al. Epineurial and perineurial fascicular nerve repairs: a critical comparison. *J Hand Surg Am*. 1976;1: 131–137.

17. Hayashi A, Pannucci C, Moradzadeh A, et al. Axotomy or compression is required for axonal sprouting following end-to-side neurorrhaphy. *Exp Neurol*. 2008;211:539–550.

22. Ray WZ, Mackinnon SE. Management of nerve gaps: autografts, allografts, nerve transfers, and end-to-side neurorrhaphy. *Exp Neurol*. 2010;223:77–85.
    This is an up-to-date review of the key pros and cons of reconstruction with nerve autografts, acellularized allografts, cadaver allografts, and nerve conduits. It also reviews end-to-side reconstruction and nerve transfers. Indications for each of these various techniques are provided.

24. Myckatyn TM, Mackinnon SE. Surgical techniques of nerve grafting (standard/vascularized/allograft). *Oper Tech Orthop*. 2004;14:171–178.

This review article nicely summarizes the neurophysiology of nerve regeneration and explains the surgical benefits of autograft versus vascularized autograft versus cadaver allograft.

27. Moradzadeh A, Borschel GH, Luciano JP, et al. The impact of motor and sensory nerve architecture on nerve regeneration. *Exp Neurol.* 2008;212:370–376.

35. Chiu DT, Strauch B. A prospective clinical evaluation of autogenous vein grafts used as a nerve conduit for distal sensory nerve defects of 3 cm or less. *Plast Reconstr Surg.* 1990;86:928–934.

40. Weber RA, Breidenbach WC, Brown RE, et al. A randomized prospective study of polyglycolic acid conduits for digital nerve reconstruction in humans. *Plast Reconstr Surg.* 2000;106:1036–1045; discussion 1046–8.

42. Karabekmez FE, Duymaz A, Moran SL. Early clinical outcomes with the use of decellularized nerve allograft for repair of sensory defects within the hand. *Hand (N Y).* 2009;4:245–249.

43. Whitlock EL, Tuffaha SH, Luciano JP, et al. Processed allografts and type I collagen conduits for repair of peripheral nerve gaps. *Muscle Nerve.* 2009;39: 787–799.

47. Brandt KE, Mackinnon SE. Microsurgical repair of peripheral nerves and nerve grafts. In: Aston SJ, Beasley RW, Thorne CHM, eds. *Grabb and Smiths' Plastic Surgery.* New York: Lippincott-Raven; 1997:79–90.

This book chapter nicely explains the key aspects of peripheral nerve repair and nerve graft. It is an excellent review for both residents and attendings.

23

Vascular territories

Steven F. Morris and G. Ian Taylor

SYNOPSIS

- This chapter provides an overview of the angiosome concept and reviews the vascular anatomy of the body. The historical perspective summarizes the major progress in understanding the vascular basis and clinical applications of flap in reconstructive surgery

- The anatomical basis of angiosomes, choke anastomotic vessels, arterial territories, and venous drainage of the human body are summarized. The neurovascular territories of skin and muscle are described. Comparisons with other species highlight the consistent features of vascular anatomy of the human body and illustrate the need to be aware of the vascular anatomy of animal flap models

- The vascular anatomy of skin, muscle, and bone of each region of the body is discussed with an emphasis on flap design, avoiding surgical complications and providing an overview of angiosomes of the body

- The general concepts of the vascular supply to tissues of the body are reviewed. The importance of these concepts to flap design is highlighted with clinical examples. These concepts also provide the basis for interpreting physiologic and pathologic events in skin flaps

- The overall architecture of the vasculature of the human body is consistent but there is significant variability which requires a versatile operative plan for successful flap design. Methods of preoperative assessment of vascular anatomy and types of flaps, including skin, fasciocutaneous, musculocutaneous and perforator flaps, are reviewed. The basis of the delay phenomenon and procedure is explored.

Access the Historical Perspective section online at
http://www.expertconsult.com

Introduction

The angiosome theory has become well accepted in the field of plastic and reconstructive surgery and allows the conceptualization of the vascular supply to all tissues of the human body. An angiosome is a composite block of tissue supplied by a main source vessel. The adjacent angiosomes are linked either by reduced-caliber choke anastomotic vessels or vessels without reduction in caliber – the true anastomoses on the arterial side. The latter are seen in many muscles or in the skin, especially where vessels accompany cutaneous nerves. Flaps designed along an axis of vessels linked by true anastomoses have a longer survival length similar to a flap that has been delayed. On the venous side the anastomotic arteries are matched by veins devoid of valves that allow bidirectinal flow. The entire human body consists of innumerable arcades of interconnecting vessels which supply all tissues.

In 1977, Converse[1] stated that "there is no simple and all-encompassing system which is suitable for classifying skin flaps." It is now generally agreed that the anatomical vascular basis of the flap provides the most accurate approach for classification. Specific, anatomically based nomenclature simplifies communication between surgeons and allows for the advancement of the field of plastic and reconstructive surgery. The main

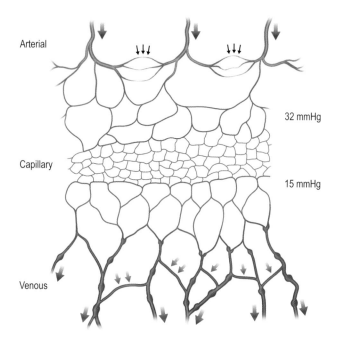

Fig. 23.1 Schematic representation of the arterial supply and venous drainage of the capillary bed. Note the choke arteries (small arrows) and bidirectional avalvular veins (small shaded arrows) that allow equilibration of flow and pressure to and from the capillary bed.

named source vessels throughout the body provide a useful road map for the description of flaps.

The vascular architecture of the body is arranged anatomically as a continuous series of vascular loops, like the tiers of a Roman aqueduct, that increase in number while their size and caliber decrease as they approach the capillary bed *(Fig. 23.1)*. The reverse situation occurs on the venous side. This anatomic arrangement of the vascular "skeleton" is shown beautifully in the corrosion cast studies of newborn babies performed by Tompsett[2] that reside in the Hunterian Museum at the Royal College of Surgeons in London *(Fig. 23.2)*. Note how the main arterial loops hug the bony framework and the secondary arcades follow the intermuscular and intramuscular connective tissue framework. The "keystones" of these arcades are represented usually by reduced-caliber (choke anastomotic) arteries and arterioles, matched on the venous side by avalvular (oscillating) veins that permit bidirectional flow. Choke arteries and avalvular veins have an essential role in controlling this pressure gradient across the capillary bed *(Fig. 23.1)*. FIGS **23.3, 23.4** APPEARS ONLINE ONLY

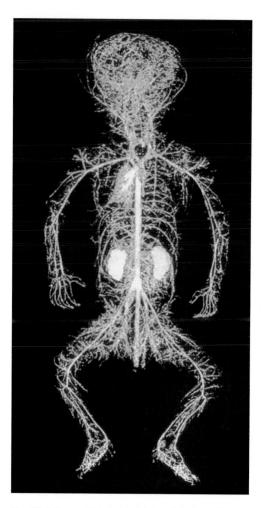

Fig. 23.2 Tompsett's arterial skeleton of the body. This corrosion cast of the newborn body shows the arterial architecture of the body. (From Taylor GI, Palmer JH. The vascular territories [angiosomes] of the body: experimental study and clinical applications. Br J Plast Surg. 1987;40:113.)

Vascular anatomical research

Angiosome

The angiosome (from the Greek *angeion*, meaning vessel, and *somite*, meaning segment or sector of the body derived from *soma*, body) is defined as a composite block of tissue supplied by a main source artery. The source arteries (segmental or distributing arteries) that supply these blocks of tissue are responsible for the supply of the skin and the underlying deep structures. When pieced together like a jigsaw puzzle, they constitute the three-dimensional vascular territories of the body (see section on the angiosome concept, below). In this section we present the basis of the anatomical studies which are the foundation of the angiosome concept.

The angiographic studies produced by Salmon using lead oxide, gelatin, and water were exceptional, however, modifications of the technique have further improved results.[41,42] In particular, reducing the concentration of lead oxide has improved computed tomographic (CT) angiographic anatomic studies.[43] A review of vascular injection techniques reveals the wide array of techniques available for investigation.[44]

Initially, cadaver injection studies to study the vascular anatomy of the human integument and other structures utilized intra-arterial injections of radiopaque substances such as barium sulfate or lead oxide or visible substances such as latex and ink. Depending on the specific study, the area of tissue of interest was then dissected and radiographed. As the radiographic film quality improved, the quality of the image of the small blood vessels improved. However, studies using simple radiographs have largely been replaced by CT techniques.[43,45,46] These investigations were conducted in fresh cadavers. In the majority of studies, the anatomical question was problem-oriented in a desire to provide a surgical solution to the individual patient's needs. We have performed a large number of fresh cadaver studies, investigating various regions, tissues, and combinations of tissues. This has included an investigation of the entire integument and underlying deep structures in a series of total body studies of the arteries,[47] which led to the angiosome concept, discussed in detail in a later section. This was followed by studies of the veins[48] and the neurovascular territories of the body[49] and detailed studies of the angiosomes of the forearm,[50] the leg,[51] and the head and neck,[52] as well as a comparative study of a series of mammals.[53] As well, we have performed detailed analyses of numerous muscle flaps including sartorius,[54] rectus femoris,[55] gracilis,[56] pectoralis major,[57] and skin flaps, including the reversed sural artery flap,[58] thoracodorsal artery perforator flap,[59] profunda femoris artery perforator flap,[60] and the superior and inferior gluteal artery perforator flaps.[61]

The investigations initially involved an analysis of various regions of the body to define possible donor sites for free skin flap transfer.[62] The studies subsequently focused on other tissues and included the anatomic basis for the transfer of bone,[63] nerve,[64] and certain muscles.[21,65] Encouraged by the success of some of the resulting clinical procedures, the authors expanded the research to investigate composite units of tissue, supplied by a single vascular system. Units of skin and tendon,[66] muscle with nerve,[67] and skin, muscle, and bone[68–70] were analyzed. It was from this work that the angiosome concept germinated. Various regions, including the anterior abdominal wall,[21,36,65,71] the anterior thorax,[72,73] the lower limb, and the upper limb, were studied. The results added strength to the angiosome concept of the blood supply and revealed the interconnections that exist at all levels between adjacent vascular territories, a relationship that is evident throughout the body.[74]

In cadaver vascular research, various techniques can be used to identify and study the area of interest. In the past, the integument (skin and subcutaneous tissue) was removed, and the sites of emergence of the dominant cutaneous perforators (0.5 mm or more) were identified on the surface of the deep fascia with lead beads. Currently, individual perforators are easily identified on CT angiography (CTA). Approximately 400 cutaneous perforators on average were identified per body.[40,47] The three-dimensional branching pattern of main source vessels can be identified. Previous workers, including Salmon, had made topographic boundary incisions to remove areas of skin, particularly in the lines of the groins, axillae, neck, and limb joints *(Fig. 23.5)*. These junctional regions are of great clinical importance, and for this reason the incisions were designed to retain their continuity wherever possible. In our current techniques, using CTA, the incisions utilized for dissection are not as crucial since the pathway and branches of individual vessels are clearly documented prior to dissection. FIG 23.5 APPEARS ONLINE ONLY

In the original studies of the vascular supply of tissues of the body, the integument was radiographed, and a montage of the entire cutaneous circulation was constructed in "plan view" *(Figs 23.6, 23.7)*.[47] Although Manchot and Salmon described the origin and course of the cutaneous arteries, and Salmon[9] made a separate study of the individual muscles, neither worker illustrated the course of the arteries between the deep tissues and the skin. Therefore, the skin and subcutaneous tissues were cut into parallel strips and placed on their side, and radiographs were taken to provide "elevation views" of the vessels in different regions of the body *(Fig. 23.8)*. Current CTA techniques allow a far more

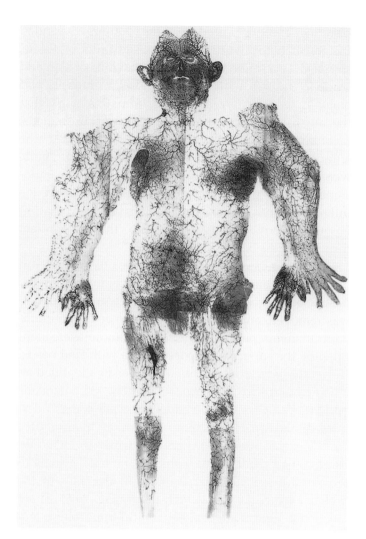

Fig. 23.7 Montage of the cutaneous arteries of the body. The skin has been incised along the ulnar border in the upper extremities, and the integument has been removed with the deep fascia on the left side and without it on the right. Note: (1) the direction, size, and density of the perforators, which are large on the torso and head and become progressively smaller and more numerous toward the periphery of the limbs; and (2) the reduced-caliber (choke) anastomotic arteries, which link the perforators into a continuous network. (From Taylor GI, Palmer JH. The vascular territories [angiosomes] of the body: experimental study and clinical applications. Br J Plast Surg. 1987;40:113.)

detailed three-dimensional appraisal of the vascular anatomy of tissues *(Fig. 23.9)*. FIG 23.6 APPEARS ONLINE ONLY

All cutaneous perforators of diameter greater than 0.5 mm were traced to their underlying source arteries. The results were averaged from each cadaveric study and plotted on a diagram of the body *(Fig. 23.10)*. Subsequently, investigations were expanded to map out the venous territories (venosomes) of the body along with the neurovascular territories of the skin and muscle.[48] These results have led to an overall picture of

the vascular territories of the entire body. The remainder of this section gives a brief overview of the arterial, venous, and nervous territories of the body.

Arterial territories

The arterial network of the body forms a continuous interlocking arcade of vessels throughout each tissue and throughout the body, linked together as loops of vessels, often of reduced caliber. The course of the cutaneous perforators depends on the proximity of the source artery to the undersurface of the deep fascia. As Michel Salmon noted in 1936,[8] arteries supply branches to each tissue that they pass, including the intermuscular and intramuscular septa, fascia, nerves, and tendons. Arteries generally fall into two groups, direct and indirect *(Fig. 23.11)*. In our anatomical dissections, it is clear that there is great variability in the exact course and size of individual vessels. The direct cutaneous vessels pass between the deep tissues before piercing the outer layer of the deep fascia. They are usually the primary cutaneous vessels, their main destination being the skin. They tend to supply the skin with larger-diameter vessels which have a large vascular territory (e.g., circumflex scapular artery). The direct branches include direct cutaneous vessels (sometimes called axial vessels) and septocutaneous vessels. The indirect vessels can be considered the secondary cutaneous supply. They emerge from the deep fascia as terminal branches of arteries which supply the muscles and other deep tissues. The majority of indirect branches are musculocutaneous perforating branches which emerge to supply the skin. In fact, there is usually significant variability in the distribution of direct and indirect vessels and their vascular territory from individual to individual. There is a vast interconnected network of direct and indirect arteries which supply the skin. The vascular territories of individual perforators vary and tend to be reciprocal with adjacent arterial vascular territories according to the so-called law of equilibrium, described by Salmon and supported by our work.

The direct cutaneous vessels arise from: (1) source arteries just beneath the deep fascia (e.g., the superficial inferior epigastric artery); (2) direct continuation of the source artery (e.g., the cutaneous branches of the external carotid artery); (3) deeply situated source artery or one of its branches to a muscle; they follow the intermuscular septa to the surface (e.g., septal cutaneous

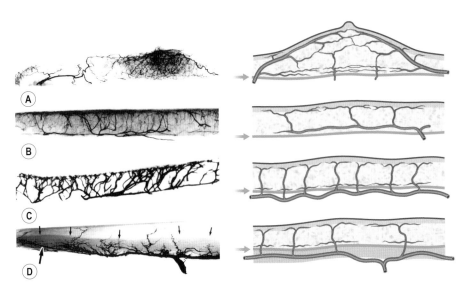

Fig. 23.8 Sectional strip radiographic studies of the breast **(A)**, thigh **(B)**, sole of the foot **(C)**, and buttock **(D)**. **(D)** includes the underlying gluteus maximus muscle. The schematic diagram illustrates the dominant horizontal axis of vessels that provides the primary supply to the skin in each case and its relationship to the deep fascia (arrow). **(A)** They predominate in the subdermal plexus. Note from left to right the internal thoracic perforator and lateral thoracic artery converging on the nipple in the radiograph of the loose skin region of the torso. **(B)** They are seen coursing on the surface of the deep fascia in this relatively fixed skin area. **(C)** The source artery itself is the dominant horizontal vessel supplying the skin, coursing beneath the deep fascia in this rigidly fixed skin region. **(D)** Small arrows define the deep fascia, and the large arrow indicates the large fasciocutaneous branch of the gluteal artery, which descends with the posterior cutaneous nerve of the thigh. (From Taylor GI, Palmer JH. The vascular territories [angiosomes] of the body: experimental study and clinical applications. Br J Plast Surg. 1987;40:113.)

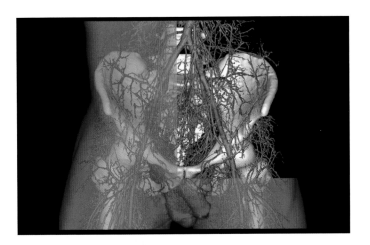

Fig. 23.9 Computed tomography angiography of a cadaver pelvis, showing bony, vascular, and skin three-dimensional anatomy. Using MIMICS software, the various anatomic structures can be included or removed. (From Morris SF, Tang M, Almutairi K, *et al.* The anatomic basis of perforator flaps. Clin Plast Surg. 2010;37:553–570.)

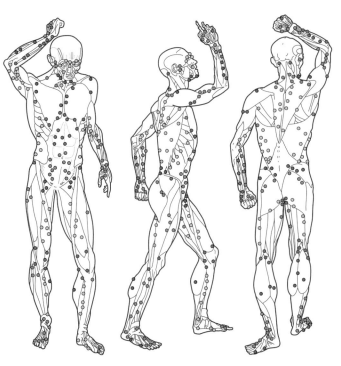

Fig. 23.10 Map of the arterial perforators of 0.5 mm or more, which are color-coded to correspond to the underlying parent arteries and course with the associated perforating veins. They provide the basis for perforator flaps. (From Taylor GI, Palmer JH. The vascular territories [angiosomes] of the body: experimental study and clinical applications. Br J Plast Surg. 1987;40:113.)

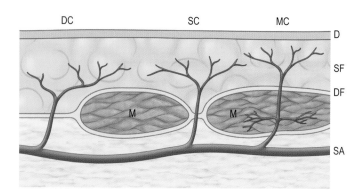

Fig. 23.11 Schematic illustration of direct and indirect cutaneous vessels. DC, direct cutaneous; SC, septocutaneous; MC, musculocutaneous; D, dermis; SF, superficial dermis; DF, deep fascia; SA, source artery; M, muscle. (From Geddes CR. MSc Thesis, Dalhousie University, Halifax, Nova Scotia, Canada.)

branches of the lateral circumflex femoral artery). Indirect cutaneous vessels generally emerge from the main source artery as it courses on the undersurface of a muscle and penetrate through the muscle; e.g., musculocutaneous perforators of the deep inferior epigastric arteries (DIEA). In the human body, there are approximately 400 perforators, about 40% of vessels are direct and 60% indirect perforators.

The direct cutaneous perforators pierce the deep fascia near where it is anchored to bone or the intermuscular and intramuscular septa (*Fig. 23.10*). These lines and zones of fixation also correspond to the fixed skin areas of the body. From these points, the vessels flow toward the convexities of the body surface, branching within the integument. The wider the distance between the cavities and the higher the summit, the longer the vessel (*Fig. 23.8*). The size and density of the direct perforators also vary in different regions. For example, in the head, neck, torso, arm, and thigh, the vessels are larger, longer, and less numerous. In the forearm, leg, and dorsum of the hands and feet, the vessels tend to be smaller, shorter, and more numerous. In the palms of the hands and the soles of the feet, where the skin is fixed, there is a high density of smaller perforators. Hence, the primary supply of each cutaneous territory varies between source arteries. Each of these territories also has indirect perforators.

The course of the cutaneous perforators between the deep fascia and the skin also varies in different regions. Regardless of their site, however, they follow the connective tissue framework of the superficial fascia, interconnecting at all levels. They ramify on the undersurface of the subcutaneous fat adjacent to the deep fascia and then branch and course toward the subdermal plexus, working their way between the fat lobules. The smaller vessels tend to course vertically toward the skin, whereas the larger vessels branch in all directions in a stellate pattern or course in a particular axis, branching as they pass parallel to the skin surface.

In the scalp and limbs, where the skin is relatively fixed to the deep fascia, the larger vessels hug that surface. They course on the deep fascia for a considerable distance in the loose areolar layer that separates them from the subcutaneous fat (*Fig. 23.8*). This is especially true when a perforator accompanies a cutaneous nerve.

In the loose skin areas of the body, the direct cutaneous vessels course for a variable distance parallel to the deep fascia. They are more intimately related to the undersurface of the subcutaneous fat, however, being plastered to it by a thin fascial sheet that separates them on their deep surface from a plexus of smaller vessels. This plexus lies in loose areolar tissue on the surface of the deep fascia. It is formed by branches that arise from the direct perforators as they pierce the deep fascia and the connections these branches make with smaller indirect perforators. The large direct perforators then pierce the subcutaneous layer. They ascend within the superficial fascia (subcutaneous fat) to reach the rich subdermal plexus, where they travel for considerable distances (*Fig. 23.8*).

Within the deep tissue, whether muscle, tendon, nerve, or bone, a pattern similar to that in the integument exists, with a three-dimensional network of vessels interlinking between vascular territories, the perimeters of which are linked by choke arteries. Within the muscles, these choke vessels often exhibit a characteristic corkscrew appearance.

Venous drainage

The cutaneous veins also form a three-dimensional plexus of interconnecting channels throughout the body (*Fig. 23.12*). There are valved segments in which valves direct flow in a particular direction, and there are avalvular segments where no valves are present. The avalvular or oscillating veins allow bidirectional flow between adjacent venous territories. They connect veins whose valves may be oriented in opposite directions, thus providing for the equilibration of flow and pressure. Indeed, there are many veins whose valves direct flow initially in a distal direction, away from the heart, before joining veins whose flow is proximal. An example of this is the superficial inferior epigastric vein that drains the lower abdominal wall integument toward the groin. In some regions, valved channels direct flow radially away from a plexus of avalvular veins, for example, in the venous drainage of the nipple–areola complex. In other areas, valved channels direct flow toward a central focus, as seen in the stellate branches of the cutaneous perforating veins of the limbs.

In general, venous anatomy parallels arterial anatomy **(Fig. 23.13)**. From dermal and subdermal venous plexuses, the veins collect either into horizontal large-caliber veins, where they often relate to cutaneous nerves and a longitudinal system of chain-linked arteries, or alternatively in centrifugal or stellate fashion into a common channel that passes vertically down in company with the cutaneous arteries to pierce the deep fascia. Thereafter, the veins travel with the direct and indirect cutaneous arteries, draining ultimately into the venae comitantes of the source arteries in the deep tissue.

In general, the origin, course, and distribution of the deep veins (vena comitantes) are a mirror image of the deep source arteries, but they are larger and more plentiful. Although the anatomy of the veins is subject to considerable variation between sides in the same individual as well as between other individuals, the pattern of venous arcades is evident throughout. These arcades generally become smaller and more numerous as the periphery of the region or the tissue is reached. The superficial veins, however, are independent of the deep arteries (e.g., greater saphenous vein, cephalic vein) and may have a different area of drainage. For example, in the forearm there are paired vena comitantes to the radial and ulnar arteries but a separate system of large-caliber subcutaneous veins, including cephalic, basilic, and antebrachial veins.

The site and density of the valves within the deep venous network are variable. The deep veins follow the bony skeleton of the body or the intermuscular septa with their associated arteries. In some regions, these veins are single; in others, they are duplicated as venae comitantes. In the limbs, the veins commence distally in the hands and feet as single channels linked by venous arcades. These arcades become progressively larger as

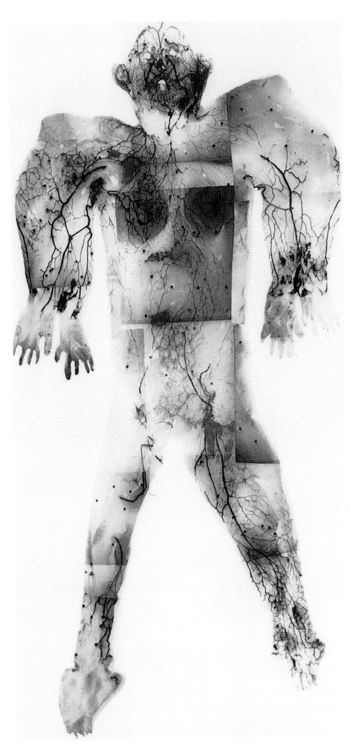

Fig. 23.12 The venous network of the integument of a female subject. This is a montage of venograms from an injection study. (From Taylor GI, Caddy CM, Watterson PA, *et al.* The venous territories [venosomes] of the human body: experimental study and clinical implications. Plast Reconstr Surg. 1990;86:185.)

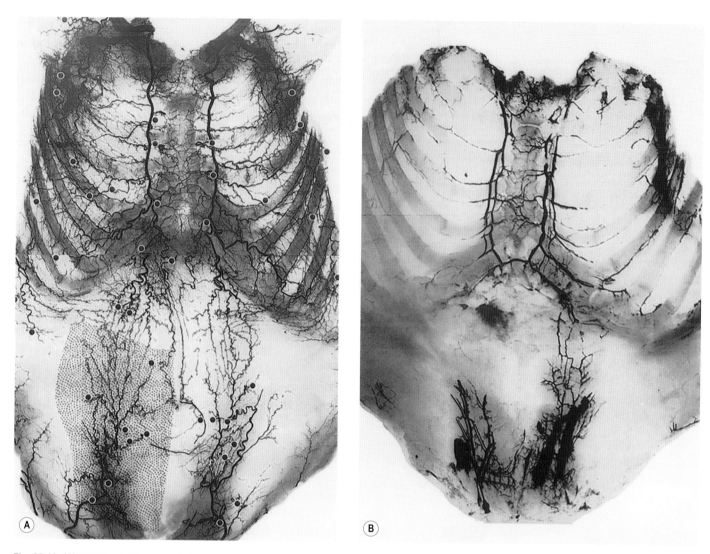

Fig. 23.13 (A) Arterial and **(B)** venous studies of the anterior torso. Note the "corkscrew" choke arteries that link adjacent territories in the arterial study and the mixture that has extruded from the deep inferior epigastric veins as a result of the resistance of the valves. Radiographic lead beads identify the origin of the cutaneous perforators from their source vessels in the arterial study. (From Taylor GI, Caddy CM, Watterson PA, *et al.* The venous territories [venosomes] of the human body: experimental study and clinical implications. Plast Reconstr Surg. 1990;86:185.)

they approach the wrist and ankle. The veins are duplicated in the forearm and leg, and each pair of veins is linked by a rich stepladder of venous channels that are usually free of valves. These venae comitantes then reunite to form single channels. In the lower limb, this occurs in the popliteal fossa, but in the upper limb, the union is most commonly in the proximal arm or even as high as the axilla.

In the torso, the pattern of arcades is conspicuous *(Fig. 23.13)*; the parent veins are oriented as longitudinal and transverse arcades that match the pattern of the source artery. Distinct territories are evident. Where

choke arteries define the arterial territories, they are matched by oscillating veins in the venous network. The existence of venae comitantes is variable.

Within the muscle, the intramuscular venous network mirrors that of the arterial side. Where arterial territories are linked by choke arteries or true anastomotic arteries without changing caliber, the venous territories of the muscles, which drain in opposite directions, are linked by avalvular oscillating veins. Broadly, the muscles can be classified into three types on the basis of their venous architecture. Type I muscles have a single venous territory that drains in one direction. Type II

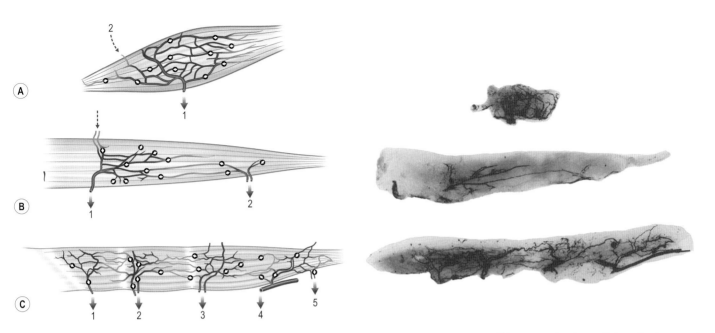

Fig. 23.14 Illustrations and radiographs of venous injection studies of the supraspinatus **(A)**, gracilis **(B)**, and sartorius **(C)** muscles. Note the oscillating veins that separate them into type I, II, and III muscles and the efferent veins entering the supraspinatus and gracilis muscles (dashed arrows). (From Taylor GI, Caddy CM, Watterson PA, *et al*. The venous territories [venosomes] of the human body: experimental study and clinical implications. Plast Reconstr Surg. 1990;86:185.)

muscles have two territories that drain from the oscillating vein in opposite directions. Type III muscles consist of three or more venous territories that drain in multiple directions *(Fig. 23.14)*.

The extramuscular veins are of two types. The first group consists of the efferent veins. They contain valves and drain the muscles to their parent veins. The other group consists of the afferent veins. They are derived from the overlying integument as musculocutaneous perforators or from adjacent muscles *(Fig. 23.14)*.

Neurovascular territories

In our anatomical studies of neurovascular territories, fresh human cadavers were injected with a radiopaque lead oxide mixture, and the nerves were dissected and labeled with fine computer wire.[49] The nerves and vessels were then segregated by subtraction angiography.

The most obvious feature seen throughout the skin and muscle is the linear arrangement of the nerves and their branches, compared with the looping arcades of the interconnecting vessel network, with the nerves taking the shortest route between two points. In general, the orientation of cutaneous nerves is longitudinal in the limbs, transverse or oblique in the torso, and

radiating from loci in the head and neck. Of particular note is that the cutaneous nerves, like the arteries, pierce the deep fascia at fixed skin sites.

Each cutaneous nerve is accompanied by an artery, but the relationship is variable. Some of the arrangements seen in the integument are shown in *Figure 23.15*. In each case, either a long artery or a chain-linked system of arteries "hitchhikes" with the nerve.

When the cutaneous nerve and artery appear at the deep fascia together, their relationship is often established early (e.g., the lateral intercostal neurovascular perforators on the torso or the saphenous system in the lower limb). However, the nerve sometimes pierces the deep fascia at a point remote from the emergence of its associated artery (e.g., the lateral cutaneous nerve of the thigh and the superficial circumflex iliac artery below the inguinal ligament; *Fig. 23.16*). Alternatively, the nerve leaves one vascular system with which it is traveling in parallel to cross the path of another (e.g., the lateral intercostal nerve, which courses initially with its artery and then leaves it to meet the superficial inferior epigastric vessel). In many of these cases, secondary or tertiary branches of the artery often peel off to accompany the nerve *(Fig. 23.16)*. Sunderland noted that each peripheral nerve is abundantly vascularized by a

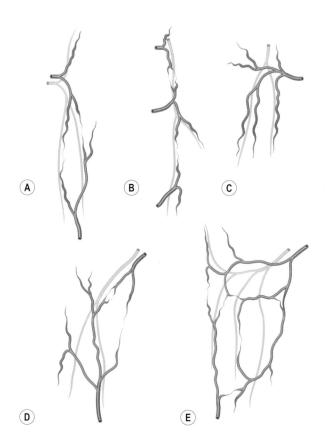

Fig. 23.15 The neurovascular patterns found in the integument. **(A)** A long artery connected to its neighbor by a true anastomosis courses with the nerve. **(B)** A chain-linked system of arteries hitchhikes with the nerve. **(C)** The nerve and artery pierce the deep fascia at separate sites. Branches of the vessel peel off to accompany the nerve as it crosses the main arterial trunk. **(D)** The nerve at first courses parallel to an artery and then approaches the neighboring artery from its periphery to descend along its branches toward the main trunk. **(E)** The nerve crosses the primary and secondary arcades of the artery before coursing parallel to the vascular network. (From Taylor GI, Gianoutsos MP, Morris SF. The neurovascular territories of the skin and muscles: anatomic study and clinical implications. Plast Reconstr Surg. 1994;94:1.)

"vascular net" of a series of nutrient arteries entering the nerve at different levels.[75] ⚲ FIG 23.16 APPEARS ONLINE ONLY

The vascular architecture of the intramuscular veins and arteries, as has been discussed previously, is almost identical for each muscle. Therefore, to simplify the description of the nervous supply to the muscles, only the arterial relations of the nerves are discussed and illustrated. The intramuscular branches of the nerves were dissected to, but not within, the individual muscle bundles. The following observations were made:

1. The nerves follow the connective tissue framework. Dissection showed the motor nerves coursing in the connective tissue sheath from its origin at the nerve trunk to the neurovascular hilum of the muscle. Thereafter, the nerve and its branches follow the intramuscular connective tissue to reach the muscle bundles.

2. The nerves are economical. As in the integument, the direct course of the motor nerves is in stark contrast to the wandering pattern of the vessels. The nerves take the shortest extramuscular and intramuscular routes compatible with the function of each muscle.

3. Neurovascular relations vary with the muscle, the extramuscular course, and the intramuscular branching of the nerves and the vessels. Some muscles have a single nerve supply; others receive multiple motor branches. All receive multiple arterial pedicles. However, despite the variables, certain observations can be made:

   - Each motor nerve is accompanied by a vascular pedicle, but the reverse does not apply.
   - The motor nerve is usually accompanied by the dominant vascular pedicle. There are exceptions to this, however. For example, the nerve supply to sternomastoid is usually accompanied by a minor vascular pedicle.
   - The nerve may enter the muscle before branching.
   - Once within the muscle, the nerve divides early, and its branches sweep rapidly into position, parallel to the muscle fibers. The vessels, however, branch and form primary and secondary arcades, often crossing the muscle bundles and nerves before tertiary and quaternary branches are provided to the muscle fibers.

Ultimately, the terminal branches of the vessels and nerves come into close contact and course together in the connective tissue framework parallel to the muscle bundles.

Neurovascular anatomy of muscles of the body

Several methods have been used to classify muscles on the basis of morphology, function, blood supply, or nerve supply *(Table 23.1)*. We have classified muscles of the body according to their most common pattern of innervation *(Fig. 23.17)*. The pattern of neurovascular

Table 23.1 Classification of muscles based on their nerve supply

Type I	Type II	Type III	Type IV
Latissimus dorsi	Deltoid	Gastrocnemius	Rectus abdominis
Extensor indicis	Gluteus maximus	Sartorius	Levator scapulae
Extensor pollicis longus	Trapezius	Tibialis anterior	Internal oblique
Abductor pollicis longus	Vastus lateralis	Flexor digitorum superficialis	Digastric
Palmaris longus	Serratus anterior	Subscapularis	Erector spinae
Teres minor	Flexor carpi ulnaris	Teres major	
Extensor hallucis longus	Biceps brachii	Triceps	
Plantaris	Brachialis	Extensor carpi ulnaris	
Popliteus	Flexor pollicis longus	Extensor digitorum longus	
	Flexor hallucis longus	Gluteus medius	
	Pectineus	Gluteus minimus	
	Adductor longus	Vastus medialis	
	Adductor brevis	Vastus intermedius	
		Peroneus longus	
		Soleus	
		Tibialis posterior	

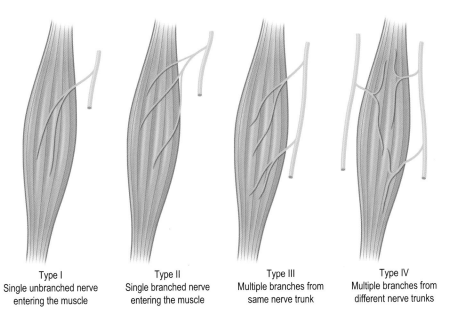

Type I
Single unbranched nerve
entering the muscle

Type II
Single branched nerve
entering the muscle

Type III
Multiple branches from
same nerve trunk

Type IV
Multiple branches from
different nerve trunks

Fig. 23.17 Classification of muscle on the basis of nerve supply. (From Taylor GI, Gianoutsos MP, Morris SF. The neurovascular territories of the skin and muscles: anatomic study and clinical implications. Plast Reconstr Surg. 1994;94:1.)

anatomy of the muscles influences the way a whole muscle or segment of muscle can be harvested as a functioning muscle microvascular transfer. It is possible to subdivide certain muscles, based on the neurovascular anatomy, into separate neurovascular units if each segment has an individual vascular pedicle. Clinically, serratus anterior, latissimus dorsi, gracilis, and rectus femoris are often used in this way, taking a portion of the muscle with their motor nerve and blood supply.[55,56]

• Type I. The muscle is supplied by a single motor nerve that divides usually after entering the muscle *(Fig. 23.18)*. Multiple vascular pedicles supply each

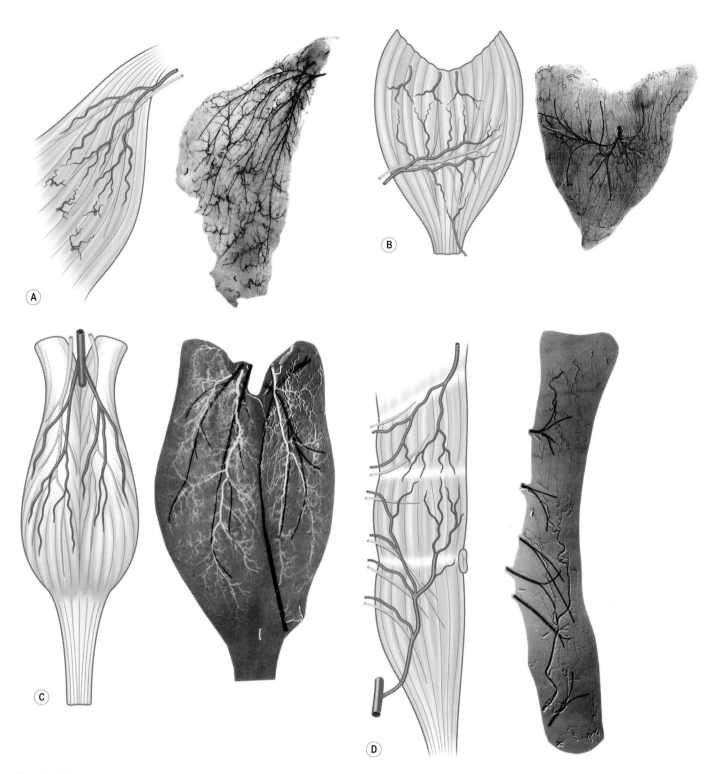

Fig. 23.18 Schematic diagram (left) of **(A)** type I (latissimus dorsi), **(B)** type II (deltoid), **(C)** type III (gastrocnemius), and **(D)** type IV (rectus abdominis) muscles to match radiograph (right) of each muscle. Nerves and vessels are seen together in the radiographs. The nerves are straight, whereas the vessels are spiral. The nerves, labeled with computer wire, appear black and the vessels pale and "ghost-like" in this subtraction study. (From Taylor GI, Gianoutsos MP, Morris SF. The neurovascular territories of the skin and muscles: anatomic study and clinical implications. Plast Reconstr Surg. 1994;94:1.)

muscle and form a continuous network throughout the tissue. It is possible in each case to remove a vascularized segment of muscle with its nerve supply and yet leave viable muscle *in situ*.

- Type II. A single motor nerve supplies each of the muscles in this group, but this time the nerve divides before entering the muscle. Muscles in this group include the deltoid *(Fig. 23.18)*, gluteus maximus, trapezius, vastus lateralis, serratus anterior, and flexor carpi ulnaris.

- Type III. Multiple motor nerve branches derive from the same nerve trunk *(Fig. 23.18)*. Once again, it is possible to subdivide each muscle into separate functional units because of the multiple vascular pedicles as well as the several nerve branches. Gastrocnemius is often split in this way, taking one head for reconstruction, leaving behind the other functional unit with its neurovascular supply attached.

- Type IV. Multiple motor nerves are derived from different nerve trunks *(Fig. 23.18)*. It is apparent that each muscle can be subdivided anatomically into several functional units because of the multiple, often segmental neurovascular pedicles. Indeed, several of these muscles are formed developmentally by the fusion of adjacent somites (e.g., rectus abdominis and internal oblique).

FIGS **23.19, 23.20, 23.21** APPEARS ONLINE ONLY

The angiosome concept

Following a review of the works by Manchot and Salmon, along with the results of our total body studies of blood supply to the skin and the underlying deep tissues, it has been possible to segregate the body anatomically into three-dimensional vascular territories named angiosomes. These three-dimensional anatomic territories are supplied by a source (segmental or distributing) artery and its accompanying vein or veins that span between the skin and the bone *(Figs 23.22–23.24)*. Each angiosome can be subdivided into matching arteriosomes (arterial territories) and venosomes (venous territories). Forty of these territories were initially described,[73] but subsequent investigation has led to many of these territories being subdivided further into smaller composite units and revealed some

that do not reach the skin surface. In a later study, 61 vascular territories were identified.[40] Recent work has illustrated no fewer than 13 angiosomes of the head and neck, originally mapped as eight supplied by branches of the external carotid, internal carotid, and subclavian arteries.[52] The angiosome concept indicates that the three-dimensional block of tissue is supplied by a major source artery and its accompanying vein(s), but it is important to note that the angiosome itself is divisible depending on the branching pattern of the source vessel.

These composite blocks of skin, bone, muscle, and other soft tissues fit together like the pieces of a jigsaw puzzle, to make up the body. In some of the angiosomes, there is a large overlying cutaneous area and a relatively small deep tissue region; in others, the reverse pattern exists. Each angiosome is linked to its neighbor at every tissue level, either by a true (simple) anastomotic arterial connection without change in caliber of the vessel or by a reduced-caliber choke anastomosis. A similar pattern with avalvular (bidirectional or oscillating) veins on the venous side defines the boundaries of the venosome *(Fig. 23.24)*.

The angiosome concept has several important clinical implications:

1. Each angiosome defines the safe anatomic boundary of tissue in each layer that can be transferred separately or combined on the underlying source vessels as a composite flap. Also, the anatomic territory of each tissue in the adjacent angiosome can usually be captured with safety when it is combined in the flap design.

2. Because the junctional zone between adjacent angiosomes usually occurs within muscles of the deep tissue, rather than between them, these muscles provide an important anastomotic detour (bypass shunt) if the main source artery or vein is obstructed.

3. Because most muscles span two or more angiosomes and are supplied from each territory, one is able to capture the skin island from one angiosome by muscle supplied in the adjacent territory. As we shall see later, this fact provides the basis for the design of many musculocutaneous flaps. FIGS **23.25, 23.26, 23.27, 23.28, 23.29, 23.30, 23.31, 23.32, 23.33, 23.34, 23.35, 23.36, 23.37** APPEARS ONLINE ONLY

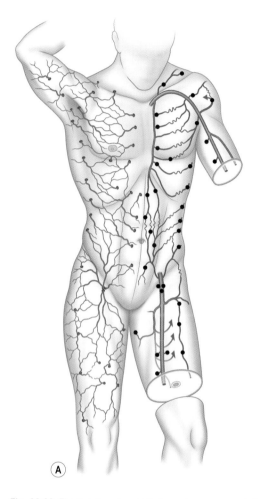

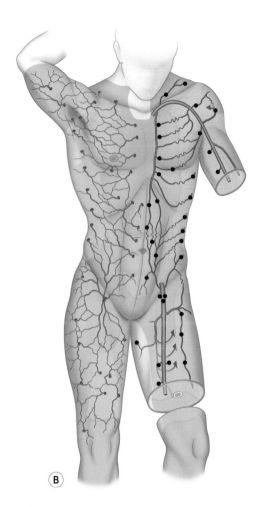

Fig. 23.22 The technique by which the angiosomes were defined. **(A)** The cutaneous perforators with their choke connections are depicted on the left. The origin of the perforators from their underlying source arteries and their muscle branches is shown on the right. **(B)** The vascular territories of each source artery are illustrated in the integument (left) and deep tissues (right) by lines drawn through the choke connecting vessels. Note that the territories correspond in these two layers and how they appear as sectors in the limbs. (From Taylor GI, Palmer JH. The vascular territories [angiosomes] of the body: experimental study and clinical applications. Br J Plast Surg. 1987;40:113.)

Anatomic concepts related to flap design

The following concepts provide an overview of the blood supply to the integument and to the deep tissues *(Box 23.1)*. They are fundamental to the mapping of the vascular territories and to the planning of incisions and flaps. They help explain the anatomic variations that exist between the vessels of different regions of the body and allow better understanding of the various classifications of the cutaneous blood supply that have appeared in the literature. Finally, these anatomic concepts provide the basis for interpreting many physiologic and pathologic processes, including the delay phenomenon and the necrosis line of flaps.

Box 23.1 Anatomic concepts

Vessels follow the connective tissue framework of the body

Arteries radiate from fixed to mobile areas and veins converge from mobile to fixed areas

Vessels "hitchhike" with nerves

Vessel size and orientation are the product of tissue growth and differentiation

Vessels interconnect to form a continuous three-dimensional network of vascular arcades

Vessels obey the law of equilibrium

Vessels have a relatively constant destination but may have a variable origin

Venous networks consist of linked valvular and avalvular channels that allow equilibrium of flow and pressure

Muscles are the prime movers of venous return

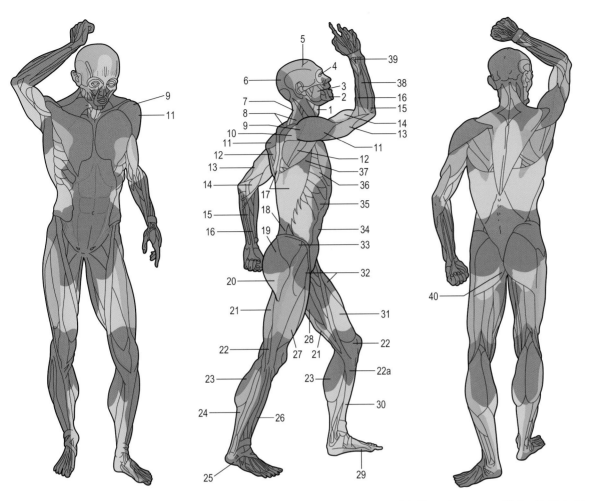

Fig. 23.23 The angiosomes of the source arteries of the body shaded to correspond to Figure 23.9. The angiosomes are: (1) thyroid; (2) facial; (3) buccal (internal maxillary); (4) ophthalmic; (5) superficial temporal; (6) occipital; (7) deep cervical; (8) transverse cervical; (9) acromiothoracic; (10) suprascapular; (11) posterior circumflex humeral; (12) circumflex scapular; (13) profunda brachii; (14) brachial; (15) ulnar; (16) radial; (17) posterior intercostals; (18) lumbar; (19) superior gluteal; (20) inferior gluteal; (21) profunda femoris; (22) popliteal; (22a) descending genicular (saphenous); (23) sural; (24) peroneal; (25) lateral plantar; (26) anterior tibial; (27) lateral femoral circumflex; (28) adductor (profunda); (29) medial plantar; (30) posterior tibial; (31) superficial femoral; (32) common femoral; (33) deep circumflex iliac; (34) deep inferior epigastric; (35) internal thoracic; (36) lateral thoracic; (37) thoracodorsal; (38) posterior interosseous; (39) anterior interosseous; and (40) internal pudendal.

Vessels follow the connective tissue framework of the body

This concept is fundamental to the design of flaps in general and to fasciocutaneous and septocutaneous flaps in particular. The connective tissue framework of the body is a continuous syncytium, like the walls of a honeycomb, calcified in some areas to form the bony skeleton, which houses, permeates, and supports the specialized tissues. The vessels follow this framework down to the microscopic level. Embryologically, vessels develop with connective tissue in the mesoderm and, through development, remain closely related. The

clinical application of this is the septocutaneous or fasciocutaneous flap.

In general, if the connective tissue is rigid, such as intermuscular septa, periosteum, or deep fascia, the vessels travel beside or on it. If the connective tissue is loose, they travel within it. The vessels occasionally travel in a fibrous sheath or a bony canal, but this tunnel always contains loose areolar tissue, physiologically, to allow the veins to dilate and the arteries to pulsate.[82]

The pattern is well illustrated if the arterial network is traced from the heart to the periphery. The major arteries are closely related to the bones of the axial skeleton *(Fig. 23.2)*. Their branches at first follow the

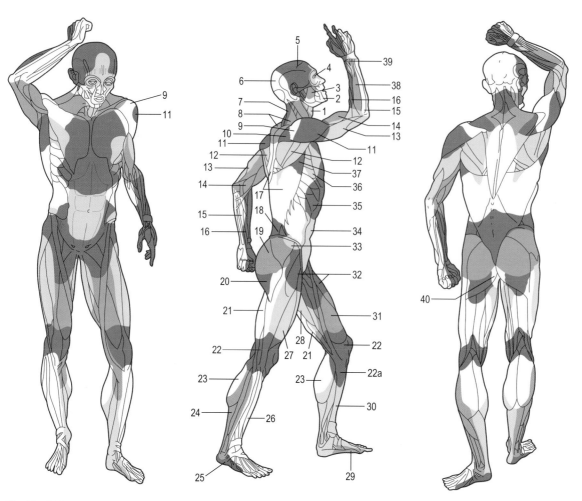

Fig. 23.24 The venosomes of the body. Compare with Figure 23.22. (From Taylor GI, Caddy CM, Watterson PA, *et al.* The venous territories (venosomes) of the human body: experimental study and clinical implications. Plast Reconstr Surg. 1990;86:185.)

intermuscular septa. In the deep tissues, they penetrate the muscles (usually on their deep surface), tendons, bones, nerves, and deep fat deposits. As the vessels divide and subdivide within the specialized tissues, their branches again follow the connective tissue framework to reflect the architecture of the tissue in question. The arterial framework is beautifully illustrated in the corrosion cast studies of Last and Tompsett.[2,83]

The cutaneous perforators exhibit the same pattern. They arise from their source artery (segmental or distributing artery) or one of its muscle branches and follow the intermuscular or intramuscular septa toward the surface *(Fig. 23.8)*. They pierce the deep fascia, branch, and ramify on its surface and ascend in the connective tissue framework of the superficial fascia, traveling between the fat locules to reach the subdermal plexus. During their course, the cutaneous vessels provide branches to the adjacent tissues, whether they are muscle, nerve, bone, fascia, or fat.

The cutaneous perforating veins can be traced in a retrograde fashion by means of the intermuscular and intramuscular septa to the outer layer of the deep fascia, where they usually form rich plexuses on either side of its surface. From there, they can be followed along the connective tissue framework of the superficial fascia, worming their way between the fat locules until they meet and become continuous with the horizontal plexus of large superficial veins near the dermis.

Arteries radiate from fixed to mobile areas and veins converge from mobile to fixed areas

Few arteries cross mobile tissue planes. Instead, they cross where tissues are anchored and radiate parallel to the plane of mobility, often for long distances. The cutaneous vessels pierce and emerge from the outer layer of the deep fascia near where it is anchored, either to its deep septa or to bone. The overlying integument is fixed also to the deep fascia at these sites. The fixed skin regions are seen easily in a well-muscled individual as grooves and valleys. They can be seen around the perimeter of muscles, especially where they interdigitate; over well-developed intermuscular septa; over the flexor surface of joints; adjacent to the dorsal and ventral midline of the body; around the base of the skull; and in the region of some bone prominences *(Fig. 23.16)*.

From the grooves and valleys in the deep fascia, the arteries flow toward the convexities of the body surface, branching within the integument. The wider the distance between the concavities and the higher the summit, the longer is the vessel. This pattern is well demonstrated in the blood supply to the integument of the scalp, nose, ears, breasts, and genitalia; the extensor surface of the joints; and the bulging surface of muscles *(Fig. 23.8)*.

Where the skin is relatively fixed to the deep fascia over a wide area (e.g., in the scalp and many areas of the limbs), the vessels remain close to the surface of the deep fascia for a considerable distance. In the loose skin areas of the body, especially over the pectoralis major muscle, the iliac fossa, and the extensor surface of joints, the vessels course for a short distance adjacent to the deep fascia. Soon they are plastered to the undersurface of the subcutaneous layer by a thin glistening sheet of fascia, and they then pierce the fat obliquely to reach the subdermal plexus, where they travel for long distances.

The veins course parallel to the plane of mobility, often for long distances, and cross where the tissues are anchored to fascia or bone. This is seen at the same site as the arteries.

Within the subdermal plexus and in the subcutaneous fat, the veins and arteries often travel nearby at a distance and only come together when they pierce the outer layer of the deep fascia. Veins leave the subcutaneous tissue and pierce the deep fascia where the integument is anchored to it. This occurs around the perimeter of muscles, in particular where they interdigitate, over well-developed intermuscular septa. This is especially true in the limbs, where they are concentrated in longitudinal rows over the flexor surfaces of joints (e.g., the cubital fossa, axilla, popliteal fossa, and groin); adjacent

to the dorsal and ventral midlines of the body; around the base of the skull and orbital margins where the galea is anchored; and where the deep fascia is fixed to bone, such as the subcutaneous border of the tibia *(Fig. 23.10)*.

In the deep tissues, veins leave muscles usually near their attachments to bone or fascia, most commonly on their deep surfaces. If a group of muscles has a common origin, for example, where the flexor and extensor muscles arise from the epicondyles of the humerus, the venous drainage of each is frequently collected into a large venous arch that courses in the muscle mass close to the bone.

It follows that, where a tissue is mobile over a long distance, whether muscle, skin, tendon, or nerve, large flaps are available for transfer and should be based on the fixed margin or end of that tissue. There are numerous situations in which this observation is used in everyday clinical practice. For example, the large axial skin flaps based on the fixed area of the groin, the paraumbilical region, and the parasternal region use the mobile skin areas over the anterior abdominal and chest walls. The commonly used muscle and tendon transfers are also based on this principle. If mobility exists between tissue planes, this provides a relatively avascular plane.

Vessels "hitchhike" with nerves

There is an intimate relationship between nerves and blood vessels throughout the deep tissues and the skin and subcutaneous tissues of the body, especially where a cutaneous nerve courses on the surface of the deep fascia. An artery may accompany the nerve for a considerable distance, often connecting with its neighbor in chain-link fashion to provide the basis for an axially oriented neurovascular flap. The cutaneous vessels and the nerve are occasionally in juxtaposition; in other situations, they course parallel to each other but at a distance. When the cutaneous nerve crosses a fixed skin site, it frequently "picks up" its next vascular companion *(Figs 23.15, 23.16)*.

There are numerous instances throughout the body where this pattern of distribution of nerves and vessels exists to supply the integument. This includes the supraorbital, infraorbital, and occipital neurovascular bundles in the head; the supraclavicular nerves collecting branches of the suprascapular and supraclavicular vessels as they cross the clavicle on to the chest; the intercostal neurovascular bundles on the torso; and the cutaneous nerves of the arm, forearm, thigh, leg, and digits, which are accompanied by long named or unnamed vessels or a chain-linked system of vessels.

The cutaneous nerves are accompanied by a longitudinal system of arteries and veins that are often the dominant blood supply to the region. The veins in company with the nerves are frequently large venous freeways, such as the cephalic, basilic, long saphenous, and short saphenous systems. The arteries either are long vessels (e.g., the supraorbital, lateral intercostal, or saphenous arteries) or exist as a chain-linked system of cutaneous perforators, often joined in series by true anastomoses without change in caliber *(Fig. 23.16)*.

The nerves pierce the deep fascia together with the vessels, they emerge separately and cross the vessels at an angle, or they approach the vessels from opposite directions. The main trunk of the vessel or some of its branches peels off to course parallel *(Fig. 23.15)* to the nerve. These vessels either course in proximity to the nerve or travel nearby *(Fig. 23.16B)*.

This neurovascular relationship presents another basis for the design of long flaps with the added potential of providing sensation at the repair site. Many of the current "axial" or "fasciocutaneous" flaps are in fact neurovascular flaps. The original long and short saphenous flaps described by Pontén are cases in point.

Vessel growth and orientation are products of tissue growth and differentiation

Two centuries ago, John Hunter[77] suggested that at some stage of fetal development, and certainly at birth, there are a fixed number of arteries in the body. This has been the authors' impression in comparing the number of cutaneous perforators encountered while raising the same flap in a child and in an adult.

If this concept is correct, it provides a plausible explanation for the density and morphology of the cutaneous arteries in different regions of the body. It explains why vessels radiate from concavities and converge on convexities and why the vessels in some areas are small and close together, whereas in others they are large and spaced well apart *(Fig. 23.38)*.

There are numerous examples to support this hypothesis. The sternomastoid and trapezius muscles split

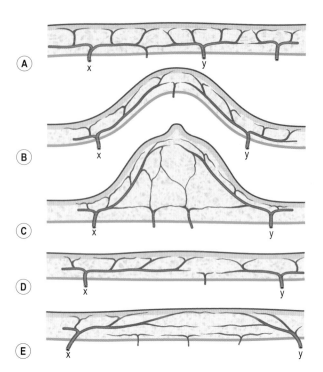

Fig. 23.38 Diagram showing how the size and course of the direct cutaneous perforators *x* and *y*, which emerge from fixed points in the deep fascia, could be modified by growth either before or after birth. **(A)** The perforators, which are fixed in number and position, form a major connecting network on the surface of the deep fascia in the "resting state." **(B)** They are stretched with the deep fascia by the expansion of underlying tissues (e.g., the scalp vessels as the brain and skull expand during fetal development). **(C)** As the breast develops within the integument, the vessels are displaced toward the dermis and lengthened as they converge on the nipple. **(D)** They are stretched apart in the limbs as the long bones grow, but they still retain their original relationship to the deep fascia. **(E)** The vessels are again stretched apart by growth, but the mobile relationship between the undersurface of the integument and the deep fascia is responsible for their oblique course. This pattern is characteristic of the loose skin areas of the torso. (From Taylor GI, Palmer JH. The vascular territories [angiosomes] of the body: experimental study and clinical applications. Br J Plast Surg. 1987;40:113.)

from the same somite.[84] The trapezius "drags" its supplying transverse cervical artery (and nerve) across the root of the neck to the back, together with a large band of skin that it nourishes. Manchot[4,5] suggested that the long course and the direction of the superficial superior and inferior epigastric arteries are brought about by the extension of the fetal torso. If one remembers that the cutaneous perforators pierce the deep fascia at fixed points and that they all interconnect, this would explain why, as the brain and skull expand, the scalp vessels hypertrophy and are stretched from the base of the calvaria toward its vertex.

The primitive cutaneous perforators in the fetus branch in all directions after piercing the deep fascia and have a stellate appearance. This pattern is retained

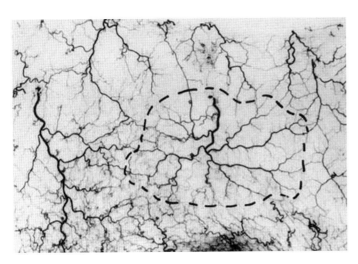

Fig. 23.39 Dotted line through choke connecting vessels of a large acromiothoracic perforator to define its anatomic territory. Compare with Figure 23.19, left side of chest. (From Taylor GI, Palmer JH. The vascular territories [angiosomes] of the body: experimental study and clinical applications. Br J Plast Surg. 1987;40:113.)

into adulthood in many regions of the body. When a perforator departs from this pattern and becomes oriented in one direction, it highlights the differential increase in growth that has occurred along that axis or the influence of a developing cutaneous nerve. Where small perforators are clustered close together, this pattern suggests that, by comparison, the growth and hypertrophy in the area are less than at those sites where the perforators are large and spaced well apart. This is well demonstrated by comparing the perforators in the proximal and distal regions of the limbs.

Vessels interconnect to form a continuous three-dimensional network of vascular arcades

Arteries

Throughout the body, each vessel and its branches are connected with adjacent vessels and branches of neighboring vessels to form arches. The keystones in these arcades are formed sometimes by true anastomoses without change in caliber. More commonly, they are represented by reduced-caliber choke arteries and arterioles. The perimeter of choke or anastomotic vessels defines the anatomic territory of each artery *(Fig. 23.39)*. Each vascular territory is surrounded by reduced-caliber choke anastomotic vessels. Thus, each tissue is supplied by a series of linked arterial territories, some small and some large.

The concept is three-dimensional and was documented by Hunter in 1794.[77] He cited the vascular arcades in the hands and the feet as examples and stated that the arcades are smaller and occur more frequently as the arteries become more distal *(Fig. 23.40)*. Thus, like a Roman aqueduct, the arterial framework consists of tiers of vascular arcades that commence from the aorta and become progressively smaller as the capillary bed is approached. In general, the large arcades are formed by the segmental or distributing source arteries (e.g., the intercostal, radial, ulnar, and deep epigastric arteries) that course between the tissues. Successive tiers of arcades are formed by the arteries, arterioles, and capillaries that supply those tissues. FIGS **23.40, 23.41, 23.42** APPEARS ONLINE ONLY

Veins

Commencing at the capillary bed, the venous arcades have a design similar to that of the arteries but in reverse, with the tiers becoming larger and less numerous until the ultimate arcade is reached – the arcade represented by the superior and inferior venae cavae, with the heart situated at the keystone. These arcades link adjacent venous territories in and between tissues.

Within this network, there is a basic venous module that is repeated in the tiers of the venous network, modified in size and shape by the structure and function of the tissue and the embryologic growth and differentiation that have given rise to its adult form *(Fig. 23.43A)*. It is stellate or medusoid in form and consists of a number of collecting veins that converge on a pedicle. A good example of this arrangement is the cartwheel of superficial veins that converge on the saphenous bulb in the groin. In some areas, the tributaries are polarized from one direction, like a tree that has been blown by the wind *(Fig. 23.43B)*; this is true in the scalp, in muscles, and in the leg where the short saphenous vein approaches the popliteal fossa.

The branches within each "venous tree" are linked by channels, often free of valves, that are oriented like the rungs of a ladder or the circumferential loops of a cobweb. These arcades are well demonstrated in the hands, in the feet, in the cubital fossa, and between the venae comitantes that accompany the arteries. Peripherally, the radiating branches of each venous tree are linked to those of its neighbor, again by avalvular veins, to complete the network *(Fig. 23.43C)*. In the

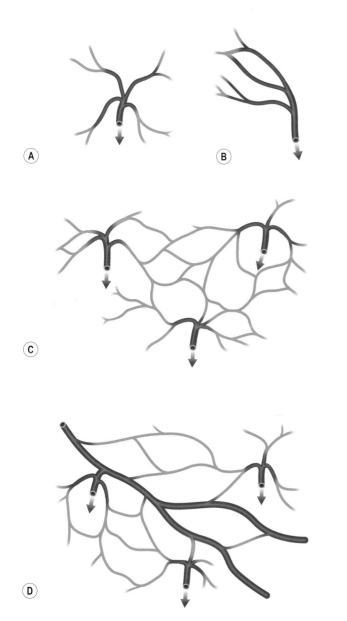

Fig. 23.43 Schematic diagrams of **(A)** the basic venous module, **(B)** its modified arrangement in different areas, and **(C)** how these modules interconnect to form a continuous network. **(D)** In the integument, this network of venous perforators is reorganized in the subdermal plexus to form longitudinal channels. The valved segments are solid blue, and the avalvular oscillating veins are light blue. (From Taylor GI, Caddy CM, Watterson PA, et al. The venous territories [venosomes] of the human body: experimental study and clinical implications. Plast Reconstr Surg. 1990;86:185.)

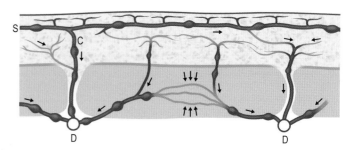

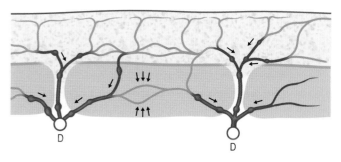

Fig. 23.44 Top, Schematic diagram of the integument and underlying muscle (shaded) in a limb illustrating the superficial (S) and deep (D) venous systems with their interconnecting network. A large vena communicans (C) connects these systems, and the alternative pathways of four venae comitantes are shown. The valved veins are dark blue, and the oscillating veins are light blue. Bottom, Similar diagram representing other regions where the predominant venous drainage is by means of the venae comitantes. Note in each diagram that oscillating veins link adjacent territories in the integument and deep tissues. (From Taylor GI, Caddy CM, Watterson PA, et al. The venous territories [venosomes] of the human body: experimental study and clinical implications. Plast Reconstr Surg. 1990;86:185.)

integument, large horizontal channels have developed within this reticular framework to subserve the specialized function of thermoregulation *(Fig. 23.43D)*. Their connections with the deep veins are retained as large channels, the venae communicantes, or by means of the smaller venae comitantes of the perforating cutaneous arteries *(Fig. 23.44)*.

Vessels obey the law of equilibrium

This concept was described by Debreuil-Chambardel and is mentioned in Salmon's description of the cutaneous arteries.[8,10] Basically, this concept states that "the anatomical territories of adjacent arteries bear an inverse relationship to each other yet combine to supply the same region." If one vessel is small, its partner is large to compensate, and vice versa. This is well illustrated by the relative size of the superficial epigastric artery and the perforators of the DIEA. When the superficial inferior epigastric artery territory is noted to be large, the DIEA territory is relatively smaller, and vice versa *(Fig. 23.7)*. This is an important observation since, if a large superficial inferior epigastric vein is noted, the drainage of the inferior portion of the DIEAP flap may be dependent on the superficial venous drainage system.

Vessels have a relatively constant destination but may have a variable origin

This is typical of the vessels that emanate from the groin to supply the skin of the lower abdomen and upper thigh. The superficial inferior epigastric and the superficial circumflex iliac arteries, for example, may arise either separately from the common femoral artery or as a combined trunk from that vessel or from one of its branches. Whatever the case, their destination is constant to supply the integument of the lower abdomen and the hip *(Figs 23.7, 23.16)*.

Venous networks consist of linked valvular and avalvular channels that allow equilibrium of flow and pressure

The venous network of the body is relatively poorly studied, compared to the arterial system. It consists of segments which have consistent valves and numerous venous channels, large and small, that are free of valves and allow flow within their lumens in either direction. Conversely, there are many small veins that have valves at or near their ostia (sentinel valves) as they enter large channels *(Fig. 23.43)*.

Directional veins

Directional veins are valved veins which exist either as longitudinal channels, well developed in the subcutaneous and deep tissues of the limbs, or as a stellate pattern of collecting veins, which converge on a pedicle. The cutaneous perforators and the pedicle draining muscles are good examples of the latter arrangement. Because many of their tributaries have valves oriented distally as they converge on the pedicle, they provide the anatomic basis for distally based flaps *(Fig. 23.43)*.

Oscillating avalvular veins

Oscillating avalvular veins are avalvular vessels which are numerous and may reach large dimensions. They connect and allow free flow between the valved channels of adjacent venous territories, territories whose valves are oriented in the opposite direction *(Figs 23.43, 23.44)*. They are also found between the valved channels of the same system; they match and accompany the choke arteries of the arterial framework. In the same way that the choke arteries define the arterial territories, oscillating veins define the perimeter of the venous territories *(Fig. 23.44)*. This is well illustrated in the study of the muscles *(Fig. 23.14)* and in some areas of the integument, especially the torso, head, and neck. In the skin of the limbs, this pattern is overshadowed by the large superficial channels in the subdermal plexus but is apparent in cross-sectional studies. If one mentally subtracts the long, large venous channels from the picture in the limbs, the remaining stellate pattern of the perforating veins matches that of the perforating arteries. It is noteworthy that there is a rich network of large oscillating veins in the anterior thigh. This may provide an explanation for arterialized venous free flaps.

Muscles are prime movers of venous return

Most surgeons have been preoccupied with the arterial supply of the various muscles used for transfer. The efferent veins that accompany the arteries and drain the muscles have been noted and assumed, quite correctly, to be sufficient to provide an adequate venous return.

However, this is but half the picture. There are afferent veins entering almost every muscle in the body that arise from the overlying integument, adjacent muscles, and underlying bone where muscles are attached. When the muscles contract, valves in the efferent veins direct flow toward the heart. During "diastole," valves direct flow into the muscles by means of their afferent veins. If the valves in the muscles in the leg become incompetent (e.g., as the late result of deep venous thrombosis), it would not be difficult to envision the back-pressure effect on the afferent cutaneous veins entering the muscle and their role in the pathogenesis of varicose veins and venous ulceration.

Many veins connect muscle pairs or groups of muscles as arcades. It is noteworthy that the muscles with the richest afferent supply were those that filled most readily with our injection studies. Notable examples are the gastrocnemius–soleus complex, the quadriceps muscles, the triceps, and the shoulder girdle muscles, especially the deltoid.

Superficial veins follow nerves and deep veins follow arteries

The venous drainage of the skin following investigation has been found to consist of two parts.

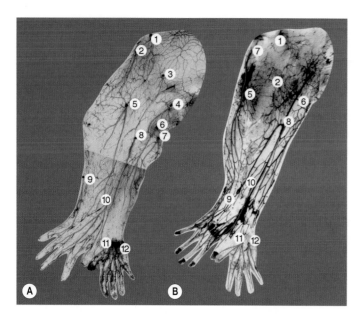

Fig. 23.45 **(A)** Arterial and **(B)** venous studies of the integument of the upper limb with: (1) the axillary; (2) lower lateral brachial; (3) supraclavicular; (4) intercostobrachial; (5) posterior antebrachial; (6) medial antebrachial; (7) medial brachial; (8) lateral antebrachial; (9) dorsal branch of ulnar; (10) superficial radial; (11) median; and (12) ulnar nerves labeled. (From Taylor GI, Gianoutsos MP, Morris SF. The neurovascular territories of the skin and muscles: anatomic study and clinical implications. Plast Reconstr Surg. 1994;94:1.)

1. A subdermal horizontal network tends to follow the cutaneous nerves. This is seen in the limbs in particular, with named cutaneous nerves following named superficial veins *(Fig. 23.45)*.

2. Where perforating veins pass through the deep fascia in a perpendicular fashion, this occurs with accompanying arteries. As stated in previous concepts, this usually occurs at fixed sites *(Fig. 23.38)*.

Applications of angiosome concept

The vascular anatomical information contained in this chapter is an overview to provide the reader with general information important for the design of flaps. From our extensive anatomical studies, we have determined that the general vascular architecture of the body is consistent but variation between different individuals and from side to side in the same individual is the rule. As our understanding of the vascular anatomy of the human body improves, our ability to design and transfer flaps successfully is also improving. Although much

is now known about the arterial framework of the body, the venous framework, and the nervous network, there are still gaps in our knowledge. Although knowledge of vascular anatomy can be applied to all aspects of surgery, the primary focus in plastic and reconstructive surgery is usually dedicated to successful flap design. Therefore, the clinical applicability of this chapter pertains primarily to the identification of cutaneous perforators, their inclusion in flap design, and augmenting the blood flow of the vessels supplying the flap when necessary.

Preoperative assessment of the cutaneous vascular supply

Flap design

It has been determined clinically and experimentally that flaps can be safely designed by identifying a cutaneous perforator and an adjacent perforator; a line drawn between the two perforators should represent the axis of a viable flap.[85–87] In the simplest situations, this approach can work well; however, the technique depends on a very accurate assessment of the cutaneous perforators.

Dopplers

A variety of Doppler ultrasound devices have been utilized to identify cutaneous vessels. The simplest Doppler probes are handheld pencil Doppler probes.[85] These are easy to use, inexpensive, portable, and provide limited information *(Fig. 23.46)*. All Dopplers require insight into their limitations. Dopplers may pick up background vessels, may not determine the course of vessels accurately, and tend to be operator-dependent. However, a simple Doppler is a handy tool to identify cutaneous vessels accurately.   FIG **23.46** APPEARS ONLINE ONLY

The Doppler probe allows surgeons to locate cutaneous perforators with precision in individual cases. Using the knowledge that most cutaneous arteries emerge from fixed skin sites, as already outlined in the section on anatomic concepts *(Fig. 23.10)*, their expected origin can be anticipated and located rapidly. There is considerable interobserver variability with the use of the Doppler. The handheld Doppler is portable, inexpensive, and can be readily utilized by the surgeon to confirm cutaneous perforators. However, the course of the perforator is difficult to determine and there is a significant learning curve associated with the use of a handheld Doppler. There are also some limitations in its use. Obese patients in particular may limit its efficiency for two reasons. First, the thick cutaneous layer may preclude detection of the perforator as it emerges from the deep fascia. Second, as adipose tissue increases, the integument stretches into folds, and the course and destination of the perforators become distorted. There is therefore an increased margin for error in siting the base and axes of the skin flap.

The use of the Doppler probe to locate the origin of cutaneous perforators is not new and has been used by many in the past.[85] It is not necessary in every case, for obvious reasons. However, its application in free-flap transfer has been found to be invaluable, especially in siting a small flap. A good example of this is the osteocutaneous fibular flap, where just a small skin paddle is required either to monitor the vascular anastomosis or as part of the reconstruction. The Doppler probe is a quick, simple method for defining the perforators.

Color duplex Doppler

The more sophisticated Doppler devices are color duplex Dopplers which have greater resolution, cost, and inconvenience but provide much more detail on examination.[88–90] The color duplex ultrasound can accurately detect vessel diameter and flow velocity.[90] Color duplex Doppler has advantages over CTA, including no intravenous contrast, lower cost, and no radiation exposure.[90] The color duplex Doppler is usually already present in the radiology department of many hospitals but it generally requires training of a technician to obtain reliable and consistent results.

CT angiography

The most accurate method to determine the position, diameter, and course of perforators to the skin is CTA. Masia *et al.* initially reported the use of a multidetector CT scanner to map perforators prior to DIEAP flap harvest.[91] The CTA technique has become very popular and is now used around the world to define preoperatively the size, course, and details of individual perforators *(Fig. 23.47)*. We have compared the accuracy of Doppler versus CTA and found CTA to be more accurate and more useful *(Fig. 23.47)*.[92] The high-resolution images of CTA provide extensive information for the surgeon regarding individual perforators as small as 0.3 mm. In DIEAP flap reconstruction of the breast, we have developed a system to report individual perforators using a grid, thus enhancing communication between radiologist and surgeon *(Fig. 23.25C)*. Also, in freestyle, perforator free-flap surgery,[93] knowledge of the perforator course prior to flap harvest can save a great deal of operating room time. The main disadvantages of CTA include cost and radiation exposure. Proponents of CTA highlight the savings gained by reducing operating room time. Also radiation can be minimized by targeted examinations of the flap donor site. In addition, allergic reactions to contrast dye and claustrophobia are potential patient problems with CTA.[90]

Axes of skin flaps

The cutaneous arteries of the skin have provided the basis of "axial" flaps used extensively in plastic and reconstructive surgery. *Figure 23.48* shows details of the origin, course, size, density, and interconnections of the cutaneous perforators. It therefore provides for the logical planning of the base and axis of a skin flap. Cross-sectional studies confirm the reason for including the outer layer of the deep fascia with flaps raised in the scalp and in the extremities; in these situations, the vessels hug the fascia for considerable distances. If a flap is designed along the course of the cutaneous nerve, such as the saphenous or the sural nerve, long safe flaps can be and have been elevated. Pontén's[28] original flaps were designed in this way, and the saphenous neurovascular flap was planned in a similar manner.[94] In the loose skin areas of the torso, it is unnecessary to include deep fascia because the cutaneous arteries course at an early stage within the integument. They frequently correspond with the course of the cutaneous nerve.[95]

Distally based skin flaps

Arterial perforators radiate in stellate patterns, and this includes branches that course proximally. The accompanying veins converge from the same directions. Hence, if a flap is based distally over such a perforating system, it will contain arterial branches that radiate proximally from it and valved veins that return to that point.

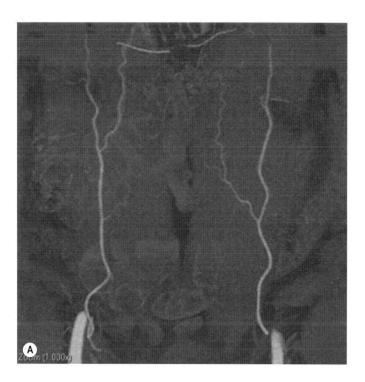

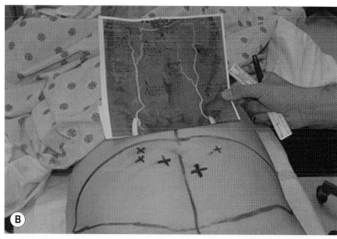

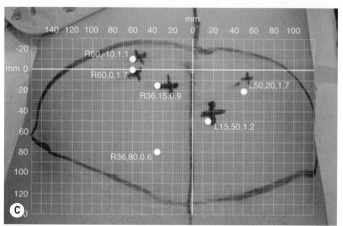

Fig. 23.47 Use of computed tomography angiography (CTA) in the planning of deep inferior epigastric artery perforator flaps. **(A)** Axial view of abdomen in patient preoperatively before deep inferior epigastric artery flap reconstruction of the breast. Arrows indicate cutaneous perforators. **(B)** Using CTA to plan surgery. Markings show perforators detected with handheld Doppler. **(C)** Grid overlay with white dots reflects radiologist's description of cutaneous perforators based on CTA using coordinates: R/L, distance from midline in millimeters, distance inferior to umbilicus, size of perforator in millimeters. (From Al-Dhamin A, Berry R, Prasad MA, *et al.* Coding system for CTA of the inferior epigastric artery perforators in DIEAP flap. Plast Reconstr Surg (in press).)

Therefore, it has been noted that the presence of the perforator in the base of the flap is important and allows distally based flaps.[96–98] An extension of this is the so-called propeller flap *(Fig. 23.49)*, which is a local island fasciocutaneous flap based on a single dissected perforator.[99] The propeller concept is an extension of the perforator flap concept. Basically, the most crucial element to the design of an adequately vascularized flap is the inclusion of a sufficient cutaneous perforator and its corresponding vein in the base of the flap. The flaps can be designed throughout the body in a wide variety of orientations as long as the vessel included as the flap vascular supply is not injured prior to or during the flap elevation and is not kinked. Therefore, gentle tissue handling and surgical technique are important to the success of propeller flaps and other local perforator flaps as well as releasing the deep fascia around the perforator to prevent kinking as the flap is rotated.

Skin flap dimensions

Because the blood supply of the integument, both venous and arterial, has been shown to be a continuous system of linked vascular territories, the survival length of a skin flap must depend on: (1) the caliber and length of the dominant vessels on which the flap is based; (2) the caliber and span of the adjacent captured artery or arteries, vein or veins; (3) the caliber and length of the connecting choke vessels; and (4) an anatomically favorable or unfavorable venous return.

Where the arterial perforators are large and widely separated, the territory of each is large and a long flap can be raised with safety. These flaps are characteristic of the loose skin areas of the torso and the scalp. Conversely, if the perforators are diminutive and close together, the territory of each is small. The viable length of the flap is short unless the supplying source vessel is included in the design. This is evident in the fixed skin area of the sole of the foot.

If very large flaps are required or if vessels of a large caliber are necessary for microvascular anastomoses, the requirements can be satisfied by chasing the perforators through the intermuscular septa or the intramuscular septa to include the underlying source vessels. The intelligent use of a delay also allows safe capture of adjacent vascular territories.

When we consider the venous drainage, the large longitudinal veins in the subcutaneous tissue of the limbs offer an excellent drainage for proximally based flaps because their valves are oriented in that direction. However, in the lower abdomen, the drainage of proximally based flaps may be anatomically unfavorable because the valves of the superficial inferior epigastric veins are directed distally toward the groin. The undermined flap of a transverse abdominal lipectomy is a case in point, and perhaps fortuitously, the area of the flap in question is amputated in the procedure.

The scalp veins are mostly free of valves, and hence flaps based in any direction will drain favorably. In many regions, however, the venous network consists of territories of valved veins oriented in different directions that are linked by oscillating veins.

The precise mechanism of the necrosis line of a flap is unknown, although the opening-up of arteriovenous

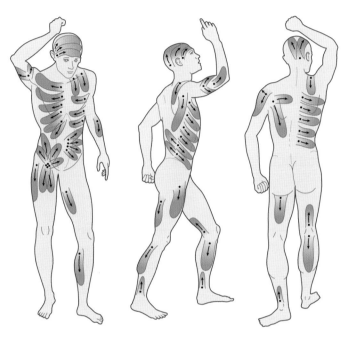

Fig. 23.48 Some of the large axial cutaneous flaps that have been used or are available based on specific perforating arteries and their accompanying perforating veins, as defined by radiographic studies of the integument. In the scalp and the limbs, they should include the deep fascia. Compare with Figures 23.9 and 23.16. (From Taylor GI, Palmer JH. The vascular territories [angiosomes] of the body: experimental study and clinical applications. Br J Plast Surg. 1987;40:113.)

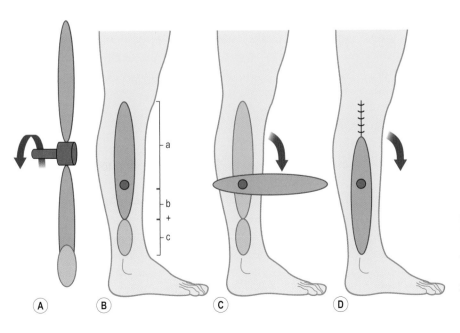

Fig. 23.49 Propeller flap. **(A)** The flap is likened to the blades of a propeller. **(B)** The flap is designed based on the largest adjacent uninjured perforator to the wound; a = b + c + 1 cm. **(C)** The flap is elevated based on the perforator. **(D)** The portion of the flap b is used to cover the donor site and the flap a is used to cover the wound. (From Teo TW. The propeller flap concept. Clin Plast Surg. 2010;37: 615–626.)

shunts provides a plausible theory. Whatever happens, it has been shown that the choke vessels on the arterial side and some of the valved territories of the venous return provide a potential mechanical obstruction to flow.

Fasciocutaneous flaps

The deep fascia should be included in the design of the fasciocutaneous flap in those sites where the skin is relatively fixed to the deep fascia, for example, in the limbs or the scalp. In these instances, the dominant cutaneous vessels course on or lie adjacent to the deep fascia. Although they can be dissected free in some cases, it may be simpler and safer to include the deep fascia with the flap. However, where the skin and subcutaneous tissues are mobile over the deep fascia, for example, in the iliac fossae or the breast, it is unnecessary to include this fascial layer because the major cutaneous vessels have already left its surface. To some extent, the initial enthusiasm for fasciocutaneous flaps has been tempered by increased anatomical understanding and there are relatively few indications for the inclusion of deep fascia in a cutaneous flap.

The term "septocutaneous" is sometimes misleading, especially when it is used to describe a surgically created entity rather than a true anatomic structure. This may occur, for example, where the cutaneous perforators of a radial or ulnar flap are dissected within an envelope of loose areolar tissue. Furthermore, the septocutaneous flap may provide traps for the unwary surgeon. In some cases, the cutaneous artery and its accompanying vein leave the underlying source vessels and course toward the surface in a surgically favorable position, adjacent to a true white fibrous intermuscular septum. This is typical of the blood supply to the skin of the lateral arm flap, where cutaneous perforators arise from descending branches of the profunda brachii vessels and follow the lateral intermuscular septum toward the skin. This pattern of supply usually exists where the muscles glide on either side of the intermuscular septum.

However, if the muscles attach to either side of the intermuscular septum, the cutaneous perforator may have a variable course. This variability is seen in particular in the lateral aspect of the upper calf. If a compound skin and bone flap is designed at this site over the lateral intermuscular septum based on the cutaneous perforators of the peroneal vessels, either these skin vessels may course directly to the surface, traveling in a favorable position, either adjacent to the septum or within the substance of the soleus or flexor hallucis longus muscles, close to their attachments to the fibula, or alternatively, they may arise indirectly from branches to the soleus or flexor hallucis muscles as terminal twigs of muscle branches that have arisen from the peroneal vessels at considerable distance from the lateral intermuscular septum. In these cases, a long and laborious intramuscular dissection of the cutaneous supply will be required to raise the flap successfully.

Musculocutaneous flaps

The musculocutaneous flap initially became popular when it was recognized that the large vessels supplying muscle were more reliable than the much smaller cutaneous vessels, and as a result the skin overlying the muscle was reliably transferred.[23–26] Musculocutaneous flaps remain preferable in cases where large vascularized tissue bulk is required. However, it is now understood that the musculocutaneous perforators can be harvested without the bulk of the muscle as perforator flaps. When skin and deep fascia are firmly bound to the underlying muscle (e.g., the gluteus maximus and latissimus dorsi), the blood supply to the overlying skin is ensured. At each fixed site over the muscle, vessels emerge to supply the integument. However, when the muscle is mobile beneath the deep fascia (e.g., the gracilis muscle), the cutaneous supply is at most tenuous.

In general, musculocutaneous flaps can be raised safely if the skin paddle is placed over the perforators of the feeding muscle artery or those in the adjacent muscle territory. Attempts to capture territories beyond this, without previous delay, frequently result in vascular insufficiency. This situation may prevail, for reasons already outlined, in the pectoralis major and the lower TRAM flaps.

Depending on the muscle type and the site of the skin paddle, the venous pathway once again may become anatomically favorable or unfavorable. In each case, the venous drainage is thrust on perforators that drain to the intramuscular plexus of veins. In type I muscles, the drainage is favorable regardless of the site of the skin paddle over the muscle because the venous drainage is in one direction. If the skin paddle is placed over the distal territory of type II and type III muscles, the valves of this territory are oriented in the opposite direction to those of the draining pedicle, and the pathway is anatomically unfavorable. This problem was highlighted by Costa *et al.*[100] in their investigations of the venous drainage of the lower TRAM flap.

Many of the musculocutaneous flaps are being replaced by local or free microvascular perforator flaps based on the musculocutaneous perforators. These musculocutaneous perforators are variable in size and position and require a flexible operative approach. These "perforator flaps" are used to provide large vessels for microvascular transfer; to eliminate the bulk of muscle, when appropriate; and to preserve muscle function, for example, in harvesting a lower transverse abdominal skin flap on one or more perforators of the DIEA.[38,39]

However, all cutaneous flaps are based on cutaneous perforators, whether direct or indirect, and regardless of whether they pass between or through the muscles to reach the overlying integument. Hence, to confine the term "perforator flap" to those instances in which the cutaneous vessel emerges from muscle to perforate the overlying deep fascia is misleading. The term "perforator flap" therefore should include any island skin flap, based on a cutaneous perforator, whether it arises from a source vessel between or within a muscle or other deep tissue. Some of the early free flaps, for example, the groin flap, are true perforator flaps, in this instance based on the superficial circumflex iliac or superficial inferior epigastric artery.[22]

Perforator flaps

A perforator flap has been variously defined as a cutaneous flap based on a musculocutaneous perforator or any cutaneous flap based on any vessel supplying the skin.[30,101,102] However, this is a semantic discussion which is not as important as the concept of perforator flaps, which represent the continuing evolution of tissue transfers. Initial pioneering reports of perforator flaps demonstrated that it was possible to harvest a skin flap reliably based on musculocutaneous perforators.[38,103,104] Perforator flaps have the advantage of the large vessel size of vessels supplying muscles of the body without the disadvantages of unnecessary muscle bulk and the

loss of function of unnecessary muscle sacrifice. The popularity of perforator flaps has increased exponentially, as evidenced by publications in the world's plastic surgical literature, since the initial reports of this surgical technique.

Anatomical understanding has laid the groundwork for the success of perforator flaps.[47] Without detailed knowledge of the underlying vasculature, perforator flap surgery would be difficult. We have compiled an atlas of the perforators of the human body and subdivided their distribution into 61 vascular territories *(Fig. 23.50)*.[39,40,105] There are approximately 400 cutaneous perforators to the skin, about 60% musculocutaneous and 40% septocutaneous.[39,40,105] The field has opened up significantly due to increased enthusiasm of surgeons to learn the "perforator flap technique" and increased flap options. Ultimately, perforator flaps have become more popular because patient outcomes have improved. Moreover, the emphasis on perforator flaps has focused attention on the vascular anatomy of the skin. Many of the 400 perforators to the skin can be used as a local or free-flap vascular supply, thus expanding the possible flap options dramatically. The use of the perforator flap technique allows clever and customized reconstructions which can provide optimal patient outcomes. However, perforator flaps are simply more flaps in the armementarium of the plastic surgeon and good clinical judgment is still required to choose the best flap or technique for a specific application.[106]

The early pioneers of perforator flap named flaps in a descriptive fashion which led to a wide array of terms to describe the flaps.[101,106] In some cases, several terms were used for the same flap, which led to confusion and sometimes delayed meaningful communication about the flaps.[101,106] In an effort to standardize descriptions of perforator flaps, we introduced a nomenclature in which all perforator flaps are named according to the source vessel supplying the flap.[30] The letters AP are added to indicate artery perforator and the initials of the muscle through which the perforators travel are added as a suffix *(Fig. 23.51)*. Hence, in the case of a DIEAP flap, DIEAP-ra (rectus abdominis). The suffix with muscle initials is only necessary when the perforating vessels can pass through different muscles. The suffix -s indicates that the perforator flap is a septocutaneous flap.

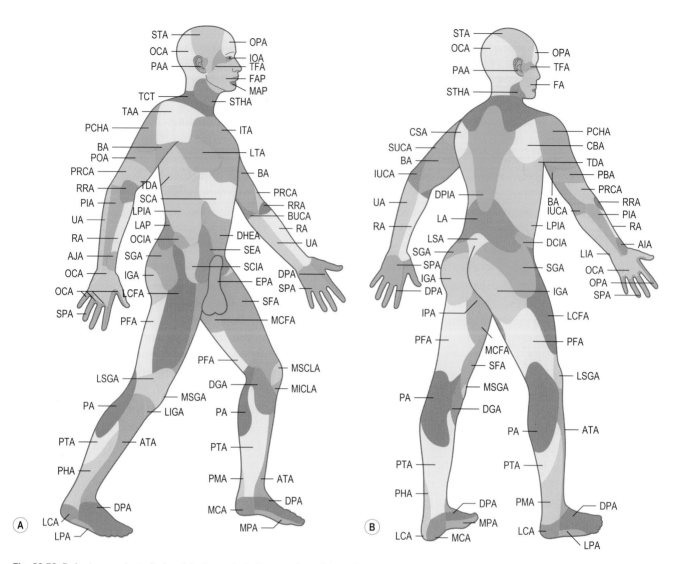

Fig. 23.50 Perforator vascular territories of the human body. The vascular territories of the body which correspond to regions of musculocutaneous and septocutaneous perforators to the skin. (From Geddes CR. MSc thesis, Dalhousie University, Halifax, Nova Scotia, Canada.) AIOA, anterior interosseous artery; ATA, anterior tibial artery; BA, brachial artery; CSA, circumflex scapular artery; DCA, dorsal carpal arch; DCIA, deep circumflex iliac artery; DGA, descending genicular artery; DIEA, deep inferior epigastric artery; DPA, dorsal pedis artery; DPAA, deep palmar arch; DPIA, dorsal branch of posterior intercostal artery; EPA, external pudendal artery; FA, facial artery; IGA, inferior gluteal artery; IOA, infraorbital artery; IPA, internal pudendal artery; ITA, internal thoracic (mammary) artery; IUCA, inferior ulnar collateral artery; LA, lumbar arteries; LCA, lateral calcaneal artery; LCFA, lateral circumflex femoral artery; LIGA, lateral inferior genicular artery; LPA, lateral plantar artery; LPIA, lateral branches of posterior intercostal artery; LSA, lateral sural artery; LSGA, kateral superior genicular artery; LTA, lateral thoracic (mammary) artery; MA, mental artery; MCA, edial calcaneal artery; MCFA, medial circumflex femoral artery; MIGA, medial inferior genicular artery; MSA, medial sural artery; MSGA, medial superior genicular artery; OCA, occipital artery; OPA, ophthalmic artery; PA, popliteal artery; PAURA, posterior auricular artery; PBA, profunda brachial artery; PCHA, posterior circumflex humeral artery; PFA, profunda femoris artery; PIOA, posterior interosseous artery; PNA, peroneal artery; PRCA, posterior radial collateral artery; PTA, posterior tibial artery; RA, radial artery; RRA, radial recurrent artery; SCIA, superficial circumflex iliac artery; SEA, superior epigastric artery; SFA, superficial femoral artery; SGA, superior gluteal artery; SIEA, superficial inferior epigastric artery; SMA, submental artery; SPA, superficial palmar arch; STA, superficial temporal artery; STHA, superior thyroid artery; SUCA, superior ulnar collateral artery; TAA, thoracoacromial artery.

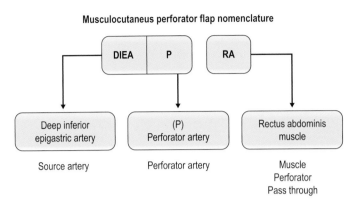

Fig. 23.51 Perforator flap nomenclature. (From Geddes CR, Morris SF, Neligan PC. Perforator flaps – evolution, classification and applications. Ann Plast Surg. 2003;50:90–99.)

The choice of a suitable perforator and the dissection of the pedicle of a musculocutaneous perforator flap through a muscle require training, expertise, and gentle operative skills. Generally, the perforator flap is planned preoperatively using a handheld Doppler, a color duplex Doppler, or CTA.[90,107] The largest perforator is usually chosen for the flap. As the flap dissection begins, each perforator over 0.5 mm in diameter is preserved until the pedicle is clearly visualized. As the dissection proceeds, gentle surgical technique is required, particularly at the fascial level, to avoid traction injuries to the small perforating vessels. Generally, the surgical technique is to skeletonize the vascular pedicle and keep the field dry.[107,108]

Dozens of new perforator flaps have been described in the past decade. However, there is a core group of very useful perforator flaps which have become standard, including DIEAP flap,[38,103,104] anterolateral thigh flap (based on the descending branch of the lateral circumflex femoral vessels through vastus lateralis, LCFAP-vl),[109] submental artery flap (SMAP),[110] posterior interosseous flap (PIOAP-s),[111] thoracodorsal artery perforator flap (TAP-ld),[112] superior gluteal artery (SGAP-gm),[113] and inferior gluteal artery perforator flap (IGAP-gm).[114] Depending on surgeon experience and preference, a number of these have replaced conventional flaps. The anterolateral thigh flap, in particular, has been called the ideal free flap, because of its usefulness in a wide variety of clinical applications.[115] The perforator flaps are thoroughly described in a textbook on perforator flaps.[39] As Pribaz and Chan state, "The use of perforator flaps is a new and exciting paradigm in reconstructive surgery."[116]

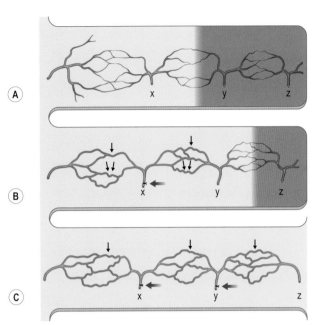

Fig. 23.52 Diagrammatic representation of the same flap raised with and without a surgical delay to illustrate the necrosis line and the changes in the choke vessels. **(A)** The adjacent territory x is captured with safety, and the necrosis line occurs at the choke–vessel interface with vessel y or the one beyond. **(B)** Vessel x had been delayed. Note the effect on the choke vessels and the site of the necrosis line. **(C)** Vessels x and y have been delayed in this bipedicled flap. Vessel z is divided and the tip of the flap elevated at a second stage to provide the longest flap. (From Callegari PR, Taylor GI, Caddy CM, *et al.* An anatomic review of the delay phenomenon I: experimental studies. Plast Reconstr Surg. 1992;89:397–418.)

The delay phenomenon

The only documented method to increase skin flap survival is the delay procedure. A delay procedure can be done in a variety of ways, from a partial incision around the margin of a planned flap, ligation of nonpedicle vessels supplying the flap, to partial or complete flap elevation *(Fig. 23.52)*. The delay can be done in one or many stages and can lead to greatly improved skin flap survival. The physiologic effect of delay is an enlargement of the existing arteries along the axis of the flap, which has been well documented in experimental animal models *(Figs 23.53, 23.54)*.[86,117,118] One adjacent anatomic vascular territory can be captured with safety on the cutaneous artery at the flap base. Anastomotic vascular keystones, usually formed by reduced-caliber choke arteries that link adjacent cutaneous perforators, play an integral role in the delay phenomenon. When a flap is elevated, these choke vessels, which initially reduce flow from one arterial territory to the next

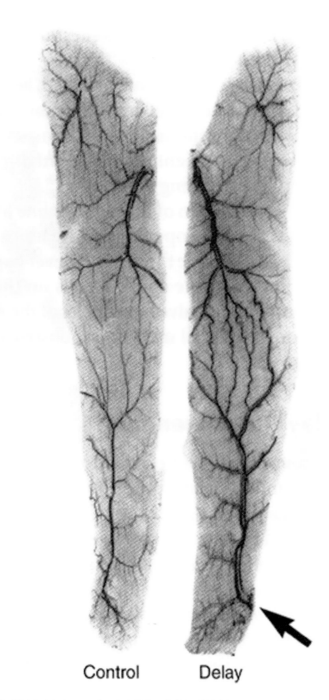

Control   Delay

Fig. 23.53 Arteriogram of control (left) and delayed (right) rectus abdominis muscles of a dog 7 days postoperatively. Note the dilated choke vessels in the delayed flap by ligation of the deep inferior epigastric artery (arrow). (From Dhar SC, Taylor GI. The delay phenomenon: the story unfolds. Plast Reconstr Surg. 1999;104:2079.)

along the flap, enlarge to the caliber of the cutaneous arteries they connect. However, this process of vessel enlargement is an active event and takes time. It is a permanent and irreversible process involving multiplication and hypertrophy of the cells in each layer of the vessel wall, with its maximal effect occurring between 48 and 72 hours after operation *(Fig. 23.55)*.[117] It has been observed that necrosis usually occurs at the level of the next choke anastomosis in the arterial network or the one beyond. Surgically, flap survival can be extended by the strategic division of vascular pedicles at various time intervals along the length of the proposed flap – the "flap delay" procedure. FIG **23.54**
APPEARS ONLINE ONLY

Composite flaps

A knowledge of the vascular supply of all the tissues that constitute each angiosome provides the basis for the transfer of composite units of skin, muscle, nerve, tendon, and bone supplied by a single arteriovenous system. This knowledge has been applied extensively in free composite tissue transfer. The vessels within the angiosome interconnect between the various layers. This interconnection is well illustrated with the transfer of composite tissue from the groin region. The direct cutaneous perforators of the superficial circumflex iliac artery interconnect with the indirect perforators of the deep circumflex iliac artery. When a composite osteocutaneous flap is based on the deep system, the perforators of the deep circumflex iliac artery capture the territory of the superficial circumflex iliac artery to perfuse the skin.[66] When the superficial system is used, the reverse applies to perfuse the anterior segment of iliac crest and the attached muscles.[68]

Angiosome concept and flap design

In this chapter, we have presented a variety of anatomical information which supports the angiosome concept and which provides a blueprint for successful flap design. As always in the course of surgical evolution, the ideas and concepts will gradually change to reflect new discoveries and the pioneering efforts of creative surgeons. Surgical advances move as the pendulum in an undulating course, ever closer to the true course.

Bonus images for this chapter can be found online at **http://www.expertconsult.com**

Fig. 23.3 Carl Mancot's vascular territories of the human integument. **(A)** Cutaneous vascular territories, ventral surface. **(B)** Cutaneous vascular territories, dorsal surface. (From Manchot C. Die Hautarterien des menschlichen Körpers. Leipzig: FCW Vogel, 1889.)

Fig. 23.4 Michel Salmon's vascular territories of the human integument, 1936. Summary of the cutaneous arterial territories of the ventral surface of the body. (From Salmon M. Artères de la peau. Paris: Masson, 1936.)

Fig. 23.5 Cadaver with body landmarks and incision lines marked. (From Taylor GI, Palmer JH. The vascular territories [angiosomes] of the body: experimental study and clinical applications. Br J Plast Surg 1987;40:113.)

Fig. 23.6 Lateral view of one female subject **(A)** and anterior view of another **(B)**. **(A)** The arm has been removed. Note the network of large vessels that sweep laterally from the ventral and dorsal midlines, ascend from the groins, descend from the shoulder girdle, and converge on the summits of the scalp and the breasts. This demonstrates the principle that vessels radiate from fixed concave zones and radiate to mobile convex areas. **(B)** A lower midline scar interrupts the vessels with compensatory opening of a large choke vessel above the umbilicus (arrow) to re-establish the flow across the midline. (From Taylor GI, Palmer JH. The vascular territories [angiosomes] of the body: experimental study and clinical applications. Br J Plast Surg 1987;40:113.)

Fig. 23.16 Arterial injection of the right upper limb and torso. **(A)** Note the chain-linked systems of arteries (arrows) that course with the cutaneous nerves in the upper limb. **(B)** On the torso, the nerves are marked on the arterial study. They course with the cutaneous arteries, cross them at angles and collect arterial branches, or approach the arteries from opposite directions (arrows). (From Taylor GI, Palmer JH. The vascular territories [angiosomes] of the body: experimental study and clinical applications. Br J Plast Surg 1987;40:113; and Taylor GI, Gianoutsos MP, Morris SF. The neurovascular territories of the skin and muscles: anatomic study and clinical implications. Plast Reconstr Surg 1994;94:1.)

Fig. 23.19 (A) Arteriogram of the skin of the pig. Note numerous small perforators on lateral torso, a superficial vein that has filled in the study (arrow), the larger segmental vessels near the ventral and dorsal midline, and the large perforator of the deep circumflex iliac artery near the hip. **(B)** Angiogram of the dog. Note the large perforator of the deep circumflex iliac artery and the thoracodorsal artery (arrows) near the hip and shoulder, respectively. **(C)** Arteriogram of the rabbit.

Note the very large perforators of the deep circumflex iliac artery and thoracodorsal arteries dorsally and the superficial inferior epigastric artery and lateral thoracic arteries ventrally. Note also the large vessels supplying the ear. **(D)** Arteriogram of the duck. Note the discrete territories bounded by choke arteries and the long, stretched-out perforator of the transverse cervical artery in the mobile skin area of the neck (arrow). (From Taylor GI, Minabe T. The angiosomes of the mammals and other vertebrates. Plast Reconstr Surg 1992;89:181.)

Fig. 23.20 Injection studies of the anterior torso with the integument removed and umbilicus located (large dot). The studies of the human and dog **(A and C)** are almost identical, with the deep inferior epigastric artery larger than the deep superior epigastric artery. In the rabbit and pig **(B and D)**, the reverse applies. (From Taylor GI, Minabe T. The angiosomes of the mammals and other vertebrates. Plast Reconstr Surg 1992;89:181.)

Fig. 23.21 Comparative study of the rectus abdominis muscle from the various mammals studied. There is a striking similarity between the studies. However, in all animals except the pig, the muscle extends on to the thorax more cranially than in the human, and this region of the rectus receives additional branches from the internal thoracic artery. The reciprocal size relationship of the deep superior epigastric artery and deep inferior epigastric artery between species is a good example of the law of equilibrium. (From Taylor GI, Minabe T. The angiosomes of the mammals and other vertebrates. Plast Reconstr Surg 1992;89:181.)

Fig. 23.25 The cutaneous perforators of the forearm, color-coded to match the angiosomes. Large and small skin perforators are indicated by size of the colored markers. Compare with Figure 23.22. (From Inoue Y, Taylor GI. The angiosomes of the forearm: anatomic study and clinical applications. Plast Reconstr Surg 1996;98:195.)

Fig. 23.26 The vascular territories of the **(A)** superficial, **(B)** middle, and **(C)** deep forearm flexor muscles. Note that the junctional zone between angiosomes occurs primarily within the muscles and that most muscles cross at least two angiosomes. Compare with Figures 23.2 and 23.24. (From Inoue Y, Taylor GI. The angiosomes of the forearm: anatomic study and clinical applications. Plast Reconstr Surg 1996;98:195.)

Fig. 23.27 The vascular territories of the **(A)** superficial and **(B)** deep forearm extensor muscles, showing once again that the junctional zone lies primarily within the muscles. (From Inoue Y, Taylor GI. The angiosomes of the forearm: anatomic study

and clinical applications. Plast Reconstr Surg 1996;98:195.)

Fig. 23.28 Cross-sectional studies of the forearm at the level of **(A)** the head of the radius, **(B)** insertion of the pronator teres, and **(C)** midforearm, showing the angiosomes of the forearm: brachial (yellow), radial (blue), ulnar (red), anterior interosseus (green), and posterior interosseous (orange) arteries. Note that the junctions of the angiosomes occur within the skin, within the muscles, and within the bone. (From Inoue Y, Taylor GI. The angiosomes of the forearm: anatomic study and clinical applications. Plast Reconstr Surg 1996;98:195.)

Fig. 23.29 Vascular territories of the lower leg. The colored spheres represent cutaneous perforators emerging from the deep fascia and depict relative size of the vessels. (From Taylor GI, Pan WR. The angiosomes of the leg: anatomic study and clinical applications. Plast Reconstr Surg 1998;102:599.)

Fig. 23.30 Vascular territories of the lower leg. **(A)** Illustration of the anterior muscle group that lies totally within the anterior tibial angiosome (blue). This angiosome extends to include part of the peroneal muscles. **(B)** Illustration of the lateral muscles and their supply from the anterior tibial (blue) and peroneal (green) angiosomes. (From Taylor GI, Pan WR. The angiosomes of the leg: anatomic study and clinical applications. Plast Reconstr Surg 1998;102:599.)

Fig. 23.31 Vascular territories of the lower leg. **(A)** The superficial muscle group with its supply from the arteries of the popliteal (purple), sural (orange), posterior tibial (yellow), and peroneal (green) angiosomes. All muscles cross at least two angiosomes and receive branches from the source arteries of each. **(B)** The deep muscles and their supply form the source arteries of each angiosome. (From Taylor GI, Pan WR. The angiosomes of the leg: anatomic study and clinical applications. Plast Reconstr Surg 1998;102:599.)

Fig. 23.32 (A–C) Vascular territories of the lower leg. Anterior view of the leg with cross-sections at three levels, viewed distally. The figures show angiosomes of the anterior tibial (blue), posterior tibial (yellow), peroneal (green), and sural (orange) arteries. Note in each case that the angiosome territories extend from the skin to the bone and that their borders, defined by anastomotic vessels, meet usually within tissues, especially within the muscles, rather than between them. (From Taylor GI, Pan WR. The angiosomes of the leg: anatomic study and clinical applications. Plast Reconstr Surg 1998;102:599.)

Fig. 23.33 Fresh cadaver lead oxide arterial study of the lateral **(A)** and anterior **(B)** view of the composite skin and superficial musculoaponeurotic system (SMAS) unit in the head and neck. The occipital (a), superficial temporal (b), and ophthalmic (c) arteries have been labeled. Note that the facial vein (v) runs a more direct course and at some distance to its arterial counterpart, the facial artery (d). **(C)** The skin layer alone reveals a vast arterial "blush" zone of the skin and SMAS shown in sagittal view. Note: (1) the rich arterial anastomotic "waves" formed between the branches of the occipital, superficial temporal, and ophthalmic arteries in the scalp; (2) the cluster of small vessels supplying the fixed skin area over the parotid gland and masseter muscle compared with the large branches of the facial artery that supply the mobile anterior face; and (3) the relative paucity of large vessels in the neck except in the anterior triangle. The SMAS layer is seen only in **(D)** with the muscles of facial expression outlined. (From Houseman ND, Taylor GI, Pan WR. The angiosomes of the head and neck: anatomic study and clinical applications. Plast Reconstr Surg 2000;105:2287.)

Fig. 23.34 (A) Lead oxide arterial study of the blood supply of the ear and adjacent tissues. Note the arcades formed between the superficial temporal and posterior auricular arteries, highlighted with arrows. **(B)** Schematic picture shows the branches of the superficial temporal (dark) and posterior auricular (light) supply to the front and back of the ear, respectively. Note also the true and choke anastomoses between these two arteries in the scalp. **(C and D)** Close-up examination of the arterial anatomy of the external nose. Note the arcades that occur

around the alar dome between the columella branch of the superior labial artery and the facial artery. The facial vein has also been partially filled with lead oxide and highlighted by the arrows. (From Houseman ND, Taylor GI, Pan WR. The angiosomes of the head and neck: anatomic study and clinical applications. Plast Reconstr Surg 2000;105:2287.)

Fig. 23.35 Angiosomes of the muscles of facial expression and mastication in the face. (From Houseman ND, Taylor GI, Pan WR. The angiosomes of the head and neck: anatomic study and clinical applications. Plast Reconstr Surg 2000;105:2287.)

Fig. 23.36 (A–D) The angiosomes of the head and neck colored and numbered to match Figures 23.22 and 23.34. The sagittal section **(B)** shows the three angiosomes. (From Houseman ND, Taylor GI, Pan WR. The angiosomes of the head and neck: anatomic study and clinical applications. Plast Reconstr Surg 2000;105:2287.)

Fig. 23.37 Radiograph of the tongue; note the almost avascular midline. (From Houseman ND, Taylor GI, Pan WR. The angiosomes of the head and neck: anatomic study and clinical applications. Plast Reconstr Surg 2000;105:2287.)

Fig. 23.40 Radiographs of the integument of the upper limb and hand. **(A)** The skin has been incised along the ulnar border. It has been removed **(B)** with the deep fascia and **(C)** without it. (From Taylor GI, Palmer JH. The vascular territories [angiosomes] of the body: experimental study and clinical applications. Br J Plast Surg 1987;40:113.)

Fig. 23.41 The interconnecting arcades of the small intestine. (From Crosthwaite GL, Taylor GI, Palmer JH. A new radio-opaque injection technique for tissue preservation. Br J Plast Surg 1987;40:497.)

Fig. 23.42 (A) The wing of a moth and **(B)** the leaf of a tree, showing their interconnecting arcades of "veins." (From Taylor GI, Palmer JH. The vascular territories [angiosomes] of the body: experimental study and clinical applications. Br J Plast Surg 1987;40:113.)

Fig. 23.46 Doppler probe for the design of skin flaps. The handheld Doppler can be used to identify cutaneous perforators for the design of skin flaps. In this case, the Doppler is used to design a flap based on perforators of the deep inferior epigastric vessels.

Fig. 23.54 Arteriogram of control (left) and delayed (right) rectus abdominis muscle of a dog 12 weeks after reanastomosis of the previously ligated deep inferior epigastric artery (arrow). Note that the choke vessels remain tortuous and dilated, revealing that the effect of the delay is permanent and irreversible. (From Dhar SC, Taylor GI. The delay phenomenon: the story unfolds. Plast Reconstr Surg 1999;104:2079.)

Fig. 23.55 Time sequence of delay. Immediately after the surgical elevation of a flap, the overall vascular diameter is reduced by vasoconstriction. Following this, gradual dilation occurs during the first 48 hours, and then dramatic dilation occurs from 48 to 72 hours. The rate of vessel enlargement then begins to plateau, and gradually, vessels increase thereafter.

Access the complete references list online at **http://www.expertconsult.com**

10. Taylor GI, Tempest M. *Salmon's arteries of the skin.* Edinburgh: Churchill Livingstone; 1988.

21. Taylor GI, Daniel RK. The free flap: composite tissue transfer by vascular anastomosis. *Aust N Z J Surg.* 1973;43:1.

    This is the authors' first report of vascularized free tissue transfer. A free flap was required for coverage of a lower-extremity wound unsuited to then-more-common techniques.

26. Mathes SJ, Nahai F. *Clinical atlas of muscle and musculocutaneous flaps.* St. Louis: Mosby; 1979.

    This landmark reference offers detailed schematics of key flaps for reconstructive procedures. Vivid photos enhance the text.

30. Geddes CR, Morris SF, Neligan PC. Perforator flaps – evolution, classification and applications. *Ann Plast Surg.* 2003;50:90–99.

    The authors provide a historical review of the evolution of perforator flaps, and the advantages of these flaps are described. A system of perforator flap nomenclature is offered.

31. Taylor GI, Corlett RJ, Dhar SC, et al. The anatomical (angiosome) and clinical territories of cutaneous perforating arteries: development of the concept and designing safe flaps. *Plast Reconstr Surg.* 2011;127: 1447–1459.

39. Blondeel PN, Morris SF, Hallock GG, et al. *Perforator flaps. Anatomy, technique and clinical applications.* St. Louis: Quality Medical Publishing; 2006.

40. Morris SF, Tang M, Almutairi K, et al. The anatomic basis of perforator flaps. *Clin Plast Surg Oct.* 2010;37;553–570.

   This report stresses the importance of understanding the cutaneous blood supply in designing perforator flaps. While individual perforator anatomy may be variable, source artery anatomy is relatively consistent.

47. Taylor GI, Palmer JH. The vascular territories (angiosomes) of the body: experimental study and clinical applications. *Br J Plast Surg.* 1987;40:113.

48. Taylor GI, Caddy CM, Watterson PA, et al. The venous territories (venosomes) of the human body: experimental study and clinical implications. *Plast Reconstr Surg.* 1990;86:185.

49. Taylor GI, Gianoutsos MP, Morris SF. The neurovascular territories of the skin and muscles: anatomic study and clinical implications. *Plast Reconstr Surg.* 1994;94:1.

   Extensive human and animal cadaveric studies were performed to characterize the anatomy of fasciocutaenous skin flaps. Cutaneous and motor nerves were found to be accompanied by a vascular system which often provided the regions' dominant blood supply.

24

Flap classification and applications

Scott L. Hansen, David M. Young, Patrick Lang, and Hani Sbitany

SYNOPSIS

- The use of flaps with an intact blood supply has revolutionized the field of plastic surgery. Today, the reconstructive surgeon faced with a soft tissue defect has a surplus of options.
- The muscle flap, the musculocutaneous flap, fasciocutaneous flap, perforator flap and the various techniques of microvascular composite tissue transplantation have made possible major advances in the field of plastic surgery.
- By applying a precise knowledge of the anatomy of skin, muscle, bone and fascia in planning reconstructive procedures, the surgeon has the ability to restore form and function in congenital and acquired defects in most topographic regions.
- Modifications and refinements in flap design offer considerable variety and versatility in the techniques available for use in reconstructive surgery.
- By applying the principles of flap design and technique, it is possible to simplify the approach to the surgical defect.
- Soft-tissue coverage, form and function are the three most important factors in determining a successful outcome.
- Through careful analysis of each individual surgical defect, the most appropriate method of reconstruction can be selected. This chapter reviews flap classification and gives examples of their applications.

 Access the Historical Perspective section online at
http://www.expertconsult.com

Flap classification

A flap consists of tissue that is mobilized on the basis of its vascular anatomy. Flaps can be composed of skin, skin and fascia, skin and muscle or skin, muscle and bone. Because the circulation to the tissue to be mobilized is crucial for flap survival, the development of flap techniques has depended on defining the vascular anatomy of the skin and underlying soft tissue. An early concept of vascular anatomy as it pertained to flap surgery was the thought that skin circulation was based on the longitudinal subdermal plexus. A random pattern flap based on this subdermal plexus was designed to allow elevation of a rectangular-shaped flap of skin and subcutaneous tissue with a length: width ratio in the range of 2–1.5:1. Milton subsequently disproved the concept of length-to-width ratios.[30] Although limited in its reach, the random pattern flap can be elevated and rotated to provide viable skin and subcutaneous tissue to cover an adjacent wound. Common flaps based on the subdermal plexus include the bipedicle flap, advancement flaps (i.e., V–Y), and rotation or transposition flaps (*Fig. 24.1*).

Historically, attempts to use a random pattern flap based on subdermal circulation distant from the wound location eventually resulted in the introduction of the tubed pedicle flap. Through a series of delays using the initial bipedicle flap design, the arc of rotation of the skin flap was increased. Alternatively, the flap was attached to an arm carrier, which later required transferring the arm carrier of the random pattern flap from one body region (donor site) to another (recipient site). This use of the random pattern flap with multiple delays or

Bipedicle flap delay

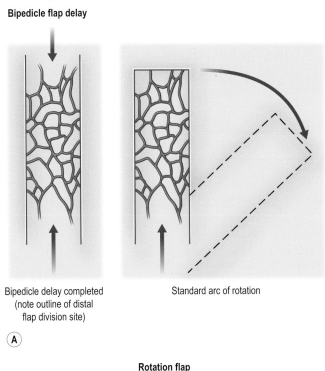

Bipedicle delay completed
(note outline of distal
flap division site)

Standard arc of rotation

(A)

Advancement flap

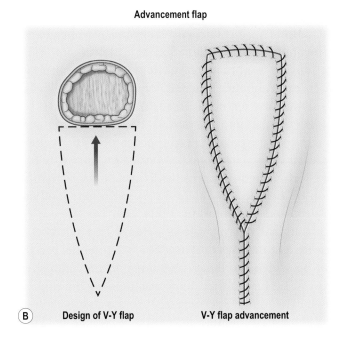

(B)   **Design of V-Y flap**   **V-Y flap advancement**

Rotation flap

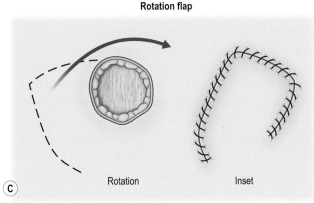

Rotation   Inset

(C)

Fig. 24.1 (A) Bipedicle flap delay. **(B)** Advancement flap. **(C)** Rotation flap.

the arm carrier allowed reconstruction of distant complex defects, particularly in the head and neck region, and for coverage of composite wounds when local tissue was unavailable or severely damaged. Despite this, the random pattern flap provided no new source of circulation when transferred to a distant site. Thus, the success of these flaps ultimately depended on the local wound environment for nourishment.

Other restrictions of random flaps include the limited arc of rotation, the proximity of the flap to the wound and the associated zone of injury and decreased bacterial resistance.[31] Given the vascular limitations of the random pattern flap, investigators attempted different

means by which to maximize the potential area of a flap, which led to the concept of flap delay. Although the delay procedure has been used for several hundred years, it was not until the early 1900s that the concept was recognized. Blair introduced the term *delayed transfer* in 1921.[32] In the 16th century Tagliacozzi delayed his upper arm flaps by making parallel incisions through the skin and subcutaneous tissue overlying the biceps muscle. In 1965, using the pig model, Milton investigated the effectiveness of four different methods of delaying a flap. He found that in developing a bipedicled flap, the best form of delay was by making two incisions and undermining the skin between the incisions.[33] The goal of a delayed flap is to enhance flap circulation, ensuring flap survival after advancement, transposition, or transplantation to a defect site. Flap delay may be used to increase circulation to the muscle or fascia or to enhance vascular connections to the overlying cutaneous territory or adjacent structures to be included during flap elevations (tendon, fascia, and bone). Although delay may be accomplished by biochemical means to improve flap perfusion, currently the most effective method to ensure delay is surgical manipulation of the flap. To date, no pharmacologic method has surpassed the reproducibility and the degree to which surgical delay protects against flap necrosis.[34] There are two theories that describe the potential mechanism by which the delay phenomenon prevents skin necrosis. The first is that delay acclimatizes the flap to ischemia (tolerance), permitting it to survive with less blood flow than would normally be required. This theory suggests that vascular delay cause adaptive metabolic changes at a cellular level within the tissue.[35] The second theory is that delay improves vascularity by increasing flow through preexisting vessels, reorganizing the pattern of blood flow to more ischemic areas.[36,37] On the basis of experimental data, it appears that both of these mechanisms, either directly or indirectly, contribute to the beneficial effects of surgical delay. Regardless of the underlying mechanisms, most experimental work on surgical delay demonstrates changes at the microcirculatory level.[38,39]

Surgical flap delay is accomplished in two ways: standard delay, with an incision at the periphery of the cutaneous territory or partial flap elevation; and strategic delay, with division of selected pedicles to the flap to enhance perfusion through the remaining pedicle or pedicles.

The technical aspects of standard surgical delay to enhance circulation are straightforward. The flap cutaneous territory is outlined and incisions are made through all or part of the border of a planned cutaneous territory *(Fig. 24.2)*. Minimal to partial flap undermining is performed. The incisions are then closed. The flap is then elevated after 10–14 days. It has been shown that after 1 week, the blood flow into the area of delay reaches a maximum.[40]

Strategic pedicle delay is accomplished by making incisions at the border of the planned flap cutaneous territory. The dissection is either deep to muscle or

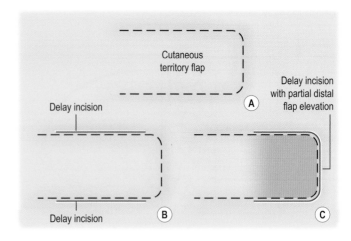

Fig. 24.2 Standard delay flap modification. **(A)** Cutaneous territory of flap. **(B)** Delay incision. **(C)** Delay incision with partial distal flap elevation.

fascia, depending on the flap type, to reach pedicles entering the flap territory. These pedicles are divided and the incision is closed. Second-stage flap elevation is performed after a 2-week period. Effectiveness of strategic delay based on ligation of the dominant vascular pedicle was initially demonstrated in the converse model of the gracilis musculocutaneous flap.[21] This type of delay is usually advocated in patients with risk factors for flap ischemia (i.e., smoking history, obesity, radiation therapy, abdominal scar). An example of an indication for surgical delay would be a patient who is to undergo breast reconstruction with a TRAM flap. It has been shown that high-risk patients benefit from surgical delay.[41] In addition, it has been shown that delay potentially reduces the incidence of abdominal wall complications.[42] New techniques for strategic delay are designed to minimize incision length and procedure-related morbidity. Endoscopic techniques allow access and division of pedicles with minimal incisions. Interventional radiology techniques may also be used to occlude dominant or secondary pedicles to the flap territory to enhance perfusion to the remaining flap pedicles.

Although important historically, the delay technique is used less frequently because of the development of better techniques, including axial, musculocutaneous, fasciocutaneous, transposition, perforator and microvascular free flaps. As with the random-pattern flap, the limitation of the delayed flap is that a parallel blood supply is not efficient. Flap delay also has disadvantages: a preliminary operation is required; inadvertent injury to the desired pedicle for flap design is possible; and resultant scar tissue at the site of flap delay may impair subsequent manipulation and inset of the flap at the recipient site.

The delay phenomenon may result in part from a sympatholytic state that results from cutting the sympathetic innervation to the vasculature and the subsequent vasodilatation. Drugs that block vasoconstriction or those that vasodilatate may be of theoretic value. Attempts have been made to stimulate the delay phenomenon pharmacologically by manipulating the autonomic nervous system.[43] Although pharmacologic delay is of theoretical importance, additional studies need to be done to prove its effectiveness.

The erroneous concept that skin circulation is based on a longitudinal vascular network independent of deeper structures delayed the progress of flap discovery. A few isolated areas with direct cutaneous vessels allowed flap elevation without the 2:1 length-to-width ratio restriction (e.g., median forehead flap). However, the need for longer flaps without a requisite delay procedure resulted in the identification of flaps with specific vascular territories based on the course of the superficial vascular pedicles with an axial alignment *(Fig. 24.3)*. Axial flaps based on this concept include the lateral forehead (superficial temporal artery), deltopectoral (internal mammary branches), superficial groin (superficial circumflex iliac artery), and dorsal foot (dorsalis pedis artery) flaps. The development of these axial flaps has had a tremendous impact, particularly in the head and neck and upper extremity reconstruction.

The longer, nondelayed axial flaps made immediate reconstruction of defects possible in the head and neck, groin, and upper extremity spurred the search for new flaps based on consistent vascular pedicles in the trunk and extremities. Muscle was soon identified as a source of tissue that could be detached from its normal origin or insertion and transposed as a flap based on its major (dominant) vascular supply. Further analysis of skin circulation revealed that there were important musculocutaneous perforator vessels supplying the overlying skin, altering the approach to flap design.[12–14] This eventually led to the concept that muscles and fascia have distinct vascular pedicles. The success of muscle flaps in reconstructive surgery is based on reliable blood supply. With knowledge of the location and subsequent preservation

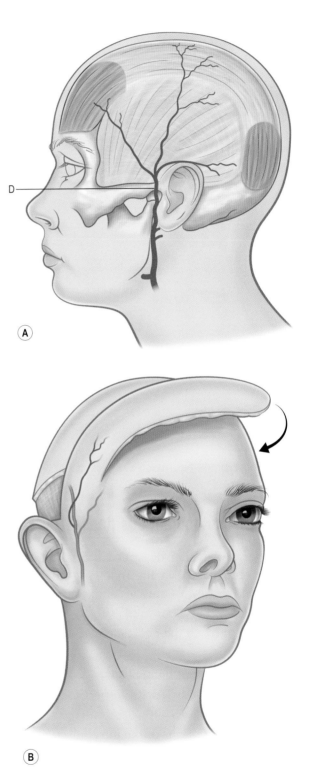

Fig. 24.3 Axial pattern flap. **(A)** Based on the superficial temporal artery. **(B)** Arc of rotation of temporoparietal flap.

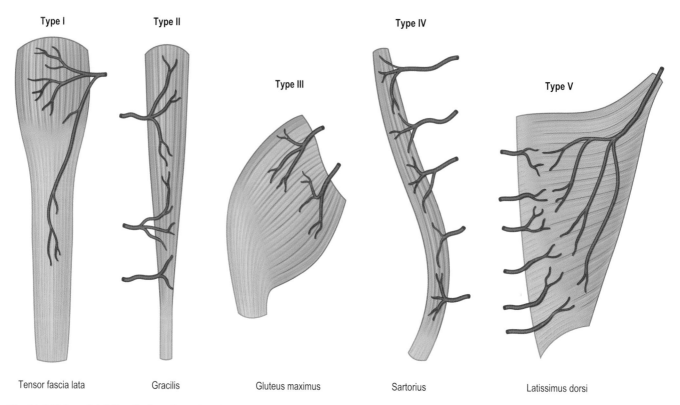

| Type I | Type II | Type III | Type IV | Type V |

Tensor fascia lata   **Gracilis**   **Gluteus maximus**   **Sartorius**   **Latissimus dorsi**

Fig. 24.4 Mathes–Nahai Classification of muscle and musculocutaneous flaps.

of the vascular pedicles to muscles, every muscle may be rotated as a flap.

Muscle and musculocutaneous flaps

In 1981, Mathes and Nahai described a classification system for muscles based on the following anatomic relationships between the muscle and its vascular pedicles:

1. The regional source of the pedicle entering the muscle
2. The number and size of the pedicle
3. The location of the pedicle with respect to the muscle's origin and insertion
4. The angiographic patterns of the intramuscular vessels.

This classification system enables the surgeon to categorize the various muscle and musculocutaneous flaps into distinctly different, clinically applicable groups based on the vascular anatomy. There are five different vascular patterns by which the various muscles are categorized *(Fig. 24.4)*.[15]

Type I: one vascular pedicle

Type I muscles are supplied by a single vascular pedicle *(Table 24.2)*.

Type II: dominant vascular pedicle and minor pedicle

Type II muscles are supplied by both a dominant and minor vascular pedicle. The larger dominant vascular pedicle will usually sustain circulation to these muscles after the elevation of the flap when the minor pedicles are divided. This is the most common pattern of circulation observed in human muscle *(Table 24.3)*.

Type III: two dominant pedicles

Type III muscles possess two large vascular pedicles from separate vascular sources. These pedicles have either a separate regional source of circulation or are located on opposite sides of the muscle. Division of one pedicle during flap elevation rarely results in loss of muscle within its vascular distribution. The muscle will usually survive on one its two dominant vascular

Table 24.2 Type I vascular pattern muscles

Abductor digiti minimi (hand)
Abductor pollicis brevis
Anconeus
Colon
Deep circumflex iliac artery
First dorsal interosseous
Gastrocnemius, medial and lateral
Genioglossus
Hyoglossus
Jejunum
Longitudinalis linguae
Styloglossus
Tensor fascia lata
Transversus and verticalis linguae
Vastus lateralis

Table 24.3 Type II vascular pattern muscles

Abductor digiti minimi (foot)
Abductor hallucis
Brachioradialis
Coracobrachialis
Flexor carpi ulnaris
Flexor digitorum brevis
Gracilis
Hamstring (biceps femoris)
Peroneus brevis
Peroneus longus
Platysma
Rectus femoris
Soleus
Sternocleidomastoid
Trapezius
Triceps
Vastus medialis

Table 24.4 Type III vascular pattern muscles

Gluteus maximus
Intercostal
Omentum
Orbicularis oris
Pectoralis minor
Rectus abdominis
Serratus anterior
Temporalis

pedicles. This vascular pattern allows the muscle to be split, allowing the use of only part of the muscle as a muscle or musculocutaneous flap *(Table 24.4)*.

Type IV: segmental vascular pedicles

Type IV muscles are supplied by segmental vascular pedicles entering along the course of the muscle belly.

Table 24.5 Type IV vascular pattern muscles

Extensor digitorum longus
Extensor hallucis longus
External oblique
Flexor digitorum longus
Flexor hallucis longus
Sartorius
Tibialis anterior

Table 24.6 Type V vascular pattern muscles

Fibula
Internal oblique
Latissimus dorsi
Pectoralis major

Each pedicle provides circulation to a segment of the muscle. Division of more than two or three of the pedicles during elevation as a flap may result in distal muscle necrosis *(Table 24.5)*.

Type V: one dominant vascular pedicle and secondary segmental vascular pedicles

Type V muscles are supplied by a single dominant pedicle and secondary segmental vascular pedicles. These muscles have one large dominant vascular pedicle near the insertion of the muscle with several segmental pedicles near the origin. The internal vasculature can be supplied by either the dominant or the segmental pedicles, and therefore the muscle may be elevated as a flap on either vascular system *(Table 24.6)*.

Fascia and fasciocutaneous flaps

A growing knowledge of the source of skin circulation after the recognition of the muscle and musculocutaneous system led to the identification of vascular pedicles emerging between muscles (septocutaneous pedicles) and entering the deep fascia. Elevation of the skin with its deep fascia represented a new vascular basis for flap design.

A fascial flap consists of fascia detached from its normal origin or insertion and transposed to another location. Without the overlying skin and fat, this represents a delicate flap. A fasciocutaneous flap, originally called an axial flap, includes the skin, subcutaneous tissue, and underlying fascia, which may be distinct from the fascia covering the underlying muscle. The vascular supply is derived at the base of the flap from musculocutaneous perforators or direct septocutaneous branches of major arteries.

The first fascia and fasciocutaneous flaps were described by Ponten in 1981 for lower extremity reconstruction and Tolhurst in 1983 for trunk and axillary reconstruction.[22,44] Investigations have shown that that the fasciocutaneous system consists of perforating vessels that arise from regional arteries and pass along the fibrous septa between muscle bellies or muscle compartments. The vessels then spread out at the level of the deep fascia, both above and below, to form plexuses, which in turn give off branches to the skin. In 1975, Schafer found three major vascular systems of the deep fascia.[45]

1. Perforating arteries from underlying muscle giving off several radiating branches, which perforate the fascia before continuing to the subdermal plexus.

2. Subcutaneous arteries running in the fat and anastomosing frequently with the superficial plexus of the deep fascia and with each other.

3. Subfascial arteries arising from the intermuscular septa and running in the loose areolar tissue beneath the deep fascia and adjoining the deep and superficial plexus.

These pedicles consist of an artery (generally a branch of the artery to the specific anatomic region of the fascia and regional musculature) and paired venae comitantes that drain into corresponding major regional veins. Direct cutaneous and septocutaneous pedicles are fairly constant in location. There is a greater variability in location of the musculocutaneous perforators. These pedicles provide a vascular basis for specific fascial or fasciocutaneous flaps. On this basis, Mathes and Nahai have classified fascia and fasciocutaneous flaps as types A, B, and C *(Fig. 24.5)*.[29]

Anatomic studies demonstrate that the *type A fasciocutaneous flaps* have a vascular pedicle to the deep fascia that emerges from a regional source coursing initially beneath the deep fascia and eventually continuing its course superficial to the deep fascia. This pedicle provides numerous fasciocutaneous perforators to the skin. Because the pedicle tends to course in a radial fashion from its regional source into its distal cutaneous distribution, the flap is often referred to as an axial flap. The long, relatively superficial course of the dominant

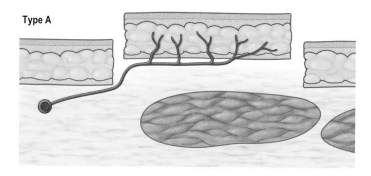

Type A

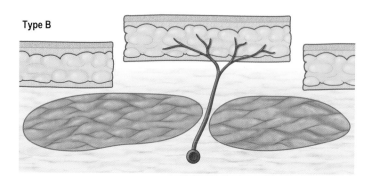

Type B

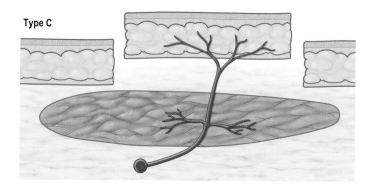

Type C

Fig. 24.5 Mathes–Nahai Classification of fascia/fasciocutaneous flaps.

pedicle permits evaluation by palpation or Doppler probe *(Table 24.7)*.

Type B fasciocutaneous flaps have a septocutaneous pedicle, which courses between major muscle groups in an intermuscular septum or between adjacent muscles. This pedicle is located within the intermuscular septum or the potential space between adjacent muscles and supplies a regional fascial vascular system. The largest septocutaneous pedicles are dominant pedicles to specific fasciocutaneous flaps and are fairly constant in location *(Table 24.8)*.

Table 24.7 Type A fascial and fasciocutaneous flaps

Deep external pudendal artery
Digital artery
Dorsal metacarpal artery
Gluteal thigh
Great toe (hallux)
Groin
Lateral thoracic (axillary)
Pudendal – thigh
Saphenous
Scalp
Second toe
Standard forehead
Superficial external pudendal artery
Superficial interior epigastric artery
Sural artery
Temporoparietal fascia

Table 24.8 Type B fascial and fasciocutaneous flaps

Anterolateral thigh
Anterior tibial artery
Deltoid
Dorsalis pedis
Inferior cubital artery (antecubital)
Lateral arm
Lateral plantar artery
Lateral thigh
Medial arm
Medial plantar artery
Medial thigh
Peroneal artery
Posterior interosseous
Posterior tibial artery
Radial forearm
Radial recurrent
Scapular
Ulnar recurrent

Table 24.9 Type C fascial and fasciocutaneous flaps

Anterolateral thigh
Deltopectoral
Nasolabial
Median forehead
Thoracoepigastric (transverse abdominal)
Transverse back

In certain regions, larger musculocutaneous perforators enter the deep fascia and contribute to both the deep fascia and cutaneous circulation. The design of a fasciocutaneous flap can be based on these dominant perforating vessels without incorporation of the underlying muscle; this vascular pattern represents the *type C fasciocutaneous flap*. However, increasing pedicle length will necessitate proximal dissection of the pedicle through muscle to its regional source or incorporation of all or part of the muscle in the flap design. Type C flaps are generally the anatomic model used for the perforator flap in microsurgical transplantation (*Table 24.9*).

Cormack and Lamberty also classified fasciocutaneous flaps based on vascular anatomy.[46] The type A flap is supplied by multiple fasciocutaneous perforators that enter at the base of the flap and extend throughout the longitudinal length. The flap can be based proximally, distally, or as an island. The type B flap has a single fasciocutaneous perforator, which is of moderate size and is fairly consistent. It is intended for use as a free flap. The type C flap is based on multiple small perforators that run along a fascial septum. The supplying artery is included within the flap. It may be based proximally, distally, or as a free flap. The type D flap is an osteomusculofasciocutaneous flap, and is based on multiple small perforators similar to the type C flap, but also include a portion of adjacent muscle and bone. It may be based proximally or distally on a pedicle or used for microvascular tissue transplantation (*Fig. 24.6*).

Perforator flaps

Further refinements in flap application have led to the development of perforator flaps. Perforator flaps have evolved from musculocutaneous and fasciocutaneous flaps without the muscle or fascial carrier. It has been shown that neither a passive muscle carrier nor the underlying fascial plexus of vessels are necessary for flap survival.[47] Advantages of perforator flaps include reduced donor site morbidity, versatility in flap design, muscle sparing (less functional deficit), and improved postoperative recovery of the patient.[48–51] Disadvantages of perforator flaps include meticulous dissection needed to isolate the perforator vessels (resulting in increased operative time, the variability in the position and size of the perforator vessels, and the ease of which the vessels can be damaged.[52–54]

The nomenclature of perforator flaps is confusing and oftentimes misstated. Perforator flaps have been designated by their location (e.g., anterolateral thigh flap), arterial supply (e.g., deep inferior epigastric artery

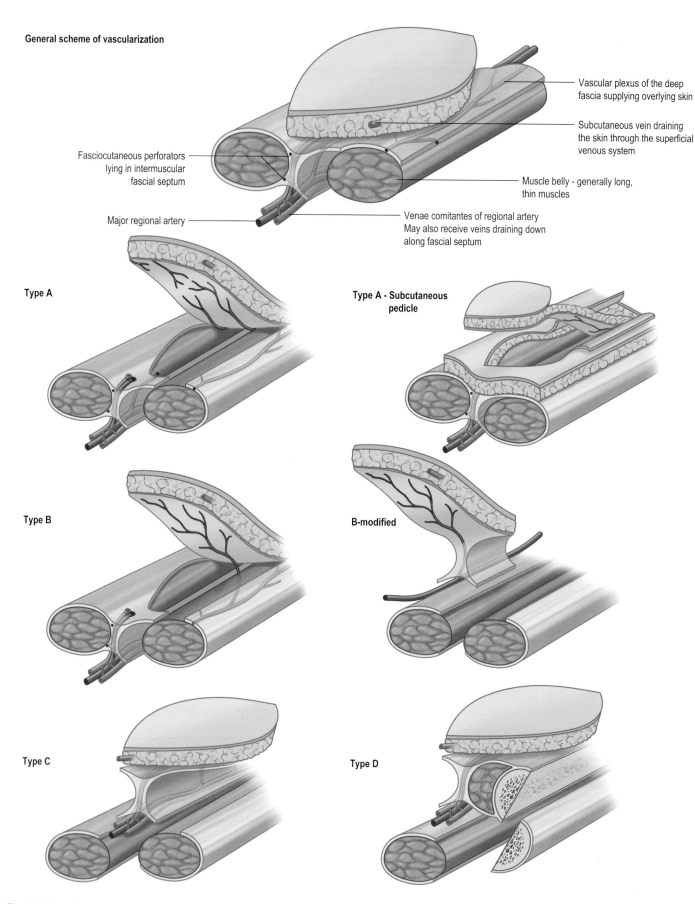

Fig. 24.6 Classification of fasciocutaneous flaps.

perforator flap), or the muscle of origin (e.g., gastrocnemius perforator flap). It has been suggested by Geddes *et al.* to standardize the nomenclature of perforator flaps by describing all perforator flaps according to the main artery of origin.[48] In this system, cutaneous flaps are divided into either cutaneous flaps or musculocutaneous perforator flaps. Cutaneous flaps include those previously described as axial, septocutaneous, and fasciocutaneous (type A and B fasciocutaneous flaps according to Mathes and Nahai). Musculocutaneous perforator flaps are the type C fasciocutaneous flaps according to Mathes and Nahai, in which the pedicle to the perforator flap is the dominant or major pedicle to the muscle with its perforator vessel passing through the muscle to the overlying fascia, subcutaneous tissue, and skin. Because the muscle is excluded from the flap, the perforator flap is anatomically a type C fasciocutaneous flap though it is confusing to subclassify these flaps in this way and it is probably best just to regard a perforator flap as such, and not as a subtype of a fasciocutaneous flap.

There are many perforator flaps currently used and others that are of theoretical value. As studied closely by Taylor and Palmer, there are many named perforating vessels to each angiosome of the body.[55] Acceptable perforator flap donor sites have four common features: (1) predictable and consistent blood supply; (2) at least one large (diameter ≥0.5 mm) perforating vessel; (3) sufficient pedicle length for the required anastomosis, unless the flap is being used as a pedicled flap; (4) ability to close the donor site primarily. Commonly used perforator flaps include the deep inferior epigastric artery perforator flap, superior gluteal artery perforator flap, thoracodorsal artery perforator flap, anterolateral thigh perforator flap, tensor fascia lata perforator flap, and medial sural artery perforator flap[47,48,56–59]

Abdominal viscera classification

The abdominal viscera are not easily classified; however, for the purposes of flap transposition or microvascular tissue transplantation, the colon, jejunum, and omentum fall conveniently into the muscle classification system *(Table 24.10)*. For microvascular transplantation, the segment of bowel (jejunum or colon) is elevated on one vascular arcade with a single dominant vessel, a type I pattern of circulation. In unusual circumstances where

Table 24.10 Abdominal visceral flap classification

Flap	Type	Circulation pattern	Size
Colon	Bowel	Type I	20–25 cm in length Lumen diameter of 8 cm
Jejunum	Bowel	Type I	7–25 cm may be transferred on one pedicle Lumen diameter of 3–5 cm
Omentum	Omentum	Type III	Variable; up to 40 × 60 cm

a longer segment of bowel extends beyond the vascular territory of one arcade, two vascular arcades must be included to ensure viability of this longer segment of bowel. In this instance, the pattern of circulation will be type III (two dominant arcades or pedicles). It is possible to reconstruct the esophagus from the base of the tongue to the stomach with a long segment of jejunum where one pedicle is revascularized in the upper chest or neck and the second pedicle is left intact. Other uses of the colon or jejunum as flaps have been for vaginal reconstruction.

The omentum may be based as a transposition flap on either the right or left gastroepiploic vessels and is thus classified as having a type III pattern of circulation. The omentum is also commonly transferred microsurgically. The omentum can be used to reconstruct a wide range of extraperitoneal defects and has been shown to have immunologic and angiogenic properties.[60–62] Although useful for reconstruction, donor site complications can be significant, including abdominal wall infection and hernia.[63,64] With the advances in minimally invasive surgery, the abdominal viscera can successfully be harvested laparoscopically obviating the need for a large midline incision providing a better cosmetic result and less donor site morbidity.[65–67]

Flap modifications

There has been considerable progress in the clinical application of muscle and musculocutaneous flaps over the years. Countless modifications and refinements in both technique and design have been described in the continuing quest for the optimal result in reconstructive surgery. These modifications include tissue expansion, segmental transposition flaps, vascularized bone flaps, distally based flaps, reverse transposition flaps, combination flaps, delayed flaps, and prefabricated flaps. The development of specialized tissue flaps has provided the surgeon with the ability to restore sensation, motor function, and bone structure in the surgical defect. With the use of complex tissues such as innervated muscle, omentum, intestine, joint, digit, iliac crest, and various long bones, the surgeon can produce, in the words of McDowell, "a few harpsichords, rather than so many logs … recognizable, new, artistic and fully acceptable noses, cheeks, chins, necks, legs, and arms rather than indistinguishable globs and blobs of transported tissue in those areas."[68]

Tissue expansion

Skin and soft tissue adjacent to the defect are preferred for the closure of the defect because of the similarity in skin color, texture, and contour. Design of local advancement flaps will frequently allow use of adjacent tissue, particularly if there is skin excess in the donor area. A rotation or advancement flap frequently requires either a back-cut or skin graft at the donor site. The size of the defect or the surrounding zone of injury often prevents the use of adjacent tissue, which is frequently not available for wound closure or composite defect reconstruction. In these circumstances, tissue expansion may allow the use of the desired adjacent tissue for reconstruction. Tissue expansion is an effective method to enlarge the cutaneous territory of superficially located muscle and fascial flaps. Although it is most commonly used to increase the cutaneous flap territory, the principle of tissue expansion may also be applied to all soft tissues, including fascia and peripheral nerve. Neumann is credited with the first modern report of this technique in 1957.[69] Radovan further described the use of this technique for breast reconstruction in 1976.[70]

Technically, the tissue expander is inserted under the skin to provide a mechanism for increasing skin dimensions to provide sufficient skin circumference for designing an advancement or transposition flap. If a fasciocutaneous flap is planned, the expander is placed below the deep fascia. If a musculocutaneous flap is planned, the expander is placed beneath the deep surface of the muscle. The expander should not be placed directly beneath the dominant vascular pedicle at its point of entrance into the flap territory to avoid injury to the pedicle during the expansion process. Although immediate skin expansion is possible, delayed expansion is usually performed prior to flap elevation. During a selected time interval, usually 6 weeks to 3 months, the expander is injected with saline at weekly intervals. Once the desired amount of expansion has been achieved, the expander is removed and the modified flap skin territory is recruited for reconstruction.

Safe tissue expansion depends on surgical judgment regarding its usefulness for a specific problem. The benefits of local surrounding tissues in reconstructive surgery are well recognized; however, this tissue is frequently injured because of its proximity to the traumatic or surgical defect obviating the ability to use this tissue. Failure of tissue expansion is usually attributable to inadequate stability of skin and associated soft tissue during the expansion process. Failure of the expander is signaled by wound dehiscence followed by expander exposure and infection. Unlike failure of flap transposition or transplantation techniques, expander failure is not generally associated with increased wound complexity or donor site problems.[71,72]

Segmental transposition flaps

A muscle can be split and a portion in continuity with the dominant vascular pedicle can be used as a transposition flap. Techniques of muscle splitting to preserve tissue and function have been described. The remaining muscle with its origin and insertion is maintained to preserve function. Alternatively, the entire muscle may be split and used to cover two defects simultaneously. Frequently, only a part of the muscle in proximity to the dominant vascular pedicle is elevated for microvascular transplantation.

The skin territory may also be modified and split into two separate skin islands or elevated with only a segment of the muscle flap. However, the skin territory must include vascular connections via musculocutaneous perforating vessels from the segmental flap (*Figs 24.7, 24.8*).

The latissimus dorsi musculocutaneous flap has been described as a muscle that can be segmentally transferred. This muscle has a consistent proximal bifurcation of its neurovascular supply into a medial and lateral subunit. For example, in the reconstruction of the cervical esophagus, the latissimus dorsi musculocutaneous

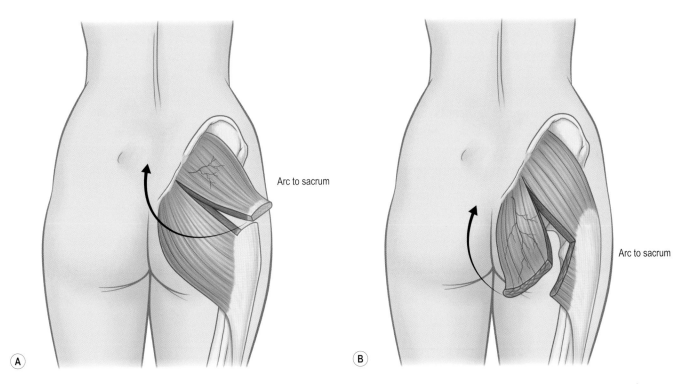

Fig. 24.7 Gluteus maximus segmental muscle transposition. **(A)** Superior half of gluteus maximus, arc to sacrum. **(B)** Inferior half of gluteus maximus muscle.

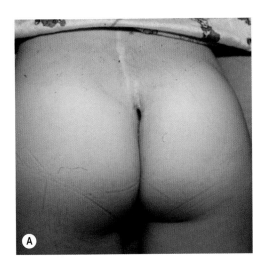
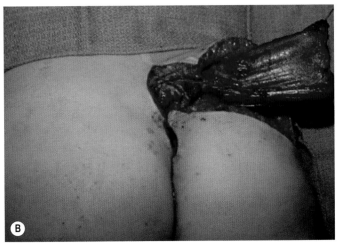

Fig. 24.8 (A–E) Function preserving muscle flap design.

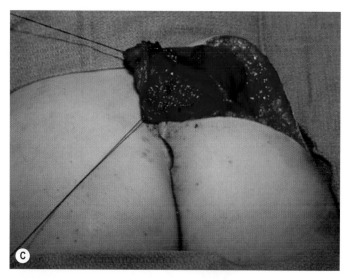

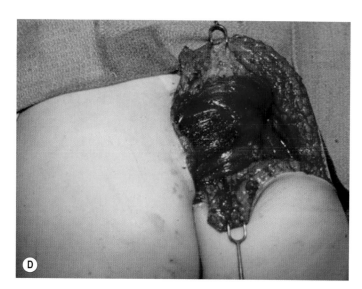

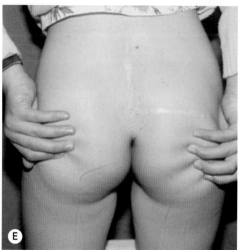

Fig. 24.8, cont'd

flap can be split into two skin paddles that can be used for lining and skin coverage.[15,28,73–75] Segmental latissimus dorsi transfer has also been used in facial reanimation and for coverage of long soft tissue defects of the lower extremity.[76–78]

The basis for splitting the pectoralis major muscle was demonstrated by Tobin in 1985.[79] The pectoralis has three segmental neurovascular subunits: the clavicular, the sternocostal, and the external subunit. These can be surgically split and independently transferred on vascular pedicles from the thoracoacromial, internal mammary and lateral thoracic vessels.[80] Splitting of the pectoralis major muscle into segments has been

performed when the segmental transfer of a single intercostal portion of the pectoralis muscle, based on a single medial perforating branch of the internal thoracic artery, is required for chest wall and neck reconstruction *(Figs 24.9, 24.10)*.[81] The concept of segmental transposition of muscle allows transplantation of independent neuromuscular units (segments of muscle innervated by a single nerve fascicle).[82]

Vascularized bone

Bone is vascularized through endosteal and periosteal sources *(Fig. 24.11)*. The complex blood supply of bone

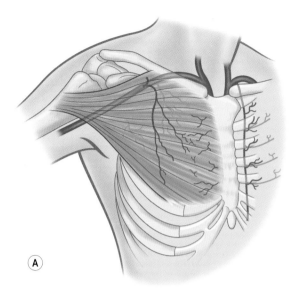

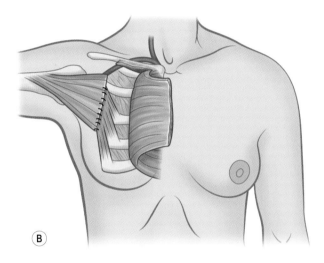

Fig. 24.9 (A,B) Pectoralis major muscle flap segmental transposition.

flap rotation. The bony attachments usually are located beyond the point of rotation. An example of a rotational bone flap is vascularized radial bone grafts based on the 1,2 or 4,5 intercompartmental suprarétinacular branches of the radial artery for carpal bone reconstruction.[83] Another example of a rotational flap including bone is the pectoralis major muscle with periosteal vascular connections to the fifth anterior rib at the site of muscle origin. Historically, this was been used for reconstruction of the irradiated mandible.[84]

Vascularized bone is useful in muscles suitable for microvascular transplantation or in those muscles designed for transposition when the vascular attachments to bone are distal to the point of rotation. The most commonly transferred bones include the fibula based on the peroneal artery *(Figs 24.12, 24.13)*, iliac crest based on the deep circumflex iliac artery *(Fig. 24.14)*, the scapula based on the circumflex scapula or thoracodorsal arteries *(Fig. 24.15)*, and the radius based on the radial artery.

The pattern of circulation to the scapula and radius are classified according to the parent flap which consists of the vascular supply and associated soft tissue component (e.g., scapular and radial forearm flaps). These bones are always transposed as an integral part of the parent flap. The fibula and the iliac crest, however, are most often transferred as bone only without a soft tissue component. Classification of the iliac crest as having a type I vascular pattern reflects its dependence on surrounding muscles as well as direct osseous vessels from the deep circumflex iliac artery. The fibula is classified as having a type V vascular pattern because of the dominant nutrient pedicle into the proximal bone from the peroneal artery and the segment at the origin of periosteal pedicles along the length of the bone (standard segmental pedicles). This type V pattern of circulation permits osteotomies to be performed to separate the bone into distinct, independently vascularized segments *(Table 24.11)*.

Certain type A and type B fasciocutaneous flaps may be elevated with bone. The regional vascular source of the flap also provides nutrient vessels to the neighboring bones. A segment of bone may be included with the fascia or fasciocutaneous flap when designed either for transposition or microvascular transplantation (e.g., the radial forearm and temporoparietal fascia flap).

is based on nutrient vessels entering the bone directly and through vascular connections between muscles and bone, typically where the muscle has a large bony origin or insertion. Muscles with all five patterns of circulation have vascular connections between the muscle fibers and the periosteum. However, the incorporation of vascularized bone with the transposition flap is generally not feasible since the point of entrance of the dominant vascular pedicle into the muscle determines the point of

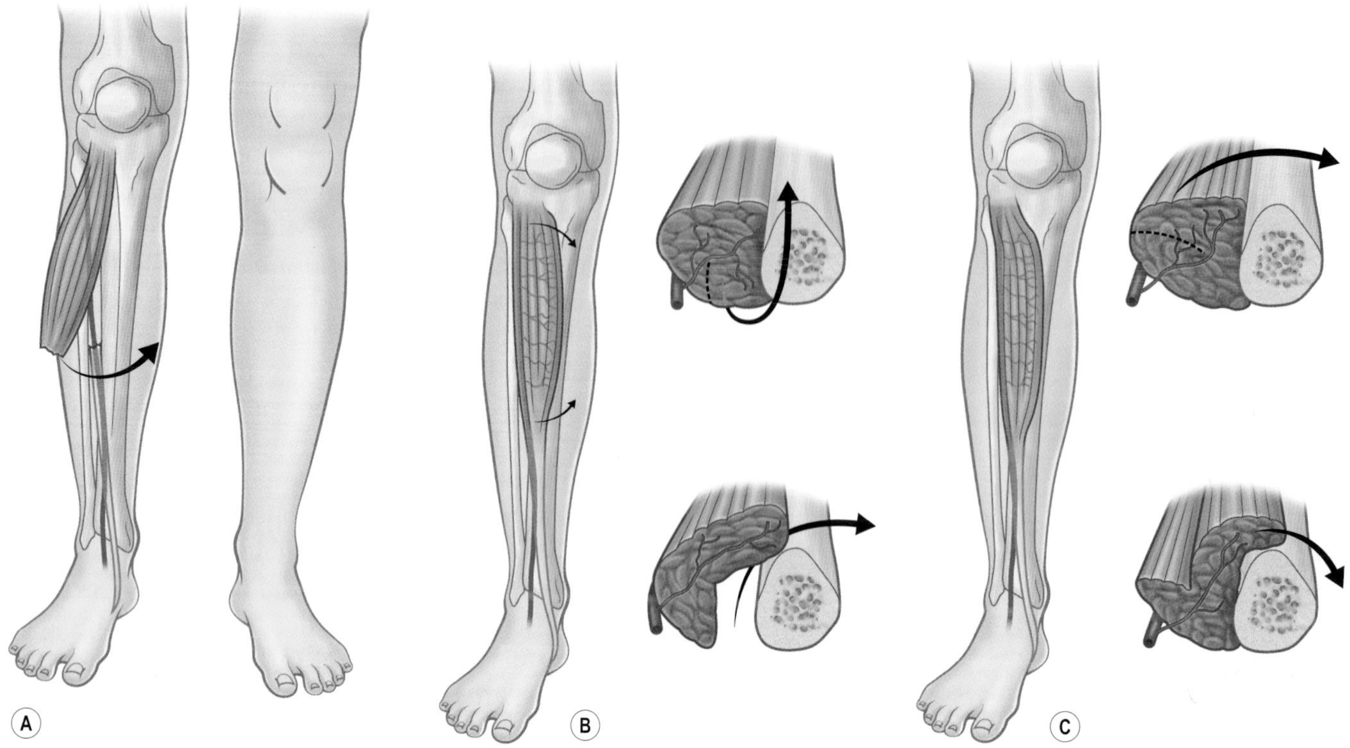

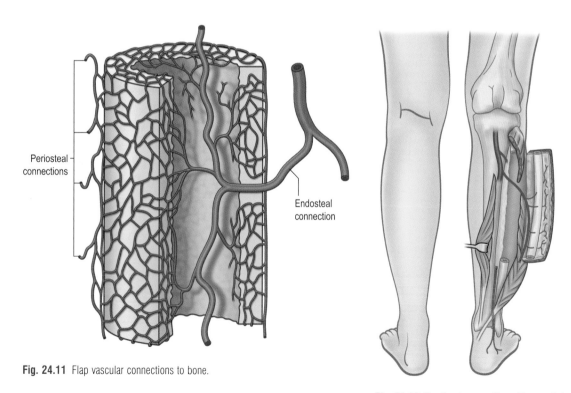

Fig. 24.10 Tibialis anterior muscle flaps split for segmental transposition. **(A)** Segmental flap. **(B)** Posterior advancement. **(C)** Anterior turnover flap.

Periosteal connections

Endosteal connection

Fig. 24.11 Flap vascular connections to bone.

Fig. 24.12 Fasciocutaneous flap with vascularized bone, fibula.

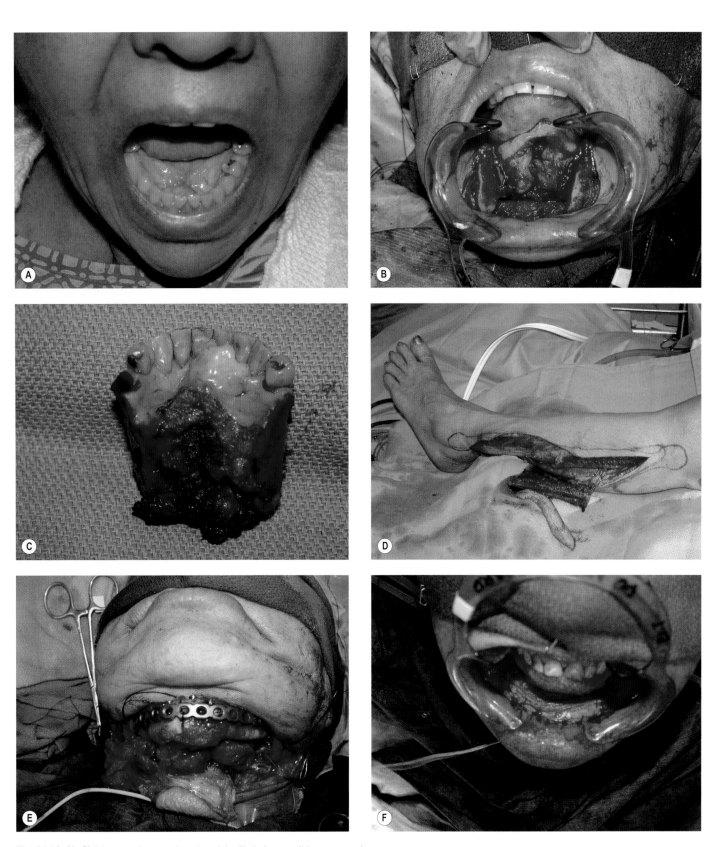

Fig. 24.13 (A–G) Microvascular transplantation of the fibula for mandible reconstruction.

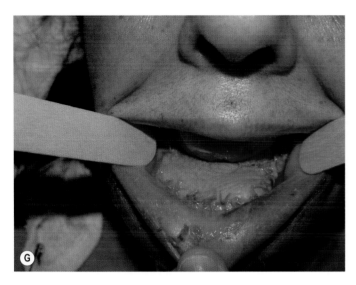

Fig. 24.13, cont'd

Table 24.11 Bone vascular classification

Bone	Blood supply	Flap type
Fibula	Peroneal artery	V[a]
Iliac crest	Deep circumflex iliac artery	I[a]
Scapula	Circumflex scapular or thoracodorsal arteries	B[b]
Radius	Radial artery	B[b]

[a]Bone associated with musculocutaneous flap. [b]Bone associated with fasciocutaneous flap.

Functional muscle flaps

Release of the origin or insertion of the muscle transposition flap will result in loss of muscle function. However, many of the muscle flaps may be designed for both coverage and functional muscle transfer. For function to be preserved, the motor nerve must be preserved along with dominant vascular supply, the muscle must be reattached to a new bone or tendon across a joint, and the muscle must exert a direct force on its new point of attachment. Muscles suitable for use as transposition flaps or microvascular composite tissue transplantation, providing both coverage and function, include the latissimus, gluteus maximus (segmental), gracilis, gastrocnemius and serratus muscles. Restoration of the original muscle length-to-width ratio and repair of the motor nerve to a suitable receptor motor nerve at the recipient site are essential for restoration of transplanted muscle function at its new inset site. The latissimus dorsi muscle flap has been used to provide neodiaphragmatic motion for repair of recurrent congenital diaphragmatic hernias, to restore knee function after resection of the quadriceps mechanism in the lower extremity, to restore elbow and shoulder motion in the upper extremity, and to restore oral and nasal function after head and neck tumor ablation.[85–88]

Sensory flap

Specific sensory nerves are identified in the cutaneous territory of many of the flaps available for reconstructive surgery. Both musculocutaneous and fasciocutaneous transposition flaps may be designed to incorporate the sensory nerve in the flap base. If the cutaneous nerve does not enter the flap base in proximity to the vascular pedicle, it is also possible to divide the sensory nerve during flap elevation and then subsequently coapt the nerve to a suitable sensory nerve at the recipient site.

Muscle flaps with intact motor nerves or with reanastomosis of the motor nerve to suitable motor or sensory nerves at the recipient site appear to retain protective sensibility, possibly through nerve fibers of proprioception. Maintenance of protective sensation is essential for hands, feet and other weight-bearing areas. Another common area in which sensate flaps are used is the oral cavity and potentially improves postoperative intraoral function.[89–91] Harris *et al.* state that reconstruction of weight-bearing areas should provide adequate contour for normal footwear, thick durable skin, protective sensation, and solid anchorage to the deep structures to resist shearing forces.[92] Studies have shown benefits of protective sensation for ankle and heel reconstruction both with rotational flaps and by microvascular tissue transfer.[93–95]

Combination flaps

Two muscle flaps frequently share a common regional source for their dominant artery and vein. Both flaps may be elevated simultaneously and either transposed as a regional flap or transplanted by microvascular surgery based on the common regional artery and vein. This technique permits a flap design with the ability to cover large defects or use of two or more flaps for specialized coverage. The subscapular artery and vein are

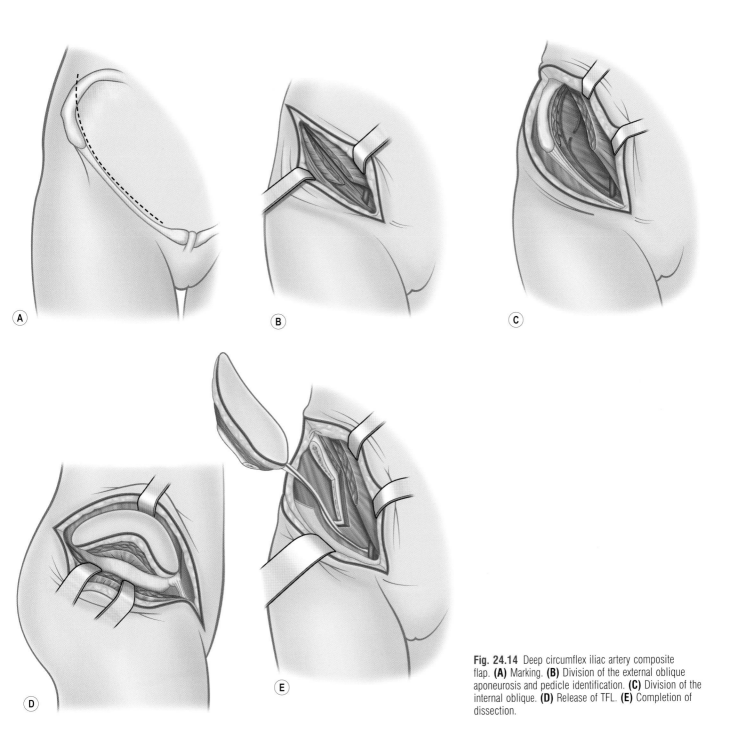

Fig. 24.14 Deep circumflex iliac artery composite flap. **(A)** Marking. **(B)** Division of the external oblique aponeurosis and pedicle identification. **(C)** Division of the internal oblique. **(D)** Release of TFL. **(E)** Completion of dissection.

a common regional source for the dominant pedicles to latissimus dorsi muscle or musculocutaneous flap, serratus anterior muscle flap, and scapular fasciocutaneous flap; all three flaps may be transposed or transplanted on this single artery and vein *(Fig. 24.16)*. Clinically, the subscapular system provides many varieties of useful combination flaps.[96,97] Another example is the gluteal thigh flap, which is an inferior gluteal musculocutaneous flap with a posterior fasciocutaneous extension.[98–100] The more subtle characteristics of each tissue component enable the surgeon to tailor the flap precisely to the specifications of the

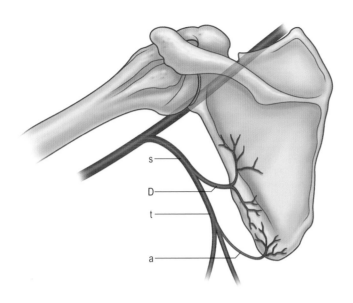

Fig. 24.15 Independent vascularized segments of the scapula based on circumflex scapular and thoracodorsal pedicles. s, subscapular artery; D, circumflex scapular artery; t, thoracodorsal artery; a, scapular arterial branch.

individual defect. Combined flaps have been further divided into Siamese, conjoint, and sequential flaps.[101] Siamese flaps have multiple flap territories, dependent on some common physical junction, yet each retaining their independent vascular supply. Conjoint flaps have multiple independent flaps, each with an independent vascular supply, but linked by a common source vessel. A sequential flap is defined as multiple independent flaps, each with an independent vascular supply artificially linked by a microanastomosis.

Prelaminated and prefabricated flaps

Flap prelamination, a term coined in 1994, involves surgical manipulation of a flap that requires partial to complete flap elevation and suturing of the flap to form structures at the site of the reconstruction.[102] This technique may also incorporate new tissues into the flap territory, establishing a multilayered flap. When these structures at the donor site have healed, flap transposition or transplantation is performed. With suture lines or various grafts healed at the time of flap inset, complex reconstructions are theoretically accomplished with less risk of complications at the recipient site. This is commonly done in flaps to be used in head and neck reconstruction. Baudet *et al.* and Pribaz *et al.* have used prelamination techniques on the forearm for nasal and central face reconstruction.[103,104] Although it is useful,

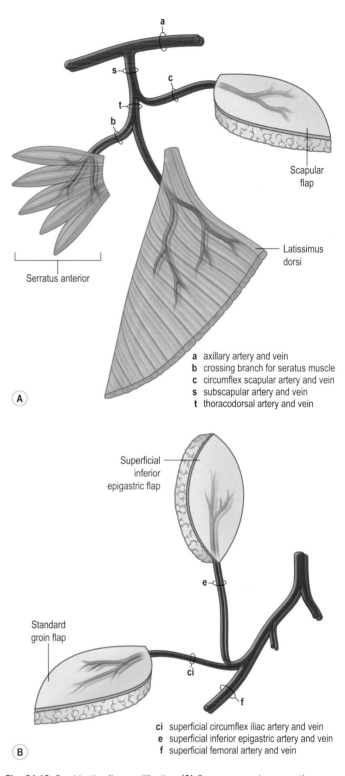

a axillary artery and vein
b crossing branch for seratus muscle
c circumflex scapular artery and vein
s subscapular artery and vein
t thoracodorsal artery and vein

(A)

ci superficial circumflex iliac artery and vein
e superficial inferior epigastric artery and vein
f superficial femoral artery and vein

(B)

Fig. 24.16 Combination flap modification. **(A)** Common vascular connections between subscapular artery and vein to dominant pedicle to latissimus dorsi, serratus anterior, and scapular flaps. **(B)** Common vascular connections between the superficial circumflex iliac artery and groin flap and the superficial inferior epigastric artery and inferior abdominal flap.

Table 24.12 Distally based flaps

Abductor digiti minimi
Anterior tibial artery
Dorsalis pedis
External oblique
Gastrocnemius
Gracilis
Hemisoleus
Peroneal artery
Peroneus brevis
Posterior tibial artery
Soleus
Vastus lateralis
Vastus medialis

many reconstructive surgeons still prefer to perform secondary procedures after successful initial flap inset rather than flap prelamination at the donor site.

Another form of flap manipulation is termed prefabrication. Prefabrication provides a new dominant vascular pedicle to structures for subsequent transposition or transplantation. A suitable artery and vein are selected and buried in fascia or subcutaneous tissue in the planned flap territory. A large pedicle to an adjacent muscle is frequently used. The pedicle and a small segment of muscle are elevated and inset beneath the proposed flap site. In 6 weeks, the flap based on the new vascular pedicle is elevated and either transposed or transplanted by microsurgery. This technique for prefabrication is not always reliable for establishing a new dominant pedicle to a flap territory. With the numerous options available for safe flap selection, this technique of flap prefabrication is rarely used.[105]

Distally based flaps and reverse-flow flaps

Certain muscles can be elevated on minor or secondary segmental pedicles. Muscles with a type II circulation can be based on the minor pedicle (*Table 24.12*). To accomplish this, one must divide the dominant vascular pedicle and transpose the muscle distally, based on the lesser pedicle. In designing a distally based flap, one must consider that the minor pedicles differ in size and location and therefore can be unreliable. Without a prior strategic delay (preliminary division of the dominant pedicle), only a segment of the muscle based on the minor pedicle will survive. If the wound requiring coverage is traumatic, the minor pedicle may be located

within the zone of injury (i.e., distal third of the lower extremity). Prior delay of the muscle by selective division of the dominant vascular pedicle will provide more reliable muscle circulation and will permit use of the cutaneous territory of the proximal muscle if a musculocutaneous flap is planned.[21]

Fasciocutaneous flaps may also be designed as distally based flaps. The deep fascia receives specific blood supply through direct cutaneous, septocutaneous, and musculocutaneous pedicles. For example, type B fasciocutaneous flaps frequently have multiple pedicles located sequentially along the axis of the intermuscular septum (e.g., posterior tibial, anterior tibial and peroneal fasciocutaneous flaps). Although the specific territory of a type B fasciocutaneous flap may have a larger pedicle proximally in the extremities, it is possible to base the flap distally on isolated septocutaneous pedicles. Similarly, the cutaneous territory of a type C fascial flap is usually based on a specific large musculocutaneous, perforating pedicle. The presence of an isolated musculocutaneous pedicle in the distal flap will allow distally based transposition of a fasciocutaneous flap.

Although distally based flaps are often termed reverse-flow flaps, not all distally based flaps have reverse flow, since perforating vessels spread out radially in the subcutaneous tissues. Thus, a flap may be oriented such that flow is antegrade and yet the pedicle may be based proximally, distally, medially, or laterally. A number of clinically useful reverse-flow flaps have been described since its original description in 1995, including the distally based radial forearm fasciocutaneous flap, posterior interosseous flap, and the reversed first dorsal metacarpal artery flap used in hand reconstruction.[106] The distally based radial forearm flap relies on retrograde flow through the deep palmar arch and associated venae comitantes with the rotation point of the reverse flap at the level of the wrist (*Fig. 24.17*). Examples of reversed flow flaps used for lower extremity reconstruction are sural fasciocutaneous flaps based on perforators from the peroneal artery, and reversed flexor hallucis longus flaps based on retrograde flow through the peroneal artery.[107,108]

Reverse transposition flap

A muscle flap based on a minor pedicle is defined as a distally based flap. However, it is possible to elevate the

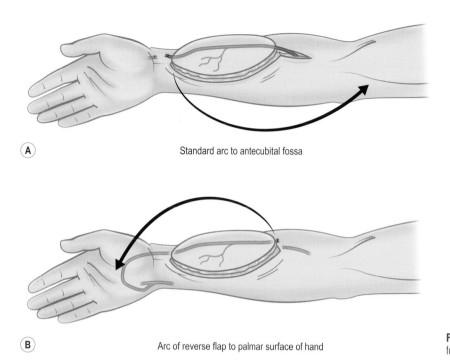

(A)   Standard arc to antecubital fossa

(B)   Arc of reverse flap to palmar surface of hand

Fig. 24.17 Radial forearm flap. **(A)** Standard arc to antecubital fossa. **(B)** Reverse arc to palmar surface of hand.

regional artery and vein with the flap, including both minor and major pedicles. With division of the proximal regional artery and vein and transposition of the flap in a distal direction opposite the standard arc of rotation, a reverse transposition is accomplished. This flap modification requires reversal of flow within the regional artery and vein to the flap and may adversely affect distal perfusion due to the division of a major regional vessel. A soleus muscle flap based on minor pedicles from the posterior tibial artery and vein located in the distal third of the lower extremity would be classified as a distally based flap. An example of a reverse flow flap is the soleus muscle flap based on the distal pedicle from the posterior tibial artery and vein. The flap is transposed distally with proximal division of the posterior tibial artery and vein. (This flap has been replaced by the sural flap, as described in Vol. IV, Ch.5.)

Type V muscles have two arcs of rotation. The standard arc is based on its major vascular pedicle (i.e., thoracodorsal artery and venae comitantes for latissimus dorsi muscle and thoracoacromial artery and venae comitantes for the pectoralis major muscle). The second arc of rotation is based on a series of secondary pedicles that provide a reverse arc of rotation (i.e., posterior intercostal and lumbar arteries and venae comitantes for the latissimus dorsi muscle and branches of the internal

mammary artery and venae comitantes for the pectoralis major muscle). The reverse arc of rotation for the latissimus dorsi muscle was described by Bostwick *et al.* in 1980.[109] The use of the latissimus dorsi muscle flap has been shown to be a reliable method of closure for complex back wounds in patients with spinal cord exposure or exposed vertebral hartdware.[110]

A direct fasciocutaneous flap (type B) may be designed as a reverse flow flap. After a dominant regional pedicle to the flap is divided, the flap is elevated with the divided dominant pedicle for transposition in the opposite direction from the source of the divided dominant pedicle. The blood supply to the flap will depend on reversal of flow in its major pedicle. For example, after division of the proximal radial artery and vein, the radial forearm flap can be elevated with its radial artery and venae comitantes and transposed distally to the hand as a reverse flap *(Fig. 24.18)*.

In a type B flap, the proximal regional source for a septocutaneous pedicle may be divided and the flap and its regional vascular pedicle rotated distally as a reverse transposition flap. This technique also requires reversal of flow within the regional pedicle. For instance, the dominant pedicles to the leg, (anterior tibial artery and venae comitantes, posterior tibial artery and venae comitantes, and peroneal artery and venae comitantes)

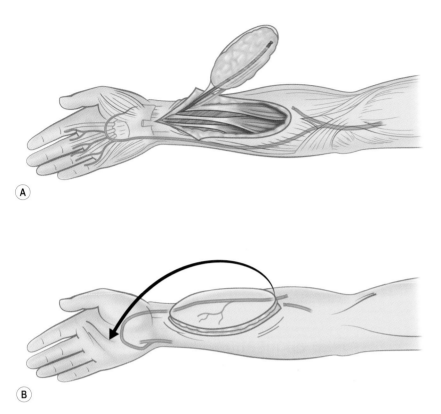

Fig. 24.18 Reverse transposition fasciocutaneous flap modification. **(A)** Radial forearm flap. **(B)** Distal flap transposition based on reverse flow.

may be divided proximal to the point of entrance of the dominant pedicle to the fasciocutaneous flap territory. Septocutaneous branches from the dominant sources of blood flow to the leg may be maintained and serve as a basis for design of a reverse transposition flap for distal coverage of leg wounds.

Venous flaps

A venous flap is defined as a composite flap of skin, subcutaneous tissue and other tissues such as nerve, tendon, and bone that uses a subcutaneous vein for the arterial inflow and venous outflow. Nakayama *et al.* first described these flaps in 1981.[111] Three types of venous flap have been identified *(Fig. 24.19)*.[112] Type I is a uni-pedicled venous flap; a single cephalad vein is the sole conduit for perfusion and drainage. These flaps can be proximally or distally based. Type II is a bipedicled venous flap with a vein entering (caudal end) as well as leaving (cephalad end) the flap. The flow of blood is from the caudal to cephalad end. Type III is an arterio-venous venous flap that is perfused by a proximal artery and drained by a distal vein. These flaps have had success in hand reconstruction. Available small, thin

flaps with defined arterial inflow and venous outflow are limited. Thus, when local flaps are not available, arterialized venous free flaps provide a good solution for successful soft tissue reconstruction *(Fig. 24.20)*.[113]

Microvascular composite tissue transplantation

With the ability to repair vessels <2 mm in diameter, it became apparent that microvascular transplantation was possible. Microvascular composite tissue transplantation has been termed free flap because the tissue is transplanted from one part of the body to another. Since flaps are now designed on known vascular pedicles, transplantation of composite tissue from the donor site to a distant site is possible by re-establishing flap circulation through anastomosis of the flap arterial and venous pedicles to suitable receptor vessels in proximity to the defect. Reliable anastomosis of vessels with external lumen diameters of 0.5–2 mm is possible with patency rates of 95% or better.[114] The ability to transplant a flap to a distant site eliminates the need to select a flap with an arc of rotation that reaches the defect. The surgeon is thus able to transfer composite tissue by flap suitability for defect coverage rather than proximity to

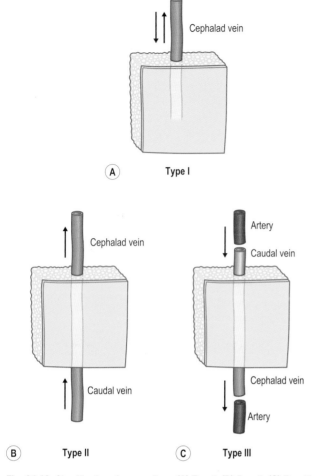

Fig. 24.19 Classification of venous flaps. **(A)** Type I. **(B)** Type II. **(C)** Type III

the defect. This technique is most suited for the type I, II, and V muscles, given the nature of the pedicles. Common muscles transferred include the latissimus, rectus abdominis, gracilis, and serratus. Common fasciocutaneous and perforator flaps transferred include the lateral arm flap, anterolateral thigh flap, deep inferior epigastric artery perforator flap and superficial inferior epigastric artery flaps.

When a microvascular anastomosis is used as part of a rotational flap, it is termed supercharging. Supercharging is a method of augmenting the blood supply to a large pedicled flap that may extend beyond the territory of a single pedicle. For example, the superiorly based unipedicled TRAM flap may be supercharged by anastomosing the inferior epigastric vessels to the thoracodorsal vessels in the axilla.[115,116]

Flap application

Whether a clinical problem is simple or difficult, the traditional approach has been to utilize the reconstructive ladder to guide surgical reconstruction **(Fig. 24.21)**. The choice of reconstructive options ranges from simple to complex.

The reconstructive ladder concept was proposed to establish priorities for technique selection based on the complexity of the technique and the defect requirements

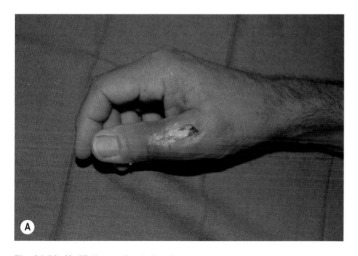

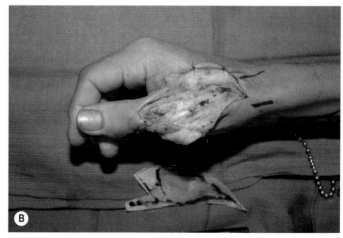

Fig. 24.20 **(A–H)** Venous flap to thumb.

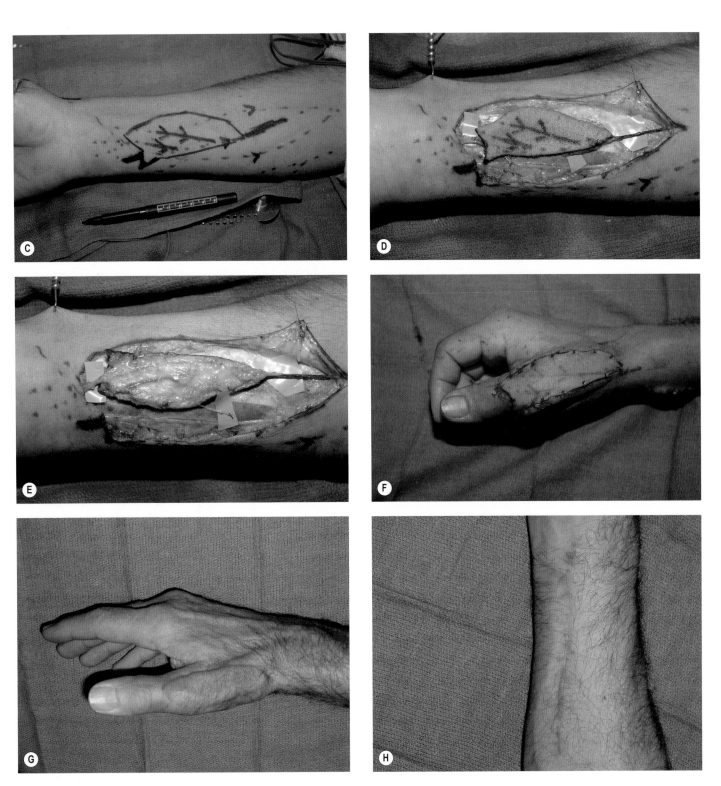

Fig. 24.20, cont'd

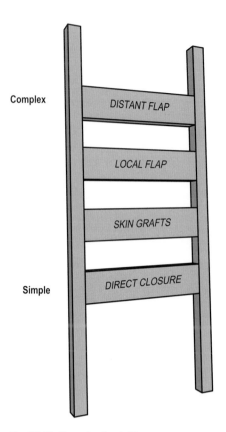

Fig. 24.21 Reconstructive ladder.

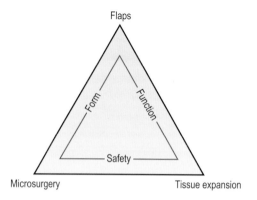

Fig. 24.22 Reconstructive triangle.

for safe wound closure. The ladder provides a systematic approach to wound closure, emphasizing selection first of simple and then complex techniques, depending on local wound requirements and complexity. Direct closure represents the simplest and most straightforward technique. Direct closure may be precluded by the size of the wound or the consequences of wound tension at the closure site resulting in malalignment of adjacent tissues. When this occurs, a more complex closure technique, such as a skin graft that uses distant skin for defect coverage, is required.

The simpler techniques, including skin grafts and local flaps, may allow defect closure. However, these techniques may not provide optimal results in terms of form and function. The more complex procedure often achieves superior results. The goals of form and function may best be served by more complex approaches, including regional or distant flaps, tissue expansion, and microvascular transplantation. A new paradigm, the reconstructive triangle, is more appropriate in the light of the more sophisticated options available today

(Fig. 24.22). This emphasizes the selection of a technique that safely achieves a successful reconstruction and restores form and function. Increased experience has led to the safe use of techniques such as flap transposition, microvascular composite tissue transplantation, and tissue expansion. The surgeon should now consider the reconstructive triangle to select the optimal technique to achieve predetermined reconstructive goals without donor site complications. Another alternative approach is the reconstructive elevator proposed by Gottlieb and Krieger.[117] Their approach is that we choose the most appropriate floor from which to choose our reconstruction, based on the specific requirements of the patient, the wound and the circumstances; for some patients choosing a more complex reconstruction even though a simpler one would achieve wound closure.

Safety in reconstructive surgery is generally measured in terms of immediate success of wound coverage or defect reconstruction. With the identification of specific vascular pedicles to muscle and fascia, flap reliability is significantly improved. However, with the introduction of perforator flaps, we are freed from those constraints, taking only the tissue that is required for the reconstruction and not sacrificing unwanted tissue simply because it acts as a carrier for the blood supply. Safe and reliable muscle or musculocutaneous and fascial or fasciocutaneous flaps and perforator flaps have been described for use in all areas of the body. When design is properly based on the precise vascular territory of their vascular pedicles, the majority of flaps survive transposition to a defect within the standard flap arc of rotation.

Certain situations will decrease flap safety. Flap loss may result when the defect is located beyond the standard arc of rotation causing excessive tension on the vascular pedicle. Defect size beyond the vascular territory of the flap pedicle may result in either an inappropriate increase in flap dimensions or excessive flap tension at the inset site. Selection of a flap with a pedicle location in the zone of injury or use in patients with preexisting vascular compromise may result in failure. Flap modifications, including segmental and distally based designs, are also subject to vascular compromise and potential loss. Thus, flap safety is determined based on anatomic design and on assessment of the specific reconstructive requirements.

The technique selected for defect closure or composite reconstruction should restore normal shape or contour. Tissue expansion is ideal for this purpose since the skin and soft tissue next to the defect have the same thickness, texture, and color. Unfortunately, this tissue is frequently damaged or unavailable for use either as an advancement or transposition flap.

Although the initial experience with the musculocutaneous flap resulted in safe wound closure, the excessive bulk was often unsightly. Frequently a muscle flap with a skin graft provided a superior restoration of form at the recipient site. With the identification of muscle and fascial units suitable for design either as a standard transposition or microvascular composite tissue transplantation, the surgeon may select the flap best suited for defect closure. When a skin island is required, the surgeon may select a flap with a thin layer of overlying subcutaneous tissue (i.e., radial forearm flap) or may plan secondary flap revision by direct excision or suction-assisted lipectomy to improve flap contour in thicker flaps. The availability of numerous flap donor sites allows selection of a technique for either standard transposition or microvascular composite tissue transplantation that best restores form for defect coverage or composite reconstruction.

Form preservation at the donor site should also influence flap selection. When possible, the donor site should be closed directly. Use of a flap that requires a skin graft for donor site closure is justified when the flap harvested is clearly superior to alternate flaps for the defect. If it is possible to stage the flap elevation with preliminary insertion of a tissue expander, an increase in both the cutaneous flap dimensions for defect closure and the adjacent skin territory for donor site direct closure may be accomplished. Although the ultimate form at the flap recipient site remains the primary basis for flap selection, deformity due to loss of form at the donor site should be avoided when possible. Thus, reconstructive balance is achieved with selection of a tissue source to restore the defect or deformity while form and function are preserved at the donor site.

In an effort to minimize donor site morbidity, many surgeons have evaluated the utility of endoscopic harvest of muscle flaps. Minimally invasive techniques for harvest of several muscles have been described. These include the latissimus dorsi, rectus abdominis, gracilis, rectus femoris, external oblique, and gastrocnemius muscles. In addition to the endoscopic harvest of muscles, laparoscopic techniques are frequently used to harvest the omentum. This has been a significant advance as the benefits include decreased scarring, less postoperative pain and theoretically less donor site morbidity.[118–120]

Stability of the closure represents the most important long-term consideration at the site of defect coverage. For this reason, flap coverage is frequently selected despite the simplicity of split-thickness skin grafts for some defects which may ultimately require a flap at a latter date. With selection of a reliable flap design and use of a standard technique for transposition or microvascular transplantation, flap coverage will provide stability at the defect site without necessarily increasing the risk or compromising safety.

Specialized functions at the site of reconstruction include hair growth, sensibility, skeletal support (bone), and motion (animation). Techniques of reconstruction must consider these specialized requirements. Although function restoration may require staged procedures, especially for a composite defect, it is often possible to restore all functional requirements with a single procedure.

Tissue expansion can increase the surface area of specialized skin, especially hair-bearing scalp. Insertion of a tissue expander at the defect edge will not interrupt the sensory innervation of the planned flap. Both skin and subcutaneous tissues of the expanded advancement or transposition flap will provide the appropriate match for defect closure with resultant optimal form and function.

The cutaneous territory flaps based whether they be muscle, fascia or perforator based, will not provide normal sensibility unless a specific cutaneous nerve to this territory is incorporated in the flap design. With the exception of defects located in weight-bearing surfaces and in areas of specialized function, including the hand, face, and oral cavity, the sensory innervated flap is not critical for stability and function. In weight-bearing areas where motor and sensory function remains intact except at the site of the defect, a well-vascularized flap without excessive bulk will generally provide stable coverage and restore function. However, a well-vascularized flap will not provide functional restoration for defects located in weight-bearing areas where sensory function is completely absent. For example, flap coverage of a pressure sore defect associated with spinal cord transaction will be subject to recurrent ulceration unless a coordinated program of patient education and pressure avoidance is instituted. Efforts to design a neurosensory flap by incorporating a sensory nerve in the flap cutaneous territory or through intervening nerve grafts following both flap transposition and transplantation may be required for functional preservation.

Restoration of skeletal support is essential for functional restoration in the head, chest, and extremities. The surgeon has the option of providing flap coverage followed by staged skeletal reconstruction or providing both flap and vascularized bone simultaneously. Studies of human vascular anatomy related to flap design have demonstrated vascular connections to adjacent bone in many body regions. Thus, both muscle and facial flaps have vascular pedicles with either periosteal or direct nutrient branches to bone. Although prosthetic materials are safely used in conjunction with flaps, vascularized bone is preferred, particularly for mandible and long bone reconstruction. However, standard bone grafting techniques are also reliable, especially if stable flap coverage is provided. Techniques involving bone osteotomy and lengthening will frequently allow skeletal restoration, especially if stable wound coverage is provided through flap coverage. Because of the complexity of flap design when vascularized bone is included, microvascular transplantation of composite flaps is preferred over regional transposition flaps with vascularized bone. When use of a vascularized bone is planned, donor site bone instability and associated loss of form and function should be avoided.

Restoration of muscle function at the site of reconstruction may also be required. After release of its origin or insertion, the muscle flap will no longer perform its intended function. However, flap technique may include preservation of the motor nerve to the muscle flap. Preservation of motor nerve innervation, along with re-establishment of the muscle origin, insertion, or both, can maintain normal muscle tension across the defect site. When local or regional muscle flaps are unavailable, a distant muscle may be transplanted by microvascular techniques that include coaptation of the muscle motor nerve with a suitable receptor motor nerve at the recipient site. Proper selection of donor muscles of appropriate size and shape can restore muscle function at the defect site.

Function preservation at the donor site represents an important consideration, particularly with use of a muscle flap or a flap with vascularized bone. A regional muscle should not be used if adjacent muscle groups are absent or injured, especially if it is feasible to transplant a distant flap microsurgically. When possible, function-preserving techniques for muscle transposition are advocated. Frequently it is possible to use a segmental muscle flap based on a reliable vascular pedicle that allows preservation of the remaining muscle with intact origin and insertion.

Advantages and disadvantages of muscle and musculocutaneous flaps

Selection of the most appropriate reconstructive method can be difficult. Careful consideration must be given to all the possible methods of repair, and the advantages and disadvantages of each technique must be weighed accordingly.

The advantages of muscle or musculocutaneous flaps include the following:

1. The vascular pedicles are specific and reliable.
2. The vascular pedicle is often located outside the surgical defect, which can be particularly important for wounds with an extensive zone of injury beyond the actual wound (e.g., after irradiation, trauma).
3. The muscle provides bulk for deep, extensive defects and protective padding for exposed vital structures (e.g., tendons, nerves, vessels, bones, and prostheses).

4. Muscle is malleable and can be manipulated (e.g., folded on itself) to produce a desired shape or volume.

5. Well-vascularized muscle is resistant to bacterial inoculation and infection.[121]

6. Reconstruction by use of muscle or musculocutaneous flaps is often a one-stage procedure.

7. Restoration of function, whether motor or sensory, is possible with certain flaps.

8. The reliability and availability of muscle and musculocutaneous flaps make them an excellent alternative means of reconstruction when the closure method of choice for a particular defect is unavailable or inadequate.

The disadvantages of muscle and musculocutaneous flaps include the following:

1. The donor defect may lose some degree of function.

2. The donor defect may be aesthetically undesirable.

3. Reconstruction with muscle or musculocutaneous flaps may provide excessive bulk, leaving an esthetically unacceptable result.

4. Muscle or musculocutaneous flaps may atrophy over time and thus fail to provide adequate coverage.

5. Removal of the muscle or musculocutaneous flap may result in contour deformities at the donor site.

The preservation of function can be extremely important when nonexpendable muscles are used as flaps. The techniques of function preservation generally involve transposing part of the muscle without completely interrupting the origin or insertion of the donor muscle. For example, the transposition of the superior half of the gluteus maximus muscle for sacral coverage in the ambulatory patient can be performed without loss of thigh extension or hip stability because the remainder of the gluteus maximus is functionally intact.[122,123]

Advantages and disadvantages of fascia, fasciocutaneous, and perforator flaps

The advantages and disadvantages of these flaps are somewhat similar to those of muscle flaps, although there are a few exceptions. The advantages include the following:

1. They are thin and pliable.

2. The blood supply is reliable and robust.

3. The donor site morbidity is minimal in regard to function.

4. They are muscle sparing.

5. They have the ability to restore sensation.

6. There are many potential donor sites.

The disadvantages of fascia, fasciocutaneous, and perforator flaps include the following:

1. There is a lack of bulk for deep defects.

2. They are technically more challenging (pedicle dissection; many require microvascular anastomosis or at least microvascular techniques).

3. There are size limitations.

4. The arc of rotation is sometimes limited though often better than the similar muscle flap because of the longer pedicle.

5. Donor site may require skin graft closure, resulting in donor site deformity.

Flap transposition and arc of rotation

Numerous pedicle flaps are available for transposition to cover or reconstruct specific defects. When a transposition flap is elevated, the dominant vascular pedicle to the flap is preserved. A factor that may prevent successful flap transposition is the flap's arc of rotation. The arc of rotation of a muscle is determined by the extent of elevation of the muscle from its anatomic bed and the ability of the muscle to reach adjacent areas without devascularization. The mobility of a muscle depends on the number of vascular pedicles and the location of the dominant vascular pedicle relative to the muscle's origin and insertion *(Fig. 24.23)*. The area covered by the arc of rotation varies among individuals. On the basis of the flap length distal to the point of rotation and the length of the vascular pedicle, a safe standard arc of rotation is measured for each flap. A modified arc of rotation is also available based on refinements in design and specific modifications of the flap. Precise knowledge of the safe standard and modified arc of rotation is necessary to avoid loss of the flap from

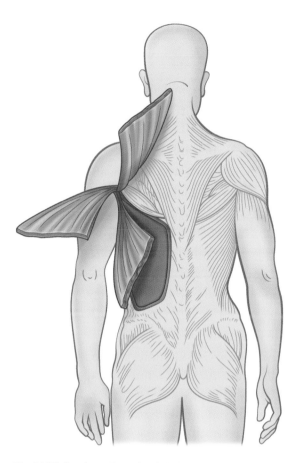

Fig. 24.23 Arc of muscle rotation (latissimus muscle).

excessive tension or damage to the pedicle from over-zealous dissection.

In general, the arc of rotation is inversely proportional to the number of vascular pedicles. If a muscle has a large number of pedicles, it usually has a limited arc of rotation. Type IV muscles, such as the sartorius and tibialis anterior, are examples of muscles with multiple segmental vascular pedicles and limited arcs of rotation. Similarly, the location of the dominant vascular pedicle relative to the muscle's origin and insertion greatly determines the arc of rotation. The closer the dominant vascular pedicle is to either the origin or insertion of the muscle, the greater the arc of rotation. The point of rotation for types I, II, III, and V muscles generally are located at one end or the proximal third of the muscle. For example, type V muscles, such as the pectoralis major and latissimus dorsi, have their major vascular pedicle near their insertion, and correspondingly have a wide arc of rotation. Certain muscles, such

as type V muscles, have two arcs of rotation. The first arc of rotation is based on the dominant blood supply, while the second is based on the secondary segmental vascular pedicles. Reverse arc of rotation refers to the degree of transposition of a flap based on its secondary segmental vascular pedicles.

The fasciocutaneous flap's standard arc of rotation is determined by the extent of elevation of the deep fascia from its normal anatomic position to reach adjacent defects. The point of rotation is based on the site of entrance of the dominant vascular pedicle into the fascia. The fascia or fasciocutaneous flap is elevated to the point of entrance of the flap pedicle, and the fascia and overlying skin distal to this point are rotated into the defect. In a type A fasciocutaneous flap, the flap is elevated to include the direct cutaneous pedicle. A standard arc of rotation is achieved with the flap elevated to the proximal edge of the flap territory. When the flap is designed as a fascial skin island, the arc of rotation can be increased with proximal dissection of the axially directed pedicle.

The standard arc of rotation for a type B flap is determined by elevating the flap to the point of entrance of the septocutaneous pedicle at the flap base. Proximal dissection of the septocutaneous pedicle to its junction with regional vessels will increase the flap's arc of rotation. This increased extension, however, is often not as great as what can achieved with a type A flap since the pedicle dissection is generally deep between muscle groups, which prevents a wider arc of rotation.

The type C flap is elevated to the muscle surface at the site of penetration of the musculocutaneous pedicle. Dissection of the pedicle through muscle to the regional vessels will increase the arc of rotation. It is also possible to include a segment of muscle with the fasciocutaneous flap design. Though the perforator flap can be thought of as a type C fasciocutaneous flap it is probably better to think of it as a separate entity. The arc of rotation of a perforator flap is purely dependent on the length of the vascular pedicle and does not depend on either muscle or fascia. For this reason, pedicled perforator flaps are very versatile.

Prediction of skin territory

The successful use of the overlying skin in a musculocutaneous flap is dependent on the skin's blood supply.

Advances in the anatomic study of the cutaneous vascular system have revealed three distinct vascular patterns supplying the skin: direct cutaneous vessels, which are specific vessels in the subcutaneous fat that run parallel to the skin surface; musculocutaneous perforators, which arise from underlying muscle; and fasciocutaneous vessels, which are specific vessels that arise from regional vasculature and extend through intermuscular spaces into the overlying fascia.

The major blood supply to the skin varies by region. Skin overlying the broad, flat muscles of the trunk (e.g., the latissimus dorsi) is largely dependent on the musculocutaneous perforating arteries. Skin overlying the thin, narrow muscles (e.g., the gracilis) is largely dependent on the fasciocutaneous perforating vessels.

Each musculocutaneous perforating artery nourishes a certain territory of skin. Saint Cyr has designated this unit as a perforasome.[124] There can be much overlap, depending on the complexity of the skin's interconnecting vascular system. By appreciating this vascular system, the surgeon can safely design the skin territory of the flap.

All muscles, with the exception of the type I group, require the division of vascular pedicles for flap transposition. Muscles with type II or type IV patterns require division of minor or segmental pedicles for flap elevation. Doing so may compromise the corresponding skin territory. Type III muscles have two large vascular pedicles arising from separate vascular sources. The entire skin overlying the muscle often survives on either of the two pedicles. Type V muscles are the most versatile because the skin islands can be based on either the proximal dominant pedicle or the secondary segmental pedicles. Type I muscles are reliable because the blood supply generally supports all the overlying skin.

In general, each superficial muscle supplies the skin lying directly over it, and the skin territory may be safely extended 3–4 cm beyond the borders of the underlying muscle. The additional skin is supported by various anastomotic networks in the subcutaneous tissues. In certain patients, there appears to be a degree of axiality in the musculocutaneous perforators that anastomose with the cutaneous vessels. This anatomic arrangement enables an even larger territory of skin to be safely elevated. For example, in the extended deep inferior epigastric musculocutaneous flap described by Taylor *et al.* in 1983, certain paraumbilical musculocutaneous perforators from the inferior epigastric artery course superolaterally in the line of the intercostal spaces, anastomosing with the lateral cutaneous branches of the intercostal system.[125] This arrangement enables the skin island to extend over the costal margin toward the tip of the scapula. Gottlieb *et al.* stated that the skin island of this flap could extend as far as the posterior axillary line, certainly a considerable distance from the borders of the underlying muscle.[126] As modifications and refinements in the musculocutaneous flap continue, it is certain that various other extended skin territories, supported by the intricate anastomoses of the cutaneous, musculocutaneous, and fasciocutaneous systems, will be discovered.

Selection of specific muscle and musculocutaneous flaps

After the decision has been made to use a muscle or musculocutaneous flap, the specific muscle must be chosen. General guidelines used to assist in the selection of a muscle include the following:

1. Ideally, the muscle should be adjacent to the defect.

2. The muscle should be of sufficient size and bulk to cover the defect. The final design of the flap should occur only after the defect is completely defined. When tumor exposure or wound debridement is required, the defect is often much larger and deeper than initially anticipated. By final design of the flap after debridement, costly errors in inadequate coverage can be avoided. If the defect is unstable or the margins are unclear (tumor pathology not available), wound packing or temporary skin graft coverage is warranted. One must also take into consideration that a significant amount of atrophy occurs if the origin, insertion, or motor nerve of the muscle is disrupted.

3. The muscle should be expendable. There are often synergistic muscles that can compensate for the loss of the selected muscle so that the donor site is not impaired. However, if no synergistic muscle groups are available, either techniques to preserve donor muscle function (e.g., muscle splitting)

should be employed or a different muscle chosen.

4. The status of the vascular pedicle that will sustain the proposed flap must be known preoperatively. Selective arteriography must be considered if there is a history of previous surgery in proximity to the vascular pedicle of the proposed muscle flap or if muscle paralysis is noted on physical examination. Earlier division of the motor nerve may also include ligation of the vascular pedicle. Examples of clinical situations when arteriography is particularly useful include the evaluation of the sural artery (gastrocnemius) after knee surgery, of the transverse cervical artery (trapezius) after neck and shoulder surgery, and of the thoracodorsal artery (latissimus dorsi) after axillary surgery.[127]

5. The donor defect must be carefully considered. Some patients do not accept the use of a skin graft at the donor site, and certain muscles are more likely than others to require grafts for closure. Likewise, some patients prefer one scar site to another (e.g., the abdominal scar of the TRAM flap versus the back scar of the latissimus dorsi flap in breast reconstruction).

6. The cutaneous territory of the proposed flap must be of sufficient size and of acceptable texture. The harvested skin should be an acceptable match to the recipient site (e.g., not hair bearing).

7. If restoration of sensation or motor function is necessary a select number of muscle, musculocutaneous and fasciocutaneous flaps are available. Common examples of muscles which provide sensation or restore function include the serratus muscle, rectus abdominis, and latissimus dorsi.[128–132]

8. Osteomusculocutaneous flaps are available for defects in need of vascularized bone in addition to soft tissue. Examples include the trapezius flap with vascularized clavicle and scapular spine,[133–135] pectoralis major flap with vascularized rib,[136,137] iliac osteomusculocutaneous flap based on the ascending and transverse branches of the lateral circumflex femoral system[138,139] and the latissimus dorsi-scapular osteomusculocutaneous flap.[140,141]

9. The operation should be technically straightforward.

Selection of specific fascia and fasciocutaneous flaps

General guidelines in choosing a specific fascia or fasciocutaneous flap are similar to those of muscle and musculocutaneous flaps, with a few exceptions.

The fascia or fasciocutaneous are must be in proximity of the defect if a rotational flap is planned. The planned flap must be of sufficient size and bulk to reconstruct the defect. Fascia and fasciocutaneous flaps are ideal for areas that do not require bulk. The vascular supply of the area must be assessed preoperatively. If a fasciocutaneous flap is planned, the perforating vessels should be assessed with a Doppler probe preoperatively so that the skin island can be designed. The presence or absence of sufficient perforating vessels determines whether a specific fasciocutaneous flap can be used. The donor defect should be considered. These can generally be closed primarily (fascial flap) but may require skin graft if skin island is large. Restoration of sensation with fasciocutaneous flaps is possible. Examples include the lateral arm flap,[142] radial forearm flap,[143] deltoid flap,[144] anterolateral thigh flap,[145] and tensor fascia lata flap.[146]

Regional application of muscle and musculocutaneous flaps

Head and neck reconstruction

Regional flaps:
1. Temporalis
2. Sternocleidomastoid
3. Platysma.

    Distant flaps:
1. Pectoralis major
2. Trapezius
3. Latissimus dorsi.

    Microvascular transplantation:
1. Radial forearm
2. Rectus abdominis
3. Latissimus
4. Scapular

5. Abdominal viscera (omentum, jejunum, colon).

6. Perforator flaps.

Radical cancer surgery or traumatic injury can produce massive defects in the head and neck. Whereas many simple defects can be adequately treated with direct closure, local scalp flaps or skin grafts, the more complicated defect requires a larger reconstruction. The muscle, musculocutaneous and fasciocutaneous flaps play a major role in these reconstructions. Historically, large surgical defects of the head and neck were managed with staged reconstruction. Currently, the most common reconstruction involves microvascular tissue transfer.

The primary applications of the muscle or musculo-cutaneous flap in head and neck reconstruction include provision of tissue bulk for a significant defect (e.g., after hemimandibulectomy); protective coverage of vital structures (e.g., the carotid artery); provision of skin for intraoral lining and coverage; and provision of skin for skull, facial, and neck defects.

The local muscle and musculocutaneous flaps for head and neck reconstruction include the temporalis, sternocleidomastoid, and platysma flaps.

The temporalis muscle is a type III, fan shaped, bipen-niform muscle. Transposition of the muscle as a turno-ver flap is especially useful for coverage of the orbit, superior maxilla, and ear.

The sternocleidomastoid is a type II muscle, first described in head and neck reconstruction by Owens in 1955.[25] This flap has historically been used for intraoral and pharyngeal reconstruction. Other uses have included augmentation of soft tissue defects of the upper neck and jaw, protective coverage of major vessels, and closure of pharyngocutaneous fistulas.[147–149] However, of all the musculocutaneous flaps used for head and neck reconstruction, the sternocleidomastoid is considered the least reliable.[19,149]

The platysma is a type II, thin, broad, sheet-like muscle extending over the entire anterior and lateral aspects of the neck. The use of the platysma as a muscu-locutaneous flap was first described in 1887 by Gersuny, who employed it in reconstructing a full-thickness defect of the cheek.[150] The platysma has been used for intraoral, lip, lower midface, and anterior neck recon-struction. Because of the thinness of the platysma muscle, the reconstructive surgeon must be particularly

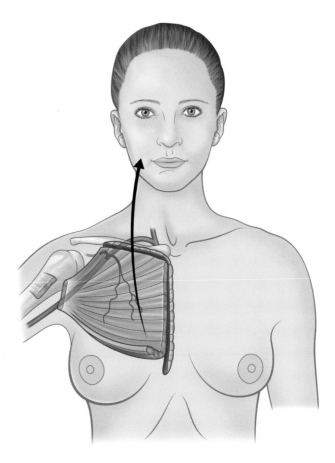

Fig. 24.24 Pectoralis major flap. Standard arc to middle third of face.

careful to avoid disrupting the muscle fibers during the dissection and placing undue tension on the vascular pedicle after transposition of the flap.

The distant muscle and musculocutaneous flaps used in head and neck reconstruction include the pectoralis major, trapezius, and latissimus dorsi flaps.

The pectoralis major is a type V, large, broad muscle. Its use as a musculocutaneous flap was first described in 1968 by Hueston and McConchie as part of a com-pound deltopectoral flap.[151] In 1977, Brown *et al.* described the use of the pectoralis major as a flap in mediastinal coverage.[17] In 1979, Ariyan introduced the pectoralis major musculocutaneous flap for head and neck reconstruction (*Figs 24.24, 24.25*).[19] During the ensuing years, the pectoralis major musculocutaneous flap proved more valuable than the deltopectoral flap and supplanted it as the primary flap (other than micro-vascular tissue transplantation) in head and neck reconstruction.

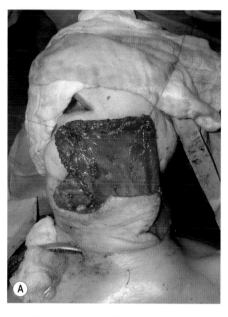
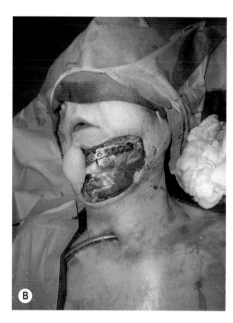
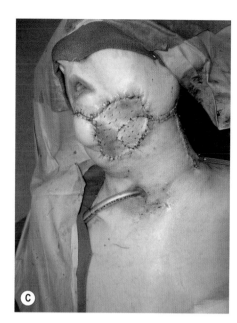

Fig. 24.25 **(A–C)** Pectoralis major flap for head and neck reconstruction.

The common applications of the pectoralis major musculocutaneous flap in head and neck reconstruction include the following: external resurfacing of the skin of the face and neck; intraoral and pharyngeal lining; carrying vascularized rib and skin in mandibular reconstruction; and reconstruction of the esophagus.[152–156] Historically, the pectoralis major musculocutaneous flap has been one of the most versatile flaps used in head and neck reconstruction.

The trapezius, a type II muscle, is less widely used than the PM muscle, yet its superior location and wide anterior arc of rotation make it a valuable musculocutaneous flap.[13,157] Modifications in design have enabled the trapezius muscle to be used as distinctly different upper and lower musculocutaneous flaps.[158] The various clinical applications of the trapezius flap have included lower facial reconstruction, especially the ear and parotid regions; lateral upper face and scalp (occipital and temporal) repair[159]; anterior and posterior neck reconstruction[160]; orbital reconstruction with the use of an extended flap[161,162]; and pharyngoesophageal reconstruction. Historically, the trapezius has also been used as an osteomusculocutaneous flap, incorporating either the lateral aspect of the clavicle or the spine of the scapula *(Figs 24.26, 24.27).*[163]

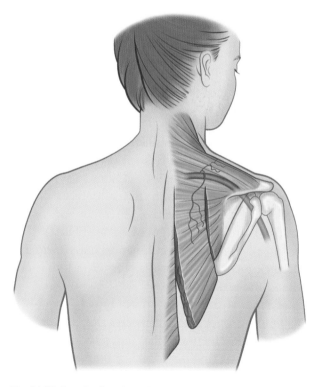

Fig. 24.26 Trapezius flap. Arc to face and anterior neck.

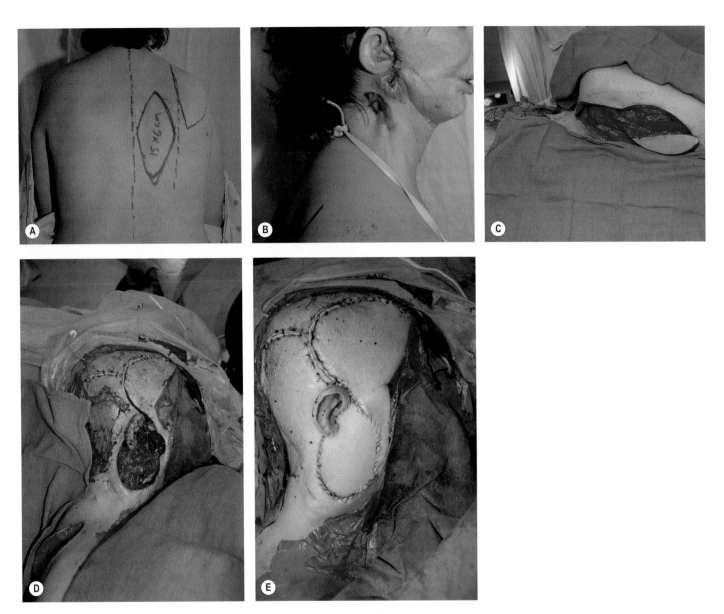

Fig. 24.27 (A–E) Vertical trapezius musculocutaneous flap for head and neck reconstruction.

The latissimus dorsi is a type V muscle originally described as a superiorly based flap by Tansini in 1896.[23] Since the first description, there have been numerous modifications and refinements of the flap. Historically, the latissimus dorsi musculocutaneous flap has been used in head and neck reconstruction for large defects or when previous radiation or surgery precluded the use of other flaps. Since Quillen *et al.* reported the use of the latissimus dorsi as a transposition island flap in 1978 to cover the mandible and neck after resection of a tumor; various other clinical applications of the muscle have been described.[164] In fact, the latissimus

dorsi musculocutaneous flap was used frequently in intraoral and pharyngeal reconstruction.[165] Other uses of the latissimus dorsi muscle in head and neck reconstruction have included reconstruction of defects of the posterior neck, shoulder, anterior neck, lower face, occipital scalp, and intraoral-pharyngoesophageal regions.

Microvascular tissue transplantation in head and neck reconstruction has become the reconstruction of choice in most centers. The use of microsurgery has allowed the surgeon to achieve superior reconstructive results with regard to form and function. Various muscle,

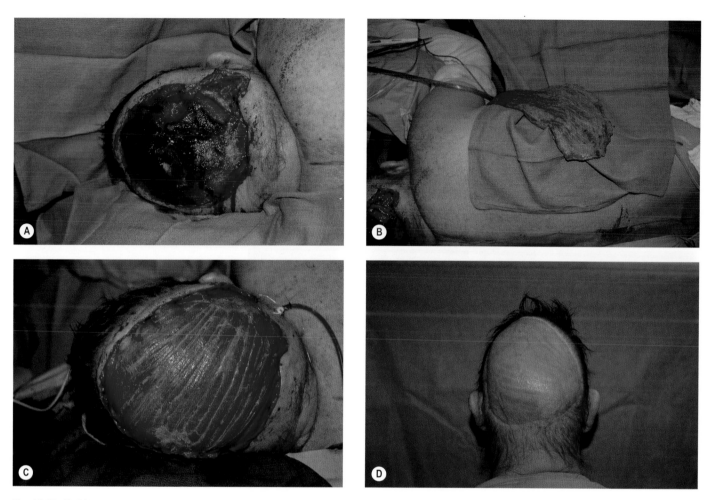

Fig. 24.28 (A–D) Latissimus dorsi flap to scalp defect.

musculocutaneous and fasciocutaneous flaps are used in head and neck reconstruction depending on the defect as well as surgeon preference. Large midface defects are often reconstructed with rectus abdominis musculocutaneous flaps.[166] The rectus provides muscle bulk to fill large three-dimensional defects in addition to providing a large skin island for external coverage.[167] Intraoral defects can often be closed with a radial forearm flap, restoring a functional oral cavity.[168] Partial or total glossectomy defects have been reconstructed with the radial forearm flap, rectus abdominis muscle flap, latissimus dorsi muscle flap, gracilis muscle flap, and anterolateral thigh flap.[169,170] Large scalp defects are effectively managed by transfer of the latissimus dorsi muscle flap or omental free flap combined with a split thickness skin graft. The latissimus has been widely used because of its large surface area, long vascular pedicle, and reliability *(Fig. 24.28).*[171,172] Although it is not commonly used, the omentum can provide stable coverage of large scalp defects.[64] The required laparotomy increases the donor site morbidity. When the patient has undergone a prior laparotomy, adhesions may complicate flap harvest.

Breast reconstruction

Regional flaps:

1. Pectoralis major
2. Serratus anterior
3. Pectoralis minor.
   Distant flaps:
1. Rectus abdominis
2. Latissimus dorsi.

Microvascular flaps:

1. Rectus abdominis

2. Deep inferior epigastric perforator

3. Superficial inferior epigastric artery

4. Superior gluteal perforator

5. Inferior gluteal perforator

6. Gluteus maximus

7. Transverse upper gracilis.

Muscle and musculocutaneous flaps have had a tremendous impact on breast reconstruction and have provided women with superior cosmetic results after mastectomy. Less aggressive surgical treatment of breast cancer such as the modified radical mastectomy, skin or nipple-sparing mastectomy, and lumpectomy have replaced the classic radical mastectomy as the treatment of choice for breast cancer. This change in approach has resulted in smaller defects and more local tissue available for use in reconstruction. In addition, more women with pre-malignant disease or with a family history of breast cancer are undergoing prophylactic mastectomy and immediate reconstruction.

Local muscles available in breast reconstruction are the pectoralis major, pectoralis minor and serratus anterior. These muscles are especially important for patients who undergo prosthetic implant or expander insertion. For patients with an intact pectoralis major muscle and adequate overlying skin, the submuscular (subpectoral or subserratus-pectoral) placement of a prosthetic implant is a common reconstructive technique.[173] The pectoralis minor and serratus muscles can also assist in implant coverage and are generally used in addition to the pectoralis major muscle.[174–176]

The distant muscles available in breast reconstruction include the latissimus dorsi, rectus abdominis and a variety of other muscles transferred microsurgically including the gluteus, and fasciocutaneous perforator flaps (deep inferior epigastric perforator, superficial inferior epigastric artery and transverse upper gracilis). Distant musculocutaneous or fasciocutaneous flaps are usually indicated for patients with inadequate local tissue, unacceptable overlying skin, or radiation damage.

Tanzini described the earliest version of the latissimus flap.[23] Since then, this muscle has become one of the most versatile flaps in plastic and reconstructive surgery. The advantages of the latissimus flap are that it has a reliable vascular supply and skin island and ultimately provides an acceptable cosmetic result.[177] The major drawback in using the latissimus dorsi muscle for breast reconstruction is that a prosthetic implant is usually required to provide adequate projection, as the musculocutaneous flap by itself is generally too thin.[178] Given this, the extended latissimus dorsi flap has been described; it provides additional soft tissue, thus obviating the need for implants.[179] In addition, the latissimus dorsi donor scar is often unsightly and the seroma rates high.[180]

The rectus abdominis is a type III muscle that commonly supplies a generous amount of abdominal fat and overlying skin. As a musculocutaneous flap the rectus abdominis has proved to be one of the most valuable options for breast reconstruction. Variations in flap design have produced different types of rectus abdominis musculocutaneous flaps (e.g., vertical, transverse, bipedicled, superiorly based, and inferiorly based flaps). The flap was initially described based on its superior pedicle, the superior epigastric artery and venae comitantes, with a vertical skin island. Subsequently, its use based on the inferior pedicle, the deep inferior epigastric artery, was reported.[181] In 1982, Hartrampf et al. described a technique that changed the entire approach to breast reconstruction.[182] By alignment of the skin island in a transverse direction, between the umbilicus and pelvis, the rectus abdominis musculocutaneous flap provided skin and soft tissue for breast reconstruction with improved abdominal contour. The transverse rectus abdominis musculocutaneous (TRAM) flap is now considered the musculocutaneous flap of choice for breast reconstruction (*Fig. 24.29*).

The indications for using the TRAM flap in breast reconstruction include a patient in need of additional soft tissue and overlying skin who has a moderate amount of lower abdominal tissue; a patient who prefers autologous tissue reconstruction without the use of a prosthetic implant; a patient who prefers a lower abdominal donor scar rather than a back scar; and a patient who has had an unacceptable result after undergoing other reconstructive methods (*Fig. 24.30*).[183]

The relative contraindications to using the TRAM flap include an extremely thin patient who has little lower abdominal tissue, a nulliparous patient in her child-bearing years, a patient with a history of abdominal wall hernia, an extremely obese patient, a heavy smoker, and a patient with lower abdominal scars. An

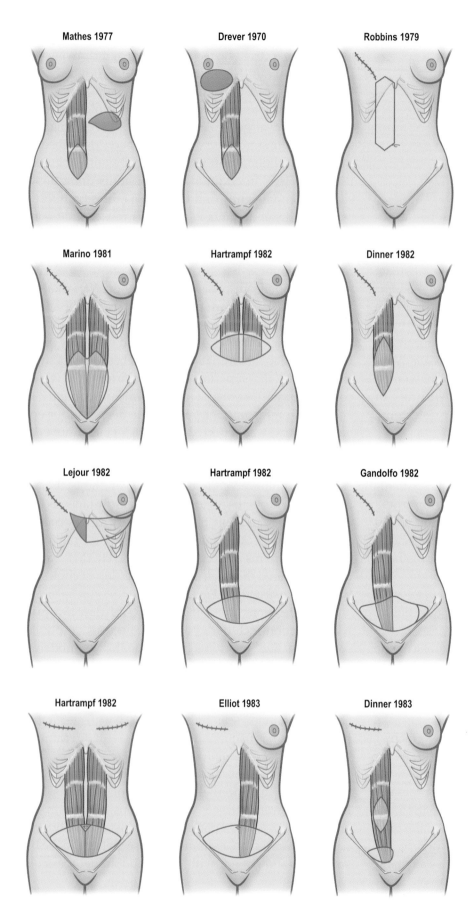

Fig. 24.29 Various designs of superiorly pedicled TRAM flaps.

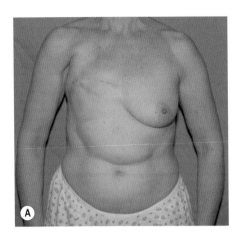
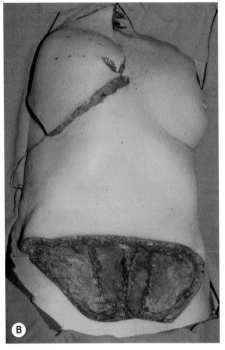
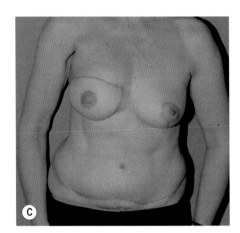

Fig. 24.30 (A–C) TRAM flap breast reconstruction.

absolute contraindication for a superiorly based transposition TRAM flap for breast reconstruction is prior division of its superior pedicle, usually related to a superior transverse laparotomy incision.

The advantages of the TRAM flap include the following:

1. It provides sufficient bulk so that a prosthetic implant usually is not required.

2. The suprapubic horizontal donor scar is esthetically acceptable.

3. Transposition of the flap can be performed with the patient in a single operative position.

4. The skin dimensions are larger than those available with the latissimus dorsi flap.

5. A simultaneous abdominoplasty is accomplished with direct donor site closure.

The major disadvantage of the TRAM flap is that there is a potential risk of abdominal hernia or weakness after the use of the unilateral or bilateral rectus muscles for flap harvest.[184]

The long-term effect of the loss of one or both rectus abdominis muscles has been the subject of many investigations.[185] Most studies report qualitative rather than quantitative data with regard to the postoperative strength of the abdominal wall. However, studies are beginning to show qualitative deficits of abdominal wall muscle loss.[186] Overall, the majority of patients resume normal activities, without physical limitations after breast reconstruction with the TRAM flap.

Reconstruction of the breast with microvascular tissue transplantation has become the primary source of breast reconstruction in some centers. Several musculocutaneous flaps have been described with the rectus abdominis being the most common.[187] In addition, the superior and inferior gluteus maximus musculocutaneous flap have been used for breast reconstruction.[188,189]

In addition to musculocutaneous flaps, perforator and fasciocutaneous flaps are being used more frequently. Perforator flaps have been advocated because of frequent use and the theoretical advantage of less morbidity at the donor site. These include the deep inferior epigastric perforator flap, superior gluteal artery perforator flap, the inferior gluteal artery perforator flap and the superficial inferior epigastric artery flap.[190–192]

Mediastinum

Regional flaps:

1. Pectoralis major.

Distant flaps:

1. Rectus abdominis

2. Latissimus dorsi

3. Omentum.

Microvascular flaps:

1. Latissimus dorsi.

The most common reason for reconstructing the mediastinum is infection after median sternotomy. Although the incidence of infection following median sternotomy is low, reported from 0.4% to 6.9%, the morbidity and mortality are significant.[193] The treatment of an infected median sternotomy wound depends on the extent of the infection and the amount of tissue necrosis. Historically, the standard therapy for an infected median sternotomy wound included debridement and closed tube irrigation. Muscle flap coverage was generally reserved for wounds recalcitrant to standard therapy. Now, it is generally accepted that early muscle flap transposition decreases morbidity, and therefore the use of a muscle flap should always be considered for the treatment of median sternotomy wounds.

The preferred local muscle for mediastinal coverage is the pectoralis major. In 1980 Jurkiewicz *et al.* described the use of the pectoralis major muscle flap to obliterate the sternal-mediastinal dead space.[194] The pectoralis major can be mobilized in several ways. The muscle can be transposed either on the dominant thoracoacromial pedicle or as a turnover flap on the segmental secondary vascular pedicles (perforating vessels from the internal mammary artery and vein). Nahai *et al.* described a modified technique of the turnover flap that preserves the lateral one-third of the muscle based on the dominant vascular pedicle and its motor nerves.[195] The advantage of this technique is the preservation of the anterior axillary fold. The pectoralis muscle flap remains the mainstay of treatment in both adults and children with sternal wound infections.[196–198]

Depending on the size of the defect, the surgeon can use one or both pectoralis major muscles for coverage.[199] If additional coverage is needed, the rectus abdominis can be used along with the pectoralis major muscles to cover the inferior aspect of the wound.[200] Used as either a muscle or musculocutaneous flap, the rectus abdominis muscle is a reliable source for inferior mediastinal coverage; as well, it provides the ability to fill a large dead space.[201,202] In considering the use of the

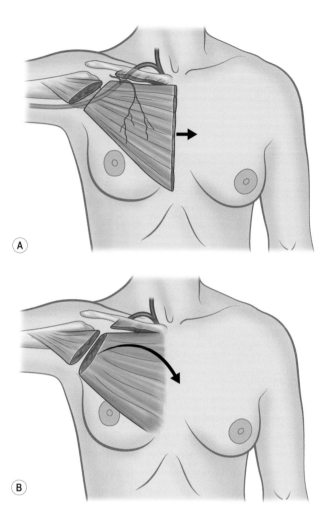

Fig. 24.31 Pectoralis major flap. **(A)** Standard flap to anterior mediastinum based on thoracoacromial pedicle. **(B)** Turnover arc to anterior mediastinum based on perforator vessels from internal mammary artery and associated veins.

rectus abdominis muscle, it must be noted that the superior epigastric artery is the continuation of the internal mammary artery inferior to the sternum that should be avoided during debridement of the sternal wound. Furthermore, the use of the internal mammary artery as a coronary artery bypass graft may adversely affect perfusion of the superiorly based rectus abdominis flap, which precludes the use of the rectus flap on that side. Collateral circulation to the internal mammary vessels distal to the site of ligation during coronary bypass will generally allow adequate perfusion through the superior epigastric artery and vein for superior transposition to the mediastinum *(Figs 24.31, 24.32)*.

The omentum is an alternative source of tissue available to be transferred for mediastinal reconstruction; it

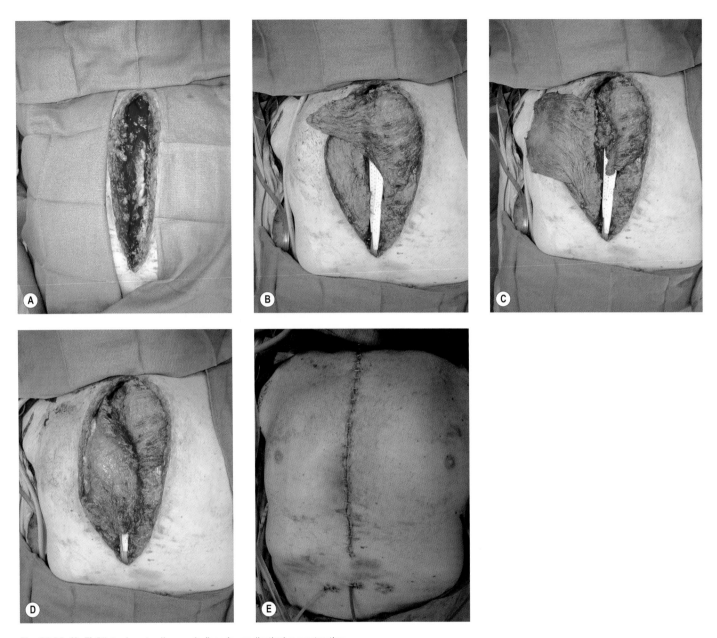

Fig. 24.32 (A–E) Bilateral pectoralis muscle flaps for mediastinal reconstruction.

may be used solely or in combination with another flap.[203] The omentum can be based on the right or left gastroepiploic vessels. In view of the risk of exposing the peritoneum to a contaminated field, however, the omentum is generally reserved for patients in whom the pectoralis major and rectus abdominis muscles are unavailable.[204] The harvest of the omentum has been achieved laparoscopically to lower the potential abdominal wall morbidity.[205]

The latissimus dorsi provides another alternative muscle or musculocutaneous flap for coverage of the upper mediastinum.[206] Its use is usually indicated when the pectoralis major is absent or damaged by previous incisions or radiation therapy.[207] The advantage of using the latissimus dorsi muscle or musculocutaneous flap is that the vascular pedicle and the donor site are distant to the infected area.[208] The disadvantages include the inconvenience of obtaining a muscle flap from the back and that the latissimus dorsi muscle may be too thin for the deeper, more extensive mediastinal defects. The latissimus dorsi can also be transferred microsurgically to sternal wound defects.[209]

Chest wall and pulmonary cavity

Regional flaps:

1. Pectoralis major
2. Latissimus dorsi
3. Serratus anterior.

   Distant flaps:

1. Rectus abdominis
2. Omentum.

   Microvascular free tissue transfer:

1. Latissimus dorsi
2. Rectus abdominis.

Reconstruction of the chest wall is challenging. Ablative surgery for neoplasm, infection, radiation, and trauma can produce extensive full-thickness chest wall defects. Furthermore, many of the patients in need of reconstruction have previously undergone some form of chemotherapy or high dose irradiation for their primary disease. Wound healing can therefore be severely compromised at the time of reconstruction.

Historically, methods of chest wall reconstruction consisted of various random and tube flaps that often required several stages before completion. Currently, the reconstruction of the chest wall is successfully accomplished without the need for delay or staged procedures. Partial thickness defects with viable muscle at the wound bed can be managed with skin grafting; larger full-thickness defects require flap reconstruction. In addition to flap reconstruction, Prolene mesh is indicated for chest wall reconstruction to provide stability and support for the overlying flap when there is significant loss of chest wall continuity.[210,211]

The pectoralis major and latissimus dorsi muscle and musculocutaneous flaps are the most commonly used in chest wall reconstruction. Larson and McMurtrey stated that the pectoralis major musculocutaneous flap is the flap of choice for defects of the lower neck and upper third of the sternum, whereas the latissimus dorsi musculocutaneous flap is preferred for wounds of the anterior chest wall that will require removal of two or

three ribs and resection of <8 cm of skin. In these authors' series of 53 flaps in 50 patients, the musculocutaneous flap alone provided adequate support and stability. Fascia, ribs, and prosthetic mesh were not needed for support.[212]

The use of the latissimus dorsi flap in a patient who has previously undergone a thoracotomy decreases the reliability of the pedicle and safety of subsequent ipsilateral flap transposition although previous thoracotomy is not an absolute contraindication. In fact, Scheflan et al. reported that a standard anterolateral thoracotomy, which separates the latissimus dorsi into an upper third and lower two-thirds, does not preclude the subsequent use of the muscle as a flap.[213] More recently, the latissimus dorsi muscle has been used successfully in patients who had undergone previous posterolateral thoracotomy.[214] The upper third of the latissimus dorsi muscle, based on the thoracodorsal pedicle, may be used to cover superior anterolateral chest wall defects. The lower two-thirds of the muscle, based on its secondary pedicles from the paraspinal perforators, can be used as a reverse latissimus dorsi flap with or without the overlying skin to cover inferolateral and posterior chest wall defects. Early work by McCraw et al. and Bostwick et al. were instrumental in the development of the reverse latissimus dorsi flap.[215,109] Latissimus dorsi muscle and musculocutaneous flaps have proved invaluable in the treatment of numerous chest wall and pulmonary cavity disorders including Poland syndrome,[216,217] spina bifida defects,[218,219] and diaphragmatic hernias.[220,221]

The serratus anterior muscle can also be useful as a local muscle flap for chest wall and pulmonary cavity reconstruction. The serratus muscle has a constant and reliable vascular pedicle and a long arc of rotation.[222] Arnold et al. described its use in reconstructing the chest wall, closing bronchopleural fistulas, and reinforcing tracheal reconstructions.[223] The serratus may be surgically split thereby utilizing only a portion for reconstruction.[80]

The rectus abdominis muscle is a distant muscle or musculocutaneous flap for chest wall reconstruction. Larson et al. showed that the rectus abdominis musculocutaneous flap is particularly useful for large chest wall defects.[212] The availability of the flap is dependent on the status of the internal mammary arteries. Miyamoto et al. favored the rectus abdominis musculocutaneous flap over the latissimus dorsi in chest wall reconstruction because of its convenience (the patient can remain in one position intraoperatively), ease of elevation and subsequent closure of the donor site.[224] In addition, it is thought that in situations when up to three ribs are removed and reconstructed with mesh, the rectus shows a distinct advantage given its thickness which minimizes the risk of creating a flail chest wall.[225] Large defects of the chest wall within the arc of rotation of the rectus can be reconstructed. The rectus abdominis muscle may be used as a transverse or vertically oriented musculocutaneous flap.[226]

If the internal mammary vessels have been manipulated the rectus flap is often transferred microsurgically.[227]

The omentum is also utilized for chest wall reconstruction. The omentum can be harvested laparoscopically, obviating the need for a large abdominal incision. When used as a transpositional flap, the omentum can be based on either the right or left gastroepiploic vessels. The omentum has a large surface area, obliterates dead space, is pliable, and contains angiogenic and immunogenic properties. The use of the omentum in chest wall reconstruction secondary to osteoradionecrosis, cancer ablation, and chronic wounds is well established.[63]

Abdominal wall

Regional flaps:

1. Rectus abdominis
2. External oblique.

Distant flaps:

1. Tensor fascia lata
2. Latissimus dorsi
3. Rectus femoris.

Microvascular free flap:

1. Tensor fascia lata
2. Latissimus dorsi
3. Rectus femoris
4. Anterolateral thigh
5. Groin.

In reconstructing abdominal wall defects, the surgical objective is to provide soft tissue coverage in addition to reestablishing the abdominal wall integrity. To plan

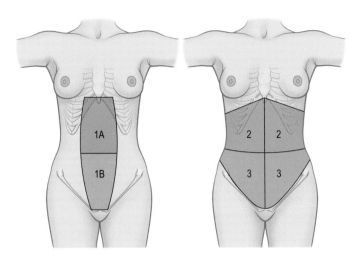

Fig. 24.33 Reconstructive zones of the abdomen.

Table 24.13 **Flaps for abdominal reconstruction by location (zone)**

Flaps	Zones			
	1A	1B	2	3
Latissimus dorsi			X	
Rectus abdominis				
Superiorly based	X		X	
Inferiorly based		X		X
Advancement	X	X		
External oblique advancement				X
Tensor fascia lata				
Transposition		X		X
Expansion	X	X	X	X
Rectus femoris		X		X

Modified from Mathes SJ, Steinwald PM, Foster RD, *et al.* Complex abdominal wall reconstruction: a comparison of flap and mesh closure. Ann Surg 2000; 232:586–596.

safe and reliable techniques for wound closure, it is helpful to classify complex wounds by location and the status of the overlying skin and soft tissue coverage. In regard to location, the abdominal wall is divided into four zones: zone 1A, upper midline defects with extension across the midline; zone 1B, lower midline defects with extension across the midline; zone 2, upper quadrant defects; and zone 3, lower quadrant defects (*Fig. 24.33, Table 24.13*).

The two muscles available for local flaps are the rectus abdominis and the external oblique. The rectus abdominis muscle or musculocutaneous flap is the flap of choice for unilateral abdominal wall defects. In 1977 Mathes and Bostwick described the use of the rectus abdominis musculocutaneous flap for reconstruction of an abdominal wall defect.[181] Parkash and Ramakrishnan reported the use of a rectus abdominis musculocutaneous island flap for coverage of an extensive radionecrotic abdominal wall ulcer that had been resistant to conservative therapy.[228] In 1983, Taylor *et al.* described the extended deep inferior epigastric flap, which consists of an inferiorly based rectus abdominis musculocutaneous flap with a superolateral fasciocutaneous extension. With this larger skin territory, extensive defects of the abdomen, as well as those of the groin and thigh, have been successfully treated.[125]

The rectus may be released from its lateral attachments to achieve midline abdominal wall closure. Several variations have been described. One variety, termed separation of components, involves separation of the external oblique fascia with an incision just lateral to the linea semilunaris allowing a plane to develop between the external and internal oblique muscles.[229] This permits medial mobility of the rectus abdominis muscle. Other variants of sliding myofascial partitions or releases have been used successfully to reconstruct the abdominal wall.[181,230] Alternatively, the rectus may be used as a turnover flap to achieve closure.[231]

The external oblique muscle may be used to reconstruct absent or deficient rectus fascia.[232] The external oblique musculocutaneous flap is alternative local flap, useful for reconstructing small, full-thickness upper abdominal wall defects.[233–235] The external oblique musculo-fascia may also be expanded and advanced centrally to repair abdominal wall defects.[236,237]

The distant muscle and musculocutaneous flaps used in abdominal wall reconstruction include the latissimus dorsi, tensor fascia lata, and rectus femoris flaps. Transposition of the latissimus dorsi musculocutaneous flap is a reliable technique that is particularly useful for superolateral abdominal wall defects.[238,239] This flap is particularly useful in traumatic defects, burn injuries and post-extirpative defects.[240–242] The latissimus dorsi can also be transferred microsurgically to cover central abdominal defects.[243] This flap may also be reinnervated and has shown enough contractile capacity and strength to adequately replace the function of the missing abdominal wall muscles.[244]

The use of the tensor fascia lata (TFL) as a musculocutaneous and musculofascial flap is indicated for lower abdominal wall reconstruction. Wangensteen initially described use of this flap for lower abdominal wall closure.[245] The unique qualities of the tensor fascia lata flap include the large amount of vascularized fascia and skin and the low donor site morbidity.[246–248] The TFL is most commonly used as a rotational flap, although success as a free flap has been demonstrated.[249] As a rotational flap, the arc of rotation is limited to the lower abdominal wall, whereas when used as a free flap, any region of the abdominal wall may be reconstructed.[250]

The rectus femoris musculocutaneous flap is a dependable alternative flap for abdominal wall reconstruction.[251,252] Variations of the rectus femoris flap, including the use of fascial extensions and tissue expansion, have been described to extend its arc of rotation.[253,254] However, it tends to be bulkier than the TFL and has greater donor site morbidity. Leg extension may be adversely affected with the use of this flap although subsequent studies show no appreciable effect.[255,253] In certain instances the rectus femoris is preferred to the TFL flap. An example would be the use of the rectus femoris to treat a radionecrotic ulcer involving the lower abdominal wall, given the need for muscle bulk to fill the defect *(Fig. 24.34).*[256]

Microvascular free tissue transfer to the abdomen, although uncommon, is a potential reconstructive option. This may be the best option for large defects and to avoid staged reconstruction. Common flaps microsurgically transferred to the abdomen include the latissimus dorsi, anterolateral thigh, groin flap, TFL flap, and rectus femoris.[257–261]

Groin and perineum

Regional flaps:

1. Sartorius.

    Distant flaps:

1. Gracilis
2. Tensor fascia lata
3. Rectus femoris
4. Rectus abdominis
5. Gluteus maximus
6. Anterolateral thigh.

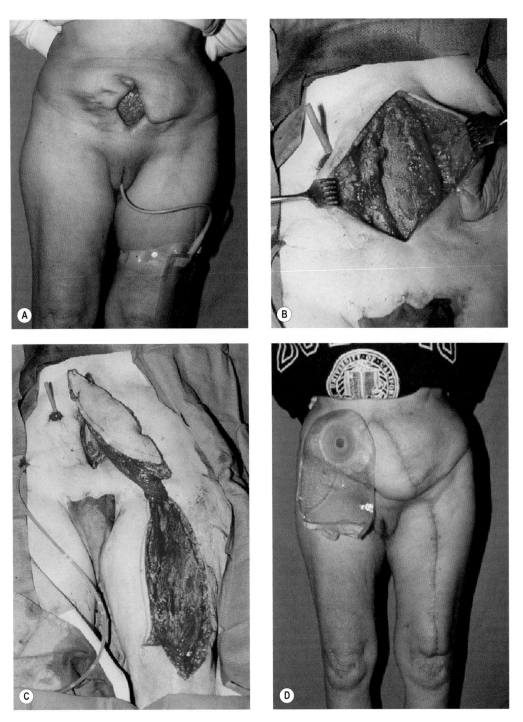

Fig. 24.34 (A–D) Rectus femoris musculocutaneous flap with intraperitoneal mesh for management of a chronic type II, zone 1B defect.

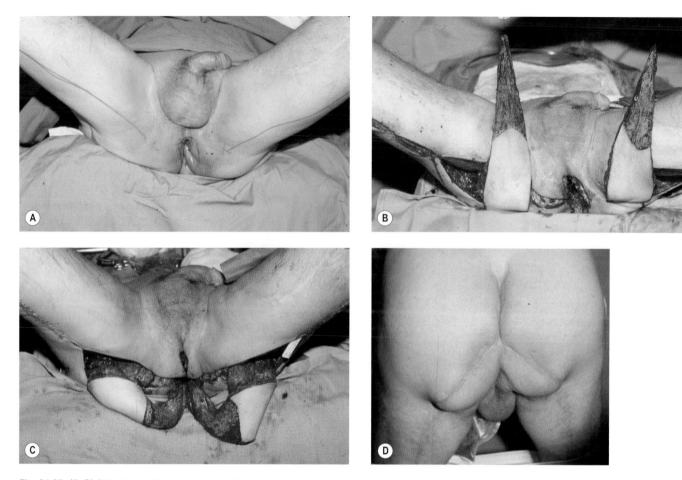

Fig. 24.35 (A–D) Bilateral gracilis and gluteal thigh flaps for reconstruction of a radiation defect of the perineum.

Reconstruction of the groin and perineum is often indicated for defects due to trauma, tumor resection and infection. The wounds can be extensive and because of their proximity to the anus and urethra, are susceptible to fecal and urinary contamination. In addition, wounds involving the groin may expose the femoral vessels. Vascular prosthetic grafts and adjunctive radiation therapy in the cancer patient can further compound the problem.

The sartorius is a type IV muscle with multiple segmental vascular pedicles that limit its arc of rotation. The division of one or two of the most proximal pedicles, however, enables the superior aspect of the sartorius muscle to be transposed medially into the groin. This technique is used for coverage of exposed femoral vessels and prosthetic vascular grafts.[262]

The gracilis is a type II muscle that has both an anterior and posterior arc of rotation. Anteriorly, the muscle can be used for groin and perineal reconstruction; posteriorly, ischial and perirectal defects can be reconstructed.[263–265] Other common uses of the gracilis muscle and musculocutaneous flap include reconstruction of the vagina, penis, scrotum, and anal sphincter **(Fig. 24.35)**.[256,266–268]

The tensor fascia lata (TFL) is particularly useful for groin and perineal reconstruction.[269,270] It can be used as either a musculocutaneous flap or a musculofascial flap. The TFL is also used in vulvar reconstruction and recurrent inguinal hernia reconstruction.[246]

The rectus femoris is useful for coverage of the groin and perineum.[271,272] It is a large, bulky muscle that has an arc of rotation similar to that of the tensor fascia lata. Despite its reliability and desirable muscle bulk, this muscle is generally used as an alternate flap in the ambulatory patient, given the potential functional deficit associated with its harvest, although more recent evidence suggests that the results of the reconstruction appear to outweigh the loss of strength.[246,273]

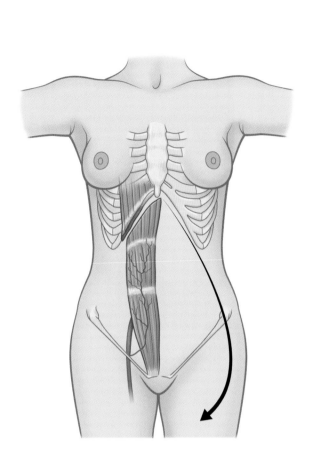
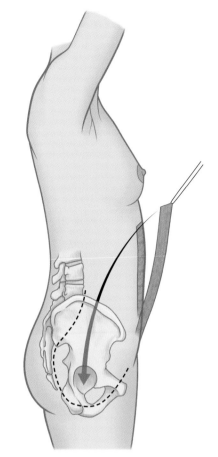

Fig. 24.36 Rectus abdominis flap. **(A)** Arc to perineum. **(B)** Arc to internal pelvis.

The rectus abdominis muscle or musculocutaneous flap based on its inferior pedicle provides a reliable flap for defects of the anterior pelvis and groin.[181,256,274] Its wide arc of rotation and abundant blood supply through the inferior epigastric vessels make it an excellent reconstructive flap for this region. The vertical rectus abdominis musculocutaneous flap is useful for large, irradiated defects in the perineum *(Figs 24.36, 24.37)*.[129,275,276]

The gluteus maximus muscle provides stable coverage for pelvic and perineal defects. Its large mass is particularly useful for obliterating pelvic dead space and covering perineal wounds; it is also useful for rectal sphincter reconstruction.[277,278] The gluteus maximus fasciocutaneous V–Y advancement flap is reliable for extensive vulvectomy and recurrent rectal cancer defects *(Fig. 24.35)*.[279,280] The gluteal thigh flap, described by Hurwitz, includes the inferior part of the gluteus maximus muscle and a large cutaneous territory of the posterior thigh that is supplied by the descending branch of the inferior gluteal artery.[98] The gluteus maximus musculocutaneous and gluteal fasciocutaneous flap is particularly useful for reconstructing deep perineal and pelvic defects.[99,281]

More recently, the anterolateral thigh flap has become a popular alternative for reconstruction of groin and perineal defects. It has the versatility of a long vascular pedicle as well as the options of including skin only, skin and fascia, or skin fascia and muscle, depending on the reconstructive requirements. By passing the pedicle under the rectus femoris muscle, the arc of rotation of the descending branch of the lateral circumflex femoral artery is greatly increased such that the flap can easily reach the perineum.[282]

Lower extremity

Regional flaps:

1. Gastrocnemius
2. Soleus.

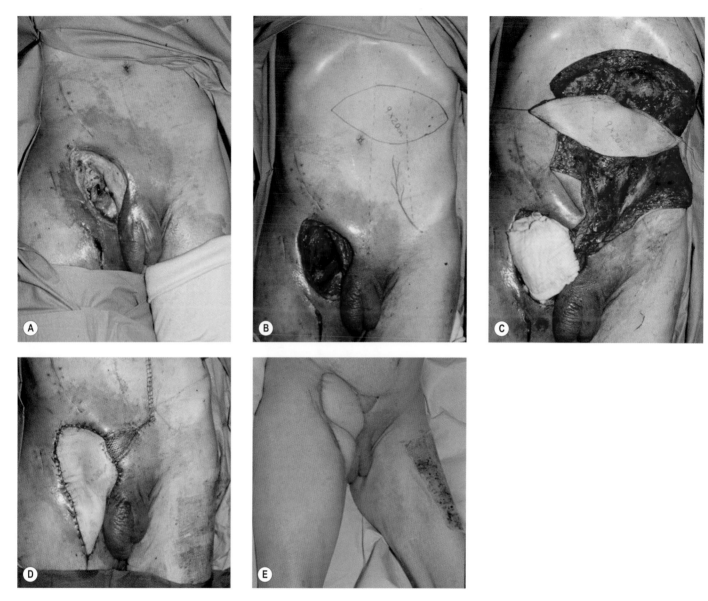

Fig. 24.37 (A–E) Rectus abdominis musculocutaneous flap for groin coverage.

Distant flaps:

1. Cross-leg.

   Microvascular free flap:

1. Latissimus dorsi
2. Rectus abdominis
3. Gracilis
4. Fibula
5. Perforator flaps.

Reconstruction of the lower extremity remains particularly challenging. Defects including exposed joints

and prostheses, infected bone, and fractures are common. Furthermore, the availability of adequate soft tissue for coverage is limited, particularly in the lower third of the leg.

There are two local sources of muscle or musculocutaneous flaps available for reconstruction of the leg, the gastrocnemius and the soleus muscles. The use of distant flaps involves microvascular transplantation of various muscles or perforator flaps depending on the size of the wound and surgeon's preference. Many muscles have been described, including the gracilis, latissimus dorsi, and rectus abdominis. In an effort to minimize donor

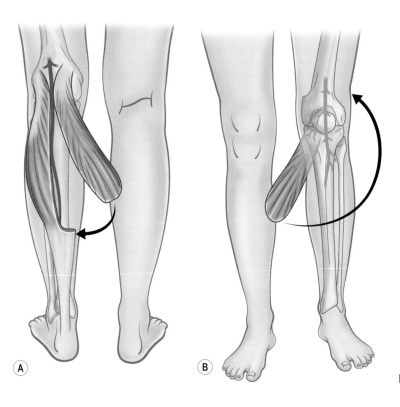

Fig. 24.38 Gastrocnemius flap. Arc to knee and upper third of leg.

site, the anterolateral thigh flap, deep inferior epigastric perforator flap and the superficial inferior epigastric artery perforator flaps may be used as well. Cross-leg flaps are also available but have largely been supplanted by either local muscle flaps or microvascular composite tissue transplantation.

The gastrocnemius is a type I muscle, consisting of a medial and a lateral head. Each head has a wide arc of rotation based on its single vascular pedicle (medial or lateral sural vessels). The gastrocnemius muscle or musculocutaneous flap is the flap of choice for coverage of the knee and for coverage of exposed bone or orthopedic hardware involving the upper two-thirds of the leg.[283,284] Defects of the middle third of the leg can also be reconstructed with the gastrocnemius muscle.[285–287] In patients with radical knee debridement and loss or disruption of the extensor mechanism, the gastrocnemius can be used to restore knee function *(Figs 24.38, 24.39)*.[288]

The soleus muscle flap is utilized for reconstructing defects involving the middle third of the leg. The soleus muscle is the prime ankle plantar flexor and it serves to stabilize the ankle in ambulation by opposing dorsiflexion.[289] Because of compensatory mechanisms, the use of the soleus muscle as a flap does not impair function. Function-preserving techniques such as muscle splitting is recommended if the soleus is used in a patient who does not have a functional medial and lateral gastrocnemius muscle.[290,291] Defects of the proximal third can be reached by the soleus, but requires extensive mobilization of the muscle.[292] In the lower third of the leg, the soleus muscle can be used as a proximally or distally based flap. In this region, however, the soleus muscle flap is generally used for smaller defects *(Fig. 24.40)*. Larger defects require microvascular tissue transplantation.

Microvascular tissue transplantation has made a significant impact on lower extremity reconstruction. Muscles such as the latissimus dorsi, rectus abdominis and gracilis have been used successfully to reconstruct extensive post-extirpative and traumatic defects.[293–295] Other useful flaps include, the fibula flap, based on the peroneal vessels to reconstruct large tibial defects, perforator flaps and the omentum which provides a

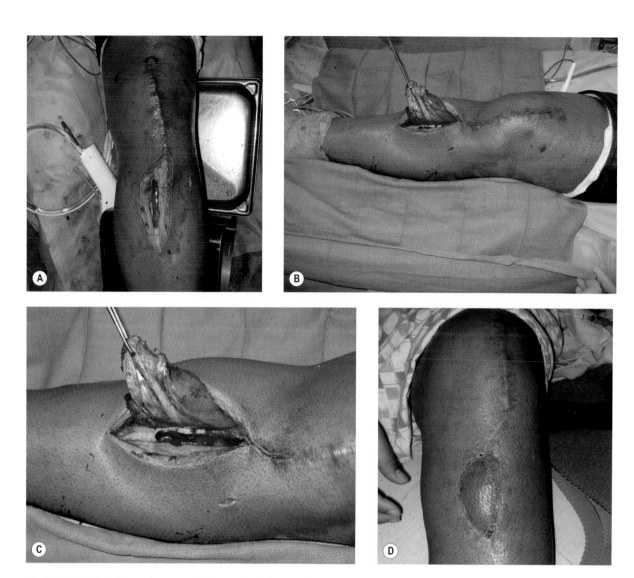

Fig. 24.39 (A–D) Gastrocnemius musculocutaneous flap for knee and proximal third of tibia defect.

large area of well-vascularized and malleable tissue.[296,297] Advances in lower extremity microsurgery now offer better functional and sensate reconstructions.[86]

In certain individuals, microvascular tissue transplantation is not possible. For those patients, alternate methods of reconstruction include the use of fasciocutaneous, random-pattern and cross-leg flaps. Various local fasciocutaneous flaps have also been identified and are of clinical utility. In 1981, Ponten described several fasciocutaneous flaps that are useful in the repair of soft tissue defects on the lower leg.[22] Examples include the anterior tibial artery flap, peroneal artery flap, sural flap (proximally or distally-based), posterior tibial artery flap, and saphenous flap.[298,299] The

distally based sural flap has proven useful in coverage of defects at the lower leg and foot in both adults and children.[300,301]

Foot

Regional flaps:

1. Flexor digitorum brevis

2. Abductor hallucis

3. Abductor digiti minimi.

   Distant flaps:

1. Cross-foot flaps.

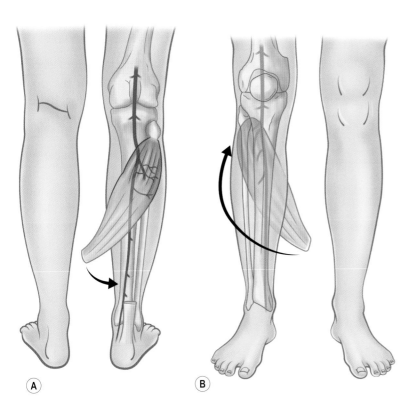

Fig. 24.40 Soleus flap. **(A,B)** Arc to middle third of leg.

Microvascular free flap:

1. Gracilis

2. Latissimus

3. Rectus abdominis

4. Serratus.

Defects of the foot are most often due to trauma or the long-standing effects of underlying systemic disorders such as diabetes mellitus and peripheral vascular disease. These wounds can be extremely difficult to treat and often are best left uncovered until the underlying disease is treated (e.g., by revascularization). For some patients with severe, irreversible underlying systemic disease, local conservative wound care may be the only appropriate form of therapy.

When reconstruction is necessary, several issues must be addressed, such as the size of the defect and the patient's vascular, neurosensory, and weight bearing status. For small defects, skin grafts are often the procedure of choice provided that there is adequate protective soft tissue within the bed of the defect. For small defects involving weight-bearing areas, axial innervated skin flaps and fasciocutaneous flaps have

been successful in providing stable coverage.[299,93] For the deeper, more extensive foot defect, the use of a muscle or musculocutaneous flap is usually necessary. The local muscles available for use as flaps include the flexor digitorum brevis, the abductor hallucis, and the abductor digiti minimi. These muscles are small and are inadequate for larger defects. The use of a distant muscle (e.g., cross-foot flap) or microvascular free tissue transfer is usually necessary for coverage of any major wound (those with excessive size and depth or with component loss).

Mathes *et al.* demonstrated the anatomy of the flexor digitorum brevis for use as a flap in 1974.[14] It is a type II muscle that measures approximately 10 × 4 cm. This muscle was then shown to be clinically useful to cover a calcaneal defect in 1974 by Vasconez *et al.*[18] In 1980, Hartrampf *et al.* described a modification of this technique, using the muscle as an island flap that increased the arc of rotation. As an island flap based on the lateral plantar artery, the flexor digitorum brevis muscle reaches the malleolus and can cover the entire posterosuperior aspect of the heel pad.[302] The authors recommended that the patency of both the dorsalis pedis and the tibialis posterior artery should be confirmed before

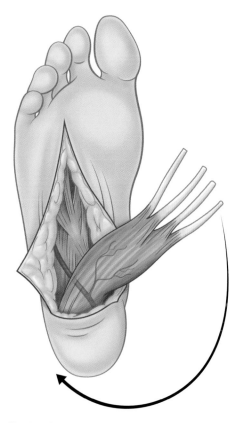

Fig. 24.41 Flexor digitorum brevis flap. Arc to heel.

the lateral plantar artery is divided. In patients who have occlusion of either the dorsalis pedis or the tibialis posterior artery, the lateral plantar artery serves as a vital conduit of collateral flow and should not be divided for flap use. The flexor digitorum brevis, when transposed as a muscle flap, may provide stable coverage and is of benefit in both diabetic and nondiabetic patients *(Fig. 24.41)*.[303,304]

The retrograde lateral plantar artery flap was described by Reiffel and McCarthy in 1980.[305] The flap is fashioned by dividing the lateral plantar vessels proximally; the plantar fascia and the flexor digitorum brevis muscle can be elevated as a flap based on distal retrograde flow. This flap is particularly useful for coverage of medial and lateral metatarsal head defects.[306]

The abductor hallucis is a type II muscle with branches of the medial plantar artery as its dominant vascular supply.[14] Based on this vascular pedicle the abductor hallucis can be elevated as a muscle or musculocutaneous flap, and it can reach defects just inferior

to the medial malleolus as well as defects of the proximal medial aspect of the dorsum of the foot. Like the lateral plantar artery, the medial plantar artery should not be divided if either the dorsalis pedis or the posterior tibial artery is occluded. The abductor hallucis muscle flap may be distally based to reconstruct forefoot defects.[307]

The abductor digiti minimi is a type II muscle with branches of the lateral plantar artery as its dominant vascular pedicle.[14] This small muscle based on its dominant pedicle can reach defects adjacent to the lateral malleolus. However, because of its size, the flap is limited in its ability to provide coverage of larger defects. In 1985, Yoshimura *et al.* reported the use of a distally based abductor digiti minimi muscle flap.[308] This muscle flap based distally on the communication between the lateral plantar artery and the plantar arch can be used to cover small defects of the distal half of the foot. The abductor digiti minimi may be harvested with the lateral calcaneal artery sensate skin flap to cover plantar heel wounds.[309]

For extensive foot defects, microvascular tissue transfer is the procedure of choice given the lack of local tissues. The gracilis, latissimus dorsi, rectus abdominis, and serratus muscle flaps have proven effective.[310–312] In addition to muscle flaps, fasciocutaneous flaps such as the anterolateral thigh flap and radial forearm flap have been used successfully.[145,313,314] Alternative methods include the use of cross-leg and cross-foot flaps *(Fig. 24.42)*.[315,316]

Pressure wounds

Regional flaps:
1. Gluteus maximus
2. SGAP flap.
   Distant flaps:
1. Tensor fascia lata
2. Gracilis
3. Hamstrings
4. Omentum.

The *gluteus maximus* is a regional flap commonly used for the surgical treatment of pressure sores. It is a type III muscle and it is the flap of choice for reconstructing deep sacral and ischial pressure sores.

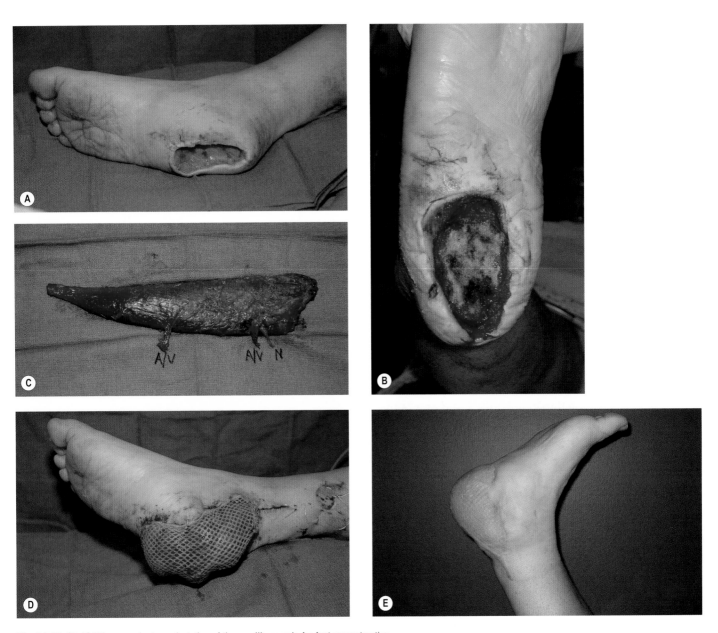

Fig. 24.42 (A–E) Microvascular transplantation of the gracilis muscle for foot reconstruction.

Function-preserving techniques such as bilateral advancement flaps using only the superior halves of the gluteus maximus for sacral coverage are recommended for the ambulatory patient.[123,317,318] Variations in technique, including the sliding gluteus maximus flap, the transposition gluteus maximus flap, and island flaps based on musculocutaneous perforating vessels (muscle preserving) have been described.[318–321] The sliding flap is indicated for small sacral defects, whereas the transposition flap (unilateral or bilateral) is generally

appropriate for larger defects because it has a greater range of coverage. For extensive pressure sores, the gluteal thigh flap has also been useful.[98,99,322,323]

More recently, the superior gluteal artery perforator flap has been used for the treatment of sacral pressure ulcers.[324] It affords the same skin as the gluteus maximus myocutaneous flap with the advantage that the muscle is completely spared and the pedicle length significantly increased. This is a particularly attractive alternative in the ambulatory patient.

Three distant muscles used in the reconstruction of pressure sores are the tensor fascia lata, gracilis, and the hamstrings. The tensor fascia lata (TFL) is a type I muscle that is useful for reconstructing trochanteric pressure sores.[247,320,325] It is also a reliable alternative flap for ischial defects because of the following advantages: there is relatively low donor site morbidity, especially in an ambulatory patient; the flap provides vascularized, durable fascia; and the flap can provide sensibility in certain instances.

Several investigators have described the use of the innervated TFL flap, based on the lateral femoral cutaneous nerve (L2–L3), for reconstruction of ischial defects. They have reported successful restoration of protective sensibility without recurrence of pressure ulceration in paraplegic patients with lesions below the L3 level.[246,326,327]

The major disadvantage of the TFL flap is its relative thinness, a problem for the deeper pressure sore. In 1981, Scheflan described a technique to increase the bulk of the TFL flap. By de-epithelializing the distal aspect of the flap and folding the inferior portion of the flap underneath, part of the flap gains bulk. Used as a "sandwich," the modified flap can usually fill the deeper defect.[328] Modifications in the design of the TFL flap have been described in an attempt to minimize the donor site morbidity. Problems such as dog-ears, excessive tension at wound closure, skin necrosis at certain wound margins, and the need for skin grafts have prompted techniques such as the use of a bilobed TFL flap[329] and the V–Y retroposition TFL flap.[330,331] These modifications appear to facilitate donor closure in certain instances.

The *gracilis* is a type II muscle, first described in 1972 by Orticochea for use as a musculocutaneous flap.[12] In the treatment of pressure sores, the gracilis is used primarily to repair the ischial defect.[332,333] Use of the gracilis does not preclude the future use of the gluteus maximus or the posterior thigh flap if the ulcer recurs. The muscle can be elevated with the patient prone, but the distal muscle should be located before the skin island is incised, in order to ensure the correct localization of the skin overlying the muscle *(Figs 24.43, 24.44)*.

The gluteus maximus muscle (type III) is well situated for coverage of both sacral and ischial pressure sores. There are a number of modifications for its design and use for both ischial and sacral pressure sores. In general, it is preferable to use segmental transposition,

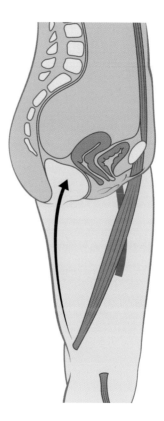

Fig. 24.43 Gracilis flap. Arc of rotation to the perineum.

reserving the superior half of the muscle based on the superior gluteal artery and associated venae comitantes for the sacral sore and the inferior half based on the inferior gluteal artery and associated venae comitantes for the ischial sore.

For the sacral sore, the cutaneous territory of the superior half of the muscle may be used as a V–Y advancement flap, or the skin island may be designed distally (near the muscle insertion) for use as a transposition flap or proximally (near the muscle origin) in V–Y advancement flap. For V–Y advancement flap, the superior half of the muscle's origin and insertion is divided so the composite of muscle plus the overlying soft tissue will cover the debridement site of the sacral decubitus. Although perforating vessels will allow bilateral V–Y advancement of the skin island with release of the muscle, adequate well-vascularized soft tissue and muscle are required to provide a long-lasting stable coverage over the sacrum *(Figs 24.45, 24.46)*. When it is used as a transposition flap, the skin island and

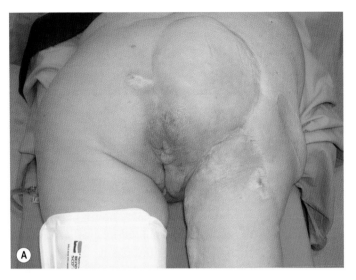

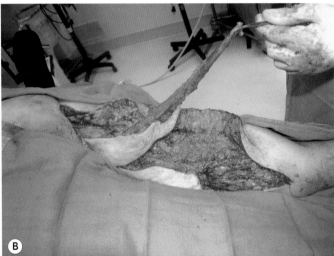

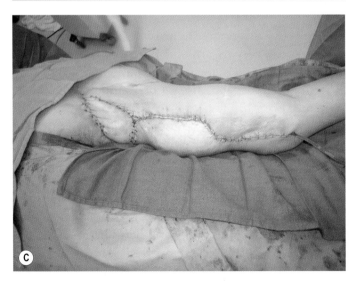

Fig. 24.44 (A–C) Gracilis musculocutaneous flap for ischial pressure sore coverage.

underlying muscle are transferred 180° to provide sacral coverage. It is not necessary to divide the superior muscle origin, although partial to complete release of the origin allows easier flap inset over the sacrum. As already mentioned, the SGAP flap has emerged as a useful alternative to the musculocutaneous flap.

The inferior half of the gluteus maximus is ideal for ischial sore coverage. The skin island is designed near the muscle insertion. After splitting of the muscle, the muscle and overlying skin island are easily rotated 90° to the ischial defect. The condensed bulk of the muscle and its specific cutaneous territory provide stable coverage at the ischial site of reconstruction **(Fig. 24.47**; see also **Fig. 24.7**).

The *hamstrings*, consisting of the biceps femoris, semi-membranous and semitendinosus, are a group of muscles of the posterior thigh. These muscles originate from the ischial tuberosity, although the biceps femoris also has a short head originating from the linea aspera of the femur. As a group, these muscles are useful in the reconstruction of ischial pressure sores. Used as a transposition flap, depending on the size of the defect, one or more of the hamstring muscles can provide ischial coverage. Hurteau *et al.* described V–Y advancement of the hamstring musculocutaneous flap for reliable coverage of the ischial pressure sore.[334] A triangular island of skin overlying the hamstring muscles is designed with the base of the triangle at the inferior margin of the ischial defect. The hamstring muscles are divided distal to the skin island, and the entire muscle group is mobilized superiorly. The origins of the hamstring muscles are detached from the ischium, thus enabling further advancement, and the flap is sutured into place. Long-term results reveal stable coverage of ischial pressure sores.[335]

Preoperative and postoperative management

Preoperative management is critical to the success of a reconstruction. Education of the patient is of particular importance. Expectations of operative outcome may differ considerably between the surgeon and patient. For example, the patient may not realize the size of the donor scar or that a skin graft will be taken. By thoroughly discussing the procedure with the patient preoperatively, the surgeon can avoid these misunderstandings.

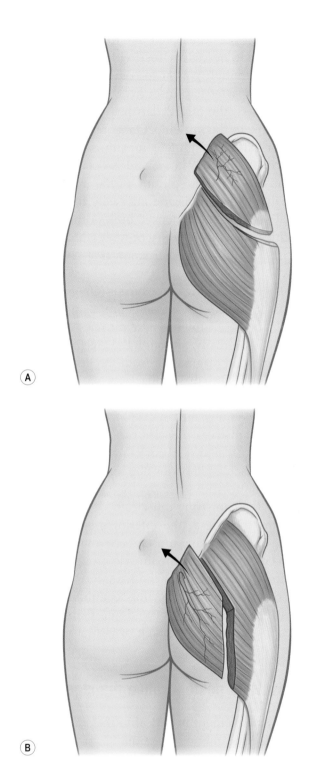

Fig. 24.45 Gluteus maximus-gluteal thigh flap. **(A)** V–Y segmental muscle advancement (superior half of gluteus maximus muscle). Flap advancement for sacral coverage. **(B)** V–Y segmental muscle advancement (inferior half of gluteus maximus muscle). Flap advancement for sacral coverage.

A complete physical exam provides valuable information. Evidence of previous incisions, muscle atrophy, co-morbid conditions, vascular supply and wound analysis may assist the surgeon in selecting the most appropriate reconstruction. Additional diagnostic measures (e.g., selective arteriography to delineate the vascular anatomy) may be indicated, depending on the physical findings.

Wound analysis includes assessment of the defect in terms of location, size and physical components. When the defect involves a significant percentage of the body surface area (e.g., burns or giant hairy nevus), the reconstructive options may be limited to skin grafts for acute coverage (e.g., burns) or sequential tissue expansion for elective reconstruction (e.g., giant hairy nevus). The components of a given defect may include one or all of the following: skin, nerves, mucosa, fascia, subcutaneous tissue, cartilage, muscle, bone, and vessels.

Each component affects function and form at the defect site. Selection of a reconstructive option is based on the feasibility and relative importance of replacing each component of the defect.

Wound analysis must also include the vascular status and bacteriology of exposed structures. Prior surgical procedures, trauma, infection, radiation therapy, or a combination of these factors may have caused vascular injury and decreased circulation in all structures within the potential zone of injury. Assessment of the vascular status may be accomplished by noninvasive means such as Doppler ultrasonography and magnetic resonance angiography, or by invasive studies, such as arteriography. Selective arteriography may be helpful to evaluate the transverse cervical artery in the patient with a history of radical neck dissection or in the patient with a history of peripheral vascular disease or trauma to the lower extremity prior to the harvest of a fibular flap.

A careful assessment should be made of the extent of debridement required to remove nonviable structures subject to bacterial invasion and impaired vascularity. Inability to accurately predict the amount of debridement required may necessitate sequential wound debridement with subsequent wound observation and bacterial culture of the wound. When regional vascular insufficiency involving the wound site is observed, preliminary or simultaneous vascular procedures may be required in conjunction with wound debridement and coverage.

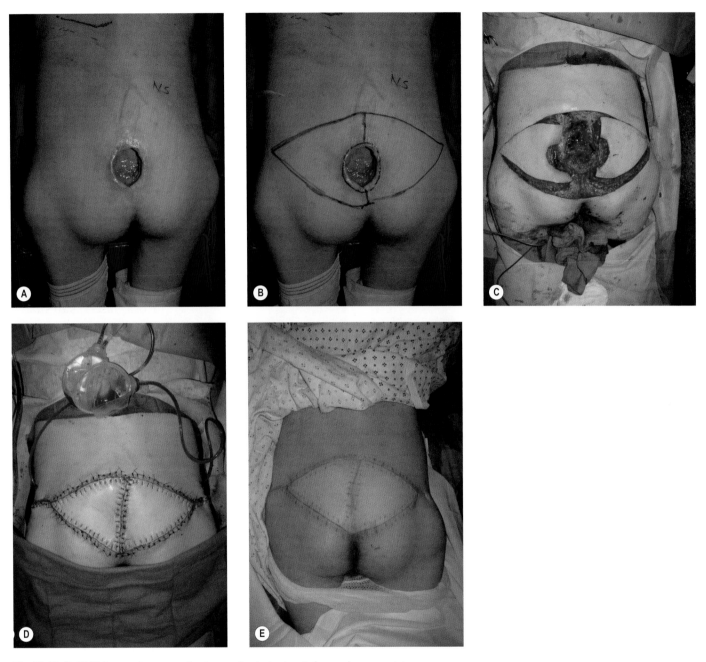

Fig. 24.46 (A–E) Gluteus maximus musculocutaneous flap for treatment of a sacral pressure sore.

The design of the flap is of paramount importance. The final design of a flap intended for standard transposition, staged expansion, or microvascular transplantation should be based on the actual defect size. The original design of the flap has an impact on future procedures if the defect should recur or require further revisions. In general, flap design is delayed until adequate wound debridement or tumor resection is accomplished. If simultaneous flap elevation and resection are performed, the flap design should allow for the maximal defect size. If tissue expansion is used, the expander advancement or transposition flap should be elevated and advanced to the potential defect site before the resection is performed. Repeat expansion will be necessary if adequate tissue is not available to cover the defect created at the resection site.

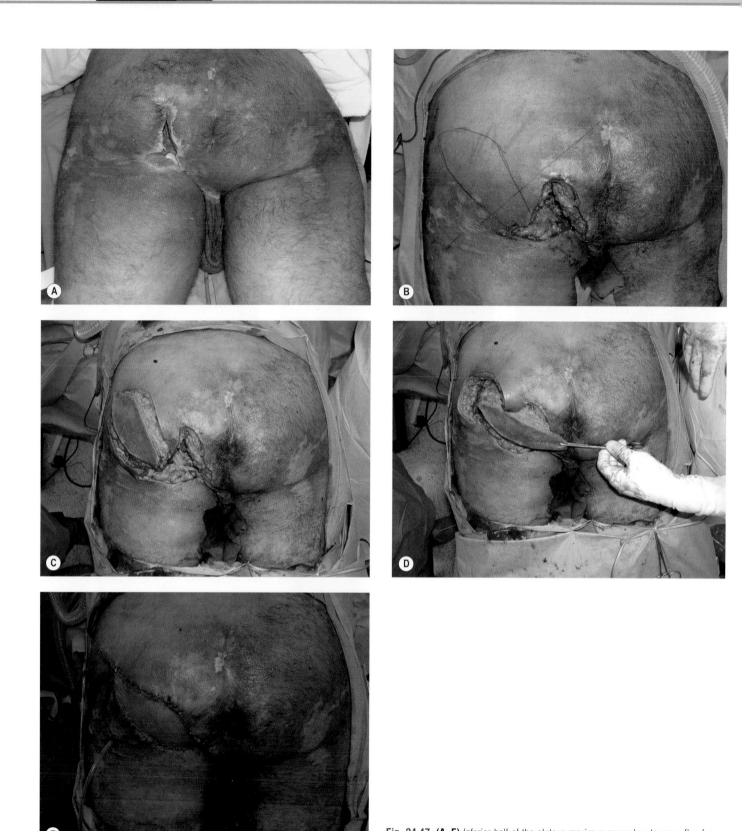

Fig. 24.47 (A–E) Inferior half of the gluteus maximus musculocutaneous flap for ischial coverage.

Prior incisions or trauma may either damage the vascular pedicle or disrupt vascular connections between the muscle or fascia and overlying skin. Selective arteriography is recommended to determine the patency of the planned flap pedicle. Prior elevation of a random cutaneous flap represents a relative contraindication to design of this skin as a musculocutaneous or fasciocutaneous flap. Experimental data have demonstrated successful elevation of a musculocutaneous flap after an interval of 3 weeks following separation of the skin territory from the underlying muscle. Although clinical use of a previously elevated rotation flap as an island musculocutaneous flap after an interval of 6 months has been reported, alternative flaps are preferred when possible. Other considerations include whether the patient has had suction lipectomy in the area of flap harvest and the reliability of the local venous drainage.

Identifying high-risk patients is important. Systemic factors such as tobacco use, obesity, cardiovascular disease (i.e., hypertension, peripheral vascular disease), immunosuppression, and pulmonary disease must be taken into account. These critical factors will influence patient and flap selection as well as the success and durability of the final result.

Tobacco use decreases skin circulation and is associated with an increased risk of flap failure. Cessation of smoking for 6–8 weeks prior to flap transportation is recommended. In patients who require an emergency flap procedure or who refuse to stop smoking, flap design should not include a skin segment extending beyond the primary territory of the muscle or fascial flap.

Obesity may result in decreased reliability of the cutaneous territory of muscle of muscle or fascia. Furthermore, the thick flap has a reduced arc of rotation. A wide skin island is recommended in the obese patient to ensure incorporation of perforating vessels between muscle or fascia and overlying skin.

In certain circumstances, flap selection may depend on the reliability of the flap. Muscles with a single vascular pedicle (type I), two dominant pedicles from different vascular sources (type III), or a dominant vascular pedicle with a secondary segmental pedicle (type V) represent the most reliable patterns of muscle flap circulation for a muscle or musculocutaneous flap. Muscles with a dominant and single or multiple minor pedicles (type II) or segmental pedicles (type IV) are less reliable because the vascular pedicles to the distal part of the muscle must be divided to achieve an adequate arc of rotation. Similarly, fasciocutaneous flaps with direct cutaneous (type A) or septocutaneous pedicles (type B) represent the most reliable pattern of circulation. The fasciocutaneous flap based on pedicles through muscle (type C) usually has several pedicles at the flap base that may be less reliable.

Design of a skin island on a broad flap base is preferable to a skin island located on a narrow flap base. Furthermore, design of the skin island at the mid-portion of the flap closer to the site of entrance of the dominant vascular pedicle is preferable to design of a skin island at the most distal aspect of the flap.

Positioning of the patient

When possible, the patient is positioned to allow visualization of both the donor and recipient sites. If this is not possible, initial positioning should provide optimal visualization of the recipient site if a major resection is required.

Careful padding of the potential pressure sites is necessary to avoid injury to normal structures. Areas subject to pressure include the scalp, elbow, breast, hip, sacrum, and feet. Use of axillary and chest padding is recommended when the patient is placed in the lateral decubitus or prone positions. A beanbag is also helpful in maintaining appropriate patient positioning without excessive pressure at sites of bony prominences. During long procedures involving microvascular composite tissue transplantation, pressure sites should be checked for proper padding midway through the procedure. Excessive abduction of the upper extremity should be avoided to prevent brachial plexus stretch injury.

Postoperative flap management is of equal importance to the success of a reconstruction. The maintenance of proper positioning, temporary immobilization, and proper dressing of the wound are critical.

Pressure on the flap base is to be avoided during the postoperative period. When possible, the area of the flap inset is elevated as in head and neck and extremity reconstruction. If the area of the flap lacks protective sensation, the site of reconstruction is placed in a nondependent position. Use of an air-fluidized bed is recommended to avoid pressure on dependent areas in patients with spinal cord injury.

Constricting bandages are avoided, particularly in the area of the flap base where pressure on the flap pedicle may compromise flap circulation. The flap is observed for potential circulatory problems during the initial postoperative period. Those patients undergoing head and neck reconstruction with microvascular tissue transfer should have strict orders to have nothing placed circumferentially around the head or neck. Nasal cannulas, oxygen masks, eye glasses, and tracheostomy collars should be avoided due to the risk of pedicle compression.

Excessive motion in the area of the flap inset is to be avoided by padding of areas adjacent to the flap inset site. In extremity reconstruction the use of a plaster splint to immobilize the joint proximal and distal to the flap inset site is recommended. Circular casts are avoided because of the risk of pressure associated with postoperative edema and difficulty in observing flap circulation.

A closed suction drain system is generally used at both the donor and recipient closure sites. Drains are not removed until the patient is mobilized since the resultant motion may temporarily increase the risk of seroma formation. Drains in proximity to a tissue expander or prosthetic implants are a potential source of infection and are removed as quickly as possible. When seroma drainage decreases to 20 mL in a 24-hour period, the closed drainage system is removed. When possible, drainage systems are removed by postoperative day 10 to avoid potential wound contamination through the drain exit site.

Perioperative antibiotics are recommended when flaps are inset at the site of contaminated defects. If an expander or permanent implant insertion site has a history of prior infection, perioperative antibiotics are also recommended. Cultures of the wound site will determine the necessity for postoperative antibiotic therapy. Continued use of postoperative antibiotic therapy should be based on wound cultures and selection of culture-specific antibiotic agents.[336]

Prolonged bed rest is avoided when possible following reconstructive surgery. With the exception of those undergoing reconstruction of the perineum and lower extremity, most patients are ambulatory after the first postoperative day. Elevation and immobilization of upper and lower extremities are generally recommended for 10 days followed by nonweight-bearing for up to 6 weeks. Weight bearing at the site of flap inset for pressure sore coverage is avoided for 4–6 weeks. Range of motion exercises at the donor site are encouraged when wound healing is complete, usually by postoperative day 7–10, to avoid joint stiffness and muscle weakness.

If the patient has difficulty regaining function at either the donor or recipient sites, a physical therapy program is recommended. Pain management for patients treated for complex defects may require consultation with a pain specialty clinic and psychiatrist. Occupational therapy is indicated for patients unable to return to their jobs. A multi-specialty approach to patients who have undergone cancer treatment is essential to provide tumor surveillance and adjuvant therapy when indicated. Patients at risk for wound recurrence, particularly following closure of a pressure sore, and patients with spinal cord injury require instruction in avoidance of pressure and shear forces at the site of flap reconstruction and assistance in obtaining devices (i.e., wheelchair with appropriate padding) to avoid future skin injury.

Postoperative use of anticoagulation is largely surgeon dependent and is usually of concern in microvascular tissue transplantation. Common postoperative regimens include daily aspirin, heparin or dextran. Aspirin inactivates platelets by blocking cyclooxygenase. Heparin is an antithrombin III inhibitor. Dextran decreases platelet adhesiveness, inhibits platelet aggregation and decreases the blood viscosity. The use of these medications varies among surgeons.

Flap monitoring techniques

Postoperative monitoring of muscle and musculocutaneous flaps is a critical component in the care of these patients. Many techniques have been developed to monitor flaps and have primarily focused on those flaps transferred microsurgically. These monitoring methods assess the patency of the small vessel microanastomosis. The goal is to discover any problem with the anastomosis early enough to salvage the flap. Musculocutaneous flaps, which have not been divided from their vascular pedicle, are generally monitored with clinical observation. Clinical observation generally involves assessment of skin color, tissue turgor, temperature, and capillary refill.

Complications

Complications with the use of muscle and musculocutaneous flaps fall into three categories: judgment, technique, and patient management. The most common complications include seroma, hematoma, superficial skin necrosis, wound separation, inadequate coverage of the defect, infection, and partial or complete loss of the flap. By analyzing these complications in relation to judgment, technique, and patient management, the surgeon should be able to understand the cause of each complication in order to prevent subsequent complications.

Errors in surgical judgment are usually due to: inadequate preparation, inadequate flap design, or inadequate knowledge of anatomy.

Inadequate preparation is characterized by proceeding with a reconstructive procedure without having sufficient resources to perform the operation. For example, a surgeon may be asked to evaluate an elderly patient who has an extensive nonhealing ulcer involving the distal third of the leg. The surgeon recommends microvascular transplantation of a muscle flap, yet foregoes a preoperative arteriogram even though the patient has significant risk factors for peripheral vascular disease. Intraoperatively, adequate recipient vessels cannot be found and the flap is therefore aborted. This underscores the importance of preoperative preparation, especially if the diagnostic study directly impacts the surgical procedure planned.

Inadequate flap design is usually due to the surgeon's failure to account for every aspect of the surgical defect. The flap should not be designed and elevated prior to debridement of the wound. This may result in a significantly larger wound and an inadequately small flap. The flap should only be designed and elevated after the defect is completely debrided.

Inadequate knowledge of surgical anatomy may result in damage to the vascular pedicle during dissection, which can lead to failure of the flap. In addition to directly injuring the vascular pedicle, the surgeon can indirectly injure a pedicle by using a flap whose vascular pedicle is within the zone of injury, as in defects involving infection and radiation necrosis. Vascular pedicles within this environment may be compromised. For example, in a distally based flap, the minor pedicle is usually close to the defect and may be affected by the underlying cause of the defect. This is one reason that a distally based flap is less reliable than the muscle flap that is based on its dominant, major, or segmental secondary vascular pedicles. Through an appreciation of these subtle anatomic differences, proper flap selection and safe flap transposition can be achieved. It is imperative that the surgeon understand the precise anatomy of the muscle and musculocutaneous flap and the relationship to its vascular pedicle(s).

Surgical technique directly affects the outcome of any procedure. The handling of tissue, particularly vascular pedicles, is of utmost importance to the success of the flap. Vessels can be injured at any stage of the operation and are subject to spasm, kinking, shearing, and twisting. One preventative measure is the placement of temporary sutures between the skin of the flap and the underlying muscle or fascia to prevent shearing of the musculocutaneous perforating vessels. Other techniques include avoidance of skeletonizing the vascular pedicle unless absolutely necessary to avoid spasm and injury. Lastly, in flaps that are tunneled beneath skin bridges, it is important to avoid a tourniquet effect produced by the potentially constrictive skin bridge.

Ultimate flap loss can be due to intrinsic or extrinsic reasons. Flap loss due to intrinsic reasons is largely caused by inadequate blood supply, which is the most common reason of flap compromise. Flap compromise due to extrinsic circumstances includes infection, hypotension, and vasoconstricting agents such as pressors. Compression or tension on the flap due to hematoma is another extrinsic cause of flap compromise. Exploration of the flap should be expeditious when failure is suspected.

Donor site complications include fluid collections due to dead space (seroma, hematoma), wound separation, infection and injury to adjacent structures during flap harvest.

Errors in patient management are a common cause of postoperative complications. For patients undergoing a muscle or musculocutaneous flap transposition, the most common errors of management include: (1) inadequate attention to the patients underlying medical conditions; (2) inadequate assessment or management of intravascular volume status; and (3) inadequate surveillance of flap viability and perfusion.

The safety and reliability of muscle and musculocutaneous flaps has been repeatedly demonstrated. Such successes now encourage surgeons to choose a more complex procedure than a simple one, especially if form and function can be improved. For example, in the reconstruction of a defect involving the lower leg, the soleus and gastrocnemius provide reliable and safe closure. However, the esthetic and functional results may be unacceptable to certain patients. In these patients, a more sophisticated technique (e.g.,

microvascular tissue transplantation) is appropriate and may be the procedure of choice.

Microvascular tissue transplantation is clearly indicated as the procedure of choice for certain defects. In fact, the use of microvascular free tissue transfer to reconstruct head and neck defects has revolutionized the field and has allowed both functional and esthetically pleasing results for large extirpative defects. The quality of the result is far greater than the risk involved.

Access the complete references list online at **http://www.expertconsult.com**

15. Mathes SJ, Nahai F. Classification of the vascular anatomy of muscles: experimental and clinical correlation. *Plast Reconstr Surg.* 1981;67:177–187.
   The classic flap vascularization classification scheme is described.

20. Ariyan S. The pectoralis major myocutaneous flap. A versatile flap for reconstruction in the head and neck. *Plast Reconstr Surg.* 1979;63:73–81.

21. Mathes SJ, Vasconez LO. Myocutaneous free flap transfer. Anatomical and experimental consideration. *Plast Reconstr Surg.* 1978;62:162–166.

53. Blondeel N, Vanderstraeten GG, Monstrey SJ, et al. The donor site morbidity of free DIEP flaps and free TRAM flaps for breast reconstruction. *Br J Plast Surg.* 1997;50:322–330.
   The DIEP flap provides the same benefits as the free TRAM in breast reconstruction. The authors analyze a clinical series to demonstrate that DIEP flaps significantly reduce donor site morbidity compared with TRAMs.

55. Taylor GI, Palmer JH. The vascular territories (angiosomes) of the body: experimental study and clinical applications. *Br J Plast Surg.* 1987;40:113–141.
   Cadaveric dissections were performed to characterize cutaneous blood supply. The angiosome concept is described.

182. Hartrampf CR, Scheflan M, Black PW. Breast reconstruction with a transverse abdominal island flap. *Plast Reconstr Surg.* 1982;69:216–225.
   The TRAM flap is introduced as an option for breast reconstruction after mastectomy.

229. Ramirez OM, Ruas E, Dellon AL. "Components separation" method for closure of abdominal wall defects: an anatomical and clinical study. *Plast Reconstr Surg.* 1990;86:519–526.
   Loss of abdominal domain is a common surgical problem. The anatomical basis and technical details of the now-ubiquitous components separation are described.

303. Attinger CE, Ducic I, Cooper P, et al. The role of intrinsic muscle flaps of the foot for bone coverage in foot and ankle defects in diabetic and nondiabetic patients. *Plast Reconstr Surg.* 2002;110:1047–1054.

25

Flap pathophysiology and pharmacology

Cho Y. Pang and Peter C. Neligan

Introduction

Flaps, both pedicled and free, are routinely used to reconstruct defects resulting from injury, excision of tumors, ulceration, or congenital malformation.[1-3] The clinical problem is that flap failure as a result of ischemic necrosis occurs in both pedicle and free flaps. In free flaps alone, ischemic necrosis occurs in 5–10% of patients, even in experienced hands.[4-10] Flap necrosis can be partial or total.[11-13] Flap failure is time-consuming and costly because it requires repeated surgery and prolonged hospitalization. In the US, the additional operating room cost ranges from about $40 000 to $68 000 for each total free flap failure, and the additional surgeon reimbursement ranges from $5000 to $35 000 for each surgery.[14,15] In addition, repeated surgery increases the incidence of donor site deformity and/or morbidity, with devastating effects on the patient. Therefore, we need to understand the pathophysiology of ischemic necrosis in flap surgery because this information may lead us to develop effective pharmacological therapies to prevent or salvage flap failure.

Pathophysiology of flap failure

Vasospasm and thrombosis in pathogenesis of pedicle and free flap failure

Clinically and experimentally, ischemic necrosis occurs mainly in the distal portion of both pedicle and free flaps. The general consensus is that vasospasm and thrombosis due to surgical trauma and insufficient distal vascularity are the main pathogenic factors in flap failure,[3] but little is known about the pathogenic mechanism. However, there are published reviews on the role of vasoactive neurohumoral substances in the local regulation of peripheral vascular tone in normal and diseased states.[16-21] These articles may provide insight into the pathogenesis of vasospasm and thrombosis in flap surgery, as illustrated in *Figure 25.1*. Briefly, endothelium-derived relaxing factors (EDRFs) such as prostacyclin (PGI_2) and nitric oxide (NO) cause relaxation of vascular smooth muscle and inhibit platelet aggregation. On the other hand, endothelium-derived contracting factors (EDCFs) such as thromboxane A_2 (TXA_2), and endothelin-1 (ET-1) raise vascular tone. Under physiological conditions, a balance of vascular

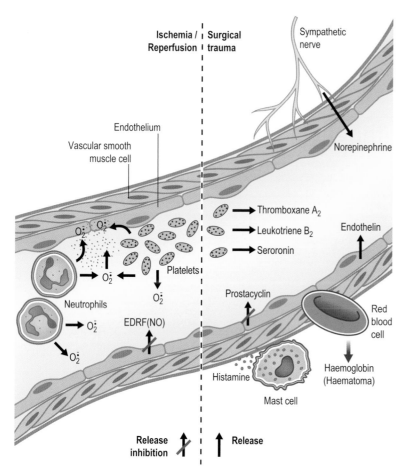

Fig. 25.1 Vasoconstriction in surgical trauma and vascular damage in ischemia–reperfusion injury. In surgical trauma, norepinephrine is released by sympathetic nerve endings and thromboxane A_2, leukotriene B_4, and serotonin are released by traumatized platelets and hemoglobin by red blood cells to cause vasoconstriction. Traumatized endothelial cells also decrease synthesis of vasodilating prostacyclin and endothelium-derived relaxing factor/nitric oxide (EDRF/NO). In reperfusion of ischemic blood vessels, superoxide radicals ($O_2^{\bullet}$) are produced by platelets and neutrophils. These free radicals can damage blood vessels.

effects between EDCFs and EDRFs maintains adequate tissue perfusion. However, an imbalance can occur as a result of surgical trauma, as shown in *Figure 25.1*. Specifically, traumatized sympathetic nerve endings release norepinephrine (NE), causing vasoconstriction and platelet aggregation. The NE released by the sympathetic nerve endings, leukotrienes, serotonin ($5HT_2$) and TXA_2 released by the platelets, and the ET-1 released by the traumatized vascular endothelial cells can cause vasoconstriction and intravascular platelet aggregation, especially in the small arteries in the distal portion of the flap where the perfusion pressure is low and the concentration of these vasoconstrictive substances is high due to the downstream effect. Hemoglobin from hemolyzed red blood cells (e.g., hematoma) is also a potent vasoconstrictor. The histamine released by the

mast cells changes the membrane permeability, resulting in edema formation. Furthermore, the synthesis and release of EDRFs such as PGI_2 and NO from the traumatized vascular endothelium are depressed. In addition, the rate of endothelial degradation of NE and $5HT_2$ by catechol-O-methyl transferase and monoamine oxidase, respectively, is reduced in situations of impaired endothelial function. The end result is that there are high local levels of vasoconstrictive and prothrombotic neurohumoral substances in surgical trauma and these substances exacerbate vasospasm and promote thrombosis in flap surgery.

In reperfusion of ischemic blood vessels, superoxide radicals ($O_2^{\bullet}$) are produced by platelets, neutrophils, and endothelial cells and these free radicals can damage vascular walls during reperfusion *(Fig. 25.1)*.

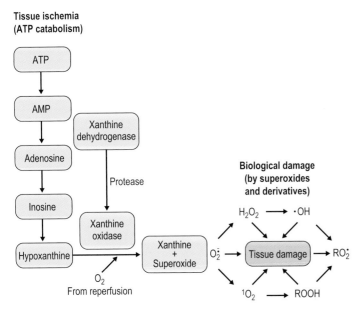

Tissue ischemia (ATP catabolism)

Biological damage (by superoxides and derivatives)

$H_2O_2 \longrightarrow \cdot OH$

$^1O_2 \longrightarrow ROOH$

O_2^- From reperfusion

Fig. 25.2 Pathogenesis of oxygen-derived free radicals in reperfusion of ischemic tissues. ATP, adenosine triphosphate; AMP, adenosine monophosphate; O_2^-, superoxide; H_2O_2, hydrogen peroxide; •OH, hydroxyl radical, $^1O_2$, singlet oxygen; RO_2^-, peroxy radicals; ROOH, hydroperoxide.

Xanthine dehydrogenase/xanthine oxidase enzyme system in pathogenesis of ischemia–reperfusion injury in free flap surgery

In free flap surgery, skin and muscle are subjected to warm (room-temperature) global ischemia under vascular clamp control during transfer from donor site to recipient site prior to reanastomosis. Human muscle and skin can withstand 2–2.5 hours and 6–8 hours of warm global ischemia, respectively.[22–26] Excessive ischemic insult can result in ischemia–reperfusion injury caused by energy depletion and formation of oxygen-derived free radicals, as shown in *Figure 25.2*. Specifically, during prolonged ischemia, adenosine triphosphate (ATP) in skin and muscle is catabolized stepwise to hypoxanthine, with concomitant increase in cytosolic Ca^{2+}.[27] At the same time, a cytosolic protease is activated by intracellular Ca^{2+} and it converts xanthine dehydrogenase to xanthine oxidase.[28,29] During reperfusion, the xanthine oxidase generates superoxide (O_2^-) by univalent reduction of molecular oxygen in the presence of hypoxanthine.[30] The unstable O_2^- forms H_2O_2 spontaneously by dismutation. Furthermore, the unstable O_2^- also interacts with H_2O_2 in the presence of a transition metal (e.g., iron) to form the most potent cytotoxic

hydroxyl radical (OH•) through the Haber–Weiss (Fenton) reaction,[31] as shown in *Figure 25.2*. There is evidence to suggest that this hypoxanthine/xanthine oxidase system is a main source of oxyradicals in ischemic rat skin and muscle.[32,33] Furthermore, inhibition of xanthine oxidase activity by allopurinol and depletion of xanthine oxidase with a tungsten diet have been shown to attenuate the microvascular damage in rat skeletal muscle subjected to 2 hours of ischemia and 30 minutes of reperfusion.[34]

There is also evidence to indicate that hypoxanthine/xanthine oxidase system is not a main source of oxyradicals in pig and human skin and skeletal muscle. Specifically, control pig and human skin samples were found to contain minimal xanthine oxidase activity, almost 40 times less than that of the rat, and xanthine oxidase activity did not rise during the first 8 hours of ischemia.[35] In pigs, intravenous allopurinol given 60 minutes before ischemia did not protect cutaneous or musculocutaneous flaps from necrosis when subsequently subjected to 8 hours of warm ischemia and 5 days of reperfusion.[36] Similarly, it was reported that xanthine oxidase activity in pig and human skeletal muscle was minute (<0.5 mU/g wet weight) compared with that of the rat.[37] In addition, 5 days of competitive xanthine oxidase inhibitor treatment (allopurinol 25 mg/kg i.v., b.i.d.) starting 2 days before ischemia or 3 days of noncompetitive xanthine oxidase inhibitor treatment (oxypurinol, 25 mg/kg, i.v., b.i.d.) starting 15 minutes before reperfusion did not attenuate pig latissimus dorsi muscle necrosis when subjected to 5 hours of ischemia and 48 hours of reperfusion.[37]

Neutrophilic nicotinamide adenine diphosphate (NADPH) and myeloperoxidase (MPO) enzyme system in pathogenesis of ischemia/reperfusion injury in free flap surgery

There is accumulated evidence to indicate that neutrophils may play an important role in ischemia–reperfusion injury in free flap surgery. Specifically, it is well known that activated neutrophils produce large amounts of O_2^- via NADPH oxidase, and these O_2^- dismutates yield high concentration of H_2O_2 and OH•, causing tissue damage.[38] MPO, which is unique and abundant in neutrophils, catalyzes the conversion of

H_2O_2 to hypochlorous acid (HOCl), a potent cytotoxic oxidizing agent ($H_2O_2 + Cl^- + H^+ \rightarrow HOCl + H_2O$).[39,40] Furthermore, it was reported that treatment with monoclonal antibodies against neutrophil–endothelium adhesion molecules attenuated ischemia–reperfusion-induced skin necrosis in rabbit ears,[41] rat epigastric island skin flaps,[42] and skin and muscle in pig latissimus dorsi musculocutaneous flaps.[43] Treatment with monoclonal antibody against neutrophil–endothelium adhesion molecules also attenuated arteriolar vasoconstriction induced by ischemia–reperfusion injury.[44] Finally, neutrophil depletion (~95%) with mechlorethamine significantly reduced necrosis in pig latissimus dorsi muscle flaps subjected to 5 hours of warm ischemia and 48 hours of reperfusion.[37] Also, neutrophil depletion attenuated vascular injury in dog gracilis muscle subjected to 4 hours of warm ischemia and 1 hour of reperfusion.[45]

On the other hand, there are arguments against the important role of neutrophils in the pathogenesis of animal or human myocardial ischemia–reperfusion injury.[46–48] Specifically, ischemia–reperfusion injury could be induced in neutrophil-free systems such as in cultured animal cardiomyocytes[49] and human atrial strips[50,51] and in isolated perfused animal hearts.[52–54] In clinical studies, free oxyradical scavengers were not effective in protecting myocardium from ischemia–reperfusion injury.[55,56] Furthermore, although monoclonal antibody to intercellular adhesion molecule-1 and anti-CD18 antibodies were effective in protecting myocardium against ischemia–reperfusion in laboratory animals,[57,58] clinical trials with these agents yielded negative results.[59–61] More recently, it was reported that ischemia–reperfusion injury was also induced in human rectus abdominis muscle strips cultured in neutrophil-free buffer.[62] There is the possibility of species difference in the role of neutrophils in the pathogenesis of ischemia–reperfusion injury. Therefore, it is important to clarify the causal role of neutrophils in ischemia–reperfusion injury in human skin and skeletal muscle.

Intracellular Ca^{2+} overload in pathogenesis of ischemia–reperfusion injury in free flap failure

Recently, experimental evidence indicates that intracellular Ca^{2+} overload plays a key role in causing cell death during myocardial reperfusion.[63] The pathogenic mechanism is summarized in **Figure 25.3**. Specifically, in sustained ischemia, mitochondrial ATP synthesis ceases and glycolysis ensues, resulting in a net breakdown of ATP and an accumulation of lactate and intracellular H^+,[64] causing intracellular acidosis. This build-up of intracellular H^+ activates the Na^+/H^+ exchange isoform-1 (NHE-1) antiporter, resulting in extrusion of H^+ and accumulation of intracellular Na^+ to restore intracellular pH. There is a further increase in intracellular Na^+ accumulation because Na^+ extrusion is limited by inactivation of the energy-dependent Na^+-K^+-ATPase pump.[65,66] Elevation of intracellular Na^+ concentration causes an increase in intracellular Ca^{2+} by activation of the Na^+/Ca^{2+} exchanger causing Ca^{2+} influx.[65,67–70] If these events

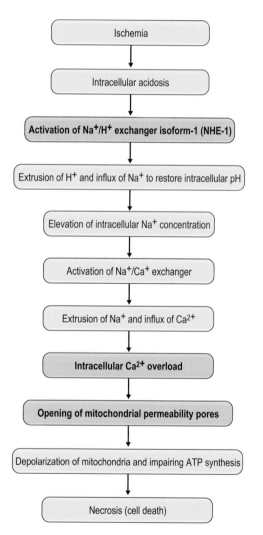

Fig. 25.3 Proposed role of intracellular Ca^{2+} overload in the pathogenesis of ischemia–reperfusion injury. ATP, adenosine triphosphate.

continue, the cystolic Ca^{2+} will be overloaded, and significant uptake of Ca^{2+} from the cytosol to the mitochondria will occur, resulting in mitochondrial Ca^{2+} overload[71] which causes depolarization of mitochondria and impairs ATP synthesis, resulting in cell necrosis[52] *(Fig. 25.3)*. However, the NHE-1 may be inhibited[72] if the extracellular acidosis is more pronounced than the intracellular acidosis after a prolonged period of ischemia.[73] At reperfusion, the rapid washout of the extracellular H^+ reactivates the NHE-1, resulting in further extrusion of intracellular H^+, and further accumulation of intracellular Na^+, causing further cystolic Ca^{2+} overload through Na^+/Ca^{2+} exchange.[74,75] Again, cytosolic Ca^{2+} overload causes mitochondrial Ca^{2+} overload, impairing ATP synthesis and resulting in cell death.[52,71] Recently, there is evidence to suggest that mitochondrial Ca^{2+} overload plays an important role in ischemia–reperfusion in skeletal muscle and this will be discussed later, along with the therapeutic treatment aimed at preventing mitochondrial Ca^{2+} overload.

Pathogenesis of no-reflow phenomenon in free flap surgery

Rabbit island epigastric skin free flaps were used to study the pathogenesis of the no-reflow phenomenon in free flap surgery.[76] It was observed that ischemia induced swelling of the endothelial and parenchymal cell, narrowing of the capillary lumen, intravascular aggregation of blood cells, and leakage of intravascular fluid into the interstitial space to form edema. This pathology increased with the increase in length of ischemic time from 1 to 8 hours and the obstruction of blood flow reached a point of irreversibility after 12 hours of ischemia, leading to no reflow and ultimate death of the flap. Three pathogenic mechanisms have been suggested to play a central role in the development of no-reflow phenomenon in the skeletal muscle of laboratory animals: (1) oxygen-derived free radicals causing damage in the endothelial and parenchymal cells; (2) this cell membrane damage allowing Ca^{2+} influx, resulting in intracellular overload; and (3) change in arachidonic acid metabolism resulting in synthesis of less vasodilating and antithrombotic PGI_2 by the endothelium and increased synthesis of vasoconstricting and thrombotic TXA_2 by platelets.[77]

Surgical manipulation for augmentation of pedicle flap viability

Clinically and experimentally, there are several surgical manipulations which have proved effective in augmenting flap viability.

Flap design in augmentation of pedicle flap viability

One of the misleading principles in plastic surgery is that the viable length of a skin flap depends on the width of the pedicle. Milton was the first to disprove this principle.[1,78–80] Using a random-pattern skin flap model in the pig, it was demonstrated that the ultimate surviving length of a pedicle flap is determined by the balance between perfusion pressure and vascular resistance. Increasing the width of pedicle flaps merely adds additional vessels of the same type and the same perfusion pressure and thus cannot increase the length of flap viability *(Fig. 25.4)*. However, in other locations of the body, increasing the width of the pedicle may increase the chance of including a large artery. Therefore, one of the surgical manipulations to augment flap viability is the conversion of a random-pattern skin flap to an arterialized skin flap by incorporating a direct artery or a larger perforator.

Surgical delay in augmentation of pedicle flap viability

Surgical delay and vascular delay are proven techniques for augmenting flap viability in human

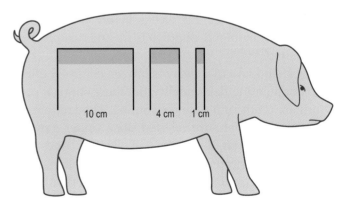

Fig. 25.4 The length-to-width ratio concept in flap design.

patients,[81–85] and in laboratory animals such as mice, rats, rabbits, and pigs.[86–99] It takes two to three stages in surgical delay of pedicle skin flaps in order to augment flap viability. Specifically, a skin flap is mapped out on the donor site and incised on its two longitudinal sides. The flap is then undermined to form a bipedicle flap and is sutured back to the donor site. Two to three weeks after construction of the bipedicle flap, the third side (distal end) is cut in one or two stages at 2–3 days apart. At the end of this stage, a single pedicle flap is completely raised and the distal portion of the flap is moved to the recipient site for wound coverage without skin necrosis.[1,100] Studies with pig random-pattern skin flaps showed that surgical delay increased skin flap capillary blood flow between 2 and 7 days of delay.[101,102] This increase in capillary blood flow was mainly in the distal random portion of the delayed skin flaps.[102]

Vascular delay in augmentation of pedicle flap viability

In mice, rats, and rabbits, vascular delay for augmenting blood flow and viability in the distal portion of latissimus dorsi muscle flaps was achieved by dividing distal perforating arteries at 1–2 weeks prior to raising of muscle flaps.[94,96,97] This phenomenon was also achieved in transverse rectus abdominis myocutaneous (TRAM) flaps in laboratory animals and human patients. Division of perforators or one or two dominant arteries that supply blood to the rectus abdominis muscle 2–3 weeks before flap surgery significantly augmented viability in TRAM flaps in rats[92,93,95,98] and augmented skin and muscle blood flow and viability in TRAM flaps in pigs.[92,93] In human patients, ligation of the deep inferior epigastric arteries 2–4 weeks before flap surgery augmented skin blood supply[84,103,104] and viability in TRAM flaps.[81,82,83,85]

Surgical and vascular delay is proven clinically effective in augmenting flap viability, but these surgical procedures are costly and time-consuming. They require at least one additional surgical step done under general anesthesia. Vascular delay by embolization does not require general anesthesia, but it requires local anesthesia and catheterization performed in the interventional radiology department.[105] Recently, "recharging" of the TRAM has been described as an alternative technique to augment flap perfusion.[106] The evolution of microsurgery saw the development of free flaps. The idea was to improve flap blood flow and viability. TRAM free flaps are a good example as the free TRAM is perfused by the more dominant deep inferior epigastric pedicle rather than the less dominant superior epigastric vessels that supply the pedicled TRAM.[106–111] However, free flap surgery is not always available and it is expensive. It requires specialized microsurgical staff and equipment and long operating room time. Furthermore, free flap surgery is not without morbidity and flap ischemic necrosis due to thrombosis and vasospasm occurs in 5–10% of patients.[4–10,111] Therefore, there is the need to understand the mechanism of the surgical delay phenomenon through research to identify pharmacological strategies to prevent/treat ischemic necrosis.

Mechanism of surgical delay in augmentation of pedicle flap viability

Many investigators have studied the surgical delay phenomenon in laboratory animals in order to gain insight into the pathogenesis and pharmacological treatment for skin flap ischemic necrosis. Several hypotheses have emerged from these studies.

Surgical delay procedure reduces arteriovenous (AV) shunt flow

Reinisch reported good correlation between postoperative fluorescein staining and the eventual skin viability in pig skin flaps. He detected warm skin temperature beyond the fluorescein dye marker in the distal portion of the pig skin flap.[112] He also demonstrated ^{51}Cr-labeled red blood cells and technetium and [85]Sr-microsphere (15 μm) activity beyond the fluorescein dye staining in acute pig skin flaps.[112] Taken together, he hypothesized that, in acute skin flap surgery, distal ischemic necrosis was caused by opening of AV shunt flow as a result of sympathetic denervation. He speculated that shunt flow occurred throughout the skin flap and the flow in the proximal areas is sufficient to supply both the AV and capillary (nutrient) blood flow, but the shunting became lethal in the distal areas of the skin flap where the total blood flow was low. In surgical delay, the bipedicle skin flap provided sufficient blood supply during the early period of sympathetic denervation and opening of AV shunts. Pearl presented data from rat abdominal arterial skin flaps, which supported Reinish's hypothesis, and also suggested that surgical delay allowed the skin flap to recover from its hyperadrenergic state before converting the bipedicle to single-pedicle skin flaps.[113] However, these observations were not supported by other investigators. For example, Prather *et al.*, using various laboratory techniques (fluorescein dye test, xenon clearance, angiograph, ^{51}Cr-tagged red blood cells and thermometry), failed to detect any evidence of vascular perfusion in the nonfluorescein distal portion of acute axial pattern skin flaps in the pig.[114] In contrast to Palmer's findings[115] in rat dorsal skin flaps, Cutting *et al.*[116,117] did not observe persistent adrenergic denervation in delayed bipedicle skin flaps. Later, Guba used 15 μm and 50 μm radioactive microspheres to measure capillary (nutrient) and total blood flow, respectively, and to calculate AV shunt flow in bipedicle axial pattern pig skin flaps. Both capillary and AV shunt flow increased between 2 and 7 days of delay in pig bipedicle skin flaps, but this increase in capillary blood flow in delayed bipedicle skin flaps was not the result of a decrease in AV shunt flow.[101]

Subsequently, using 15 μm and 50 μm radioactive microspheres as well as fluorescein dye, Kerrigan[118] found no evidence of AV shunt flow in the distal portion of acute random and arterial pig skin flaps destined to necrose, as indicated by lack of fluorescein penetration. Finally, using a similar radioactive microsphere technique, Pang *et al.* demonstrated that AV shunts played no important role in the pathogenesis of distal ischemic necrosis in random-pattern skin flaps in the pig and augmenting distal skin viability by surgical delay did not rely on closing of AV shunts, but vasodilation of existing blood vessels.[102,119] It is important to point out that there may also be species differences in the extent of AV shunt flow in the skin assessed by the radioactive microsphere technique. Specifically, Pang *et al.* observed in the pig that the AV shunt flow in the control skin and in the skin of acute and delayed random-pattern skin flaps within 6 hours postoperatively was ~60% of the total blood flow.[102] However, Sasaki and Pang[120] observed in the rat that the AV shunt flow in abdominal island skin flaps within 6 hours postoperatively was ~10% of the total skin blood flow. More recently, Kreidstein *et al.*[121] observed that the AV shunt flow in isolated perfused human paraumbilical skin was ~1%. Taken together, AV shunt flow does not seem to play an important role in the pathogenesis of distal ischemic necrosis in acute pedicle skin flaps.

Surgical delay procedure depletes vasoconstriction and prothrombotic substances in the skin flap

Local tissue content of vasoconstricting and prothrombotic substances such as NE, TXA_2, 5HT and ET-1 are known to be elevated by surgical trauma.[3,122–136] These substances are released locally by traumatized blood cells, endothelial cells, and sympathetic nerve endings *(Fig. 25.1)*. These are potent vasoconstrictors in skin vasculature.[135,137–144] There is a general consensus that vasospasm and thrombosis play an important role in the pathogenesis of ischemic necrosis in acute skin flaps and the surgical delay procedure reduces local production and also allows time to deplete the vasoconstricting and prothrombic substances before converting the bipedicle flap to single-pedicle flaps. In the past, research in skin flap surgery was focused on the use of vasodilating and antithrombotic drugs to augment skin flap viability. So far, the outcomes of pharmacological therapy for prevention or treatment of pedicle flap ischemic necrosis are disappointing and will be discussed later.

Surgical delay procedure induces vascular territory expansion by opening existing choke arteries

Pang *et al.* studied the capillary blood flow in delayed random-pattern pig skin flaps. We found that the capillary blood flow increased significantly within 2 days of delay and a maximum increase in skin flap capillary blood flow occurred between 2 and 3 days of delay, and remained unchanged between 4 and 14 days of delay without an increase in density of arteries (arteriogenesis) assessed by histology. This increase in capillary blood flow occurred mainly in the distal portion of the skin flap.[102] Similar increase in capillary blood flow was also seen in vascular delay of pig TRAM flaps within 3–4 days of delay and it is unlikely that an increase in arterial density (arteriogenesis) could have occurred during this short period of time. Therefore, these investigators described this phenomenon as vascular territory expansion by recruitment (opening) of existing

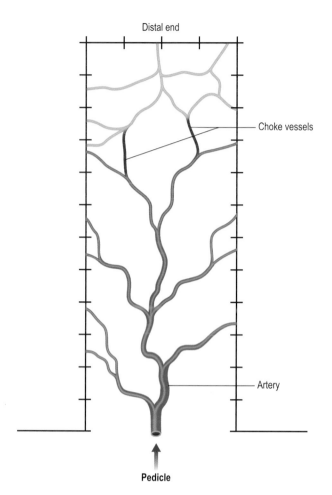

Distal end

Choke vessels

Artery

Pedicle

Fig. 25.5 Opening of existing blood vessels (choke vessels) in the distal portion of the surgically delayed skin flap.

arteries, as illustrated in *Figure 25.5*.[91] Opening of existing blood vessels was demonstrated by Taylor and colleagues in vascular delay of skin flaps in the guinea pig, rabbit, dog, pig, and human,[145–148] and by Yang and Morris in vascular delay of rat skin flaps,[149,150] and this phenomenon was labeled by these investigators as angiosome territory expansion by opening of existing choke blood vessels.

Surgical delay procedure induces angiogenesis

Lineaweaver *et al.* reported that vascular delay increased the viability of the skin paddle of rat TRAM flaps and this protective effect of vascular delay was associated with a significant increase in gene expression of vascular endothelial growth factor (VEGF) and basic fibroblast growth factor (FGF) in the skin paddle of the rat TRAM flaps within 12 hours of vascular delay. These investigators speculated that these cytokines induced vasodilation and angiogenesis to augment skin paddle viability in rat TRAM flaps.[151] The vascular mechanism of surgical delay is still unclear. However, it was previously reported that the angiogenesis inhibitor endostatin inhibited ischemia-induced microvascular density and viability of mouse dorsal random-pattern skin flaps.[152] Therefore, endostatin can be used in the future to investigate the role of angiogenesis and arteriogenesis in surgical delay in skin flap surgery in laboratory animals.

Pharmacological therapy for augmentation of pedicle flap viability

As discussed previously, the surgical delay procedure is costly and time-consuming. Therefore, much research has been focused on drug therapy for augmenting blood flow and viability in pedicle flap surgery.

Drug therapy against vasoconstriction and thrombosis in pedicle and free flap surgery

Vasoconstricting and prothrombotic substances such as NE, TXA$_2$, 5HT, and ET-1 are known to be elevated in skin flap surgery as a result of surgical trauma.[122,123,125,126,153–160] These are very potent vasoconstrictors.[135,161–168] In the past, research in skin flap surgery was focused on the use of vasodilating and antithrombotic drugs to augment skin flap viability. These studies were reviewed in detail up to 1990 by various investigators and will not be discussed here.[3,118,169,170] The categories of drugs included: α-adrenoreceptor antagonists; drugs causing depletion of catecholamine in nerve terminals; drugs preventing catecholamine release from the nerve terminal; β-adrenoreceptor agonists; direct vasodilators, calcium channel blockers, hemorrheological drugs; vasodilating eicosanoids and their synthesis inhibitors; anti-inflammatory drugs; drugs inhibiting adherence and accumulation of neutrophils; and free radical scavengers. More recently, research in drug therapy for augmenting flap viability also focused on vasodilation,[171–187] antithrombosis,[188] and inhibition of neutrophil from adherence and accumulation.[189] In general, the results with these vasodilating and anti-thrombotic drug treatments in augmenting pedicle flap viability were controversial, inconclusive, or very modest at best, compared with surgical delay. Finally, most of these studies were performed in loose-skinned laboratory animals (e.g., rats, rabbits) whose skin vasculature and anatomy are different from those of the human.[190] Using more clinically relevant pig pedicle skin flap models, Pang and colleagues tested the following drugs, which were reported to augment rat skin flap viability by other investigators. It was observed that neither skin blood flow nor viability was significantly improved by the following categories of drug: glucocorticoid,[191] α-adrenoreceptor antagonists,[192] vascular smooth-muscle relaxants,[193,194] β-adrenoreceptor agonist,[193] TXA_2 synthesis inhibitor,[195] TXA_2 receptor antagonist,[195] and vasodilating prostanoids.[196] It was observed that $5HT_2$ receptor antagonists augmented skin flap viability in the pig, but the beneficial effect was modest compared with surgical delay.[195,197] In conclusion, the mechanism of surgical or vascular delay is unclear. So far, there is no effective drug therapy which can mimic surgical or vascular delay in augmenting skin flap viability.

Angiogenic cytokine protein or gene therapy for augmentation of pedicle flap viability

Angiogenic cytokines such as VEGF, FGF, and platelet-derived growth factors (PDGF) are known to induce an increase in capillary density (angiogenesis). Recently, flap research has been focused on the use of local angiogenic cytokine protein therapy to augment flap viability. For example, improved viability was observed following local subdermal injection of $VEGF_{165}$ immediately after elevation of rat dorsal random-pattern skin flaps[198,199]; local interarterial injection of $VEGF_{165}$ immediately after raising of rat epigastric island skin flaps[200,201]; and injection of $VEGF_{165}$ into the rectus abdominis muscle 20 days before construction of TRAM flap in the rat.[202] There is also evidence to indicate that FGF can augment skin flap viability. This has been observed following intradermal injection of FGF 30 minutes before surgery in rat dorsal random-pattern skin flaps[203]; subdermal injection of FGF immediately after surgery and at 48 hours postoperatively in rat dorsal random-pattern skin flaps[204]; and subdermal injection of FGF 18 days

before construction of arterial skin flaps in mouse ears.[205] Last but not least, it was reported that local PDGF treatment mimicked the surgical delay phenomenon in augmenting latissimus dorsi muscle viability in the mouse.[206] So far none of these angiogenic cytokines has been tested on tight-skinned animals such as the pig. Since the angiogenic cytokines were effective in augmenting skin flap viability when given several days before or immediately after surgery, it is possible that vasodilation may play an important role this mechanism. Khan *et al.* used the rat dorsal random-pattern skin flap model to study the mechanism of acute local intradermal $VEGF_{165}$.[207] It was observed that subdermal injection of $VEGF_{165}$ at the time of surgery effectively attenuated pedicle skin flap ischemic necrosis in a dose-dependent manner, mainly by inducing the synthesis/release of the vasorelaxing factor NO. The mechanism by which $VEGF_{165}$ augmented skin flap viability appeared to depend on the vasodilator effect of $VEGF_{165}$ in the early stage (within 6 hours) after surgery, followed by the angiogenic effect (i.e., increase in capillary density) of $VEGF_{165}$ in the later stage after surgery. It is important to point out that $VEGF_{165}$ is a potent vasodilator in skin vasculature. Specifically, it has been reported that $VEGF_{165}$ is seven times more potent than acetylcholine in inducing skin vasodilation in isolated perfused pig island buttock skin flaps.[208]

The biological half-life of $VEGF_{165}$ is 30–45 minutes in normoxic and 6–8 hours in hypoxic conditions.[209] It is possible that the effectiveness of $VEGF_{165}$ protein therapy is limited by its short half-life and $VEGF_{165}$ gene therapy may be the key to providing a steady release of $VEGF_{165}$ perioperatively.[210] Specifically, local intradermal or subcutaneous injection of liposomal or adenoviral vectors encoding the cDNA of $VEGF_{165}$ (Ad.$VEGF_{165}$) given at 0.5, 2, 3, 7, or 14 days before surgery was shown to augment skin flap viability in the rat.[211–214] Local subcutaneous injection of $VEGF_{165}$ plasmid DNA 7 days preoperatively also increased skin viability in rat musculocutaneous (TRAM) flaps.[215] Of interest is the observation that the number of capillaries and arterioles were significantly increased in the skin of rat musculocutaneous (TRAM) flaps when Ad.$VEGF_{165}$ was injected subcutaneously 14 days before surgery.[216] However, it is important to point out that review of the data in the literature thus far indicates that the efficacy of rat dorsal skin flap viability augmentation was similar between

$VEGF_{165}$ protein and gene therapy, and the skin flap viability was about 15–20% lower than that of surgical delay.[207,217] Therefore, more than $VEGF_{165}$ is required to mimic surgical delay in augmenting flap viability.

Pharmacological therapy for augmentation of free flap viability

Vasospasm, thrombosis, and ischemia–reperfusion injury are the main causes of free flap failure. At the present time, there are relatively safe drugs which are used clinically to prevent or treat vasospasm and thrombosis in flap surgery. However, drug therapy for ischemia–reperfusion injury still remains a subject of animal research.

Drug therapy for prevention of vasospasm and thrombosis in free flap surgery

Drug therapy is used by some surgeons to prevent or treat anastomotic vasospasm and thrombosis in free flap surgery. These drugs can be classified into three categories and their dosage, efficacy, and treatment guidelines have been reviewed.[218–220]

Anticoagulant agents

Heparin, aspirin, and dextran are the three common anticoagulants used in microsurgery, but their efficacy is unclear. For example, it was reported that intravenous heparin treatment reduced the incidence of anastomotic thrombosis when given before the restoration of blood flow in the rabbit.[221] Subsequently, results from two clinical studies in free flap surgery indicated that low dosage of intraoperative heparin treatment (3000 or 5000 units intravenously) did not increase the rate of hematoma formation or intraoperative bleeding. However, these low doses of heparin treatment also did not have any significant effect on the prevention of microvascular thrombosis.[222,223] Obviously, a higher systemic dose of heparin is required. Some surgeons recommend an intraoperative bolus injection of 100–150 units/kg of intravenous heparin before cross-clamping and a supplement injection of 50 units/kg of heparin every 45–50 minutes until re-establishment of blood flow after anastomosis.[224] However this is not common

practice. More clinical research is required to identify an effective dose of heparin for the prevention of anastomotic thrombosis without hematoma formation in free flap surgery.

It was observed in the rabbit that a low dose of aspirin (10 mg/kg) caused an antithrombotic effect because it reduced TXA_2 (vasoconstrictor) formation in the platelet to a greater extent than PGI_2 (vasodilator) formation in the endothelium.[225] Low doses of aspirin were also observed to inhibit anastomotic thrombosis and improve the microcirculation in the rat.[226] In humans, low-dose aspirin (40–325 mg) was observed to inhibit platelet cyclooxygenation production of TXA_2 with minimal inhibition of endothelium-derived production of PGI_2.[227–229] However, more than 24 hours are required to achieve maximal cyclooxygenation inhibition.[227,230] It was also reported that a low oral dose of aspirin (325 mg/day) did not cause postoperative hematoma formation in clinical free flaps.[231] Furthermore, there is clinical evidence to indicate that a low dose of aspirin is effective in preventing coronary graft occlusion given preoperatively or within 24 hours of surgery.[232,233]

The low-molecular-weight dextran 40 (MW 40 000) and dextran 70 (MW 70 000) are known to have blood volume expansion and antithrombogenic effects in human.[233] Dextran 40 is the most popular dextran used to decrease platelet aggregation and to improve blood flow in free flap surgery. The effective doses have been reviewed elsewhere.[220] However, dextran 40 also has undesirable side-effects such as anaphylaxis, pulmonary and cerebral edema, and renal failure.[234] In addition, clinical evidence is accumulating to indicate that pre- or postoperative low-molecular-weight dextran treatment may not be effective in augmenting free flap viability.[235–237]

Thrombolytic agents

While early detection and re-exploration are crucial for salvaging failing free flaps, those flaps unresponsive to standard interventions may benefit from the selective use of thrombolytics for lysing formed thrombi.[238] The common thrombolytic agents that have been used successfully in clinical free flaps are streptokinase,[239–248] and recombinant tissue plasminogen activator.[249–252] The effective doses of these thrombolytic agents have also been discussed.[219,220] Results from these studies are encouraging. However, most, if not all, of these studies were small or in the form of case reports.

Antispasmodic agents

Papaverine, nifedipine, and lidocaine are the most common topical antispasmodic drugs used in clinical microsurgery. Papaverine is an opiate alkaloid, which relaxes vascular smooth muscle, especially during spasms. It inhibits phosphodiesterase, the enzyme involved in the breakdown of cyclic adenosine monophosphate (cAMP), resulting in accumulation of cAMP, causing vasodilation.[253] Nifedipine is a calcium channel blocker. The mechanism of action is inhibition of calcium influx into the arterial smooth-muscle cells, thus causing smooth-muscle cell relaxation.[254] The vasodilator effect of lidocaine is the result of its effect on the Na^+/Ca^{2+} ion exchanger pump causing a reduction in intracellular calcium content, resulting in vasodilation.[255]

Preischemic and postischemic pharmacological conditioning against ischemia–reperfusion injury in free flap surgery

In the past 20 years, research in ischemia–reperfusion injury in cardiac and skeletal muscle has been focused on the efficacy and mechanism of preischemic and postischemic conditioning against ischemia–reperfusion injury.[256] This information is important because it may provide insight into the identification of new drugs for prevention or salvage of skin and skeletal muscle from ischemia–reperfusion injury in free flap and replantation surgery.

Local preischemic conditioning against ischemia–reperfusion injury in skeletal muscle

The phenomenon of preischemic conditioning against ischemia–reperfusion injury was first recognized in dog myocardium.[257] Subsequently, Mounsey et al. demonstrated this phenomenon for the first time in pig muscle flaps.[258,259] Specifically, they reported that instigation of three cycles of 10 minutes' occlusion/reperfusion in pig latissimus dorsi muscle flaps with a vascular clamp reduced the muscle infarction by 40–50% when these muscle flaps were subsequently subjected to 4 hours of

warm ischemia and 48 hours of reperfusion. This observation was confirmed with pig gracilis muscle flaps in this laboratory.[260,261] Subsequently, other investigators reported that local preischemic conditioning also augmented ischemia–reperfusion injury tolerance in rat skeletal muscle,[262–264] and in the skin of cutaneous and musculocutaneous flaps in the rat.[265,266] Local preischemic preconditioning also attenuated vascular dysfunction in rat skeletal muscle[267] and capillary no reflow in rat and dog skeletal muscle induced by sustained ischemia and reperfusion.[268,269] However, local preischemic conditioning has clinical limitations because it requires instigation of brief cycles of ischemia and reperfusion by repeated clamping of the vascular pedicle and there is the risk of damaging the blood vessels. However, understanding the mechanism of local preischemic conditioning may provide insight into the identification of pharmacological treatment to mimic local preischemic conditioning. Using pharmacological probes, it was uncovered that the mechanism of local preischemic conditioning in pig latissimus dorsi muscle flaps involved adenosine A_1 receptor–protein kinase C–mitochondrial K_{ATP} channel-linked events.[270–275] Martou et al. demonstrated the efficacy of preischemic conditioning against ischemia–reperfusion injury in ex vivo human rectus abdominis muscle strips.[62] This model is now being used to study the pharmacological preischemic conditioning against ischemia–reperfusion injury in ex vivo human skeletal muscle strips.

Remote preischemic conditioning against ischemia–reperfusion injury in skeletal muscle

Of interest was the report from Oxman et al. that instigation of a 10-minute cycle of occlusion and reperfusion in a hind limb by tourniquet application preconditioned the heart against reperfusion tachyarrhythmia in the rat.[276] This is known as remote preischemic conditioning. Based on this technique, Addison et al. demonstrated for the first time the efficacy of noninvasive hind limb remote preischemic conditioning for global protection of skeletal muscle against ischemia–reperfusion injury.[277] Specifically, it was demonstrated that the instigation of three cycles of 10 minutes of occlusion/reperfusion in a hind limb of the pig by tourniquet application (~300 mmHg) under general anesthesia protected multiple skeletal muscles at various distant

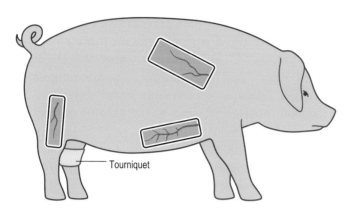

Fig. 25.6 Noninvasive remote preischemic conditioning for global protection of skeletal muscle against ischemia–reperfusion. Instigation of three cycles of 10 minutes' occlusion/reperfusion in a hind limb of the pig by tourniquet application (~300 mmHg) protected latissimus dorsi, gracilis, and rectus abdominis muscle flaps from infarction when subsequently subjected to 4 hours of ischemia and 48 hours of reperfusion.

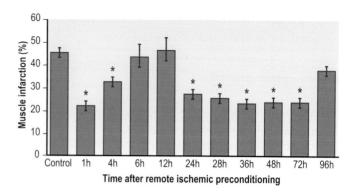

Fig. 25.7 Biphasic time course of the infarct-protective effect of remote ischemic conditioning. Muscle flaps in control and treatment groups were subjected to 4 hours of ischemia and 48 hours of reperfusion. In the treatment groups, 4 hours of ischemia began at 0, 4, 6, 8, 24, 28, 36, 48, 72, or 96 hours after remote ischemic conditioning. Infarct protection occurred at 0–4 hours and 24–72 hours after remote ischemic conditioning. Values are mean ± SEM; $n = 8$ flaps. Means with an asterisk are similar and are significantly different from the means without an asterisk ($n = 8$ flaps, $P < 0.05$).

locations from infarction when these muscles were subsequently subjected to 4 hours of ischemia and 48 hours of reperfusion *(Fig. 25.6)*. These investigators also observed that mitochondrial K_{ATP} channels play a central role in the trigger and mediator mechanisms of hind limb remote preischemic conditioning of pig skeletal muscle against infarction.[278]

Subsequently, Moses *et al.* also demonstrated that the infarct-protective effect of remote preischemic conditioning in pig skeletal muscle is biphasic[279] and the time course is similar to that seen in local preischemic conditioning in the myocardium of rabbits[280–282] and dogs[283] and in the skeletal muscle of rats.[284,285] Specifically, an early phase of infarct protection started immediately after hind limb remote preischemic conditioning, waned within 4 hours, and completely disappeared in less than 6 hours after remote preischemic conditioning *(Fig. 25.7)*. The late phase (second window) of infarct protection (re)appeared within 24 hours after hind limb remote preischemic conditioning and lasted up to 72 hours. More importantly, it was observed that sarcolemmal and mitochondrial K_{ATP} channels play a central role in the trigger and mediator mechanism, respectively.[279] The logical approach in the future is to identify a non-hypotensive prophylactic drug (e.g., sarcolemmal K_{ATP} channel opener) to be taken orally 24 hours before surgery to achieve 48 hours of uninterrupted perioperative protection of skeletal muscle from ischemia–reperfusion injury in elective microsurgery.

Postischemic conditioning for augmentation of free flap viability

Khiabani and Kerrigan reported that local intra-arterial infusion of the NO donor SIN-1 to pig latissimus dorsi myocutaenous flaps and buttock cutaneous flaps by means of a catheter for 18 hours after 6 hours of ischemia was effective in salvaging the ischemic skin and muscle from reperfusion injury.[286] However, this technique is too invasive for routine clinical use. McAllister *et al.* reported that instigation of four cycles of 30-second reperfusion/reocclusion at the onset of reperfusion after 4 hours of ischemia reduced pig latissimus dorsi muscle flap infarction by ~50%, assessed at 48 hours of reperfusion.[287] This phenomenon is known as postischemic conditioning and was first demonstrated in dog myocardium.[288] Subsequently, Park *et al.* demonstrated that postischemic conditioning also protected contractile function of rat extensor digitorum longus muscle subjected to 3 hours of ischemia and 5 days of reperfusion.[289] McAllister *et al.* also demonstrated that the mechanism of postischemic conditioning in pig skeletal muscle involved lowering of mitochondrial free Ca^{2+} content, closing of mitochondrial permeability transitional pores (mPTP), and increase in muscle ATP content. The infarct-protective effect of postischemic conditioning was mimicked by intravenous injection of the mPTP opening inhibitor cyclosporine A (10 mg/kg) at 5 minutes before reperfusion.[287] This observation suggests that cyclosporine A may be a potential clinical therapeutic agent for salvage of ischemic replants and muscle free flaps from reperfusion injury. Mowlavi et al. reported that preischemic or postischemic cyclosporine A treatment (15 mg/kg, orally) increased rat gracilis muscle viability when subjected to 4 hours of ischemia and 24 hours of reperfusion.[290] However, statistical significance was achieved in preischemic treatment but not postischemic treatment. A higher oral dose of cyclosporine A may be required for postischemic treatment because, according to McAllister et al., the effective dose of cyclosporine A for postischemic conditioning in pig skeletal muscle flap was 10 mg/kg intravenously.[287] At the present time, an in vitro model is being used to study the efficacy and mechanism of cyclosporine A in salvage of ex vivo ischemic human rectus abdominis muscle from reperfusion injury.[291]

Most recently, McAllister et al. also reported that preischemic or postischemic treatment with the Na^+/H^+ exchanger inhibitor cariporide (3 mg/kg, intravenously) induced a significant decrease in mitochondrial free Ca^{2+} content and infarct size in pig latissimus dorsi muscle flaps when subsequently subjected to 4 hours of ischemia and 48 hours of reperfusion.[292] This observation further supports their finding that the mechanism of postischemic conditioning involves lowering of mitochondrial free Ca^{2+} content and inhibition of opening of the mPTP, and the mPTP opening inhibitor cyclosporine A is effective in salvage of ischemic pig skeletal muscle from reperfusion injury.

Conclusion and future directions

Surgical and vascular delay is the only proven clinical technique for augmenting skin and muscle flap viability. However, these surgical manipulations are time-consuming and costly. Similarly, preischemic and postischemic conditioning are effective in protecting free flaps from ischemia–reperfusion injury in laboratory animals, but surgeons are reticent to conduct clinical tests on the efficacy of ischemic conditioning against ischemia–reperfusion injury in free flap surgery because these techniques are invasive and/or time-consuming. Therefore, there is the need to continue to search for pharmacological therapy to increase skin and muscle blood flow and distal perfusion in pedicle flaps and to

protect skin and muscle from ischemia–reperfusion injury in free flap and replant surgery.

The angiogenic cytokine $VEGF_{165}$ is known to cause vasodilation and increase in capillary density (angiogenesis), resulting in augmentation of skin viability in random-pattern skin flaps in the rat. However, review of the literature thus far indicates that the skin flap viability in $VEGF_{165}$ gene or protein therapy was about 15–20% lower than that of surgical delay.[207,217] Angiopoietin-2 is known to induce arteriogenesis in mouse ischemic hind limb.[293] Future studies are recommended to investigate if combined local $VEGF_{165}$ and angiopoietin-2 protein or gene therapy will synergistically increase capillary and arteriole density, resulting in maximizing skin viability in random-pattern skin flaps.

In the case of ischemia–reperfusion injury in free flap surgery, future studies are required to understand the mechanism of preischemic and postischemic conditioning in protecting skeletal muscle and skin against ischemia–reperfusion injury in laboratory animals. This probably will include studying the role of inflammation, Na^+/H^+ exchanger, mitochondrial free Ca^{2+} content, and opening of the mPTP in the pathogenesis of ischemia–reperfusion injury. This area of research will most likely lead to the identification of pharmacological agents for protection of skin and skeletal muscle from ischemia–reperfusion injury when given either before or after ischemia. Further studies are also recommended to investigate the additive effect of combined preischemic and postischemic pharmacological conditioning in protection of skin and skeletal muscle from ischemia–reperfusion injury. Last but not least, the published human skeletal strip culture technique[62] is recommended for scanning drugs for clinical studies of preischemic and postischemic pharmacological conditioning of skeletal muscle against ischemia–reperfusion injury.

Acknowledgments

The authors thank Dianne McIntyre and Luke Itani for performing the word processing and drawing the figures, respectively, for this manuscript. Cho Y Pang is the principal investigator of operating grants from the Canadian Institutes of Health Research (MOP 81149 and MOP 82833).

Access the complete references list online at **http://www.expertconsult.com**

3. Daniel RK, Kerrigan CL. Principles and Physiology of Skin Flap Surgery. In: McCarthy JG, ed. *Plastic Surgery*. Philadelphia: WB Saunders; 1990.

46. Baxter GF. The neutrophil as a mediator of myocardial ischemia-reperfusion injury: time to move on. *Basic Res Cardiol*. 2002;97:268–275.

Due to its ubiquity in toxicity in the context of reperfusion, the neutrophil has long been thought to play a key role in ischemia–reperfusion tissue damage. A thorough review is presented to demonstrate that this supposition is not as grounded in the literature as it may initially seem.

62. Martou G, O'Blenes CA, Huang N, et al. Development of an in vitro model for study of the efficacy of ischemic preconditioning in human skeletal muscle against ischemia-reperfusion injury. *J Appl Physiol*. 2006;101:1335–1342.

Ischemic preconditioning has been shown to improve tolerance to ischemia in animal models. This study demonstrates a protective effect of hypoxic preconditioning on human skeletal muscle exposed to reperfusion conditions.

145. Callegari PR, Taylor GI, Caddy CM, et al. An anatomic review of the delay phenomenon: I. Experimental studies. *Plast Reconstr Surg*. 1992;89:397–407; discussion 417–8.

This paper presents an elegant series of experiments demonstrating the arterial basis for the delay phenomenon. Subjects ranging from tissue expansion as delay phenomenon to details of delay technique are addressed.

151. Lineaweaver WC, Lei MP, Mustain W, et al. Vascular endothelium growth factor, surgical delay, and skin flap survival. *Ann Surg*. 2004;239:866–873; discussion 873–5.

It has previously been demonstrated that VEGF administration enhances skin flap survival in an animal model. VEGF is implicated as a possible mediator of pharmacologic delay in this study, which shows surgical delay to increase VEGF expression and skin flap survival.

217. Huang N, Khan A, Ashrafpour H, et al. Efficacy and mechanism of adenovirus-mediated VEGF-165 gene therapy for augmentation of skin flap viability. *Am J Physiol Heart Circ Physiol*. 2006;291:H127–H137.

277. Addison PD, Neligan PC, Ashrafpour H, et al. Noninvasive remote ischemic preconditioning for global protection of skeletal muscle against infarction. *Am J Physiol Heart Circ Physiol*. 2003;285:H1435–H1443.

This animal study demonstrates that tourniquet-based ischemic preconditioning protects against distal muscle against infarction. Direct antagonism was employed to implicate opioid receptor activation as a mechanism for this phenomenon.

279. Moses MA, Addison PD, Neligan PC, et al. Inducing late phase of infarct protection in skeletal muscle by remote preconditioning: efficacy and mechanism. *Am J Physiol Regul Integr Comp Physiol*. 2005;289:R1609–R1617.

287. McAllister SE, Ashrafpour H, Cahoon N, et al. Postconditioning for salvage of ischemic skeletal muscle from reperfusion injury: efficacy and mechanism. *Am J Physiol Regul Integr Comp Physiol*. 2008;295:R681–R689.

292. McAllister SE, Moses MA, Jindal K, et al. Na+/H+ exchange inhibitor cariporide attenuates skeletal muscle infarction when administered before ischemia or reperfusion. *J Appl Physiol*. 2009;106:20–28.

26

Principles and techniques of microvascular surgery

Fu-Chan Wei and Sherilyn Keng Lin Tay

SYNOPSIS

- Microvascular surgery refers to the surgical coaptation of small vessels usually less than 3 mm in diameter.
- This technique has evolved significantly over the last four decades, starting from replantations and revascularizations to free-flap surgery.
- The operating microscope and the development of loupes, microinstruments, and microsutures have greatly aided its widespread use.
- Various techniques have been developed for the handling of small vessels. There are several ways in which the anastomosis can be performed after careful vessel preparation. The most commonly used techniques are the end-to-end, end-to-side and the use of the anastomotic coupling devices.
- Difficult situations such as vessel diameter discrepancy and poor vessel quality with atherosclerotic plaques and loose intima can usually be overcome with special techniques. Inadequate vessel length can be managed with microvascular grafts.
- While previously considered only when simpler methods of reconstruction were unfeasible, free tissue transfers have become commonplace and are now first-line options for single-stage reconstruction, with superior functional and aesthetic outcomes.
- The disadvantages of microsurgery include the steep learning curve, lengthy operative times, and the need for technical expertise and specially trained personnel.
- In free-flap surgery, indications, contraindications, and timing are critical. Good preoperative planning is required, including the selection of the appropriate flap and recipient vessels.
- Experience is vital in postoperative monitoring of free flaps; early detection of a failing free flap with prompt intervention greatly improves the salvage rates.

- The majority of complications are related to vascular compromise and many relate to pedicle thrombosis due to kinking, compression, or technical error.
- Early detection and prompt surgical exploration are mandatory if vascular compromise is suspected. Pharmacological agents such as aspirin, heparin, and dextran are also useful adjuncts.
- Despite the improvements in techniques and postoperative care, flap failure rates remain around 3%. Managing these cases can be one of the most challenging aspects of reconstructive microsurgery.
- Microsurgery has indeed revolutionized our approach to reconstructive challenges. With further refinements, we will see an even wider application, particularly in the fields of supramicrosurgery, freestyle free flaps, composite tissue allotransplantation, and tissue engineering.

 Access the Historical Perspective section online at **http://www.expertconsult.com**

Introduction

Microsurgery refers to surgery that takes place under microscope magnification. Within the field of plastic surgery, it encompasses microvascular, microneural, microlymphatic, and microtubular surgery. Specifically, microvascular surgery refers to the surgical coaptation of small vessels performed under magnification and illumination. In a clinical setting, it is often used synonymously with the term "reconstructive microsurgery," and is implied in replantations and free tissue transplantations.

The introduction of the operating microscope in 1960 heralded the beginnings of the era of microsurgical reconstruction and it is generally used with vessels which are 3 mm or less in diameter in conjunction with specially designed fine instrumentation and microsutures. As an alternative, surgical loupes with magnifications of 2.5×–8× can be used.

Over the last four decades, microvascular surgery has become an indispensable tool for the reconstruction of complex defects. While previously considered only when simpler methods of reconstruction were unfeasible, free tissue transfers have become commonplace and are now being considered as a first-line option to provide superior outcomes, both functionally and aesthetically. Other benefits include time effectiveness and better economy in breast, head and neck, and extremities reconstruction, with even psychological advantages.

There are, of course, also disadvantages of microsurgery, including the steep learning curve, lengthy operative times, need for special resources, technical expertise, and considerable investment in instruments and specially trained personnel. Despite improvements in techniques and postoperative care, there is a small but not insignificant risk of flap failures of 2–3% even in the best surgical units.

This chapter details the tools and techniques used to maximize microvascular surgical outcome. Also discussed are the principles of microvascular surgery particularly with respect to free-flap surgery, options available when failure occurs, and the future of microvascular surgery. Replantations are highlighted in a separate chapter.

Tools

Since the introduction of vessel repair by Carrel, the diameter of vessels that can be anastomosed has become progressively smaller, due largely to developments in surgical techniques, surgical instrumentation and microsutures, and improved optics in present-day microscopes.

Magnification under adequate illumination allows more accurate perception of operative anatomy and positioning of instrumentation, with improved outcomes and facilitation of procedures that would be impossible to undertake without assisted vision.

Intraoperative magnification also reduces surgeons' fatigue as a result of improved ergonomics. Two types of optical system are used by surgeons to produce magnification – the surgical microscope and loupes.

Surgical microscopes

The modern operating microscope, with its refined optics, provides up to 40× magnification with a variable working distance. Zoom and focus can be adjusted with a foot control panel, although newer models have the controls in the handles used to adjust the position and angle of the scope. When using the microscope, choosing the appropriate level of magnification is important in order to maneuver the instruments and perform the anastomosis efficiently. Low magnification (6×–12×) can be used for vessel preparation and suture tying while middle magnification (19×–15×) can be used for suture placement. High magnification is usually only required for very small vessel anastomosis and inspection of the anastomosis. A further advantage over loupes is that the surgeon and assistant can view the same field and most operating microscopes can be attached to an external monitor for wider audience viewing and teaching and recording purposes.

Unfortunately however, the microscope is big and clumsy with space requirements which often restrict the surgeon's choice of positioning. Ceiling-mounted microscopes require less space but are confined to a single operating room and are often impractical in busy centers. For tips for use, see *Box 26.1*.

Loupes

Loupes can provide magnifications of 2.5×–8× and may be mounted on glasses or headbands. They are cost-effective, portable, and offer operator freedom.[23] They enhance visualization of the anatomy, allowing precise dissection of tissues and placement of instruments and sutures. In experienced hands, high-magnification loupes can even provide an effective alternative to the operating microscope for vessels as small as 1 mm. A retrospective study of 200 consecutive free microvascular tissue transplantations compared the performance of free tissue transplants with 3.5× loupes and the operating microscope.[20] There was no difference in outcome between the two groups, with free-flap success rates of 99% for both the loupe and the microscope groups. However, microscopes were required when performing anastomoses in children and on vessels of 1.5 mm or less in diameter. Despite these studies, most centers still use the microscope for its greater range of magnification and light sources. This is particularly important for smaller-vessel anastomoses in the era of perforator flap, freestyle, and supramicrosurgery practice.

Types

Two types of loupe are used in surgery: the compound (galilean) and prismatic loupe. In contrast to single-lens off-the-shelf magnifying reading glasses, compound loupes have significantly superior optics. These consist of two magnifying lenses separated by air, achieving higher magnification, greater depth of field, and better working distance. However, image quality tends to become distorted at magnifications above 2.5× and all such lenses create a "halo" effect at the periphery of the visual field which may disturb the surgeon. These drawbacks are counterbalanced by their relatively low cost and light weight and they are widely used and available from most manufacturers.[24]

Prismatic loupes provide higher optical quality because of a Schmidt prism, which lengthens the path of light through a series of mirror reflections inside the loupe. They can provide improved magnification, wider fields of view, and longer depths of field or working distance, but are 30–40% heavier, more expensive than compound loupes, and more easily damaged.[24]

Choosing loupes

While choice of magnification is largely dependent on the surgeon's preference, as a rough guide, a 2.5× magnification is often sufficient for hand surgery and flap harvesting. If the loupes are to be used for perforator dissection or anastomoses, 3.5–4.5× magnifications may be more suitable. It is important to note that both the field of view and depth of field decrease with increasing magnification, while the weight of the loupes increases. Loupes with a magnification higher than 4.5× tend to be cumbersome and too heavy for daily use (especially if they are prismatic), resulting in neck tension and increased fatigue. In such instances, opting for the microscope might be a better option.

Once the magnification has been chosen, other features such as lens design, working angle, and distances need to be considered. Some might choose to have the loupes mounted on glasses or headbands, while others might prefer through-the-lens (loupes mounted to the lenses of the frames) over the flip-up or snap-fit type. The latter permits cheaper changing of the magnification and the ability to change the lens prescription more conveniently. Some manufacturers can also supply headlights for use where additional lighting may be required – particularly useful with the use of higher magnifications.

Microsurgical instruments

Even with excellent optical systems, it would not have been possible for microsurgical techniques to have evolved without parallel refinements in microsurgical instruments and suture materials. Many fine instruments have been available for many years from jewelers but most have been developed during research on vascular, lymphatic, and neural microsurgery. A confusing array of instruments and supplies for microsurgery is now available, but with experience, most microsurgery can be done with surprisingly few instruments and most surgeons will become proficient with a reasonably small set.

Essential features in all microsurgical instruments include fine tips to spread, hold, or cut delicate tissue and suture, a nonreflective surface and comfortable handles that close easily to prevent fatigue.[25] Many of the instruments used in microvascular surgery will also be spring-loaded, and choosing the right spring tension is important – too weak and the tips will close all the way just by holding the instrument; too firm and your hand will fatigue after a short period of use.

Most microinstruments are made of heat-hardened stainless steel, which is more resistant to wear and tear. They are prone to magnetization and should be stored on demagnetized or nonmagnetic shelves. If an instrument becomes magnetized, placing it in a coil demagnetizer attached to a regular alternating current supply and withdrawing it slowly will help. Antimagnetic materials such as titanium are becoming popular, promising to be rust-free and lighter in weight. In reality, however, they too can become magnetized. Most microinstruments are available with a round or flat handle, and range from 10–18 cm in length depending on surgeon preference and depth of working field. In general, shorter instruments are used when the anastomosis is closer to the surface, for example, in hand surgery, while instruments longer than 18 cm are used for procedures involving free tissue transfer. Longer instruments may also be balanced such that the balance point rests in the webspace. The slight counterweight at the end of the instrument reduces fatigue and allows better control and precision.

All instrument manufacturers give instructions for maintenance, and it is extremely important to follow these instructions to ensure maximal performance of the microinstruments. It is advisable to store the microinstruments in specially designed instrument cases and to protect their fine tips with silicone or rubber tubes. To be effective, they need to be fine-tipped with the jaws meeting precisely. The user should therefore minimize damaging them by not using them for anything other than handling vessels and nerves. Blood and contaminants should be regularly cleaned off by the scrub nurse during the course of surgery and finally rinsed with distilled or deionized water to avoid staining of the instruments. High chloride concentrations should be avoided as they lead to pitting and corrosion.

Types

Scissors

Microvascular scissors should be spring-loaded with sharp but gently curved blades and slightly rounded tips. When held closed, they can be used safely as a dissecting probe without the danger of damaging the vessel. Those designed for trimming the adventitia off the vessel end have straight blades with sharp tips and are also good for stitch-cutting.

Needle holders

Spring-loaded microvascular needle holders are held like pencils, resting on the first web. The handle is ideally rounded to allow the instrument to be rolled between the index and middle fingers and the thumb during the passing of the needle. Flat handles are also available. The jaws should be thin and gently curved with narrow shoulders to be able to grasp the microsutures. Some needle holders come with a ratchet lock to facilitate the parking and passing of the needle; however, in inexperienced hands, the locking and locking maneuvers easily damage the needle and can cause significant trauma to the tissues handled.

Forceps

The jeweler's forceps were originally designed by the Swiss Dumont factory and is characterized by a flat handle and sharply narrowing tips. These tips must be aligned with a precision of 1/1000 inch, the diameter of the 10-0 nylon. When closed with moderate pressure, the jaws should meet evenly over a length of 3 mm so that the suture can be easily handled. They are further classified by the width of the contact surface, the narrowness, and the overall configuration. No. 2 forceps has wide jaws and can be used as needle holders. No. 3 forceps is straight and fine-pointed and no. 5 forceps has very fine tips. These are suitable for tissue handling and thus are commonly used in microsurgery. They are used almost continually in the nondominant hand for tissue handling, receiving the needle, and suture tying. No. 7 forceps has curved jaws. Microforceps are also available with round handles, although the flat handle is the preferred style. The most commonly used forceps are smooth-tipped, but the forceps can also be toothed, curved, angled, or equipped with a hole in the tip for better grasping. The angled forceps allows a grip that is parallel or perpendicular to the working surface and is useful for reaching under vessels, tying knots, and performing patency tests. A modified jeweler's forceps with a slender, smoothly polished nontapering tip can be used to dilate vessels gently.

Vascular clamps

The vascular clamps that are commonly used today have evolved significantly since the bulldog clamps that Jacobson used in his historical first microanastomoses, and many of the earlier models are now obsolete. The clamps developed by Henderson et al.[26] in 1970 required a small key and screw mechanism for adjustments and were not suitable for vessels less than 1.5 mm. In 1974, Acland[27] developed a double microvascular clamp with a small wire frame and a stay suture-holding device. Although it is still available today, it has largely been superseded by modifications of the design by Tamai[28] with the two clamps incorporated into a sliding bar.

Clamps are ideally atraumatic and have sufficient closing pressure to prevent bleeding and slippage but not damage the vessel wall. They are available as single clamps or double approximator clamps. In general, clamps are divided into those used on veins or arteries. Those designed for veins have a smaller closing pressure and usually a flat jaw all the way to the end. Those designed for arteries have greater closing pressure with a slight incurve at its tip to prevent crushing of the vessel wall. Generally, clamps marked with a V may be used for veins and most arteries, although particularly thick-walled veins may require the use of clamps marked with A.

To optimize closing pressure, clamps are available in a variety of sizes for different vessel diameters (i.e., the external diameter of the vessel in the natural state of full dilation). Pressure is inversely proportional to the vessel size – the smaller the vessel inside the clamp, the higher the pressure exerted on the vessel by the clamp. Ideally, a clamp exerts a pressure of 5–10 g/mm^2 and 15–20 g/mm^2 when used on the largest and smallest vessels in its size range, respectively. Where possible, use the smallest appropriate clamp to minimize crushing the vessel with too large a clamp. Although they can be applied by hand or artery forceps, special clamp applicators for the smaller clamps are available to ensure the accurate placement and removal of the clamps without damaging the vessels and to the calibration.

Bipolar coagulator

The development of the bipolar coagulator in 1956 promoted further development of microsurgery because a completely bloodless field was now attainable. The bipolar coagulator conducts current between the tips of the jeweler's forceps, producing heat damage only within a very small area between the instrument tips, allowing precise coagulation of small branches as close

as 2 mm to the main vessel in place of vascular clamps.[29,30] Its power setting must be optimized as too much power results in spreading of the heat with inadvertent damage to the surrounding tissues. Some surgeons prefer to use this for dissection instead of a knife or scissors, and bipolar scissors are now commercially available.

Irrigation and suction

Having a clear view of the vessel walls is imperative for successful anastomosis and even a small amount of blood may obscure the field. Constant irrigation with Ringer's lactate or heparinized saline and the use of suction are useful.[31–33] Irrigation serves several purposes: to prevent desiccation of vessels, sticking of suture to tissue, to wash away blood and clots to provide a good view, and to wash away any prothrombotic factors that might act as a nidus for thrombus formation and to improve patency.[34–36] This may be performed through a continuous irrigation system[37] with a smooth and blunt irrigation tip or more simply with a 5–10-mL syringe and a lacrimal cannula or 24-gauge angiocath.

There have been many suggested ways of suction, varying from suction through small segments of moistened hydrocellulose sponge or gauze, to suction tubes that drain through a perforated background plate and to homemade suction tips with an intravascular catheter attached to a 10-mL syringe placed over the normal suction tubing.[38] On occasion, when there is only a small amount of ooze, cellulose spearheads (eye sponges) on a polypropylene handle afford precise control and immediate absorption.

Anastomotic devices

Microsutures

Buncke[39] described making his first microneedle by drilling a hole in a 75-mm stainless steel wire. This needle held a single strand of silk and was used to replant a rabbit's ear by anastomosis of 1-mm vessels. Soon a commercially available needle was developed by Acland,[40] working with the Springler-Tritt company.

Since then, microsurgical sutures have been available in combinations of different materials, suture sizes (8-0 to 12-0), tensile strengths, and needle configurations.

The microsuture is considered to be the standard means of vascular anastomosis. The most widely used sutures are 9-0 monofilament nylon on a 100-μm curved needle and 10-0 nylon on a 75-μm needle. The choice is usually made based on the vessel wall thickness and diameter, with 9-0 sutures used for vessels of 2 mm or more in diameter and 10-0 for those between 1 and 2 mm in diameter. Smaller suture–needle combinations are available but reserved for use by experienced microsurgeons with very fine instruments, for very distal fingertip replantations, anastomoses in small children, and in lymph vessel anastomosis. Microneedles are typically shaped as three-eighths of a circle but are also available as a half-circle or straight (rarely used now), with round, tapered, or spatula-shaped tips to prevent damage to the fragile vessel wall. The commonest suture used in microsurgery is nonresorbable nylon which has low tissue reactivity and knot-holding ability, although polypropylene is preferred by some as it slides and handles better within the tissue.

Anastomotic devices

Despite the fact that microsutures are nowadays relatively inexpensive, reliable, and readily available, they do not fully meet the criteria of an "ideal" anastomosis. Many nonsuture techniques have developed in the search for faster and less traumatic anastomosis.

In 1962, Nakayama et al.[41] introduced an anastomotic device consisting of two metallic rings and interlocking pins that remain in situ as a permanent implant. The Unilink system developed by Östrup and Berggren in 1986,[42] the 3M and ACE coupling devices that were adaptations of this ring–pin device, is currently marketed under the name microvascular anastomotic system. This system consists of two disposable rings made of high-density polyethylene with a series of six to eight evenly spaced 0.16-mm diameter stainless steel pins that are implanted with a reusable anastomotic instrument.

The ring–pin device is a simple, efficacious, and faster technique of anastomosis and has the added advantage of not disturbing the intima in the anastomosis. It is the most successful and commonly used coaptation device. It has yielded excellent patency rates of up to 100%, even in fields that have been previously irradiated.[43–45] The rings come in a variety of sizes from 1–4 mm in diameter, allowing the coaptation of vessels ranging from 0.8–4.5 mm with a maximal wall thickness of 0.5 mm, and the device is suitable for both end-to-end and end-to-side anastomosis. It is contraindicated in peripheral vascular disease, areas with ongoing radiation therapy, active infection, concurrent diabetes, and corticosteroid therapy.

In an experimental comparison of venous anastomosis with use of this device, the sleeve technique, and the standard end-to-end technique, patency rates were 100%, 80%, and 95%, respectively. In an analysis of 1000 consecutive venous anastomoses with this method in breast reconstruction, Jandali et al.[46] reported an anastomotic time of 2–6 minutes with a 99.4% patency rate. No total flap losses were encountered. It has also been used effectively in end-to-side anastomosis of veins in head and neck free-flap reconstruction, with 99–100% patency.[45,47] To resolve the problems of a permanent rigid ring, an absorbable anastomotic coupler was developed and has been used experimentally and clinically, achieving patency rates of 92.9–100%[48–50] and 95%, respectively.[51] The ring was completely absorbed at 70 days to 30 weeks after anastomosis. Although used mainly for venous anastomoses, the mechanical coupling device has been also been used successfully in performing arterial anastomoses, with up to 100% patency rate,[52–55] proving to be expeditious, safe, and reliable. Contraindications of using this device on arterial anastomosis include thick-walled vessels that do not adequately evert, diameter discrepancies of more than 1.5:1 ratio, nonpliable vessels stiffened by prior radiotherapy or calcification, and any artery less than 1.5 mm in diameter.[52]

The nonpenetrating microvascular stapler, available as a disposable device (VCS clip applier system), reported by Kirsch et al.,[56] uses nonpenetrating titanium clips applied in an interrupted, everting fashion. The clips come in four sizes, ranging from 0.9 to 3.0 mm, and demonstrate a reduced anastomotic time and higher patency rate. In an end-to-end anastomosis, two stay sutures are first placed at 180° degrees to facilitate the eversion of vessel walls during clip placement and a special everting forceps and experienced assistant are needed. In an end-to-side anastomosis, four sutures are recommended with sutures at the heel and toe and two stay sutures at the 3 and 9 o'clock positions. Yamamoto et al.[57] reported clinical use of these staples with a mean anastomosis time of 12 minutes and Cope *et al.*[58] reported a 100% patency rate of 153 anastomoses of both veins and arteries. A comparative scanning electron microscopic study demonstrated no major differences between sutured and stapled anastomoses.[59]

All anastomotic devices are essentially for use on healthy vessels only; the veins should be pliable, the arteries soft to allow eversion,[44] and the vessel ends minimally size-discrepant.

Other nonsuture methods

Methods to glue or to weld a union of two vessels seem attractive and have been intensively studied experimentally.

Two adhesives have been studied for use in anastomoses: fibrin glues, and cyanoacrylate glues. To prevent the glue entering the vessel lumen, it was essential first to approximate the vessel walls with conventional sutures, thereby reducing the total number of sutures required for an adequate seal. Fibrin glue is now commercially available as two components, one with fibrinogen, factor XIII, and plasma proteins and a second with thrombin, aprotinin, and calcium chloride. When mixed together, it imitates the final pathway in coagulation. Fibrin glue has been used to seal anastomoses, both experimentally[60] and clinically.[61,62] In a comparative study of fibrin glue in free flaps,[63] the application of fibrin glue reduced the number of sutures required to complete the anastomosis and significantly reduced the anastomotic, but not ischemic, times with a slightly lower survival rate in the suture-only group. Although these demonstrate a faster union without compromising patency rate,[62,63] fibrin has not achieved clinical popularity, partly because of concerns that glue might inadvertently enter the vessel lumen, and the potential allergic reactions and anaphylaxis.[64–66] Cyanoacrylates have been used experimentally, but have been plagued by findings of histotoxicity,[67] marked foreign-body granulomatous response, extreme thinning of the vessel wall, splitting of the elastic lamina, and calcification of the media.[68,69] 2-Octyl-cyanoacrylate, however, might be less toxic.[70,71]

Welding with thermal[72,73] or laser[74] energy has long been advocated but, despite intensive experimental investigation, its clinical application remains scarce. There are no clinical reports of thermal welding to date.

Different laser types (neodymium : yttrium-aluminum-garnet,[74] carbon dioxide,[75,76] argon and, most recently, diode lasers[77,78]) have been used, showing up to 100% patency rates and better blood flow in veins when compared to conventional suturing techniques. Laser-activated protein solders have been introduced to achieve more strength.[79] In an experimental setting, a diode laser-assisted carotid artery end-to-end micro-anastomosis provided an equal survival rate as a contralateral suture anastomosis, with a shorter anastomosis time, and scanning electron microscopy showed faster healing on the laser side.[78,80] Although later studies have shown promising results on tensile strength, the fear of possible weakening at the site of the anastomosis with consequent pseudoaneurysm formation has so far prevented the clinical use of laser welding. In a study of 27 patients with laser-assisted microvascular anastomosis, there was a 96.6% overall success rate with one rupture of the arterial anastomosis and three hematomas requiring surgical evacuation.[81]

Other experimentally studied methods of anastomosis have included cylindrical or T-shaped intravascular stents.[82,83] An external metallic ring has been suggested to keep the cylindrical form of a sutured anastomosis and to avoid through-stitching.[84–86]

General principles of microvascular surgery

Having discussed the tools necessary for micro-surgery, there are a few principles and requirements that are critical to ensure a successful outcome. After all, and despite all its advances, clinical success in microsurgery relies ultimately on attention to detail, good decision-making, and technical skill in vessel anastomosis.

Basics

The prerequisites of good microsurgical work are a calm disposition and patience. The surgeon must be able to concentrate on the procedure without unnecessary interruptions and should not be hurried. It is inadvisable to work too long at a stretch and it is perfectly justifiable to take a break during long sessions under the microscope or when using surgical loupes. Undoubtedly, the presence of a competent assistant and a knowledgeable specialized scrub nurse makes a big difference to the speed and ease of the operation.

While some have the natural ability and dexterity for the fine movements requisite of a microsurgeon, training and practice will go a long way to refine technique. Because of the inherent complexity and the increased dexterity and hand–eye coordination required, the traditional apprenticeship model of surgical training cannot be as readily applied to microsurgery. Although trainees can learn the techniques from senior surgeons in a clinical setting, training should ideally begin in the laboratory,[87,88] with novices starting by familiarizing themselves with instrument handling under magnification, progressing from suturing stretched surgical gloves[89] or silicone tubes[90] and then to live anastomoses in a rat model.[91–94] Only when trainees have achieved patency in arterial anastomoses should they go on to venous anastomoses.

Planning and positioning

In surgery, time spent planning and positioning is never wasted and this is especially true for microsurgery. In the right position, movements will be easier and the procedure will progress faster. It is important to be comfortable as comfort often relates directly to success,[29] while poor planning and positioning result in fatigue, frustration, and even failure.

Choosing the right incisions and the right positioning of the patient becomes easier with experience. A two-team approach can reduce the operating time and proper patient positioning alleviates the need to reposition the patient during surgery.

The surgeon should position him- or herself comfortably. If seated, preferably on a self-adjustable stool, legs should be under the operating table with feet flat on the ground. This provides a stable base that can be maintained for prolonged periods of time. The forearms should rest on folded drapes such that they are approximately at the same level as the anastomosis. These small details will minimize tremor and fatigue.

Next the microscope should be positioned so that it does not obstruct movement, while providing maximum control and maneuverability. However, the location of the anastomosis often dictates where the microscope is ultimately placed. The microscope base is then fixed to

allow the surgeon sufficient room to maneuver the microscope into the exact position.

Securing the flap or flap inset

The inset of the flap should be considered before the anastomosis is performed. After circulation is restored, the flap swells and bleeds from the edges and this can make insetting the flap in deep recesses particularly difficult. This is especially true in head and neck surgery where the flap may be required in tight, hard-to-reach areas with limited visibility. The inset should be performed first, ensuring that good hemostasis has been achieved before the pedicle is divided after flap harvest. Partial or complete inset of the flap before the anastomosis also allows for a more accurate judgment of pedicle length, avoiding problems resulting from tension or redundancy. It also allows for tailoring and thinning of the flap in a bloodless field before circulation is restored. In some cases, such as in breast surgery, where the anastomosis lies deep to the inset, there is no choice but to inset the flap after the anastomosis is completed. In such instances, the flap is just secured near the defect, allowing adequate exposure and positioning of the vessels.

Choice and dissection of recipient vessels

Another important factor in ensuring success of free-flap surgery is the use of healthy recipient vessels of appropriate size with good outflow. Ideally they should be away from zones of trauma and sites of irradiation. A healthy vessel has a soft wall and a vascular sheath that can be easily dissected, while traumatized vessels may be encased in fibrotic tissue which is prone to bleeding during dissection. It is sometimes necessary to assess the presence and quality of the recipient vessels, particularly following lower extremity trauma or in patients with longstanding diabetes or atherosclerotic disease before flap harvest. Preoperative angiography is indicated when one or both pedal pulses is not palpable. However, it might not add relevant information if at least one pedal pulse is palpable,[95] and normal findings may not always translate into healthy usable vessels. When there is clinical suspicion of vessel damage, ankle/brachial pressure index, systolic toe pressure, and hand-held Doppler auscultation may determine the need for formal angiography. Other considerations in deciding which recipient vessels to use include a single-vessel leg, multiple previous free flaps, and the availability and adequacy of recipient veins.

Once the recipient vessel has been adequately exposed and identified, dissection of the vascular pedicle proceeds under loupe magnification to free sufficient length to allow a tension-free anastomosis. The total length of dissection ultimately depends upon the length of the chosen flap's pedicle, depth at which the recipient vessels are situated, the size of the vessels, and the technique of anastomosis to be used. Vein grafts have been shown to reduce success rates and can usually be avoided if proper preoperative planning has been made. If the recipient vessels are deep, a greater length of vessel needs to be dissected in order to orientate them in a more desirable position or even more superficially to allow an unobstructed view that will facilitate the anastomosis *(Fig. 26.1)*. Gross trimming of the adventitia is performed around the area of the anastomosis, allowing sufficient length of trimmed vessel for application of the vascular clamp. The quality of the artery and vein must then be checked. Under microscope magnification, the vessels are inspected for signs of damage that indicate the need for more proximal dissection.

It is vital to check the flow within the artery. Expansile pulsation of the vessel usually indicates adequacy but should be confirmed by healthy spurting from the divided vessel. If a healthy-looking vessel does not spurt well, check that the patient is normotensive. Steps to relieve vasospasm should be taken and are discussed later in this chapter. If there is still no relief, the vessel should be cut back until healthy spurting is encountered. Once this is confirmed, a vascular clip can be applied while waiting for the flap to be harvested or to be inset.

The ideal recipient vein should be at least as wide as the flap vein. If the recipient vein is smaller in diameter, it may produce a bottle-neck effect and compromise drainage of the flap. The vein is divided to assess its quality and good backflow from the vein indicates a fairly health vessel. If there is any doubt, a small catheter may be introduced into the lumen and heparinized saline flushed into the vein. If there is little or no resistance, the vein is likely to drain well. If high pressure is required to flush the vein, tying off tributaries near the site of anastomosis may help reduce the backflow. A

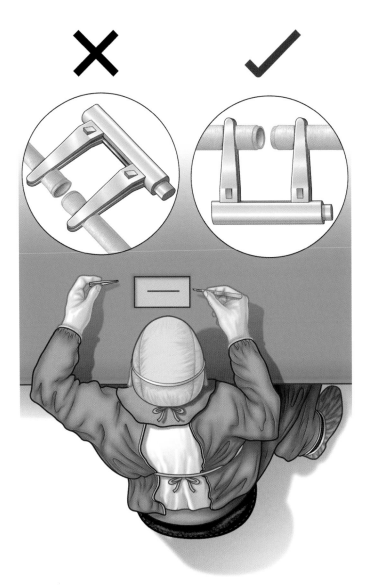

Fig. 26.1 Horizontal vessel orientation allows both lumens of the vessel to be adequately visualized.

single or double clamp is then applied in preparation for anastomosis.

The vessels should be irrigated during and after dissection with heparinized saline and, on completion of the dissection, it is common practice to cover the vessels with 2–4% lidocaine or 3% papaverine-soaked gauze pieces to prevent desiccation and vasospasm.

When the flap is ready for revascularization, the vessel ends to be anastomosed are placed in a double approximating clamp under microscope magnification. An appropriate-sized clamp is chosen to allow an

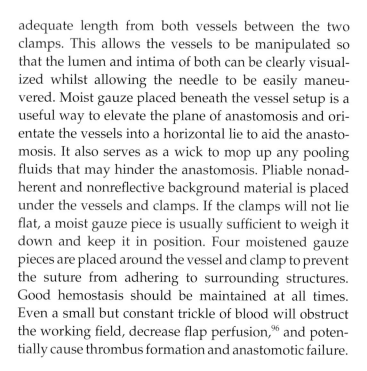

Friable walls

Separation of medial walls

Separation of intimal walls

Intraluminal valves, clots, flaps, tears

Branches near anastomosis

Fig. 26.2 Loose intima.

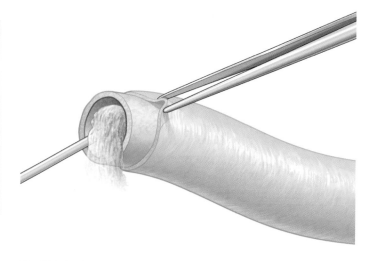

Fig. 26.3 Intraluminal irrigation of vessels.

adequate length from both vessels between the two clamps. This allows the vessels to be manipulated so that the lumen and intima of both can be clearly visualized whilst allowing the needle to be easily maneuvered. Moist gauze placed beneath the vessel setup is a useful way to elevate the plane of anastomosis and orientate the vessels into a horizontal lie to aid the anastomosis. It also serves as a wick to mop up any pooling fluids that may hinder the anastomosis. Pliable nonadherent and nonreflective background material is placed under the vessels and clamps. If the clamps will not lie flat, a moist gauze piece is usually sufficient to weigh it down and keep it in position. Four moistened gauze pieces are placed around the vessel and clamp to prevent the suture from adhering to surrounding structures. Good hemostasis should be maintained at all times. Even a small but constant trickle of blood will obstruct the working field, decrease flap perfusion,[96] and potentially cause thrombus formation and anastomotic failure.

Preparation of vessels

The lumens of the vessels must be inspected for irregularities such as intimal tears or separation from the media, thrombi, atherosclerotic plaques, and friable calcified walls *(Fig. 26.2)*. Any debris is gently irrigated away *(Fig. 26.3)* or atraumatically removed with microforceps. Failing this, the vessel should be cut back, without compromising the flap pedicle length, to attain a healthier vessel segment. Occasionally, a suboptimal

vessel intima has to be accepted and a successful outcome is then dependent on meticulous anastomotic technique. Some surgeons will choose to cut the vessel back to a healthy level at the expense of length, opting to use an interpositional vein graft in such situations since inadequate debridement of vessels is often a major cause of flap failure.

The vessel wall consists of three principal layers. The innermost tunica intima is formed by a single layer of endothelium resting on a basal lamina. External to this is a thin subendothelial layer consisting of connective tissue adjacent to the internal elastic lamina that separates the tunica intima from the tunica media. The tunica media consists mainly of smooth-muscle cells and is the thickest layer of the arterial wall. In veins, however, this layer is much thinner and, sometimes in lesser veins, almost indistinguishable. The tunica media is covered by the external elastic membrane, and the outermost layer of the vessel wall is the tunica adventitia. This comprises loose areolar connective tissue that contains the vasa vasorum, which nourishes the vessel wall.[97] Veins consist of the same layers as arteries, but the layers are less defined, particularly with regard to the tunica media which in some lesser veins is almost indistinguishable *(Fig. 26.4)*.

Loose adventitia can be peeled off the vessel wall using microforceps or sharply trimmed by pulling it towards the lumen and cutting parallel to the luminal edge *(Fig. 26.5)* to a distance of 3–4 mm from the anastomotic site. It has been shown that neither method

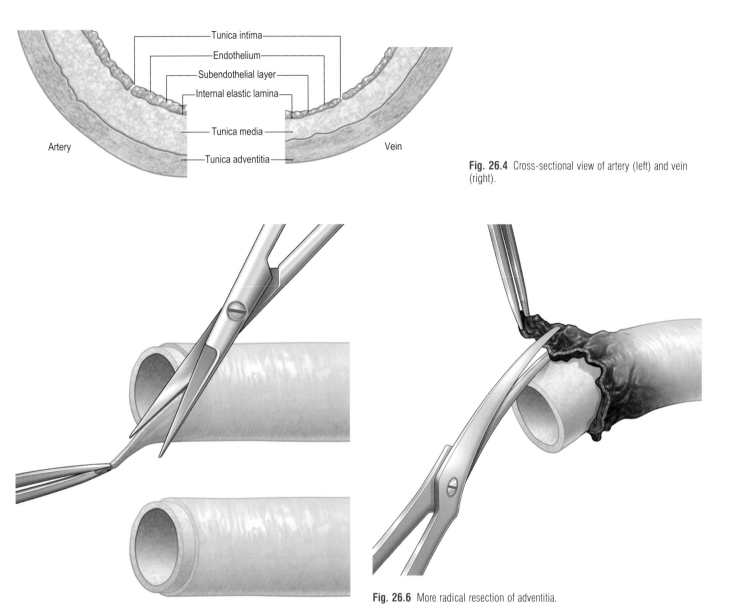

Fig. 26.4 Cross-sectional view of artery (left) and vein (right).

Tunica intima
Endothelium
Subendothelial layer
Internal elastic lamina
Tunica media
Tunica adventitia
Artery
Vein

Fig. 26.5 Sharp trimming of adventitia.

Fig. 26.6 More radical resection of adventitia.

completely removes all the adventitia and that sharp dissection appears to cause less damage to the vessel.[98,99] The main purpose is to improve visualization of the vessel ends and prevent the adventitia from falling into the lumen while tying the knot. Alternatively, a more radical trimming is performed by cutting the tented adventitia parallel to the length of the vessel, meticulously avoiding injuring the tunica media *(Fig. 26.6)*. Avoid overly aggressive adventitial stripping as this may cause necrosis of the vessel wall at the anastomotic site with resultant false aneurysms. In smaller veins

with thin tunica media, it is advisable to remove only the adventitia that overhangs the vessel ends.

The vessel lumens are gently dilated with a vessel dilator and the stretch maintained for a second *(Fig. 26.7)*. This will aid the suturing process, prevent vasospasm, and allow intraluminal blood to be flushed out with heparinized saline. Blood beyond the clamps, in undamaged vessels, is not in contact with wound thromboplastins and is not at risk of clotting. A hemostat artery forceps is used to bring the two clamps towards each other so that the vessel ends are just touching or with minimal overlap *(Fig. 26.8)*.

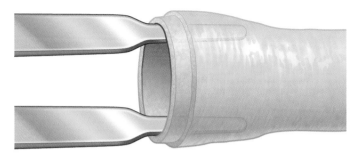

Fig. 26.7 Gentle luminal dilatation of the vessel end.

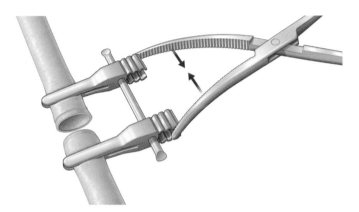

Fig. 26.8 Using artery forceps to bring the clamps together.

Anastomotic sequence

There is no consensus regarding optimal anastomotic sequence. In reality, the relative vessel position will dictate whether the artery or vein is first anastomosed, with the deeper, more-difficult-to-reach vessel being repaired first.

If the anatomy does not restrict the choice, arterial repair first may be a sensible choice as it will shorten the warm ischemia time. The re-establishment of circulation may also reveal the more dominant venous drainage and aid the selection of which donor vein to use. There are disadvantages, however, as the flap may start bleeding and affect the anastomosis of the vein. Subsequent venous congestion may increase bleeding from the flap edges and allow a buildup of free radicals. To avoid this, the artery may be left clamped proximal to the anastomosis (risking vessel injury from prolonged clamping) or the second vein may be intermittently released to allow drainage of the flap. Alternatively, the venous anastomosis could be performed first, which additionally allows for better adjustment of the pedicle

length, although this will delay revascularization of the flap.

An early experimental study showed that flap failure in straightforward cases was highest if the arterial anastomosis was performed first and immediately unclamped. This was attributed to venous congestion.[100] However other studies have failed to show an optimal sequence of anastomosis in both skin and muscle flaps.[101,102] In our practice of more than 800 free flaps per year, we routinely repair the artery first and leave it unclamped as the vein is being repaired and have not noticed major problems related to the temporary venous congestion. If there is a second comitant vein, however, we avoid venous congestion by allowing the less dominant vein to drain freely into gauze away from the operating field.

Some surgeons advocate two venous anastomoses where possible to avoid complications of venous insufficiency, and Khouri *et al.* reported a significantly higher failure rate when only one venous anastomosis was performed (4.3% versus 0% if two anastomoses).[103] A single venous anastomosis to a suitable recipient vein however will provide adequate drainage and reduce operative time without increasing morbidity. Futran and Stack showed equivalency of single and dual venous anastomosis with respect to flap survival in a series of 43 free radial forearm flaps.[104] This too is our clinical experience. Sound judgment is required and, if the first vein is less reliable or if its patency is uncertain, a second venous anastomosis should be performed to secure venous drainage of the flap.

Microvascular anastomosis techniques

Having discussed the general principles of setup, vessel preparation, and common pitfalls, this section now focuses on how these principles can be applied to the different anastomotic techniques to achieve success.

Suturing techniques

End-to-end anastomosis

The method of performing the anastomosis depends largely on personal preference. The end-to-end anastomosis using interrupted sutures is by far the most

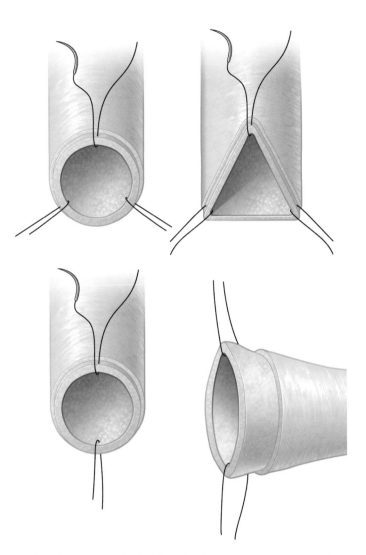

Fig. 26.9 Interrupted suturing techniques by placement of three stay sutures at 120° or at 180° to ease subsequent placement of sutures.

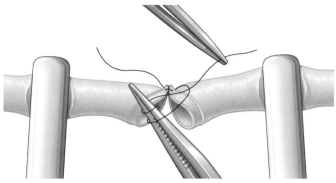

Fig. 26.10 Knot tying with a double throw.

common method used. It is simple and appropriate for most arterial and venous anastomoses. A halving, triangulation, or "back wall-up" technique can be used to perform this anastomosis *(Fig. 26.9)*.

Carrel recommended avoiding luminal narrowing at the anastomotic site, avoiding the creation of folds and a rough inner surface of the vessel, and opposing the two intimal edges closely. These principles still hold true today. In his original description,[104a] three stay sutures were placed at 120° from each other. Cobbett modified this, using only two stay sutures at 120° from each other, and found that, when tensioned apart, the longer back wall fell away from the shorter front wall and reduced the chance of taking a through stitch, where the intima of the posterior wall is incorporated into the

suture. Another alternative to this is placing the two stay sutures at 180° angle to ensure even spacing between the sutures.

The first two sutures are both the most important and the most difficult. The bite should incorporate all the layers of the vessel, especially including a good bite of the intima. The size of the bite is determined by the thickness of the wall and the suture and should be maintained throughout. The first throw should be a double one to ensure that it maintains the intended tension *(Fig. 26.10)*, and then two single throws follow to complete the knot. The knots are snugged down by sight and not by feel and should stop when the two vessel edges meet and slightly evert. If the sutures are too tight, small tears in the vessel wall may expose the subendothelium and allow platelet aggregation and thrombus formation.[105] Additionally, sutures that are too tight can damage the media of the arterial wall and if at least a third of the vessel wall undergoes necrosis, re-endothelialization does not occur and occlusion of the lumen invariably follows.[106,107]

Sutures are placed in between the stay sutures, aiming to place the smallest number of sutures to achieve a leakproof anastomosis, and the approximator clamp is turned over. The back wall can now be sutured by either placing a suture exactly midway between the two existing stay sutures or, with experience, sutures can be accurately placed to complete the anastomosis. As the anastomosis progresses, it becomes increasingly difficult to visualize the lumen and it is advisable to leave the last few stitches untied, leaving the ends loose until the last suture is placed. These sutures are then tied in turn. It is better to leave any apparent gaps alone until the clamp is released and the vessel refills in order to

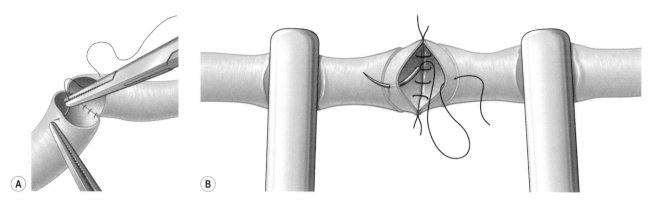

Fig. 26.11 (A, B) Placing a halving suture may facilitate accurate stitch placement when performing end-to-end anastamosis with interrupted suturing.

prevent through stitching. If the vessel configuration does not allow the clamp to be turned over, the back wall-up technique must be employed. The first suture is placed posterocentrally and subsequent sutures are placed on either side of the first knot, working around the circumference and spacing them appropriately apart. Once the back wall is completed, the anterior wall can be sutured using the interrupted, continuous, or open-loop suture techniques *(Figs 26.11, 26.12)*.

Continuous suturing is a technique suitable for minimally size-discrepant vessels larger than 2 or 3 mm and not only can significantly reduce anastomosis time by nearly half but is more hemostatic[108] *(Fig. 26.13A)*. However, there are problems with suture entanglement; the sutures must be placed meticulously and the final tying of the knot must be accurate to prevent purse-string constriction of the lumen. It is advisable to place two or three stay sutures, leaving one suture end long. Starting from the last stay suture, running sutures are placed at regular intervals and tied to the next stay suture. Then the needle is passed under the vessel and the double clamp turned over and suturing continued. This reduces the likelihood of creating a purse-string effect *(Figs 26.13B)*. With meticulous attention to detail, patency rates of 97.5–100% can be achieved[109–111] in both veins and arteries and end-to-end and end-to-side repairs.

Open-loop suturing is a technique that combines the convenience of the continuous running suture with the advantages of interrupted suturing technique. First a running suture is performed leaving the loops small enough that they do not flop to the side. Then the first suture is tied and the suture ends cut short. The next loop is pulled through and tied in a similar fashion until

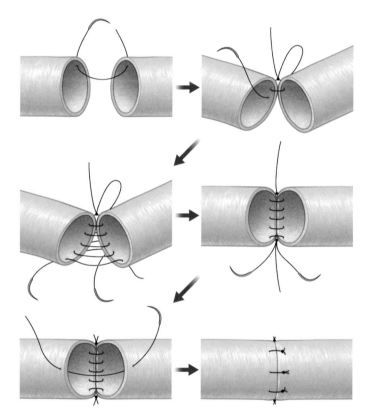

Fig. 26.12 Back wall first.

all the loops have been tied *(Fig. 26.14)*. This technique reduces the number of maneuvers and the need to handle the needle constantly after each suture. Maximal lumen visualization is maintained throughout and the risk of purse-stringing is eliminated. This method needs practice, however, as the loops can easily become entangled and time may be wasted untangling them.

Sleeve anastomosis, introduced by Lauritzen[112] in 1978, is a variant of the end-to-end technique, "end-in-end," and entails telescoping the vessels by using two extraluminal sutures that pull one vessel inside the other *(Fig. 26.15)*. Fewer sutures are required, resulting in reduced anastomosis time and less vessel trauma, but low patency rates reported by Sully *et al.*[113] prevented this technique from gaining popularity, despite contradictory results by others. The sleeve technique was suggested to be limited to vessels with size discrepancy. A modification of "hemi-invagination" by Riggio *et al.*[114] improved patency rates to 95–100% by placing a side cut on the overlapping vessel and adding a stitch at its apex, thus effectively dilating the vessel to facilitate anastomosis of vessels of equal size.

End-to-side

The end-to-side anastomosis is particularly useful when there is significant vessel size or wall thickness discrepancy[115] or when there is a need to preserve the distal circulation, as in a single-vessel leg.

In order to perform an end-to-side anastomosis, an arteriotomy or venotomy has to be made in the recipient vessel. This may be triangular or elliptical or a simple longitudinal slit that will open up due to contraction of the muscle in the vessel wall. The hole should not have irregular edges as this may weaken the wall and facilitate thrombus formation. A sufficient length of recipient vessel is dissected to allow placement of two clamps on either side of the anastomotic site and the adventitia trimmed nearly circumferentially between the two clamps. A baby Satinsky clamp is useful for clamping the recipient vessel to facilitate the anastomosis and is less traumatic than bulldog clamps. Alternatively, vascular slings may be double-looped around both ends and tightened to act as stabilizers and to cut off the blood flow to the segment of vessel. A single stitch is taken transversely at the anastomotic site and used as a stay suture. Holding this suture up, the vessel around the suture is excised using microvascular scissors and extended as necessary with a no. 11 blade *(Fig. 26.16)*. Alternatively, the Acland–Banis arteriotomy clamp can be used to pick up and hold part of the vessel wall that is to be excised. The blade is then held close against the clamp tip, allowing an ellipse to be excised. Ideally

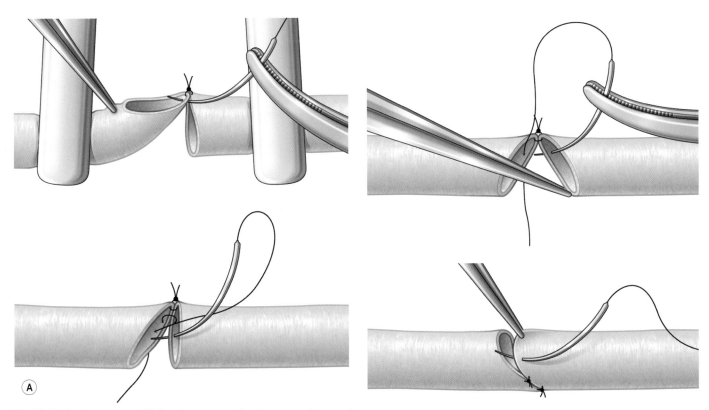

Fig. 26.13 Continuous suture. **(A)** Complete anastomosis using one continuous suture.

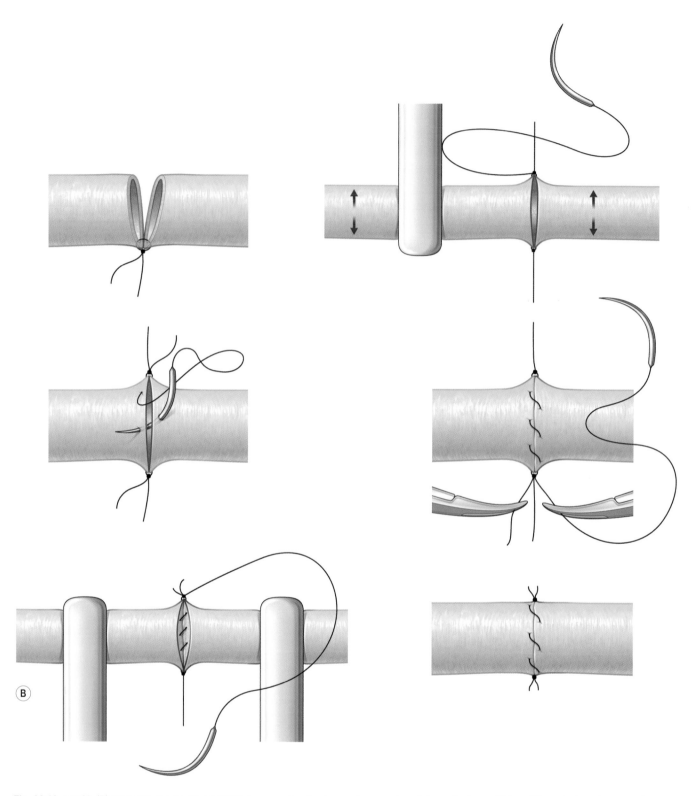

Fig. 26.13, cont'd (B) Using stay sutures placed at 180 degrees and performing continuous sutures between the two and tying off to each stay suture prevents purse-stringing of the lumen. (From Chen YX, Chen LE, Seaber AV, Urbaniak JR. Comparison of continuous and interrupted suture techniques in microvascular anastomosis. J Hand Surg Am 2001;26:530-539.)

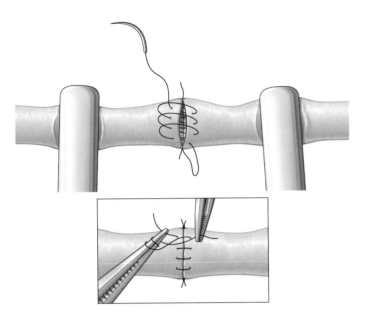

Fig. 26.14 Open-loop suture.

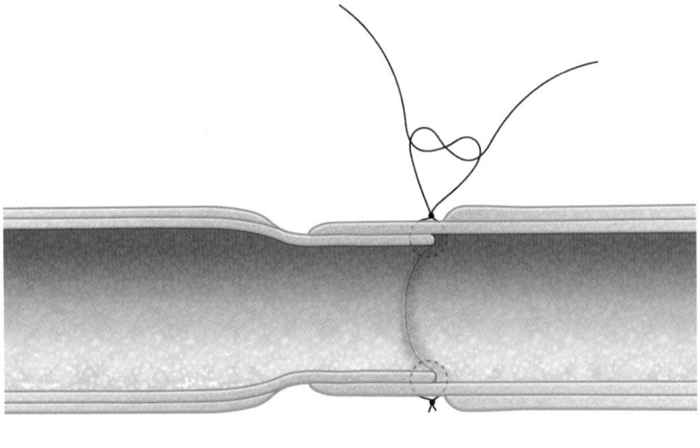

Fig. 26.15 Sleeve anastomosis.

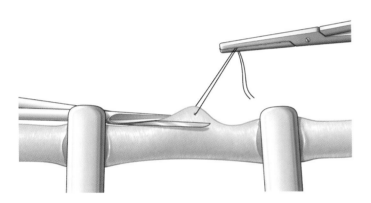

Fig. 26.16 End-to-side anastomosis. Making the arteriotomy.

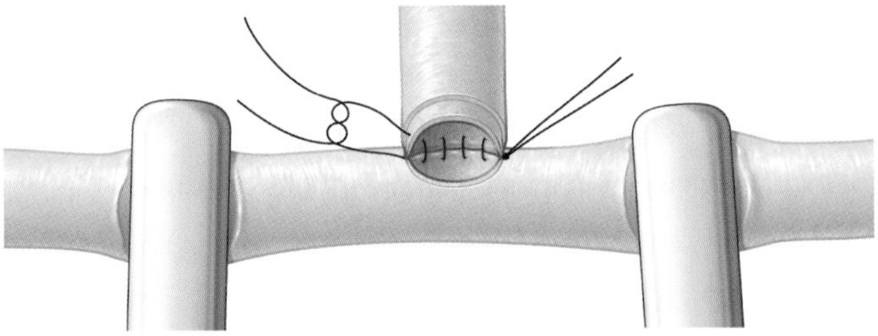

Fig. 26.17 End-to-side anastomosis. In cases where there is insufficient length to rotate the vessel, the back wall needs to be sutured first.

this opening should not be longer than the diameter of the donor vessel as it will stretch once the clamps are released.

If the flap vessel is long enough, the anastomosis can be performed with stay stitches at the distal and proximal ends of the arteriotomy and the "front" wall be completed before pulling the vessel towards you and performing the "back" wall. If there is insufficient length to manipulate the donor vessel, then the wall further from you must be performed first *(Fig. 26.17)*. The sutures are then placed radially to the center of the arteriotomy. Persistent leakage from the distal and proximal ends may be severe if the sutures are placed transversely.

According to Godina, the additional advantages of this anastomosis included a higher success rate, greater freedom of operative planning, and technical simplicity in terms of access to the vessels and it was his anastomotic technique of choice.[116] However, in a study of over 2000 microvascular anastomoses in more than 900 tissue transplants, end-to-end and end-to-side microvascular techniques were found to be equally effective when properly applied. Patency approached 100%.[117] Although arterial anastomosis patency was similar to end-to-end anastomosis, end-to-to side venous anastomosis had a higher success rate in a study of 90 rats.[118] In a further experimental study, while there were no differences in vessel patency between an end-to-side hole and an

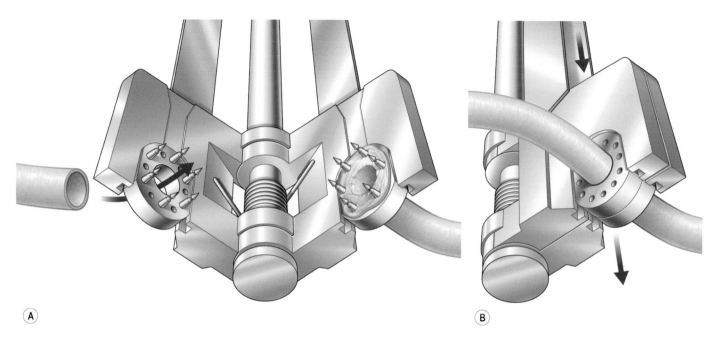

Fig. 26.18 Application of the coupler device. **(A)** The vessel is orientated at 90° to the applicator and the vessel end impaled evenly on the pins. **(B)** The vessel is anastomosed and released by turning the applicator handle.

end-to-side slit technique, the latter was easier to perform in vessels less than 1.5 mm in diameter.[119]

Use of the coupler

The use of the anastomotic coupling device is the most common alternative to the conventional suture. It is a time-saving alternative that consistently produces equivalent patency rates to conventional methods. The outer diameter of each vessel is measured after gentle dilatation against the vessel-measuring gauge. In size discrepancy vessels, a coupler is chosen such that the internal diameter of the device is the same as the measured outer diameter of the smaller vessel.

The coupling device is loaded on to the anastomotic instrument, ensuring that it is well seated. The anastomotic instrument is placed perpendicular to the vessels, and the vessel end threaded through the ring. The edges of the vessel are impaled securely on to the first pin, taking a bite that is approximately 1–2 pin diameters with an adequate intimal bite. The vessel is impaled on every other pin first before completing the intermediate pin placements to ensure it is evenly spaced. Draping the flap vessel first allows easier position of the coupler than the less mobile recipient vessel. The rings are then brought together by turning the applicator handle clockwise and reinforced using hemostat artery forceps. The applicator handle is turned counterclockwise to eject the device *(Fig. 26.18)*.

Difficult, less commonly encountered microvascular anastomosis

Anastomosis between size-discrepant vessels

Despite careful planning, size-discrepant vessels are commonly encountered. Fewer problems are encountered if the inflow from the recipient is small and the flap artery is big, or if the outflow of the flap is small and the recipient vein is large; however, the sudden change of caliber may still cause turbulence that predisposes to thrombosis. Various techniques are used to deal with this, and vessel mismatches of up to 4:1 can be safely anastomosed end-to-end. The simplest method is gently to stretch the smaller vessel mechanically to match the larger one, placing interrupted sutures further apart on the larger vessel. Alternatively, placing a fish-mouth incision or obliquely cutting the smaller vessel can reduce the discrepancy. Angles of more than 30° of the oblique cut may cause kinking, and should be avoided.

Another technique involves performing the anastomosis just distal to a side branch and opening up the distal wall so that the V shape of the branch is now the vessel end. When the discrepancy is greater than 3:1, consider an end-to-side anastomosis, a vein graft to graduate the discrepancy, or using a side branch of the larger vessel, which may be a better size match. As a last resort, the smaller vessel is dilated maximally and sutured as widely as possible to the larger vessel. The remaining vessel can be directly sutured to itself and an obliquely placed surgical clip will taper the vessel and minimize turbulence *(Fig. 26.19)*.

A discrepancy between the vessel walls may also be encountered but does not usually pose a problem. Gentle dilation will serve to thin the wall but if a significant discrepancy persists, the key is to take equal bites of the intima from both vessels, incorporating less of the media and adventitia of the thicker-walled vessel.

Vertically oriented anastomosis

This is the most challenging configuration of vessels. If possible, change the position of the body part, and adjust your position or table to make the anastomosis more horizontally oriented. Freeing up more of the vessel length will allow the vessel to be manipulated into a more horizontal plane using properly placed gauze pieces. If the position cannot be changed and there is limited space to rotate the vessel, reduce the magnification of the field as this would increase the depth of field, reducing the need to alter the focus of the microscope constantly on each vessel end.

Atherosclerosis and loose intima

Atherosclerotic vessels are commonly encountered given that free-flap surgery is increasingly extended to those with cardiac disease and the elderly. If a significant plaque is found, cutting back the vessel to healthier intima or even choosing another vessel altogether may be necessary. It is important to ensure that the inside of the vessel is clean and that there are no intimal flaps. The vascular clamp should not exert too much tension as this can fracture the calcified walls or plaques.

A round needle is useful and meticulous placement of interrupted sutures using the smallest microsuture should be ensured. The intima must be visualized at all times and the suture should ideally be passed from the

inside of the lumen of the atherosclerotic vessel to the outside to avoid further separation of the intima from the vessel wall. This is possible if only one vessel is diseased. But when both recipient and donor are diseased, a double-needle suture may be useful. If unavailable, then careful counterpressure from forceps placed within the vessel as the needle is passed will minimize intimal separation *(Fig. 26.20)*. Vessel dilation should be avoided and careful vessel wall eversion avoids leaving raw areas exposed to the blood flow. Too much tension, however, may erode the plaque and tear the vessel wall.

Microvascular grafts

An increased storehouse of flaps with various pedicle lengths, technical refinements, and proper planning has been key to diminishing the need for vein grafts.[18,120] Despite this, they are still sometimes necessary, particularly in the trauma setting. There is an association between interposition vein grafting and free-flap complication and failure[103,121,122]; however this may be a reflection of the complexity of the case and other factors such as vessel quality[123] and hematoma formation[124] that can independently lead to flap failure rather than the actual use of the vein grafts. Indeed, other studies have shown that patency and flap survival are not reduced by the use of vein grafts,[125,126] which can be performed quickly and safely if certain principles are followed.

The indications for vein grafts include a gap resulting from a short pedicle, tension at the site of anastomosis, considerable size mismatch, and the need to place the anastomosis outside the zone of injury. Occasionally the judicious use of a y-shaped vein graft will serve a further function of being able to restore circulation to the distal stump.[127]

The harvest of the graft is just as important as the subsequent anastomosis and should be done with loupe magnification. Ideally, the vein graft should match the caliber of the vessels to be anastomosed.[128] If possible, upper limb defects are bridged with upper limb veins. The cephalic and saphenous veins are by far the commonest source of vein grafts but may need predilatation to allow a better wall thickness match. If there is a concurrent lack of soft-tissue cover, a narrow venous flap for arterial gaps may solve both problems at once.[129] The vein should be handled minimally during the dissection

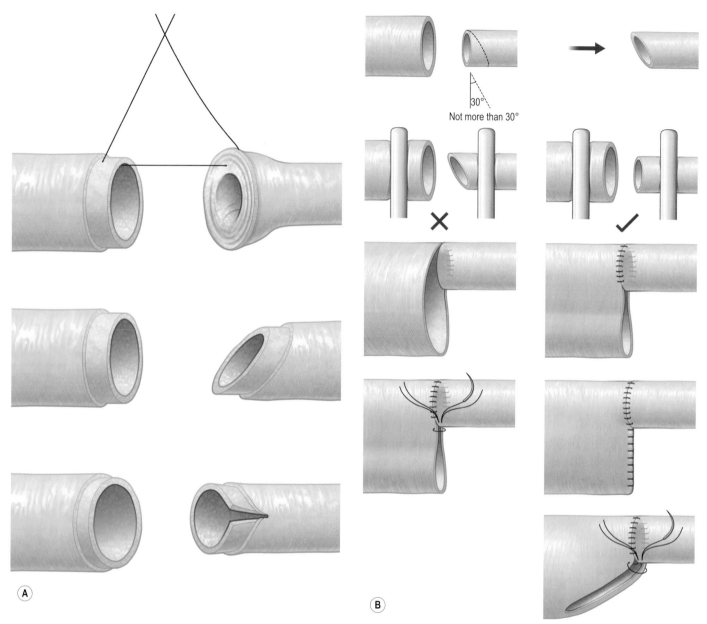

Fig. 26.19 Size-discrepant vessels. **(A)** The smaller vessel end can be dilated and stretched to match the larger one, cut obliquely to increase the diameter or a longitudinal side cut of the smaller vessel can be made. **(B)** The smaller vessel can be sutured as widely to as much of the larger vessel. A clip can be brought across obliquely to taper the remaining end of the larger vessel and may help to reduce turbulence.

and all tributaries ligated or coagulated. The length required should be marked out, remembering that vein grafts contract after division only to lengthen considerably, with the potential risk of kinking, after restoration of high-pressure flow.

Since even short segments of veins may contain valves, the direction of the vein is crucial and must always have antegrade flow. In our practice, the proximal end is marked with a surgical clip. This facilitates

hydrodilation of the vessel which stretches the graft out to length, untwists the vein, relieves vasospasm, and allows visualization of potential bleeding points. The open end is then anastomosed first and the clamp released for a final check that the direction is correct and the length not redundant.

Arterial grafts have significant advantages over vein grafts, such as the absence of valves, an anatomical taper, similar luminal and wall thickness profiles, and

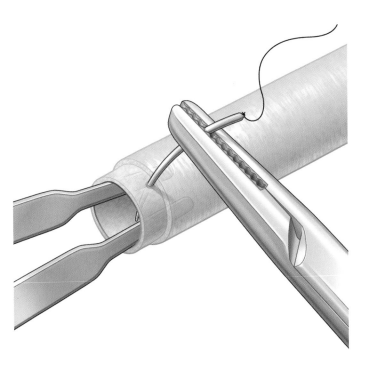

Fig. 26.20 Use of forceps to provide counterpressure to minimize trauma and separation of the intima.

better handling characteristics. Arterial grafts maintain their endothelium and have less subintimal hyperplasia. They also produce more prostacyclin relative to vein grafts in the first 3 weeks, resulting in greater antithrombogenic activity.[130] However they have not been shown to have significant advantages in the context of microvascular surgery.[131] They may be harvested from the subscapular tree,[132] anterior and posterior interosseous arteries,[133] radial or ulnar arteries, the deep or superficial inferior epigastric artery,[134] and the dorsalis pedis artery.

Testing patency

Patency should be assessed after the completion of each anastomosis and the flap assessed for adequate perfusion periodically through the operation. This can be done by simple observation or by conducting a patency test.

The characteristics of the arterial pulsation are important and can be expansile or longitudinal. The latter occurs in the long axis of the vessel and is a sign of partial or complete thrombosis. The flap will show no evidence of return of circulation and the anastomosis should be redone. Other signs of patency of the artery include good flow from the vein. If the recipient vein fills well and has a natural round diameter it is likely to be patent. If it is engorged and the blood column is darker than that in the recipient vessel, it is thrombosed and will require reanastomosis. Other signs of a nonpatent venous anastomosis will include engorgement of secondary veins within the flap, and continuous dark bleeding from the edges of the flap.

If in doubt, two simple tests can be performed distal to the anastomosis. The first is an "uplift" test by gently hooking up a thin-walled vessel until the column of blood is almost occluded. If the vessel is patent, alternate filling and collapsing with each pulse will be evident. The second is the empty-and-refill test[29] *(Fig. 26.21)*. This test is slightly more traumatic and should only be performed when needed. Gently occlude the vessel distal to the anastomosis, and, with a second pair of forceps, empty a segment of the vessel by occluding the vessel next to the first pair and running it in the direction of the flow. The first pair of forceps is released and the emptied segment refills immediately. If the refill is sluggish or absent, the vessel is not patent.

General aspects of free-flap surgery

Although the first clinical application of microvascular surgery was in replantation, this soon evolved into free-flap surgery, opening up a new era in reconstructive surgery, allowing the reconstruction of previously unreconstructable defects. The concept of the reconstructive ladder was introduced as a series of reconstructive options with increasing complexity and this approach to wound management has served us well for the past three decades. With the advent of microsurgery and subsequent refinements, the grounds beneath the ladder and the goals above it have changed. Increasingly complex wounds are created through more radical ablative surgery, for either tumor extirpation or trauma debridement. The answer to the call for a more elegant, direct, and effective reconstruction to replace like-for-like tissues in a single-stage procedure came with the invention of microsurgery.

It is perhaps safe to say, at least for the present, that microsurgery has opened up the boundaries of reconstructive surgery to new and almost limitless possibilities. For some defects, especially where function is as

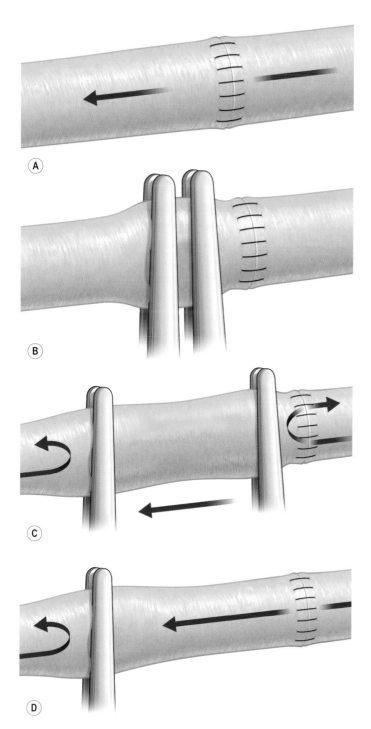

Fig. 26.21 Empty-and-refill test. **(A)** Direction of flow across the anastomosis. **(B)** Two atraumatic forceps are placed downstream of the anastomosis. **(C)** The forceps furthest away from the anastomosis is used to empty the vessel downstream. **(D)** The proximal forceps is released whilst the distal one continues to occlude the vessel. The vessel should immediately refill confirming patency.

important as wound cover, the "reconstructive elevator" (proceeding directly to a more complex option like microsurgery) is now employed regularly rather than the old "reconstructive ladder." This paradigm shift, together with increased technical sophistication and the multiplicity of donor flaps currently available, has enabled microsurgery to be the option of choice in certain selected units, even when local or regional options are available. This ultimately provides a superior functional and aesthetic reconstruction, with an acceptable donor site, thus greatly benefiting the patient.

Advantages and disadvantages

The advantages of free microvascular tissue transfers over more conventional methods of reconstruction have been well documented. Free-flap surgery offers freedom of choice of donor tissue components to achieve a superior functional and aesthetic result by replacing "like for like," especially when local or regional tissue is inadequate. The flap can be tailored to meet specific requirements of the recipient site in size, form, tissue components, and even function. In contrast to regional or distant pedicled flaps that may require a multistage reconstruction, the use of free flaps is often a single-stage procedure that allows earlier mobilization, reduced hospitalization and overall costs. The new tissue has better cutaneous blood flow[135] and vascularity that may enhance wound healing and reduce infection. With an increasing repertoire of flaps and refinements in their harvest, a donor site which can be primarily closed with minimal donor morbidity can often be used.

When both operation and recovery proceed to plan, the advantages of free tissue transfer are clear. However, these benefits have to be weighed against the risks of long operation and anesthetic times, donor site morbidity, the potential lack of available quality recipient vessels, the need for highly specific skill sets and clinical backup, steep learning curves and, of course, the most feared complication – flap failure.

Preoperative evaluation

Patient factors

Free tissue transfer is feasible and often successful in the presence of patient factors once considered to be high-risk for flap failure. However, it is important to evaluate fully the fitness of the patient for free-flap surgery to identify and reduce the risk factors associated with poor outcome.

As with all major surgery, cardiac and respiratory fitness should be optimized before free tissue transfer. This encompasses good preoperative hypertensive and diabetic control. Age, in itself, is not a contraindication to free-flap surgery as long as the patient is in otherwise acceptable health and deemed fit for anesthesia. The outcomes of free tissue transfer in the extremes of ages are comparable to those in the general population,[103,136–141] although there is an increase in postoperative medical complications in the elderly.

Smoking has not been shown to affect significantly vessel patency, flap survival, and reoperation rates, but increases donor site complications with poorer wound healing at the flap–wound bed interface.[142–145] However, patients should be advised to stop smoking preoperatively as their risk of complications approaches that of the nonsmoker if they stop smoking 4 weeks before surgery.

Obesity clearly increases the risks of microvascular surgery and is associated with increased hemorrhage and hematomas.[103] In 936 transverse rectus abdominis myocutaneous (TRAM) flap breast reconstructions, the incidence of total flap loss, hematomas, seromas, and overall donor site complications was higher in patients with a body mass index of over 30.

Alcohol withdrawal is also related to increased flap failure[146] and nonflap-related complications[147] and patients at high risk for postoperative alcohol withdrawal syndrome should be identified and treated prophylactically.

Evaluation of recipient and donor sites

Irradiation impairs the quality of local tissues and vessels and may predispose to complications at the recipient site.[148,149] Khouri et al. found that reconstruction in an irradiated recipient site was a significant predictor of flap failure, with increased odds of failure of 4.2,[103] but many others have failed to show that radiation significantly affects flap survival.[148–150] In our experience of 145 patients with reconstruction in an irradiated field, radiation and time between surgery and radiotherapy had no bearing on overall flap survival but

increased the risk of reoperation and complications.[151] Careful dissection and meticulous attention to surgical technique should be undertaken when performing the anastomoses. Where possible, however, site the anastomosis outside the area of irradiation.

Infected or traumatic wounds should be adequately debrided and, if necessary, reconstructive surgery postponed until adequate control of the wound is achieved. The zone of injury needs to be taken into consideration and the anastomosis placed outside this zone where possible. Preoperative angiography is recommended in patients with abnormal distal pulses,[152] and in those in whom both pedal pulses are not palpable.[95] Normal angiographic findings do not guarantee the presence of vessels suitable for anastomosis, and routine angiography is unjustified.[153]

Harvesting a free flap requires an intimate knowledge of the anatomy of the vessels, and their variations, supplying the transferred tissues. The design of the flap may be centered on perforators that are mapped out by the bedside using a hand-held Doppler device[154] or more accurately through color duplex ultrasound,[155–157] computed tomography angiography with or without three-dimensional reconstruction[158–160] or magnetic resonance imaging angiograms.[161–163] Accurate preoperative mapping has been shown to aid perforator selection, increase the safety of perforator dissection, and reduce operative time.[157,160,163]

Choice of flap

Preoperative planning, selection, and design of the flap are more important than the harvest itself. There is no flap ideal for all circumstances and the surgeon must accept some compromises and choose the most appropriate available flap for the patient. Chosen well, the patient comes away with an optimal result; chosen badly, and the entire reconstruction is set up to fail.

The first question to answer is: "Does this defect need a free flap?" If the answer is yes, then other factors to be considered include the size and tissue components of the defect and the goals of reconstruction. For example, for a young patient with a benign tumor of the mandible, in whom functional outcome is as important as aesthetic outcome, a flap that incorporates vascularized bone for immediate or delayed osteointegration of dental implants should be chosen *(Fig. 26.22)*.

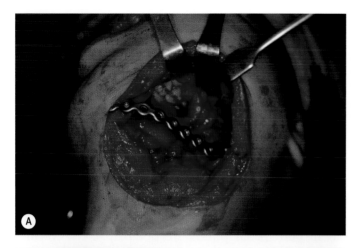

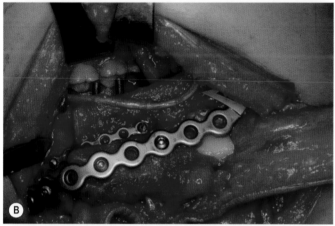

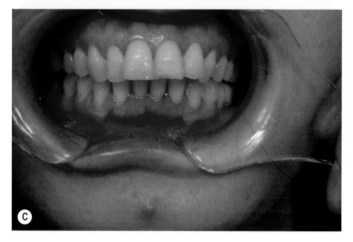

Fig. 26.22 Osteointegrated teeth in a fibula osteoseptocutaneous flap reconstructed neo-mandible. **(A)** Segmental defect of the mandible after tumor excision. **(B)** Double-barreled fibula inset. **(C)** Final appearance of the mandible after osteointegrated teeth implantations.

Conversely, an elderly patient with a poor-prognosis mandibular cancer may benefit from a more straightforward operation with a reconstruction plate and fasciocutaneous flap such as the anterolateral thigh flap that addresses the primary goal of uncomplicated wound healing.[164] Appropriately sized recipient vessels must be available and must be considered in deciding the length and caliber of the flap pedicle. This may ultimately decide the suitability of one flap over another in order to minimize the need for interpositional vein grafts.

An important consideration is the potential donor site, such as the cosmetic result of the donor site that requires skin grafting and reduced muscle power and potential herniation following muscle flap and even perforator flap harvest. Consideration should also be given to the logistics of the flap harvest, patient positioning, and the feasibility of using a two-team approach to streamline the operation.

Timing

The timing of posttraumatic lower extremity reconstruction has been the subject of ongoing debate since Godina first recommended that they be performed within 72 hours of injury.[164a] Today, when the free flap is actually performed is largely determined by the surgeon's experience and assessment and the local healthcare system, logistics, and facilities. The definitions of the ideal time periods also vary significantly, with some defining acute reconstruction as the interval ranging from emergency or immediate procedures within 24 hours to urgent procedures done within 72 hours, and others suggesting that the first 24 hours be termed "primary free-flap closure."[165] There are those who advocate reconstruction within 72 hours[166,167] or 5 days,[168] but proponents of delaying the reconstruction argue that the viability of an extremity can be better assessed, the reconstructive procedure better planned, and performed under better operating conditions. In our practice, we have found that adequate debridement results in a fresh surgical wound that can be reconstructed at any time and that actual timing has little to do with the final outcome of the flap. However, we agree that immediate cover must be considered if vital structures are exposed and that, on occasion, emergency free-flap transfer may salvage a devascularized limb or a finger, in addition to improving the functional and aesthetic results and shortening the hospital stay.[169] In oncological reconstructions, immediate reconstruction is performed at the same time as the ablative surgery to achieve uncomplicated wound healing. Reconstruction at the same time has been shown to delay the delivery of adjuvant therapy modestly.[170] In reconstruction of the breast where the final aesthetic outcome is of significant importance, delayed reconstruction can be performed on completion of adjuvant chemo- or radiotherapy but is reliant on the ability to close the defect primarily. Alternatively, in patients for whom postmastectomy radiation therapy required is undecided, "delayed immediate" reconstruction with a temporizing expander avoids the difficulties associated with radiation delivery after immediate reconstruction and maintains the skin envelope.[171]

Microvascular anesthesia

The importance of stable anesthesia by an anesthetic team familiar with microsurgery should not be underestimated. Good pain, temperature, and sympathetic control should be maintained throughout to prevent vasospasm and vasoconstriction. Finetuning of blood pressure will help in ensuring that the operation proceeds smoothly; during flap dissection, the blood pressure should be kept adequately low to keep a bloodless field, but brought up gradually when hemostasis is being secured and the anastomosis being performed to ensure good recipient inflow and flap perfusion. Adequate fluid management includes slight hemodilution to maintain high cardiac output and low systemic vascular resistance.[172]

Special techniques and flap modifications

Increasing familiarity with the principles and techniques of microsurgery has encouraged various innovations and refinements in the pursuit of excellence. The goal now is not only simply to achieve closure, but to do so with the least amount of donor morbidity, in the shortest operative time, and with the best results in terms of function and appearance.

Endoscopic harvest

Endoscope-assisted harvest of free flaps allows the use of smaller incisions and improved donor site appearance. However this requires special instrumentation and a steep learning curve that may initially increase the operative time. Flaps harvested with endoscope assistance include gracilis,[173] rectus abdominis,[174] and latissimus dorsi[175] muscle flaps, temporoparietal fascial flaps,[176,177] and jejunal segments.[178] Although the complication rates are not dissimilar, incision lengths are shorter, donor site morbidity and pain are reduced, and patient satisfaction is higher when the flaps are harvested endoscopically.

Perforator flaps, freestyle flaps, and supramicrosurgery

A perforator flap is defined as a flap based on a musculocutaneous perforating vessel that is directly visualized and dissected free from the surrounding muscle until adequate pedicle length is obtained (*Fig. 26.23*). This minimizes donor site morbidity and allows the harvest of only the specific components required for the reconstruction. In areas where the anatomy of the cutaneous vessels has not been studied extensively or with flaps with considerable variations in anatomy of their blood supply, the detection of an audible perforator with a hand-held Doppler probe may form the basis of flap harvest.[156] The vessel is identified at the level of the fascia, through an exploratory incision, and if sizeable (0.5 mm with good visible pulsation), then dissection in a retrograde fashion will follow its course to the parent vessel on which the flap may be raised as a free flap. This concept has been termed "freestyle free flaps"[179] and these flaps can be designed almost anywhere as long as small-caliber vessels are acceptable.

To reduce donor site morbidity further, Koshima *et al.* advocate supramicrosurgery,[180–182] the dissection and anastomosis of vessels with diameters of less than 1 mm. This allows flaps based on vessels harvested without breaching the deep fascia, facilitating a quick operative harvest time without intramuscular dissection, but yields a very short pedicle that requires highly honed surgical skills and extremely fine instruments and sutures.

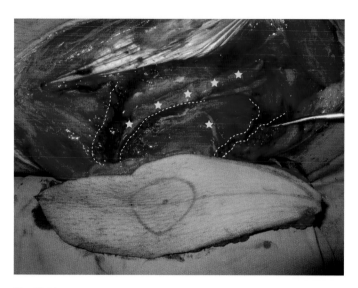

Fig. 26.23 Perforator flap harvest via an intramuscular dissection of the perforators. * Perforator. ***** Source artery of the perforators: descending branch of the circumflex iliac artery. ----- Edge of the dissected vastus lateralis muscle.

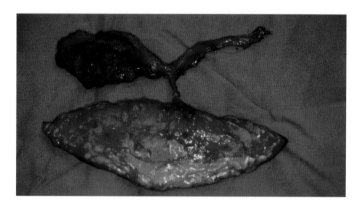

Fig. 26.24 Chimeric flap with muscle and skin component.

Chimeric flaps

A chimeric flap refers to a flap with separate components that can be independently maneuvered but are ultimately linked to each other by a common source vessel.[183] This allows the freedom of placement of each component and often results in an optimal one-stage reconstruction of compound defects[184,185] *(Fig. 26.24)*.

Thinned flaps

Flaps that are thick and bulky often require a secondary revision in order to improve final outcome. However, with better understanding of the vascular supply and from increasing experience with perforator flaps,

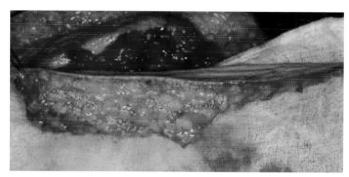

Fig. 26.25 Thinning of a thick cutaneous flap. —— Shows the edge of the flap where flap has been excised safely to thin the flap according to requirements.

one-stage flap thinning has become possible. Skin is nourished by a subdermal plexus arising from branches of the main pedicle midadipose layer and thinning can be performed safely to about 3–4 mm in thickness, except for 2 cm around the pedicle.[186] This reduces the need for secondary revisions.[187] Another method of thinning is microdissection of blood vessels in the adipose layer under microscopic magnification and removal of the adipose tissue surrounding the vessel[188–190] *(Fig. 26.25)*.

Prefabricated/prelaminated flaps

Some defects require complex reconstructions of various components that cannot be met by conventional flaps. Flap prefabrication and prelamination have been applied to areas where specific contours and structures are desired, for example, in reconstruction of the esophagus, penis, and certain head and neck defects.

Prefabrication involves a two-stage process, the first of which implants an axial vascular pedicle into the donor tissue that is required,[191] thus allowing it to be transferable once neovascularization has occurred. The second stage, about 8 weeks after the implantation, involves the transfer of this neovascularized tissue, based on its recently implanted pedicle, to reconstruct the defect on its recently implanted pedicle. This allows the creation of large, thin skin flaps that retain the qualities of the donor site and can be modified with various combinations of vascular pedicles, donor tissues, and geographic locations for different clinical needs.[192,193]

Prelamination is another two-stage process where one or more tissues are added to a reliable vascular bed to create a multilayered composite flap. In the second stage, once matured in approximately 2 weeks, the composite flap is transplanted to the defect. This delayed procedure allows the best chance for the prelaminating layers to heal, stabilize, and assume their expected structures and positions. By laminating the vascular bed with skin, bone, cartilage, or mucosa, prelaminated flaps have been used to reconstruct the oral lining,[194] ear,[195] nose,[196,197] neourethra,[198] penis,[196] and neoesophagus.

Postoperative management, complications, and outcomes

Intraoperative free-flap success does not always translate into overall free-flap success and clinical management of the patient and monitoring of the flap are essential in the initial postoperative period.

The postoperative management of the patient is crucial in preventing major morbidity and mortality. Patients should be kept warm, adequately fluid-filled (hematocrit <0.3), and painfree. Blood pressure should be normalized based on preoperative blood pressure and tachycardia avoided as sympathetic overdrive may cause vasospasm. Good hyperglycemic control reduces the incidence of complications in the surgical patient who may require insulin therapy. Prophylactic antibiotics are routinely prescribed to prevent wound infection and low-molecular-weight heparin is used to prevent deep-vein thromboses.

Monitoring

Monitoring begins on the re-establishment of blood flow into the flap. The flap should constantly be assessed on release of the microvascular clamps, during closure, on completion of inset, when the patient transfers from the table, and on admission into the ward.[199] Early detection and intervention of flap problems can improve overall flap salvage[200–202] and many methods of flap monitoring are now available, although none has been completely effective or uniformly accepted. The ideal monitor should be reliable, noninvasive, objectively repeatable, promptly reactive to blood flow changes, appropriate for continuous monitoring in all types of free tissue transfers, usable for the unskilled, and economically available.[203]

There is no substitute for experienced nursing and medical staff, whether in a dedicated intensive care unit or on the general ward. Clinical observation of the flap is the gold standard for monitoring and should be performed at hourly intervals for the first 24 hours. This can be extended to 2-hourly for the next 24 hours, then 4-hourly for the next 48 hours. Signs to be noted are color, capillary refill, turgor, and surface temperature. If capillary refill is not obvious, pinprick testing can be used to observe the color and speed of bleeding. However, this pinprick should just scratch the dermis and not penetrate too deeply and risk injury to the underlying pedicle. This form of monitoring may not be as suitable for flaps in aesthetically important areas. Surface temperature measurement with a surface temperature probe is easy and inexpensive[204] and a recorded difference of 1.8°C between flap and control sites is 98% sensitive and 75% predictive of vascular compromise.[205] The trend of the temperature of the flap over time is also a useful guide to the failing flap[199] and temperatures below 30°C are indicative of flap failure.[206]

A hand-held pencil Doppler probe (low-frequency continuous ultrasonography)[204] applied on to the flap over a cutaneous perforator location is another method of monitoring. This point should be marked intraoperatively away from the pedicle to prevent false-positive results. An implantable Doppler probe can be used to monitor flaps without a perforator to the skin or buried flaps.[207] This small probe is attached to a polymer sleeve that is placed around the pedicle vessel (most accurate on the vein) adjacent to the anastomosis with a probe lead wire exiting through the incision. This lead is removed by gentle traction which leaves the sleeve in place when monitoring is no longer required. The signals have a characteristic pattern that can differentiate arterial from venous thrombosis. Laser Doppler measures the reflected waveforms of light, from a helium-neon laser, by the red blood cells moving within the capillaries, and provides an objective measurement for flap perfusion. Interpretation of the results of laser Doppler requires experience but can be very accurate, detecting vascular compromise with no false positives or negatives[208] and distinguishing venous obstruction from arterial occlusion.[209]

Other available adjuncts less commonly used include pulse oximetry to identify both a pulsatile flow and arterial saturation in replanted or revascularized digits or toe-to-hand transfers,[210] photography, tissue oxygen tension measurement, tissue pH levels, microdialysis, fluorescein dye mapping, near-infrared spectroscopy, thermodilution technology, photoplethysmography, and nuclear medicine studies.[211] Clinical monitoring is currently the gold standard and, regardless of which adjunct is additionally used, close flap monitoring should be a standard part of the postoperative care of these patients during the first 72 hours after surgery at the minimum.

Buried flaps

Monitoring buried flaps postoperatively is a challenge and many techniques have been used to assess the flaps, either directly or indirectly. Implantable Doppler probes have been used routinely, as covered previously. Part of the flap may be externalized, for example, a jejunal stump may be brought to the surface to observe peristalsis and color or a skin paddle may be externalized. This should be used with some caution as this only monitors the common source vessel and may not accurately reflect the buried component, especially if the two components are based on different perforators.[212] The distal end of the pedicle that is usually ligated close to the supply of the skin can also be externalized and its pulsations observed directly under a transparent film dressing. This can then be tied off in the follow-up clinic.[213]

Flap outcomes

With maturation of microsurgical technique, failures have thankfully become rarer and success rates of free tissue transfers now range from 96% to 100%.[18,58] Failures can be attributed to poor planning, poor choice of flap or vessels, poor timing, or poor technique. However, many of the failing flaps may be salvaged and the success of the salvage (54–100%[103]) is in part dependent on good patient management, highly trained staff, and early detection and intervention.

When a flap begins to fail, the likely causes must be identified and rectified. Although the majority of the complications are related to vascular compromise, simple measures should be taken by the bedside first to avoid unnecessary explorations. Systemic factors such as hypotension, hypovolemia, hypothermia, and

sympathetic overdrive due to pain should be resolved. Once the blood pressure is normalized and the patient warmed up, the flap should be reassessed for the need to return to the operating room. Local factors include the release of external compression secondary to compressive surgical dressing, hematoma, or a tight wound closure. Releasing some sutures or loosening the dressings may relieve the compression, solving the problem or at least temporizing the immediate threat to the flap before the formal salvage procedure. If the flap does not improve, a prompt return to the operating room to assess the patency of the vessels under the microscope is mandatory. Resection and reanastomosis or the use of a Fogarty thrombectomy[214] may be required. Intraoperative lysis with streptokinase, urokinase or tissue-type plasminogen activator may also help.[215–217]

Causes of a failing flap

Anastomotic failure

There are many causes of anastomotic failure, such as those related to technical errors in the anastomosis, or intrinsic factors predisposing to vasospasm or thrombogenesis.

The principal faults leading to anastomotic failure are tearing, leaking, narrowing of the lumen, through-stitching, and inclusion of the adventitia.[29] Tearing occurs when there is too much tension at the site of the repair. It can also be caused by too meticulous stripping of adventitia: the veins of the head and neck region are especially fragile. Leaking occurs when there is too big a gap between sutures, or there is a tear or a tiny unnoticed branch near the anastomotic site. Even a small leak will precipitate intraluminal thrombus formation[218] and narrowing of the lumen can also be caused by oversized bites, entangling knots with one another, or continuous suturing that is too tight. Through-stitching entails taking a bite of the back wall with the suture, causing luminal obstruction. This can be avoided by always visualizing the lumen of the vessel through constant luminal irrigation by an assistant or by raising the anterior wall with the tops of microforceps to separate it from the back wall. Inclusion of adventitia as a result of inadequate vessel preparation should be avoided as the prolapsed adventitia is another nidus for thrombus formation. Finally, desiccation of the vessel may also lead to failure.

Vasospasm

Vasospasm occurs in 5–10% of microsurgical procedures and plays an important role in the pathogenesis of hypoperfusion, promoting thrombosis, which may lead to partial or total flap loss. It may be seen intraoperatively and up to 72 hours postoperatively, with the former often being more problematic. The pathophysiology of vasospasm is not clear, but is thought to occur secondary to both general and local factors. General factors include low core temperatures, hypotension, and sympathetic response to pain, while local factors include trauma to the vessel, tight adventitia, myogenic response to local hemorrhage, desiccation of the tissues, and vascular disease. Surgical dissection may induce sympathetic nerve endings to release vasoactive compounds, and impair release of vasodilators,[219] compounding the vasospasm and thrombosis. Veins appear to be more susceptible to vasospasm than arteries and, once established, harder to resolve[220] and more detrimental.

If the vessel is left untouched for a few minutes, it may vasodilate to its natural diameter. However, a variety of antispasmodic agents or mechanical dilation can be used to aid relief of the vasospasm.

Most of the antispasmodic agents available are locally applied to avoid systemic complications. The most commonly used agents are papaverine, lidocaine, and calcium channel blockers such as nifedipine, verapamil, and nicardipine. Papaverine (30 mg/mL) is an opium alkaloid that functions as a phosphodiesterase inhibitor and has a direct action on smooth muscle through the release of cyclic adenosine monophoshate. Lidocaine is a local anesthetic agent that has a biphasic response with low and high concentrations potentiating contraction and dilatation, respectively.[221] Its vasodilatory mechanism remains unclear but is thought to be related to sodium–calcium exchange pump. Some studies suggest that its concentration should be increased up to 20% or be combined with papaverine.[222] The benefit of lidocaine continues after the drug is washed out with heparinized saline solution and, as it is not significantly absorbed from the wound, systemic effects are unlikely.[223] In practice however, common concentrations of lidocaine used vary between 2 and 4%.[224] Calcium channel blockers work by blocking voltage-gated calcium channels in vascular smooth muscle. This blocks the calcium influx required for muscle contraction and may even be more effective than papaverine.[225] Sympathetic blockade using brachial plexus blocks has also been reported to be effective.[226–228]

Mechanical treatments of vasospasm include gently dilating healthy vessel ends with a specially designed blunt-ended vessel dilator forceps or with microneedle holders. Metallic standard-sized dilators or intraluminal irrigation through the passage of a fine intracath may also be used. This should be done with caution, especially in arteriosclerotic vessels, as catheters can strip endothelium and expose the thrombogenic subendothelium.[229] Surgical stripping of adventitia is an effective method of relieving vasospasm because of a sympathectomy effect and mechanical thinning of the vessel walls allows them to dilate more freely.[230] If the spasm is intractable, the vessel should be aggressively resected until normal vessel is reached. Occasionally this may require an additional vein graft or turning to another recipient vessel for anastomosis.

Stable and thorough anesthesia is an important requirement: hypovolemia, pain, and low core temperature (<36°C) can all result in vasospasm. The patient's temperature should be constantly monitored and adequate hydration maintained, and the wound should not be allowed to dry out.

Thrombogenesis

Many free-flap complications relate to pedicle thrombosis (4–80% within the first 48 hours) caused by changes in the intraluminal blood flow, endothelial damage, and the state of coagulability. Changes in flow can be due to external mechanical compression from bandages, closure of the wound under tension, the weight of the flap, tension, twisting, kinking, or vasospasm of the vascular pedicle after the anastomosis is completed. Intraluminal turbulence may be caused by irregularities in the intima from technical error, suture material, and the result of size mismatch.

Hypercoagulability may be systemic or local. Hypercoagulable states such as pregnancy, active cancer, and recent trauma should be identified preoperatively as far as possible and warrant thromboprophylaxis. Hypercoagulation disorders like activated protein C,[231] hyperfibrinogenemia,[232] antiphospholipid syndrome,[233] and reactive thrombocytosis[234] should be treated preoperatively, although routine screening for these is not cost-effective. Thromboplastins are soluble in water and present in abundance in the surgical wound. When blood is contaminated by this, clotting will occur and periodic irrigation with heparinzed saline will minimize this risk. Even a smooth and streamlined microvascular anastomosis will produce some thrombus, and when blood flow is restored, the thrombus continues to grow for 5 minutes, starts to disintegrate by 10 minutes, and disappears nearly completely by the end of an hour. If the anastomosis is irregular, the thrombus will grow rapidly and occlude the vessel. Endothelial cells are critical in local blood flow control and produce vasoconstrictors such as endothelin-1[235,236] and vasodilator substances, nitric oxide and prostacyclin. Damaged endothelium produces a highly thrombogenic state, resulting in platelet aggregation and the initiation of a complex clotting cascade, and surgical precision is vital to minimize vessel damage.[237]

The risk of thrombosis is greatest within the first 48 hours and decreases to 10% after 72 hours.[202] Arterial and venous thrombi present at different times and form through different mechanisms. The majority of arterial thromboses occur during the first 24 hours and are related to platelet aggregation at the anastomotic site.[238] Venous thrombosis is more often responsible for flap compromise, presents later, and is related to the formation of a fibrin clot. The goals of anticoagulant phrophylaxis are therefore to interfere with platelet function and aggregation, counter the effects of thrombin on platelets and fibrinogen, and reduce blood viscosity or increase blood flow.[239] While the use of anticoagulants to lower the incidence of anastomotic thrombosis is widely practiced, literature regarding the efficacy of one treatment over another is sparse and largely based on the individual surgeon's preference and preconceptions. Protocols differ not only in the agents used, but also the dose, combination, timing, and duration. Heparin, dextran, and aspirin are the most commonly used prophylactic antithrombotics today.

Heparin reduces platelet aggregation, activates antithrombin III (thereby directly deactivating clotting factors II, IX, X, XI and, indirectly, factors V and VIII), lowers blood viscosity, and has[240] direct vasodilatory properties. This polyglycosaminoglycan was the first anticoagulant described and has been in clinical use for over 50 years to prevent both arterial and venous

thromboses, even at subtherapeutic levels[241] and independent of rate of blood flow. As a washout solution, it may have a protective effect against ischemia/reperfusion injury through a direct effect on microvascular endothelium.[242] Intravascular heparin improves flap salvage rates[243] and clinically reduces the rate of thrombotic events.[103] Its use, however, may be more important in patients with atherosclerotic or injured vessels, when vein grafts have been used and with thrombosis of an anastomosis, than in patients with healthy vessels and straightforward anastomoses.[244] The use of intravascular unfractionated heparin may increase the risk of hematoma formation,[245,246] but both Chien et al.[247] and Kroll et al.[248] have found that flap survival was equivalent to that with other regimens without increased incidence of hematoma. Low-molecular-weight heparins, which inhibit clotting factor Xa with less of an effect on thrombin inactivation, may be just as effective in improving patency without the risk of hematoma formation.[249] Unfractionated heparin is used universally to irrigate vessels during microvascular surgery and has been shown experimentally to improve patency when administered at high concentrations[36,250,251] while minimizing the systemic complications. Heparin binds to the endothelium and has a half-life of 5 hours[252] and should be applied as soon as the vessels are divided. Clinically, however, Khouri showed no increase in patency regardless of concentration[103] and Yan suggested that high-pressure local irrigation might even cause intimal and endothelial damage.[253] Nevertheless, together with another important side-effect of heparin-induced thrombocytopenia, systemically administered heparin should be used judiciously.

Dextran is a polysaccharide synthesized from sucrose and produced synthetically as a 40- or 70-kDa molecular weight polymer. Its antithrombotic effect is mediated through increasing the electronegativity of erythrocytes, platelets, and endothelium and therefore platelet aggregation, decreasing factor VIII-Ag and thereby platelet function and fibrin structure, and, finally, as a volume expander that reduces blood viscosity. Dextran-40, the more popular dextran for anticoagulation in microsurgery,[103,248,254] is excreted more effectively by the kidneys and has a shorter action than dextran-70. No randomized controlled studies have shown a cause-and-effect relationship between the use of dextran and flap loss or prevention of thrombosis. In particular, it has not been shown to be more effective than other anticoagulants and its benefits of improved vessel patency are not seen beyond a week.[255,256] Although it has relatively few side-effects, these can be serious and include anaphylaxis, volume overload, pulmonary or cerebral edema, platelet dysfunction, and even acute renal failure.[257,258] A comparison of dextran and aspirin-related complications in head and neck patients with free-flap reconstructions showed that both were equally effective in preventing flap failure, but dextran was associated with a 3.9- and 7.2-fold increased relative risk of systemic complications after 48 and 120 hours of dextran infusion respectively.[259]

Aspirin is an antiplatelet agent that inhibits cyclooxygenase and reduces the breakdown of arachidonic acid to thromboxane, a potent vasoconstrictor and platelet aggregator, and prostacyclin, a vasodilator that inhibits platelet aggregation. Low-dose aspirin (75 mg/day) has been shown to inhibit thromboxane selectively at the site of the anastomosis[260] while preserving prostacyclin production of the endothelium. Experimentally, it has been shown to improve anastomotic patency and capillary perfusion and may be related to the timing of administration.[261,262] It is, however, less effective than heparin[262,263] and, despite the lack of clinical evidence for its effect on free-flap patency, it is still used widely. The adverse effects of aspirin such as gastric hemorrhage, renal failure, and prolonged bleeding are a direct result of the mechanisms that make its use attractive in microsurgery and have been minimized with the use of low-dose aspirin. The newer cyclooxygenase II inhibitors are also associated with fewer renal and gastric side-effects but do not prevent platelet aggregation and are therefore not used in microsurgery.[264]

Other antithrombotic agents tested in animal models to determine their efficacy in augmenting flap survival include pentoxifylline,[265] hirudin,[251] nonsteroidal anti-inflammatories,[266,267] other antiplatelets such as dipyridamole and ticlopidine,[268] and prostaglandin E₁.[269]

Thrombolytics such as streptokinase, urokinase, and tissue plasminogen activator have been advocated for flaps not responding to standard salvage techniques[215] and may be effective in reversing microvascular thrombosis,[216,217] but clinical evidence is sparse and anecdotal.[270–273] A retrospective multi-institutional study even reported no significant improvement in patency with the use of thrombolytic therapy in free-flap salvage.[274] Streptokinase enhances the conversion of plasminogen to plasmin with subsequent fibrinolysis, whilst urokinase and tissue-type plasminogen activator, which activate plasminogen directly, are less antigenic and have fewer systemic effects. There is a significant risk of bleeding following systemic exposure to thrombolytics but this can be minimized by local intra-arterial administration of the thrombolytic and drainage of the venous effluent.[275]

When surgical and pharmacological salvage fails, medicinal leeches (Hirudo medicinalis) have been used effectively to treat venous congested flaps.[276] When applied to the flap, they bite into it, injecting a local anesthetic, vasodilator, and anticoagulant, hirudin, which is present in their saliva. Leeches increase perfusion within congested flaps by feeding on the blood. They then fall away when full, but the bleeding continues for up to 10 hours with the combination of vasodilator and anticoagulant.[277] New leeches can be applied when the bleeding slows or the flap appears congested again. Therapy is continued until the flap re-establishes an effective venous drainage through new vessel ingrowth around the flap margins. As there can be significant blood loss with leech therapy, this is usually limited to small- to medium-sized flaps and the patient's hemoglobin should be monitored daily. Prophylactic antibiotics should also be give against Aeromonas hydrophila from the leeches' digestive tract.

Ischemic tolerance, ischaemia–reperfusion injury, and no-reflow phenomenon

Prolonged periods of warm ischemia (the time between interruption and re-establishment of the circulation) concern microsurgeons as they predispose to tissue necrosis and flap failure. Primary ischemia occurs when the anastomosis is being performed and can be kept to a minimum by donor site and vessel preparation before flap pedicle division and an accurate anastomosis, whilst secondary ischemia occurs later as a result of pedicle obstruction.

The tolerance to ischemia varies from tissue to tissue depending on their metabolic requirements, with skin, nerve, bone, muscle, and then intestine being increasingly tolerant. Within a composite flap, the overall tolerance is equal to that of the least tolerant component. A study of 700 free flaps failed to show a statistical difference in ischemic times between successful and failed flaps and concluded that ischemic time was irrelevant to flap survival provided ischemia was not prolonged beyond 3 hours or to the point of "no-reflow phenomenon."

While the goal of microsurgical anastomosis is to restore flow and reperfuse the flap, after a prolonged period of ischemia, this reperfusion may compound insult to the flap through local and systemic inflammatory responses. This is known as ischemia–reperfusion injury and is thought to be a result of the buildup of oxygen radicals during the ischemic period. These cause tissue injury, specifically of cellular membranes through their powerful oxidizing and reducing potentials. They also stimulate an intense inflammatory reaction by recruiting inflammatory cells such as leukocytes, neutrophils, and platelets, and other inflammatory mediators and cytokines,[278] while suppressing protective molecules such as nitric oxide synthase, prostacyclin, and thrombomodulin.

Severe ischemia–reperfusion injury results in irreversible vasoconstriction, and the resulting inability to reperfuse the flap despite patent anastomoses is known as the "no-reflow phenomenon."[279] This is a result of ischemia-induced endothelial injury, which leads to cellular swelling, interstitial swelling, exposure of subendothelial collagen, platelet–leukocyte aggregation, reduction in blood flow and, if not rectified, thrombosis and flap failure.

Experimental studies have shown a protective function of intravascular administration of heparin,[242,280] vasodilators, prostaglandin E_1, nitrendipine and prostacyclin, thrombolytics, urokinase and streptokinase, nonsteroidal anti-inflammatory drugs, and free radical scavengers deferoxamine and superoxide dismutase.[281,282] Inhibiting the action of selectins, integrins, and intercellular adhesion molecules with monoclonal antibodies to prevent inflammatory cell adhesion may also prevent ischemia–reperfusion injury, but these have not translated clinically.[283,284]

Donor site complications – dependent again on flap choice

Every flap harvested leaves a donor site of varying morbidity, therefore the benefits of the reconstruction must outweigh its sequelae. The incidence of donor site complications varies between 5.5% and 31%, with early donor problems associated with wound healing (hematoma, seroma, and wound dehiscence).[285,286] These are more likely in obese patients, diabetics, and smokers. Hematomas may occur with any flap harvest and meticulous hemostasis with a normotensive (for the patient) blood pressure must be performed. Seromas occur when extensive dissections leave large dead spaces, for example, with a latissimus dorsi or deep inferior epigastric perforator harvest, and wound dehiscence occurs with tight closure, which can be avoided with good preoperative planning.

Long-term problems are usually that of poor cosmesis, reduced function, and chronic pain. If the donor site has to be grafted, this causes a significant cosmetic disadvantage and patient dissatisfaction.[286–289] Suprafascial dissection reduces the size of the donor defect, allows preservation of the superficial nerves, prevents tenting of tendons, and improves skin graft take. This allows a full-thickness skin graft with superior cosmesis to be applied with confidence and reduces potential tendon exposure from delayed healing.[289–291] Muscle flaps may cause weakness and functional impairment, for example, serratus anterior muscle elevation may cause scapular winging and the TRAM flap is associated with hernia formation.[292,293] Harvesting vascularized bone may result in impaired function of a fracture-susceptible donor site, requiring troublesome splinting for a prolonged period,[285,294] and even affecting gait. Cutaneous nerves may be sacrificed, leaving painful neuromas or unacceptable numbness.[294–296] Temporary or permanent palsies may result from injured motor nerves and compartment syndrome from overzealous closures.[297]

Management of failed flaps

Flap failure has profound implications for both patient and surgeon and represents one of the most challenging aspects of reconstructive microsurgery. Despite the increased experience and refinements in microsurgical techniques and perioperative management, a small number of flaps still fail. With the low incidence of flap failure, there are few articles in the literature that address the management of flap failure and no guidelines regarding the best approach to this problem exist.

Many questions are raised immediately when a flap fails. Why did it happen? What defect requires reconstruction? How and when should the defect be reconstructed? These questions invariably form the basis of a systematic approach to the problem at hand and should be considered when managing a failed flap. Analyzing 54 failed flaps, Oliva et al.[21] recommend that three issues must be considered when the initial flap is declared nonviable – the reasons for failure, the indications for the free-flap reconstruction, and the current status of the resultant wound.

It is important to identify the reasons for the failure as subsequent attempts at reconstruction might be plagued with the same issues and be doomed to fail. If the cause is reversible or preventable, then this bodes well for a repeat attempt with another free flap. Examples include technical errors, suboptimal postoperative management, and delay in diagnosis and salvage. Irreversible patient factors like systemic vascular disease, radiation injury, and lack of healthy recipient vessels do not preclude a further attempt but the decision to proceed with a second microsurgical reconstruction should be weighed carefully against the risks. If the risks outweigh the benefits, a nonmicrosurgical procedure may be the sensible option, although this may be just as complicated.

The need for further reconstruction is then evaluated. Factors to be considered include the extent of the failure,[298] exposure of vital structures, and the effect of an open wound on subsequent therapy. An important question to address is whether the initial goal of a sophisticated reconstruction should be pursued or if a downgraded reconstruction is an acceptable compromise between achieving wound closure and the aesthetic and functional goals. Partial loss of a flap secondary to necrosis may be amenable to conservative treatment with conventional dressings, vacuum-assisted closure, or skin graft. Complete failures, such as those due to arterial insufficiency, are more catastrophic and require more aggressive treatment while venous failures deserve a more expectant management with the use of medicinal leeches or by allowing the flap to bleed out slowly to allow partial salvage. This may support a skin graft after tangential debridement.[298] If the flap loss results in exposure of vital structures such as the great vessels of the neck, skull base, metal plates or bare bone, the situation may be life-threatening and mandates prompt coverage with another flap.[299] For breast reconstruction, it is reasonable to consider primary or

secondary closure if the patient can accept the cosmetic implications. In extremity reconstruction, where the threat is isolated to the extremity involved, a more expectant approach can be taken, provided metal plates or vital structures are not exposed. Less aggressive management may however result in higher rates of limb amputation.[300] In oncological reconstruction, the primary goal is uncomplicated wound healing in order that adjuvant therapy can proceed. In these circumstances a second flap will expedite wound healing and should be considered early. A pedicled muscle or cutaneous flap might be a reasonable alternative to a free flap.

Once the decision has been made to proceed, the course of action needs detailed planning. Factors to be considered include the timing of the repeat surgery, the type of reconstruction required for the resulting defect, and if there is a need for a second free flap. If a second free flap is needed, then what donor sites are available and what recipient vessels can be reliably dissected and safely used? Importantly, are the goals of reconstruction the same as they were initially?

The timing of the surgery is dependent on several factors. If the patient is unstable, then reoperation is ideally delayed. Infection-free, the flap may act as a temporizing biological dressing until the patient is fit for further surgery. The recipient site and exposure of vital structures may dictate the urgency of the surgery. If the patient is fit enough, the same second free flap should be performed at the time of adequate debridement.[21] In our experience of 101 failed free flaps, 34% received a second free flap[299] and we feel a second free flap should be attempted in any case in which failure may lead to loss of the injured limb, leave exposed major neck vessels, or cause delay in adjuvant chemo- or radiotherapy. Restoration of function should also be attempted in a previous functional muscle transfer. The success rate of second free flaps is higher in the head and neck region (94.1%) compared to that in the extremity (82.2–87.5%).[299,301] A downgrade of reconstruction should only be considered if the patient is not in optimal condition or in the presence of overwhelming infection as this often results in poorer cosmetic and functional outcomes.

The second free flap needs to be chosen and designed carefully. It should have good vascularity and a longer pedicle as debridement may leave a larger defect, and the new recipient vessels are likely to be further from the defect. Where possible, do not reuse the previous recipient vessels as they are likely to be inflamed and friable. Interpositional vein grafts may be required but have been associated with a higher incidence of flap failure and vascular complications.[302,303] If the same flap is available on the contralateral side, this is our flap of choice and was most commonly used.[299] However, as it is generally accepted that a flap with an osseous component poses additional difficulties during flap elevation and inset and has been associated with a higher failure rate,[122] a safer option should be considered. Other indications for choosing a different type of flap (for example, choosing a myocutaneous, fasciocutaneous, or even pedicled flap with reconstruction plate over an osteocutaneous flap) include the absence (abdominal flaps) or unavailability of the contralateral side (already used or in the zone of injury) or a downgrading of the reconstructive goals due to patient fitness, altered prognosis, or the need to ensure survival.

Future of microsurgery

Technology is constantly evolving and its presence is very much part of the advances that we see in microsurgery. One area is robotics. While already applied and embraced in other areas of surgery, robotic-assisted microsurgery has only been used experimentally.[304] Despite good vessel anastomotic patency, elimination of hand tremors, increased range of motion and enhanced three-dimensional visualization, the additional time required and prohibitive costs have delayed their adoption into routine practice.[305]

Composite tissue allotransplantation (CTA) is an emerging field that is showing great promise. It represents the ultimate reconstruction, replacing like for like when autotransplantation is not enough, and takes free-flap surgery another leap forward. However there are many barriers that limit their widespread use and these can be divided into four main categories – ethical, functional, psychological, and immunological issues. Of these, the most intensely studied is the immunological burden that mandates lifelong immunosuppression with its attendant risks and complications that CTA places on the recipient. The induction and maintenance of transplantation tolerance are the "holy grail" of transplantation and the closer we come to solving this issue, the closer we will be to CTA becoming a commonplace reality.

There is also a role for microvascular surgery in the exciting field of tissue engineering and it is now possible to engineer large blocks of single or composite tissue. To allow these to maintain their viability and be useful in reconstruction, vessel implantation will be required, and with that the need for microsurgery to coapt these vessels to the recipient site.

In the last 40 years, free-flap surgery has gained a strong foothold in our reconstructive armamentarium. Whilst its application has grown considerably and is now considered a relatively routine option, the basic principles and techniques have changed little. Many surgeons still use the original techniques of microsurgery pioneered in the early 1900s and, given their good results, few see the need to change them. New flaps and improving donor sites build on our increasing knowledge and understanding of anatomy and wound healing, but the fundamental techniques still apply to all. Finally, with the continued refinements to improve donor site morbidity and final outcomes, the field of microsurgery will continue to flourish with an ever-expanding application of free-flap surgery.

Access the complete references list online at **http://www.expertconsult.com**

1. Tamai S. History of microsurgery – from the beginning until the end of the 1970s. *Microsurgery*. 1993;14: 6–13.

7. Kriss TC, Kriss VM. History of the operating microscope: from magnifying glass to microneurosurgery. *Neurosurgery*. 1998;42:899.

13a. Anonymous. Replantation surgery in China: Report of the American Replantation Mission to China. *Plast Reconstr Surg*. 1973;52:476–489.

15a. Antia NH, Buch VI. Transfer of an abdominal dermo–fat graft by direct anastamosis of blood vessels. *Br J Plast Surg*. 1971;24:15–19.

17. Daniel RK, Taylor GI. Distant transfer of an island flap by microvascular anastomoses. A clinical technique. *Plast Reconstr Surg*. 1973;52:111–117.

22. International Registry on Hand and Composite Tissue Transplantation – World Exp., 2009. Accessed 31.12.2009, at www.handregistry.com.

30. O'Brien BM, Henderson PN, Bennett RC, et al. Microvascular surgical technique. *Med J Aust.* 1970;1:722–725.

103. Khouri RK, Cooley BC, Kunselman AR, et al. A prospective study of microvascular free–flap surgery and outcome. *Plast Reconstr Surg.* 1998;102:711–721.

104a. Carrel A. Anastomose bout a bout de la jugulaire et de la carotide primitive. *Lyon Medical.* 1902;99: 114–116.

164. Wei FC, Jain V, Celik N, et al. Have we found an ideal soft–tissue flap? An experience with 672 anterolateral thigh flaps. *Plast Reconstr Surg.* 2002;109:2219–2226; discussion 27–30.

164a. Godina M. Early microsurgical reconstruction of complex trauma of the extremities. *Plast Reconstr Surg.* 1986;78:285–292.

174. Lin CH, Wei FC, Lin YT, et al. Endoscopically assisted fascia–saving harvest of rectus abdominis. *Plast Reconstr Surg.* 2001;108:713–718.

197. Pribaz JJ, Weiss DD, Mulliken JB, et al. Prelaminated free flap reconstruction of complex central facial defects. *Plast Reconstr Surg.* 1999;104:357–365; discussion 66–67.

305. Siemionow M, Ozer K, Siemionow W, et al. Robotic assistance in microsurgery. *J Reconstr Microsurg.* 2000;16:643–649.

27

Principles and applications of tissue expansion

Malcolm W. Marks and Louis C. Argenta

SYNOPSIS

- Tissue expansion is a time-tested, proven, simple technique to generate tissue to reconstruct defects.
- The technique stretches skin and soft tissue that have the same color and texture as the adjoining skin where expanded tissue is needed.
- In the breast, expansion is particularly useful in stretching existing anatomy to accommodate a permanent prosthesis.
- Use of the tissue expansion technique can be encouraged.

 Access the Historical Perspective section online at
http://www.expertconsult.com

Introduction

The plastic nature of the human integument can be witnessed whenever the skin must allow for growth underneath it. The surgeon can take advantage of this plasticity when either medical need or aesthetic surgery would benefit from the creation of new, autogenous skin. Tissue expansion can be observed in a variety of developmental, medical, and cultural concepts. For example, basic methods of tissue expansion can be seen in some tribal practices in which wooden and metallic rings are purposely and gradually used to increase the size of lips and earlobes. Just as development of a fetal brain will cause the overlying skull to grow, growth of the skeleton will cause all normal skin and soft tissues that envelope bone to respond and expand. Similarly, the growth of other structures inside the body will cause skin and subcutaneous tissues to expand, as shown by the serial growth of the abdomen with successive pregnancies. Whether the growth is caused by benign or malignant tumors under histologically normal skin or is experienced in the gravid abdomen, there is a clear response to nongenetic stimuli for the necessary growth to accommodate underlying structures.

The benefits of this strategy have caused a significant evolution of therapeutic techniques since the early 1980s: donor tissue can be generated *in situ* and used for reconstruction without compromise of innervation, vascularity, or external physical appearance.

There are various methods for expansion of skin, bone, and other tissues. Placement of a prosthesis under soft tissues allows the surgeon gradually to add saline and expand subcutaneous and cutaneous tissues. External hardware is used by surgeons to expand fractured bone gradually through the application of distraction force. The techniques have been applied to the craniofacial skeleton as well as to most of the long bones of the body.[1,2] Vacuum-assisted closure (VAC) uses this principle of applying force to the cells surrounding a wound to stimulate the induction of new tissue that will subsequently close the wound.[3]

Knowledge advances in tissue expansion principles are discussed below.

Biology of tissue expansion

Extensive information is available regarding the biology of tissue expansion. After animal experiments were completed,[9,16] studies on human tissue examined the process of tissue expansion that occurs both during the period of expansion and postoperatively.[17] Studies of the effects of tissue expansion on nerve, muscle, and bone have also been published.

Skin

Statistical analysis of multiple sites over the implant and its periphery has revealed a significant increase in epidermal thickness during the process of expansion. Early after placement of the prosthesis, significant thickening of the epidermis is evident. This is also seen in sham controls and may represent, in part, postoperative edema. Within 4–6 weeks, epidermal thickness generally returns to initial levels, but some increase in thickness persists for many months.

The increased area of skin over the expander includes not only normal skin recruited from adjacent areas but also new skin generated by increased mitosis.[18] Hair follicles are not reproduced in humans, so individual follicles are distracted during expansion. Distractions between follicles are less noticeable in blonds than in dark-haired individuals. Melanocytic activity is increased during expansion but returns to normal levels within several months after completion of the reconstruction. Although hair follicles and accessory skin structures are compressed by tissue expansion devices, they show no evidence of degeneration.

During expansion, the dermis decreases rapidly in thickness over the entire implant. Thinning is most pronounced in the first several weeks after implant placement and persists for the entire period of expansion. Dermal thinning persists at least 36 weeks after expansion is completed in human tissue.[19]

Capsule

A dense fibrous capsule that becomes less cellular over time forms around the implant. The capsule is thickest at 2 months of expansion. Progressive collagenization with well-organized bundles develops over 3 months.

Molecular studies have demonstrated upregulation in the wingless signaling pathway in the pathogenesis of fibroproliferation in the capsule; this proliferation may contribute to the capsular contracture seen after radiation therapy in breast cancer patients. Such increases have not been demonstrated in nonirradiated tissue. No evidence of dysplastic changes or loss of normal cell maturation has been observed. Dystrophic calcification may occur when a hematoma resolves or when the prosthesis is repeatedly traumatized. The capsule resolves after the prosthesis is removed and little clinical or histologic evidence of it remains over time. Histological examination of capsular tissue demonstrates an extensive vascular plexus within collagen. The capsule itself can be harvested as a local flap because of this induced vascularity.

Muscle

Muscle atrophies greatly during the process of expansion, whether the prosthesis is placed above or below a specific muscle. The effects on human muscle after expansion during breast reconstruction have shown occasional histologic ulceration. Focal muscle fiber degeneration with glycogen deposits and mild interstitial fibrosis has been noted. Some muscle fibers show disorganization of the myofibrils in the sarcomeres.[20] Animal studies on the histomorphologic changes in skeletal muscle suggest that the expansion of skeletal muscle is not a stretching process but is rather a growth process of the muscle cell accompanied by an increase in the number of sarcomeres per fiber. Expanded skeletal muscle repairs normal muscle architecture, vasculature, and function after the prosthesis is removed.[21] Muscle mass returns to normal levels after removal of the device in humans.

Bone

The effect of expansion on underlying cranial bone has been studied in the animal model.[22] Decreases in both bone thickness and volume in cranial bone are evident beneath the expander, where osteoplastic bone resorption occurs. In contrast, there is an increase in these predominantly at the expander periphery, where a periosteal inflammatory reaction is seen. Bone density is unaffected.

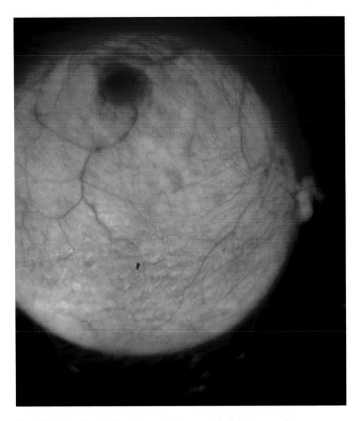

Fig. 27.1 Transillumination of expanded human skin that shows an intense increase in arterioles and venules as well as a dense, interconnecting capillary bed. The proliferation of capillary bed renders the overlying skin erythematous.

Expansion over the cranium in children under a year of age should be done judiciously and slowly. An unclear association between craniosynostosis and expansion over the anterior skull has been seen in one patient. Depression of cranial bone during expansion may occur before 1 year of age, but usually corrects itself once the expander is removed. Cranial bone appears to be measurably more affected in thickness than long bone is. Long-bone remodeling begins within 5 days after removal of the expander, and the long bone is completely normal within 2 months. Remodeling in cranial bone is complete in 2–3 months.

Vascularity of expanded tissue

The robust vascularity of expanded tissue was clinically in evidence long before laboratory work measured it *(Fig. 27.1)*. It has been clinically and histologically demonstrated that a large number of new vessels are formed adjacent to the capsule.[23]

The content of collagen fibers in existing vessels initially decreases after expansion, while elastic fibers in existing blood vessels initially increase in response to mechanical stress.

Angiogenesis occurs in response to induced ischemia of the expanded tissues. The number of cells expressing vascular growth factor is significantly higher in expanded tissue than in nonexpanded, similar tissue.[22] Expanded fascial flaps show a measurable increase in vascularity between the fascia and subcutaneous tissue. Increased perfusion to the distal and peripheral areas of the flap also increases the robustness of the flap[23] and the possibility of harvesting a larger flap. Similar studies on prefabricated, expanded, pedicled flaps have shown increased vascularity within the pedicle, as well as in the surrounding, adjacent, random area.

The increase in vascularity affords the expanded tissue important functional benefits. Animal studies have shown that flaps elevated in expanded tissue have significantly greater survival areas than acutely raised and delayed flaps *(Fig. 27.2)*.[24] Similar studies employing labeled microspheres have demonstrated an increase of flap survival, as well as increased blood flow in the expanded tissue.[15]

Cellular and molecular basis for tissue expansion

The application of mechanical stress to living cells affects various cell structures and signaling pathways that are highly integrated *(Fig. 27.3)*.[25,26] These closely integrated cascades are theorized to explain the generation of new tissue through mechanical stimulation.[26] Several *in vitro* stretching systems have been used to understand better the molecular events that occur.[27]

Mechanical deformation forces involve several cellular mechanisms including the cytoskeleton system, extracellular matrix, enzyme activation, secondary messengers, and ion channels. The cytoskeleton plays a critical role in mediating the transformation of extracellular mechanical force to intracellular events. A system of microfilaments within the cytoplasm not only maintains intracellular tension and cell structure but also transduces signals to adjacent cells and initiates transduction cascades within the cell *(Fig. 27.4)*.[26]

Protein kinase C plays a pivotal role in signal transduction. Mechanical strain on cell walls activates

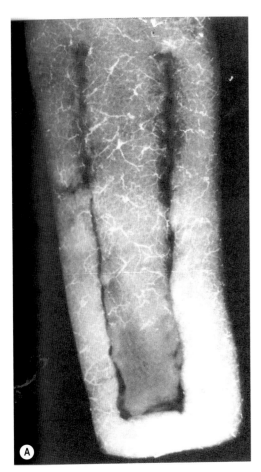
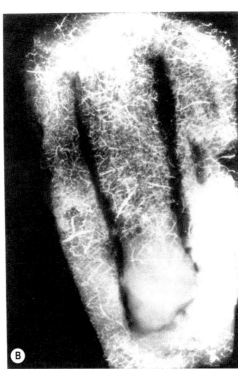

Fig. 27.2 Barium-injected radiograph of vessels in a random-pattern skin flap in a pig **(A)** and an expanded flap in the same animal model **(B).** A dramatic increase in the vascularity of the expanded flap is evident. (From Cherry GW, Austad E, Pasyk K, *et al.* Increased survival and vascularity of random-pattern skin flaps elevated in controlled, expanded skin. Plast Reconstr Surg 1983;72:680–687.)

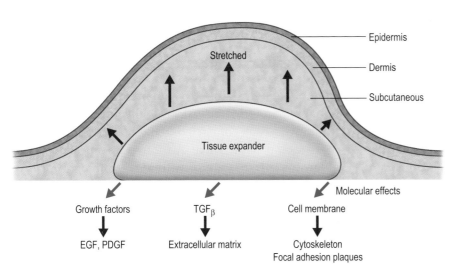

Fig. 27.3 Effects of tissue expansion on surrounding tissue. Strain-induced responses are mediated by growth factors such as platelet-derived growth factor (PDGF) that are known to stimulate cutaneous cell proliferation. Other growth factors such as transforming growth factor-β (TGF-β) may stimulate extracellular matrix production. Membrane-bound molecules including protein kinase play a key role in regulating intracellular signaling cascades. EGF, epidermal growth factor. (Adapted from Takei T, Mills I, Arai K, *et al.* Molecular bases for tissue expansion: clinical implications for surgeon. Plast Reconstr Surg 1998;102:247–258.)

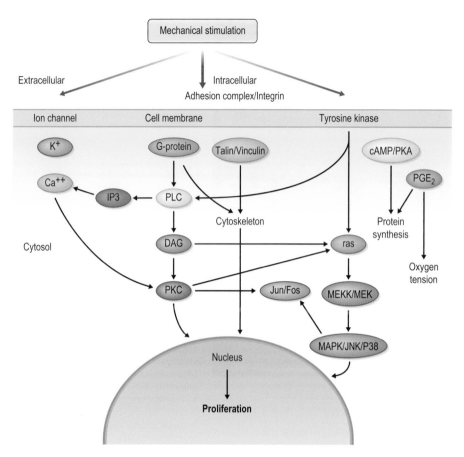

Fig. 27.4 Schematic of possible signal transduction pathways induced by mechanical strain. Transduction pathways are activated by numerous strain-induced signals transmitted through various membrane receptor or membrane ion channels. Terminal enzymes that are activated by these intracellular cascades transduce these signals into the nucleus. cAMP, cyclic adenosine monophosphate; DAG, diacylglycerol; IP$_3$, inositol 1,4,5-triphosphate; JNK, c-Jun amino-terminal kinase; MAPK, mitogen-activated kinases; MEK, MAPK kinase; MEKK, MAPK kinase; PGE$_2$, prostaglandin E$_2$; PKA, protein kinase A; PKC, protein kinase C; PLC, phospholipase C.

inositol phosphatase, phospholipase A$_2$, phospholipase D, and other messengers. Activation of these components leads to activation of protein kinase C, which is, in turn, associated with activation of proteins; presence of this protein activation cascade suggests that intracellular signals can be transmitted to the nucleus. Protein kinase C activation has been noted in human cells subjected to strain *in vitro*.[26]

Many growth factors, including platelet-derived growth factor and angiotensin II, play a role in strain-induced cell growth.[28] Extensive laboratory studies now underway are attempting to quantify and determine the interrelationships of these two, complex molecules. Downstream of the cellular membrane molecules, several common pathways are activated by expansion via both growth factors and mechanical strain; these pathways affect both the cytoskeletal system and protein kinase families.

Implant types

A wide variety of off-the-shelf and custom implants of any shape is available from manufacturers. Radovan's initial expander consisted of a silicone prosthesis with two valves, each connected to the main reservoir by silicone tubing. One valve was used to inject fluid; the other was used to withdraw fluid. Technologic improvements produced a single valve that serves both purposes. There are also expanders that have integrated valves and those that self-inflate, a technology that has received renewed interest since biologically safe hydrocolloids became available.

Expanders with distal ports

Remote filling ports have the advantage of minimizing the risk of implant puncture during inflation. The distal, self-sealing injection port and inflation reservoir are connected to the prosthesis by a length of tubing. This allows the injection port to be placed away from the expander pocket and is advantageous when the overlying skin and soft tissues are thin or when the pocket is too tight to hold an expander with an integrated valve safely.

It is also possible to move the inflation port of a distant reservoir to the exterior of the body; this location facilitates inflation, particularly when the expansion is accomplished by ancillary help or family. Concerns about colonization risk can affect both selection of an implant and management of complications.

Early implants carried a high risk of various types of failure, but improvements in the design of expanders and associated ports have significantly reduced the incidence of mechanical failure.

Expanders with integrated ports

The inflation reservoir may be incorporated directly in the prosthesis. Such devices have the advantage of avoiding the remote port and its associated mechanical problems. However, the risk of inadvertent perforation of the prosthesis during inflation is higher with integrated valves because the valve and integrated prosthesis can be difficult to palpate. Magnetic and ultrasonic devices can be useful when the valve is difficult to locate and metal finding devices have been designed. Expander prostheses with integrated valves are particularly popular for breast reconstruction where adequate soft tissue and pocket can accommodate the added projection of the injection port.

Self-inflating expanders

Self-inflating expanders have become available largely through Europe; these contain osmotic hydrocolloids that cause migration of extracellular water through the silicone membrane of the device. The first such expander was devised by Dr. Austad and was used experimentally; however, it was not approved by the Food and Drug Administration and is not available in the US.[8]

An osmotically active hydrogel expander has been developed and used in expansion of the orbit for management of microphthalmia and anophthalmia.[29] Chummun and associates recently reported their experience using the osmotic tissue expander in patients. Their implant draws sufficient water from the adjacent tissues, spontaneously expanding the prosthesis up to 10 times its original volume.[30]

These devices have the theoretical benefit of continuous slow inflation of the prosthesis. Further benefits may include reducing the number of office visits, lessened pain, and more rapid expansion. Such prostheses have the downside of potential continued expansion even if overlying tissue becomes compromised.

Prosthesis shape, texture, and surface treatment

Prostheses that expand differentially into any specific shape, rather than the usual round, are available. Differential expanders have found the most use in reconstruction of the breast, where ptosis and projection are desired. Low-profile implants that accordion on themselves were designed to eliminate fold-flaw erosion early in the expansion process.

Attempts have been made to incorporate surface textures and geometrics on the expander surface to immobilize the expander and to decrease capsular contracture. Textured silicone expanders have the theoretical advantages of allowing less capsule formation and achieving more rapid expansion. New expanders with surface-bound macromolecules are in development and will attempt to speed expansion by minimizing adjacent scar formation; these will probably become available in the future. Molecules that will form a bacteria-hostile environment are also being devised. These will decrease the development of "slime" around implants in which bacteria live, thus decreasing microbial ability to resist systemic antibiotics.

Basic principles

Tissue expansion is a protracted procedure that may involve temporary, but very obvious, cosmetic deformity. In general, emotionally stable patients of all ages tolerate tissue expansion well. Noncompliant or mentally impaired patients are poor candidates. Smokers have a higher risk of complications. Tissue expansion is generally best performed as a secondary reconstructive procedure rather than in the acute trauma period. Expansion can be performed adjacent to an area of an open wound before definitive closure, but such a procedure carries the risks of infection, extrusion, and less-than-optimal results. Tissue expansion is best suited to those patients who require definitive, optimal coverage when time is not of the essence.

Incision planning and implant selection

The key to successful expansion is meticulous planning before any incision is made. The proposed type of flap – advancement, rotation, or interpositional – that is to be expanded should be carefully planned: the simpler the flap, the less the potential for complication. Ideally, planning is done so that: (1) incisions are incorporated into tissue that will become one margin of the flap; (2) aesthetic units are reconstructed; (3) scars are in minimally conspicuous locations; and (4) tension on suture lines is reduced. The length and position of resultant scars play a major role in determining the overall cosmetic postoperative result. Careful planning allows the prosthesis to be placed through an incision that will both minimize the risk of compromise during flap development and optimize cosmetic reconstruction.

Incisions should be planned to minimize tension on the suture line and risk of extrusion. Tension from the initial inflation on the suture line will be greater when incisions are parallel to the direction of expansion than when they are perpendicular to it. Undermining of the prosthesis should be sufficient enough that the prosthesis can be easily accommodated and the wound can be closed in multiple layers. The inflation valve and tubing should be maintained at a site away from the incision.

Choice of an implant with an external distal port may affect surgical planning. Cultures of implants with external valves revealed that 82% of these prostheses had colonized the expander capsule and had some infection present; this constitutes an infection risk that is slightly higher than that of totally buried prostheses.[31] Although patients tolerate this colonization well and experience few complications, externalized ports are contraindicated when a permanent prosthesis or bone grafts are to be used after expansion is complete.

The size of the implant selected should closely relate to the size and shape of the donor surface. An implant equal to or slightly smaller than the donor area is selected. Because there is minimal risk in hyperinflating the prosthesis to several times the manufacturer's designated volume, less importance is placed on the implant's specific volume than on its overall base size. On occasion, a custom-fabricated implant may be necessary.

In general, the use of multiple small expanders is better than the use of one large expander. Inflation of multiple prostheses proceeds more rapidly and complications are fewer. Multiple expanders also allow the surgeon to vary the plan for reconstruction after expansion has been achieved.

Because of the variety of functional, medical, and surgical considerations, the choice between an integrated valve and a distal inflation port should be considered on a case-by-case basis, without neglecting plans for infection control and the possible need for nonmedical personnel to inflate the implant.

Implant and distal port positioning

If a remote or distal filling port and reservoir is chosen, it must be placed superficially in subcutaneous tissue, where even an extremely small port is easily palpable under stable skin. To minimize discomfort, it is occasionally possible to position a filling port in an area that is relatively less sensitive. The port should be placed in a location that will not be subjected to pressure when the patient is lying in a position that could put direct pressure immediately over the fill port. Bony prominences are avoided.

Care must be taken to avoid kinking of the tubing so that the injected saline will flow readily to the prosthesis. The prosthesis tubing should avoid the incision through which the implant is placed and should not traverse joints. If placement of an external valve is chosen, the connecting tubing should be tunneled a significant distance from the prosthesis.

Expanders are usually placed beneath the skin and subcutaneous tissue above fascia. When the subcutaneous tissue is thin or the risk of extrusion is significant, prostheses may be placed under muscle.

Implant inflation strategy and technique

Implants should be partially inflated immediately after wound closure. This allows closure of "dead space" to minimize seroma and hematoma formation. It also smoothes out the implant wall to minimize risk of fold extrusion. Enough saline is placed to fill the entire dissection space without placing undue tension on the suture line.

Serial inflation usually starts 1–2 weeks after initial placement, although inflation schedules can be individualized to the specific case and the tolerance of the patient. Inflation reservoirs seal best when a 23-gauge or smaller needle is used. A 23-gauge butterfly intravenous needle is especially useful; it allows the patient to move slightly without dislocating the needle.

Frequent small-volume inflations are better tolerated and are physiologically more suited to the development of adequate overlying tissue than are large infrequent inflations. For practical purposes, most prostheses are inflated at weekly intervals. On occasion, accelerated inflation schedules may be followed.[32] In children who have devices with external ports, small-volume inflation at 2–3-day intervals is well tolerated. Individual inflations proceed until the patient experiences discomfort or blanching of the overlying skin. In hypoesthetic areas, objective changes in flap vascularity must be evaluated with particular care. Although a variety of devices such as pressure transducers and oxygen tension monitors are available to help determine proper inflation; an objective inspection of the patient's response is usually a reliable indicator of appropriate inflation. Serial inflations proceed until an adequate amount of soft tissue has been generated to accomplish the specific surgical goal.

Tissue expansion in special cases

Burns

The use of tissue expansion in reconstruction of burns, particularly about the scalp and face, has revolutionized the treatment of burn patients. Because there is almost always inadequate tissue after burns, reconstruction should be carried out after all burns have thoroughly healed and scars have matured. Planning is particularly important in these cases so that a minimum number of suture lines is produced and that these suture lines do not cross aesthetic units. Significant late distortion and contracture may result in excessive scars placed in burned tissue, particularly in the facial area.

Skin that has suffered a partial-thickness burn or that has been scarred by adjacent burns is attenuated and is more amenable to expansion.[33] Incisions can be placed in previous scars, but the scar should be mature and relatively thick so that extrusion does not occur. Using an access incision within normal tissue that is peripheral to the burned area further minimizes the risk of extrusion. The principle of using multiple, smaller-volume prostheses is especially appropriate in burn patients. Perioperative antibiotics and meticulous preparation are always used because the incidence of infection is higher in burn patients.

Tissue expansion in children

Skin and soft tissue are always thinner in children than in adults. These tissues are probably better vascularized but less resistant to trauma. Tissue expansion has a higher complication rate in children than in adults.[34] Rather than using excessively large prostheses or expanding tissue aggressively, accomplishing serial repeated expansions may be helpful in children. This is done with the understanding that major complication risk – particularly extrusion – is more common at the second, third, and fourth serial expansion.[35] This is particularly true in the head and neck (with the exception of the scalp). Expansion of the facial areas and neck can be particularly difficult.

After age 5, most children are able to cooperate adequately, so complication rates decrease. In many children, an external reservoir is used to minimize the amount of emotional trauma caused by injections. Application of EMLA to the skin over the buried injection port is also helpful in minimizing discomfort. Small-volume inflation at frequent intervals is especially useful in children because the amount of pain generated is considerably less.

As in all cases, planning should be meticulous so that the flaps generated will result as much as possible in reconstruction of anatomic units. With growth, contracture may occur, particularly about the mouth and around the orbits, and revision will be required.

Expansion of myocutaneous, fascial, and free flaps

Myocutaneous flaps are the standard of care for the treatment of large defects, particularly when bone and vital structures are involved. The territories of standard flaps are well described. These territories can be considerably enlarged by placing an expander beneath the standard myocutaneous flap, and an extremely large flap can be developed over a short period. Expansion increases the vascularity of the flap and allows a large, adjacent random area to be carried with the original flap.[36] The vascular pedicle of such flaps remains intact and may in fact be elongated, thus allowing flaps to be transferred farther.

Myocutaneous flaps such as the latissimus dorsi and pectoralis can be expanded to almost double their surface area, allowing coverage of almost any defect on the abdomen or thorax.[37] Expanders of up to 1000 mL can be placed beneath such flaps and rapidly expanded. For example, bilateral latissimus dorsi myocutaneous flaps can be expanded and moved to the midline to cover large meningoceles or the vertebral column. The expansion prostheses in these cases are placed under the latissimus dorsi muscle through incisions in the lateral margin of the muscle.

In the procedure one edge of the myocutaneous flap is selected for implant placement, and care is taken not to injure the vascular pedicle. The expanded myocutaneous flap generated can then be transferred as either a pedicled flap or a free flap. Such expanded flaps not only provide coverage of other donor defects but also preserve the function of the muscle.

Fasciocutaneous flaps can be expanded either before or after transposition. When flaps are expanded before transfer, it is best to keep the prosthesis as far away from the pedicle as possible, thus preferentially expanding the random area of the flap. Within 6 months of transfer of these flaps, the random blood supply is usually sufficiently established to allow placement of the expander anywhere under the flap.[38]

Total facial reconstruction with an extraordinarily large flap has been accomplished using a pre-expanded bilateral parascapular free flap. Use of this strategy allows one large aesthetic unit to be moved.[39,40]

Expanded full-thickness skin grafts

Because a donor defect is usually created by harvesting full-thickness grafts, their use is infrequent. The placement of a large tissue expander beneath the donor site can result in a large full-thickness graft that is particularly useful in resurfacing large areas of the face or the entire hand or foot. Expanded full-thickness grafts are extremely resilient and have been shown to grow in children over time. The rate of contracture is significantly less than that of split-thickness grafts.

The best color matches are generated when the full-thickness graft is expanded and harvested as close as possible to the recipient site. The periorbital area and the area around the mouth are particularly well suited to reconstruction with expanded full-thickness grafts harvested from the supraclavicular area. Expanded full-thickness grafts are very helpful in reconstructing defects of the forehead that encompass more than 70% of its surface area. A single full-thickness graft can be harvested from the supraclavicular area or from under the breast fold. Care must be taken that hair-bearing tissue is not transferred to an area that normally has no hair.

Expanders with a surface area equal to that of the donor site are placed through peripheral incisions. The prosthesis is then inflated to an adequate volume. After sufficient donor tissue is generated, a template is made of the recipient site and transferred to the expanded donor area. The full-thickness graft is harvested so that it is approximately 10–15% larger than the recipient area, allowing for some contracture. The prosthesis is then removed, leaving the capsule intact, and the donor site closed primarily. Closing of the donor site should be done so that the resulting scar is as innocuous as possible. In the recipient site, expanded full-thickness skin grafts require more immobilization than split-thickness skin grafts do. A bolster dressing or, ideally, a VAC sponge dressing is required. The graft is sutured in place and a VAC sponge placed over the graft; 125 mmHg of negative pressure is maintained for 4 days. Successful take of such grafts placed with this technique is extremely high.

Reconstruction in the head and neck

The head and neck area contains many specialized tissues that must be matched appropriately to achieve optimal aesthetic reconstruction. Aesthetic reconstruction is maximized by mobilization of adjacent local tissues rather than by transfer of distant tissues with poor match of color, texture, or hair-bearing capability. Tissue expansion therefore allows optimal aesthetic reconstruction by use of a similar adjacent tissue area to reconstruct a defect without creation of a donor site.[11,41]

The skin of the face can be subdivided into five tissue-specific areas:

1. The scalp is unique in that it contains specific hair-bearing qualities that cannot be mimicked by any other tissue of the human body.

2. The forehead is a continuation of the scalp, but it is distinguished from the scalp by its thick skin, large number of sebaceous glands, and lack of hair.

3. The nose is embryologically related to the forehead, so it closely mimics the forehead in color, texture, and sebaceous gland content.

4. The lateral cheek areas, neck, and upper lip have fewer sebaceous glands; the skin is thinner, and the hair-bearing pattern is significantly different in quality and quantity from that on the remainder of the body.

5. The skin of the periorbital areas is extremely thin and pliable, containing a minimal number of sebaceous glands.

There is a limited amount of tissue on the human face, so procedures must be planned carefully and reconstruction accomplished correctly at the first attempt. Correct planning should take into consideration the area and shape of the defect, quality of the remaining tissue of the aesthetic unit, pre-existing scars, and reconstructive needs of other areas of the head and neck. Because of the risk of complications, it is prudent to plan alternative reconstructive strategies before any prostheses are placed. If there is a chronic infection, the presence of fistulas, or the need to reconstruct facial mass, other reconstructive alternatives may achieve a better final result.

Scalp

Tissue expansion is the ideal procedure for the reconstruction of scalp defects *(Fig. 27.5)*.[42] Expansion of the scalp is well tolerated and is the only procedure that allows development of normal hair-bearing tissue to cover the areas of alopecia. The amount of scar and deformity generated is considerably less than with previous procedures such as serial reduction and complex multiflap procedures.

While some animal studies have demonstrated an increase in hair follicles during tissue expansion, our clinical experience suggests that humans do not form a significant number of new follicles. Rather, existing follicles are redistributed to a larger surface area. Because of the finite number of follicles, attempts should be made to redistribute them as homogeneously as possible. To accomplish this, large or multiple expanders, expanding large areas of the remaining scalp, produce the best results. Hair follicles can be separated by a factor of 2 without producing noticeable thinning. The darker the hair, the more visible the thinning is. Individuals who have large defects and require extreme expansion may achieve better results by lightening the hair with dyes.

Although there is considerable overlap in the vascular territories of the scalp, the incorporation of one or more major vessels of the scalp optimizes reconstruction. Flaps should be well vascularized to ensure maximum growth of hair. Planning is therefore of importance, as is consideration of scar and previous areas of trauma. Advancement or rotation flaps achieve the best results, particularly when the anterior hairline is reconstructed. Simultaneous expansion and mobilization of the forehead may also help achieve a normal hairline.

Previous scars and incisions can be used for placement of the prosthesis. Once the galea is encountered, dissection can proceed widely with a blunt dissector. It is not unusual to mobilize most of the remaining scalp so that the prosthesis is well accommodated. Individual pockets are not necessary for multiple expanders, but care should be taken to fix the inflation reservoirs so that they do not migrate into a common pocket. Prostheses with incorporated inflation reservoirs can also be used, but patients often find them bulky and uncomfortable. Inflation reservoirs can be

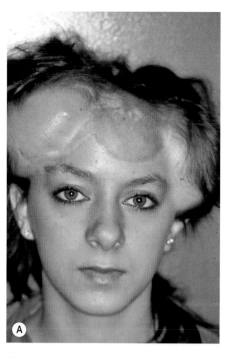
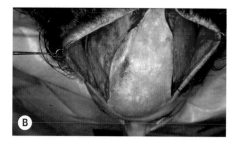
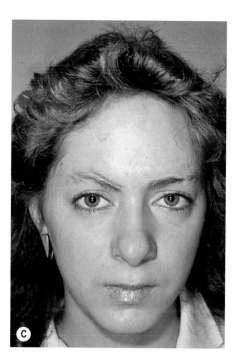

Fig. 27.5 (A) Young woman with avulsion injury to the right scalp, which had been covered with a transposition flap from the left scalp that resulted in a scalp and forehead skin graft. Two expanders were placed, one on either side, encompassing as much of the hair and forehead as possible. **(B)** Expanders removed and advancement flaps ready for repositioning. **(C)** Patient shown postoperatively with a normal hairline, normal brow, and normal hair-bearing scalp.

placed at the vertex of the scalp or in the forehead. Care should be taken not to place them where pressure is applied during sleep.

Expansion of the scalp is initially uncomfortable. It is better to use frequent small saline injections than to use infrequent large injections. After several weeks, the scalp loosens, and large amounts of saline can be infused without difficulty. Most scalp expansions can be accomplished in 6–8 weeks, particularly when multiple expanders are used.[43]

Once adequate expansion has been achieved, the prostheses are removed through the incisions through which they were originally placed or at the margin of the flap to be moved. Flaps should be designed for advancement, transposition, or rotation. Every attempt should be made to minimize transection of the major vessels of the scalp; care in this regard will allow faster healing and better regeneration of hair follicles. Removal or cutting of capsule and galea should be avoided in order to preserve blood supply. Large areas of the scalp are mobilized and positioned by temporary staples. (Dog-ears are left in place because they subside over time.) The wounds are then closed.

It may be impossible to gain an adequate amount of tissue with one expansion when large areas of the scalp must be resurfaced, in which case serial expansion is used *(Fig. 27.6)*. After the initial expansion, flaps are advanced as far as possible. Lesions or areas of alopecia are excised only after the flap has been advanced. The expander is then left in place under the flap and, after several months, the scalp is re-expanded. Adults tolerate three or four sequential expansions without difficulty. Infants and children may thin excessively after two expansions; an interim period of 8–12 months is optimal for a later expansion.

In growing children, scars frequently widen over time. These require revision when they become a cosmetic problem, optimally after 16–18 years of age. Scalp that has been vigorously expanded may lose some hair follicles, but these usually regrow hair. Twelve months should pass before any areas of alopecia are considered permanent.

Some erosion and depression of the skull may be seen in children radiographically and, occasionally, clinically. The thickness of the periosteum and subcutaneous tissue at the margins of the expander

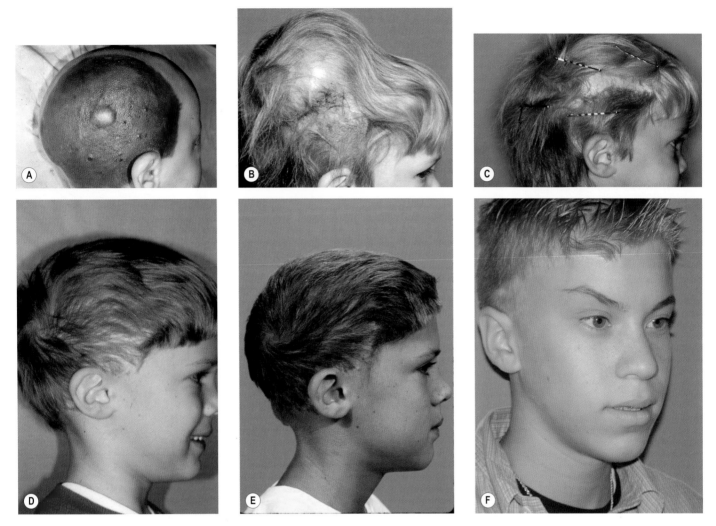

Fig. 27.6 (A) Child born with a giant hairy nevus occupying one-third of the scalp. **(B)** The remaining normal scalp was expanded, allowing removal of more than half of the lesion. **(C)** The original expander was left in place and 4 months later re-expanded, generating tissue that allowed removal of the remaining lesion. **(D)** The patient is shown 1 year after expansion. **(E)** The patient 10 years after expansion with stable hairline and normal hair distribution. **(F)** Patient shown at age 18. No revisions have been required.

may be obvious, but will resolve once the device is removed. Expansion should best be delayed in children until they are approximately 1 year of age. By this time, the skull is solid enough that significant erosion is not a cause for concern. Long-term studies have demonstrated no detrimental growth of the skull in children who have undergone scalp expansion in infancy *(Fig. 27.7)*.

Male-pattern baldness

Tissue expansion can be used to develop hair-bearing flaps that will replace skin that is affected by male-pattern baldness.[44–46] Expansion allows the homogeneous distribution of the remaining hair follicles and reduces the tension that can be caused by excision of scalp.

In patients with vertex baldness, the remaining temporal and occipital scalp can be expanded for 2 months. Expanders are placed through incisions that would normally be used for scalp reduction. Cosmetic deformity during this process may be significant after the first several weeks. At the second procedure, the scalp is advanced as far as possible and the area of alopecia removed.

Patients who are unable to accept the deformity that occurs with single large expansions can be serially expanded and undergo serial scalp reduction. In these

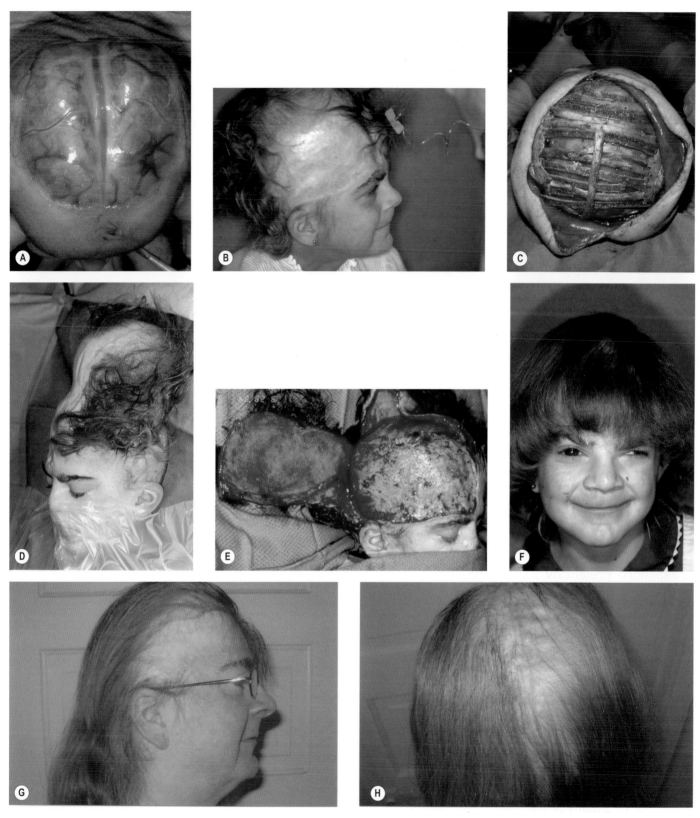

Fig. 27.7 (A) An infant born with severe aplasia cutis congenita involving the scalp, skull, and derma that left exposed brain. **(B)** The brain was covered immediately after birth with two, large, scalp–forehead advancement flaps. Absence of the cranium prevented the patient from attending school. **(C)** At age 4 years, the flaps were separated from the underlying brain; a reinforced polyethylene sheet was secured to the cranial defect, an expander was placed over the sheet, and the scalp was expanded for 3 months. **(D)** The cranium was reconstructed with multiple split-rib grafts within the expanded capsule. **(E)** One year later, the scalp was re-expanded to more than 1000 mL over the reconstructed cranium. The skin graft was excised and the scalp and forehead flaps were repositioned appropriately. The reconstructed skull suffered no ill effect during the re-expansion. **(F)** Patient shown 1 year after reconstruction. **(G)** The patient at age 36 with an intact skull, normal scalp, and minor alopecia. **(H)** Posterior scalp showing thinning of hair-bearing tissue, but a resilient, pliable scalp over an intact cranium. (From Argenta LC, Dingman RO. Total reconstruction of aplasia cutis congenita involving scalp, skull, and dura. Plast Reconstr Surg. 1986;77:650–653.)

patients, the prosthesis is inflated until deformities become visible. The expanders are deflated and the hair-bearing flaps advanced as far cephalad as possible. The prostheses are left in place, and a second or third expansion is carried out until the entire bald area is removed.

Expansion can also be used to increase the size of standard transposition flaps greatly. Anterior baldness that affects the hairline can be modified into a new, natural-looking hairline with Juri transposition flaps. However, these flaps are limited in size and may require multiple delays to ensure adequate hair viability.[47] Expanders placed beneath the temporoparietal area can dramatically increase the size of Juri flaps and increase their safety. Bilateral flaps, one transposed behind the other, will cover the entire forehead and a significant portion of the scalp behind it. The bilateral advancement transposition flap is especially efficacious in transposing a large amount of hair to the forehead.[48]

Forehead

The forehead is anatomically and histologically identical to the scalp except for its different numbers of sebaceous glands and hair-bearing follicles. Reduction or increase of the surface area of the forehead by 20–25% is not usually readily apparent after appropriate hair styling. By expanding the scalp in conjunction with expanding the forehead, better symmetric brow positioning is achieved while maintaining the normal hairline.

In individuals with very high hairlines, the scalp can be expanded posteriorly and brought forward to the junction of the forehead and scalp. Generally, a lateral movement of scalp tissue is less visible postoperatively. When defects involve tissue lateral to the orbit, expansion of the cheek area with cephalad movement of the exposed tissue may be helpful. The temporal hairline and the lateral hairline that lies anterior to the ear can be reconstructed with an advancement or transposition of scalp flap.

Prostheses are usually placed in the forehead through an incision in the scalp. The prostheses are placed beneath the frontalis muscle because this plane is safe and a well-vascularized flap can be developed. Multiple expanders are usually needed both to generate adequate tissue to be mobilized and simultaneously to allow the brows to remain in an appropriate symmetric position.

Expansion is at first difficult and uncomfortable, but as in the scalp, the expansion proceeds rapidly after several weeks. Flaps may be developed in any direction but are usually simple advancements. The adjacent scalp should be mobilized at the same time so that a normal hairline can be reconstructed.

Expansion of the forehead is useful in many craniofacial anomalies with low hairlines. Expansion of the remaining forehead is accomplished and moved into a cephalad direction. The intervening hair-bearing scalp is excised. Fixation of the expanded forehead to the underlying skull with small screws reduces the amount of retraction.

If the entire forehead must be reconstructed, the optimal choice is the use of an expanded full-thickness graft from the neck. These grafts must be secured in place with negative-pressure devices for at least 4 days.

Lateral face and neck

The type of skin on the lateral facial areas and neck is essentially the same. This skin has hair-bearing potential and is relatively thin, but contains numerous oil and sebaceous glands. It is much thinner than skin on the forehead and nose.

A large Mustardé expanded rotation flap can be developed on the neck for use in facial reconstruction. In children, there is a higher risk of extrusion problems in the expansion of this area of the face (*Fig. 27.8*). In adults, such reconstruction can be accomplished with relative ease. The flap is based inferiorly and medially.

The prosthesis is inserted through a preauricular facelift-type incision. The platysma should not be incorporated because doing so exposes the marginal mandibular nerve to trauma and restricts flap advancement. Distal reservoirs are usually placed in the neck or behind the ear. The prosthesis is then inflated as tolerated by the patient. Despite placement of the prosthesis over the carotid artery and jugular vein, few complications have been encountered.

Once an adequate amount of tissue has been generated, the Mustardé flap is elevated. This is done through a preauricular incision that is carried in front of the hair-bearing scalp and then on to the lateral orbital area above the lateral canthus. The flap is then rotated medially and superiorly to cover whatever areas of the cheek require resurfacing. In general, it is best to rotate this

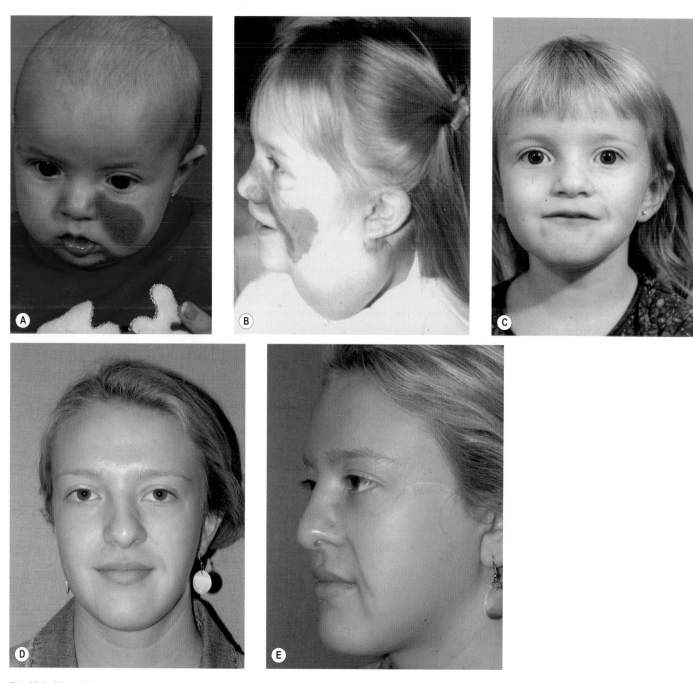

Fig. 27.8 (A) An infant with a giant hairy nevus of the face. **(B)** The neck and lateral face were expanded by placing a prosthesis through an incision in the nevus. An expanded Mustardé cheek rotation flap was rotated as an aesthetic unit over the lateral face. **(C)** The patient at 5 years of age. **(D)** The patient at 18 years of age with minimal scars that are easily amenable to makeup. **(E)** Lateral view demonstrating no ectropion and an aesthetic reconstruction.

flap and secure it in place with temporary staples before the recipient area is excised. It is best not to carry the medial scar in this flap beyond the lateral commissure because scars below that feature tend to distort the mouth. The flap is suspended both medially and laterally at a level above the canthi; this prevents development of later ectropion. If coverage is required for the periorbital area, this is done as a separate aesthetic unit graft, usually a full-thickness graft from the supraclavicular area.

The lower half of the face and the neck are aesthetically the same unit. Hair distribution, sebaceous gland density, and skin thickness are similar. Defects of the lower face and neck can be interchangeably reconstructed by expanding either the lower face or the neck. Most frequently, the neck is expanded and the flap advanced into the lower face. If necessary, bone grafts that are placed beneath the expanded flap can reconstruct the mandible and maxilla.

The prosthesis should be placed in the neck superficial to the platysma muscle; despite its placement directly above major arteries and veins, complications are few. Bilateral expanders usually have a volume of 400–500 mL. Once an adequate amount of tissue is generated, the flaps can be brought superiorly to cover the lower edge of the face, medially to cover the central portion of the neck, or laterally in the neck as needed (*Fig. 27.9*). When flaps are brought from the neck into the face, it is important to secure the flap with permanent sutures to the deep muscles at the commissures of the mouth. If this is not accomplished, oral incontinence may develop later. Form-fitting neck collars may be necessary to secure the expanded flap in place over the neck after a portion of it has been brought on to the face.

Nose

Reconstruction of major defects of the nose, including total nose reconstruction, may be facilitated by pre-expanding the forehead skin. Before the use of tissue expansion, having both inadequate amounts of tissue and difficulty closing the forehead could be anticipated. However now, when total nose reconstruction is performed, expansion of the entire forehead with a 400–600-mL prosthesis generates an adequate number of large, well-vascularized flaps to accomplish both total nose reconstruction and closure of the donor site. Because the color and texture of the forehead are ideally suited to reconstruction of the nose, this procedure makes reconstruction of any nasal defect possible.

Any of the standard forehead flaps can be employed in conjunction with expansion. If reconstruction of the nasal lining is also necessary, expansion of a forehead or Converse scalping flap develops enough tissue to allow folding of the expanded tissue on itself.

The supraorbital and supratrochlear vessels are located by Doppler examination, and the nasal flap is based on the location of either of these axial vessels. Prostheses are best placed beneath the frontalis muscle through an incision above the hairline. At the second procedure, the expander is removed and the flap, including the capsule, is rotated inferiorly. Approximately 2 cm above the supraorbital rim, the posterior capsule is incised, and development of the flap is continued in a subperiosteal plane. This allows mobilization of the flap into the orbit, almost down to the canthus.

Having sufficient bony and cartilaginous supporting structures of the nose is critical to avoiding contraction of the expanded tissue. Early experience in use of expanded forehead tissue was unsuccessful because the underlying bony and cartilaginous structure was not adequate. A cranial bone or rib graft is taken to reconstruct the dorsum of the nose. This is either secured to the remaining nasal bone or attached by a plate to the skull. The nasal cartilage is reconstructed bilaterally with cartilage from the conchal bowl. Thinly carved rib cartilage is also useful if the ear cartilage is inadequate. Nasal stents are used for 3–4 months to maintain a patent airway while the flap matures.

The forehead flap is divided and inset approximately 2 weeks after rotation. Some swelling and contracture of tissue may occur, but major touch-ups are infrequently needed (*Fig. 27.10*).

Ear

Most cases of microtia and traumatic ear deformities can be reconstructed without expansion. Expansion is helpful when skin and soft tissue are insufficient for reconstruction. As with all ear reconstructions, a child should be approximately 7 years of age before reconstruction is begun. A custom or rectangular expander is placed beneath the remaining non-hairbearing tissue that is adjacent to the remnant.[49] The prosthesis is then expanded and left in place for approximately 3 months.[19] This allows both significant thinning of the overlying skin and tissue maturity that will together result in minimal secondary distortion due to contracture.[49]

The expansion prosthesis is best placed through an incision in the postauricular hair-bearing tissue, preserving the temporoparietal fascia for possible later needs. Once adequate tissue has been generated, the framework is reconstructed with carved costal cartilage.

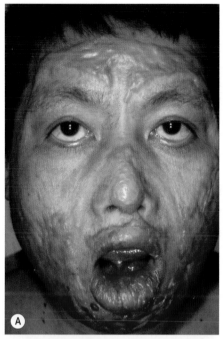
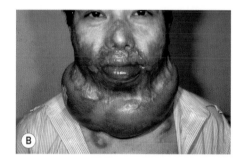
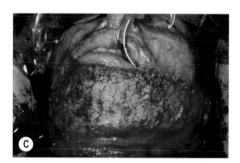
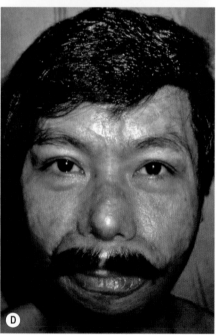

Fig. 27.9 (A) Young man who sustained extensive burns over the face, but in whom the neck was largely spared. **(B)** Bilateral large expanders were placed in the neck and the entire neck and upper chest were expanded dramatically. **(C)** The area of burned skin over the lower face was excised and the neck flap advanced superiorly. The capsule was secured firmly to the muscle on the lateral commissures to minimize later distortion of the mouth. **(D)** The patient 2 years later. The upper lip has been reconstructed as an aesthetic unit from hair-bearing, temporoparietal flaps.

Some exaggeration of the bulk of the infrastructure minimizes distortion because it conforms to the cartilage. Silicone and other synthetic frameworks give excellent initial results, but they are fraught with late complications. In general, autologous tissues are recommended for ear reconstruction.

Periorbital area with expanded full-thickness grafts

The periorbital area contains skin that is soft and pliable. It contains few glands and no hair. Unfortunately, little tissue in the periorbital area can be expanded or moved

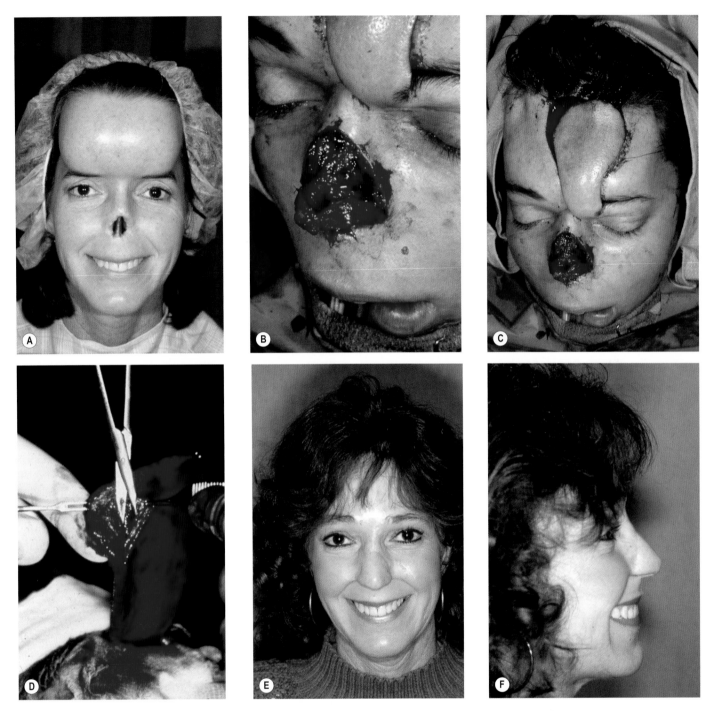

Fig. 27.10 (A) This woman had her nose resected for a mucosal melanoma. Three years later, reconstruction was begun by placement of a 450-mL expander in the forehead. **(B)** At the second procedure, the infrastructure of the nose was made with a cantilever bone graft and bilateral, conchal cartilage grafts. **(C)** The forehead flap was turned down in the subperiosteal plane to the level of the medial canthus. **(D)** The distal third of the flap was markedly thin so that the skin could be turned on itself to recreate the nasal lining. **(E)** and **(F)** The patient 11 years after reconstruction with a functional breathing nose. No further modifications have been required in the succceding 24 years.

easily. When large areas require reconstruction, full-thickness skin grafts from expanded donor sites are recommended. Replacement of aesthetic units – the entire periorbital area or the upper or lower lid – gives the best result *(Fig. 27.11)*.

The supraclavicular area contains soft pliable skin that mimics orbital skin. Therefore, this is a good site for expanding, templating, and harvesting tissue subcutaneously, above the platysma. After harvesting, the expanded skin graft is thinned to dermis and sutured to the recipient site (see section on expanded full-thickness skin grafts, above). Long-term results have been remarkable in that this tissue grows with children, scar is minimal, and secondary reconstruction is infrequent.

Reconstruction in the breast, chest, trunk, and extremities

Postmastectomy breast reconstruction

Tissue expansion was introduced by Chemar Radovan in 1982 to facilitate breast reconstruction in postmastectomy patients because these patients were found to have insufficient chest wall tissue for placement of the implant.[7] Originally, the expanders were placed subcutaneously, but results from these reconstructions tended to be firm and round with a less-than-ideal cosmetic appearance. As the procedure became more widely accepted, surgeons preferred subpectoral and submuscular placement of implants. Breast reconstruction techniques have continued to evolve over the last 30 years and, with refinements in the techniques for autologous tissue transfer, the aesthetic standards for breast reconstruction have increased. Tissue expansion allows ideal color and texture match of the reconstructed breast with the remaining chest wall because the breast is generated from existing chest wall skin. Tissue expansion is a much simpler option for breast reconstruction than the more complex procedures used in autologous tissue transfer.

In a 2007 survey, the American Society of Plastic Surgeons reported 57 102 breast reconstructions, of which 60% were expander reconstructions.[50] Use of tissue expansion and breast implants remains the most common method for postmastectomy reconstruction in the US. Four factors account for widespread use of this technique: (1) continued refinements in surgical technique for mastectomy; (2) preservation of the pectoralis major muscle and its innervation; (3) less radical excision of skin with skin-sparing mastectomy; and (4) preservation of the inframammary fold. Because of these practical techniques, more reconstruction cases in patients with qualitatively good chest wall skin and soft tissue are suited to expansion techniques.

Placement of an expander prosthesis for breast reconstruction is a simple, straightforward procedure. In the case of immediate reconstruction, it adds little operative time after mastectomy and does not prolong the postmastectomy hospitalization. Delayed reconstruction with a tissue expander can be done as an outpatient procedure or with minimal hospitalization; it is ideally suited to both elderly patients and those who wish to have a minimal postoperative recovery.

Breast reconstruction with the tissue expansion technique usually requires two operative procedures. In the first procedure, the tissue expander is placed through the original mastectomy scar, thus avoiding additional scarring. Removal of the tissue expander and placement of the permanent implant are also accomplished through a straightforward approach and can be done under general or local anesthesia in an outpatient setting. However, if the expander is less than ideally positioned, the second procedure will be more complicated, requiring capsulotomy or capsulectomy. The reconstructed breast will experience some shifting and settling after placement of the permanent implant, so it is usually best to delay nipple reconstruction for several months.

Recreation of the inframammary fold and natural breast ptosis remains a difficult aesthetic goal. The location of the expander – whether it is better placed subpectorally or entirely submuscularly – is therefore a frequently debated topic. The use of acellular dermal matrices to cover the lower pole of the implant expander was introduced in 2005[51] and has gained in popularity in recent years because it obviates the need for dissection of the serratus anterior. This results in less implant displacement during expansion.

The frequent visits required to inflate the expansion device fully create some inconvenience for patients, who are seen every 7–14 days; this process usually

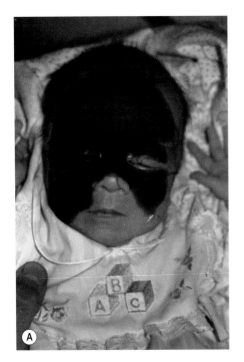
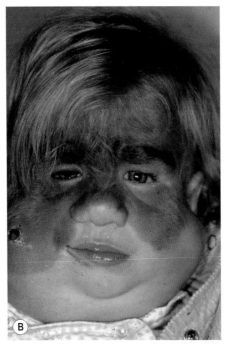
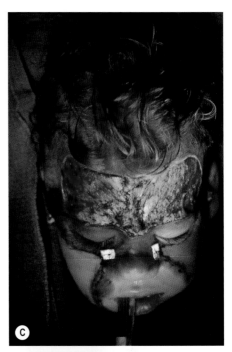
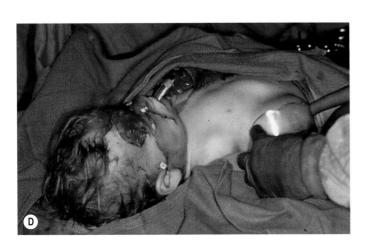
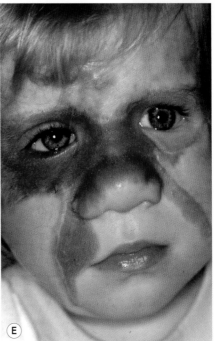

Fig. 27.11 **(A)** A complex midface giant hairy nevus in a newborn. Reconstruction was undertaken in multiple stages at 2.5 years of age. **(B)** Bilateral expanders were placed in the neck area to reconstruct the lateral face and a third expander was placed in the lateral thoracic wall to generate an expanded, full-thickness skin graft. **(C)** Bilateral Mustardé cheek flaps were advanced as aesthetic units. Note that the nevus outside the anatomical aesthetic unit was left in place to be resected later. **(D)** and **(E)** The forehead was excised and a full-thickness skin graft was harvested from the expanded right thoracic wall.

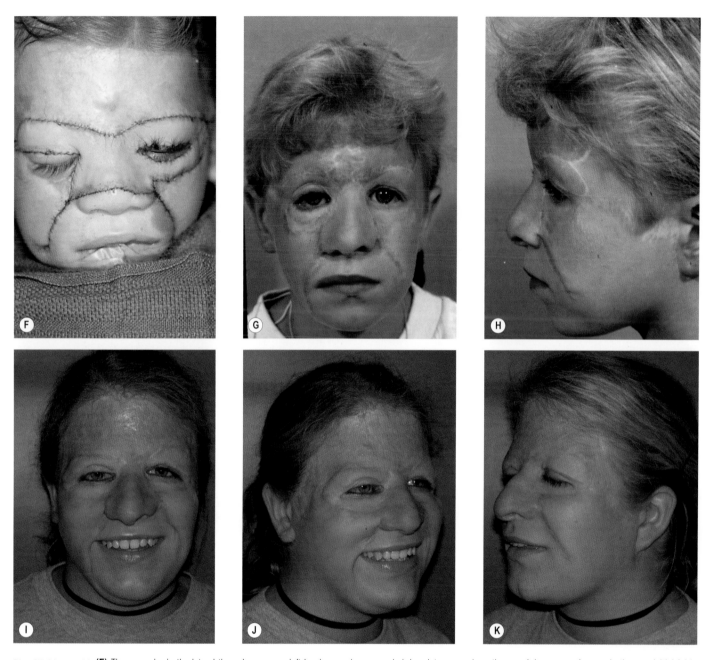

Fig. 27.11, cont'd (F) The expander in the lateral thoracic area was left in place and re-expanded. In a later procedure, the remaining areas of nevus in the nasolabial folds on each side were excised. The entire periocular and nasal area was then excised and grafted with full-thickness, expanded graft. **(G)** and **(H)** The patient 5 years after reconstruction with a stable result. **(I–K)** The patient at 21 years of age. Note that the face has grown normally and symmetrically and that facial nerve function has been maintained. The patient is able to hide remaining scars with minimal makeup.

continues for 2–3 months, depending on the desired final size of the implant. Overinflation is helpful when permanent breast implants are to be placed. Inflation of breast expanders by 20% over capacity is commonly performed so that after the permanent implant is placed, some ptosis of the breast can be developed.

The expander device

The original expanders were smooth-walled silicone devices with a remote port. Placement of the remote valve often proved tedious and, if not perfectly placed, resulted in mechanical filling difficulty.

In recent years, expanders with integrated valves have become the expanders of choice in breast reconstruction.[52,53] The valve is located in the upper pole of the breast. Because an inflation needle can puncture an expander, the valve is easily palpable and has a metal backing to prevent injury to the attached expander. The integrated valve avoids the need to create a separate lateral pocket and subcutaneous tunnels for the connecting tube. It avoids the complications associated with a distal port, including rotation and extrusion of the port, and mechanical problems related to the connecting tubing such as kinking and leaking.

The textured silicone implant has been an important advance in breast reconstruction with tissue expansion. A textured surface enables tissue ingrowth and adherence of the capsule, which, in turn, immobilizes the implant. It is imperative that the textured expander be ideally positioned. The immobility of the textured implant enables development of two aesthetic benefits: a more anatomic expansion of the overlying tissue and more expansion in the inframammary fold area that helps establish a fold with some degree of ptosis.

Expander devices are generally described as round or anatomic. There is a myriad of expander shapes and sizes: In the last 10 years, McGhan, Medical (Allergan), Mentor, and PMT have developed anatomic expanders of varying projection and height.[53–55] Each device is designed to allow for a more natural breast reconstruction by providing unique differential expansion of the upper, middle, and lower poles of the breast. In our experience, however, two other factors determine the final outcome more than the expander shape does: the quality of the skin and subcutaneous tissue and the preservation of the inframammary fold after mastectomy.

Immediate postmastectomy breast reconstruction

The inframammary folds should be marked with the patient sitting in an upright position before general anesthesia is induced for mastectomy and placement of the expander. The mastectomy should be accomplished in a fashion that maximizes local control, with careful attention, however, to preservation of skin and subcutaneous tissue, especially in the inframammary fold area. In recent years, with the advent of skin-sparing mastectomy, general surgeons are much more conscientious in preservation of the skin. If too much skin is spared, the plastic surgeon will need to trim excess skin that could cause dog-ears and sagging; this is done after placing the expander.

After completion of the mastectomy, the expander device is placed in one of three locations, depending on the surgeon's preference and experiences. These are the submuscular position, the subpectoral (dual-plane) position, and the subpectoral position with supplementation with an acellular allogenic dermal matrix (ADM).

Complete muscle coverage is more important in immediate than in secondary breast reconstruction because it completely isolates the implant from the overlying mastectomy wound. Should there be skin necrosis with a loss of mastectomy flaps, wound dehiscence, delayed healing – especially in previously irradiated chest walls – or cellulitis, a totally submuscular implant may be salvaged, whereas a partially submuscular implant will be lost.

After placement of the implant by one of these three methods, suction drains are placed in the subcutaneous space and in the axilla if a lymph node dissection has also been accomplished. The wounds are closed and the expander filled with enough fluid to obliterate dead space, but avoiding excessive tension on the wound closure.

Submuscular position

When the submuscular position is used for expansion, a submuscular pocket is dissected for placement of the tissue expander. The muscle incision can be made in one of two locations. If a musculofascial layer has been preserved after mastectomy, the incision can be made parallel to the pectoralis major fibers. Using sharp and blunt dissection, the pectoralis major muscle is lifted off the underlying chest wall and the pectoralis minor muscle. Dissection is continued inferiorly beneath the origin of the rectus abdominis muscle and laterally beneath the serratus interior muscle.

Alternatively, an incision can be made at the lateral boarder of the pectoralis major or parallel to the fibers of the serratus anterior muscle. This dissection is continued down to the rib, and from the lateral position, a pocket is dissected inferiorly, superiorly, and medially, lifting the pectoralis major origin off the rectus abdominis muscle and the origin of the serratus anterior muscle.

It is important to avoid dissecting the serratus anterior muscle too far laterally, regardless of the location of the muscle incision, for this would allow displacement of the implant into the axilla. If the fascia at the junction at the pectoralis major and rectus abdominal muscles has been violated during mastectomy, complete submuscular closure can be difficult. In general, a small exposure of the implant is of no consequence. A large exposure can be covered with a transposition or rotation of anterior rectus abdominis fascia.

Subpectoral (dual-plane) position

Only the upper two-thirds of the expander in the subpectoral (dual-plane) position is covered by muscle. Advantages include less postoperative discomfort and less discomfort during expansions. Criticisms of this technique include the risk of upward migration of the pectoralis major, which results in even less coverage of the lower portion of the implant. If there is a wound breakdown at the mastectomy incision, the implant, rather than muscle, will be exposed.

The inferior border of the pectoralis major is identified, the pectoralis fascia is incised if it has been preserved, and the muscle is elevated while preserving the origin of the serratus anterior rectus abdominis muscle. The expander is introduced so that it lies in a dual plane with its upper pole covered by muscle and its lower pole by subcutaneous tissue.

Subpectoral position with an acellular allogenic dermal matrix

An acellular ADM can be used to extend the subpectoral pocket, creating a hammock effect below the implant that provides, ideally, an aesthetic inferior pole and inframammary fold, as well as soft-tissue coverage *(Fig. 27.12)*.[56–63] The hammock, or sling, holds the expander in place, minimizing the risk of downward migration of the implant. Further, the expander is less restricted than when it is completely submuscular, so expansion can progress more rapidly before placement of the permanent implant. In nonirradiated patients, human acellular dermis is revascularized and remodeled into the host tissues.[64] A number of human acellular dermal matrices are commercially available, including AlloDerm (Life Cell) and Neoform (Mentor).

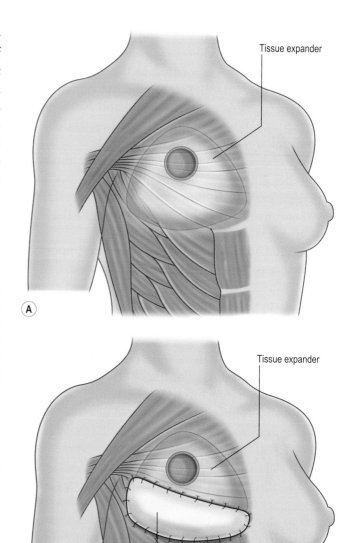

Fig. 27.12 (A) Tissue expanders for breast reconstruction are usually placed beneath the pectoralis and serratus muscles. **(B)** It is possible to place the prosthesis under the pectoralis major, where the muscle covers only the top half of the prosthesis, when a dermal matrix is sutured to the lower half of the pectoral muscle and the chest wall to cover the lower half of the prosthesis.

The ADMs are expensive: their cost must be considered when planning the best reconstructive course. Another disadvantage of using ADMs is that they also promote serous drainage, requiring drains to be maintained until serous drainage is less than 30 cc/day.

The pectoralis major muscle is elevated as described above. A sheet of dermal matrix is sutured to the fascia overlying the rectus abdominis muscle at the planned inframammary fold. The size of the matrix is determined by the diameter of the chest wall and elasticity of the chosen dermal matrix. Typical sheet sizes vary from 4×12 cm to 6×16 cm. The expander is introduced beneath the pectoralis superiorly and the ADM inferiorly; then the muscle and superior edge of the ADM are approximated. Drains are placed to accommodate serous drainage.

If there is breakdown of the mastectomy wound, the underlying matrices will become exposed. Our preferred management of this complication is early excision of ischemic skin and reclosure of the wound.

Secondary breast reconstruction with tissue expansion

As with immediate reconstruction, it is important to mark the inframammary fold and the extent of undermining in permanent ink while the patient is sitting in an upright position, before induction of anesthesia. The tissue expander may be placed in one of the three pockets described for immediate placement after mastectomy, above.

Inflation follows the general plan for expansion as previously described. Inflation of the expander is initiated 10–14 days after placement. The patient returns weekly or biweekly for serial percutaneous inflations. A 23-gauge butterfly needle is used with a distal port and a 21-gauge needle is used with an integrated port. Care is taken at each inflation not to overinflate the expander, causing unnecessary discomfort. The expander should be inflated until the overlying skin and subcutaneous tissues feel firm. If the patient experiences significant discomfort, saline is withdrawn until the patient is comfortable. With each inflation, the overlying skin frequently becomes hyperemic, but the problem usually resolves after inflation has been completed. After volumetric symmetry with the opposite side is achieved, hyperinflation of the expander is often carried out. If a large amount of ptosis is to be developed or extensive repositioning of the breast is necessary, additional hyperinflation may be required. Expanders may be left in place for many months or even years before being exchanged for permanent implants; this principle is also applied in the management of adolescent hypomastia.[65]

Immediately before follow-up surgery is undertaken to place a permanent silicone or saline implant, sufficient saline is removed from the expansion prosthesis to achieve symmetry with the contralateral breast.

Repositioning of the inframammary fold can influence breast ptosis and definition. Increased ptosis is created by infolding and uplifting the expanded tissue and advancing a lower abdominal flap.[66,67] After removing excess saline to determine the appropriate, symmetrical volume of the reconstructed breast, the inframammary fold is moved up or down so that the apices of the breasts are at an equal level. The new position of the fold is marked so that the reconstruction can be accomplished through an incision at the desired inframammary fold *(Fig. 27.13)*. The capsule is left intact unless the prosthesis needs to be repositioned. Stable reconstruction of the inframammary fold can be achieved by tacking the interior capsule to the posterior chest wall capsule at the same level where the earlier, symmetrical marking was made. The abdominal skin is undermined above the fascia and is advanced superiorly into the inframammary cleavage to close the posterior wall defect *(Fig. 27.14)*.

Tissue expansion in cases of chest wall irradiation

Studies suggest that previous chest wall irradiation negatively affects success with tissue expansion and subsequent implant placement.[68,69] The complication rate due to infection, extrusion, and wound complications is higher; furthermore, the final aesthetic result is compromised by capsular contracture and firm, uncomfortable results.

Two groups of patients are probably best managed with autologous tissue transfers instead of with tissue expansion. They are those undergoing: (1) mastectomy for recurrence of disease after previous lumpectomy and radiation; and (2) secondary reconstruction after mastectomy and radiation. In selected patients with excellent-quality chest wall skin and soft tissue, tissue expansion may be considered even though the incidence of complications and a compromised aesthetic result are high.

Chest wall irradiation is being done with increasing frequency in postmastectomy patients. A large number of women who have undergone placement of a tissue expander at the time of mastectomy now have to deal

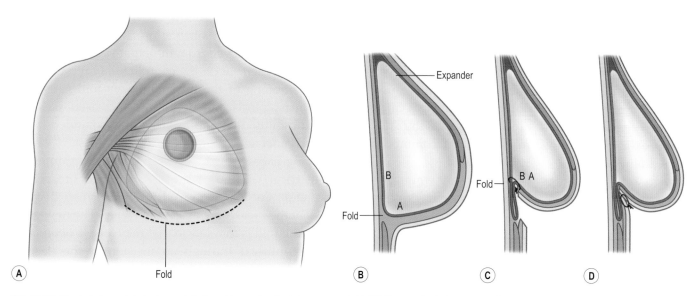

Fig. 27.13 The technique of designing a ptotic breast by moving the inframammary fold. **(A)** The prosthesis is overexpanded to make an excess amount of tissue. **(B)** The position of the desired breast fold (point B) is determined on the thoracic wall. **(C)** Through an inframammary incision at point C, the expander is removed and a permanent device is placed. The skin and soft tissue (point A) are moved superiorly and sutured to point B. **(D)** The abdominal wall is undermined above the fascia and advanced into the inframammary defect.

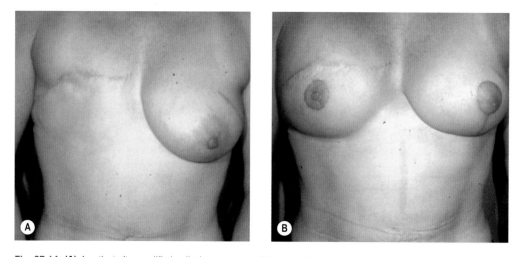

Fig. 27.14 (A) A patient after modified radical mastectomy with preservation of the pectoralis muscle. **(B)** An expander was placed beneath the pectoralis and serratus muscles and then gradually overexpanded. At a second procedure, a permanent implant was placed and a ptosis procedure was performed on the opposite side.

with postoperative radiation. There is no consensus at this time on how to manage these patients. Alternatives that have been presented include the following:

1. Continue expansion until the time of irradiation, but cease inflating the expander during and for several months after irradiation; then resume expander inflation once the radiation dermatitis has resolved and follow with placement of the permanent implant.

2. Complete expansion and exchange with the permanent implant and then proceed with radiation.

3. Remove the fluid in the expander, initiate and complete radiation therapy, then reinflate the expander once tissues have begun to heal.

4. Remove the tissue expander and make plans for autologous tissue reconstruction after radiation is complete.

More than 50% of patients are reported to have satisfactory results if tissue expansion is completed despite treatment with radiation.[69] Our approach is to continue tissue expansion and secondary, permanent implantation in patients who are determined to need radiation therapy after expander placement. We will convert strategy to an autologous tissue reconstruction in those patients with complications or disappointing aesthetic outcomes.

Patient education about risks and alternatives is critical: there must be an understanding of strategy before any reconstruction is initiated in patients receiving radiation for breast cancer treatment.

The hypoplastic breast

Tissue expansion has played an important role in the reconstruction of both acquired and congenital breast hypoplasia. Management of the deformity depends on the degree of breast asymmetry, the nature of the deformity, the quality of the chest wall soft tissue, and the age of the patient at presentation.

Unilateral hypoplasia varies from a smaller, well-formed breast to total absence of the breast; these cases further have variable hypoplasia or aplasia of the nipple and areola. If a hypoplastic nipple–areola complex is present, it will usually lie in a cephalad position relative to that of the contralateral breast.

The degree of breast hypoplasia is determined and characterized as minor hypoplasia with a normal nipple–areola complex, moderate to severe hypoplasia, or total breast aplasia. The nipple–areola complex is characterized separately as normal, hypoplastic, displaced, or aplastic. Mild breast hypoplasias may be corrected with simple placement of a breast implant, but more severe hypoplasias and aplasias with nipple–areola displacement are best treated with initial placement of a tissue expander. If presurgical examination reveals that the pectoralis muscle is absent, the deformity is probably associated with Poland syndrome (see below).

A tissue expander is placed through either an inframammary or axillary incision into the subpectoral space. The surgeon may choose from many expanders: these include smooth and textured-wall implants, implants with integrated valves, and expanders with distal ports. The prosthesis is initially expanded at 2-week intervals. As the expander is inflated and the overlying skin relaxes, the cephalad-displaced nipple–areola complex will descend. The more slowly the expander is inflated, the better the nipple–areola will descend. A slow expansion also minimizes development of striae. The expander is ultimately overinflated to a volume that is at least 40% larger than the desired volume of the permanent implant. The expander is left in place for several months after the final inflation to allow development of additional ptosis.

The permanent implant is introduced at a second procedure. An incision is made through the original incision that was made to place the expander. The expander is removed, and a capsulectomy is carried out, if needed. If capsulectomy is not needed, the inferior portion of the capsule may be tacked to the rib periosteum to delineate the inframammary fold better. A permanent implant is selected to achieve symmetry with the contralateral side.

Reconstruction with a permanent expander prosthesis is also possible. This prosthesis is inflated to a size several hundred milliliters larger than the desired final volume. The expander prosthesis is allowed to remain overinflated for several months. In the office, saline is then withdrawn to achieve symmetry with the contralateral breast. When desired, the port with its attached tubing is removed through an incision made over the distal port.

The tuberous breast

Expansion is a useful technique in the correction of the hypoplastic tuberous breast. Through an inframammary or periareolar approach, the tuberous breast is lifted off the underlying pectoralis fascia. Radial cuts are made through the breast tissue to expand the base of the breast, and a tissue expander is introduced in the submammary plane. Inflation and expansion are achieved as previously discussed. Once adequate expansion has been achieved, the expander is removed and replaced with the permanent prosthesis. Alternatively, a permanent expander device is used and overinflated by several hundred milliliters. Several months after completion of the inflation, fluid is removed to achieve symmetry with the contralateral side, and the port and attached tubing are removed.

The immature breast

The use of tissue expanders has been beneficial in the management of young adolescents presenting with breast asymmetry.[70] Adolescence is a critical time that is characterized by intense social pressures and self-awareness of a developing physique, so failure to address the problem of breast asymmetry can result in psychological problems. These patients do not need full maturity for reconstruction.

A subpectoralis muscle plane is elevated through a small axillary incision. An expander prosthesis with an integrated valve or distal port is placed in the subpectoral plane beneath the hypoplastic breast. If a distal-port prosthesis is used, the inflation reservoir is placed in the lateral thoracic wall or in the upper abdomen below the inframammary fold. The prosthesis is then inflated at intervals appropriate to maintain symmetry with the developing breast on the contralateral side. The slow expansion will cause the areola to enlarge, and the nipple–areola complex will progressively be displaced caudally to a more normal position. The adolescent can continue with normal activities, participation in sports, and other physical endeavors.

Once development of the contralateral breast has stabilized, usually between 18 and 19 years of age, the expander is removed. Definitive reconstruction is achieved as previously described for correction of the mature breast.

Correction of Poland syndrome

Poland syndrome involves not only abnormal development of the breast but also thoracic wall deformities, deformities of the upper extremity, and vertebral anomalies. Poland syndrome exhibits a uniform absence of the sternal head of the pectoralis major muscle. Further structural problems may be seen and include abnormalities in the anterior ribs and costal cartilages and deficiencies of the muscles of the scapular area, including the latissimus dorsi. Other findings include deficiency of subcutaneous tissue; hypoplasia, aplasia, or malposition of the nipple–areola complex; and deficiency of breast tissue.

A mild deformity characterized by breast hypoplasia or aplasia is corrected with the initial placement of a tissue expander through a transaxillary approach. A 700-mL or larger expander is used to achieve full expansion over a 3–4-month period. Then the tissue expander is removed and a permanent breast implant is placed. Ideally, if there is an adequate latissimus dorsi muscle, it may be transposed to cover the breast prosthesis. Its insertion is taken down and transposed anteriorly on the humerus to form an anterior, axillary fold. Alternatively, the tissue expander can be placed at an initial operation and covered immediately with a latissimus dorsi muscle transposition. Once expansion has been completed, the expander is removed and the permanent breast implant introduced.

More severe cases of Poland syndrome that are characterized by contour depression of the ribs will require either an osteotomy and repositioning of the ribs or the use of a custom, solid, Silastic implant. The anterior axillary fold is reconstructed by transposition of the insertion of the latissimus dorsi muscle over the custom Silastic implant. The breast contour is reconstructed with tissue expansion and the subsequent use of a permanent breast implant.

In the immature girl with Poland syndrome, expanders are placed at the onset of contralateral breast development through a small incision in the axilla. To maintain aesthetically pleasing symmetry, the implant is gradually inflated until development of the contralateral breast has stabilized. In the final months of treatment, the expander is overinflated by 200–300 mL and then replaced with the permanent implant. If a latissimus dorsi muscle is available, it is transposed at this time to cover the breast prosthesis *(Fig. 27.15)*.[70]

Expansion of the trunk

The trunk and abdomen are well suited to tissue expansion in individuals of all ages. Because of the large adjoining surface area from which tissue can be recruited, large prostheses can be placed and flaps quickly expanded *(Fig. 27.16)*. Expansion of the trunk with large prostheses may produce significant deformity and discomfort. Expansions of the back and buttocks are particularly difficult for the patient because of their interference with everyday functions of living. Fortunately, using multiple prostheses in such areas produces sufficient tissue for completion of the reconstruction, minimizes distortion, and allows rapidly expedited expansion.

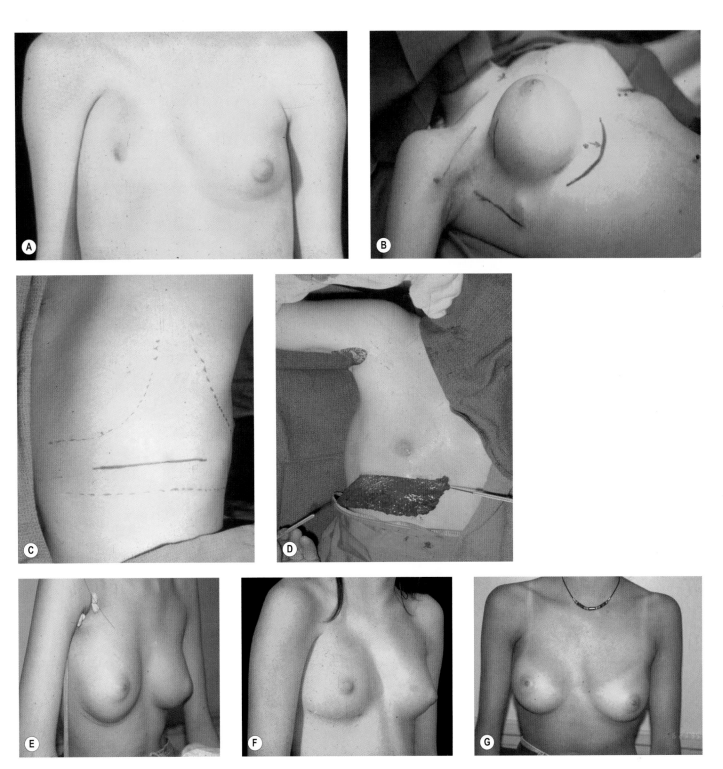

Fig. 27.15 **(A)** This 17-year-old patient presented with severe right breast hypoplasia with nipple hypoplasia and superior malposition of the right nipple as a feature of her Poland syndrome. **(B)** She underwent the subcutaneous placement of a tissue expander beneath the skin and soft tissues of the right breast to expand the soft-tissue envelope and increase the distance from the clavicle to the nipple. A latissimus dorsi muscle flap was harvested using two small incisions on the back and single incisions in the axilla and inframammary region of the breast. **(C, D)** The muscle was transposed to the chest through a high axillary tunnel and placed beneath the expanded soft-tissue envelope and anchored to the parasternal area and inferior aspect of the expanded breast envelope. **(E)** An implant was placed beneath the muscle to provide the necessary volume to the breast reconstruction, producing an immediate and **(F)** long-term improvement of the breast appearance at 3-year postoperative follow-up. **(G)** This produced an excellent change in the breast appearance at 3-year follow-up after surgery. (This case courtesy of Julian J. Pribaz MD.) (Reproduced from: Hall Findlay E, Evans G. Aesthetic and Reconstructive Surgery of Breast. Elsevier Saunders, 2010. Copyright Elsevier 2010.)

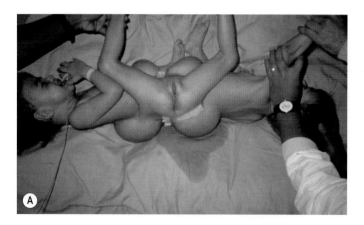

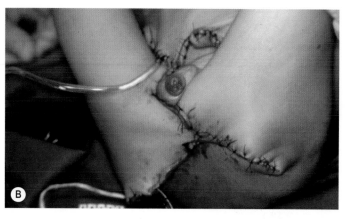

Fig. 27.16 (A) Separation of ischiopagus twins was aided by first expanding both the anterior and posterior trunk skin. **(B)** At a second procedure, the hemipelvis of each side was brought together with the opposite side by closing the pelvic ring over expanded soft tissue. Soft tissue was adequate to achieve total closure in both infants. The children have now survived over 10 years since separation and are doing well.

Large prostheses can be either placed above the fascia or incorporated between fascia and muscle planes in the abdomen or on the back. Incorporation of any of the latissimus dorsi, pectoralis major, or rectus muscles allows development of an expanded myocutaneous flap. Prostheses placed between layers of the abdominal wall have been used to develop large flaps for abdominal wall reconstruction *(Fig. 27.17)*.[71]

Large deformities, such as burns, giant hairy nevi, and other congenital anomalies, may require multiple serial expansions. In such cases as these, the expanders are inflated maximally and the flaps are advanced. The prostheses are left in place and re-expansion is carried out in the subsequent weeks. In the abdomen, two or three serial expansions are usually well tolerated, even in children.

Expansion in the extremities

Skin and soft tissues of the extremities tolerate tissue expansion well,[72] so tissue defects resulting from congenital abnormalities, tumor, or trauma can be corrected. The capsule that develops adjacent to the expander has a resilient surface that can be transposed over joints and tendons to decrease adhesions.

The use of multiple expanders in the extremity has the advantages of less distortion, less compromise of everyday life activity, and more rapid development of tissue. Standard rectangular and round prostheses usually suffice; they are best placed axially to the defect. Functional impairment, even when the prostheses are placed directly over vessels and nerves, is unusual.

Occasional transitory neurapraxias have been described in the lower extremity but are uncommon in the upper extremity. If such discomfort or neurapraxia develops, the prostheses should be deflated and then reinflated at a much slower rate.

In areas such as the hand or foot, custom implants can be fabricated. The dorsum of the hand or foot lends itself well to expansion, whereas the palm and plantar areas are particularly painful during, and resistant to, expansion. Expanded full-thickness grafts harvested from the abdomen are extremely versatile in reconstruction of the foot and hand. These grafts are stable and can be harvested as a single graft. Reasonable protection and sensation return to these grafts over time.

The upper leg is easily expanded because of the thickness of skin and its underlying subcutaneous tissue: one large expander or multiple smaller expanders may be used. Complications are infrequent. However, below the knee, inflation carries major risks. Clean, isolated defects, such as those that follow local tumor excisions, are more amenable to expansion than sites where large areas of previously traumatized skin surround the defect. Multiple small expanders are recommended to minimize the risks of implant loss. If cellulitis or tissue compromise occurs during expansion, the prosthesis should be deflated or removed.

Lower leg expansion after crush injuries carries particularly high risk. Individuals who have suffered major crush or degloving trauma to the extremity are better treated with function-restoring microvascular and myocutaneous flaps than with attempts at excessive aesthetic reconstructions using tissue expansion.

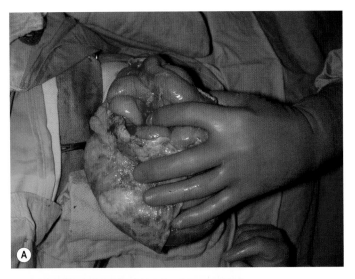
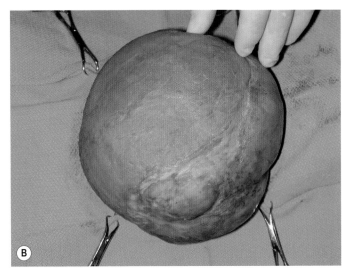
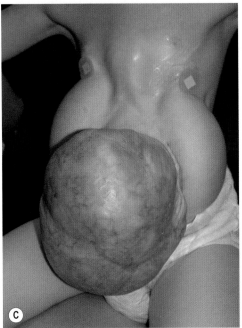
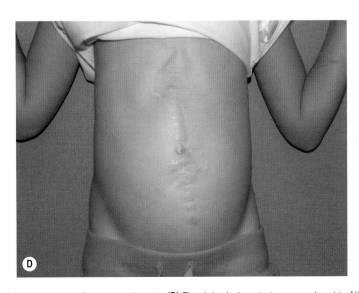

Fig. 27.17 **(A)** A ruptured omphalocele including the liver had failed reconstruction on two attempts. **(B)** The abdominal contents were enclosed in Alloderm and a vacuum-assisted closure dressing placed over it to colonize it with granulation tissue. When adequate granulation tissue had been developed, a cultured split-thickness skin graft was placed over the entire defect. **(C)** At 4 years of age, expanders were placed beneath and lateral to the rectus muscle to generate adequate skin and muscles for abdominal closure. **(D)** The viscera was reduced to the abdominal cavity and the rectus muscles were brought together in the midline to create a stable abdominal wall. The patient has remained stable for 7 years without further surgery.

Complications and their management

Initial attempts at tissue expansion were associated with a high rate of complication; these included, but were not limited to, implant failure due to either puncture during inflation or mechanical problems. As more experience accumulated, however, the incidence of complications dramatically decreased. Complication rates are directly proportional to the number of expansion procedures performed and the experience of the individual surgeon.[73] Most complications incurred during tissue expansion are relatively minor and do not interfere with completion of multistage procedures.

Implant failure

Despite design improvements, the use of an excessively large needle or the inadvertent puncture of the implant can lead to implant deflation. To maximize sealing of the valve, the implant reservoir should be entered at a 90° angle. If there is any question about the location of the inflation reservoir, radiologic or sonographic techniques may be helpful.

Infection

As with the placement of any prosthesis in the human body, infection is possible. The introduction of bacteria to the wound in the perioperative period is the most common cause of early infection. The area to be reconstructed should be stable, and there should be no open wounds at the time that the procedure is undertaken. Areas susceptible to lymphedema, such as traumatized lower extremities, carry a significantly higher rate of infection. An area of copious lymphatic drainage, such as the neck or the groin, also tends to accumulate lymphatic fluid around a prosthesis and is more susceptible to infection. These areas should be drained with suction drains until all excess drainage stops. Antibiotics are given as long as the drain remains in place.

Late infections are usually caused by iatrogenic introduction of bacteria during the course of inflation. The inflation procedure should be performed under sterile conditions in the office. Povidone-iodine (Betadine) is used to prepare the injection site. Externalized distal ports carry a high colonization rate, but the resultant contamination produces little complication. Many infections can be difficult to detect and can be tolerated well by the patient.[74]

Some erythema may occur over all expansion prostheses; however, pain, warmth, and systemic symptoms such as fever and chills suggest clinical infection. If the infection occurs in the perioperative period or early course of expansion, the prosthesis should be removed and the wound irrigated. The procedure is aborted, and a second attempt is made 3 or 4 months after healing.

If infection occurs late in the course of expansion, the prosthesis can be removed and the expanded tissue advanced after irrigation of the infected cavity. Permanent implants should not be placed when Gram stain of the expander space reveals bacteria.

Implant exposure

Implant exposure can occur both early in the postoperative period and after a protracted course of expansion. Treatment of the exposed implant depends on the timing of exposure. Exposure early after placement is usually related to inadequate dissection or use of an excessively large prosthesis that abuts on wound closure. If the prosthesis becomes exposed soon after placement, it is best to remove it and reoperate 3–4 months later.

Late exposure is usually related to excessively rapid or overzealous inflation. Rapid expansion is medically necessary only in few instances. Tissue expansion should be carried out judiciously to achieve optimal cosmetic results. If minimal or late exposure occurs during the course of expansion, the procedure can continue with the use of antibiotic creams on the exposed area: In this situation, multiple, rapid fillings are done to generate adequate tissue. Reinforcement of the compromised overlying skin with paper tape is sometimes helpful. Most flaps survive and do well even with some exposure of the implant.

In compromised tissues such as grossly traumatized lower extremities or irradiated and burned tissues, the use of tissue expansion can more easily result in implant exposure – a cautious approach is warranted.

Compromise and loss of flap tissue

Tissue expansion exerts changes on living tissue similar to those seen in the phenomenon of conventional flap delay.[24] Expanded flaps are almost universally more robust than nonexpanded flaps. To ensure vascularity, one should attempt to maintain a major axial vessel in the expanded tissue.

Access the complete references list online at **http://www.expertconsult.com**

6. Neumann CG. The expansion of an area of skin by the progressive distention of a subcutaneous balloon. *Plast Reconstr Surg*. 1957;19:124–130.

   This classic article describes mystoid skin expansion as a first stage in the reconstruction of an amputated ear. It is a landmark case report more than 20 years before tissue expansion became an accepted reconstructure modality.

7. Radovan C. Breast reconstruction after mastectomy using the temporary expander. *Plast Reconstr Surg*. 1982;69:195–208.

   This article is a follow-up to Dr. Radovan's original article on tissue expansion and breast reconstruction and a review of his experience in 68 patients.

11. Argenta LC, Watanabe MJ, Grabb WC. The use of tissue expansion in head and neck reconstruction. *Ann Plast Surg*. 1983;11:31–37.

12. Manders EK, Schenden MJ, Furrey JA, et al. Soft-tissue expansion: concepts and complications. *Plast Reconstr Surg*. 1984;74:493–507.

    This is an article by Dr Manders, one of the earliest surgeons to review a large series of patients treated with tissue expansion in multiple areas. It is an excellent overview of the technique and a look forward to its use for the next 25 years.

30. Chummun S, Addison P, Stewart KJ. The osmotic tissue expander: a 5-year experience. *J Plast Reconstr Aesthet Surg* 2011;63:2128–2132.

    Inflation through a port is a cumbersome technique requiring multiple office visits for the patient. Since Dr. Austald first reported the self-inflating tissue expander in 1982 there has been little progress. Drs Chummun, Addison and Stewart present an excellent experience on the modern use of self-inflating expanders.

42. Manders EK, Graham 3rd WP, Schenden MJ, et al. Skin expansion to eliminate large scalp defects. *Ann Plast Surg*. 1984;12:305–312.

53. Spear SL, Pelletiere CV. Immediate breast reconstruction in two stages using textured, integrated-valve tissue expanders and breast implants. *Plast Reconstr Surg*. 2004;113:2098–2103.

    This is an excellent article and follow-up to the 1998 article on immediate breast reconstruction using integrated valve tissue expanders. It presents the refinements and improved aesthetic results now achievable.

69. Cordeiro PG, Pusic AL, Disa JJ, et al. Irradiation after immediate tissue expander/implant breast reconstruction: outcomes, complications, aesthetic results, and satisfaction among 156 patients. *Plast Reconstr Surg*. 2004;113:877–881.

70. Argenta LC, VanderKolk C, Friedman RJ, et al. Refinements in reconstruction of congenital breast deformities. *Plast Reconstr Surg*. 1985;76:73–82.

74. Adler N, Dorafshar AH, Bauer BS, et al. Tissue expander infections in pediatric patients: management and outcomes. *Plast Reconstr Surg*. 2009;124:484–489.

28

Therapeutic radiation: Principles, effects, and complications

Gabrielle M. Kane

SYNOPSIS

- Radiation therapy (RT) can be used as a primary or adjuvant treatment for many cancers.
- The unit of dose measurement is the gray (Gy).
- Side-effects are characterized as acute and late toxicities.
- Acute toxicities are temporary and reversible.
- Late toxicities are permanent.
- The primary mechanism of action of radiation is through breakage of DNA strands.
- Treatment planning is achieved through use of three-dimensional computed tomography (CT) planning.
- Delivery of radiation can be very precise with the use of intensity-modulated radiation therapy (IMRT) as well as with image-guided radiation therapy (IGRT).

 Access the Historical Perspective section online at
http://www.expertconsult.com

Introduction

Radiation therapy (RT) requires an understanding of physics. A multidisciplinary team, including radiation oncologists, physicists, dosimetrists and radiotherapists, is required for the delivery of radiation. Delivery of radiation can be achieved using different modalities, including kilovoltage, orthovoltage, megavoltage, electron therapy using a linear accelerator, proton therapy, and brachytherapy.

RT is the use of ionizing radiation to treat malignant tumors and some benign disorders. Nearly two-thirds of cancer patients receive RT as part or all of their treatment. Radiation oncology is the discipline of medicine that addresses the causes, prevention, and treatment of human cancer with special emphasis on the role of ionizing radiation.[4] Radiation oncologists work in a multi-professional context with radiation therapists, nursing, dosimetry and medical physics, along with dieticians, social workers, and counselors. Radiation therapists are the technologists who deliver the RT. Unlike their counterparts in diagnostic radiology, they spend not only considerable time on the technical components of treatment (treatment delivery, quality assurance, and verification), but also interact with and support cancer patients throughout the duration of their therapy. The radiation oncologist is also part of a multidisciplinary team, with specialized surgical and medical oncologists, along with diagnostic radiology and pathologists, which advocates for the best evidence-based care for their cancer patients. However, outside the immediate team, it is rare for other physicians to know much about the process, rationale, and issues around RT, and even less about the risks and causes of toxicity, let alone the technology involved. This chapter is designed as a primer, or virtual elective in the topic, and aims to help improve communication and understanding between plastic surgeons and radiation oncologists so that they can better appreciate some of the common issues that they have to deal with. This chapter starts with a brief description of the basics of radiation technology, modalities, medical physics, and radiobiology. It then outlines practical applications, with a description of RT planning and process, and clinical treatment issues. The final section describes specific toxicity syndromes.

Radiation technology

RT has always been totally dependent on technology. Although much of the equipment that has been the mainstay of RT is being replaced by newer technology, some of it remains in effective and efficient use. For example, kilovoltage therapy can be effectively used for very superficial treatments. It delivers 100% of the prescribed dose at the skin, has rapid fall-off below the skin, and a tight penumbra (edge). In the 50–150-kV range, penetration provides useful coverage only to a depth of 5 mm; orthovoltage therapy (150–500 kV) provides better penetration, but is not capable of treating much more than 3 cm below the skin. With kV energies, skin dose becomes the rate-limiting step. At the orthovoltage range of energy, interaction between radiation and matter is strongly dependent on the atomic number (Z) of the attenuating material – in other words, in this process, known as the photoelectric effect, tissue such as bone, which has a high Z, attenuates more radiation; fat and soft tissue (lower Z) attenuate less; and air (for example, in the lungs) hardly at all, thus producing the contrast necessary for diagnostic imaging. Unfortunately, this higher absorbed dose in bone resulted in many more problems from ORN.

Megavoltage radiotherapy allows even greater penetration of tissue, resulting in better skin-sparing and improved dose homogeneity. Cobalt units deliver MV radiation, and have a ^{60}Co source that generates gamma (γ) rays with average megavoltage energy of 1.3 MV. ^{60}Co has a half-life of 5.26 years, and, because of this decay and subsequent drop in output, the source needs to be replaced every few years. Maximum dose (D_{max}) is not achieved until 0.5 cm beyond the surface of the skin and the intrinsic scatter of the beam and ionized particles means that the penumbra, or dose fall-off at the edge of a beam, is not very tight. Despite this, cobalt is still the most prevalent and important external-beam radiotherapy modality in the world. Although affluent countries have mostly replaced their cobalt units with linear accelerators, cobalt still provides an excellent low-maintenance, reliable, safe, and effective alternative in many low- and middle-income countries.

The linear accelerator, or linac, produces high-frequency electromagnetic waves to accelerate charged particles – electrons – to a very high energy through an accelerator tube and a beam transport system. When the electrons hit a target at the end of this, they produce megavoltage X-ray beams that have sharper edges and can penetrate deep tissue. Typical photon energies produced by linacs are 4, 6, 10, and 18 MV that result in increasing maximum depth doses. The machines can also be set so that the high-energy electrons exit the accelerator without hitting the target to produce electron beams, which are less penetrating than photons, with a faster fall-off, that can be used for superficial treatments. Most linacs can produce a range of electron energies from 4 to 17 MeV.

Particle therapy

Electrons are the most commonly used particle therapy. As described above, they deposit their energy superficially, sparing structures deeper in the body, with fairly steep dose distribution curves. Electrons produce more side scatter than photons and have wider penumbras. They are typically used to treat skin cancers and "boosts" to breast tumor cavities. They are also used to spare sensitive organs that may otherwise reach maximum tolerance, for example, protecting the spinal cord when treating posterior neck nodes.

Other particle therapies are less commonly available. Protons have similar biologic activity as photons; their advantage is that they have a unique shape to their dose distribution, with low steady-dose deposition until near the end of their clearly defined range when the dose peak then falls sharply to nearly zero. This is the Bragg peak phenomenon, which allows very precise dose distribution, protection of critical structures, and dose intensification. Protons are ideal for treating structures in the base of skull, such as the clivus, especially for chordomas, where the necessary dose is far above the tolerance of the sensitive optic chiasm and other sensitive structures in that region, and would otherwise cause severe toxicity. Another indication for protons is to deliver pediatric craniospinal irradiation for cancers such as medulloblastoma, because the proton dose distribution significantly reduces the exit dose through structures anterior to the spine (kidneys, bowel, lungs) when compared to conventional treatment with photons. The most common use of protons currently is in the treatment of prostate cancer, allowing the prostate to receive a higher dose of radiation, but causing less damage to the rectum and bladder. Many new proton facilities are opening, but they are expensive and cumbersome to construct and maintain, requiring a cyclotron or a synchrotron to accelerate protons, and a large space.

Neutron RT offers the advantage of high linear energy transfer, a property that allows the delivery of 20–100 times more energy along their path than photons, thus being biologically more effective in treating radioresistant tumors such as sarcomas and salivary gland tumors. Their use requires a careful balance of risk and benefit as they can lead to more severe long-term side-effects, due to relatively high effective entrance and exit doses.[5]

Carbon, neon, and heavier ions hold promise as they combine the radiobiological advantages of neutrons with the dose distribution and Bragg peak of protons, but are only available in very specialized units.

Brachytherapy

Brachytherapy is a method of delivering radiation treatment over very short distances using radioactive sealed sources. There are three main ways of delivering this type of radiation: (1) an applicator can be used to deliver dose to the surface of a thin tumor, for example, an eye plaque used to treat ocular melanoma; (2) intracavitary – inserting the sealed source into the cavity of an organ, e.g., in the treatment of cervical cancer, a combination (tandem) apparatus is used consisting of a cylindrical rod inserted into the cervical os and through the cervical canal into the uterus, with two ovoids placed in the lateral fornices; and (3) interstitial, when the source is either implanted directly into the tumor or postoperative bed, for example, for postoperative treatment of sarcoma, or when radioactive gold seeds are implanted directly into an organ, e.g., in the treatment of early-stage prostate cancer. Brachytherapy is often used in

conjunction with external beam, usually to increase the total dose to a smaller volume at the site of greatest risk of recurrence. For example, after partial mastectomy, the whole breast receives external-beam treatment followed by implantation of a source to provide a boost to the tumor bed.

Originally, following the work done by Marie Curie and others, radium needles were used, until the importance of radioprotection was realized. In the modern era, artificially produced radionuclides are used, most commonly those derived from cesium (^{137}Cs), iridium (^{192}Ir), iodine (^{131}I), palladium (^{103}Pd), and gold (^{198}Au). The activity of these radionuclides is still calculated relative to that of radium. To protect health professionals and the patient, the process of using high-energy sources, such as ^{137}Cs and ^{192}Ir, has evolved considerably, most notably with the use of after-loading. This means that the empty cylinders (for intracavity) or catheters and trocars (for interstitial brachytherapy) are inserted in the operating room, and loaded with inert metal "dummy" sources that are easily visible on radiologic imaging; this is done to verify the position and calculate the dose distribution. The patient is not treated until in a shielded room, either as an inpatient, when treatment is delivered over several days, or in a brachytherapy suite, when the treatment is a short one, such as when high dose rate is used. The radioactive sources are housed in a shielded safe in a remote-controlled after-loading unit, which looks very much like a small heating furnace. After a final verification of positioning, the applicator, catheters, cylinders, or trocars are connected with tubes to the after-loading unit, and, after all personnel have left the room, the active sources, which look like small beads, are remotely loaded through a pressurized system. The unit is programmed to control the position of the sources and the duration of the sources in any position to achieve the prescribed dose in a homogeneous fashion over the three-dimensional dose distribution. When protracted treatments are used, for example, with low-dose-rate brachytherapy, or when a high dose rate is given just in short pulses of time, the units can be paused, and the active sources retract temporarily into the safe within the after-loading unit, making it possible for personnel to enter the room to provide care.

Low-energy radionuclides such as ^{131}I, ^{103}Pd, and ^{198}Au do not pose the same concerns for health workers, and thus are used as permanent implants in the form of seeds, most commonly for prostate cancer.

Physics

An explanation of RT techniques and dosimetry requires a basic understanding of physics. The photon generated by the linac is a very high-energy X-ray that does not have any charged particles in it. However, when it enters the body, it passes through tissue faster than the speed of light. As it goes through the skin and enters the tissue, it uses the Compton process to deposit energy. This means that it interacts with biological tissue by colliding with an electron on the more loosely bound outer shell of an atom *(Fig. 28.1)*. The photon continues along its path, but the electron is knocked off, like a billiard ball, at an angle that depends on the speed and angle with which it was hit. The electron travels (scatters) a distance that is proportional to the energy with which it was hit, meaning that higher photon energies propel electrons more in a forward direction than lower energies can do, before the electron is deposited, and the dose absorbed into the tissues. This triggers downstream free radical interactions, and these can cause DNA single-strand or double-strand breaks, or other injuries, including damage to basepairs and protein cross-links. The chromosomal aberrations that result from double-strand breaks mean that the cancerous cell cannot repair or duplicate at the end of its life cycle, and this is the principal cause of cell death.

If all of these electron energy deposits are added up, then a distribution curve showing absorbed dose and depth can be plotted *(Fig. 28.2A)* that shows that skin

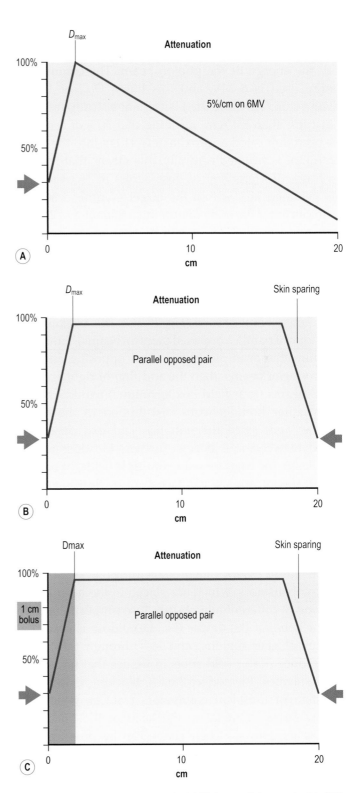

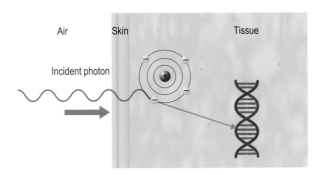

Fig. 28.1 Incident photon knocks an electron off the outer ring and scatters it along a pathway through a distance before the electron energy is absorbed.

Fig. 28.2 (A) Depth dose distribution for 6-MV photons. Only approximately 30% of the dose is absorbed at the skin surface; the maximum dose (100%) is absorbed at a depth of 1.5.cm, and then attenuates by approximately 5% per cm. **(B)** When two beams are opposed, depth doses can be added, resulting in an even distribution across the target volume. **(C)** If a higher dose is required at the skin surface, a strip of bolus material is placed on the skin.

absorbed dose is less than 40%, and 100% or D_{max} occurs some distance into the skin at a depth that is consistent with the energy of the photon beam. The commonest energy used is 6 MV, and this has a D_{max} of 1.5 cm beyond skin. The dose then falls off at a steady rate that is just less than 5%/cm, meaning that 50% of the dose has been deposited approximately 11 cm into the body. If a tumor is situated centrally, this means that there is too much of a gradient of dose across it. To overcome this heterogeneity within the target volume, a second beam can enter the body (assuming a diameter of 20 cm) from the opposite side, again depositing its maximal energy at 1.5 cm, then attenuating at <5%/cm. The energy deposits from each side are added, a homogeneous distribution is achieved across the target volume *(Fig. 28.2B)*, and the skin does not receive a therapeutic dose, unless bolus is used *(Fig. 28.2C)*. This explains the technique of parallel-opposed pairs (of beams). Similarly, assuming the example, above used opposing anterior and posterior beams, then the addition of right and left lateral beams (four-field box technique) would give an even tighter homogeneous distribution to the target volume, and, since the entrance and exit doses are shared between four beams, further skin dose reduction. This is the basis for using multiple fields, or beams, from different angles, to "focus" (a misleading term, since the beam does not focus on a spot, as light does through a lens) and deposit maximal dose to a target.

In conventional RT, most beams are delivered with uniform intensity across the field. Beam-modifying devices are accessories such as shielding blocks, wedges, and compensators, which are placed in the head of the machine to differentially absorb dose proportionally to the thickness of the device (i.e., more dose is absorbed through thicker regions, and less through thin), and thus reduce hot or cold spots in tissues that have non-square shapes. In modern linacs, blocking is done by a system of multileaf collimators (MLCs), which are narrow strips of metal in the head of the linac that act like miniblocks. Their shape can be programmed for shielding *(Fig. 28.3)*. Three-dimensional conformal therapy uses multiple beams to be shaped in such a way that a significant amount of normal tissue can be excluded.

MLCs can also be programmed to move dynamically in and out of the beam, so that the amount of time in each position is adjusted to allow a variable amount of

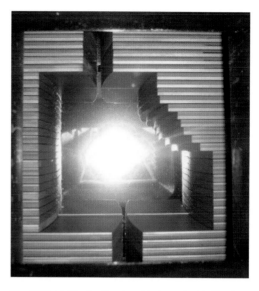

Fig. 28.3 Multileaf collimators (photographed looking into the head of the machine) are used to provide static shielding, or, when programmed dynamically, differential dose absorption for intensity-modulated radiation therapy.

dose through each leaf, compensates for irregular shapes with great precision, and can control the dose to specified targets within a volume. This is the basis for IMRT, which involves identifying doses for individual or multiple target volumes and constraints for normal organs that need to be protected from the effect of radiation, and then using a sophisticated RT planning program that modulates the intensity across multiple individual beams or arcs with dynamic MLC, using an inverse planning system. This allows the creation of a very conformal plan that can even have convex and concave shapes to avoid a critical structure, for example, avoiding the spinal cord in a way that conventional beams would not be able to do *(Fig. 28.4)*. It is also possible to "dose paint" so that different areas receive different doses at the same time, and also to reduce volumes, adapting to reduction in the tumor size. A similar result is obtained with tomotherapy, which uses principles of CT scanning to deliver intensity-modulated beams slice by slice. An advantage of IMRT over this system is that IMRT is delivered on a normal linac rather than a dedicated machine.

With the move to increasing high precision in RT delivery, consistent reproducibility of treatment position has become increasingly important. Electronic portal imaging (digital MV X-rays taken on the RT machine) can take both orthogonal views of the target, e.g., anterior and lateral beams, and beam's eye view

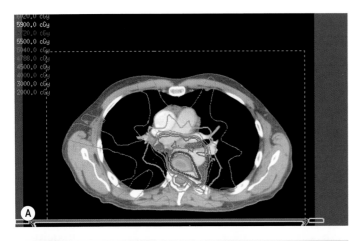

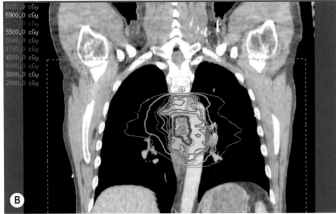

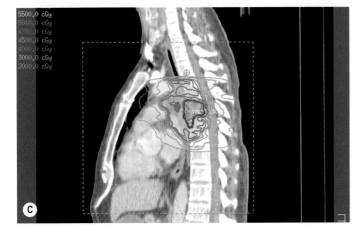

Fig. 28.4 (A) Axial intensity-modulated radiation therapy plan of a sarcoma involving the mediastinum extending into a thoracic vertebral body. The technique allowed a radical dose (66 Gy) to be delivered to the target volume, but constrained the cord dose to a safe dose of 52 Gy. **(B, C)** Coronal and sagittal distributions.

images. The utility of this is enhanced when there are recognizable and stable landmarks, for example, some part of the bony anatomy. However, when the target is somewhat mobile, then fiducial markers, such as seeds placed in the prostate gland, can greatly help to match up the target. The cone beam CT uses kV three-dimensional imaging to verify positioning for IGRT.

Stereotactic techniques have been used in structures such as the brain for many years. A linac-based process involves the use of multiple very small beams that cover a small target (2–5 cm) to a large dose of RT, delivering a therapeutically radical equivalent dose in just a few, or even just one, fraction. It has primarily been used on central nervous system tumors, including benign conditions such as arteriovenous malformations or schwanommas, immobilizing the head in a frame. The gamma knife uses a ^{60}Co source with similar principles. With the advent of IGRT, this principle is now applied to sterotactic body RT for sites elsewhere in the body, such as lung, liver, and paraspinal tumors. Large doses, for example 5 Gy, are given in five fractions twice a week to a total of 25 Gy, which is the equivalent of an ablative dose, but with much greater precision, and far less toxicity. It is well tolerated even by frail and ill patients.

Intraoperative RT is not a modern idea. It is used to treat small areas (4–10 cm) of the body that are at high risk for recurrence after the tumor has been removed. It is especially used to treat the retroperitoneum while the patient is asleep. Electrons are used most commonly, and electron-shaping cones that are attached to the head of the machine are positioned into the wound and lined up against the tissue at risk for residual disease by the radiation oncologist and surgeon together. Personnel then leave the room, the beam is switched on, and the dose is delivered in less than 2 minutes, the cones are removed, and the surgeon can close the wound.

Radiobiology

Radiation injury can be viewed from two perspectives: the radiation effect on tumor cells, and the radiation toxicity on normal cells. The therapeutic ratio is a dose–response relationship between tumor control and normal tissue complications, and helps balance the two perspectives. In an ideal world, the curves representing tumor response and normal tissue complications would be well separated *(Fig. 28.5A)*. Far too often, they are so close together that it is not possible to achieve a high enough dose to eradicate the tumor without causing harmful complications *(Fig. 28.5B)*. Usually in clinical practice there is some degree of compromise, and

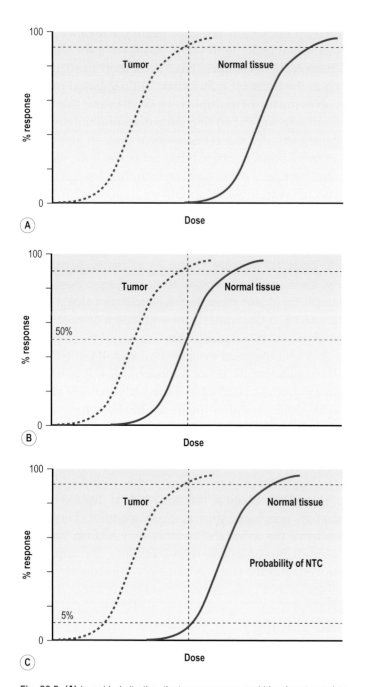

Fig. 28.5 (A) In an ideal situation, the tumor response would be almost complete before causing any normal tissue reaction. **(B)** More commonly, the dose required to achieve adequate tumor response also causes an unacceptably high risk of normal tissue reaction. **(C)** An acceptable trade-off is one that allows adequate tumor control and a 5% (or less) probability of normal tissue complications.

traditionally, a 5% risk of normal tissue complications is accepted *(Fig. 28.5C)*, taking into account the specific risks of the situation.

Radiation toxicity is expressed during mitosis of normal cells. Acute toxicity occurs during treatment or shortly afterwards. It is related to the total dose, the size of the volume irradiated, and radiosensitizing drugs such as chemotherapy. It occurs in cells with a rapid turnover, such as oral mucosa or skin epithelium, where cell division is necessary to maintain function. Even though these cells may be affected within a few days of starting fractionated treatment, their damage does not become manifest for at least 2 weeks as the progenitor stem cells do not have as rapid a turnover. Examples are skin erythema and desquamation, oral mucositis, and esophagitis. These reactions usually start to heal 2 weeks after the completion of treatment. Even quite brisk reactions can heal fast *(Figs 28.6, 28.7)*. Acute toxicity is reversible, and does not predict for permanent damage. The exception is if there is consequential damage, i.e., there is persistent injury due to the destruction of the basement membrane zone with complete depletion of stem cells due to very high dose, and usually an additional factor such as chemotherapy, infection, or trauma. This can be found in chronic ulcers in the skin, bladder, or gastrointestinal tract. Delayed acute toxicity occurs 6 weeks to 6 months after the completion of treatment; it is also reversible. As with acute toxicity, it is dose-, volume-, and drug-related. Examples are radiation pneumonitis and L'Hermitte's syndrome (a transient demyelination syndrome of the spinal cord, which does not predict subsequent radiation myelitis).

Late toxicity occurs 6 months or later after the completion of X-ray therapy (XRT). It represents damage that is expressed at the end of the life cycle of parenchymal cells that have slow cell renewal and a relative inability to repopulate from stem cells. It occurs in organs that have less dependence on cell turnover and have both proliferative and functional cell populations, primarily connective and nervous tissue. Examples are the endothelium of blood vessels, and osteoblasts and chondroblasts of bone. These injuries are characterized by fibrosis, often over many years, and are not reversible, thus of serious consequence. It is therefore essential to factor these risks into dose limitations. They are strongly correlated with fraction size.

A method of quantifying the risk of permanent tissue damage is the concept of TD5/5, which is the total dose, given in standard fraction sizes, that produces a 5% risk of damage to a specified organ at 5 years.[6] These figures have been updated to reflect modern conformal treatments[7] and provide a guide for constraining the dose to

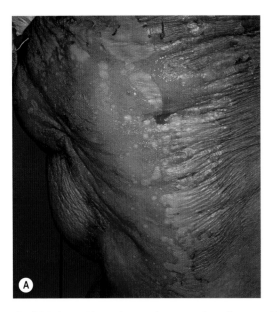 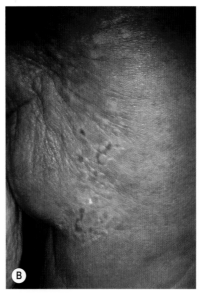 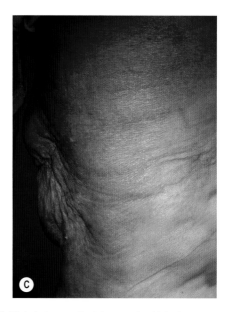

Fig. 28.6 Acute skin reactions can be severe, depending on multiple factors, including the volume and total dose. **(A)** Clinical photograph of the posterior thigh of a woman with a large sarcoma, treated with postoperative radiation to a total dose of 66 Gy. She had a history of over 240 lb (109 kg) intentional weight loss, and had marked skin redundancy, resulting in multiple folds, exacerbating her acute reaction. **(B)** Rapid improvement after just 7 days of conservative management with application of saline soaks and aloe vera gel. The white patches are healthy islands of new skin. **(C)** 14 days postcompletion of X-ray therapy.

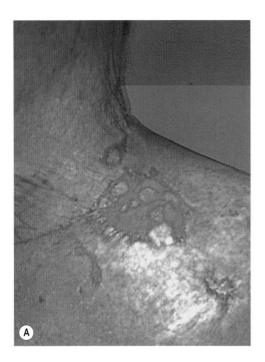 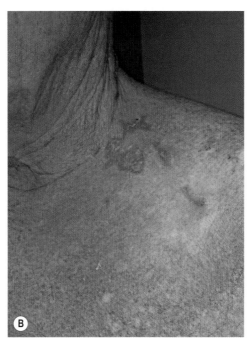

Fig. 28.7 (A) An acute skin reaction at the base of the neck at a completion dose of 70 Gy, and **(B)** 1 week later, again demonstrating rapid recovery and skin islands. This reaction at the base of the neck is fairly typical, and is a result of the obliquity of the surface and narrowness of the shoulder.

an organ at risk during the treatment-planning process, as well as for guiding informed consent.

Ionizing radiation kills cells by damaging DNA either directly or indirectly. A direct hit can cause lethal double-strand breaks, or, more commonly, the damage is caused by the release of oxygen-derived free radicals from water associated with absorption of energy into the cellular tissue. Cell death can take several forms. Lethal chromosome damage can result in apoptosis, which is a type of programmed cell death associated with activation of the tumor suppressor gene p53. Apoptosis is rapid, inducing no inflammatory response, and although it has been described in many different tissues, only certain types of tumors, for example, hemopoietic ones, undergo apoptotic death. The commonest mechanism is senescence, in which cells survive and continue to function, but lose their capacity to reproduce and proliferate.

All organized tissues mount repair in response to injury. Radiation injury prompts the body to respond in a similar way as it does to other trauma, for example, surgery. However, there are three important differences. Firstly, radiation delivers a repetitive, daily injury during the course of fractionated treatment. Secondly, the injury caused by the release in the tissue of free radicals affects all cellular and extracellular components within the volume of tissue irradiated. Thirdly, radiation causes damage to the DNA.

Response to radiation injury causes a signal transduction pathway that is mediated by the ataxia telangectasia mutated (ATM) gene to instigate DNA repair and to regulate cell cycle checkpoints, giving the cells additional time to repair. A cascade of cytokines is an immediate response, and may lead to both radiosensitization and protection.[8] Interleukin-1 and 6, and tumor necrosis factor-α cause an inflammatory response and coagulation effect. Transforming growth factor-β (TGF-β) is one of the most widely studied radiation-induced cytokines, and plays multiple roles. It causes fibroblast differentiation as well as stimulating the production of collagen. It is involved in the synthesis and regulation of extracellular matrix molecules. Following radiation, the extracellular matrix is both quantitatively and qualitatively modified – degrading progresses are altered and production of collagen synthesis increases. TGF-β also down-regulates thrombomodulin activity in endothelium, leading to platelet aggregation, and, from the platelets, release of more TGF-β, thus setting up a self-perpetuation production of TGF-β that contributes to the chronicity of radiation injury. However, it is primarily the sustained activity of TGF-β-driven myofibroblasts that causes the fibrotic reactions to radiation. Fibrosis is not an endpont, but a dynamic process of fibroblast activity. In traumatic wounds, remodeling happens over years, but this capacity to remodel in lost in irradiated tissue and instead there is self-perpetuating reactive fibrosis.[9]

Irradiated skin and soft tissue are susceptible to minimal trauma, creating a problem for surgical intervention. Radiation causes delayed wound healing, with decreased wound-breaking strength because of the

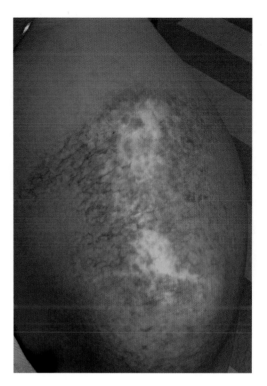

Fig. 28.8 A severe late skin reaction as a result of fast neutron therapy following excision of a large dermatofibrosarcoma protuberans tumor from the shoulder 22 years earlier. It demonstrates characteristic telangiectasia, hypopigmentation, subcutaneous fibrosis and, medially, delayed healing of a minor skin abrasion.

damage to the microvasculature and the decreased cellular elements.[9] These problems are related to the total dose, the dose per fraction, the timing of the surgery, and the extent of the surgery. The optimal time to operate on irradiated skin is the window provided once the acute reaction has resolved and before the development of excessive fibrosis, generally 3–10 weeks after completion of XRT *(Fig. 28.8)*.

Applications

Radiation treatment-planning and process

The preparation for radiation treatment, or planning, starts with a decision on the intent to treat – curative, palliative, or optimization of local control (complex palliation) – and the probable dose prescription. Following informed consent, the patient is simulated for the treatment. Two-dimensional planning with fluoroscopy has now been mostly replaced by a three-dimensional approach, using diagnostic quality CT scan with contrast (intravenous and oral as necessary). The scanners

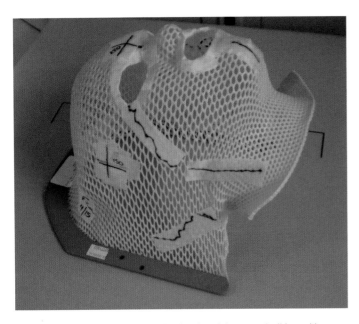

Fig. 28.9 A mask to immobilize the head and neck in a reproducible position.

are equipped with a flat, as opposed to concave, couch, and the bore is often extra-wide, to accommodate some of the positions, such as arms above the head, or legs separated in a frog-leg position, to suit the proposed treatment best. To achieve a reproducible position, some form of immobilization device is made. The type of device depends very much on the area to be treated. To treat the head and neck region, a mesh acrylic mask, similar to the type of mask worn by burn patients requiring compression treatment, is formed exactly to the patient's face and head with eye, nares, and mouth openings *(Fig. 28.9)*. This not only allows reproducible positioning but obviates the need for tattoos or other skin markings in visible areas. Extremities are immobilized using casts of the same material and body immobilization is achieved with the use of vacuum splints and bags. All of these devices are referenced to the couch position. Once the position is confirmed, immobilized, and referenced, the patient then has a CT scan in this position and goes home. The CT scan images are imported into a radiation treatment-planning system.

Using the original diagnostic scans, and often fusing them with the planning CT, the radiation oncologist starts contouring, which is a process of delineating all the structures of interest on every CT slice as it is displayed on the workstation. Any visible tumor is delineated as one or several gross tumor volumes (GTV). These are then encompassed by one or more clinical target volumes (CTV), which include normal-looking tissue considered by the radiation oncologist to be at high risk of containing tumor cells, such as the margin immediately beyond the GTV and the lymph node draining areas. Defining this volume and deciding on its dose require considerable judgment of risks and benefits, and are considered to be central to the discipline of radiation oncology. It is possible to have several CTVs that require different doses, depending on likelihood of tumor burden. The CTV is then expanded to a form a planning target volume that accounts for measured movement of the tumor or organs, for example, to account for a lung mass moving with the lungs on respiration, as well as other calculated variations.

The next step is to identify and contour all organs at risk (OAR), that is, those normal tissues that are sensitive to radiation – examples would be kidneys, spinal cord, and femoral head. Each of these sensitive structures is identified with a dose limit, or constraint. The result is a three-dimensional digital representation of the patient, tumor, and organs at risk. Working with dosimetrists, a treatment technique is decided by placing multiple beams through a series of protocols to determine the optimal arrangement of beams that will cover the target volumes homogeneously to the prescribed dose or doses, and spare critical structures. Generating dose volume histograms can help approve constraints for the OAR, by calculating the percentage of any OAR that receives a particular dose. For example, in the thorax, the V_{20} refers to the percentage of cancer-free lung (i.e., without the CTV) lung that receives >20 Gy; if this is above 35%, it is strongly predictive for radiation pneumonitis. This aspect of radiation treatment planning, rather than just positioning the patient on the CT bed, is the heart of the simulation process.

Once the radiation treatment plan has been designed, it is checked by a physicist for quality assurance to ensure that the plan is technically feasible on the treatment unit, and that no further beam modification is necessary. The patient returns for a dummy run of the plan, ironically referred to as a "virtual simulation." During this session the patient is repositioned in the immobilization device on the treatment machine, and, using light beams, the geometric parameters are checked, then verification films are taken using X-rays generated by the treatment machine and these are compared to the digitally reconstructed radiographs to ensure that the isocenter of the fields, the field shapes, and the shielding are all consistent with the plan. If all parameters set up correctly, the patient is tattooed to facilitate accurate placement on the machine on subsequent visits. If there are any problems, adjustments are made before the patient returns the next day for the start of actual treatment. Further verification is done with electronic portal imaging on the machine (ports films) or, more frequently, especially with high precision treatments, three-dimensional images are taken using a CT scanner that is mounted on the machine, e.g., cone beam CT, and adjustments, or shifts, are made as necessary. Together this imaging process is referred to as IGRT, which verifies that highly conformal plans are delivered not only accurately, but also with precision.

Clinical applications

Units of radiation

The unit of absorbed radiation dose is the gray (Gy), and corresponds to 1 joule of energy per kilogram of tissue. One gray equals 100 cGy. SI units that are named after people are, by SI convention, lower case when the whole name is used, but capitalized when the abbreviation is used. The gray replaced the older unit rad. One rad is equivalent to 1 cGy.

Treatment intent

Radiation can be used as the primary modality of therapy, or combined with other modalities such as surgery and chemotherapy. When the treatment intent is curative, radical doses, such as 66 Gy for early (and 70 Gy for late) laryngeal cancer or 80 Gy for prostate cancer, are delivered in standard fractionation sizes of 1.8–2.0 Gy per daily fraction, 5 days a week, over periods of 7 weeks or more. Typically, the maximum dose is applied to known tumor, but lower doses (45–50 cGy) are used to treat tissues that have the potential for microscopic, or occult, disease, for example, the supra-clavicular lymph nodes when three or more positive axillary lymph nodes have been resected for breast cancer, in other words, the CTV. However, when resection margins are histologically positive, i.e., there is known residual disease, a higher dose is needed, and the context is no longer adjuvant.

In noncurative situations, treatment may be used to palliate symptoms such as pain or bleeding, employing hypofractionated regimens that use smaller total doses but a larger dose per fraction. A common palliative course would be 30 Gy delivered in 10 fractions of 3 Gy. However, there are also noncurative situations when a patient has known metastatic disease, but bulky or aggressive tumor at the primary site that is, or will shortly become, very symptomatic and impair quality of life. Radical radiation approaches are used to optimize local control, for example, an unresectable fungating breast cancer even in the presence of bone metastases.

Patient selection

As in any branch of medicine, careful patient selection is very important, and informed consent essential. However, patients are often referred to radiation oncology when surgery or chemotherapy options are not feasible because of comorbidities or poor performance status. There are some basic principles to follow. For all patients, but particularly for young people, potential benefit of radiation must be weighed against the late sequelae of radiation, including the risk of second malignancy. Poor performance status and patient preferences can shift a potentially curative scenario into one of observation, or nonradical radiotherapy. However, chromosomal fragility syndromes such as Li–Fraumeni syndrome and Rb or ATM gene carriers are contraindications to radical or curative RT. Previous RT is only a relative contraindication, in that it may be possible to give a palliative dose, or even to treat to radical doses using stereotactic techniques to treat small volumes.

Hints and tips

For all patients, but particularly for young people, potential benefit of radiation must be weighed against the late sequelae of radiation, including the risk of second malignancy

Chromosomal fragility syndromes such as Li–Fraumeni syndrome, and Rb or ATM gene carriers, are contraindications to radical or curative radiation therapy

Previous radiation therapy is a relative contraindication

Breast cancer

Until 1997, it was widely believed that XRT for breast cancer only offered local control, and that any improvement in survival was related to the effect of adjuvant systemic therapy. Any survival advantage of radiation was negated by deaths that may have been caused by cardiotoxicity from large fractions and older, less precise techniques. Two landmark studies from Denmark in 1997 and 1999, and one from British Columbia (BC) published in 1997, changed breast cancer practice dramatically.[10–12] All studies examined women who were node-positive and had undergone mastectomy (in the Danish studies, over 1700 premenopausal women were treated with chemotherapy, and over 1300 postmenopausal women were treated with hormonal therapy, and in the BC study, 318 premenopausal women were treated with chemotherapy) and were then randomized to chest wall and regional lymph node radiation or no radiation, with survival as an endpoint. Both studies found an improvement in survival. The Danish study showed that patients with positive lymph nodes had a significant survival advantage with radiation, although the total number of lymph nodes sampled per patient was smaller than in current practice. Subsequently, a subgroup analysis conducted of 1152 patients who had 8 or more lymph nodes removed showed that those who had 1–3 positive lymph nodes had a 15-year overall survival of 57% after radiation, in comparison to 48% of those who did not, and those with 4 or more positive nodes improved their 15-year overall survival to 21% from 12%. A 20-year update on the BC study found that nodal irradiation conferred a 32% reduction in breast cancer mortality, and a 27% increase in overall survival. The impact on overall survival has been confirmed in subsequent meta-analyses.[13,14] These findings led to a marked increase in the number of women undergoing more extensive radiation to include the regional lymphatics. The results of a National Cancer Institute of Canada study (MA 20) are awaited to know the effects of nodal RT on local control, survival, and quality of life in women with conserved breasts who were randomized to breast RT alone or breast and nodal RT.

Breast conservation

Adjuvant breast irradiation allows breast conservation by reducing the risk of breast cancer recurrence. The evidence for the effectiveness of postlumpectomy radiation is strong, and derived from many randomized clinical trials.[15] It is one of the commonest radiotherapy treatments in North American practice. Cosmesis was also found to be satisfactory in a large European study that used rigorous assessment methods.[16] It is contraindicated when there has been previous radiation treatment to the breast or chest wall (e.g., in the treatment of Hodgkin's lymphoma), during pregnancy, or when the margins are positive. Women with active connective tissue disease, especially scleroderma,[17] may have an increased risk of acute and late toxicities, and woman with large tumors may have poorer cosmesis as a result of a larger defect. These, however, are only relative contraindications.

Although not as dramatic a finding as for nodal XRT, radiation to the intact breast alone confers benefit. Meta-analysis of mature data indicates that not having breast RT after lumpectomy confers a relative risk (RR) of local recurrence of 3.0, and that the risk of death increases by 8.6% (RR 1.086), showing that RT of the breast alone also confers a small survival advantage.[18]

Indications for postmastectomy radiation (PMRT)

National Comprehensive Cancer Network (NCCN) guidelines advise that PMRT is indicated for circumstances where the tumor is 5 cm or larger; when the margins are positive, or closer than 1 mm; or where there are regional lymph node metastases, since these are all strong predictors of chest wall recurrence. Radiation should also be considered when the lymph node status is uncertain, and the histology shows that the tumor has evidence of lymphovascular involvement, which predicts for local recurrence.[19,20] Conversely, it is not indicated when the tumor size is less than 5 cm with negative margins and without spread to the lymph nodes. There is even evidence to suggest that tumors of 5 cm that are N0 do not benefit from PMRT.[21]

Radiation of the nodal draining areas

Nodal irradiation is indicated when four or more lymph nodes are positive; RT for 1–3 nodes is still a grey area, even though it has become fairly routine practice. When there has been an adequate sampling, the upper axilla is usually not included in the volume, although the supraclavicular area, i.e., the next echelon of nodes, is included. Internal mammary (IM) nodal RT is controversial, and subject to institutional bias.[22] IM nodal involvement is known to be more common in medial and central breast cancers, and to be present when axillary lymph nodes are positive,[23] although IM clinical failure is rare. Positive IM nodes detected on imaging such as positron emission tomography (PET) fludeoxyglucose scan are rarely resectable, unlike axillary nodes, and thus need a higher dose of RT,[24] as this situation is no longer one of adjuvant therapy.

RT techniques

The target volume includes the breast, subcutaneous tissues, and chest wall. In any technique used to cover these tissues, the lower axilla is usually within the high dose volume. The classic technique is breast "tangents," using medial and lateral beams *(Fig. 28.10)* that are either angled or blocked to reduce the dose to the heart and lungs. The beam can be modified with a wedge-shaped device to reduce the "hot spot" of radiation dose that can result from this technique. IMRT and other conformal approaches are frequently used now, obviating the need for wedges, providing homogeneous dose distribution and reducing treatment time.

The same techniques are used to treat the chest wall, although the scar and drains have traditionally been in the high-dose volume, necessitating bolus to ensure that the scar receives an adequate dose

(Fig. 28.11). The use of bolus on the entire chest wall is debatable, except in the case of inflammatory breast cancer, where tumor cells, by definition, invade the dermis, and so it is essential to achieve full dose on the chest wall skin.

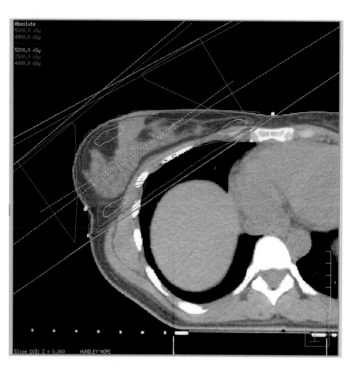

Fig. 28.10 Conserved breast treated with classic breast tangents; internal mammary lymph node chain not covered.

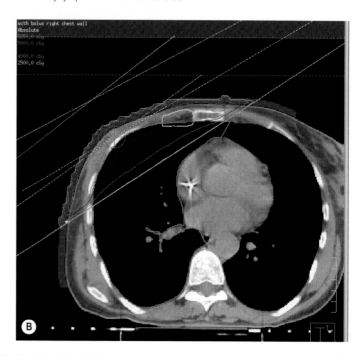

Fig. 28.11 (A) Postmastectomy X-ray therapy plan, including the internal mammary lymph node chain nodal area using a wide tangent technique, resulting in a larger volume of irradiated lung. **(B)** The use of bolus to bring the surface dose to 100%, losing the skin-sparing effect.

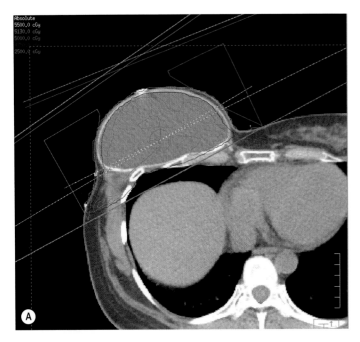 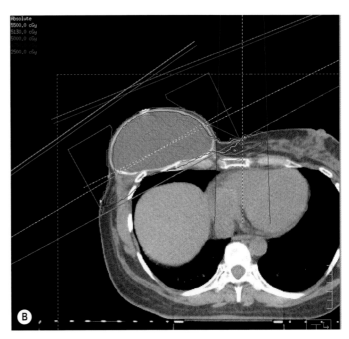

Fig. 28.12 (A) Treating a right breast mound with inflated expander in place can mean that the medial aspect of the contralateral breast may be "splashed." **(B)** The expander *in situ* is more problematic for the contralateral breast when the internal mammary lymph node chain lymph nodes are treated.

Apart from the lower axilla, which is incidentally covered in breast or chest wall techniques, additional planning is required to ensure that the targeted lymph node areas match carefully to the breast/chest wall volumes to avoid overlap and increased toxicity to the normal tissues, including the brachial plexus. The apex of the ipsilateral lung receives a full dose when treating the supraclavicular lymph node. Luckily, the total volume of sensitive lung parenchyma is small, due to the geometry and pyramidal shape of the lung. However, if overlap of fields happens, a portion of the brachial plexus may receive almost a double dose of radiation, and thus be at very high risk of brachial plexopathy. If treating the IM nodal chains, there are two main techniques: the first uses an extra-wide tangent arrangement, which can result in a significantly larger volume of lung tissue being damaged. The addition of an electron field patched on to the medial aspect of the tangent fields delivers a fairly homogeneous dose over the IM nodes, despite increasing lung, and also cardiac dose, if the tumor is located on the left side. Getting adequate dosing into the IM nodes, and avoiding critical structures, can be especially challenging when an expander has already been placed in the chest wall prior to using this technique *(Fig. 28.12)*, sometimes causing the electron dose to "splash" on to the contralateral breast. This

does not happen often on the flat chest wall of PMRT, or when the breasts are natural and fall to the side, leaving the ipsilateral parasternal area flat.

The standard adjuvant dose to the chest wall or breast ranges from 45 to 60 Gy, given in 1.8–2 Gy/fraction, depending on practice, with the same dose used for the nodal areas. As a result of a Canadian study in early-stage breast cancer, hypofractionated RT prescribing 42.5 Gy at 2.66 Gy/fraction provides the same local control as more prolonged treatment schedules. Despite the larger dose per fraction, cosmesis remains acceptable on long-term follow-up.[25,26]

Even in the absence of positive margins, local recurrence is most likely to occur in the operative bed, or tumor cavity. The use of a boost to this volume can reduce this risk, and is recommended in patients at higher risk for local failure (age <50 years, positive axillary nodes, lymphovascular invasion, or close margins). A European Organisation for Research and Treatment of Cancer (EORTC) study[27] showed that women aged 40 or younger benefited significantly from extra treatment to the tumor cavity, halving their risk of local recurrence from 19.5% to 10.2%. The benefit was less striking in women aged over 40. Boost doses of 2 Gy/fraction usually bring the total dose to the tumor cavity to a minimum of 60 Gy, and can be delivered with photons, including using conformal or IMRT techniques, electrons, a combination of photons and electrons, or brachytherapy. Although debates rage over the best way to deliver a boost dose, the evidence is not conclusive, and the technique again depends on institutional experience and operator skill. Addition of a boost can result in fibrosis and compromise cosmesis.[27]

Another approach has been to treat only the area most at risk, i.e., the cavity plus a margin, and not treat the whole breast. Accelerated partial breast irradiation remains the subject of clinical trials, although it seems to provide equivalent local control in patients over age 60 years, with low risk features, in a very convenient fashion with 10 b.i.d. treatments of either brachytherapy (total 34 Gy) or external-beam photon therapy (total 38.5 Gy) to the tumor bed.

Sequencing with systemic treatment

Many chemotherapy agents, including Adriamycin and epirubicin, and all the taxanes, act as radiosensitizing agents, and concurrent use can cause marked acute toxicity. This can result in chemotherapy dose reduction, or interruption of RT, thus substandard use of both treatments, and potentially compromised outcomes. It is now more common to use these modalities sequentially, rather than concurrently, with chemotherapy sequenced before radiation. The evidence on neoadjuvant chemotherapy (i.e., chemotherapy given before surgery) can result in downstaging of the disease at the time of surgery. However, the RT should still be planned dependent on the original clinical staging evidence.[28] Common hormonal therapies can be given concurrently with RT, although practice is often to wait until the completion of adjuvant XRT. The same applies to trastuzumab (which is marketed under the brand name Herceptin).

Although there is much evidence on this topic, it is often unclear and open to much interpretation. Institutional experience still tends to drive clinical practice.

Head and neck cancer

Head and neck cancers are mostly squamous cell carcinomas (SCCs) and radiation has an important role in the primary, postoperative, and palliative aspect of their management. Previously, a general principle of minimizing toxicity by using either surgery or radiation, and keeping the other modality for salvage, was preferred. However, increasingly, especially in locally advanced disease, combined modality, particularly postoperative radiation treatment, is used because it has been shown to reduce the incidence of recurrence, particularly in the cervical lymph nodes. The use of concurrent chemotherapy has also changed the practice over the last 10–15 years. Several studies have shown a benefit in both survival and local control[29]; as a result, cisplatinum-based therapy has become the standard of care in the management of all but the most favorable – early disease that has a high cure rate with RT alone. However acute toxicity is considerably worsened by concurrent chemotherapy.

SCC head and neck cancers have lower local control rates if treatment time is extended, due to repopulation of tumor cells.[30] To overcome this effect, efforts have to be made to deliver five fractions per week even if it requires treating twice a day to do so. Approaches that intensify the course of treatment by giving it over a shorter period of time (accelerated fractionation) or giving treatment more than once a day using a smaller dose per fraction over the same time period (hyperfractionation) can improve outcome but result in severe acute toxicity so that breaks in treatment may be necessary, thus negating the benefit of altering the fractionation schedule.

Doses used for gross tumor are in the 66–72-Gy range. Areas at risk are treated to 50 Gy, although postoperatively, this is in the 56–60-Gy range. Before the introduction of IMRT, these areas were usually treated sequentially, covering the larger volume to a "microscopic" dose, before boosting the smaller volume or volumes containing gross disease, although a concomitant boost was sometimes used. However IMRT allows a technique of "dose painting" or differential dosing so that the areas at higher risk are programmed to receive a slightly higher dose per day than the areas of low risk. It can also reduce the dose to the parotid, reducing the risk of permanent xerostomia.

Acute toxicities occur during the course of treatment and resolve 2–3 months following completion of treatment. They are reversible unless the acute damage is confluent, causing damage to the basal membrane and depleting the supply of stem cells. Mucositis, which is exacerbated by smoking and alcohol, starts during weeks 2–3, becoming confluent by the end. It affects the mucous membranes within high-dose volume and mucositis in the mouth, oropharynx. and hypopharynx results in difficulty in swallowing. Because of concerns about nutritional status, percutaneous endoscopic gastrostomy tubes are inserted before the start of treatment. Mucositis is painful and mouthwashes containing local anesthetic help this, but usually narcotics are also required. The skin develops erythema by weeks 3–4, even with the aggressive use of topical aloe vera gels and other unguents and steroids. Reaction is inevitably brisk with moist desquamation by completion of treatment. Because of dose to the parotid, patients will also experience change in taste; radiation causes xerostomia, changing the consistency of saliva by drying the water component, which results in thick mucoid secretions that are difficult to clear. During treatment patients often lose weight and experience fatigue.

Late toxicities depend on the size of dose per fraction given. They occur 6 months to 3 years following the completion of treatment and unfortunately are permanent and progressive. The primary problem is fibrosis that can affect the subcutaneous tissues, musculature, and joints. The patient can experience trismus, neck stiffness, aching, and swallowing difficulties as a result. If the parotid has been treated to more than 26 Gy the patient may be left with permanent xerostomia, which can exacerbate dental problems. The patient may also experience voice changes due to chronic laryngeal edema and/or cartilage damage. Patients are also at risk of ORN.

Soft-tissue sarcoma

Sarcomas comprise a heterogeneous group of more than 50 bone and soft-tissue mesenchymal subtypes. Soft-tissue sarcomas (STS) are rare mesenchymal malignancies arising from connective tissue. They can arise anywhere in the body but most commonly affect the extremities and trunk. In the pediatric population, 7% of tumors are STS, with half of these being rhabdomyosarcoma, and, especially in younger children, these tumors are more responsive to chemotherapy, so radiation is either spared or used in much lower doses, as much as possible to avoid arresting growth or increasing the risk of a second malignancy.

Because of the rarity of STS (only about 10 000 are diagnosed per year in the US) and the numerous locations and subtypes, they are best managed in specialized multidisciplinary groups. Radiation treatment is also best conducted in a specialized facility, not only because of the radiation oncologists' expertise, but also so that they can work with the surgeon in delineating target volumes. Even more importantly, the other members of the radiation team, including therapists, dosimetrists and nursing, need to be experienced with the fine details of immobilization, set-up, verification, and the management of acute toxicities related to the very large volumes that are often necessary. Prognosis depends on size, grade, histological subtype, and superficiality of the tumor. Location is also important; retroperitoneal sarcomas have an independently worse outcome, but usually do not present until tumors are very large.

Generally, sarcomas in adults are not very chemosensitive, the exceptions being historically osteosarcoma, and more recently, gastrointestinal stromal tumors, which respond well to therapy with imatinib (Gleevec), a protein-tyrosine kinase inhibitor. Chemotherapy is also useful in palliative situations, and there is increasing information on the usefulness of neoadjuvant chemotherapy, although the advantage may be considered marginal.[31] Since sarcoma patients frequently develop lung metastases, further development in this area is important.

Although the primary treatment of STS is surgery, adjuvant radiation is important for limb and function conservation in extremity sarcoma and reducing the risk of local recurrence. Overall, local control rates are approximately 80% at 5 years.[32] If the patient is unfit for surgery, primary RT can provide useful local control. The role of XRT in adjuvant treatment of osteosarcoma, chondrosarcoma, and chordoma is minimal, although it can be a useful modality for palliation.

Doses and techniques in adults

Postoperative adjuvant XRT is indicated after resection of high-grade or large tumors with negative margins, or any tumor with positive margins. NCCN guidelines use 10 cm to define large STS, although, in practice, many feel that this should be as small as 5 cm.

Standard adjuvant postoperative radiation doses for STS are 60–66 Gy in 30–33 fractions, or higher if any gross disease remains, with reduction in the size of the volume after 50 Gy. The CTV is often large, encompassing the entire operative bed, which is determined with postoperative magnetic resonance imaging (MRI) to visualize the operative "footprint," or by reconstructing preoperative imaging (e.g., fusing with diagnostic MR scan) and using surgical clips, operating room report and guidance from the surgeon to determine the extent of the volume, and to identify those areas most at risk. Generous margins are used to cover any uncertainty.

The standard preoperative neoadjuvant XRT dose is 50 Gy given in 25 fractions of 2 Gy over 5 weeks. The GTV covers the radiologically visible tumor and the CTV covers peritumoral edema as seen on MRI T2 imaging, or CT or PET CT volume plus 2–3 cm. If the margins are positive after resection, a further 16–20 Gy is usually given, although recent work suggests that this practice is not necessary.[33]

Optimal immobilization is important in the RT planning process. It is also necessary to delineate bones, joints, and sensitive structures such as the vulva so that dose to these sites can be minimized. It is also necessary to spare a longitudinal strip of skin and subcutaneous tissue so that lymphatic drainage remains intact to reduce the risk of chronic lymphedema. Conformal techniques, including IMRT, are often needed to meet these constraints when possible, without risking tumor recurrence.

The issue of whether pre- or postoperative XRT is used remains controversial. Certainly the preoperative advantages of an early start of XRT, a smaller irradiated volume and likely lower dose, and, as a result of these features, less fibrosis and better functional outcome[34] are compelling. However, the delay to definitive surgical treatment and the doubling of risk of wound complications (17–35% in the Canadian randomized trial) are also serious issues to consider.[34]

Skin cancers

Nonmelanoma skin cancers

This group encompasses basal cell carcinoma (BCC), SCC, Merkel cell carcinoma, and cutaneous angiosarcoma. Of these, the commonest are BCC and SCC. The majority are radiation-related, albeit mostly solar radiation! Due to their chronic immunosuppression, patients who have undergone transplantation are more likely to develop SCC, which tends to behave more aggressively. The role of radiation is in primary treatment when the patient is not a surgical candidate (comorbidities, anticoagulation, patient preference) or when surgery may risk function or cosmesis. It is used in the adjuvant setting to reduce the risk of local recurrence and palliatively for locally advanced and unresectable disease. In this situation high doses are often used to optimize local control. Radiation can be used for definitive treatment of SCCs or after recurrence when further surgery is not possible. The important issue is the risk of lymph node metastases and inclusion of the regional nodes in situations of high risk. An important consideration is the presence of perineural invasion, which may involve treating extended volumes along neural pathways. In all, 30–40% of incompletely incised BCCs recur but they can be salvaged equally with surgery or radiation.[35] Doses for the primary treatment of BCC are in the range of 40–50 Gy delivered in 10–20 fractions with margins of 5 mm on gross disease.

When delivering radiotherapy for skin cancers one has to be able to achieve a high dose superficially. One of the best ways to do this is to use superficial kV equipment that provides 100% of the dose at the surface and a very tight penumbra resulting in smaller fields. However this equipment has now been largely supplanted by electrons which have a larger penumbra due to their propensity to scatter. Furthermore, low-energy electrons do not provide 100% of the dose at the surface and this needs to be corrected with the use of bolus. Photons and cobalt gamma rays can also be used with bolus to achieve a high dose at surface but, unlike kV or electrons, their dose does not fall off quickly.

Although treatment with XRT is highly curative, late toxicities of treatment result in cosmetic changes related to change in pigmentation, fatty necrosis, subcutaneous fibrosis, and dermal telangectasia formation. These tend not to arise for 2 years or more after treatment and not all patients suffer these effects. These risks are increased with larger volumes and larger fraction size. Luckily, since many of these cancers are small, and the patient population is, by and large, elderly and frail, one can still get away with using hypofractionated treatment over a shorter period of time.

Merkel cell carcinoma is a rare neuroendocrine skin tumor that has a lethal potential for spread. Both the local disease and the regional lymph nodes need to be treated. Inclusion of nodal areas means that radiotherapy volumes become larger and smaller fraction sizes are necessary.

Angiosarcoma is mainly treated with surgery but when this is not possible or when there is recurrence or the presence of positive margins, radiation is necessary. Higher doses, between 66 and 70 Gy, are needed. Tumor location can be an important issue in planning treatment. A common radiation problem, for example, is how to treat the entire scalp without causing excessive toxicity to healthy tissues, in this case the brain. To overcome this, one can use a technique called "German helmet," in which a combination of photons and electrons is used in such a way as to minimize penetration to the brain, and subsequent cognitive dysfunction.

Malignant melanoma is generally thought of as being radioresistant. *In vivo* studies show that the cell survival curve has a very broad shoulder, indicating that these cells have a large capacity to repair sublethal damage. The way to overcome this is to hypofractionate and use large doses per fraction.

Adjuvant radiation can reduce the risk of local recurrence in high-risk adjuvant situations. At the MD Anderson Cancer Center, criteria for this include desmoplastic histology, depth >4 mm with ulceration or satellite lesions, positive margins, or recurrent disease.[36] Radiation to involved or high-risk but clinically negative lymph nodes can improve control. Hypofractionated radiotherapy is effective, albeit with a high risk of lymphedema, improving local control from 50% to 87%[37] without affecting survival. Radiation also plays a major role in palliation of brain and bone metastases, and uncontrolled tumor. When possible, hypofractionated regimens such as 6 Gy twice a week for a total of 30–36 Gy are commonly used.[38]

Benign disorders

RT was historically used to treat many benign conditions, such as ankylosing spondylitis, tinea capita, and eczema, that fortunately now are treated with systemic therapies. However, it is still used in the treatment of noncancerous conditions such as prevention of heterotopic ossification after hip replacement surgery and keloid scars.[39] The doses used are low, so unlikely to cause significant problems with fibrosis. However, especially in a younger person, the concerns about development of a radiation-induced malignancy must be weighed against the potential gain of using radiation for benign disease.

Specific toxicities and complications

Bony injury

ORN is a necrotic wound manifested in irradiated bone that persists without healing for 3–6 months, in the absence of tumor recurrence.[40] It presents as clinically exposed bone, sometimes without any pain, and radiologic evidence of necrosis on both CT and MRI between 1 and 3 years following radiation. Radiologic findings may mimic disease recurrence. ORN is mostly seen as a result of treating head and neck cancer, especially floor-of-mouth tumors, and affects the mandible more than the maxilla. It can also develop at other bony sites, such as the sternum or pelvis. Radiation-related risk factors include fraction size (>200 cGy), the volume of bone irradiated, a total dose to the bone of >6000 cGy, and re-irradiation. The type of radiation is also important, because particle therapy (electrons, neutrons, protons), brachytherapy, and kilovoltage energy can result in higher absorbed doses within bone than from megavoltage photons or gamma-rays from cobalt. The use of three-dimensional treatment-planning systems, improvements in immobilization, as well as conformal techniques such as IMRT and higher precision with IGRT for localization, helps to minimize the volume of bone in the target, as well as the dose. Other risk factors in the head and neck region include poor oral hygiene and dental extraction, making careful dental preparation an integral part of treatment planning. Concurrent chemotherapy causes mucositis and xerostomia, further increasing the risk, as does the xerostomia resulting from relatively low doses to the parotid. ORN arising in other sites can also be associated with trauma and surgery.

Although ORN in the head and neck region had an incidence of 6.8% in 1968,[41] it is fortunately now quite rare, with recent series reporting incidences of 0–2%.[42,43] Bisphosphones can cause osteonecrosis without radiation,[44] but it is still unclear what increased risks are incurred with concurrent radiation and bisphosphonate therapies.

Radiation-related bone fractures are more common. Rib fractures tend to be the result of coughing. Limb fractures can happen with minimal or no trauma. No intervention is necessary for clavicles or ribs, but long bones usually require an intramedullary nail and there can be long delays in union. An analysis of fractures associated with STS identified that the total dose to the bone and the volume irradiated were critical factors, leading to recommendations that the maximum dose to the bone should be 5900 cGy, and that the volume of bone receiving >4000 cGy be limited to 64%.[45]

Bone growth in children

Radiation can impede bone development in children, leading to limb shortening, asymmetry (including scoliosis), deformity and functional impairment, and thus is a dose-limiting step in RT. This effect was noticed soon after the use of radiotherapy became widespread, since radiotherapy was a significant modality in the treatment of pediatric tumors, although it was difficult to quantify risks as treatments and dosimetry were very heterogeneous. Radiologically, changes on the growth plate that resemble rickets can be seen, including metaphyseal sclerosis, metaphyseal fraying, and epiphyseal plate widening, reflecting the radiosensitivity of rapidly proliferating cells in this region. The child's age at the time of radiation is important, since most bone growth occurs in the first 5 years. The most important radiotherapy factors are the total dose and volume of bone irradiated. Although 30 Gy is considered the tolerance threshold dose, growth effects are seen with as low a dose as 15 Gy, suggesting a very steep dose–response curve in this range.[46] The use of orthovoltage therapy can significantly increase the absorbed dose in bone, and thus markedly increase the risk.

Craniofacial growth is different to long bones, since these bones develop through intramembraneous ossification, resulting in a complex three-dimensional pattern of growth.[47] Disruption of this growth by radiation in all or any part of the head and face can cause significant clinical problems, including distorted appearance and functional problems related to eating. Dentition is also affected.

Cranial irradiation is used for prophylaxis again central nervous system relapse in leukemia. Not only can this affect cognition and bone growth, it can also impair the production of growth hormone, and this results in decreased bone mineralization.[48] Genetic factors are important, for example, in the treatment of retinoblastoma, where there may be much greater sensitivity to XRT. Biological factors that are disrupted by XRT include remodeling of the extracellular matrix in response to paracrine and endocrine signaling that affects chondrocyte production. Radioprotective agents, such as amifostine, have been studed *in vivo* and found to protect a number of cell lines, such as osteoblast-like, endothelial, and fibroblastic, from harmful effects of radiation.[49]

Lymphedema

When assessing lymphedema in someone who has had a previous cancer diagnosis, it is important to exclude recurrent disease before assuming that the edema is related to treatment. However, lymphedema after breast cancer is common. Norman *et al.* identified 42% 5-year accumulative incidence in a 5-year prospective, population-based study of breast cancer survivors. However, the majority (23%) described only mild lymhedema, and only 2% had developed chronic, severe edema.[50]

Independent risk factors for breast cancer-associated lymphedema include radiation treatment of the axilla, the extent of axillary lymph node dissection, the type of breast surgery, and the presence of regional lymph node metastases.[51] A history of infection and injuries, and the patient's body mass index are also associated factors. The combination of XRT and axillary lymph node dissection confers the greatest risk.[50] A large series from Massachusetts General Hospital reported lymphedema rates of 10% in women who had breast-conserving surgery and XRT to the axilla,[51] although historically, higher rates have been reported. It has also been suggested[49] that, with survival and longevity, this late toxicity becomes more prevalent. However, as sentinel lymph node dissection becomes the standard of care in early breast cancer, this will result in a lower risk of lymphedema than conventional axillary lymph node dissection risks.[52] The mechanics of RT-related lymphedema are due to the radiation-induced fibrosis causing compression of the lymph vessels.

Brachial plexopathy

Brachial plexopathy is most commonly due to metastatic disease involving the brachial plexus, and it can be very difficult to distinguish between the late side-effect of XRT versus recurrence. PET has been reported to be helpful.[53] However, it is also a rare (1%) complication of radiation treatment.[54] Its development is dependent not just on total dose, with a marked increase above 5000 cGy, but also on the dose per fraction. RT technique is also a very important factor, as older breast RT techniques that extended to the lymph nodes could result in overlapping fields just above the clavicle immediately above the brachial plexus, meaning that the plexus received up to twice the prescribed dose. Concurrent chemotherapy also increased the risk.

Radiation-induced malignancies

Radiation has been shown to induce malignant transformation *in vitro*, for example, in laboratory mice, and *in vivo*, for example, from atom bomb survivors, as well as long-term follow-up studies. Three mechanisms for radiation-induced malignancy have been suggested: (1) DNA damage and subsequent mutation; (2) disturbances of multiple defense or control mechanisms within the cell at the molecular level; and (3) the chronic ongoing damage of irradiated tissue.[55]

Radiation-induced malignancies are rare within the first 5 years after treatment, and usually present many (20–40) years after treatment. As more cancers are cured, and the number of long-term survivors increases, so does the risk of radiation-induced malignancies.[56] Although a second malignancy rate of 1 per 100 000 patients treated is often cited, this figure is only an estimate, and may be misleading. Many different mathematical models are used to standardize the doses, dose per fraction and quality of radiation, as well as the volume of the target, the organs treated, and the age of the patient. Second primary tumors are more common in those who have already had a malignancy, with a RR of 1.12, regardless of treatment. Chemotherapy, especially alkylating agents, is also carcinogenic, although more likely to induce leukemia than a solid tumor, and within a much shorter latent period. The addition of chemotherapy during RT also increases the risk. Some of the best data come from follow-up of childhood survivors,[57] although also identifying large variations in findings. In children, susceptibility varies according to age and the type of tissue irradiated, with leukemia developing after 5–8 years, and solid tumors, the commonest of which are thyroid cancer, breast cancer and bone and central nervous system malignancies, usually occurring many years later.[58,59] Some second primary malignancies, especially carcinomas, arise around the periphery of the high-dose volume. Concerns have been expressed about the risk of techniques such as IMRT: although they have very conformal high-dose volumes and can minimize dose to critical structures, there is a large lower-dose volume from the multiple-beam entry through normal tissues.[59,60] Thyroid cancer is unlikely when the gland has received doses over 30 Gy. Conversely, sarcomas tend to arise in heavily irradiated tissues, and appear to have a dose–response effect. Survivors of Hodgkin's disease treated with mantle radiation (i.e., mediastinal, cervical, and axillary nodal XRT and shields over the lungs) have four times the risk of developing breast cancer. The woman's age at the time of XRT is extremely important: adolescent girls aged 10–16 years have a 136-fold greater risk of developing breast cancer than their nonirradiated peers.[61] Factors such as smoking can markedly increase the risk, even in parts of the lung that received only a tiny scattered dose. Some genetic predispositions, such as Li–Fraumeni syndrome, which is linked to germline mutations of the p53 suppressor gene, or ATM and RB gene carriers, are exquisitely susceptible to any form of radiation.

Exposure to radiation

Radiation accident studies have shown that there is a proportional relationship between the amount of radiation exposure and the risk of developing cancer.[62] The sievert (Sv) is the SI unit that measures the biological effect of absorbed dose, taking into consideration the relative biological effectiveness of the radiation (e.g., 1 for photons and electrons, 20 for high-dose neutrons) and the biological effect on different organs. When all of these weightings are 1, then 1 Sv = 1 Gy. The gray is a unit of absorbed dose in any material defined only by physical, not biological, properties of radiation. The sievert is used to quantify risk of radiation damage, including cancer. To put this into perspective, on average, a chest X-ray is 0.34 mSv, mammogram 0.48 mSv, and CT thorax

6 mSv. There is background cosmic radiation of 0.24 mSv per year, and on a return flight between Seattle, WA and Toronto, ON would be exposed to 0.085 mSv. Radiation oncologists are limited to an occupational exposure of 20 mSv per year, excluding medical and background sources of radiation, but after the March 2011 earthquake and subsequent explosion in a nuclear reactor, the emergency nuclear workers at Fukushima, Japan were exposed to up to 400 mSv per hour. The Japanese public already has a 20–25% lifetime risk of cancer, and exposure to 400 mSv increases that risk by 2–4%. Survivors of the atom bombs in Hiroshima and Nagasaki have an excess risk of cancer (RR 1.42 at 1 Sv) that persists through their lifetime. Exposure to 1 Sv increases the lifetime risk of fatal cancer by approximately 5%. The most sensitive organs to this sort of accidental exposure are bone marrow and thyroid, and leukemia is the most common resulting malignancy. Radiation sickness is an acute effect of radiation exposure, causing nausea, headache, and bone marrow suppression, and is rarely experienced at exposures of less than 1 Sv.

Regardless of the regulatory safety requirements, the ALARA (as low as reasonably achievable) principle is the mantra of all who work with ionizing radiation in their efforts to reduce the risk of harm.

Conclusion and future trends

Radiation treatment uses ionizing radiation to treat malignancies as a primary therapy, or, more importantly now, as part of a planned collaborative multidisciplinary approach, used in combination with systemic therapy and surgery. Like surgery, it is a local therapy, and has a curative, adjuvant, or palliative role in managing most cancers. Although acute toxicities are reversible, late toxicities are not, and are related mostly to the loss of normal fibrosis mechanisms. The risk of radiation-induced malignancy, as well as other late side-effects, becomes more important as more cancers are cured, and the proportion of survivors grows.

Dramatic advances in radiation treatment planning, delivery, and verification technology have increased the accuracy and precision of treatment, allowing higher doses to tumor, and reducing the risk of radiation injury by sparing more normal tissue. Improvements in RT-planning systems provide not only the ability to apply dose constraints to specified structures, but also to provide data that help quantify risk of toxicity, in tandem with better reporting and collection of data and outcomes. These approaches all contribute to improving the prevention of radiation injury. Radioprotection also occurs by reducing risk of radiation damage through modification of delivery techniques, but modulating radiation cellular response is of greater importance. Although this concept has been studied for years, clinical results have been disappointing; nevertheless, the new generation of biological modifiers offer greater hope. However, the future of radiation oncology lies in biology, and specifically bioengineering and tissue regeneration, and the imperative to repair the damage that has already been caused.

 Access the complete references list online at **http://www.expertconsult.com**

6. Emami B, Lyman J, Brown A, et al. Tolerance of normal tissue to therapeutic irradiation. *Int J Radiat Oncol Biol Phys*. 1991;21:109–122.

7. Bentzen SM, Constine LS, Deasy JO, et al. Quantitative analyses of normal tissue effects in the clinic (QUANTEC): an introduction to the scientific issues. *Int J Radiat Oncol Biol Phys*. 2010;76(3 Suppl): S3–S9.

8. Devalia HL, Mansfield L. Radiotherapy and wound healing. *Int Wound J*. 2008;5:40–44.

   This review article discusses basic radiation physics and effects of radiation on wounds. It examines various postulated hypotheses on the role of circulatory decrease and radiation-induced direct cellular damage. The new concept related to the radiation pathogenesis proposes that there is a cascade of cytokines initiated immediately after the radiation. Sustained activation of myofibroblasts in the wound accounts for its chronicity. Recent advances highlight that transforming growth factor-β₁ is the master switch in the pathogenesis of radiation fibrosis. This article overviews its role and summarizes the available evidence related to radiation damage. The goal of this article was to provide its modern understanding, as future research will concentrate on antagonizing the effects of cytokines to promote wound healing.

9. Denham JW, Hauer-Jensen M. The radiotherapeutic injury – a complex "wound". *Radiother Oncol.* 2002;63: 129–145.

   Radiotherapeutic normal tissue injury can be viewed as two simultaneously ongoing and interacting processes. The first has many features in common with the healing of traumatic wounds. The second is a set of transient or permanent alterations of cellular and extracellular components within the irradiated volume. In contrast to physical trauma, fractionated RT produces a series of repeated insults to tissues that undergo significant changes during the course of radiotherapy. Normal tissue responses are also influenced by rate of dose accumulation and other factors that relate to the RT schedule. This article reviews the principles of organized normal tissue responses during and after RT, the effect of RT on these responses, as well as some of the mechanisms underlying the development of recognizable injury. Important clinical implications relevant to these processes are also discussed.

14. Van de Steene J, Soete G, Storme G. Adjuvant radiotherapy for breast cancer significantly improves overall survival: the missing link. *Radiother Oncol.* 2000;55:263–272.

   The influence of surgical adjuvant radiotherapy on overall survival of patients with operable breast cancer is still a controversial subject. The negative result of the EBCTCG meta-analysis of clinical randomized trials on adjuvant radiotherapy in breast cancer is in strong contrast with the Danish 82B, 82C, and British Columbia trials showing an impressive survival benefit. This paper tries to fill in the gap between the conflicting results. The results of this study stress the importance of reducing cardiovascular and other late toxicity in adjuvant radiotherapy for breast cancer.

22. Taghian A, Jagsi R, Makris A, et al. Results of a survey regarding irradiation of internal mammary chain in patients with breast cancer: practice is culture driven rather than evidence based. *Int J Radiat Oncol Biol Phys.* 2004;60:706–714.

   This paper examines the self-reported practice patterns of radiation oncologists in North America and Europe regarding radiotherapy to the internal mammary lymph node chain (IMC) in breast cancer patients. The results of this study revealed significant international variation in attitudes regarding treatment of the IMC. The international patterns of variation mirror the divergent conclusions of studies conducted in different regions, indicating that physicians may rely preferentially on evidence from local studies when making difficult treatment decisions.

55. Tubiana M. Can we reduce the incidence of second primary malignancies occurring after radiotherapy? A critical review. *Radiother Oncol.* 2009;91:4–15; discussion 1–3.

   Second primary malignancies (SPMs) occurring after oncological treatment have become a major concern during the past decade. Their incidence has long been underestimated because most patients had a short life expectancy after treatment or their follow-up was shorter than 15 years. This paper concludes that efforts should be made to base SPM reduction on solid data and not on speculation or models built on debatable hypotheses regarding the dose–carcinogenic effect relationship. In parallel, radiation therapy philosophy must evolve, and the aim of treatment should be to deliver the minimal effective radiation therapy rather than the maximal tolerable dose.

57. Robison LL, Green DM, Hudson M, et al. Long-term outcomes of adult survivors of childhood cancer. *Cancer.* 2005;104(Suppl):2557–2564.

60. Brenner DJ. Extrapolating radiation-induced cancer risks from low doses to very low doses. *Health Phys.* 2009;97:505–509.

62. Preston DL, Ron E, Tokuoka S, et al. Solid cancer incidence in atomic bomb survivors: 1958–1998. *Radiat Res.* 2007;168:1–64.

29

Vascular anomalies

Arin K. Greene and John B. Mulliken

SYNOPSIS

- Vascular anomalies are divided into tumors or malformations.
- Vascular tumors are comprised of proliferating endothelium, the endothelial lining of malformations is more quiescent.
- Infantile hemangioma is the most common tumor of infancy; it grows rapidly after birth and involutes during childhood.
- Most infantile hemangiomas are observed; problematic lesions are treated pharmacologically or by resection.
- Vascular malformations are present at birth, although not always obvious; they may slowly enlarge during childhood and adolescence.
- Vascular malformations are managed by observation, laser, sclerotherapy, embolization, or resection; pharmacotherapy is not available.

Introduction

Vascular anomalies is a newly evolved field that incorporates several surgical and medical specialties. Because these disorders usually involve the skin, the initial consultation is often with a plastic surgeon (or a pediatric dermatologist). Development of this field has been impeded by a lack of standardized terminology. For centuries, it was believed that vascular birthmarks were imprinted on the unborn child by a mother's emotions or diet. This was reflected in words for brightly colored foods to describe vascular anomalies. Adjectives such as "cherry," "strawberry," and "port-wine" have their roots in these traditional beliefs.[1] Physicians usually preferred the Latin term *naevus maternus* for vascular birthmarks, but their understanding was little advanced beyond folklore.

In the 19th century, the first attempt was made to categorize vascular anomalies histologically by Virchow, the father of cellular pathology. Virchow's *angioma simplex* became synonymous with "capillary" or "strawberry" hemangioma. His term *angioma cavernosum* was used indiscriminately for subcutaneous hemangiomas (that regress) and venous malformations (that never regress). *Angioma racemosum* was modified to racemose (cirsoid) aneurysm or "arteriovenous hemangioma", referring to an arteriovenous malformation, a vascular lesion that expands over time.[2] His student, Wegener, developed a comparable histomorphic subcategorization for "lymphangioma".[3] This nomenclature persisted well into the 20th century. Often the same word was applied to entirely different vascular anomalies. This confusing nosology has been responsible for improper diagnosis, illogical treatment, and misdirected research.

A biologic classification system, introduced in 1982,[4] cleared the terminologic confusion that had long obscured the field. This scheme evolved from studies that correlated physical findings, natural history, and cellular features.[4] The key to this biologic classification is proper use of the Greek nominative suffix -*oma* which once meant "swelling" or "tumor". In modern times -*oma* denotes a lesion that arises by upregulated cellular growth. There are two major categories of vascular

Table 29.1 Classification of vascular anomalies

Tumors	Malformations	
	Slow-flow	Fast-flow
Infantile hemangioma (IH)	Capillary malformation (CM) 　Cutis marmorata telangiectatica congenita (CMTC) 　Telangiectasias	Arterial malformation (AM) 　Aneurysm 　Atresia 　Ectasia 　Stenosis
Congenital hemangioma (CH) 　Rapidly involuting congenital 　hemangioma (RICH) 　Noninvoluting congenital 　hemangioma (NICH)	Lymphatic malformation (LM) 　Microcystic 　Macrocystic 　Primary lymphedema	Arteriovenous malformation (AVM) 　Capillary malformation-arteriovenous 　malformation (CM-AVM) 　Hereditary hemorrhagic telangiectasia (HHT) 　PTEN-associated vascular anomaly
Hemangioendotheliomas 　Kaposiform hemangio- 　endothelioma (KHE) 　Other	Venous malformation (VM) 　Cerebral cavernous malformation (CCM) 　Cutaneomucosal venous malformation (CMVM) 　Glomuvenous malformation (GVM) 　Verrucous hemangioma (VH)	Combined malformations 　Capillary-arteriovenous malformation (CAVM) 　Capillary-lymphatic arteriovenous 　malformation (CLAVM)
Pyogenic granuloma (PG)	Combined malformations 　Capillary-venous malformation (CVM) 　Capillary-lymphatic malformation (CLM) 　Capillary-lymphatic-venous malformation (CLVM) 　Lymphatic-venous malformation (LVM)	

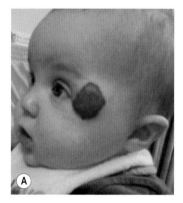 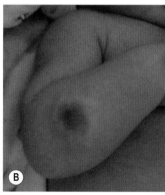 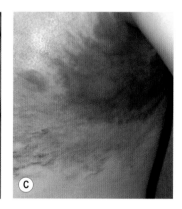 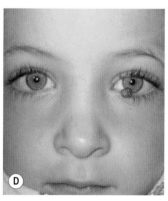

Fig. 29.1 Vascular tumors of infancy and childhood. **(A)** A 3-month-old female with enlarging infantile hemangioma of the cheek first noted at 1 week of age. **(B)** A 6-week-old male with a rapidly involuting congenital hemangioma (RICH). Note purple color and peripheral halo. **(C)** A 1-year-old male with a kaposiform hemangioendothelioma complicated by Kassabach-Merritt phenomenon. **(D)** A 5-year-old male with a two month history of bleeding pyogenic granuloma of left lower eyelid.

anomalies, tumors and malformations *(Table 29.1)*. *Vascular tumors* are endothelial neoplasms characterized by increased endothelial turnover *(Fig. 29.1)*. Infantile hemangioma is the most common, a tumor that arises in infants. Other vascular tumors are congenital hemangioma, hemangioendotheliomas, tufted angioma, hemangiopericytomas, angiosarcoma, and pyogenic granuloma. *Vascular malformations* are the result of abnormal development of vascular elements during embryogenesis *(Fig. 29.2)*. They are designated according to the predominant channel type as: *capillary malformation, lymphatic malformation, venous malformation, arteriovenous malformation*, and complex forms such as capillary-lymphatic-venous malformation. Malformations with an arterial component are rheologically fast-flow; the remainder are slow-flow.

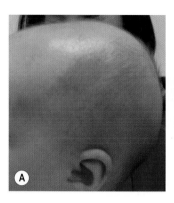 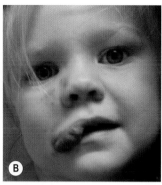 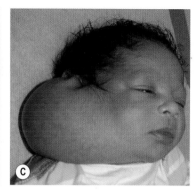 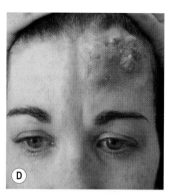

Fig. 29.2 Vascular malformations. **(A)** A 4-month-old male with capillary malformation of the scalp. **(B)** A 3-year-old female with an expanding venous malformation of the lip first noted at birth. **(C)** Infant male with macrocystic lymphatic malformation. **(D)** A 39-year-old female with a bleeding, ulcerated arteriovenous malformation of the forehead.

Table 29.2 Incorrect terminology commonly used to describe vascular anomalies

Tumors		Malformations	
Biological name	Incorrect term	Biologic name	Incorrect term
Infantile hemangioma	"Capillary hemangioma" "Cavernous hemangioma" "Strawberry hemangioma"	Capillary malformation	"Port-wine stain" "Capillary hemangioma"
Hemangioendothelioma	"Capillary hemangioma"	Lymphatic malformation	"Cystic hygroma" "Lymphangioma"
		Venous malformation	"Cavernous hemangioma"
		Arteriovenous malformation	"Arteriovenous hemangioma"

This biologic classification was accepted by the International Society for Vascular Anomalies in 1996.[5] Differences that distinguish between hemangiomas and vascular malformations were confirmed by imaging[6,7] and by immunohistochemical markers.[8,9] It is critical to underscore that vascular malformations, although fundamentally structural disorders, can exhibit endothelial hyperplasia, possibly triggered by clotting, ischemia, embolization, partial resection, or hormonal influences.

History and physical examination should give diagnostic accuracy of more than 90% in distinguishing between vascular tumors and vascular malformations *(Fig. 29.3)*.[10] The most likely error in assigning a clinical diagnosis continues to be an inaccurate, imprecise use of terminology *(Table 29.2)*. Perhaps the most egregious example is "hemangioma", so often applied generically and indiscriminately to vascular lesions that are entirely different in histology and behavior. There is no such entity as "cavernous hemangioma". The lesion is either a deep infantile hemangioma or a venous malformation.

The terms congenital and acquired should be used with caution in describing vascular anomalies. The word "congenital" should be restricted to a vascular lesion that is completely expressed at birth. Hemangioma can be nascent or fully grown in a neonate. Vascular malformations, although present at birth at a cellular level, may not manifest until childhood or in adult life. "Acquired", a term often used for cutaneous lesions that appear after 1 year of life, is inappropriate for a vascular anomaly that is present, but not clinically apparent, at birth.

Vascular tumors

Infantile hemangioma

Pathogenesis

Infantile hemangioma (IH) is a benign endothelial tumor with a biologic behavior that is unique because it grows rapidly, slowly regresses, and never recurs.

2 Months   12 Months   2.5 Years

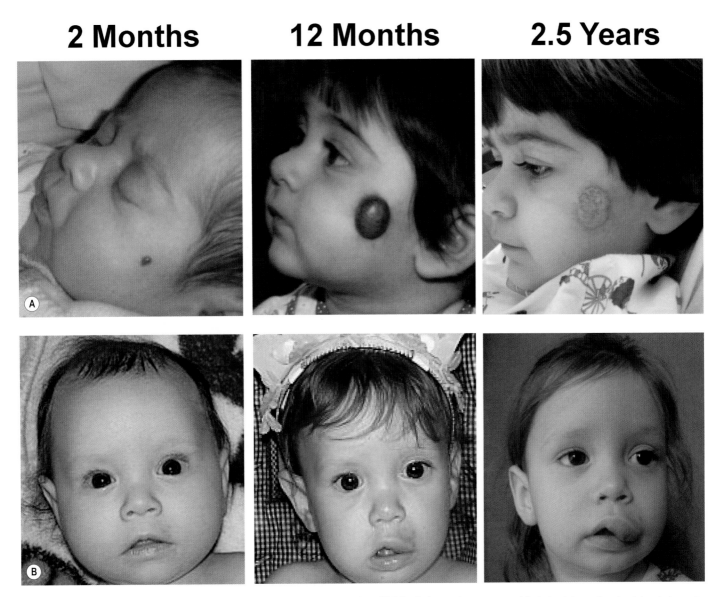

Fig. 29.3 Natural history of infantile hemangioma compared to a vascular malformation. **(A)** Infantile hemangioma grows rapidly during infancy, then involutes during early childhood. **(B)** Venous malformation slowly enlarges over time and does not involute.

There are three stages in its life cycle: the proliferating phase (0–1 year of age), the involuting phase (1–4 years of age), and the involuted phase (after 4 years of age). During the proliferating phase, the histopathologic examination shows clusters of plump endothelial cells with small vascular channels and minimal connective tissue.[11,12] During involution, mature blood vessels are formed. Vascular channels enlarge and are lined by flattened endothelial cells. Increased extracellular matrix, multi-laminated basement membranes, and pericytes are deposited around the vessels. After involution, the majority of the IH is replaced with adipocytes and

connective tissue. All that remains are thin-walled vessels with multi-laminated basement membranes and larger feeding and draining vessels.[13,14]

Recent findings suggest that IH arises from vasculogenesis (formation of blood vessels from progenitor cells) rather than angiogenesis (blood vessel formation from pre-existing vasculature).[15] Because hemangioma endothelial cells (HemECs) are clonal, a somatic mutation in a precursor cell may be responsible for the tumor.[16,17] It is likely that IH begins as an intrinsic (genetic) alteration in a stem cell; its life cycle may be influenced extrinsically, by up or downregulated local angiogenic factors. The precursor cell for IH may be a multipotent hemangioma-derived-stem cell (HemSC), which has been isolated.[18] HemSCs express CD90, a mesenchymal cell marker, and can differentiate into multiple cell lineages. They produce human GLUT1-positive microvessels after clonal expansion in immuno-deficient mice.[18] They differentiate into endothelium and express CD31. HemECs share similarities with placental endothelium,[19,20] and it has been postulated that the precursor cell for IH might have embolized from the placenta. Genetic studies, however, have shown that HemECs are derived from the child and not the mother.[21,22]

Several mechanisms may contribute to the rapid enlargement of IH. Hypoxia may stimulate circulating hemangioma-derived endothelial progenitor cell (HemEPC) recruitment to the growing tumor.[15] Increased circulating endothelial progenitor cells have been found in children with IH.[23-26] HemEC have been shown to have defective NFAT activity that causes decreased VEGFR-1 expression. Because VEGFR-1 acts as a decoy receptor, more VEFG-A becomes available to bind to VEGFR-2, which stimulates endothelial proliferation.[27] Local factors, such as a reduction in anti-angiogenic proteins, also may potentiate tumor growth during the proliferating phase.[28]

The mechanism for IH involution is unknown. As endothelial proliferation slows, apoptosis increases, and the IH is replaced by fibrofatty tissue. Apoptosis begins before 1 year of age and peaks at 24 months causing a reduction in tumor volume.[29] Decreasing circulating maternal estrogens, which are pro-angiogenic, may contribute to involution. Alternatively, increased angiogenesis inhibitors in the epidermis overlying the hemangioma may promote involution.[28] The source of adipocytes during involution are HemSCs, which also may differentiate into pericytes.[15,18]

Clinical features

Infantile hemangioma occurs in approximately 4–5% of Caucasian infants.[30] IH is more frequent in premature children and in females (4 : 1).[31,32] The tumor is typically single (80%) and involves the head and neck (60%), trunk (25%), or extremity (15%).[10] The median age of appearance is 2 weeks; 30–50% are noted at birth as a telangiectatic stain, pale spot, or ecchymotic area.[33] IH

grows faster than the child during the first 9 months of age (*proliferating phase*); 80% of its size is achieved by 3.2 (±1.7) months.[34] IH is red when it involves the superficial dermis. A lesion beneath the skin may not be appreciated until 3–4 months of age when it has grown large enough to cause a visible mass; the overlying skin may appear bluish. By age 9–12 months, growth of IH reaches a plateau. After 12 months, the tumor begins to regress (*involuting phase*); the color fades and the lesion flattens. Involution ceases most of children by age 4 years (*involuted phase*).[35] After involution, one-half of children will have: residual telangiectasias, scarring, fibrofatty residuum, redundant skin, or destroyed anatomical structures. There is no strong evidence for Mendelian inheritance of IH;[36] however, autosomal dominant transmission has been reported with a locus on 5q.[37,38]

Head and neck hemangiomas

The majority of IH are small, harmless lesions that can be monitored under the watchful eye of a pediatrician. However, 10% of proliferating IH cause significant deformity or complications, usually when located on the head or neck. Ulcerated lesions may destroy the eyelid, ear, nose or lip. IH of the scalp or eyebrow can result in alopecia. Periorbital hemangioma can block the visual axis or distort the cornea causing amblyopia. Subglottic hemangioma may obstruct the airway.

Multiple hemangiomas

Approximately 20% of infants have more than one IH.[33] The term *hemangiomatosis* designates five or more small (<5 mm) tumors. These children are more likely to have IH of internal organs, although the risk is low. The liver is most commonly affected; the brain, gut, or lung are rarely involved. Ultrasonography should be considered to rule-out hepatic IH.

Hepatic hemangiomas

The liver is the most common extracutaneous site for IH. Some 90% of fast-flow hepatic lesions are IH.[39] The differential diagnosis includes arteriovenous malformation, hepatoblastoma, and metastatic neuroblastoma, none of which demonstrate significant shunting on imaging.[39] There are three subtypes of hepatic hemangioma: *focal*, *multifocal*, or *diffuse*.[40] Although most hepatic IHs are nonproblematic and discovered incidentally, large tumors can cause heart failure, hepatomegaly, anemia, or hypothyroidism. Focal hepatic hemangioma is usually asymptomatic and not associated with cutaneous lesions. There is evidence that solitary hepatic hemangioma is a variant called "rapidly involuting congenital hemangioma (RICH)".[40] Occasionally, this tumor can cause cardiac overload and thrombocytopenia; however, these symptoms resolve as the tumor regresses. Multifocal hepatic IH are often accompanied by cutaneous lesions. Although usually asymptomatic, intrahepatic multifocal lesions can cause high output cardiac failure which is managed by corticosteroid or embolization.[40] Diffuse hepatic IH can cause massive hepatomegaly, respiratory compromise, or abdominal compartment syndrome. Infants also are at risk for hypothyroidism and irreversible brain injury because the large tumor volume expresses enough deiodinase to inactivate thyroid hormone.[41] Patients require thyroid stimulating hormone monitoring and, if abnormal, intravenous thyroid hormone replacement until the IH begins to regress.

Hemangiomas and structural anomalies

There are uncommon presentations of IH with malformations in the head/neck or lumbosacral regions. PHACE association affects 2.3% of patients with IH, and consists of a plaque-like IH in a regional distribution of the face with at least one of the following anomalies: Posterior fossa brain malformation; Hemangioma; Arterial cerebrovascular anomalies; Coarctation of the aorta and cardiac defects; Eye/Endocrine abnormalities.[42] When ventral developmental defects (Sternal clefting or Supraumbilical raphe) are present, an "S" is added (PHACES).[42] Of infants, 90% are female and cerebrovascular anomalies are the most common associated finding (72%).[43] Because 8% of children with PHACE association have a stroke in infancy, these patients should have an MRI to evaluate the brain and cerebrovasculature.[44] Infants are referred for ophthalmologic, endocrine and cardiac evaluation to rule-out these associated anomalies.

Reticular hemangioma is an uncommon variant of IH that most commonly affects the lumbosacral area and lower extremity; 83% of these infants are female.[45] Unlike typical IH, reticular tumors are likely to ulcerate; they rarely can cause cardiac overload. Reticular hemangiomas are associated with ventral-caudal malformations (omphalocele, recto-vaginal fistula, vaginal/uterine duplication, solitary/duplex kidney, imperforate anus, tethered cord lipomyelomeningocele).[46–50] Ultrasonography (US) is obtained to rule-out associated anomalies in infants less than 4 months of age. MRI is indicated in older infants or when US is equivocal. After involution small veins usually remain; these can be treated by sclerotherapy.

Diagnosis

Most IH are easily diagnosed by history and physical examination. Fast-flow is confirmed using a hand-held Doppler device. By formal ultrasonography, IH appears as a soft-tissue mass with fast-flow, decreased arterial resistance, and increased venous drainage.[51] On MRI, the tumor is isointense on T1, hyperintense on T2, and enhances during the proliferating phase.[52] Involuting IH exhibits increased lobularity and adipose tissue; the number of vessels and flow is reduced. Rarely, biopsy is indicated if malignancy is suspected or if the diagnosis remains unclear following imaging studies. Tumors or fast-flow lesions that may be confused with IH include: arteriovenous malformation, congenital hemangiomas, cutaneous leukemia (chloroma), hemangioendotheliomas, infantile fibrosarcoma, infantile myofibromatosis, lymphoma, metastatic neuroblastoma, PTEN-associated vascular anomaly, and pyogenic granuloma. If biopsy is needed, positive erythrocyte-type glucose transporter (GLUT 1) immunostaining differentiates IH from other vascular tumors and malformations.[9]

Nonoperative management
Observation

Most IH are simply observed because 90% are small, localized, and do not involve anatomically important areas. Infants are followed closely, on a monthly basis, during the proliferative phase if a lesion has the potential to cause obstruction, destruction, or ulceration requiring intervention. Once the IH has stabilized in growth, patients are followed annually during the involuting phase if it is possible surgical intervention may be necessary in childhood for excess skin, residual fibrofatty tissue, or reconstruction of damaged structures.

Wound care

During the proliferative phase, at least 16% of lesions ulcerate, the median age is 4 months.[53] Superficial IH is prone to ulceration because the skin is damaged by the tumor. In addition, arteriovenous shunting reduces oxygen delivery to the skin, causing ischemia. Consequently, desiccation or minor injury can cause skin breakdown. Tumors located in trauma-prone areas are at greater risk for ulceration; the lips, neck, and anogenital region are the most common locations. To protect against ulceration, IH in these areas should be kept moist with hydrated petroleum during the proliferative phase to minimize desiccation and shearing of the skin. IH in the anogenital area may be further protected by using a petroleum gauze barrier to prevent friction from the diaper.

If ulceration develops, the wound is washed gently with soap and water at least twice daily. Small, superficial areas are managed by the application of topical antibiotic ointment and occasionally with a petroleum gauze barrier. Large, deep ulcers require damp-to-dry dressing changes. To minimize discomfort, a small amount of topical lidocaine may be applied no more than 4 times daily to avoid toxicity. EMLA (eutectic mixture of local anesthetics) contains prilocaine and should not be used in infants less than three months of age because of the risk of methemoglobinemia.

Bleeding from an ulcerated IH is usually minor, and is treated by applying direct pressure. All ulcerations will heal with local wound care; usually healing takes at least two weeks. Intralesional or oral corticosteroid may accelerate regression and thus promote healing.

Topical corticosteroid

Topical corticosteroid is relatively ineffective; especially if IH involves the deep dermis and subcutis.[54–56] Ultrapotent agents may be effective for a very superficial IH. Although lightening may occur, if there is deep component it will not be affected. Adverse effects include hypopigmentation, cutaneous atrophy, and even adrenal suppression.[57]

Intralesional corticosteroid

Small, well-localized IHs that obstruct the visual axis or nasal airway, or those at risk for damaging important structures (i.e., eyelid, lip, nose) are best managed by intralesional corticosteroid *(Fig. 29.4)*. Triamcinolone (3 mg/kg) stabilizes the growth of the lesion in at least 95% of patients; 75% of tumors will decrease in size.[58] The corticosteroid injection lasts 4–6 weeks, and thus infants may require 2–3 injections during the proliferative phase. Intralesional corticosteroid may cause subcutaneous fat atrophy. Blindness has been reported following injection of deep periorbital hemangioma due to embolic occlusion of the retinal artery.[59,60]

Systemic pharmacotherapy

Problematic IH that is larger than 3–4 cm in diameter is managed by oral prednisolone or propranolol. Interferon is no longer recommended in children less than 12 months of age because it can cause neurologic sequela, particularly spastic diplegia.[61] Vincristine may be considered as a second-line option in the unlikely event that a child has failed or has a contraindication to prednisolone and propranolol.[62,63]

Oral corticosteroid has been used to treat IH for over 40 years and has proven to be very safe and effective *(Fig. 29.4)*.[64-70] Patients are given prednisolone 3 mg/kg/day for one month; the drug is then tapered by 0.5 cc every 2-4 weeks until it is discontinued between 10-12 months of age when the tumor is no longer proliferating. The drug is given once a day in the morning, and infants have monthly outpatient follow-up. Using this protocol, all tumors will stabilize in growth and 88% will become smaller (accelerated regression).[70] Treatment response usually is evident within 1 week of therapy by signs of involution: decreased growth rate, fading color, and softening of the lesion. Patients do not require prophylaxis against gastric irritation or prophylactic antibiotics. There are no adverse effects on neurodevelopment.[68] Twenty per cent of infants will develop a cushingoid appearance that resolves during tapering of therapy.[70] Approximately 12% of infants treated after 3 months of age exhibit decreased gain in height, but return to their pretreatment growth curve by 24 months of age.[65]

Propranolol has recently proved to be another effective treatment for problematic infantile hemangioma, but its efficacy and safety, compared to corticosteroid has not been studied.[71,72] Partial and non response to propranolol has been reported, and potentially serious

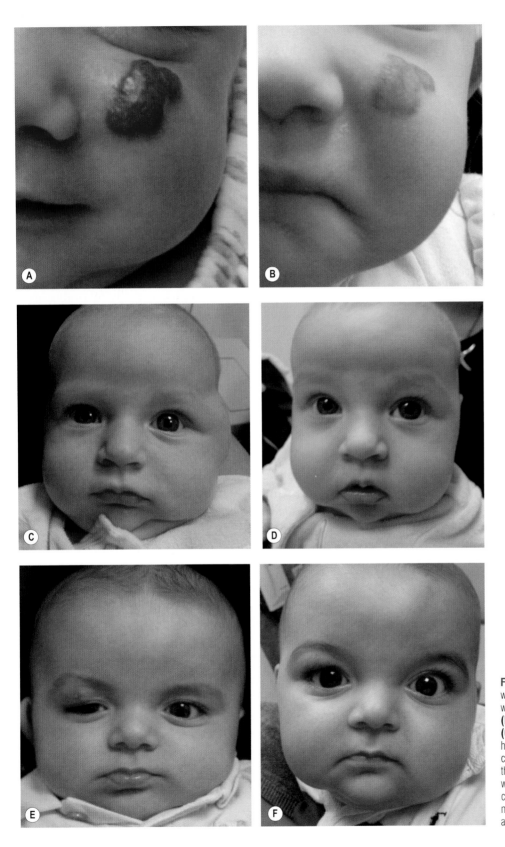

Fig. 29.4 Management of infantile hemangioma with pharmacotherapy. **(A)** Cheek lesion injected with triamcinolone at three months of age. **(B)** Accelerated regression at 12 months of age. **(C)** A 3-month-old female with deep infantile hemangioma of left face prior to initiation of oral corticosteroid. **(D)** After 1 month of drug treatment, the tumor has regressed. **(E)** 4 month-old female with diffuse infantile hemangioma of upper eyelid causing astigmatism and obstruction. **(F)** After 2 months of drug treatment, the lesion has regressed and astigmatism has diminished.

side effects have occurred: bronchospasm, bradycardia, hypotension, hypoglycemia, seizures, and hyperkalemia.[72-78] Propranolol may conceal symptoms of congestive heart failure caused by a large infantile hemangioma, and may further worsen cardiac function.[73] Children with asthma/reactive airway disease, blood glucose abnormalities, congenital heart disease, and cerebrovascular malformations (PHACES association) may not be candidates for propranolol.[73] Infants receiving propranolol are monitored closely for potential drug toxicity. Patients undergo cardiology consultation, electrocardiogram, echocardiogram, glucose/electrolyte measurements, and frequent blood pressure, heart rate, and respiratory examinations. Children with airway disease, prematurity, or less than 3 months of age undergo inpatient initiation of propranolol.[73,77]

Based on our present risk-benefit analysis, we prefer corticosteroid for problematic infantile hemangioma because: (1) the tumor will consistently respond to 3 mg/kg/day of prednisolone; (2) we believe prednisolone is safer than propranolol; and (3) the infant receiving prednisolone does not require complicated/expensive monitoring for an acute, life-threatening adverse drug event (unlike the child receiving propranolol).

Embolic therapy

Large IH, usually multifocal hepatic lesions, can cause high-output congestive heart failure. Embolization may be indicated for the initial control of cardiac overload while systemic corticosteroid therapy takes effect. Cardiac failure often recurs even after initial improvement, and drug therapy should be continued after embolization until the child is approximately 10–12 months of age when natural involution begins.

Laser therapy

There is little, if any, role for pulsed-dye laser treatment for proliferating IH. The laser penetrates only 0.75–1.2 mm into the dermis, and thus only affects the superficial portion of the tumor. Although lightening may occur, the mass is not affected.[79,80] These patients have an increased risk of skin atrophy and hypopigmentation.[80] The thermal injury delivered by the laser to the ischemic dermis increases the risk of ulceration, pain, bleeding, and scarring.[81] Nevertheless, pulsed-dye laser is indicated during the involuted phase to fade residual telangiectasias.

Operative management

Proliferative phase (infancy)

Resection of IH generally is not recommended during the early growth phase. The tumor is highly vascular during this period and there is a risk for blood loss, iatrogenic injury, and an inferior outcome, compared to excising residual tissue after the tumor has regressed.[70,82-84] Nevertheless, in experienced surgical hands, there are indications for operative intervention during this phase: (1) failure or contraindication to pharmacotherapy; (2) well-localized tumor in an anatomically favorable area; (3) if resection will be necessary in the future and the scar would be the same *(Fig. 29.5)*.[33] Circular lesions located in visible areas, particularly the face, are best removed by circular excision and purse-string closure.[85] This technique minimizes the length of the scar as well as distortion of surrounding structures. Lenticular excision of a circular hemangioma results in a scar as long as three times the diameter of the lesion. In comparison, a two-stage circular resection followed by lenticular excision/linear closure 6–12 months later will leave a scar approximately the same length as the diameter of the original lesion.[85] Lenticular excision and linear closure is preferred in certain facial locations, such as the lips and eyelids.

Involuting phase (early childhood)

Resection during involution is much safer because the lesion is less-vascular and smaller. Because the extent of the excision is reduced, the scar is less noticeable. Approximately 50% of IH leave behind fibrofatty tissue or damaged skin after the tumor regresses causing a deformity *(Fig. 29.6)*.[33] Sometimes a child requires reconstruction of damaged structures (i.e., nose, ear, lip). Staged or total excision should be considered during this period, rather than waiting for complete involution if: (1) it is clear that the lesion will require resection (e.g., post-ulceration scarring, destroyed structures, expanded skin, significant fibrofatty residuum); (2) the length of the scar would be similar if the procedure was postponed to the involuted phase; (3) the scar is in a favorable location. Another advantage of

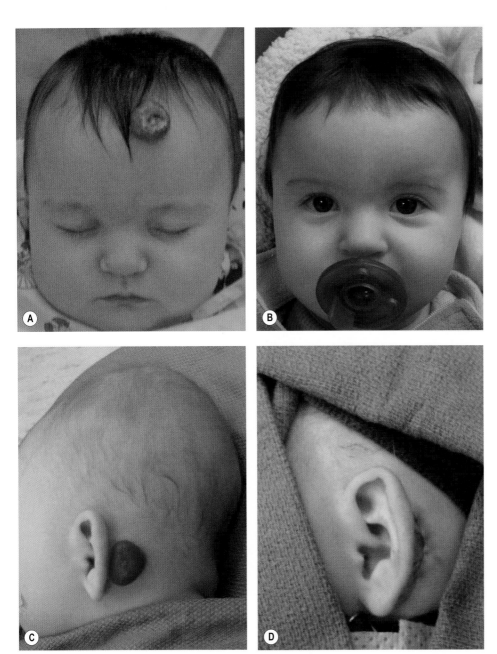

Fig. 29.5 Operative management of proliferating infantile hemangioma **(A)** A 7-month-old female with a well-localized, ulcerated lesion in an anatomically favorable area. The tumor was removed by transverse lenticular excision and linear closure because of its location near the hairline. **(B)** Six weeks postoperatively. **(C)** A 4-month-old female with a rapidly growing, ulcerated retroauricular tumor at risk for causing a prominent ear deformity. **(D)** Following resection and linear closure in retroauricular sulcus.

operative intervention during this period, compared to late childhood, is that reconstruction is underway prior to the child's development of memory or awareness of a facial difference.

Involuted phase (late childhood)

Waiting until IH has fully involuted prior to removal ensures that the least amount of fibrofatty residuum and excess skin is resected, resulting in the smallest possible scar. Postponing intervention until complete involution has occurred must be weighed against the possible psychosocial implications of maintaining a deformity until late childhood. Allowing for full involution is recommended for lesions when it is unclear if a surgical scar would leave a worse deformity than the appearance of the residual hemangioma.

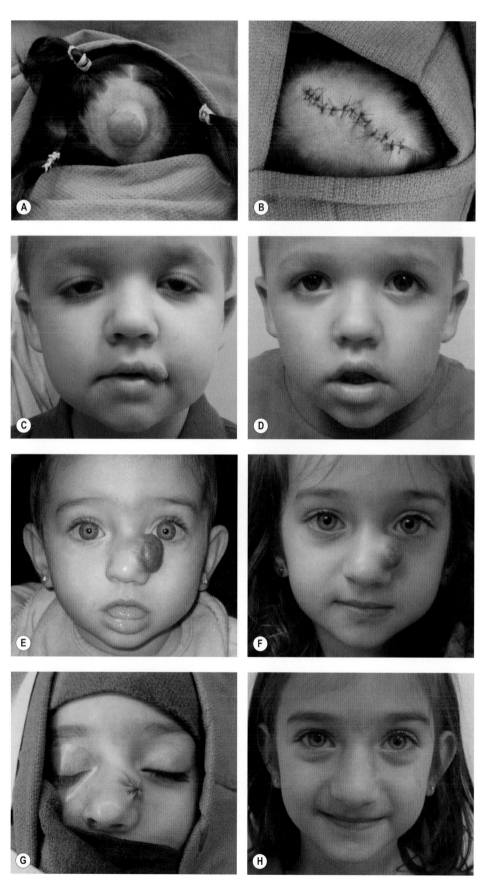

Fig. 29.6 Operative management of involuting phase infantile hemangioma. **(A)** A 2-year-old female with residual fibrofatty residuum and alopecia. A one-stage lenticular excision was chosen because the scalp is an unfavorable location for circular closure, and the linear scar is concealed by hair. **(B)** Note that the length of the scar is approximately three times the diameter of the tumor. **(C)** A 3-year-old male with residual fibrofatty tissue of the upper lip. **(D)** The lesion was removed using a lenticular excision with placement of the scar along the vermilion-cutaneous junction. **(E)** An 8-month-old female with a large nasal hemangioma. **(F)** The same patient at 3 years old. The tumor has involuted facilitating the operative procedure. **(G)** Following circular excision and purse-string closure to limit the length the scar. **(H)** Three months following second-stage circular excision and purse-string closure.

Congenital hemangiomas

Clinical features

There are rare hemangiomas that arise in the fetus, are fully-grown at birth, and do not have postnatal growth.[86–88] These congenital hemangiomas are red-violaceous with coarse telangiectasias, central pallor, and a peripheral pale halo. These lesions are more common in the extremities, have an equal sex distribution, and are solitary with an average diameter of 5 cm.[86–88] There are two forms: *rapidly involuting congenital hemangioma* (RICH) and *noninvoluting congenital hemangioma* (NICH). RICH involutes rapidly after birth and 50% of lesions have completed regression by 7 months of age; the remaining tumors are fully involuted by 14 months.[86,88] RICH affects the head or neck (42%), limbs (52%) or trunk (6%). RICH does not leave behind a significant adipose component, unlike common IH. NICH, in contrast, does not regress; it remains unchanged with persistent fast-flow.[87] It involves the head or neck (43%), limbs (38%), or trunk (19%).[87]

Management

RICH usually does not require resection in infancy because it regresses so quickly. Occasionally, RICH is complicated by congestive heart failure, and this is controlled by corticosteroid or embolization as the lesion involutes. After regression, RICH may leave behind atrophic skin and subcutaneous tissue. Reconstruction with autologous grafts (fat, dermis) or acellular dermis may be indicated. NICH is rarely problematic in infancy; it is observed until the diagnosis is clear. Resection of NICH may be indicated to improve the appearance of the affected area, as long as the surgical scar will be less noticeable than the lesion.

Kaposiform hemangioendothelioma

Clinical features

Kaposiform hemangioendothelioma (KHE) is a rare vascular neoplasm that is locally aggressive, but does not metastasize.[89–92] Although one-half of lesions are present at birth, KHE may develop during infancy (58%), between age 1–10 years (32%), or after 11 years of age (10%);[93] adult-onset is rare.[94] KHE has an equal sex distribution, is solitary, and affects the head/neck (40%), trunk (30%), or an extremity (30%).[93,95] The tumor is often >5 cm in diameter and appears as a flat, reddish-purple, edematous lesion.[91,96] KHE causes a visible deformity as well as pain. Over half the patients have Kasabach–Merritt phenomenon (KMP) (thrombocytopenia <25 000/mm^3, petechiae, bleeding).[90–92,96] KHE does not exhibit rapid postnatal growth; however, the tumor can expand with the onset of KMP. KHE partially regresses after two years of age, although it usually persists long-term causing chronic pain and stiffness.[97] KHE has overlapping clinical and histopathological features with another tumor, tufted angioma, suggesting they are on the same neoplastic spectrum. KMP also may complicate *tufted angioma*, which has a similar anatomic distribution as KHE, but is more erythematous and plaque-like.[98]

KHE is diagnosed by history, physical examination, and imaging. MRI is indicated for diagnostic confirmation and to asses the extent of the tumor. MRI shows poorly-defined margins, small vessels, and invasion of adjacent tissues. There is T2-hyperintensity, postgadolinium enhancement, and signal-voids also may be present. Histologically, KHE has infiltrating sheets or nodules of endothelial cells lining capillaries.[90,99] Hemosiderin-filled slitlike vascular spaces with red blood cell fragments, as well as dilated lymphatics, are present. Tufted angioma is distinguished from KHE by small tufts of capillaries ("cannonballs") in the middle to lower third of the dermis.[98]

Management

Most lesions are extensive, involving multiple tissues, and well beyond the limits of resection. Patients with KMP require systemic treatment to prevent life-threatening complications. Large, asymptomatic tumors without KMP are also managed with pharmacotherapy to minimize fibrosis and subsequent long-term pain and stiffness. Vincristine is first-line therapy, the response rate is 90%.[62] KHE does not respond as well to second-line drugs, interferon (50%) or corticosteroid (10%).[62,96] Thrombocytopenia is not significantly improved with platelet transfusion because the platelets are trapped in the tumor. Platelet transfusion also worsens swelling and should be avoided unless there is active bleeding or a surgical procedure is planned. By 2 years of age, the tumor usually has undergone partial involution and the platelet count normalizes. There is evidence that KHE never totally regresses.

Pyogenic granuloma

Pyogenic granuloma (PG) is neither "pyogenic" nor "granulomatous". Some pathologists call it *lobular capillary hemangioma*.[100] PG is a solitary, red papule that grows rapidly on a stalk. It is small, with an average diameter of 6.5 mm; the mean age of onset is 6.7 years.[101] The male to female ratio is 2:1. PG is commonly complicated by bleeding (64%) and ulceration (36%).[101] PG primarily involves the skin (88%), but can also involve mucous membranes (11%). It is distributed on the head or neck (62%), trunk (19%), upper extremity (13%), or lower extremity (5%).[101] In the head and neck region, affected sites include: cheek (29%), oral cavity (14%), scalp (11%), forehead (10%), eyelid (9%), or lips (9%).[101]

Once established, PG rarely spontaneously heals. PGs require intervention to control likely ulceration and bleeding. Numerous methods have been described: curettage, shave excision, laser therapy, and excision.[101,102] Because the lesion extends into the reticular dermis, it may be out of the reach of the pulse-dye laser, cautery or shave excision. Consequently, these modalities have a recurrence rate of 43.5%.[101] Full-thickness excision is more definitive treatment.

Vascular malformations

Capillary malformation

Pathogenesis

Capillary malformation (CM) is the modern term for the antiquated "port-wine" stain. Its pathogenesis is not understood. The 19th century "neurovegetative theory" asserted that the primary embryonic defect occurs in the developing autonomic nervous system.[1] There are several clinical findings that support this hypothesis. The geographic patterns of CMs are often regional or dermatomal (particularly with branches of the trigeminal nerve), suggesting a relationship to the developing peripheral nervous system. The occasional finding of

hyperhidrosis in an area of CM supports such an association. Neuroectoderm is known to contribute to the pericytic and smooth muscle layers of vascular walls.[103,104] The neurogenic hypothesis also is supported by the finding of decreased perivascular neural density in CMs and abnormal patterns of innervation of leptomeningeal vessels in Sturge–Weber syndrome.[105,106] The cutaneous flush of a CM may, in part, be due to an inability of these vessels to constrict secondary to diminished sympathetic innervation.

Clinical features

CMs occur anywhere on the body; they can be localized or extensive. Rarely, they are multiple and generalized, such as in Sturge–Weber syndrome. CM should not be confused with a *nevus flammeus neonatorum*, the most common vascular birthmark, seen in 50% of white neonates. These macular stains are popularly referred to as "angel kiss" on the forehead, eyelids, nose, and upper lip or "stork bite" in the nuchal area. These predictably fade by 2 years of age, representing a minor transient dilatation of dermal vessels. If they persist, such a birthmark must be relabeled CM.

CMs have an equal gender distribution; the birth prevalence is 0.3%.[107] The cutaneous discoloration is usually, but not always, evident at birth because the stain may be hidden by the erythema of neonatal skin. CM often causes psychological concerns as the pink color of childhood darkens and the skin thickens, sometimes with raised fibrovascular cobblestoning. Facial CMs often occur in a dermatomal distribution; 45% are restricted to one of the three trigeminal dermatomes.[108] Conversely, 55% of facial CMs are noted to overlap sensory dermatomes, crossing the midline or occurring bilaterally. The mucous membranes often are contiguously involved. Pyogenic granuloma may develop in CM, causing ulceration and bleeding. CM also can lead to soft-tissue and skeletal overgrowth below the stain. When located on the face, hypertrophy of the lip, cheek, or forehead can occur; the lip is most commonly affected.[109] Enlargement of the maxilla or mandible can result in an occlusal cant (vertical maxillary overgrowth) with increased dental show and malocclusion.

An extensive CM in an extremity is often associated with increased circumference and limb length discrepancy. CMs in truncal or extremity distributions rarely demonstrate the evolution of textural and color changes seen in facial CMs. CMs often accompany developmental defects of the central neural axis. An occipital CM, often with an associated hair tuft, can overlie an encephalocele or ectopic meninges. A capillary stain on the posterior thorax can signify an underlying arteriovenous malformation of the spinal cord (Cobb syndrome).[110–112] A CM over the cervical or lumbosacral spine is a red flag for occult spinal dysraphism, lipomeningocele, tethered spinal cord, and diastematomyelia.[33]

Management

In patients with an upper facial CM, as well as V_1–V_2 distribution, the possibility of Sturge–Weber syndrome should be considered. Pulse-dye laser therapy can improve the appearance of CM by lightening the color; the head and neck region responds better than the extremities.[113–115] Outcome also is superior for smaller lesions and those treated at a younger age.[116,117] Of the patients, 15% achieve at least 90% lightening, 65% improve 50–90%, and 20% respond poorly.[118] Improvement is less in Asian patients with facial CMs; only 13.6% of Asian patients show 50% or more lightening.[119] A higher rate of complications, including pigmentary changes and hypertrophic scarring, is reported in individuals with darker skin.[119,120] After pulse-dye laser treatment, CM often re-darkens over time.[121]

Facial CM is best treated with pulse-dye laser early in childhood, before memory or self-awareness begins. Intervention in infancy may achieve superior lightening of the lesion, as well as reduce the risk of subsequent darkening and hypertrophy, compared with photocoagulation in later childhood.[117] Infants can be treated with pulse-dye laser while awake (using topical anesthesia), depending on the size and location of the CM. After infancy, it is more difficult to restrain an awake child and general anesthesia is preferred, unless the lesion is small. Adolescents generally tolerate laser treatment while awake, depending on the location and extent of the CM. Multiple treatments, spaced 6 weeks apart, are often required until the CM fails to improve with additional treatments. Some families may elect to wait to treat CM of the trunk or extremities until the child is old enough to make the decision. Similarly, patients may wish to undergo laser therapy only if their lesion darkens and becomes more visible over time.

Because overgrowth often is not present at birth and is progressive, most patients do not require contouring, usually labial, until adolescence or adulthood (*Fig. 29.7*). Cutaneous fibrovascular hypertrophy occurs over many years, requiring intervention in adulthood. Malocclusion can be corrected in adolescence with orthodontic manipulation. If orthodontics is insufficient, an orthognathic procedure is considered when the jaws are completely grown, usually at age 16 years in females and age 18 years in males. Le Fort I osteotomy

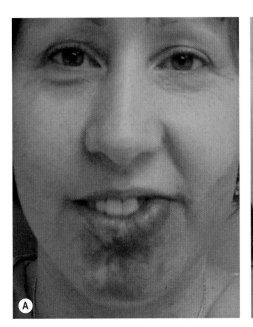
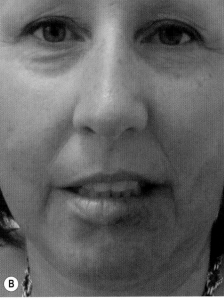

Fig. 29.7 Management of capillary malformation. **(A)** A 48-year-old female with a capillary malformation of the lower face causing labial overgrowth. **(B)** The appearance after pulsed-dye laser treatment of the chin and contouring of the hypertrophied lower lip using a transverse mucosal excision.

or bimaxillary procedure may be necessary. Facial asymmetry caused by overgrowth of the zygoma, maxilla, or mandible can be improved by contour burring.

Trunk or extremity soft tissue overgrowth can be associated with increased subcutaneous adipose tissue. Suction-assisted lipectomy can improve contour while avoiding a large incision. Small fibrovascular nodules or pyogenic granulomas are easily excised. Severe cutaneous thickening and cobblestoning can be resected and reconstructed by linear closure, skin grafts, or local flaps.

Cutis marmorata telangiectasia congenita

Cutis marmorata telangiectasia congenita (CMTC) manifests as congenital cutaneous marbling, even at normal temperatures, that becomes more pronounced with lower temperatures or with crying.[122] The involved skin is depressed in a serpiginous reticulated pattern and has a deep purple color. Differential diagnosis includes cutis marmorata (or livedo reticularis) and reticular hemangioma. Cutis marmorata is merely an accentuated pattern of normal cutaneous vascularity. It is seen as a transient mottling pattern when the child is placed in a low-temperature environment but disappears on warming.

CMTC occurs sporadically in an equal gender distribution.[122,123] CMTC can cause ulceration and may be localized, segmental, or generalized. It most frequently involves the trunk and extremities; it is typically unilateral (65%) and involves a lower extremity (69%).[122] The affected extremity is often hypoplastic.[124,125] Almost all infants show improvement during the first year of life which continues into adolescence.[1,126] Atrophy, pigmentation, and ectasia of the superficial veins often persist into adulthood. CMTC may be associated with hypoplasia of the iliac and femoral veins.[127]

Macrocephaly-capillary malformation (M-CM) is a clinically discrete condition.[128,129] The vascular lesions are patchy, reticular CM (not CMTC or cutis marmorata). The stains commonly occur on the nose and philtrum, and may be present on the trunk or extremities. Unlike CMTC, the vascular malformation in M-CM does not ulcerate or fade. In addition, the lower limb is often hypertrophied.[129] These children have a high risk for neurologic abnormalities, including developmental delay, mental retardation, megalencephaly, and hydrocephalus.[128]

Lymphatic malformation (LM)

Pathogenesis

The lymphatic system develops during the 6th week of embryonic life.[1] Paired jugular lymph sacs appear, followed by mesenteric, cisterna chyli, and posterior lymph sacs. These enlarge and become connected to the thoracic duct. A second stage of maturation involves the transformation of the sacs into primary lymph nodes and the centrifugal spread of peripheral lymphatics.[130] Investigations support the venous origin of lymphatics,[130–132] rather than derivation from mesenchymal structures. One etiologic theory for LMs is that either anlagen of the sacs or their sprouting lymphatic channels become "pinched off" from the main lymphatic system, leading to aberrant collections of lymphatic fluid-filled spaces. Another theory attributes LMs to abnormal budding of the lymphatic system with a loss of connection to the central lymph channels or to development of lymphatic tissue in aberrant locations.[1]

Understanding the molecular basis for LMs is in its infancy. The VEGF receptor 3 (VEGFR3, also called Flt4) is restricted to the lymphatic endothelium during development.[131] VEGF3 knockout mice die at embryonic day 9 with major venous anomalies, just before lymphatics sprout.[133] No genetic basis has been determined for LMs. Lymphedema, a generalized type of lymphatic anomaly in the limbs, can be hereditary, and mutations in *VEGFR3, FOXC2, SOX18, CCBE1* are responsible for some primary forms *(Table 29.3)*.[134]

Clinical features

LM is characterized by the size of the malformed channels: microcystic, macrocystic, or combined. Macrocystic lesions are defined as cysts large enough to be punctured by a needle and treated by sclerotherapy. Because the lymphatic and venous systems share a common embryological origin, lymphatic-venous malformation (LVM) also can occur. LM is usually noted at birth or within the first 2 years of life. On occasion, LM first becomes evident in later childhood, adolescence, or even adulthood. Prenatal ultrasonography can detect

Table 29.3 Vascular anomalies with known genetic mutations

Condition	Mutated gene	Inheritance
Venous malformations		
Sporadic venous malformation (VM)	TIE2 (40–50%)	
Glomuvenous malformation (GVM)	Glomulin	Dominant
Cutaneomucosal venous malformation (VMCM)	TIE2	Dominant
Cerebral cavernous malformation (CCM)	KRIT1	Dominant
Lymphatic malformations		
Familial congenital primary lymphedema	VEGFR3	Dominant
Lymphedema-distichiasis	FOXC2	Dominant
Lymphedema-hypotrichosis-telangiectasia	SOX18	Recessive
Hennekam syndrome	CCBE1	Recessive
Arteriovenous malformations		
Capillary malformation-arteriovenous malformation	RASA1	Dominant
Hereditary hemorrhagic telangiectasia type 1 (HHT1)	ENG	Dominant
Hereditary hemorrhagic telangiectasia type 2 (HHT2)	ACVRLK1	Dominant
PTEN-associated vascular anomaly	PTEN	Dominant

relatively large lesions as early as the 2nd trimester. LMs are frequently misdiagnosed prenatally as other pathologic entities, such as teratoma.[135] True LMs seen antenatally must be differentiated from "posterior nuchal translucency" or "cystic hygroma", obstetric terms reserved for nuchal fluid accumulations in the 1st trimester. Fetuses with posterior nuchal translucency and fetal hydrops have a poor prognosis. Most are aneuploid; they frequently die in utero and may have Turner or Noonan syndrome.[136,137]

LM is most commonly located on the head and neck; other common sites are the axilla, chest, and perineum. Lesions are soft and compressible. The overlying skin may be normal, have a bluish hue, or be studded with pink-red vesicles. LM typically causes deformity and psychosocial issues, especially when it involves the head and neck. The two most common complications associated with LM are bleeding and infection. Intralesional bleeding occurs in up to 35% of lesions causing ecchymotic discoloration, pain, or swelling.[138] Infection complicates as many as 70% of lesions and can progress rapidly to sepsis.[138] Cutaneous vesicles can bleed and cause malodorous drainage. Oral lesions may lead to macroglossia, poor oral hygiene, and caries. Swelling due to bleeding, localized infection, or systemic illness may obstruct vital structures. Two-thirds of infants with cervicofacial LM require tracheostomy.[138,139] Bony overgrowth is another complication; the mandible is most commonly involved resulting in

an open bite and prognathism. Thoracic or abdominal LM may lead to pleural, pericardial, or peritoneal chylous effusions. Periorbital LM causes a permanent reduction in vision (40%), and 7% of patients become blind in the affected eye.[140] Generalized LM presents with multifocal or osteolytic bony lesions, splenic involvement, as well as pleural and/or pericardial effusions. So-called "lymphangiectasia" of the bowel with protein-losing enteropathy also may be present. Other terms for the generalized skeletal presentation include Gorham–Stout syndrome, disappearing bone disease, and phantom bone disease.[141]

A total of 90% of LM are diagnosed by history and physical examination.[10] Small, superficial lesions do not require further evaluation. Large or deep LMs are assessed by MRI to: (1) confirm the diagnosis; (2) define the extent of the malformation; (3) plan treatment. LM appears as either a macrocystic, microcystic or combined lesion with septations of variable thickness. It is hyperintense on T2-weighted sequences and does not show diffuse enhancement.[142] Although US is not as accurate as MRI, it may provide diagnostic confirmation or document intralesional bleeding. US findings for macrocystic LM include anechoic cysts with internal septations, often with debris or fluid-fluid levels.[51] Microcystic LM appears as ill-defined echogenic masses with diffuse involvement of adjacent tissues.[142] Histological confirmation of LM is rarely necessary. LM shows abnormally walled vascular spaces with eosinophilic, protein-rich fluid, and collections of lymphocytes. Immunostaining with the lymphatic markers D2–40 and LYVE-1 are positive.[143]

Management

LM is a benign lesion; intervention is not mandatory. Small or asymptomatic lesions may be observed. An infected LM often cannot be controlled with oral antibiotics and intravenous antimicrobial therapy may be required. Intervention for LM is reserved for symptomatic lesions that cause pain, significant deformity, or threaten vital structures.

Sclerotherapy

Sclerotherapy is first-line management for large or problematic macrocystic/combined LM *(Fig. 29.8)*. Cysts are

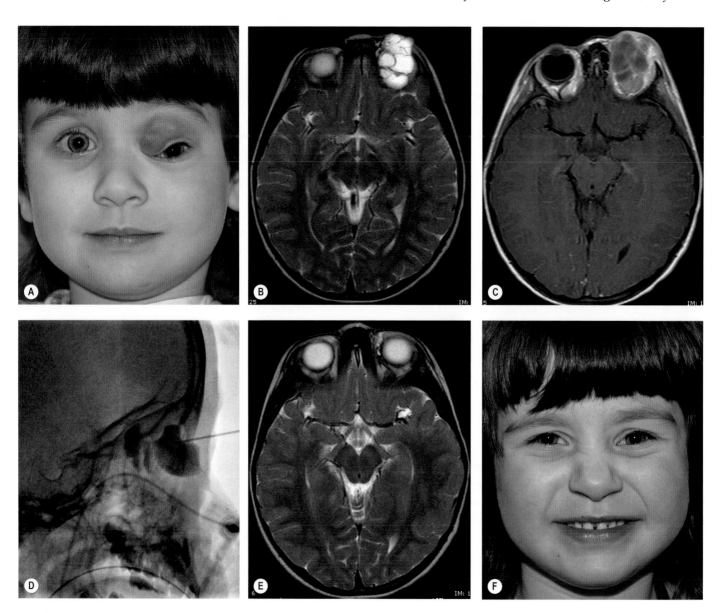

Fig. 29.8 Management of macrocystic lymphatic malformation. **(A)** A 3-year-old female with lymphatic malformation of the left orbit causing exotropia and ptosis. **(B)** Axial T2 MR shows a large hyperintense lesion with multiple, thin internal septations in the superolateral compartment of the orbit. **(C)** Postcontrast T1 MR depicts septal enhancement. There are two different signal intensities due to fluid-fluid levels from intralesional bleeding. **(D)** Fluoroscopic image following needle aspiration and the injection of opacified doxycycline. **(E)** Post treatment MR demonstrates almost complete resolution of the lymphatic malformation. **(F)** The patient is asymptomatic four months following sclerotherapy. (Reprinted from Greene AK, Perlyn CA, Alomari AI, Management of Lymphatic Malformations, *Clinics in Plastic Surgery*, 2011:38(1):77, with permission from Elsevier.)

aspirated followed by the injection of an inflammatory substance which causes scarring of the cyst walls to each other. Sclerotherapy is preferred and has a lower complication rate than attempted resection.[144] Several sclerosants are used to shrink LM: doxycycline, sodium tetradecyl sulfate (STS), ethanol, bleomycin, and OK-432. We prefer doxycycline because it is effective (83% reduction in size) and safe (<5% risk of skin ulceration).[142,145,146] STS is our second-line agent. Ethanol is an effective sclerosant but has the highest complication rate. It can be used for small lesions, but large volumes should be avoided to reduce the risk of local and systemic toxicity. Ethanol can injure nerves, and thus should not be used in proximity to important structures. The use of OK-432 is limited because it is not widely available.

The most common complication of sclerotherapy for LM is cutaneous ulceration (<5%).[142] Ethanol is associated with additional systemic toxicity: CNS depression, pulmonary hypertension, hemolysis, thromboembolism, and arrhythmias.[142] Extravasation of the sclerosant into muscle can cause atrophy and contracture. LM often re-expands over time; 9% recur within 3 years following OK-432 treatment and most will re-expand with longer follow-up.[144,147] Consequently, patients often need repeated sclerotherapy over the course of their lifetime. If a problematic LM recurs and macrocysts are no longer present, resection is the next alternative.

Resection

Attempts at extirpation of LM can cause significant morbidity: major blood loss, iatrogenic injury, and deformity.[138,139,148] For example, resection of cervicofacial LM can injure the facial nerve (76%) or hypoglossal nerve (24%).[138] Excision is usually subtotal because LM involves multiple tissue planes and important structures; recurrence is common (35–64%).[147,149] Resection is reserved for: (1) symptomatic microcystic LM causing bleeding, infection, distortion of vital structures, or significant deformity; (2) symptomatic macrocystic/combined LM that no longer can be managed with sclerotherapy because all macrocysts have been treated; (3) small, well-localized LM (microcystic or macrocystic) that may be completely excised *(Fig. 29.9)*. When considering resection, the postoperative scar/deformity following removal of the LM should be weighed against the preoperative appearance of the lesion.

For diffuse malformations, staged resection of defined anatomic areas is recommended. Subtotal excision of problematic areas, such as bleeding vesicles or a hypertrophied lip, should be carried out rather than an attempting "complete" resection that might result in a worse deformity than the malformation itself. Macroglossia may require reduction to return the tongue to the oral cavity or to correct an open-bite deformity. Bony overgrowth is improved by osseous contouring and malocclusion may require orthognathic correction, usually after skeletal maturity.

Bleeding or leaking cutaneous vesicles can be controlled by resection if they are localized and the wound can be closed by direct approximation of tissues. Vesicles often recur through the scar. Large areas of vesicular bleeding or drainage are best managed by sclerotherapy or carbon dioxide laser; alternatively, wide resection and skin graft coverage is required. Microcystic vesicles involving the oral cavity respond well to radiofrequency ablation.[150] Patients and families are counseled that LM can expand following any intervention, and thus additional treatments are often required in the future.

Venous malformation

Pathogenesis

Venous malformation (VM) results from an error in vascular morphogenesis. Lesions are composed of thin-walled, dilated, sponge-like channels of variable size and mural thickness.[1] There is a normal-appearing endothelial lining; it is the smooth muscle architecture that is abnormal. Smooth muscle alpha-actin staining demonstrates decreased smooth muscle cells that are arranged in clumps rather than concentrically.[1] This mural abnormality probably accounts for the tendency of these malformations to gradually expand over time. In addition, intralesional clotting often occurs, ranging from simple fibrin deposition to the later-appearing pathognomonic calcified "phleboliths". Varying degrees of fibrovascular ingrowth may be noted in these mural thrombi.

Molecular causes for VMs are known. For example, 50% of patients with a sporadic VM will have a somatic mutation in the endothelial receptor *TIE2*.[151] Approximately 10% of patients with VM have multifocal, familial lesions. *Glomuvenous malformation* (GVM) is

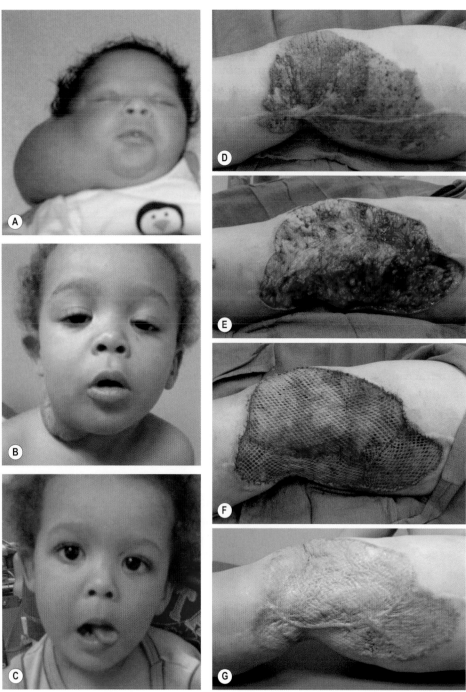

Fig. 29.9 Operative management of lymphatic malformation. **(A)** Newborn male with a large macrocystic lymphatic malformation of the right face and neck. **(B)** Age 2 years. Following sclerotherapy the child has residual skin excess with microcystic lymphatic malformation. **(C)** Six weeks following neck-lift to remove redundant skin and malformation using a peri-auricular incision. **(D)** A 7-year old-male with diffuse, bleeding microcystic lymphatic vesicles of the lower extremity. **(E)** Following resection. **(F)** Split-thickness skin graft coverage of wound. **(G)** Healed graft six months postoperatively.

the most common type; *cutaneomucosal-venous malformation* (CMVM) is rare.[134,152] GVM is an autosomal dominant condition with abnormal smooth muscle-like glomus cells along the ectatic veins. It is caused by a loss-of-function mutation in the *glomulin* gene.[153,154] CMVM is an autosomal dominant condition caused by a gain-of-function mutation in the *TIE2* receptor.[155] *Cerebral cavernous malformation* (CCM) results from mutations in CCM1/(*KRIT1*), CCM2, and CCM3 genes.[156–159]

Clinical features

VMs are blue, soft, and compressible; calcified phleboliths often can be palpated. VM range from small, localized cutaneous lesions to diffuse malformations involving multiple tissue planes, vital structures, and internal organs. VM is typically sporadic and solitary in 90% of patients.[151,152] Sporadic VM is usually greater than 5 cm (56%), single (99%), and located on the head/neck (47%), extremities (40%), or trunk (13%).[152] Almost all lesions involve the skin, mucosa, or subcutaneous tissue; 50% also affect deeper structures (i.e., muscle, bone, joints, viscera).[152]

GVMs are typically multiple (70%), small (two-thirds <5 cm), and located in the skin and subcutaneous tissue; deeper structures are uncommonly affected.[152,154] GVM involves the extremities (76%), trunk (14%), or head/neck (10%).[152,154] Lesions are more painful than typical VM.[152,154] CMVM are multifocal mucocutaneous lesions; they are less common than GVM. Lesions are small (76% <5 cm), multiple (73%), and located on the head/neck (typically tongue or buccal mucosa) (50%), extremity (37%), or trunk (13%).[152] CCM is a rare familial disorder with VM involving the brain and spinal cord; patients also may have hyperkeratotic skin lesions.[134,157] Patients are at risk for development of new intracranial lesions and hemorrhage.[157–159]

Blue rubber bleb nevus syndrome (BRBNS) is a rare condition characterized by multiple, small (<2 cm) VMs involving the skin, soft tissue, and gastrointestinal tract.[160–162] Morbidity is associated with gastrointestinal bleeding requiring chronic blood transfusions. *Diffuse phlebectasia of Bockenheimer* is an old eponym to specify an extensive extremity VM involving skin, subcutaneous tissue, muscle, and bone.[163] *Sinus pericranii* refers to a venous anomaly of the scalp or face and transcalvarial communication with the dural sinus. *Verrucous hemangioma* (VH) is a low-flow vascular malformation that is clinically similar to a hyperkeratotic VM ("verrucous VM").[164] Lesions range from 2–8 cm and are located on an extremity (91%) or trunk (9%).[164] VH involves the skin and subcutis, becomes more hyperkeratotic over time, and frequently causes bleeding.

Maffucci Syndrome denotes the coexistence of cutaneous venous malformations with bony exostoses and enchondromas.[165] Osseous lesions appear first, most often in the hands, feet, long bones of the extremity, ribs, pelvis, and cranium. Recurrent fractures are common.[166] VMs are most commonly located on distal extremities, but may occur anywhere.[167] Malignant transformation, usually chondrosarcoma, occurs in 20–30% of patients at an average age of 40 years (range 13–69 years)[166–168]

A majority of the chondrosarcomas are low grade and often cured by resection.[168,169]

Complications of VM include pain, swelling, and psychosocial issues. Head and neck VM may present with mucosal bleeding or progressive distortion leading to airway or orbital compromise. Extremity VM can cause leg-length discrepancy, hypoplasia due to disuse atrophy, pathologic fracture, hemarthrosis, and degenerative arthritis.[148] VM of muscle may result in fibrosis and subsequent pain and disability.[170] A large VM involving the deep venous system is at risk for thrombosis and pulmonary embolism. Gastrointestinal VM can cause bleeding and chronic anemia. Stagnation within a large VM results in a localized intravascular coagulopathy (LIC) and painful phlebothromboses.

At least 90% of VMs are diagnosed by history and physical examination.[10] Dependent positioning of the affected region usually confirms the diagnosis. Small, superficial VM do not require further diagnostic work-up. Large or deeper lesions are evaluated by MRI to: (1) confirm the diagnosis; (2) define the extent of the malformation; and (3) plan treatment. VM is hyperintense on T2-weighted sequences.[142] In contrast to LM, VM enhances with contrast, often shows phleboliths as signal-voids, and is more likely to involve muscle.[142] US may be used for some localized lesions; findings include compressible, anechoic-hypoechoic channels separated by more solid regions of variable echogenicity.[51] Phleboliths are hyperechoic with acoustic shadowing.[142] CT is occasionally indicated to assess osseous VM. Histological diagnosis of VM is rarely necessary, but may be indicated to rule out malignancy or if imaging is equivocal.

Management

Patients with an extensive extremity VM are prescribed custom-fitted compression garments to reduce blood stagnation and minimize expansion, LIC, phlebolith formation, and pain.[171–173] Patients with recurrent pain secondary to phlebothrombosis are given prophylactic daily aspirin (81 mg) to prevent thrombosis. Large lesions are at risk for coagulation of stagnant blood, stimulation of thrombin, and conversion of fibrinogen-to-fibrin.[173] LIC can become disseminated intravascular coagulopathy (DIC) following trauma or therapeutic intervention. The chronic consumptive coagulopathy can cause either thrombosis (pheboliths) or bleeding (hemarthrosis, hematoma, intraoperative blood loss).[173] Low molecular weight heparin (LMWH) is considered for patients with significant LIC who are at risk for DIC.[174] Patients who develop a serious thrombotic event require long-term anticoagulation or a vena caval filter.

Sclerotherapy

Intervention for VM is reserved for symptomatic lesions that cause pain, deformity, obstruction (i.e., vision, airway), or gastrointestinal bleeding. First-line treatment is sclerotherapy, which is safer and more effective than resection *(Fig. 29.10)*.[175] Good to excellent results are obtained in 75–90% of patients, including reducing the size of the malformation and alleviating symptoms.[142,175,176] Diffuse malformations are managed by targeting specific symptomatic areas, often the entire lesion is too extensive to treat at one time. Sclerotherapy is repeated until symptoms are alleviated or when injectable vascular spaces are no longer present. Although sclerotherapy effectively reduces the size of the lesion and improves symptoms, the malformation remains. Consequently, patients may have a mass or visible deformity after treatment that may be improved by resection. In addition, VM usually re-expands after sclerotherapy, and thus patients often require additional treatments.

The preferred sclerosants for VM are sodium tetradecyl sulfate (STS) and ethanol; STS is the most commonly used. Although ethanol is more effective than STS, it has a higher complication rate. Most patients, especially children, are managed under general anesthesia using US or fluoroscopic imaging. The most common local complication of sclerotherapy for VM is cutaneous ulceration (<5%).[175,176] Extravasation of the sclerosant into muscle can cause atrophy and contracture. Post-treatment swelling may necessitate close monitoring. Compartment compression is a serious consequence of sclerotherapy for extremity VM. Systemic adverse events following sclerotherapy, including hemolysis, hemoglobinuria, and DIC, are more common with large lesions. Patients with low fibrinogen levels are given LMWH 14 days before and after the procedure.[173] Anticoagulation is held for 24 h perioperatively (12 h before and after the intervention) to prevent bleeding complications.

Resection

In contrast to sclerotherapy, resection is rarely primary treatment because: (1) the entire lesion is difficult to remove; (2) the risk of recurrence is high because hidden channels adjacent to the visible lesion are not excised; (3) the risk of blood loss and iatrogenic injury is greater. Resection should be considered for: (1) small, well-localized lesions that can be completely removed, or (2) persistent mass or deformity after completion of sclerotherapy (patent channels are no longer accessible for further injection) *(Fig. 29.11)*. When considering resection, the postoperative scar/deformity following removal of the VM should be weighed against the preoperative appearance of the lesion. Subtotal resection of a problematic area, such as labial hypertrophy, is indicated, rather than attempting "complete" excision of a benign lesion that might result in a worse deformity than the malformation itself. Patients and families are counseled that VM can expand following excision, and additional operative procedures may be required in the future.

Almost all VMs should have sclerotherapy prior to operative intervention. After adequate sclerotherapy, the VM is replaced by scar and thus the risk of blood loss, iatrogenic injury, and recurrence is reduced. In addition, fibrosis facilitates resection and reconstruction. Because GVM is usually small and less amenable to sclerotherapy, first-line therapy for painful lesions may be resection. Nd : YAG photocoagulation can be an adjuvant to sclerotherapy for the management of difficult airway lesions.[177] Gastrointestinal VM with chronic bleeding, anemia, and transfusion requirements is typically managed by resection. Solitary lesions can be treated by endoscopic banding or sclerotherapy. Multifocal lesions of BRBNS require removal of as many lesions as possible through multiple enterotomies, instead of bowel resection, to preserve intestinal length.[162] Diffuse, problematic colorectal VM may require colectomy, anorectal mucosectomy, and endorectal pull-through.[178]

Arteriovenous malformation

Pathogenesis

Arteriovenous malformation (AVM) is believed to result from an error of vascular development between the 4th

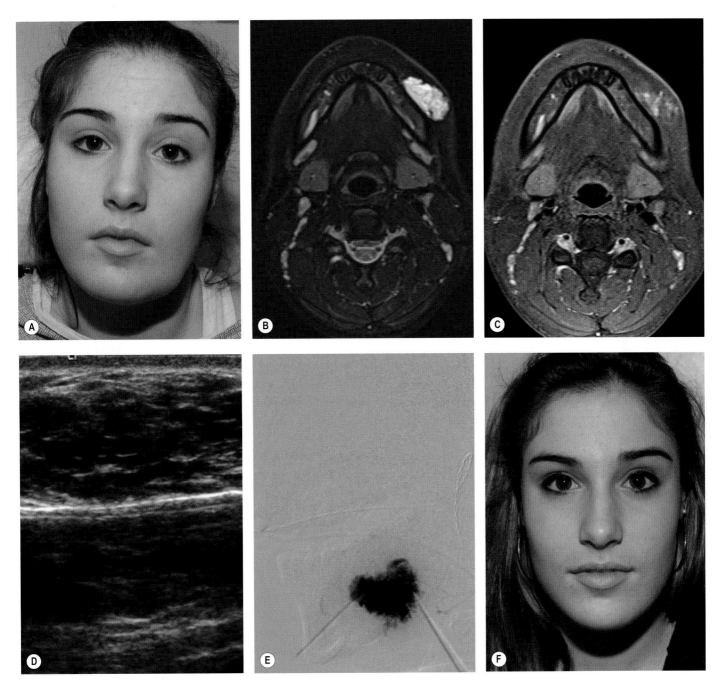

Fig. 29.10 Management of venous malformation with sclerotherapy. **(A)** A 15-year-old female with an enlarging lesion of the left cheek. **(B)** Axial T2 MR with fat suppression illustrates a localized lesion involving the cheek. **(C)** Axial T1 MR exhibits heterogeneous enhancement of the lesion with contrast. **(D)** Ultrasound shows compressible hypoechoic venous spaces with echogenic walls. **(E)** Venogram of the spongiform venous malformation with a minor draining vein. **(F)** Resolution of facial asymmetry two months following sclerotherapy with sodium tetradecyl sulfate. (Reprinted from Greene AK, Alomari AI, Management of venous malformations, *Clinics in Plastic Surgery*, 2011:38(1):87, with permission from Elsevier.)

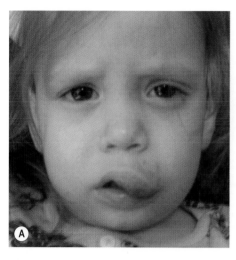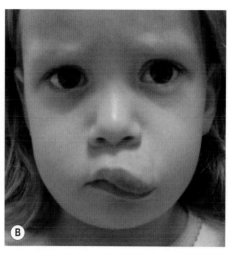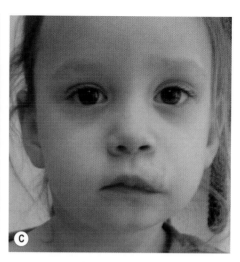

Fig. 29.11 Management of venous malformation with sclerotherapy followed by resection. **(A)** A 2.5-year-old female with an enlarging venous malformation of the upper lip. **(B)** Reduction of the venous malformation after two sessions of sclerotherapy. Further sclerotherapy was not possible because venous spaces had been replaced by fibrosis. **(C)** Improved contour three months after resection of residual scarred venous malformation using a transverse mucosal incision.

and 6th weeks of gestation.[1] Halsted wrote that it results from failure of arteriovenous channels in the primitive retiform plexus to regress.[179] This may explain why AVM is 20 times more common in the central nervous system, where apoptosis is rare.[180] An absent capillary bed causes shunting of blood directly from the arterial-to-venous circulation, through a fistula (direct connection of an artery to a vein) or nidus (abnormal channels bridging the feeding artery to the draining veins).

Genetic abnormalities cause certain types of familial AVM. *Hereditary hemorrhagic telangiectasia* (HHT) results from mutations in endoglin and activin receptor-like kinase 1, which affect transforming growth factor-beta signaling.[181–183] *Capillary malformation-arteriovenous malformation* (CM-AVM) is caused by a mutation in *RASA1*.[184]

AVM may enlarge because of increased blood flow causing collateralization, dilatation of vessels (especially venous ectasia), and thickening of adjacent arteries and veins.[1,185] Latent arteriovenous shunts may open, stimulating hypertrophy of surrounding vessels from increased pressure.[1,186] Alternatively, aneurysms may increase the size of these lesions.[187,188] *Angiogenesis* (growth of new blood vessels from pre-existing vasculature) and *vasculogenesis* (*de novo* formation of new vasculature) also may be involved in AVM expansion.[189] Although neovascularization may be a primary stimulus for AVM growth, it also could be a secondary event. For example, ischemia, a potent stimulator of

angiogenesis, causes enlargement of AVM after proximal arterial ligation or trauma.[1,190–191] Alternatively, increased blood flow due to arteriovenous shunting may promote angiogenesis; vascular endothelial growth factor (VEGF) production and endothelial proliferation are stimulated by increased blood flow.[192,193] Both males and females have a two-fold risk of progression in adolescence; increased circulating hormones during this period may promote AVM expansion.[189]

Clinical features

The most common site of extracranial AVM is the head and neck, followed by the limbs, trunk, and viscera.[33] Although present at birth, AVM may not become evident until childhood. Early lesions present as a pink-red cutaneous stain, without a palpable thrill or bruit. Often they are initially mistaken as a capillary malformation or infantile hemangioma. Arteriovenous shunting reduces delivery of capillary oxygen causing ischemia. In time, the patient is at risk for pain, ulceration, and bleeding. AVM also may cause disfigurement, destruction of tissues, and obstruction of vital structures. High-pressure shunting of blood may lead to venous hemorrhage; ruptured arteries can form in weakened areas, such as aneurysms. Arterial bleeding most commonly occurs at skin or mucosal surfaces from erosion into a superficial component of the lesion. AVMs can cause cardiac enlargement and result in high-output

Table 29.4 Schobinger staging of arteriovenous malformation (AVM)

Stage	Clinical findings
I (Quiescence)	Warm, pink-blue, shunting on Doppler
II (Expansion)	Enlargement, pulsation, thrill, bruit, tortuous veins
III (Destruction)	Dystrophic skin changes, ulceration, bleeding, pain
IV (Decompensation)	Cardiac failure

cardiac failure by the direct communication between the high-resistance, high-pressure arterial system and the low-pressure, low-resistance venous system. While the presence of an AVM may be troublesome, it is the *expansion* of the lesion that is the primary cause of morbidity. AVM can be classified according to the Schobinger staging system *(Table 29.4)*.[190]

Most AVMs are diagnosed by history and physical examination. Hand-held Doppler reveals fast-flow and excludes a slow-flow vascular anomaly. If AVM is suspected, the diagnosis should be confirmed by US with color Doppler examination. MRI also is necessary to: (1) confirm the diagnosis; (2) determine the extent of the lesion; (3) plan treatment. To adequately assess the anomaly, MRI with contrast and fat suppression, as well as a T2-weighted sequences, is necessary.[194] MRI shows dilated feeding arteries and draining veins, enhancement, and flow-voids.[194] If the diagnosis remains unclear after US and MRI, angiography is sometimes needed. Usually angiography only is indicated prior to embolization or when resection is planned. Characteristic features are tortuous, dilated, arteries with arteriovenous shunting and dilated draining veins.[194] The nidus is angiographically seen as tortuous, small vessels, with occasionally ill-defined larger contiguous vascular spaces. CT may be indicated if the AVM involves bone. Histopathological diagnosis of AVM is rarely necessary, but may be indicated to rule out malignancy or if imaging is equivocal. Biopsy of an AVM can cause bleeding and reactive expansion of the lesion.[189]

Management

Because AVM is often diffuse, involving multiple tissue planes and important structures, cure is rare. The goal of treatment usually is to *control* the malformation. Intervention is focused on alleviating symptoms (i.e., bleeding, pain, ulceration), preserving vital functions (i.e., vision, mastication), and improving deformity. Management options include embolization, resection, or a combination. Resection offers the best chance for long-term control, but the re-expansion rate is high and extirpation may cause a worse deformity.[189] Almost all AVMs will re-expand after embolization.[189] Consequently, embolization is used to reduce blood loss during resection or sometimes for palliation of unresectable lesions.

Asymptomatic AVM should be observed unless it can be completely removed with minimal morbidity; embolization or incomplete excision of an asymptomatic lesion may stimulate it to enlarge and become problematic. Intervention is determined by: (1) the size and location of the AVM; (2) the age of the patient; (3) Schobinger stage. Although resection of an asymptomatic Stage I AVM offers the best chance for long-term control or "cure", intervention must be individualized based on the deformity that would be caused by resection and reconstruction. For example, a large Stage I AVM in a nonanatomically important location (i.e., trunk, proximal extremity) can be resected without consequence, before it progresses to a higher stage where resection is more difficult, and the recurrence rate is greater. Similarly, a small, well-localized AVM in a more difficult location (i.e., face, hand) may be excised for possible "cure" before it expands and complete extirpation is no longer possible.

In contrast, a large, asymptomatic AVM located in an anatomically sensitive area is best observed; especially in a young child who is not psychologically ready for major resection and reconstruction. Although the recurrence rate is lower when Stage I AVM is resected, it is still high, and thus even after major resection and reconstruction the malformation can recur. Some patients (17.4%) do not have significant long-term morbidity.[189]

Intervention for Stage II AVMs is similar to Stage I lesions. The threshold for treatment is lower if an enlarging lesion is causing a worsening deformity or if functional problems are occurring. Stage III and IV AVMs require intervention to control pain, bleeding, ulceration, or congestive heart failure.

Embolization

Embolization is the delivery of an inert substance, through a catheter into the AVM nidus to occlude blood flow and/or fill a vascular space. Scarring reduces arteriovenous shunting, shrinks the lesion, and diminishes symptoms. Embolization is used either as a preoperative adjunct to resection or as monotherapy for lesions not amenable to extirpation. Because the AVM is not removed, almost all lesions eventually re-expand after treatment. Stage I AVM has a lower recurrence rate than higher-staged lesions.[189] Most recurrences occur within the first year after embolization, and 98% re-expand within 5 years.[189] Despite the high likelihood of re-expansion, embolization can effectively palliate an AVM by reducing its size, slowing expansion, and alleviating pain and bleeding. Preoperative embolization also reduces blood loss during extirpation, but not the extent of resection.

Substances used for embolization are either liquid (*n*-butyl cyanoacrylate (n-BCA), Onyx) or solid (polyvinyl alcohol particles (PVA), coils). The goal of embolization is occlusion of the nidus and proximal venous outflow. The embolic material is delivered to the nidus, *not* to the proximal arterial feeding vessels. Occlusion of inflow will cause collateralization and expansion of the AVM; access to the nidus also will be blocked preventing future embolization.[194] For preoperative embolization, temporary occlusive substances (Gelfoam powder, PVA, embospheres) that undergo phagocytosis are used. Permanent liquid agents capable of permeating the nidus (n-BCA, Onyx) are employed when embolization is the primary treatment.[194] The most frequent complication of embolization is ulceration.

Resection

Resection of AVM has a lower recurrence rate than embolization alone; it is considered for a well-localized lesion or to correct deformity (i.e., bleeding or ulcerated areas, labial hypertrophy) *(Fig. 29.12)*.[189] Wide extirpation and reconstruction of large, diffuse AVM should be exercised with caution because: (1) cure is rare and the recurrence rate is high; (2) the resulting deformity is often worse than the appearance of the malformation; (3) resection is associated with significant blood loss, iatrogenic injury, and morbidity. When excision is planned, preoperative embolization will facilitate the procedure by reducing the size of the AVM, minimizing blood loss, and creating scar tissue to aid the dissection. Multiple embolizations, spaced 6 weeks apart, may be required prior to resection. Excision should be done 24–72 h after embolization, before recanalization restores blood flow to the lesion.

Resection margins are best determined by assessing the type of bleeding from the wound edges. Some defects can be reconstructed by advancing local skin flaps. Skin grafting ulcerated areas has a high failure rate because the underlying tissue is ischemic; excision with regional flap transfer may be required. Free-flap reconstruction permits wide resection and primary closure of complicated defects, but does not appear to improve long-term AVM control.[189] Despite sub-total and presumed "complete" extirpation, most AVMs treated by resection recur. The majority of recurrences occur within the first year after intervention and 86.6% re-expand within 5 years of resection.[189] Nevertheless, many of these patients remain asymptomatic. Patients and families are counseled that AVM is likely to re-expand following resection, and thus additional treatment may be required.

Capillary malformation-arteriovenous malformation

Capillary malformation-arteriovenous malformation (CM-AVM) is an autosomal dominant condition caused by a loss-of-function mutation in the *RASA1* gene; the prevalence is 1 in 100 000 Caucasians.[184,195] Patients have atypical capillary malformations (CMs) that are small, multifocal, round, pinkish-red, and often surrounded by a pale halo *(Fig. 29.13)* (50%).[184,195] A total of 30% also have an AVM: Parkes Weber syndrome (PWS) (12%), extracerebral AVM (11%), or intracerebral AVM (7%).[195] A patient presenting with multiple CMs, especially with a family history of similar lesions, should be evaluated for a possible AVM. Because 7% of patients with CM-AVM will have an intracranial fast-flow lesion, brain MRI should be considered.[134] Exploratory imaging of other anatomical areas is not necessary because extracranial AVM have not been found to involve the viscera.[195] Although the CM is rarely problematic, associated AVMs can cause major morbidity.

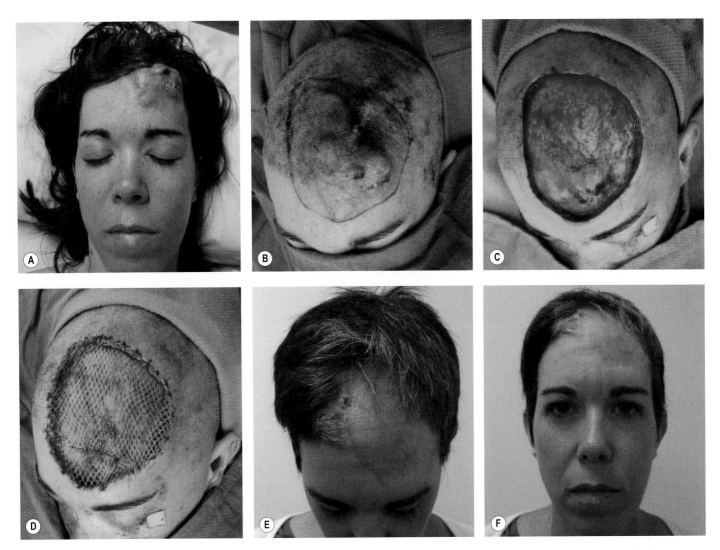

Fig. 29.12 Management of arteriovenous malformation. **(A)** A 39-year-old female with an enlarging, bleeding, ulcerated stage 3 lesion of the forehead and scalp. **(B)** Intraoperative view following preoperative embolization. **(C)** Wound after extirpation. **(D)** Split-thickness skin graft coverage of periosteum. **(E,F)** Healed graft four months postoperatively.

Eponymous vascular anomalies with overgrowth

Sturge–Weber syndrome

Sturge–Weber syndrome (SWS) is a sporadic neurocutaneous disorder estimated to occur in 1 in 50 000 live births *(Fig. 29.14A).*[196–198] The three cardinal features are capillary malformation (CM) in the upper trigeminal neural distribution, ocular abnormalities (glaucoma, choroidal vascular anomalies), and leptomeningeal vascular malformation.[199] Patients also commonly have soft tissue and/or bony overgrowth (60–83%); the frequency is similar to that for glaucoma (65–77%) and for neurological sequelae (87–93%).[109]

In all patients with an upper facial CM, a diagnosis of Sturge–Weber syndrome should be considered on initial presentation. The capillary stain can be in the ophthalmic (V1), extend into the maxillary (V2), or involve all three trigeminal dermatomes. Patients with maxillary or mandibular involvement alone are at low risk for SWS. The leptomeningeal anomalies can be capillary, venous, or arteriovenous malformations. Small foci may be silent, but extensive pial vascular lesions can cause refractory seizures, contralateral hemiplegia, and delayed motor and cognitive development. The

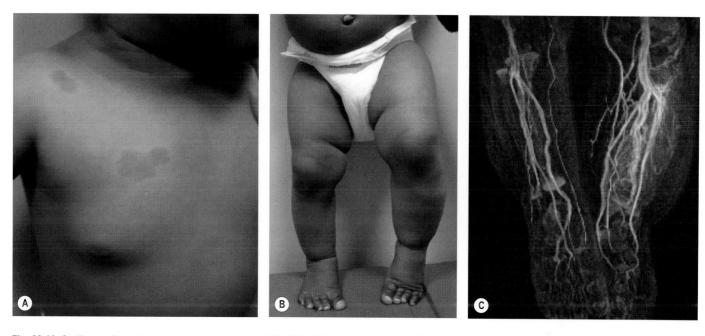

Fig. 29.13 Capillary malformation-arteriovenous malformation (CM-AVM). **(A)** A 1-year-old female with multifocal capillary malformations of the chest and shoulder. **(B,C)** Arteriovenous malformation of left lower extremity with overgrowth.

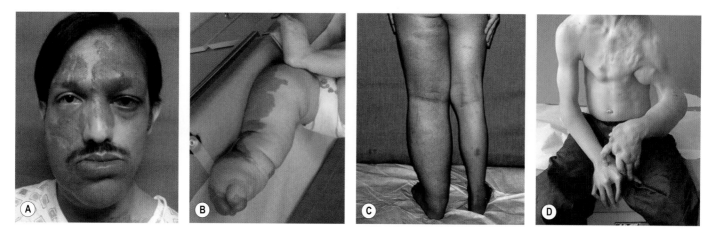

Fig. 29.14 Eponymous vascular anomalies with overgrowth. **(A)** A 36-year-old male with Sturge-Weber syndrome. **(B)** Infant female with Klippel-Trenaunay syndrome. **(C)** A 7-year-old male with Parkes Weber syndrome. **(D)** An 11-year-old male with CLOVES syndrome.

anomalous choroidal vascularity can lead to retinal detachment, glaucoma, and blindness. Ophthalmic examination should be performed every 6 months until the age of 2 years and yearly thereafter. MRI best demonstrates pial vascular enhancement in an infant or child thought to have Sturge–Weber syndrome.

In addition to facial capillary staining; extra-craniofacial CMs (29%) and extremity hypertrophy (14%) are frequently present.[109] In the past, SWS patients with extra-craniofacial CM and limb hypertrophy often have been erroneously labeled as having either "Klippel–Weber–Trénaunay syndrome", Klippel–Trénaunay syndrome (extremity capillary-lymphatico-venous malformation with overgrowth) or Parkes Weber syndrome (extremity capillary-arteriovenous malformation with overgrowth). In contrast to Klippel–Trénaunay or Parkes Weber syndromes, patients with SWS do not have combined venous, lymphatic, or arterial anomalies in an extremity, although simple diffuse venous varicosities can occur.

Klippel–Trénaunay syndrome

Klippel–Trénaunay syndrome (KTS) denotes a slow-flow, capillary-lymphatic-venous malformation (CLVM) of an extremity in association with soft tissue and/or skeletal overgrowth *(Fig. 29.14B)*. Unfortunately, it is often incorrectly called "Klippel–Trénaunay–Weber", invoking Parkes Weber syndrome, a fast-flow vascular malformation. There is tremendous variability in the presentation of this disorder, from a slightly enlarged extremity with a capillary stain to a grotesquely enlarged limb with malformed digits. KTS affects the lower extremity in 95% of patients, the upper extremity in 5% of patients, and least commonly the trunk. Sometimes the contralateral foot or hand is enlarged, often with a macrodactylous component and frequently in the absence of a capillary stain. In 10% of patients with KTS, the involved limb is hypoplastic. Pelvic involvement is common with CLVM of the lower extremity. It is usually asymptomatic, although hematuria, bladder outlet obstruction, cystitis, and hematochezia can occur. Upper extremity or truncal CLVM can involve the posterior mediastinum and retropleural space, although this is rarely symptomatic. The capillary malformation is distributed in a geographic pattern over the lateral side of the extremity, buttock, or thorax. Whereas the capillary malformation is typically macular in a neonate, later it becomes studded with hemolymphatic vesicles. The venous component of CLVM manifests as abnormal drainage of the affected area. The lymphatic abnormalities are typically macrocystic in the pelvis and thighs and microcystic in the abdominal wall, buttock, and distal limb.

MRI is obtained to confirm the diagnosis and determine the extent of the anomalies. A large, embryonal vein in the subcutaneous tissue (the marginal vein of Servelle) is often located in the lateral calf and thigh and communicates with the deep venous system. Complications include thrombophlebitis (20–45%) and pulmonary embolism (4–24%).[200–203] Unlike some other hemihypertrophy syndromes, patients with KTS are not at increased risk for Wilms tumor and screening ultrasonography is unnecessary.[204] By 2 years of age, radiologic surveillance of leg length by plain radiography is indicated. If the discrepancy is >1.5 cm, a shoe-lift for the shorter limb can prevent limping and scoliosis. Epiphysiodesis of the distal femoral growth plate is typically done around 11 years of age. Enlargement of the foot may require a ray, midfoot, or Syme amputation to allow the use of footwear. Management of the VM component is conservative with compressive stockings for insufficiency and aspirin to minimize phlebothrombosis. Symptomatic varicose veins may be removed or sclerosed. Sclerotherapy may be necessary for focal macrocystic lymphatic malformation or to treat cutaneous vesicles. Excision and grafting is occasionally necessary for diffuse bleeding and/or oozing cutaneous vesicles. Circumferential overgrowth may be managed by staged contour resection. Venous insufficiency does not occur following staged subcutaneous excision or removal of the marginal vein of Servelle. A functioning deep venous system is present, although it is often difficult to visualize because of predominant flow in the superficial veins.

Parkes Weber syndrome

Parkes Weber syndrome (PWS) is a diffuse AVM in an overgrown extremity with an overlying CM *(Fig. 29.14C)*. PWS involves the lower extremity approximately twice as often as the upper extremity; patients have microshunting in muscle. The malformation is evident at birth with symmetric enlargement and pink staining of the involved limb. The cutaneous stain tends to be confluent rather than patchy and is typically warmer than a banal capillary malformation. The diagnosis is confirmed by the detection of a bruit or thrill. MRI is obtained to evaluate the extent of the malformation. Overgrowth in an affected extremity is subcutaneous, muscular, and bony with diffuse microfistulas. The enlarged limb muscles and bones exhibit an abnormal signal and enhancement. Angiography demonstrates discrete arteriovenous shunts.

Treatment is predicated on symptoms. In rare instances, an infant presents with high-output congestive heart failure secondary to shunting through arteriovenous fistulas. This situation mandates emergent embolization with permanent occlusive agents, often followed by repeated procedures. Children are observed annually with careful monitoring for axial overgrowth and development of cutaneous problems. Embolization may be useful for pain or cutaneous ischemic changes. Occasionally, amputation is necessary.

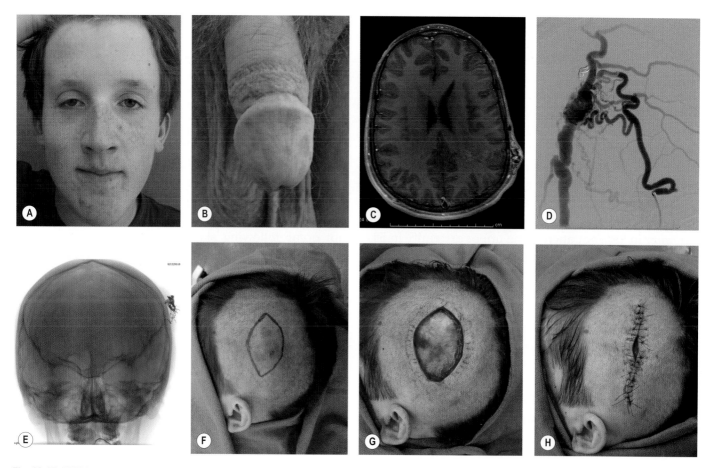

Fig. 29.15 PTEN hamartoma-tumor syndrome (Bannayan-Riley-Ruvalcaba syndrome). **(A)** A 16-year-old male with enlarging, painful scalp lesion. **(B)** Penile freckling associated with the syndrome. **(C)** Axial T1 MR image shows enhancing soft tissue lesion consistent with PTEN-associated vascular anomaly. **(D)** Angiogram illustrates arteriovenous shunting without a nidus. **(E)** Onyx cast of lesion following preoperative embolization. **(F)** Intraoperative view. **(G)** A 9 cm × 4.5 cm wound following resection. **(H)** Linear closure after wide scalp undermining and subgaleal scoring.

PTEN hamartoma-tumor syndrome (Bannayan–Riley–Ruvalcaba syndrome)

Patients with *PTEN* mutations, a tumor suppressor gene, have PTEN hamartoma-tumor syndrome (PHTS) *(Fig. 29.15)*. This autosomal dominant condition is also referred to as Cowden syndrome or Bannayan–Riley–Ruvalcaba syndrome.[205,206] Males and females are equally affected, and approximately one-half (54%) of patients have a unique fast-flow vascular anomaly with arteriovenous shunting, referred to as a PTEN-associated vascular anomaly.[206] Patients may have multiple lesions (57%), and 85% are intramuscular.[206]

Suspicion of a PTEN-associated vascular anomaly usually is initiated after reviewing the MRI or angiographic study of a patient suspected of having an AVM. Unlike typical AVM, these lesions may be multifocal, are associated with ectopic adipose tissue, and have disproportionate, segmental dilation of the draining veins.[194,206] If a patient is suspected of having a PTEN-associated vascular anomaly on imaging, a physical examination is performed. All patients with PHTS have macrocephaly (>97th percentile), and all males have penile freckling.[206] In addition, PHTS is associated with mental retardation/autism (19%), thyroid lesions (31%), or gastrointestinal polyps (30%).[206] Biopsy may aid the diagnosis of a PTEN fast-flow lesion. Histopathology shows skeletal muscle infiltration with adipose tissue, fibrous bands, and lymphoid aggregates. In addition, tortuous arteries with transmural muscular hyperplasia and clusters of abnormal veins with variable smooth muscle are present.[206] Genetic testing is confirmative, although a germline mutation is not found in 9% of families clinically diagnosed with PHTS.[207]

If physical examination is consistent with PHTS, molecular testing is necessary because this mutation is associated with multiple benign and malignant tumors which require surveillance. Patients are followed closely for the presence of tumors, particularly endocrine and gastrointestinal malignancies. In addition, the patient and family are counseled about the risk of transmitting the gene to their offspring. Symptomatic lesions are managed similarly to nonsyndromic AVM, with embolization or resection. It is our experience that the recurrence rate after these interventions is even higher than for nonsyndromic AVM, possibly because the loss of the tumor suppressor protein favors a more proliferative environment.

CLOVES syndrome

Congenital Lipomatosis Overgrowth, Vascular malformations, Epidermal nevi, and Scoliosis (CLOVES) represents a newly described overgrowth syndrome.[208,209] Many of these patients previously were thought to have "Proteus syndrome". Unlike Proteus syndrome, patients with CLOVES do not have skeletal involvement and the soft-tissue component is not progressive. All patients have a truncal lipomatous mass, a slow-flow vascular malformation (most commonly a CM overlying the lipomatous mass), and hand/foot anomalies (increased width, macrodactyly, first web-space sandal gap) *(Fig. 29.14D)*.[208,209] Patients also may have AVM (28%), neurological impairment (50%), or scoliosis (33%).[208,209] Treatment for the lipomatous lesions is resection, but the recurrence rate is high.

Conclusion

Patients with vascular anomalies all too often have been medical "nomads". During infancy and childhood, their parents took them from one physician to another, because no one seemed to understand the condition. The problem usually was that these anomalies lay in the interface between several medical and surgical disciplines. No single specialist had sufficient knowledge to treat the wide variety of disorders.

Terminologic confusion has been replaced with a common language. Interested specialists can now communicate with one another. Vascular anomaly teams, composed of various disciplines on the basis of local interest, enthusiasm, and capabilities, continue to form in many major referral centers. These teams are in a unique position because the collective knowledge of such a group provides a forum for problems that otherwise appear "too complicated" or "insoluble". In addition, they serve as a focus for clinical and basic research in this field.

The future of the field of vascular anomalies is exciting because a significant opportunity exists to improve the lives of these patients. Plastic surgeons are well-positioned to make progress because of their training; management of these lesions requires creativity, surgical problem-solving skills, and a mastery of operative principles. Plastic surgeons, in collaboration with other specialists, will continue to be primary caretakers of patients with vascular anomalies.

 Access the complete references list online at **http://www.expertconsult.com**

4. Mulliken JB, Glowacki J. Hemangiomas and vascular malformations in infants and children: a classification based on endothelial characteristics. *Plast Reconstr Surg.* 1982;69:412–422.

    Forty-nine tissue specimens from various vascular lesions were analyzed histologically and by tritiated thymidine uptake. Hemangiomas showed endothelial hyperplasia during the proliferative phase while malformations had quiescent endothelium. This landmark study clarified the field of vascular anomalies by proposing a binary classification: hemangiomas and malformations.

9. North PE, Waner M, Mizeracki A, et al. GLUT1: a newly discovered immunohistochemical marker for juvenile hemangiomas. *Hum Pathol.* 2000;31:11–22.

    This is a retrospective immunohistochemical study of 143 hemangiomas, 66 vascular malformations, 20 pyogenic granulomas, and five hemangioendotheliomas. GLUT1 (erythrocyte-type glucose transporter) only was expressed in infantile hemangioma (during proliferation and involution). GLUT1 is a sensitive marker to differentiate infantile hemangioma from congenital hemangiomas, other vascular tumors, and vascular malformations.

10. Finn MC, Glowacki J, Mulliken JB. Congenital vascular lesions: clinical application of a new classification. *J Pediatr Surg*. 1983;18:894–900.

41. Huang SA, Tu HM, Harney JW, et al. Severe hypothyroidism caused by type 3 iodothyronine deiodinase in infantile hemangiomas. *N Engl J Med*. 2000;343:185–189.

42. Freiden IJ, Reese V, Cohen D. PHACE syndrome. The association of posterior fossa brain malformations, hemangiomas, arterial anomalies, coarctation of the aorta and cardiac defects and eye abnormalities. *Arch Dermatol*. 1996;132:307–311.

62. Haisley-Royster C, Enjolras O, Frieden IJ, et al. Kasabach-Merritt phenomenon: a retrospective study of treatment with vincristine. *J Pediatr Hematol Oncol*. 2002;24:459–462.

    This is a multi-institutional review of 15 patients with kaposiform hemangioendothelioma/tufted angioma treated with vincristine. The response rate was greater than 90%, which was superior to corticosteroid or interferon. This study established vincristine as the first-line therapy for patients with hemangioendotheliomas.

66. Bennett ML, Fleischer AB, Chamlin SL, et al. Oral corticosteroid use is effective for cutaneous hemangiomas. *Arch Dermatol*. 2001;137:1208–1213.

    This is a meta-analysis of published series describing the treatment of infantile hemangioma with oral corticosteroid.

Corticosteroid was shown to be a very effective (85% response rate) and safe treatment for problematic infantile hemangioma. 3.0 mg/kg per day became the accepted dose of prednisolone; it had superior efficacy compared to lower doses.

88. Berenguer B, Mulliken JB, Enjolras O, et al. Rapidly involuting congenital hemangioma: clinical and histopathologic features. *Pediatr Dev Pathol*. 2003;6:495–510.

91. Sarkar M, Mulliken JB, Kozakewich HP, et al. Thrombocytopenic coagulopathy (Kasabach–Merritt phenomenon) is associated with kaposiform hemangioendothelioma and not with common infantile hemangioma. *Plast Reconstr Surg*. 1997;100: 1377–1386.

155. Vikkula M, Boon LM, Carraway KL, et al. Vascular dysmorphogenesis caused by an activating mutation in the receptor tyrosine kinase TIE2. *Cell*. 1996;87: 1181–1190.

    Two families with inherited multiple venous malformations were found to have an activating mutation in the endothelial receptor tyrosine kinase TIE2, suggesting that the TIE2 signaling pathway is critical for endothelial-smooth muscle cell interaction. This was the first mutation implicated in the pathogenesis of vascular anomalies; the disorder is called cutaneous-mucosal venous malformation.

30

Benign and malignant nonmelanocytic tumors of the skin and soft tissue

Rei Ogawa

SYNOPSIS

- All typical skin and skin-associated soft-tissue tumors, apart from malignant melanocytic tumors (malignant melanoma), are described from the point of view of a plastic surgeon.
- Biopsies should only be performed for a clear purpose, such as for the differential diagnosis of benign tumors or to analyze the stage and grade of malignant tumors, which would allow the area to be resected to be determined.
- One current and useful model is the reconstructive matrix, which helps plastic surgeons to determine the best reconstructive solutions for their patients in the context of particular medical and socioeconomic environments by considering aspects of surgical complexity, technological sophistication, and patient surgical risk.

Introduction

The skin consists of the epidermis, which is derived during ontogeny from the superficial ectoderm, and the dermis, which is derived from the mesenchyme. Starting in the first 3–4 weeks of human ontogeny, cells derived from the neural crest migrate into the epidermis *(Fig. 30.1)* where they become melanocytes and Schwann cells; the latter associate with peripheral nerves in the skin. Later, the cutaneous appendages develop. These include hair, which originates from epidermal cells, and hair papillae, which are filled with mesenchyme; vessels and peripheral nerve endings also develop in the papillae. Other cutaneous appendages are the sebaceous glands, which are derived from the epithelial wall of the hair papillae, and the eccrine and apocrine sweat glands, which are also epidermal in origin. There are also soft tissues that are associated with skin, namely fat, muscles, and blood vessels (all of which have a mesenchymal lineage) and nerves (derived from neural crest cells). Thus, skin and skin-associated soft-tissue tumors can be classified simply into those that are of epithelial, cutaneous appendage, neural crest, and mesenchymal origin *(Fig. 30.2)*.

In this chapter, all typical skin and skin-associated soft-tissue tumors apart from malignant melanocytic tumors (malignant melanoma) are described from the point of view of the plastic surgeon.

Diagnosis

Inspection and palpation

The diagnosis of skin tumors starts with inspection and palpation. The following information should be recorded: the number of lesions (solitary or multiple), the shape of the lesions (e.g., round, oval, polygonal, geographic, linear, annular), its size, its elevation status (e.g., narrow-pedicled, wide-pedicled, dome-like, hemispherical, flat elevated, umbilicated), its surface status (e.g., smooth, rough, papillary, granular, transudatory, xerophily, ulcerative, erosive, atrophic,

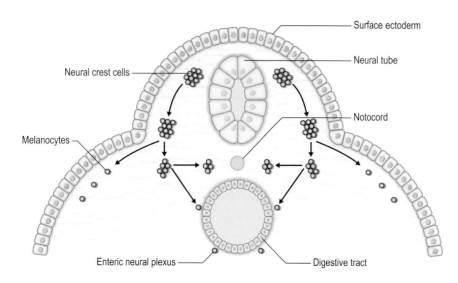

Fig. 30.1 The human embryo at 3–4 weeks.

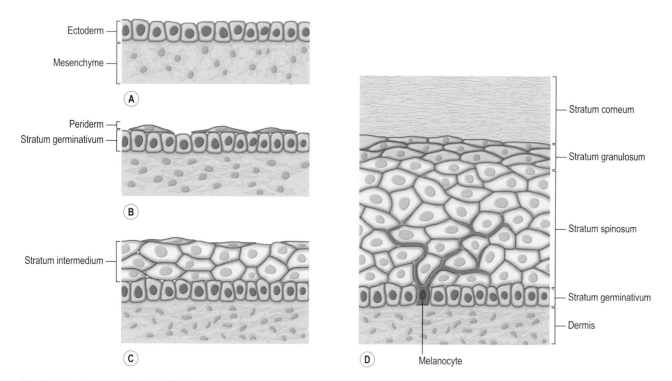

Fig. 30.2 Development of the skin. **(A)** The fifth week of fetal life; **(B)** the seventh week of fetal life; **(C)** the fourth month of fetal life; **(D)** at birth.

lustrous, necrotic), its color (e.g., normal, yellow, pale yellow, erythematous, blackish brown, black, blue, depigmented, pigmented, hyperemic, livid), its hardness (e.g., soft, elastic soft, elastic hard, hard, bone-like hard, fluctuating), its alignment (e.g., localized, disseminated, centrifugal, systematized, singular, symmetric, asymmetric, bilateral), its site, whether there are any

subjective symptoms (e.g., pain, itch, contracture sensation, numbness, burning sensation, cold sensation), and the time course of the appearance of the lesion (e.g., acute, subacute, chronic, temporary, recurrent). Color plays a particularly important role in the diagnosis of skin lesions *(Box 30.1)*. The possibility of malignant tumors should be suspected at all times. If the shape, size, elevation status, or color of a lesion changes rapidly, a biopsy should be considered.

Dermoscopy

Dermoscopy is a specialized technique that employs a binocular microscope to observe the skin surface. It is useful for diagnosing pigmented lesions and is necessary for differentially diagnosing malignant melanoma and nevus. It is also required for the diagnosis of seborrheic keratosis, basal cell carcinoma (BCC) and vascular lesions. The Consensus Net Meeting on Dermoscopy 2000[1] has recommended the use of a two-step diagnostic algorithm, in which the first step is to differentiate melanocytic from nonmelanocytic pigmented lesions by using specific dermoscopic criteria. The second step is to differentiate between the various nonmelanocytic lesions by using other specific dermoscopic criteria *(Fig. 30.3)*. The dermoscopic criteria that are used to diagnose melanocytic lesions, seborrheic keratosis, BCC, and vascular lesions are shown in *Box 30.2*.

Ultrasound and Doppler imaging

To observe skin lesions, high-frequency ultrasound around 20–50 MHz is needed.[2] However, if the lesion shows extension perpendicular to the skin surface that exceeds a depth of 20 mm, the standard ultrasound

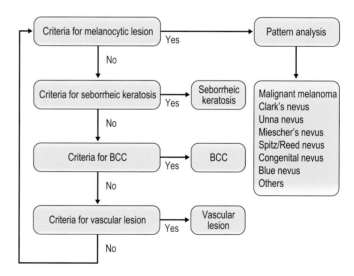

Fig. 30.3 Two-step diagnosis using dermoscopy. BCC, basal cell carcinoma. (Modified from Consensus Net meeting on Dermoscopy. Available at http://www.dermoscopy.org/consensus/.)

(3–10 MHz) should be used. In such cases, computed tomography (CT) and magnetic resonance imaging (MRI) can provide additional information. Ultrasound can be used to determine tumor thickness, its relationship with adjacent structures, and the presence of lymph node metastasis. A variety of ultrasound devices are suitable for this purpose, including mechanical or electron scanning, one-dimensional A-mode, two-dimensional B-mode, and three-dimensional C-mode devices.

Doppler imaging using color Doppler imaging (CDI) or power Doppler imaging is useful for the differential diagnosis of benign and malignant skin tumors, assessing inflammatory reactions, and detecting lymph node metastases. This is because 90% of malignant skin tumors exhibit a high blood flow rate of 3–20 cm/s that is not observed in more than 95% of benign skin tumors. The resolution of power Doppler imaging is higher than that of CDI. M-mode and duplex (a combination of B- and M-mode) scanning are useful for observing hemangiomas or vascular malformations.

X-ray, CT, MRI, angiography, scintigraphy, and positron emission tomography (PET)

X-ray analysis is useful for detecting calcifying lesions such as pilomatricoma and malignant tumors that have necrosis-induced calcifications. Moreover, bone deformation associated with malignant or nonmalignant tumor invasion into bones can be observed by using X-rays.

CT detects metastatic lesions in the bone, lymph nodes, and lungs better than MRI. Helical CT or multidetector low CT can generate three-dimensional and high-resolution images. Contrast-enhanced CT and CT angiography are useful for detecting malignant tumors, vascular regions, and adjacent vascular structures.

MRI detects soft tissues better than CT. In general, malignant tumors present with low-iso signal intensity on T2-weighted images (T2WI) and low signal intensity on T1-weighted images (T1WI), while benign tumors exhibit high signal intensity on T2WI and low signal intensity on T1WI. Magnetic resonance angiography is superior to MRI in determining the nidus and exact nature of the collateral structures in hemangiomas and vascular malformations.

Angiography is an invasive imaging method that was frequently used in the past to investigate vascular lesions. While it detects hemangiomas and vascular malformations readily, its use with pediatric patients requires general anesthesia.

Scintigraphy can be used for metastatic lesion screening. ^{67}Ga and ^{201}TiCl are used in tumor- or inflammation-seeking scintigraphy, while ^{99}Tc-MDP and ^{99m}Tc-HMDP are used in bone scintigraphy. Scintigraphy suffers from low resolution, and this makes it difficult to detect lesions that are less than 2 mm in diameter by this method.

PET is also useful for detecting the metastatic lesions of malignant skin tumors.[3] 2-deoxy-2-[^{18}F] fluoro-D-glucose (FDG) PET (FDG-PET) has been used for the diagnosis and staging of cancers and for monitoring treatment, particularly with regard to Hodgkin's lymphoma, non-Hodgkin lymphoma, and lung cancer. PET can also sometimes detect many other types of solid tumors that occasionally show up as very highly labeled lesions. FDG-PET is particularly useful for searching for tumor metastasis, or for recurrence after the removal of a primary tumor that was known to be highly active. However, since PET can also detect inflammatory lesions, it will be necessary to exclude the possibility that a PET-detected apparent tumor is not an inflammatory, erosive, or ulcered area.

Pathologic diagnosis

A definitive diagnosis requires a pathologic diagnosis. However, biopsies should only be performed for a clear purpose, such as for the differential diagnosis of benign tumors or to analyze the stage and grade of malignant tumors, which would allow the area to be resected to be determined. Moreover, biopsies should only take place after careful inspection, palpation, and imaging analyses. Depending on the purpose of a biopsy and the lesion characteristics, the surgeon can choose from a range of different biopsy techniques, including punch, incisional, excisional, and mapping biopsies. In the case of incisional biopsies, normal skin should be excised together with early-stage lesions and the characteristic areas of lesions (e.g., inflammatory, erosive, or ulcered areas).

In the case of a possible malignant tumor, an excisional biopsy is recommended to prevent malignant cell dissemination into blood. However, surgeon judgment is needed to determine the amount of normal skin that should be removed. In general, the normal skin margin of an excisional biopsy should be as minimal as possible, especially if the tumor is suspected to be benign. However, if the margins of an excisional biopsy of a malignant tumor are wide enough, such biopsies could actually serve the same purpose as radical resections. Such extensive excisional biopsies could also reduce the number of operations that are needed to treat a tumor. Thus, if a low-grade malignant tumor (e.g., BCC) is suspected, an excisional biopsy that includes several millimeters of normal skin margin may be considered. For high-grade malignant tumors, excisional biopsies will often lead to a pathologic diagnosis that indicates the need for additional wide resection, radiation therapy, and/or chemotherapy.

A way to detect lymph node metastasis that is increasingly being used is to perform sentinel node biopsy, which shows whether the cancer has spread to the very first lymph node.[4] If the sentinel lymph node does not contain cancer, it is highly likely that the cancer has not spread to any other area of the body. However, this technique is only of therapeutic value for patients with positive nodes: for patients who have negative nodes, the possibility that the lymph node has undetectable cancerous cells should be considered. In addition, there is no compelling evidence that the survival of patients who have a full lymph node dissection as a result of a positive sentinel lymph node biopsy is better than that of those patients who do not have a full dissection until later in the disease, when the lymph nodes can be felt by a physician. Thus, such patients may be subjected unnecessarily to full dissection, which is associated with lymphedema.

The TNM clinical classification system and the pTNM pathologic classification system

The TNM clinical classification[5,6] applies only to malignant tumors *(Figs 30.4, 30.5)*. T indicates the size of the tumor and whether it has invaded nearby tissue, N indicates whether regional lymph nodes are involved, and M indicates the presence of distant metastasis. The TNM classification system is based on clinical evidence

acquired before definitive treatment. Once intraoperative and surgical pathologic data become available, the pathologic TMN (pTNM) classification system can be used. The pT, pN, and pM categories correspond to the T, N, and M categories.

Regional lymph nodes are those that drain the site of the primary tumor *(Fig. 30.6)*. The pN assessment of the regional lymph nodes requires that a sufficient number of lymph nodes are removed for histologic examination (usually six or more). If the examined lymph nodes are negative but fewer than six lymph nodes were resected, the pN classification is designated pN0.

Box 30.3 shows examples of the TNM classification system, namely the systems used for eyelid, vulva, penis, and soft-tissue sarcomas.

Clinical staging

The TNM system[5,6] is used to show the anatomical extent of malignant tumors. For purposes of tabulation and analysis, it is useful to condense these categories into stages *(Table 30.1)*. To be consistent with the TNM system, carcinoma *in situ* is categorized as stage 0. In general, tumors that are localized to the organ of origin are categorized as stages I and II, while those that exhibit extensive local spread, particularly to the regional lymph nodes, are classified as stage III. The tumors that have distant metastasis are classified as stage IV. For pathological stage groups, if sufficient tissue has been removed for pathological examination to evaluate the highest T and N categories, M1 may be either clinical (cM1) or pathological (pM1). However, if only a distant metastasis has had microscopic confirmation, the classification is pathological (pM1) and the stage is pathological.

Treatment

Wide excision

With regard to wide resection of malignant tumors of skin, the horizontal and vertical margins vary depending on the type of tumor. Retrospective histopathologic studies have supported reductions in the horizontal margin in recent years. The horizontal margins that are

T – Primary tumor*

TX	Primary tumor cannot be assessed
T0	No evidence of primary tumor
Tis	Carcinoma in situ
T1	The greatest dimension of the tumor is 2 cm or less
T2	The greatest dimension of the tumor is more than 2 cm but less than 5 cm
T3	The greatest dimension of the tumor is more than 5 cm
T4	The tumor invades deep extradermal structures such as cartilage, skeletal muscle, or bone

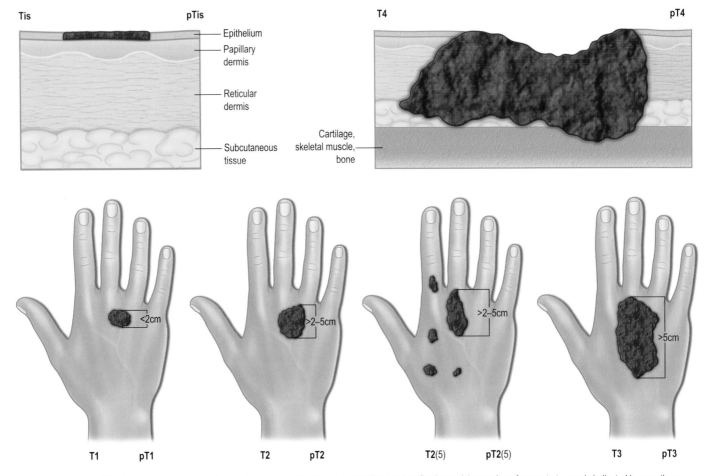

* In the case of multiple simultaneous tumors, the tumor with the highest T category is used for the classification and the number of separate tumors is indicated in parentheses (e.g., T2 (5))

Fig. 30.4 The T factor of the TNM classification system, as described by the International Union for Cancer (UICC). (Used with the permission of the Union for International Cancer Control (UICC), Geneva, Switzerland. The original source for this material is TNM Atlas: Illustrated Guide to the TNM/pTNM Classification of Malignant Tumours 5th edition. Edited by Christian F. Wittekind, Frederick L. Greene, Robert V.P. Hutter, Martin Klimpfinger, Leslie H. Sobin. Springer, 2004, ISBN: 9783540442349.)

recommended for particular tumor types are listed in *(Box 30.4)*. In the case of malignant soft-tissue tumors, the type of excision can vary with regard to the extent of the margins around the tumor: curative wide, wide, and marginal excisions indicate margins that are at least 5 cm outside the tumor-reactive layer, less than 5 cm outside the tumor-reactive layer, and within the tumor-reactive layer, respectively. Moreover, Mohs micrographic surgery, where tumors undergo histologic analysis during surgery in such a way that almost all of the surgical margins can be examined for tumor extensions, can help to obtain complete margin control during the removal of a skin cancer and soft-tissue sarcoma.[7]

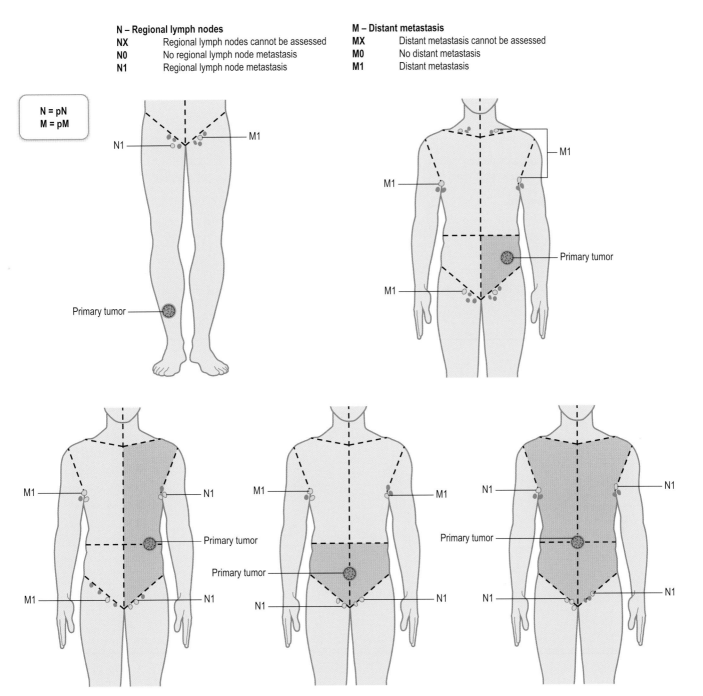

Fig. 30.5 The N and M factors of the TNM classification system, as described by the International Union for Cancer (UICC). (Used with the permission of the Union for International Cancer Control (UICC), Geneva, Switzerland. The original source for this material is TNM Atlas: Illustrated Guide to the TNM/pTNM Classification of Malignant Tumours 5th edition. Edited by Christian F. Wittekind, Frederick L. Greene, Robert V.P. Hutter, Martin Klimpfinger, Leslie H. Sobin. Springer, 2004, ISBN: 9783540442349.)

Unilateral tumors

Head, neck	Ipsilateral preauricular, submandibular, cervical, and supraclavicular lymph nodes
Thorax	Ipsilateral axillary lymph nodes
Upper limb	Ipsilateral epitrochlear and axillary lymph nodes
Abdomen, loins, and buttocks	Ipsilateral inguinal lymph nodes
Lower limb	Ipsilateral popliteal and inguinal lymph nodes
Anal margin and perianal skin	Ipsilateral inguinal lymph nodes

Tumors in the boundary zones

Between
Right / left midline

Head and neck / thorax	Clavicula-acromion-upper shoulder blade edge
Thorax / upper limb	Shoulder-axilla-shoulder
Thorax / abdomen, loins, and buttocks	Front: middle between the navel and the costal arch. Back: lower border of the thoracic vertebrae (midtransverse axis)
Abdomen, loins, and buttocks / lower limb	Groin-trochanter-gluteal sulcus

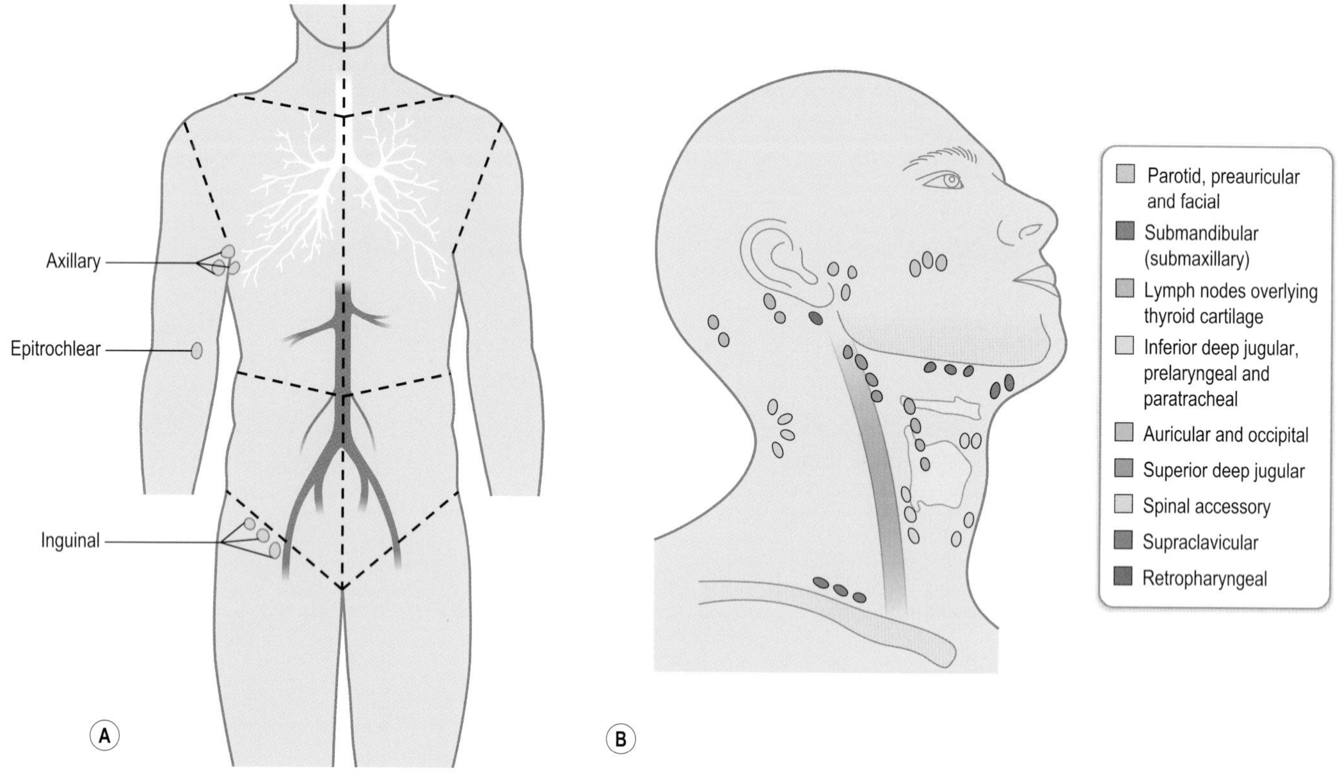

Fig. 30.6 The regional lymph nodes, as described by the International Union for Cancer (UICC). (Used with the permission of the Union for International Cancer Control (UICC), Geneva, Switzerland. The original source for this material is TNM Atlas: Illustrated Guide to the TNM/pTNM Classification of Malignant Tumours 5th edition. Edited by Christian F. Wittekind, Frederick L. Greene, Robert V.P. Hutter, Martin Klimpfinger, Leslie H. Sobin. Springer, 2004, ISBN: 9783540442349.)

Lymph node dissection

Axillary lymph node dissection

Since sentinel lymph node biopsy is now a widely practiced technique, there are fewer occasions where preventive axillary lymph node dissection is necessary. Metastatic squamous cell carcinoma (SCC) is an example of a malignant nonmelanocytic skin tumor that warrants axillary lymph node dissection. Axillary lymph nodes can be classified into levels I, II, and III, which relate to the lateral and internal edges of the pectoralis minor muscle. Level I is the bottom level and lies below the lower edge of the pectoralis minor muscle. Level II lies underneath the pectoralis minor muscle, while level III is above the pectoralis minor muscle. Structures that

Box 30.3 The TNM classification systems for eyelid, vulva, penis, and soft-tissue sarcomas (International Union for Cancer)

Carcinoma of the skin of the eyelid

TX Primary tumor cannot be assessed

T0 No evidence of primary tumor

Tis Carcinoma *in situ*

T1 The tumor is of any size and does not invade the tarsal plate; or the tumor is at the eyelid margin and its greatest dimension is 5.0 mm or less

T2 The tumor invades the tarsal plate; or the tumor is at the eyelid margin and its greatest dimension is more than 5.0 mm but less than 10.0 mm

T3 The tumor involves the full eyelid thickness; or the tumor is at the eyelid margin and its greatest dimension is more than 10.0 mm

T4 The tumor invades adjacent structures, including the bulbar conjunctiva, sclera/globe, soft tissues of the orbit, perineural invasion, bone/periosteum of the orbit, nasal cavity/paranasal sinuses, and central nervous system

N1 Regional lymph node metastasis

Carcinoma of the skin of the vulva

TX Primary tumor cannot be assessed

T0 No evidence of primary tumor

Tis Carcinoma *in situ*

T1 The tumor is confined to the vulva, or the vulva and the perineum, and its greatest dimension is 2 cm or less

T1a The tumor is confined to the vulva, or the vulva and perineum, its greatest dimension is 2 cm or less, and it exhibits stromal invasion that is no greater than 1.0 mm

T1b The tumor is confined to the vulva, or the vulva and the perineum, its greatest dimension is 2 cm or less, and it exhibits stromal invasion that is greater than 1.0 mm

T2 The tumor is confined to the vulva, or the vulva and the perineum, and its greatest dimension is more than 2 cm

T3 The tumor invades the lower urethra, vagina, and/or anus

T4 The tumor invades the bladder mucosa, rectal mucosa, and/or upper urethral mucosa, or is fixed to the pubic bone

NX Regional lymph nodes cannot be assessed

N0 No regional lymph node metastasis

N1 Unilateral regional lymph node metastasis

N2 Bilateral regional lymph node metastasis

Carcinoma of the skin of the penis

TX Primary tumor cannot be assessed

T0 No evidence of primary tumor

Tis Carcinoma *in situ*

Ta Noninvasive verrucous carcinoma

T1 The tumor invades the subepithelial connective tissue

T2 The tumor invades the corpus spongiosum or cavernosum

T3 The tumor invades the urethra or prostate

T4 The tumor invades other adjacent structures

NX Regional lymph nodes cannot be assessed

N0 No regional lymph node metastasis

N1 Metastasis in a single superficial inguinal lymph node

N2 Metastasis in multiple or bilateral superficial inguinal lymph nodes

N3 Metastasis in deep inguinal or pelvic lymph nodes, unilateral or bilateral

Soft-tissue sarcoma

TX Primary tumor cannot be assessed

T0 No evidence of primary tumor

T1 The greatest dimension of the tumor is 5 cm or less

T1a The tumor is superficial*

T1b The tumor is deep*

T2 The greatest dimension of the tumor is more than 5 cm

T2a The tumor is superficial

T2b The tumor is deep

N1 Regional lymph node metastasis

*Superficial tumors are located exclusively above the superficial fascia and do not invade the fascia, while deep tumors are either exclusively beneath the superficial fascia, or are superficial to the fascia but invade into or through the fascia. Retroperitoneal, mediastinal, and pelvic sarcomas are classified as deep tumors.

(Modified from Sobin LH, Gospodarowicz MK, Wittekind C (eds) TNM Classification of Malignant Tumours (UICC: International Union Against Cancer), 7th edn. New Jersey: Wiley-Blackwell, 2009; and Wittekind CF, Greene FL, Hutter RVP et al. (eds) TNM Atlas: Illustrated Guide to the TNM/pTNM Classification of Malignant Tumours, 5th edn. Heidelberg: Springer, 2004.)

should be preserved during axillary lymph node dissection are the pectoral nerves, the long thoracic nerve, the intercostobrachial nerves, the axillary artery and veins, the thoracoacromial artery and veins, and the subscapular artery and veins.

Inguinal lymph node dissection

Widespread use of sentinel lymph node dissection has also reduced the frequency of inguinal lymph node dissection. Representative indications for inguinal lymph node dissection are metastatic SCC and extramammary Paget's disease (EMPD). Traditionally, the area of dissection is a triangle composed of the inguinal ligament, the internal edge of the sartorius muscle, and the internal edge of the long adductor muscle. In the wide resection of inguinal lymph nodes, the femoral vein is identified along with the saphenous vein. After clamping the saphenous vein, the adductor longus muscle is identified and should be cleaned of all fatty nodal tissue by retracting the saphenous vein en bloc with the lymph nodes until the adductor canal is reached.

Table 30.1 Clinical staging (International Union for Cancer)

Carcinoma of the skin (general staging system)

Stage	T	N	M
Stage 0	Tis	N0	M0
Stage I	T1	N0	M0
Stage II*	T2	N0	M0
Stage III	T3		
	T1, 2, 3	N1	M0
Stage IV	T1, 2, 3	N2, 3	M0
	T4	AnyT	M0
	AnyT	AnyN	M1

*The American Joint Committee on Cancer considers stage I tumors that have more than one high-risk feature to be stage II tumors.

Merkel cell carcinoma of the skin

Stage	T	N	M
Stage 0	Tis	N0	M0
Stage I	T1	N0	M0
Stage IA	T1	pN0	M0
Stage IB	T1	cN0	M0
Stage IIA	T2, 3	pN0	M0
Stage IIB	T2, 3	cN0	M0
Stage IIC	T4	N0	M0
Stage IIIA	AnyT	N1a*	M0
Stage IIIB	AnyT	N1b*, 2	M0
Stage IV	AnyT	AnyN	M1

*N1a: Microscopic metastasis (clinically occult: cN0 + pN1)

N1b: Microscopic metastasis (clinically occult: cN1 + pN1)

Carcinoma of the skin of the eyelid

Stage	T	N	M
Stage 0	Tis	N0	M0
Stage IA	T1	N0	M0
Stage IB	T2a*	N0	M0
Stage IC	T2b*	N0	M0
Stage II	T3a*	N0	M0
Stage IIIA	T3b*	N0	M0
Stage IIIB	AnyT	N1	M0
Stage IIIC	T4	N1	M0
Stage IV	AnyT	AnyN	M1

*T2a: >5–10 mm in its greatest dimension or located at the tarsal plate or lid margin

T2b: >10–20 mm in its greatest dimension or located in the full-thickness eyelid

T3a: >20 mm in its greatest dimension, located in adjacent ocular/orbital structures, or showing perineural invasion

T3b: Needs enucleation, exenteration, or bone resection

Carcinoma of the skin of the vulva

Stage	T	N	M
Stage 0	Tis	N0	M0
Stage I	T1	N0	M0

Stage	T	N	M
Stage IA	T1a	N0	M0
Stage IB	T1b	N0	M0
Stage II	T2	N0	M0
Stage IIIA	T1, 2	N1a, 1b*	M0
Stage IIIB	T1, 2	N2a, 2b*	M0
Stage IIIC	T1, 2	N2c*	M0
Stage IVA	T1, 2	N3*	M0
	T3	AnyT	M0
Stage IVB	AnyT	AnyN	M0

*N1a: 1–2 lymph node metastases, each with a greatest dimension less than 5 mm

N1b: 1 lymph node metastasis whose greatest dimension is 5 mm or greater

N2a: 3 or more lymph node metastases, each with a greatest dimension less than 5 mm

N2b: 2 or more lymph node metastases whose greatest dimensions are 5 mm or greater

N2c: Lymph node metastasis with extracapsular spread

N3: Fixed or ulcerated regional lymph node metastasis

Carcinoma of the skin of the penis

Stage	T	N	M
Stage 0	Tis	N0	M0
	Ta	N0	M0
Stage I	T1a	N0	M0
Stage II	T1b	N0	M0
	T2	N0, 1	M0
	T3	N0	M0
Stage IIIA	T1, 2, 3	N1	M0
Stage IIIB	T1, 2, 3	N2	M0
Stage IV	T4	AnyN	M0
	AnyT	N3	M0
	AnyT	AnyN	M1

Soft-tissue sarcoma

Stage	T	N	M	Grade
Stage IA	T1a	N0	M0	Low-grade
	T1b	N0	M0	Low-grade
Stage IB	T2a	N0	M0	Low-grade
	T2b	N0	M0	Low-grade
Stage IIA*	T1a	N0	M0	High-grade
	T1b	N0	N0	High-grade
Stage IIB	T2a	N0	M0	High-grade
Stage III	T2b	N0	M0	High-grade
Stage IV	AnyT	N1	M0	AnyG
	AnyT	AnyN	M1	AnyG

*Extraskeletal Ewing and primitive neuroectodermal tumors are classified as high-grade. If grade cannot be assessed, classify the tumor as low-grade.

(Modified from Sobin LH, Gospodarowicz MK, Wittekind C (eds) TNM Classification of Malignant Tumours (UICC: International Union Against Cancer), 7th edn. New Jersey: Wiley-Blackwell, 2009; and Wittekind CF, Greene FL, Hutter RVP et al. (eds) TNM Atlas: Illustrated Guide to the TNM/pTNM Classification of Malignant Tumours, 5th edn. Heidelberg: Springer, 2004.)

Box 30.4 **Recommended surgical margins of wide excisions of nonmelanocytic tumors of the skin and soft tissues**

Horizontal margin

3–5 mm
Bowen's disease, solar keratosis, basal cell carcinoma

10–30 mm
Squamous cell carcinoma, malignant appendage-origin tumors, extramammary Paget's disease, Merkel cell carcinoma, malignant mesenchymal-origin tumors

50 mm
Malignant soft-tissue tumors

Vertical margin

With fat layer
Tumors that are limited to the dermis

With deep fascia
Tumors that extend into the fat layer

With skeletal muscle
Tumors that extend into the deep fascia

With the membranes of deeper structures such as cartilage or bone
Tumors that extend into skeletal muscle

With deeper structures like cartilage or bone
Tumors that extend into membranes of deeper structures like cartilage or bone

Others
The margins of wide tumor excisions that occur in anatomically complicated and special regions (e.g., eyelid, vulva, penis, finger/toe tip, and ear) will vary on a case-by-case basis. This is also true for soft-tissue tumors. In general, at least one layer of barrier structure should be excised. For example, for tumors that are limited to the fat layer, the deep fascia of skeletal muscle is considered as the barrier structure and should be removed with the tumor upon wide excision.

Reconstructive surgery

Reconstruction via skin grafting is a basic surgical technique that is used to reconstruct the tissue defects that occur after tumor extirpation, that is also useful for early detection of local recurrence. The most ideal approach after tumor extirpation is to suture the wound margins directly together. However, this can only be performed if the wound is not too big and the adjacent skin can be extended sufficiently. One concern with this approach is that malignant cells may be left in the deep margins of the wound. Recent developments in reconstructive techniques, including thin flap-based techniques and wound coverage materials, mean that plastic surgeons can now choose from a wide and rapidly evolving variety of primary and aesthetic secondary reconstruction methods. Given this constantly altering medical (and

social) environment, it is difficult to develop up-to-date reconstructive algorithms, and indeed, previous algorithms such as the reconstructive ladder, elevator, and triangle quickly lose favor. Consequently, the techniques that are chosen for primary and secondary reconstruction are largely determined on a case-by-case basis. However, one current and useful model is the reconstructive matrix,[8] which helps plastic surgeons to determine the best reconstructive solutions for their patients in the context of particular medical and socioeconomic environments by considering aspects of surgical complexity, technological sophistication, and patient surgical risk.

Radiation therapy

Malignant tumors vary in their sensitivity to radiation-induced damage, which directly affects the success of radiation therapy. For example, malignant melanomas are less sensitive to radiation and are therefore rarely treated with radiation therapy. Malignant skin tumors that are relatively sensitive to radiation and are therefore commonly treated with radiation therapy include BCC,[9] SCC,[10] and Merkel cell carcinoma of the skin.[11] Acute skin reactions to radiation therapy occur during the first 7–10 days after treatment and are characterized initially by erythema that then progresses to pigmentation, epilation, and desquamation; this is particularly the case when higher doses are used. Subacute and late complications occur several weeks after radiation therapy and can progress for long periods of time. These complications include scarring, permanent pigmentation, depigmentation, atrophy, telangiectasis, subcutaneous fibrosis, and necrosis.

Chemotherapy

Chemotherapy can be either adjuvant or primary, and all chemotherapies can be administered either systemically or topically. Adjuvant chemotherapy is mainly used for malignant melanoma, while primary chemotherapy is indicated for SCC,[12] angiosarcoma,[13] and EMPD.[14] However, the radical chemotherapy with which malignant skin tumors are generally treated can sometimes be seen as neoadjuvant chemotherapy before surgery for advanced-stage cancer. Single-agent chemotherapies include peplomycin sulfate and CPT-11[15] for

SCC, pacitaxel for angiosarcoma, and docetaxel for angiosarcoma and EMPD. Multiagent chemotherapies includes cisplatin + doxorubicin and cisplatin + 5-fluorouracil (5-FU) + bleomycin for SCC; mesna + doxorubicin + ifosfamide + dacarbazine for angiosarcoma; and 5-FU + mitomycin C, 5-FU + carboplatin + leucovorin, and 5-FU + carboplatin + mitomycin C + epirubicin + vincristine for EMPD.

Laser therapy

Dye lasers or neodymium-doped yttrium aluminum garnet (Nd: YAG) lasers can be used for lesions that are characterized by neoplastic changes or malformations in capillary vessels or their overgrowth, such as hemangiomas,[16] vascular malformations,[17] and keloid/hypertrophic scars.[18] Ruby and alexandrite lasers can be used to treat superficial pigmented lesions whose colors range from brown to black, while Q-switched ruby and alexandrite lasers are useful for intradermal pigmented lesions such as the nevus of Ota.[19] CO_2 lasers and erbium yttrium aluminum garnet (Er: YAG) lasers target the water contents of a lesion,[20] which makes them suitable for lesions with various colors like seborrheic keratosis, telangiectatic granuloma, xanthoma, and fibroma.

Others (including immunotherapy, cryotherapy, electrocoagulation therapy, and sclerotherapy)

At this stage, the only indication for immunotherapy is malignant melanoma. Cryotherapy and electrocoagulation therapy induce the freezing and melting of the tumor tissues, which results in their necrosis and/or apoptosis; these methods are suitable for superficial benign or malignant tumors like seborrheic keratosis, fibroma, and BCC. Sclerotherapy, where a sclerosant like ethanol, ethanolamine oleate, polidocanol, or OK-432 is injected into affected vessels, can be used to treat vascular malformations. Promising technologies that may become useful in the near future include: hyperthermic infusion therapy, where the tumor is infused with a substance that makes it more susceptible to locally applied heat; molecular target therapy, which involves drugs or other substances that block the growth and spread of the tumor by interfering with specific tumor growth and progression molecules; and gene therapy and gene cell therapy, where genes are manipulated in target healthy cells (to enhance their cancer-fighting properties) or in target cancer cells (to kill them or inhibit their growth).

Benign cutaneous and soft-tissue tumors

Benign epithelial-origin tumors

Epidermal nevus (e.g., verrucous epidermal nevus and linear epidermal nevus)

This nevus is composed of skin cells that normally occur at the affected site but show hyperkeratosis and papillomatosis (*Fig. 30.7*). It can be considered to be a hamartoma, which is a benign focal, tumor-like malformation that is composed of a mixture of the cells that characterize the tissue of its origin; such nodules grow at the same rate as the surrounding tissues. The dermis below the epithelial nevus is usually normal. Epithelial nevi sometimes exhibit a diffuse or extensive distribution that affects a large area of the patient's body (termed systematized epidermal nevus); careful observation is necessary in these cases. Systematized epidermal nevus often occurs together with abnormalities in other organ systems. This condition is termed epidermal nevus syndrome,[21] and has been described as a sporadic neurocutaneous linkage of congenital ectodermal defects in the skin, brain, eyes, and/or skeleton. Laser therapy, cryotherapy, electrocoagulation, surgical abrasion, and excision are suitable for treating epithelial nevi. If abrasion therapy is used, it should be remembered that these lesions are usually limited to the epidermis; thus, to prevent heavy scarring, only the epidermis and the superficial layer of the dermis should be removed.

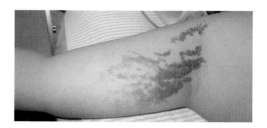

Fig. 30.7 Epidermal nevus of the upper arm.

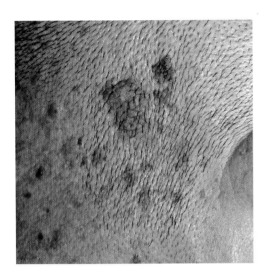

Fig. 30.8 Seborrheic keratosis on the temporal region.

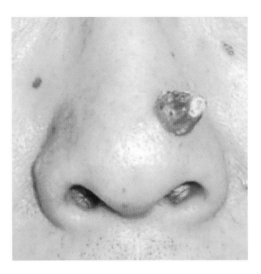

Fig. 30.9 Keratoacanthoma on the nose.

Seborrheic keratosis (also known as senile wart)

This is a benign skin growth that originates from the basal and squamous cells in the epidermis *(Fig. 30.8)*. It should be differentiated from nevus cell nevus, senile keratosis, BCC, and malignant melanoma. The sign of Leser–Trélat, which is the dramatic, sudden appearance of multiple seborrheic keratoses, can be a paraneoplastic syndrome, namely an ominous sign of an internal malignancy.[22] In such cases, not only do new lesions suddenly appear, pre-existing lesions also frequently increase in size and become symptomatic. This sign should not be overlooked and screening for internal malignancy should be recommended to the patient. Laser therapy, cryotherapy, electrocoagulation, surgical abrasion, and excision are all suitable treatments for seborrheic keratosis. However, if the tumor invades the dermis, which can occur, surgical excision is recommended.

Keratoacanthoma

Keratoacanthoma has been a controversial entity for many years, mainly because it closely resembles SCC[23] *(Fig. 30.9)*. It grows rapidly and can sometimes self-heal. Upon histopathology, atypical squamous cells can be detected, which makes it difficult to distinguish from SCC. For this reason, excisional biopsy should be considered despite the fact that this lesion occasionally self-heals. If the lesion is on the nose and face, Mohs micrographic surgery is particularly suitable since it

facilitates good margin control along with minimal tissue removal.

Epidermoid cyst (also known as epidermal cyst and atheroma)

Epidermal cyst is a smooth, dome-shaped, freely movable, somewhat fluctuant subcutaneous swelling that is sometimes attached to the skin by a central pore *(Fig. 30.10)*. It is covered with a stratified squamous epithelium that resembles the epidermis or the follicular infundibulum; thus, there is a granular cell layer adjacent to the keratin-containing cyst lumen. Epidermoid cysts can rupture spontaneously or be ruptured by external mechanical forces. Extremely large epidermoid cysts, also known as giant atheromas *(Fig. 30.11)*, should undergo pathology to rule out malignant change,[24] although such changes are rare. Epidermoid cysts that exhibit inflammation or recur should be removed by simple excision. In the case of large cysts, the contents can be removed first, after which the cyst walls can be removed with minimal incision *(Fig. 30.12)*. In cases where pus and blood are excreted, the surgeon should consider incising the cyst and draining it first, and then excising it completely 1–2 weeks later.

Milia

Milia are a smaller version of an epidermoid cyst (less than 4 mm in diameter). They may derive from the outer root sheath of vellus follicles. There are primary

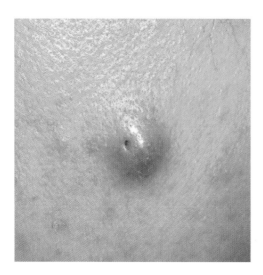

Fig. 30.10 Epidermoid cyst with a central pore.

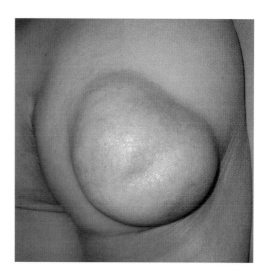

Fig. 30.11 Giant atheroma.

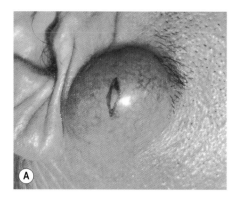
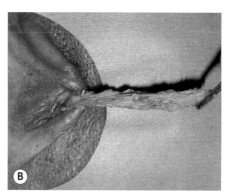
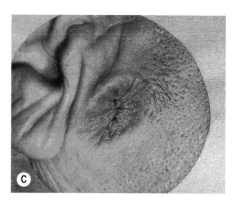

Fig. 30.12 An epidermoid cyst **(A)** and the removal of the cyst with a minimal incision **(B, C)**.

and secondary milia.[25] Primary milia include congenital milia, benign primary milia of children and adults, milia en plaque, nodular grouped milia, multiple eruptive milia, nevus depigmentosus with milia, and genodermatosis-associated milia. Secondary milia are the disease-, medication-, and trauma-associated milia. Milia can be treated easily by making small holes in the surface with a needle or CO_2 laser and then extruding the contents.

Dermoid cyst

A dermoid cyst is a congenital subcutaneous cyst that develops along the embryonic lines of closure *(Fig. 30.13)*. It is most common on the head and neck area, particularly the supraorbital region, brow, upper eyelid, glabella, and scalp. These cysts can be easily removed surgically, but care should be taken not to injure the temporal branch of the facial nerve. The cyst lumen contains keratin debris and hair shaft fragments. Preoperative X-rays should be taken to distinguish it from pilomatricoma on the head and neck region, especially in pediatric patients. Since it has been reported that dermoid cysts can exhibit malignant changes, complete surgical removal is recommended.[26]

Others

Rare benign epidermal-origin skin tumors include clear cell acanthoma, large cell acanthoma, acantholytic acanthoma, warty dyskeratoma, traumatic inclusion cyst, human papillomavirus-associated cyst, proliferating epidermal cyst, and cutaneous keratocyst. The preoperative diagnosis of these tumors can be difficult, but many can be treated radically with a simple excision and suture.

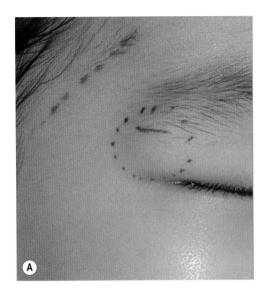
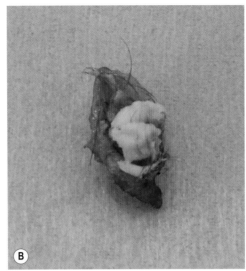

Fig. 30.13 (A) Dermoid cyst on the supraorbital region; **(B)** the excised cyst.

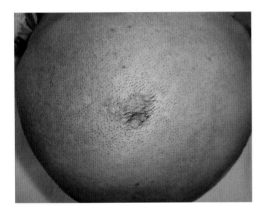

Fig. 30.14 Nevus sebaceous on the scalp.

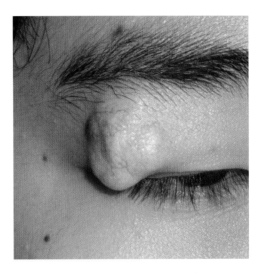

Fig. 30.15 Pilomatricoma on the upper eyelid.

Benign appendage-origin tumors

Nevus sebaceous

Nevus sebaceous is a hamartoma rather than a neoplasm *(Fig. 30.14)*. It is essentially confined to the head and neck regions, and can be found not only in the sebaceous gland but also in the epidermis, dermis, hair follicles, and sweat glands. Consequently, it is also referred to as organoid nevus. In appearance, it resembles an epidermal nevus. Since other tumors like BCC and trichilemmoma can arise from nevus sebaceous over time,[27] complete surgical excision is recommended. If it is located in the hair, the hair stream should be carefully considered while performing the excision and suturing; moreover, dehairing caused by unnecessary buried or dermal sutures should be avoided.

Pilomatricoma (also known as calcifying epithelioma and pilomatrixoma)

This is a cystic nodule that tends to occur on the head and neck regions of young patients *(Fig. 30.15)*. Multiple pilomatricoma may be seen in a familial setting in patients who also have myotonic dystrophy. A calcified region can be seen by ultrasound, X-ray, CT and MRI. This region will appear as a high-intensity signal on ultrasound, while on MRI it will show up as a low-intensity signal on both T1WI and T2WI. Since malignant tumors sometimes have a calcified lesion that is caused by necrosis, it is necessary to exclude this possibility when making a diagnosis of pilomatricoma. It is not associated with a clear capsule and thus should be excised carefully and completely to prevent recurrence. Malignant pilomatricoma has been reported,[28] but there have been less convincing reports of the carcinomatous transformation of pre-existing benign pilomatricoma.

Trichilemmal cyst

This is a subcutaneous cyst that is derived from the outer root sheath of the hair follicle and arises most frequently on the hairy region on the head *(Fig. 30.16)*. Clinically, it resembles an epidermoid cyst. Multiple cysts on the head are seen in 70% of cases. Complete excision is recommended. The conservative approach involves a small punch biopsy of the cyst that allows the cyst cavity to be entered. The contents of the cyst can then be emptied, leaving an empty cyst wall that can be grasped with a forceps and pulled out of the small incision. This method often results in a very small scar and very little, if any, bleeding. Proliferating trichilemmal cyst is an uncommon lesion that is characterized histologically by trichilemmal keratinization. It is thought to originate from a trichilemmal cyst and to have the potential for malignant transformation, at which point it is termed a malignant proliferating trichilemmal cyst.[29]

Syringoma

Syringoma is the result of intradermal eccrine proliferation that is malformative rather than neoplastic in most cases. It occurs mainly on the eyelids and presents as a 1–2-mm nodule. Since the main reason for treating syringoma is cosmetic, the tumor should be destroyed in such a way that there is minimal scarring and no recurrence. For this purpose, electrocoagulation, dermabrasion, CO_2 lasers, Er:YAG lasers, and fractional photothermolysis[30] can be used, although attention should be paid to preventing pigmentation and scarring.

Apocrine cystadenoma (also known as apocrine cysthidroma)

Apocrine cystadenoma is characterized by the dilatation of an apocrine duct and secondary proliferation of the ductal epithelium that is architecturally bland *(Fig. 30.17)*. Apocrine cystadenomas appear most commonly as solitary, soft, dome-shaped, and translucent papules or nodules. They are located most frequently on the eyelids, especially the inner canthus. They grow slowly and usually persist indefinitely. They can be incised and drained, but electrosurgical

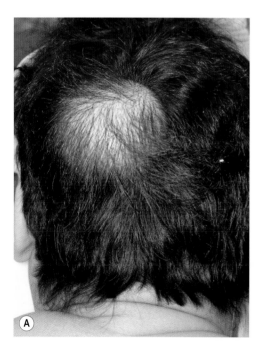
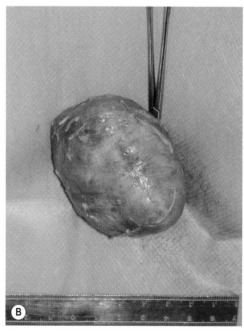

Fig. 30.16 Solitary trichilemmal cyst on the scalp **(A)** and after its excision **(B)**.

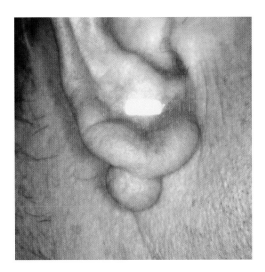

Fig. 30.17 Apocrine cystadenoma on the earlobe.

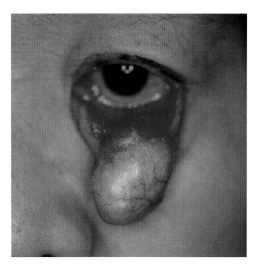

Fig. 30.18 Chondroid syringoma on the lower eyelid.

destruction of the cyst wall is often needed to prevent recurrence. Punch, scissors, or elliptical excision can also remove these tumors. Multiple cystoadenomas can be treated with a CO_2 laser. Trichloroacetic acid[31] has also been used.

Chondroid syringoma (also known as cutaneous mixed tumor)

Chondroid syringoma derives from the sweat glands and is most frequently seen on the head and neck, where it presents as an unexceptional dermal or subcutaneous nodule *(Fig. 30.18)*. The tumor consists of a gland-like epithelial component that is set in a chondromyxoid stromal component. It is believed that there are both eccrine and apocrine variants. Hirsch and Helwig[32] proposed the following five histologic criteria for diagnosis: (1) nests of cuboidal or polygonal cells; (2) intercommunicating tubuloalveolar structures lined with two or more rows of cuboidal cells; (3) ductal structures composed of one or two rows of cuboidal cells; (4) occasional keratinous cyst; and (5) a matrix of varying composition. Since malignant forms have been reported, although they are rare, complete surgical excision is recommended.[33]

Others

Other benign appendage-origin tumors include steatocystoma multiplex *(Fig. 30.19)*, trichofolliculoma, trichoepithelioma, poroma folliculare, trichilemmoma,

sebaceous adenoma, eccrine nevus, and apocrine nevus. Moreover, hair follicles, sebaceous glands, and sweat glands (apocrine and eccrine glands) can undergo hyperplasia that results in a hamartoma; these skin appendages can also develop adenomas, benign epitheliomas, and primordial epitheliomas.

Benign neural crest-origin tumors

Pigment cell nevus (also known as pigmented nevus and nevus cell nevus)

These are acquired and congenital nevi that originate from melanocytes. It has been suggested that healthy adults have on average 5–10 nevi. Dome-like elevated nevi sometimes bear hair. If an acquired nevus has a diameter of more than 7 mm and it is still growing, the possibility of malignant melanoma should be considered. It seems now that malignant melanomas do not originate from pigment cell nevus (except in the case of congenital giant nevus) but rather derive directly from epidermal melanocytes; this is known as the *de novo* carcinogenesis theory.[34] There are five types of pigmented nevi, as follows.

Lentigo simplex

Lentigo simplex is a black-brown pigmented nevus, 2–3 mm in diameter. It is believed to be an acquired pigment cell nevus that is at an early stage *(Fig. 30.20)*. Its margins can be either jagged or smooth. It is the

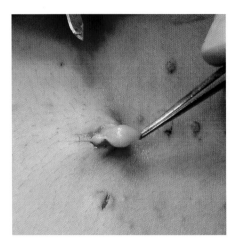

Fig. 30.19 Steatocystoma multiplex on the trunk.

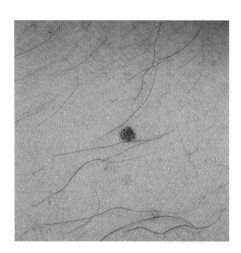

Fig. 30.20 Lentigo simplex on the forearm.

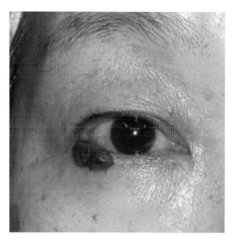

Fig. 30.21 Intradermal nevus on the lower eyelid.

result of the proliferation of melanocytes in the basal layer of epidermis. It is not induced by sun exposure and is not associated with systemic disease. The lesions are few in number and may occur anywhere on the skin or mucous membranes. They usually first appear in early childhood around 3 years of age, but they can also be present at birth or develop later. Cryosurgery, lasers,[35] and simple excision can be tried.

Acquired pigment cell nevus

Acquired pigment cell nevi are due to the proliferation of melanocytes and can be divided into three types according to the location of the melanocytes. In junction nevi, the melanocytes are mainly located at the junction between the epidermis and dermis. In compound nevi, the melanocytes are located in the dermis as well as at the junction between the epidermis and dermis. In intradermal nevi *(Fig. 30.21)*, the melanocytes are in the dermis only. Laser treatment is ineffective for melanocytes located in the deeper layer of dermis because these cells lack the melanin pigment. Thus, simple surgical excision is recommended to prevent recurrence. The nevus that has a depigmented area around it is called Sutton's halo nevus.[36]

Congenital pigment cell nevus

The congenital pigment cell nevus is present at the time of birth and increases in size as the body grows, although its shape does not change. It is divided according to size into the small type (less than 1.5 cm in diameter), medium type (1.5–20 cm in diameter), and large or giant

type (over 20 cm in diameter) *(Fig. 30.22)*. Histology shows that the nevus cells tend to be diffusely distributed in the deep layer of the dermis. Careful observation is needed because malignant melanomas can arise from giant congenital pigmented cell nevi.[37] Nevi that present on both the upper and lower eyelids are called divided nevi, while hairy giant nevi are called animal-skin nevi *(Fig. 30.23)*. Giant nevi should be removed and reconstructed by the serial excision method, skin grafting, local flaps, or a combination of these.

Dysplastic nevus (also known as Clark's nevus and atypical mole)

Clinically, dysplastic nevus resembles an early-stage malignant melanoma.[38] It was initially thought to be a prodrome of malignant melanoma but is now suggested to be a type of acquired pigment cell nevus. Complete excision and pathologic examination should be performed. The US National Institutes of Health Consensus Conference on the diagnosis and treatment of early melanoma defined the familial atypical mole and melanoma syndrome,[39] the criteria for which are the occurrence of malignant melanoma in one or more first- or second-degree relatives, the presence of numerous (often >50) melanocytic nevi, some of which are clinically atypical, and the presence of certain histologic features in many of the associated nevi.

Juvenile melanoma (also known as Spitz nevus)

This is a dome-like nodule that is about 1 cm in diameter and occurs on the face or legs of young patients

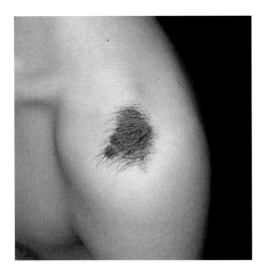

Fig. 30.22 Medium-type congenital pigment cell nevus on the back.

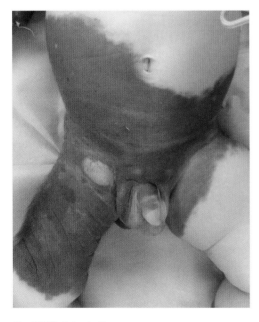

Fig. 30.23 Animal-skin nevus.

(Fig. 30.24).[40] The surface is smooth and sometimes exhibits telangiectasia. It may be nonpigmented or have a color that ranges from pink to orange-red. Some lesions are pigmented, especially those on the lower extremities. After its appearance, the lesion tends to grow rapidly and may reach a size of 1 cm within 6 months. After this rapid initial growth phase it tends to become static, although color changes may be observed. Bleeding and pruritus are rare. Complete excision and pathologic examination should be performed.

Nevus spilus (also known as café-au-lait spot)

This is a benign tumor of melanocytes that is characterized by the increased accumulation of melanin granules rather than the proliferation of melanocytes *(Fig. 30.25)*. The whole nevus has a uniform café-au-lait color. The presence of six or more nevus spilus lesions that are greater than 5 mm in diameter in prepuberty and over 15 mm in diameter in postpuberty is indicative of neurofibromatosis type 1 (NF1), also known as von Recklinghausen's disease *(Fig. 30.26)*. NF1 is caused by a mutation of the chromosome band 17q11.2, which encodes neurofibromin. Neurofibromatosis type 2 (NF2) patients rarely have nevus spilus lesions and do not demonstrate the cutaneous neurofibromas that typically result in the early diagnosis of NF1, although they may have cutaneous schwannomas that resemble skin tags. Moreover, because symptoms from cranial nerve VIII schwannomas usually begin in the third decade of life, patients with NF2 are typically diagnosed later in life than patients with NF1.[41]

Becker's melanosis (also known as Becker's pigmented hairy nevus)

This lesion is characterized by the slight proliferation of melanocytes in the basal layer of the epidermis, the increasing accumulation of melanin granules, and the presence of hair. It mainly occurs in males and develops at puberty, which suggests that androgens may play a role in its development. This is supported by the fact that it is associated with hypertrichosis, the occasional development of acneiform lesions within the patch, and, albeit rarely, with an accessory scrotum in the genital region. In addition, it has been reported that Becker melanosis lesional skin has significantly more androgen receptors than the normal surrounding skin. Ruby lasers, CO_2 lasers, and Er:YAG lasers can be used to treat Becker's melanosis.[42]

Nevus of Ota (also known as nevus fuscoceruleus ophthalmomaxillaris and oculodermal melanocytosis)

This is a blue nevus that arises from the first and second branches of the trigeminal nerve *(Fig. 30.27)*. It is common in Asians and rare in Caucasians. Women are

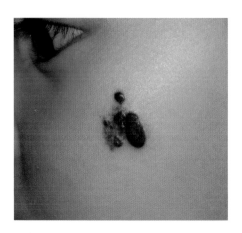

Fig. 30.24 Spitz nevus on the cheek.

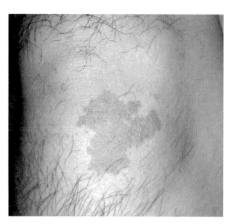

Fig. 30.25 Solitary nevus spilus on the knee.

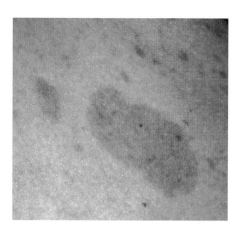

Fig. 30.26 Nevus spilus on the thigh of patient with neurofibromatosis type 1.

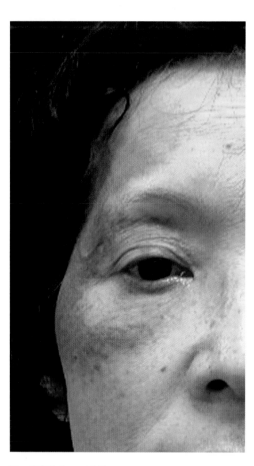

Fig. 30.27 Nevus of Ota.

nearly five times more likely to be affected than men. It is not congenital but appears during early infancy and puberty.[43] It is caused by the proliferation of melanocytes in the dermis. Bilateral nevus of Ota also exists:

this is called acquired bilateral nevus of Ota-like macules or late-onset dermal melanocytosis. It has been suggested that nevus of Ota may be derived from melanocytes that have not migrated completely from the neural crest to the epidermis during embryogenesis. The variable prevalence among different populations suggests a genetic influence, but familial cases of nevus of Ota are exceedingly rare. The two peak ages of onset in early infancy and early adolescence suggest that hormones are a factor in the development of this condition. Q-switched ruby or alexandrite lasers have been used to treat nevus of Ota.[44] After 4–8 treatments, the degree of skin pigmentation is reduced dramatically. Cryotherapy, dermabrasion, or peeling can also be used as a multimodal therapy on a case-by-case basis.

Nevus of Ito

This dermal melanocytosis can be considered as a subtype of nevus of Ota *(Fig. 30.28)*. It occurs on the acromiodeltoid region.[45] Its pathogenesis is unclear, but the fact that the dermal melanocytes of the nevus of Ito are in close proximity with nerve bundles suggests the nervous system may be a factor in its development. Recommended treatments are the same as those for nevus of Ota.

Mongolian spot (also known as congenital dermal melanocytosis)

More than 90% of Native American, 80% of Asian, and 70% of Hispanic infants have this proliferative disorder

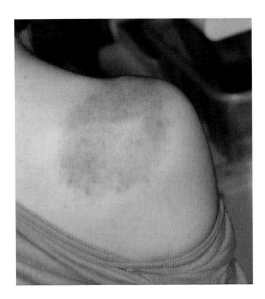

Fig. 30.28 Nevus of Ito.

of dermal melanocytes, which presents as bluish-gray spots on the sacral and coccygeal region *(Fig. 30.29)*. Fewer than 10% of Caucasian infants have mongolian spots. These spots disappear before the age of 10 years. The blue-gray color is due to the melanocytes that are deep in the skin. It usually presents as multiple spots or one large patch covering the lumbosacral area (lower back), buttocks, flanks, and/or shoulders *(Fig. 30.30)*. It results from the entrapment of melanocytes in the dermis during their migration from the neural crest to the epidermis during embryonic development.[46] Treatment is usually not necessary, but Q-switched alexandrite laser can be used for severe cases.

Blue nevus

Like the nevus of Ota and the mongolian spot, this is a dermal melanocytosis. However, it involves more cells, which means it has a nodular form. There are three types: common, cellular, and combined.[47] The cellular lesion is usually larger than the common lesion and tends to invade the subcutaneous tissue. The combined lesion is a blue nevus that is combined with a pigment cell nevus or a juvenile melanoma. A biopsy should be performed to determine the proper diagnosis. For a solitary lesion, simple excision is usually curative. There are rare cases of persistent blue nevi that manifest as satellite lesions around the original excision site. These must be distinguished from malignant blue nevus and re-excision is recommended.

Neuroma

Neuromas are hamartomas composed of peripheral nerve components, namely Schwann cells, fibroblasts, and axons; they arise as a result of ineffective, unregulated nerve regeneration that leads to neurofiber hyperplasia. They are often the result of nerve injury, especially injuries sustained during surgery; both superficial (skin or subcutaneous fat) and deep (e.g., cholecystectomy) surgery can induce neuromas. Neuromas are often very painful. It should be noted that neuroma is often used as a general term to describe any swelling of a nerve; thus, it does not necessarily mean neoplastic tumors. An example of this more general usage of the term is Morton's neuroma, which is a mononeuropathy of the foot; to avoid confusing it with a tumor, this condition is now often referred to as Morton's metatarsalgia.[48] Surgical removal is the treatment of choice for neuromas.

Schwannoma (also known as neurilemmoma)

This is a benign proliferation of Schwann cells in the dermis or subcutaneous tissues *(Fig. 30.31)*. NF2 is associated with multiple schwannomas. Pathology shows that there are two basic histological types of schwannoma called Antoni types A and B. Type A is characterized by numerous Verocay bodies. These are acellular, eosinophilic areas that are oval, linear, or serpiginous in shape and are surrounded by parallel-lying or palisading bundles of spindled Schwann cells with blunt, elongated nuclei. In each Verocay body, the long axes of the cells are all oriented toward the acellular area. Type B lacks Verocay bodies and consists of a loose, myxomatous stroma with fewer and more randomly arranged spindle cells. Neither type appears to have neurites. Schwannomas are typically encapsulated and the associated peripheral nerve may be seen in the microscopic section. Occasionally, older lesions show degenerative changes such as hemorrhage, hemosiderin deposition, mild chronic inflammatory cell infiltration, dense fibrosis, and nuclear pleomorphism. Such ancient schwannomas[49] are benign but must be differentiated from neurofibrosarcoma and malignant schwannoma. Surgical removal is the first choice of treatment.

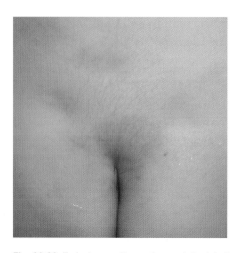

Fig. 30.29 Typical mongolian spot on an Asian infant.

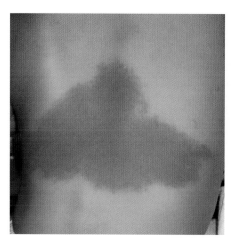

Fig. 30.30 Atypical mongolian spot on the back.

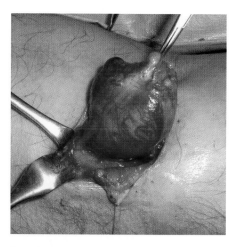

Fig. 30.31 Schwannoma on the popliteal region.

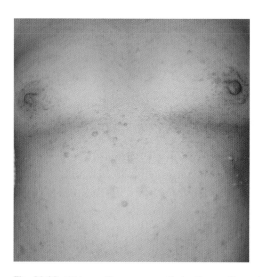

Fig. 30.32 Mild neurofibroma on a patient with neurofibromatosis type 1.

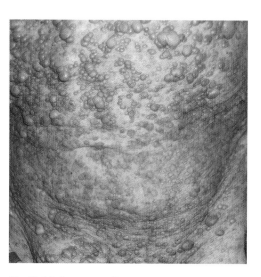

Fig. 30.33 Severe neurofibroma on a patient with neurofibromatosis type 1.

Neurofibroma

A neurofibroma is a benign tumor of the peripheral nerve sheath. It is usually found in individuals with the genetically inherited diseases NF1 and NF2, and can result in symptoms that range from physical disfiguration and pain to cognitive disability *(Figs 30.32, 30.33)*. Neurofibromas arise from Schwann cells but also incorporate many other types of cells and structural elements, which makes it difficult to identify and understand all the pathogenic mechanisms. Neurofibromas should be removed surgically or treated with a CO_2 laser. However,

once a plexiform neurofibroma[50] has undergone malignant transformation, radiation and chemotherapy can be used as adjuvant therapies.

Others

Other benign neural crest-origin tumors include the granular cell tumor and rudimentary polydactyly. The latter often have normal Merkel cells in the basal portion of the epidermis in addition to the proliferation of nerve fibers and encapsulated corpuscles. The proliferation of various neural components may be the essential feature of this condition.

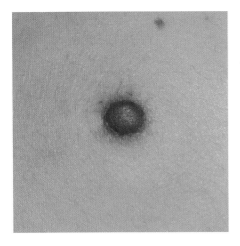

Fig. 30.34 Sclerosing hemangioma.

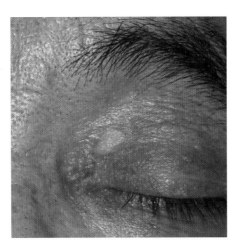

Fig. 30.35 Xanthoma on the upper eyelid.

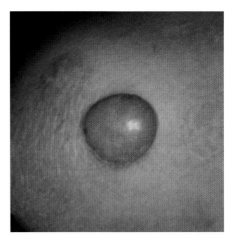

Fig. 30.36 An adult-onset juvenile xanthogranuloma on the elbow.

Benign mesenchymal-origin tumors

Dermatofibroma (also known as fibrous histiocytoma)

Dermatofibroma is a common cutaneous nodule that frequently develops on the extremities (mostly the lower legs). It is usually asymptomatic, although pruritus and tenderness are not uncommon. It is characterized by the proliferation in the dermis of both fibroblasts and other cell types, including histiocytes (skin macrophages) and vascular endothelial cells. It can be divided into the cellular type, which is mainly characterized by histiocyte proliferation, and the fibrous type, which predominantly shows fibroblast proliferation. Strong endothelial cell proliferation can sometimes be observed in both types, in which case a diagnosis of sclerosing hemangioma is made *(Fig. 30.34)*. Moreover, if the cellular components are small and the tumor is composed of hyalinized collagenous fibers, it can be called a sclerotic fibroma. There are many other special dermatofibroma forms, including hemosiderotic histiocytoma, xanthomatous histiocytoma, atypical dermatofibroma, aneurysmal dermatofibroma, myxoid dermatofibroma, and keloidal dermatofibroma.[51] Removal of the tumor is not necessary unless diagnostic uncertainty exists or particularly troubling symptoms are present.

Xanthoma

Xanthoma is characterized by the aggregation of foamy histiocytes that have phagocytized lipids *(Fig. 30.35)*.

The most common xanthoma occurs on the upper eyelid and is often associated with hyperlipidemia. Xanthomas are not always associated with underlying hyperlipidemia but when they are, it is necessary to diagnose and treat the underlying lipid disorders to decrease the xanthoma size and reduce the risk of atherosclerosis. Treatment of the hyperlipidemia initially entails dietary changes and the use of lipid-lowering agents such as statins, fibrates, bile acid-binding resins, probucol, or nicotinic acid. Eruptive xanthomas usually resolve within weeks of initiating systemic treatment, while tuberous xanthomas usually resolve after a few months. However, tendinous xanthomas take years to resolve or may persist indefinitely. While the main goal of therapy for hyperlipidemia is to reduce the risk of atherosclerotic cardiovascular disease, in patients with severe hypertriglyceridemia the goal is to prevent pancreatitis. Surgery or locally destructive modalities, including lasers, can be used for idiopathic or unresponsive xanthomas.[52]

Juvenile xanthogranuloma

This is a single or multiple dome-like tumor that occurs on the head and neck region, the body, or the limbs of young patients *(Fig. 30.36)*. Approximately 35% of cases of juvenile xanthogranuloma occur at birth, with as many as 70% of cases occurring in the first year. Most juvenile xanthogranulomas resolve by the age of 5 years. Despite the term "juvenile" in the disease name, 10% of cases manifest in adulthood. Histologic analysis can reveal the presence of Touton giant cells *(Fig. 30.37)*.

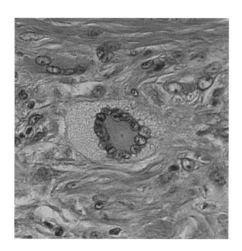

Fig. 30.37 Touton giant cell in a juvenile xanthogranuloma.

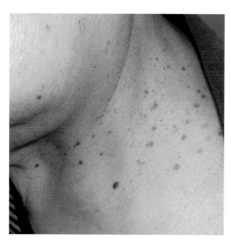

Fig. 30.38 Acrochordon.

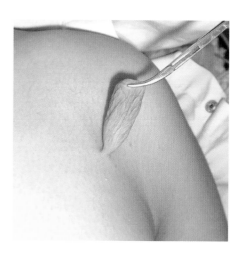

Fig. 30.39 Fibroma pendulum.

This tumor can be associated with NF1, Niemann–Pick disease, urticaria pigmentosa, and juvenile chronic myelomonocytic leukemia.[53] The lesions can be excised for diagnostic and cosmetic reasons.

Soft fibroma

There are three types of soft fibroma: (1) acrochordon (also known as a skin tag) *(Fig. 30.38)*, which occurs on the neck and axilla and increases after middle age; (2) fibroma pendulum[54] *(Fig. 30.39)*, which is a large fibroma over 10 mm in diameter that has a narrow pedicle; and (3) anything other than (1) or (2). The color can vary between normal skin color and brownish-red. Small, pedunculated soft fibromas can be removed with curved or serrated blade scissors, while larger skin tags may simply require excision. For small, soft fibromas, aluminum chloride applied prior to removal will decrease the amount of bleeding, which is usually minor anyway. Anesthesia prior to electrodesiccation is another option. Other methods of removal include cryotherapy and ligation with a suture or a copper wire; however, freezing of the surrounding skin during liquid nitrogen cryotherapy may result in dyschromic lesions. Taking hold of the acrochordon with forceps and applying cryotherapy to the forceps may provide superior results.

Keloid and hypertrophic scars

These scars are caused by the hyperproduction of collagen due to abnormal and prolonged cutaneous wound

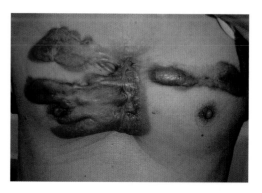

Fig. 30.40 Typical keloids on the anterior chest of an Asian patient.

healing. It has been suggested that mechanical forces such as skin-stretching tension and mechanotransduction signaling pathways are associated with their generation and growth.[55] The differential diagnosis of keloids *(Fig. 30.40)* and hypertrophic scars *(Fig. 30.41)* remains difficult; indeed, it is possible that they are manifestations of a fibroproliferative disorder of the skin[56] that expresses a continuum of features. Nevertheless, for simplicity in clinical situations, the terms "hypertrophic scars" and "keloids" can still be used: hypertrophic scars are considered to be those that improve naturally and gradually, although the full maturation process may take up to 2–5 years, whereas keloids are considered to be those that rarely resolve naturally. To prevent the development of these scars and to treat them, multimodal therapy[18] that includes steroid ointment/tape/injection, taping fixation, silicone gel sheeting, surgery, radiation,[57] cryotherapy, laser, and 5-FU is recommended.

Lipoma

Lipoma is the most common of the mesenchymal soft-tissue tumors *(Figs 30.42, 30.43)*. There are many sub-types, including lipoblastoma, angiolipoma, spindle cell lipoma, pleomorphic lipoma, and hibernoma. It was shown recently that these adipocellular tumors are characterized by specific chromosome and gene abnormalities and that these abnormalities can be used for diagnosis. Lipomas can be classified according to their location into entities such as intramuscular and inter-muscular lipoma. Systemic lipoma is termed lipomatosis *(Fig. 30.44)*. Diffuse lipomatosis sometimes affects the limbs, head and neck, and intestinal tract. Lipomatosis on the finger results in megadactyly. Multiple symmetric lipomatosis[58] mainly occurs on the upper body *(Fig. 30.45)*. Steroid-induced lipomatosis can be a side-effect of corticosteroid administration. A rapidly growing lipoma should be examined carefully to eliminate the possibility that it is actually a liposarcoma. Complete surgical excision with the capsule is advocated to prevent local recurrence.

Leiomyoma

Cutaneous or subcutaneous leiomyoma is a tumor that is derived from smooth muscles in the skin, including the arrector muscle of hair and vascular smooth muscle.[59] These tumors are localized and are associated with pain. Leiomyomas can be categorized into four types: (1) multiple piloleiomyoma; (2) solitary piloleiomyoma; (3) angioleiomyoma; and (4) genital leiomyoma. Angioleiomyomas and genital leiomyomas usually occur as solitary lesions. In contrast, piloleiomyomas may be solitary or multiple; in the latter case, there may be thousands of lesions. This is because the arrector pili muscle from which piloleiomyomas originate has multiple points of insertion, such as those located proximal to the hair follicle, those located distal to the multiple attachment points within the papillary and reticular dermis, and those located in the basement membrane. Piloleiomyomas can emerge from each of these insertion points, thus occurring as multiple tumors. Angio-leiomyoma often occurs on the distal area of the limbs, especially under the knee in women. In contrast, angi-olipoma commonly occurs on the head in men and is often not associated with pain. Surgical excision or

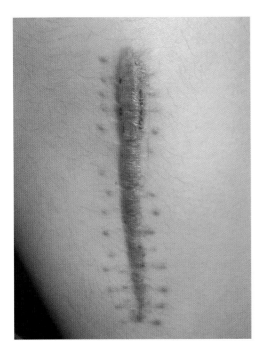

Fig. 30.41 Typical hypertrophic scars on the thigh of an Asian patient.

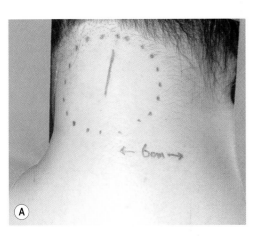

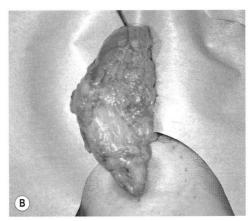

Fig. 30.42 Lipoma on the nape **(A)** and the lesion after excision **(B)**.

ablation of the leiomyoma may be helpful for some symptomatic individuals.

Rhabdomyoma

Rhabdomyoma is a benign tumor of striated muscle. It is most commonly associated with the heart and tongue but can also occasionally occur as a superficial mesenchymal tumor. There are adult, fetal, and genital types. The adult-onset type often occurs on the head and neck area, whereas the fetal type often occurs on the postauricular area of children under the age of 3 years. Patients with adult rhabdomyoma should have surgical resection of head and neck lesions, especially those lesions that compress or displace the tongue, or protrude and partially obstruct the pharynx or larynx. Fetal rhabdomyomas are usually located in the subcutaneous tissues.[60] In most instances, they can be excised without

much difficulty. Local excision is the treatment of choice for genital rhabdomyomas.

Osteochondrogenic tumors

Chondromas and osteochondromas often occur in adults on the hand and foot. Osteochondromas are sometimes associated with calcification. Osteomas are composed of mature bone but can be considered to be reactive outgrowths. Osteoma cutis[61] refers to the presence of bone within the skin in the absence of a pre-existing or associated lesion, as opposed to secondary types of cutaneous ossification that are the result of metaplastic reactions to inflammation, trauma, and neoplastic processes. Osteoma cutis can be removed by excision or laser resurfacing that ablates the overlying skin. Myositis ossificans, panniculitis ossificans, and fibrodysplasia ossificans progressiva are also reactive ossifications. Exostosis is also considered to be a reactive osteochondrogenic disorder (*Fig. 30.46*). This often occurs on the cranial and subungual regions. Exostosis can be removed easily by a chisel and hammer, and its recurrence is rare.

Accessory auricle (also known as nevus cartilagines)

This congenital nevus arises from the area between the tragus and the lateral neck (*Fig. 30.47*). Nevi that are near the ear are largely composed of cartilage, while nevi that are distant from the ear are mainly composed

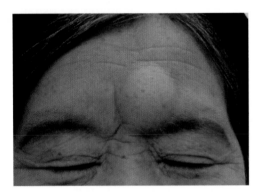

Fig. 30.43 Lipoma on the face.

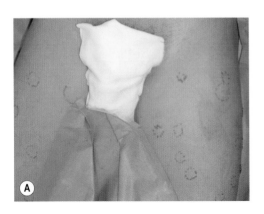
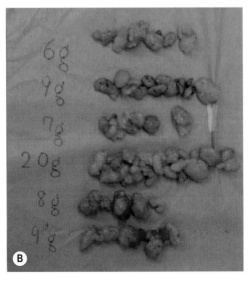

Fig. 30.44 Multiple lipomatosis **(A)** and the lesions after excision **(B)**.

of hair follicles. Multiple accessory auricles[62] are sometimes associated with hemifacial microsomia. Surgical removal may be possible. If so, sufficient skin and cartilage should be removed so that flat and linear scars are the result rather than a dog-ear deformity.

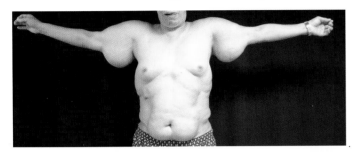

Fig. 30.45 Multiple symmetric lipomatosis.

Granuloma

Granulomas can be broadly classified as infectious *(Fig. 30.48)* and noninfectious. Almost all noninfectious granulomas are foreign-body granulomas; some of these are associated with a type IV allergy. There are a number of causes of foreign-body granuloma. These can be divided into endogenous causes such as uric acid salt, cholesterol, and sebum production, and exogenous causes such as materials injected for aesthetic surgery[63] *(Fig. 30.49)*, vaccines, surgical sutures, and materials implanted by trauma *(Fig. 30.50)*. Small pyogenic granulomas (telangiectatic granulomas) and foreign-body granulomas can be removed by surgery, but this may not be possible for large and multiple granulomas. In

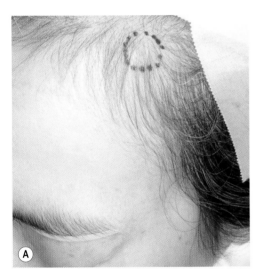

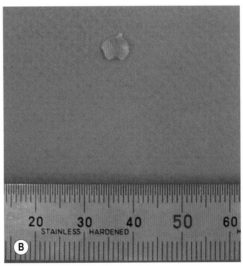

Fig. 30.46 Exostosis on the frontal bone **(A)** and the excised specimen **(B)**.

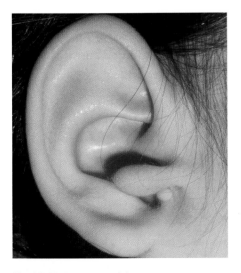

Fig. 30.47 Accessory auricle.

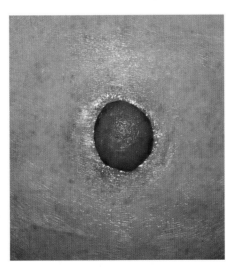

Fig. 30.48 Pyogenic granuloma on the back.

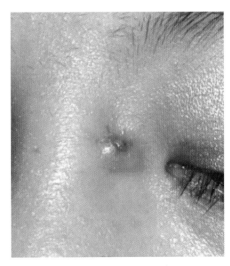

Fig. 30.49 Foreign-body granuloma caused by a nasal implant.

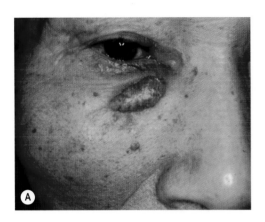
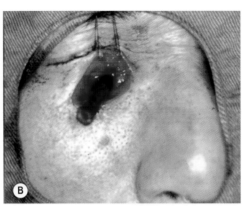

Fig. 30.50 Foreign-body granuloma caused by the implantation of a large wood splinter **(A)** and view of the patient just after surgery **(B)**.

this case, systemic or local corticosteroid administration to reduce inflammation should be considered.

Glomus tumor

Glomus tumors arise from the arterial portion of the glomus body, or the Sucquet–Hoyer canal, which is an arteriovenous anastomosis in the dermis that participates in temperature regulation. Patients with solitary glomus tumors usually have paroxysmal pain that can be severe and exacerbated by pressure or temperature changes, especially cold. Multiple glomus tumors can also be painful but are less common; the pain is also usually not severe. Two features that are useful for diagnosing glomus tumors, particularly solitary painful glomus tumors (especially those under a nail), are the Hildreth sign, which is the disappearance of pain after a tourniquet is placed on the proximal arm, and the Love test, where pain is elicited by pressing the skin overlying the tumor with the tip of a pencil. The treatment of choice for solitary glomus tumors is surgical excision. For multiple glomus tumors,[64] excision may be more difficult because of their poor circumscription and the large number of lesions. In this case, excision should be limited to symptomatic lesions.

Capillary malformation

Hemangioma simplex

This is the result of the abnormal development or differentiation of capillary vessels in the dermis.[65] According to its location, it can be classified into three types: (1) portwine stain (face, limbs, and upper body) *(Figs 30.51, 30.52)*; (2) salmon patch (medial forehead, glabella, nasal tip, and upper lip); and (3) nevus Unna

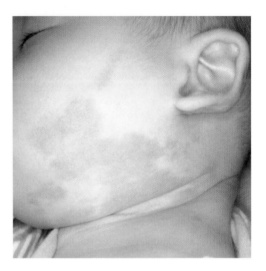

Fig. 30.51 Portwine stain on the face of an infant.

(nape). Portwine stains are sometimes associated with Sturge–Weber syndrome (face) and Klippel–Trenaunay syndrome (limb). Patients with solitary hemangioma simplex, regardless of whether they have these syndromes, should be subjected to brain examinations. Of the three types, only the salmon patch can disappear within a year after birth. A dye laser or Nd:YAG laser can be used to treat these lesions.

Strawberry hemangioma

This tumor is derived from the endothelial cells of capillary vessels in the skin. It arises around 3–4 weeks after birth and its growth peaks at 6–7 months of age *(Figs 30.53, 30.54)*. After this growth period, the volume rarely decreases naturally, although the color can become less livid spontaneously. Consequently, laser treatments with, for example, dye or Nd:YAG lasers should be performed at an early stage to prevent the capillaries from proliferating further.[66] On a case-by-case basis, surgical excision, steroid injection, and compression therapy may also be suitable.

Venous malformation

A representative type of venous malformation is a cavernous hemangioma, which is a blood-storing lesion with a low blood flow *(Fig. 30.55)*. Histology shows the absence of endothelial cell proliferation. It is seen in Klippel–Trenaunay syndrome, which is characterized by various malformations, including capillary malformation and bony and soft-tissue hypertrophy. Venous malformation is best treated with sclerosing therapy, where sclerosing agents like absolute ethanol, polidocanol, sodium tetradecyl sulfate, or ethanolamine oleate are injected into the lesion under ultrasound or digital subtraction angiography guidance.[67]

Arteriovenous fistula and arteriovenous malformation (AVM)

Arteriovenous fistula and AVM are high-flow pulsating lesions with an arteriovenous shunt; they are either acquired because of trauma or are congenital *(Fig. 30.56)*. CDI is useful for detecting the blood flow in the tumor. Patients with Parkes–Weber syndrome who have a huge limb AVM sometimes exhibit congestive heart failure. The Schobinger classification allows AVMs to be classified into four clinical stages: (I) quiescence; (II) expansion; (III) destruction; and (IV) decompensation. Patients with heart failure are considered to have stage IV AVMs. Surgical removal is the first choice of treatment but is often hampered by the diffuse distribution of the vessels and the specific anatomy in the affected region (e.g., the local presence of a facial nerve). Incomplete resection results in the rapid regrowth of the remaining lesion. In cases where surgical removal is difficult, embolosclerosing therapy can be used as a palliative therapy.[68]

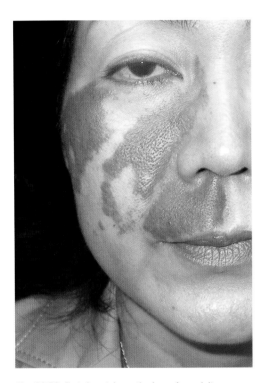

Fig. 30.52 Portwine stain on the face of an adult.

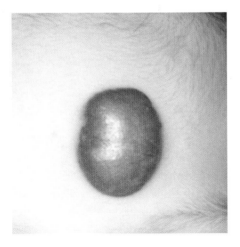

Fig. 30.53 Strawberry hemangioma on the frontal head of an infant.

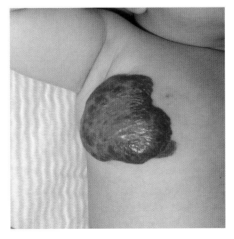

Fig. 30.54 Strawberry hemangioma on the trunk.

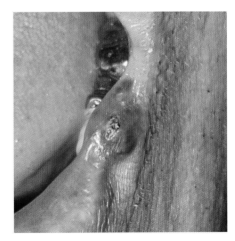

Fig. 30.55 Cavernous hemangioma on the lower lip.

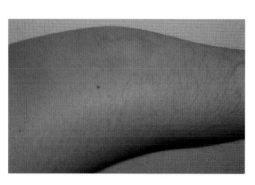

Fig. 30.56 Congenital mild arteriovenous malformation on the forearm.

Lymphatic malformation

There are two main types of lymphatic malformation: lymphangioma and cystic hygroma. Clinically, lymphatic malformation can be classified into macrocyst (cystic hygroma and lymphangioma cystoides), microcyst (lymphangioma simplex), and combined (lymphangioma cavenous) types. The microcysts can be removed surgically, while the macrocysts and combined types should be treated by surgery or sclerotherapy using OK-432[69] or absolute ethanol on a case-by-case basis.

Others

There are many other benign mesenchymal-origin tumors. These include giant cell tumor, histiocystoma, reticulohistiocystoma, fibroxanthoma, desmoid tumor, mucous cyst of the oral mucosa *(Fig. 30.57)*, cutaneous myxoma, Langerhans cell histiocytosis, Kimura disease, plasmacytosis, and mastocytosis.

Malignant cutaneous and soft-tissue tumors

Malignant epithelial-origin tumors

Actinic keratosis

Actinic keratosis is an intraepidermal early-stage SCC caused by long-term exposure to ulraviolet light *(Fig. 30.58)*. It is mostly seen in the elderly, especially fair-skinned people who have been highly exposed to the sun. The areas that bear the lesions are those that have been most exposed. Over time, actinic keratoses

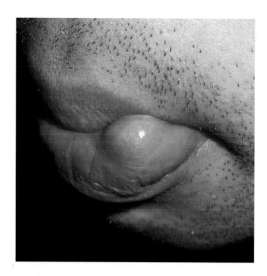

Fig. 30.57 Mucous cyst of the oral mucosa.

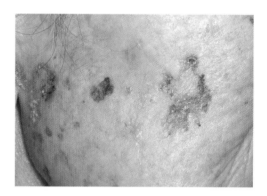

Fig. 30.58 Actinic keratosis on the cheek of an elderly patient.

develop into invasive SCC. They are epidermal lesions that are characterized by aggregates of atypical, pleomorphic keratinocytes at the basal layer that may extend upwards to involve the granular and cornified layers. Cutaneous horns[70] sometimes occur in association with a hyperkeratotic actinic keratosis. Surgical removal is recommended but cryosurgery, CO_2 lasers, 5-FU ointment, and chemical peeling may also be useful for selected cases.

Bowen's disease

Bowen's disease is an intraepidermal carcinoma since it is a malignant tumor of keratinocytes. It can progress to invasive SCC. If the invasion is deep, it is termed Bowen's carcinoma; this carcinoma can metastasize. The diagnosis of Bowen's disease is often delayed because the lesion is asymptomatic and early skin changes may be subtle and overlap with the clinical features of many

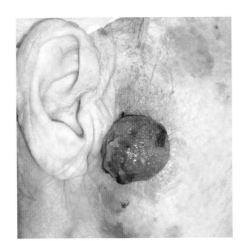

Fig. 30.59 Squamous cell carcinoma on the cheek of an elderly patient.

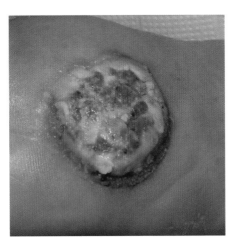

Fig. 30.60 Squamous cell carcinoma on the sole that has arisen from traumatic scars.

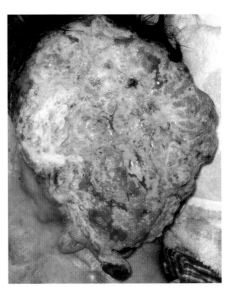

Fig. 30.61 Advanced squamous cell carcinoma on the face that shows necrosis and infection.

conditions, including tinea corporis, nummular eczema, seborrheic keratosis, Paget's disease, superficial BCC, actinic keratosis, and psoriasis. A classic feature of the clinical history is the presentation of a nonsteroid-responsive dermatosis. Surgical removal is recommended but cryosurgery, CO_2 lasers, 5-FU ointment, and imiquimode 5% cream[71] may also be suitable for selected cases.

Squamous cell carcinoma

SCC is a common cutaneous malignancy that often presents as an elevated, indurated lesion with varying degrees of ulceration and crusting (*Fig. 30.59*). SCC can arise on any site but is most common in damaged skin such as actinically damaged skin, postburn scars (Marjolin's ulcer), traumatic scars (*Fig. 30.60*), stasis ulcers, chronic radiation dermatitis, lupus erythematosus lesions, lichen planus on the oral mucosa, and human papillomavirus infection lesions. One type of SCC is verrucous carcinoma. Since SCC can resemble BCC, it is important to make a differential diagnosis. One notable characteristic of SCC is the bad smell caused by the macerated keratin and bacterially infected necrotic tissues (*Fig. 30.61*). SCC should be removed by surgery. Mohs micrographic surgery[72] is frequently used to remove SCCs. Radiotherapy given as external-beam radiotherapy or as brachytherapy (internal radiotherapy) can also be used.

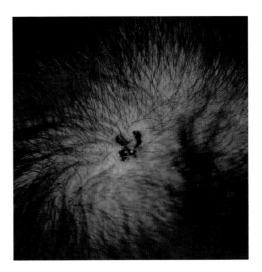

Fig. 30.62 Basal cell carcinoma on the scalp.

Basal cell carcinoma

BCC is the most common type of skin cancer (*Fig. 30.62*). It rarely metastasizes and kills, but is still considered malignant because it can invade surrounding tissues and cause significant destruction and disfigurement. It most commonly affects the head and neck, and cosmetic disfigurement is not uncommon. It can be classified into 10 types[73] (*Box 30.5*). It should be removed by surgery. Mohs micrographic surgery is frequently utilized. However, for selected cases of superficial BCC, CO_2 lasers or cryosurgery can be used.

Box 30.5 **Histological classification of basal cell carcinoma (BCC)**

1. Multifocal superficial BCC (superficial multicentric)
2. Nodular BCC (solid, adenoid cystic)
3. Infiltrating BCC
   3.1. Nonsclerosing
   3.2. Sclerosing (desmoplastic, morpheic)
4. Fibroepithelial BCC
5. BCC with adnexal differentiation
   5.1. BCC with follicular differentiation
   5.2. BCC with eccrine differentiation
6. Basosquamous carcinoma
7. Keratotic BCC
8. Pigmented BCC
9. BCC in basal cell nevus syndrome
10. Micronodular BCC

(Reproduced from LeBoit PE, Burg G, Weedon D, et al. (eds) World Health Organization Classification of Tumors. Pathology and Genetics of Skin Tumors. Lyon: IARC Press, 2006: 10–33.)

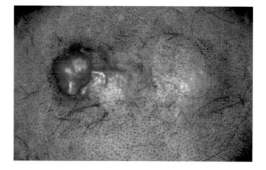

Fig. 30.64 Malignant trichilemmal cyst.

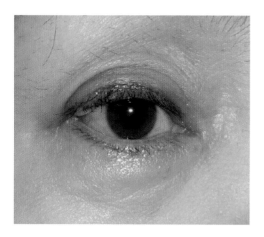

Fig. 30.63 Meibomian gland carcinoma on the upper eyelid.

Malignant appendage-origin tumors

Sebaceous carcinoma

Meibomian gland carcinoma *(Fig. 30.63)*, Zeis gland carcinoma, and Montgomery's gland carcinoma are all sebaceous carcinomas. These carcinomas often exhibit erosion and ulceration. A wide excision with a normal skin margin exceeding 5 mm is recommended. Lymph node dissection should be considered in T4 cases because of the high rate of lymph node metastasis associated with sebaceous carcinomas. Chemotherapy and radiation therapy may also be useful.[74]

Trichilemmal carcinoma

The outer hair root sheath consists of cells with clear vacuolated cytoplasm due to the presence of abundant glycogen. Trichilemmal carcinomas are malignant tumors of these cells. They include malignant trichilemmoma, malignant pilomatricoma, and malignant proliferating trichilemmal cyst *(Fig. 30.64)*. The latter is thought to be derived from proliferating trichilemmal cyst,[29] while malignant pilomatrichoma is believed to be derived from pilomatricoma. Clinically, these tumors present as pale tan or reddish papules, indurated plaques, or nodules. Wide excision should be performed as a radical therapy.

Sweat gland carcinoma

There are many types of eccrine and apocrine carcinomas. These malignant primary cutaneous tumors exhibit glandular and/or ductal features that are thought to reflect their origin as eccrine or apocrine ducts and/or glands. The diagnosis of sweat gland carcinoma requires that the tumor shows sweat gland features, as shown by extracellular ductal or intracytoplasmic lumen formation. This can be indicated by resistance to diastase, staining with periodic acid–Schiff stain, and immunohistochemical positivity for epithelial membrane antigen and carcinoembryonic antigen. The presence of S100 protein may also indicate sweat gland differentiation. Conventional surgical excision has been associated with high recurrence rates but Mohs micrographic surgery is helpful.[75] These carcinomas should be treated according to the guidelines for SCC.

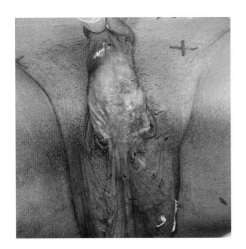

Fig. 30.65 Mapping biopsy for extramammary Paget's disease.

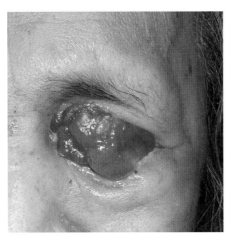

Fig. 30.66 Merkel cell carcinoma on the eyelid.

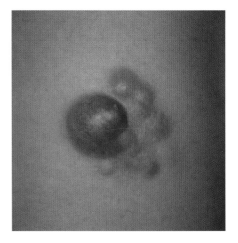

Fig. 30.67 Dermatofibrosarcoma protuberans on the abdomen.

Extramammary Paget's disease

Paget's disease is an adenocarcinoma that is limited to the epidermis. Since mammary Paget's disease is sometimes associated with invasive breast cancer, it can be considered as an intraepidermal proliferating breast carcinoma. In contrast, EMPD is only occasionally associated with an underlying invasive malignancy. It is usually found in the vulva, penis, and axilla. Since its invasive speed is relatively high, it can be difficult to detect early, especially if the lesion has been treated as eczema. Mohs micrographic surgery[76] or mapping biopsy is helpful for determining the normal skin margin for wide excision *(Fig. 30.65)*. Sentinel lymph node biopsy is also useful for deciding whether to remove the lymph nodes.

Merkel cell carcinoma

Merkel cell carcinoma is a rare and highly aggressive cancer where malignant cancer cells develop on or just beneath the skin and in hair follicles *(Fig. 30.66)*. The majority of Merkel cell carcinomas appear to be caused by the newly discovered Merkel cell polyomavirus. It occurs most often on the face, head, and neck, and usually appears as firm and painless nodules or tumors. A normal skin margin of 1–3 cm is needed for wide excision. Moreover, since this tumor tends to metastasize to lymph nodes, lymph node dissection and adjuvant radiation therapy may have to be implemented.[77] Distant metastasis cases should also receive chemotherapy.[77]

Malignant mesenchymal-origin tumors

Dermatofibrosarcoma protuberans (DFSP)

DFSP is also called giant cell fibroblastoma. Over 90% of DFSP tumors have the chromosomal translocation t(17;22) that fuses the collagen gene COL1A1 with the platelet-derived growth factor gene. Typically, DFSP occurs as multiple or solitary tumors that have a red color, hemispherical elevation, and papillary vessels on the surface *(Fig. 30.67)*. They have a keloidal appearance, which has sometimes led to misdiagnosis and treatment with corticosteroids. They metastasize rarely, but distant metastasis to the lung can result from local recurrence. Radical resection should include a normal skin margin of 5 cm. Mohs micrographic surgery with continuous histological margin control is needed to reduce local recurrence rates.[78] Adjuvant chemotherapy and radiation therapy may be useful.

Malignant fibrous histiocytoma (MFH)

There are four types of MFH: (1) storiform-pleomorphic type; (2) myxoid type; (3) giant cell type; and (4) inflammatory type. Moreover, atypical fibroxanthoma is considered to be a superficial type of MFH *(Fig. 30.68)*. Despite being called histiocytomas, these tumors are not believed to be derived from histiocytes. In fact, it is

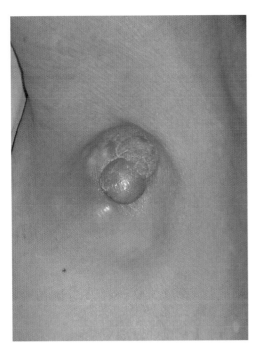

Fig. 30.68 Malignant fibrous histiocytoma on the axilla.

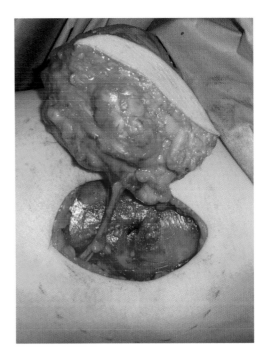

Fig. 30.69 Liposarcoma on the thigh.

currently being argued on the basis of immunohisto-chemistry and electron microscopic observations[79] that most of the storiform pleomorphic-type MFHs should be reclassified as liposarcomas, leiomyosarcomas, or rhabdomyosarcomas. Radical therapy involving wide excision is needed. Adjuvant chemotherapy and radiation therapy may also be useful.

Liposarcoma

Liposarcoma is derived from the fat cells in deep soft tissues such inside the thigh or the retroperitoneum *(Fig. 30.69)*. They are generally large and bulky tumors with multiple smaller satellites located outside the main tumor. Diagnosis requires the detection of lipoblasts, which usually have an abundant, clear, multivacuolated cytoplasm and an acentric, darkly staining, vacuole-compressed nucleus. Dedifferentiated liposarcomas exhibit a dedifferentiated area in the tumor that sometimes results in osseous metaplasia.[80] Radical therapy involving wide excision is needed. Adjuvant chemotherapy and radiation therapy may be useful.

Leiomyosarcoma

This rare malignancy mainly occurs on the limbs of middle-aged and older patients *(Fig. 30.70)*. It can be

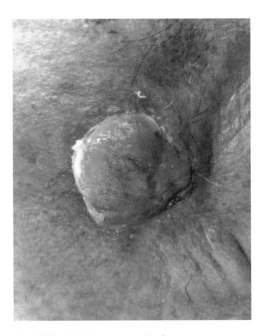

Fig. 30.70 Leiomyosarcoma on the face.

very unpredictable as it can remain dormant for long periods of time and recur after years. It is generally not very responsive to chemotherapy or radiation. However, neoadjuvant or adjuvant chemotherapies,[81] or radiation, are recommended.

Rhabdomyosarcoma

Rhabdomyosarcoma is thought to arise from skeletal muscle progenitors and occurs in many anatomic locations. Sometimes it is found attached to muscle tissue or wrapped around intestines. Mostly it occurs in areas that naturally lack skeletal muscle, such as the head, neck, and genitourinary tract. Its three most common forms are embryonal rhabdomyosarcoma, alveolar rhabdomyosarcoma, and pleomorphic rhabdomyosarcoma. Embryonal rhabdomyosarcoma is more common in younger children, where the cancer cells resemble those of a typical 6–8-week embryo. Alveolar rhabdomyosarcoma occurs more commonly in older children and teenagers, and the cells resemble those of a typical 10–12-week embryo. Pleomorphic rhabdomyosarcoma is a rare sarcoma that occurs most often in older patients. Radical therapy involving wide excision is needed. There is also evidence that rhabdomyosarcomas are the target of host immune responses.[82]

Osteosarcoma

This aggressive cancerous neoplasm arises from primitive transformed cells of mesenchymal origin that exhibit osteoblastic differentiation and produce malignant osteoids *(Fig. 30.71)*. Complete radical surgical en bloc resection is the treatment of choice.[83] Some recent studies have suggested that osteoclast inhibitors such as alendronate and pamidronate may improve the quality of life by reducing osteolysis, which decreases the pain as well as the risk of pathological fractures.

Chondrosarcoma

At presentation, nearly all chondrosarcoma patients appear to be in good health as this form of cancer usually does not affect the whole body. Indeed, the patients are generally not aware of the growing tumor until there is a noticeable lump or pain. An earlier diagnosis is generally accidental, such as when a patient undergoes testing for another problem. Occasionally, the first symptom will be a broken bone at the cancerous site. Therefore, broken bones due to mild trauma warrant further investigation, even though there are many conditions that can lead to weak bones and this form of cancer is not a common cause of such breaks. Chemotherapy or traditional radiotherapy is not very effective for most chondrosarcomas, although proton beam radiation therapy is showing promise with regard to local tumor control.[84] Complete surgical ablation is the most effective treatment but can be difficult to achieve. Proton beam radiation can facilitate the surgical removal of chondrosarcomas in awkward locations.

Angiosarcoma

Angiosarcoma is the common name for malignant neoplasms of endothelial cells *(Fig. 30.72)* but it is replaced with the terms lymphangiosarcoma and hemangiosarcoma when more clinical precision is required.

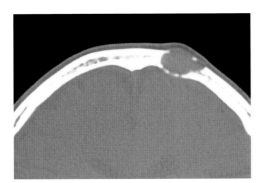

Fig. 30.71 Computed tomography of an osteosarcoma on the frontal bone.

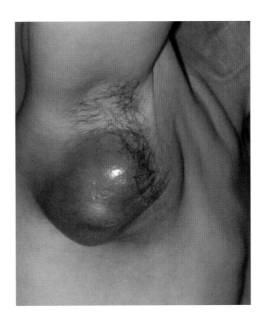

Fig. 30.72 Angiosarcoma on the axilla.

Haemangiosarcomas and lymphangiosarcomas of the skin are not uncommon. Given the location of angiosarcomas, metastasis to distant sites occurs often. Surgery, radiation therapy, chemotherapy, and immunotherapy using interleukin-2[85] should be used, but the prognosis of these tumors is poor. However, the prognosis of neoplasia of superficial vessel tissues such as those in the skin is generally better because the risk of malignancy is lower; moreover, these tumors are generally more accessible to treatment.

Kaposi's sarcoma

Kaposi's sarcoma is caused by the Kaposi's sarcoma-associated herpesvirus (KSHV), also known as human herpesvirus 8. It became widely known after its frequent appearance in acquired immune deficiency syndrome patients was noted in the 1980s. Although the viral cause of this cancer was discovered in 1994, this causal link remains poorly understood by the general populace, including by the groups that are at particular risk of contracting KSHV. Kaposi's sarcoma lesions present as red, purple, brown, or black nodules or blotches that are usually papular (i.e., palpable or raised). They are typically found on the skin but can often spread elsewhere, especially to the mouth, gastrointestinal tract, and respiratory tract. Their growth can range from very slow to explosively fast, and they are associated with significant mortality and morbidity. Radiation therapy, cryotherapy, and chemotherapy may be useful. Surgery is not the primary choice of treatment, although it may be useful as supportive therapy. Highly active antiretroviral therapy should be combined with these therapies.[86]

Others

Other malignant mesenchymal-origin tumors include epithelioid sarcoma, synovial sarcoma, extraskeletal Ewing's sarcoma, histiocytic sarcoma, and Langerhans cell sarcoma. In general, treatment consists of induction chemotherapy, wide surgical excision, and then maintenance chemotherapy. Multiagent chemotherapy has improved survival rates.

Access the complete references list online at **http://www.expertconsult.com**.

1. *Consensus Net meeting on Dermoscopy. 2000 Available online at http://www.dermoscopy.org/consensus/.

2. Jemec GB, Gniadecka M, Ulrich J. Ultrasound in dermatology. Part I. High frequency ultrasound. *Eur J Dermatol.* 2000;10:492–497.

   Basic ultrasound terminology and mechanics are discussed. A discussion of applications of this technology to dermatologic diagnosis is offered.

3. Blumer SL, Scalcione LR, Ring BN, et al. Cutaneous and subcutaneous imaging on FDG-PET: benign and malignant findings. *Clin Nucl Med.* 2009;34:675–683.

   This atlas-style article describes the appearance of cutaneous and subcutaneous lesions on FDG-PET. The authors stress that, with clinical correlation, FDG-PET can be a useful diagnostic adjunct for these lesions.

5. *Sobin LH, Gospodarowicz MK, Wittekind C, eds. TNM Classification of Malignant Tumours (UICC: International Union Against Cancer). 7th ed. New Jersey: Wiley-Blackwell; 2009.*

6. *Wittekind CF, Greene FL, Hutter RVP, et al. TNM Atlas: Illustrated Guide to the TNM/pTNM Classification of Malignant Tumours. 5th edn. Berlin: Springer; 2004.*

   This review compares the efficacy of Mohs micrographic surgery (MMS) to alternative treatment modalities for nonmelanoma skin cancer in terms of cost, initial cure rate, and recurrence rate. The authors conclude that MMS is superior in terms of these metrics.

8. Erba P, Ogawa R, Vyas R, et al. The Reconstructive Matrix – A New Paradigm in Reconstructive Plastic Surgery. *Plast Reconstr Surg.* 2010;126:492–498.

   The "reconstructive ladder" is a classic paradigm in which the simplest effective treatment modality for a given defect is identified as the most appropriate. The authors offer the "reconstructive matrix" as a new treatment model that accounts for socioeconomic issues as well as evolving medical knowledge and technology in determining the optimal reconstructive option for a given patient and defect.

18. *Ogawa R. The most current algorithms for the treatment and prevention of hypertrophic scars and keloids. *Plast Reconstr Surg.* 2010;125: 557–568.

   The author presents an algorithm for the treatment of hypertrophic scars and keloids based on a review of the literature. Differential diagnosis and prevention are also addressed.

39. *The US National Institutes of Health Consensus Conference on the diagnosis and treatment of early melanoma. Available at: http://consensus.nih.gov/1992/1992Melanoma088html.htm.

31

Melanoma

Stephan Ariyan and Aaron Berger

SYNOPSIS

- The definitive diagnosis of melanoma is based on histologic analysis. Clinical features suggestive of malignancy include: asymmetry, border irregularity, color changes, diameter >0.6 cm, and evolving changes – the ABCDE criteria.

- The four major histopathologic subtypes of melanoma are: lentigo maligna, superficial spreading, nodular, and acral lentiginous. Desmoplastic melanoma is a less common subtype of melanoma that lacks pigment and may demonstrate perineural invasion.

- Initial workup of the pigmented lesion should include excisional biopsy with a 1–2-mm margin of normal-appearing skin. If functional or cosmetic concerns prohibit removal of the entire lesion, incisional or punch biopsy may be performed.

- Histologic evaluation of the primary lesion must include: Breslow depth in millimeters, presence/absence of ulceration, mitotic rate per mm^2, peripheral and deep margin status, and Clark level (especially for lesions ≤1 mm in depth).

- Recommended excision margins are determined by Breslow depth. In situ melanoma requires a 0.5-cm margin of normal-appearing skin. For invasive melanoma, a 1-cm margin is recommended for lesions ≤1 mm in depth, a 1–2-cm margin is recommended for lesions 1.01–2.0 mm in depth (depending upon functional/cosmetic concerns), and a margin of at least 2.0 cm is recommended for lesions >2.0 mm in depth.

- Subungual melanoma of the hand should be resected at the distal interphalangeal joint to preserve function.

- Sentinel lymph node biopsy is offered to patients with melanomas >1 mm in thickness, and patients with thin melanomas (≤ 1 mm thick) that demonstrate high-risk features, including ulceration and/or high mitotic rate. The likelihood of detecting metastatic deposits in a sentinel lymph node biopsy increases with the thickness of the primary lesion.

- For patients with stage I and II disease, chest X-ray and liver function tests compose the recommended workup. Patients with regional (stage III) or systemic metastases (stage IV) should undergo a comprehensive staging workup that may include computed tomography scans with positron emission tomography imaging.

- Serum lactate dehydrogenase is used in the American Joint Committee on Cancer staging system as it portends a worse prognosis in patients with metastatic disease.

- Patients with high-risk primary tumors or metastatic disease should be considered for adjuvant treatment with interferon-alpha or enrollment in a clinical trial.

 Access the Historical Perspective section and Figs 31.1, 31.2 online at **http://www.expertconsult.com**

Introduction

Few diseases are as fascinating and as troublesome to physicians as malignant melanoma, and perhaps no other disease elicits as much fear in the patient as does this diagnosis. Although it accounts for only 4% of all malignant neoplasms, its very diagnosis suggests to some patients an aggressive, rapid progression to death. The name alone may leave some patients with a sense of hopelessness that is often unjustified. Despite some reported descriptions of rapid spread, the natural history of melanoma and its overall cure rate of 80% compare favorably with those of cancers of the breast, colon, rectum, and oropharynx and are far better than for cancer of the lung.

Epidemiologic studies demonstrate that the incidence of melanoma has been increasing faster than that of any other cancer in the US.[1] For the year 2010, in the US alone, 68 130 new melanoma cases were diagnosed and 8700 deaths were attributed to melanoma.[2] While melanoma accounts for roughly 4% of all skin cancers, it is responsible for more than 77% of skin cancer deaths. Current estimates of the lifetime risk for developing invasive melanoma is 1 in 37 for white men and 1 in 56 for white women.[2] Our understanding of melanoma continues to improve, and we can now differentiate low-risk from high-risk patients on the basis of multifactorial analyses from several series of large numbers of patients. However, despite our best attempts to understand the molecular basis of this disease, limited success has been demonstrated in terms of new medical treatments, and successful treatment of this disease relies heavily upon the surgeon. FIGS **31.1**, **31.2** APPEARS ONLINE ONLY

Clinical evaluation

Clinical diagnosis

Although an experienced clinician should be able to diagnose malignant melanoma by its appearance, the diagnosis is often not made until the specimen is examined histologically. Therefore, a review of the various pigmented lesions is essential for making a differential diagnosis.

All infants are born with nevi, but the lesions are usually not apparent at birth because they do not produce pigment. During the following few weeks or months, melanocytes produce pigment as a response to circulating hormones. As the nevi develop, they undergo maturation, which leads to the classification of the following various forms.

Junctional nevus

Junctional nevi are small flat lesions that first appear after birth and are smooth, nonpalpable, and light to dark brown or black *(Fig. 31.3A)*. They are called junctional because the nevus cells are located at the interface of the epidermis and dermis. As the person develops and matures, the nevus cells grow and push into the dermis to develop into the common adult intradermal nevus.

Compound nevus

As the nevus matures, the central portion pushes into the dermis, causing this central portion to elevate and appear thicker *(Fig. 31.3B)*. This nevus is called compound because the central portion is intradermal and thick, whereas the periphery is still junctional and flat. Compound nevi often are seen during adolescence, and the changes in such moles may cause concern to the patient, family, or primary care physician.

Intradermal nevus

The intradermal nevus is the common adult mole of the face or trunk that is elevated because of the maturation and proliferation of the nevus in the dermis, which now pushes up the overlying epidermis *(Fig. 31.3C)*. It may be light or dark, usually is elevated, and may be sessile or pedunculated.

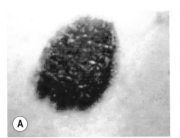 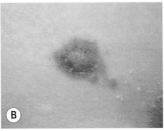 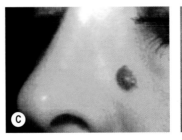 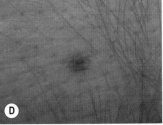

Fig. 31.3 (A) Junctional nevus is flat, smooth, and nonpalpable. **(B)** Compound nevus is developing into mature, thicker intradermal nevus in the center within a flat junctional nevus in the periphery. **(C)** Intradermal nevus is a mature mole with elevation of the surface elements due to thickening of the layer of nevus cells. **(D)** Blue nevus presents with melanin deposits deep in the dermis, reflecting the blue wavelength of light.

Blue nevus

Most nevi appear brown or black because the melanin is superficial and absorbs light. When the nevus contains melanin that is located more deeply, blue wavelengths of light pass through the less pigmented epidermis and are reflected back to the eye as a blue nevus *(Fig. 31.3D)*.

Congenital nevus

Congenital nevi differ from others in that they already produce pigment at birth *(Fig. 31.4A)*. There is some controversy about whether congenital nevi are

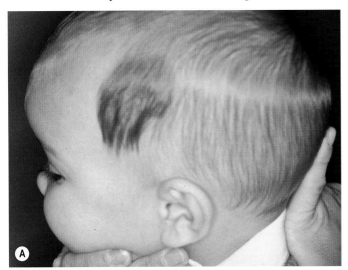

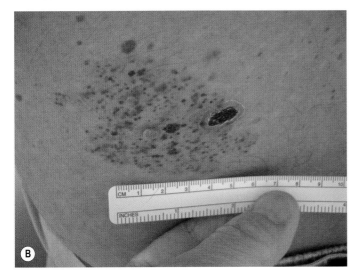

Fig. 31.4 (A) Congenital nevus is a large flat pigmented mole that had produced pigmentation *in utero* and was present as a pigmented lesion on the day of birth. It may be hairy (as in this case) or not. **(B)** Invasive (1.4-mm) melanoma developed within a congenital nevus on the trunk of a 57-year-old male.

precursors of melanoma. Kaplan's review[12] of the literature reported the transformation to melanoma to occur in 2–42% of congenital nevi *(Fig. 31.4B)*. In a retrospective study of 234 melanomas by Rhodes and Melski,[13] some of the histologic features of congenital nevi were found among 8% of the melanoma specimens. A systematic review of all studies evaluating the risk of melanoma in congenital nevi was performed by Krengel et al.[14] A total of 6571 patients with congenital nevi were followed for at least 3.4 years, and 46 patients (0.7%: range 0.05–10.7%) developed 49 melanomas. Of note, primary melanomas arose inside the nevi in 67% of cases. Using age-adjusted data from the Surveillance, Epidemiology and End Results database, they calculated that patients with congenital nevi carry an approximately 465-fold increased relative risk of developing melanoma during childhood and adolescence. Large congenital nevi *(Fig. 31.5)*, greater than 40 cm in diameter, were associated with the highest risk of developing melanoma, as well as dying from melanoma.[14,15] However, the true incidence of the development of melanoma within congenital nevi is difficult to determine as the number of patients in the general population who have congenital nevi but never consult a physician, or eventually undergo excision, is unknown.

On the basis of available information about the potential for malignant transformation, it is a good policy to remove congenital nevi if it can be done without much difficulty *(Fig. 31.5)*. Malignant transformation does not usually occur before adolescence, thus, if the lesion is to be excised, it should be done before adolescence. Because it is difficult to excise nevi from the skin of children under local anesthesia and general anesthesia is often necessary for children younger than 12 years, the risk of complications from general anesthesia should be weighed against the risk of malignant transformation before adolescence. On the other hand, patients may request removal of the lesion to improve their appearance. Despite concerns for appearance, some lesions cannot be completely removed because in doing so we may cause a greater deformity. These lesions may require staged excisions.

Atypical (dysplastic) nevus

The atypical nevus is a clinical diagnosis of a nevus with melanocytes involving the epidermis and dermis that

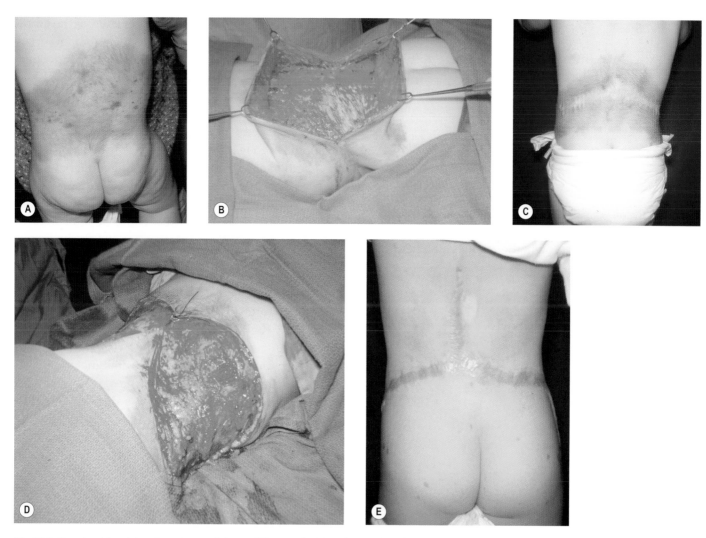

Fig. 31.5 Staged excision. A large truncal congenital nevus **(A)** was excised from the central portion of the lesion **(B)** to reduce the size of the lesion to half after one operation **(C)**. A second procedure a year later **(D)** removed the remainder of the lesion **(E)**.

have features suggestive of malignancy. Clinically, it is large (>6 mm), with a macular surface, irregular margin, and variegated color. It may have a background of erythema *(Fig. 31.6)*. These are benign lesions with histologic features that are abnormal. At various times, they have been called atypical nevi or dysplastic nevi. However, a National Institutes of Health Consensus Conference in 1992 recommended the descriptive term "atypical nevus" for the clinical diagnosis and the histologic term "dysplastic nevus" to describe the histologic degree of atypia and architectural disorder.[16]

To ensure accurate diagnosis, histologic examination of the lesion is required. Microscopically, the dysplastic nevus has melanocytic hyperplasia, with the melanocytes arranged as solitary units or small elongated nests oriented parallel to the long axes of the rete ridges. The melanocytes have nuclear atypia and abundant cytoplasm with a fine "dusty pattern" of melanin deposits.[17] Dysplastic nevi are often associated with atypical melanocytic hyperplasia, lymphocytic infiltration, and some evidence of regression. As such, patients with these lesions are believed to be at greater risk for transformation to melanomas.

Atypical (dysplastic) nevus syndrome

Studies at several institutions have found atypical nevi in association with melanoma that has no familial pattern. At the University of Pennsylvania, Elder *et al.*[18] first described this as the dysplastic nevus syndrome in

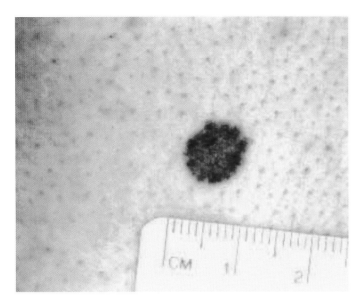

Fig. 31.6 Dysplastic nevus is a histologic confirmation of the clinical entity called atypical nevus. This is a large (>6 mm) flat mole of varying coloration.

their 1980 report. In the same year, the Yale Melanoma Unit visited the Sydney Melanoma Unit in Australia and documented the presence of atypical nevi in 37% of 296 patients with melanoma who had no known family history.[19] Similar atypical nevi were discovered in only 7% of a control population of male prison inmates without any history of melanoma.[19] Clinically, these moles were large and resembled the dysplastic nevi of familial melanoma. Biopsies showed a 90% correlation between the histologic diagnosis of dysplastic nevi and the clinical appearance of these atypical moles. The tendency to develop atypical nevi is presumed to have a genetic basis, and the diagnosis of "atypical nevus syndrome" has been applied to patients with a range of phenotypic expressions,[20] including just the presence of multiple atypical nevi and no personal or family history of melanoma, to the familial atypical multiple mole and melanoma syndrome.[21]

B-K mole syndrome

Some prospective studies have shown that melanoma may be associated with a familial distribution in 10–11% of the cases.[22] These familial melanomas tend to appear earlier and are distributed among dysplastic nevi over the body, with an excess over the trunk and a deficit over the upper extremities. Clark *et al.*[23] and Reimer *et al.*[24] suggested the role of atypical moles and dysplastic nevi in the development of hereditary melanoma when they described these moles in association with melanomas in seven families. They applied the initials of the first family, which were BK, to name this clinical entity the B-K mole syndrome.

Differential diagnosis

The clinician is faced with the task of differentiating the malignant melanoma from a number of other lesions that may clinically resemble melanoma, such as seborrheic keratosis *(Fig. 31.7A)*, pyogenic granuloma *(Fig. 31.7B)*, and pigmented basal cell carcinoma *(Fig. 31.7C)*. This differentiation may sometimes be more difficult because of a recent growth, bleeding into a lesion, or peripheral inflammation. In these instances, only microscopic examination of the tissue provides the proper diagnosis.

Extensive or radical surgical procedures should not be performed without the proper diagnosis of a melanoma because clinical impressions are not uniformly correct. Epstein *et al.*[25] reviewed 559 patients with black lesions that they believed might be melanomas. They found that their diagnosis of melanoma was correct only a third (38.7%) of the time. Indeed, the most common diagnoses were benign nevi (35%), pigmented basal cell cancer (30%), and benign angiomas or vascular lesions (13%). Only 2% of all the lesions were found to be melanoma. Dermoscopy, the use of a hand-held lens in combination with oil immersion, has been shown to improve diagnostic accuracy in skilled hands.[26,27] However, it is used routinely by only 23% of dermatologists.[28] In general, the diagnostic work-up of melanocytic lesions will precede the surgeon's involvement, unless the lesion is in a region of cosmetic concern.

Hutchinson freckle

Hutchinson freckle is a flat, brown, macular lesion that may grow at various rates and achieve different shades of pigmentation *(Fig. 31.8)*. This lesion occurs most commonly on the face, neck, and other sun-exposed surfaces of adults in middle age or later. On histologic examination, this lesion appears as an overgrowth of melanocytes at the epidermis–dermis junction. Although lentigo maligna is an *in situ* melanoma, invasive

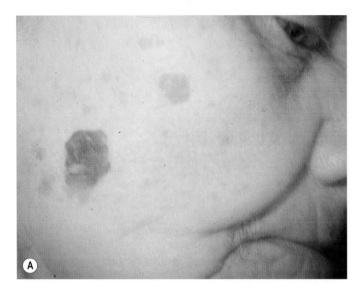

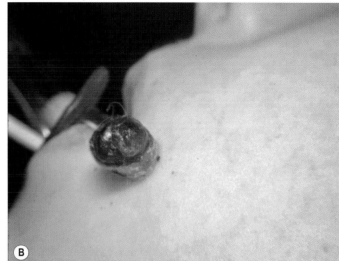

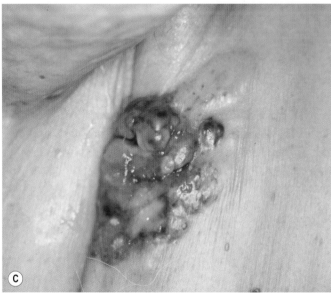

Fig. 31.7 Pigmented lesions that need to be differentiated from a melanoma. **(A)** Seborrheic keratosis of cheek is a velvety smooth keratosis that may turn dark brown to black with drying of the keratin layer. **(B)** Pyogenic granuloma with exophytic granulation tissue and darkening due to desiccation of the blood and coagulum. **(C)** Pigmented basal cell carcinoma with heaped-up "pearly" margins. Pigment may represent hemosiderin or melanin granules from melanocytes that may be incorporated into the lesion.

melanoma may develop within a Hutchinson freckle and is then called lentigo maligna melanoma.

Melanoma

The lesions of melanoma may be flat or nodular, with significant darkening, erythema, or bleeding. On histologic examination, the earliest lesions demonstrate atypical melanocytes migrating above the dermis–epidermis junction and appearing within the upper portions of hair follicles and eccrine ducts. These changes are typical of melanoma *in situ*.[29] Special staining with S100 and HMB45 may be necessary to confirm the diagnosis in cases with histologic features that may be equivocal. However, when even a single atypical melanocyte invades from the dermis–epidermis junction down into the dermis, the diagnosis is melanoma.[30]

There are clinical features of pigmented lesions that are characteristic for melanoma. These criteria have been promoted by the American Cancer Society as the ABCD Guidelines *(Fig. 31.9)*.

A asymmetry of the lesion as it grows from a round or oval lesion

B border irregularity, which is a result of irregular growth rates of different parts of the lesion

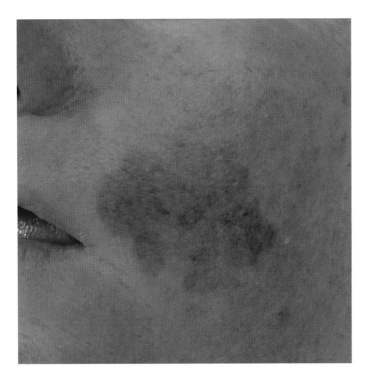

Fig. 31.8 Hutchinson freckle is a flat lesion with various shades of pigmentation.

C color changes representing pigment granules deposited at varying depths in the dermis, depending on the rate of invasion

D diameter of the lesion becoming more than ¼ inch (>6 mm).

In addition to the above ABCD criteria, a review of the literature recommended the addition of E for "evolution," in order to emphasize the significance of evolving pigmented lesions in the natural history of melanoma, especially given the existence of small-diameter (≤6 mm) melanomas.[31] In treating patients with suspicious pigmented lesions, physicians should be attentive to changes (evolving) of size, shape, symptoms (itching, tenderness), surface (especially bleeding), and shades of color. An investigation of the recognition process of melanoma by 135 dermatologists revealed that most dermatologists rely more on the lesion's overall pattern, the "ugly duckling sign" (i.e., unique appearance relative to the patient's other nevi), and recent change according to the patient, rather than the better-known ABCD algorithm.[32] This observation lends support to the addition of an E category for evolution of melanocytic lesions by the nondermatologist.

Based on existing literature, most patients who present to their dermatologist are unaware of an existing melanoma. Most melanomas (56.3%) detected in the general dermatology practice are found by the dermatologist during routine physical examination, and are not part of the presenting complaint.[33] Numerous studies[34–36] demonstrate that physicians are more likely to detect melanomas at a thinner stage than nonphysicians. In these studies, there was a significant difference between the thickness of physician-detected melanomas (0.23–0.68 mm) and those detected by patients or their spouses (0.9–1.43 mm).

An occasional, and potentially reassuring, feature of melanoma is intralesional depigmentation *(Fig. 31.10)*. This is a manifestation of immunologic regression of the tumor as a result of the destruction of the melanoma cells by the host's immune response. The histologic examination of only a section through the depigmented portion may be misread as an inflammatory reaction. However, deposits of residual melanin granules may exist in the depigmented portion *(Fig. 31.10B)*, and histologic examination of sections through the adjacent pigmented portion may reveal the true diagnosis of the melanoma.

Nevertheless, depigmentation does not always indicate melanoma: a halo nevus *(Fig. 31.11A)* is a benign lesion with a peripheral ring of depigmentation.[37] Histologic examination of the halo portion shows lymphocytic infiltration without pigment granules *(Fig. 31.11B)*. Further evaluation of the lesion and surrounding tissue shows no evidence of cells of malignant melanoma *(Fig. 31.11C)*.

Multiple primary melanomas

Multiple primary melanomas have been reported to occur among 3% of melanoma patients.[38] The risk for a second melanoma in a patient with one melanoma approaches 4–5%.[39] However, with a positive family history of melanoma, the risk for multiple primary melanomas rises to 10% or more.[40] The highest risk of all appears to be in individuals who have a family history of melanoma in one or two first-degree relatives and who have clinical evidence of dysplastic nevi, suggesting a probability approaching 100% in due time.[41] Although multiple primary melanomas may be found among 10% of the patients, Ariyan *et al.*[42] reported that

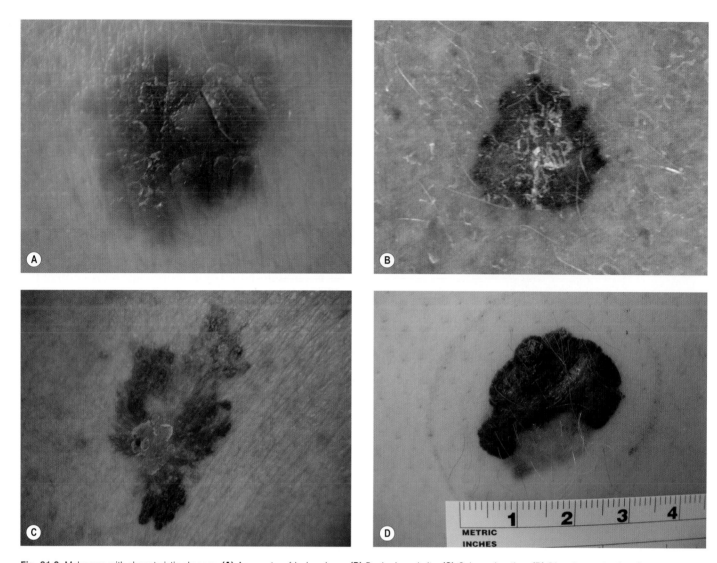

Fig. 31.9 Melanoma with characteristic changes. **(A)** Asymmetry of lesion shape. **(B)** Border irregularity. **(C)** Color variegation. **(D)** Diameter greater than 6 mm.

half of these subsequent melanomas are *in situ*, and the vast majority of the rest are less than 1.0 mm thick; thus, they did not seem to affect cure rates.

Classification/staging of disease

Melanoma is most commonly located in the skin, although it may also occur rarely in the mucosa of the oral cavity, nasopharynx, esophagus, vagina, and rectum. The staging system developed for melanoma applies to lesions arising in the skin, and thus, the discussion in this chapter is primarily limited to cutaneous melanoma.

The purpose of a classification system in malignant disease is to separate varying stages of severity to predict prognosis and to propose treatment options based on those predictions. Therefore, all classification systems have evolved from data collected over time. As such, each of these classifications needs to be re-evaluated periodically to refine the separation of stages on the basis of changes in outcome. Melanoma staging has evolved to include important data acquired from pathologic analysis of the initial biopsy (and potential biopsy of regional lymph nodes).

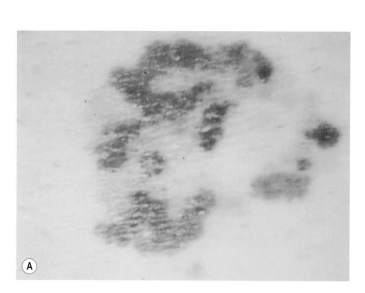

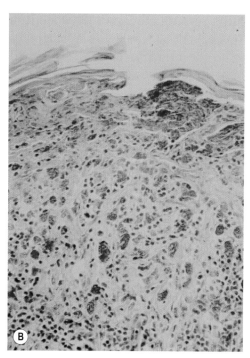

Fig. 31.10 (A) Melanoma with areas of depigmentation within the lesion. **(B)** Histologic examination of the specimen cut through the area of depigmentation shows significant lymphocytic infiltration with disrupted pigment granules leading to the colorless patches within.

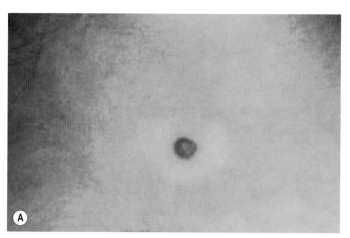

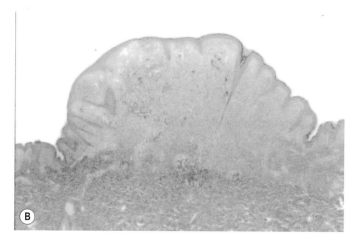

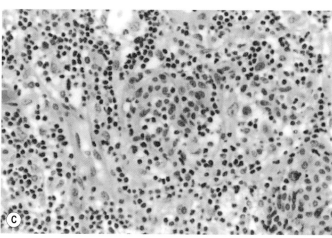

Fig. 31.11 (A) Halo nevus with a ring of depigmentation surrounding the lesion. **(B)** Histologic examination of the depigmented portion shows infiltration with lymphocytes, but **(C)** there is no evidence of pigment granules or malignant cells.

The current (2010), seventh edition of the American Joint Committee on Cancer (AJCC) staging system relies upon data related to the primary tumor (T), regional lymph nodes (N), and metastases (M). Also known as the TNM system, this staging system was developed based upon analysis of over 38 900 patients with cutaneous malignant melanoma[43,44] (*Tables 31.2, 31.3*).

Histologic subtypes of melanoma

While morphology or histologic subtype does not necessarily correlate with clinical behavior, subclassification is important for pathologic recognition and diagnosis. Melanoma may be classified morphologically into four major growth patterns: lentigo maligna, superficial spreading, nodular, and acral lentiginous types (*Fig. 31.12*). Superficial spreading melanoma (*Fig. 31.12B*) represents 50–80% of all the types and is characterized by growth in the radial (horizontal) phase for a period of years before evolution into the vertical growth phase. Nodular melanoma (*Fig. 31.12C*), on the other hand, evolves into the vertical growth phase early in its development and represents 20–30% of the group but in some series may compose the majority of the lesions.[45] Lentigo maligna melanoma (*Fig. 31.12A*) is differentiated from superficial spreading melanoma and nodular melanoma by its location on sun-exposed surfaces of the body and within pre-existing lentigo maligna (Hutchinson freckle). This morphologic type of melanoma was believed to have a better prognosis than other types by virtue of a different biologic behavior, but it has been shown to have a prognosis identical with that for superficial spreading melanoma with comparable depths of invasion.[46] It has been shown that lentigo maligna melanoma merely grows in a horizontal fashion more than in a vertical fashion, resulting in thinner lesions than superficial spreading melanoma or nodular melanoma, which is the reason for its purported better prognosis.

Acral lentiginous melanoma appears on the palms of the hands, soles of the feet (*Fig. 31.12D*), subungual areas of the fingers and toes (*Fig. 31.12E*), and webspaces.[47] The importance of subungual melanoma is that it is often erroneously believed to be a fungal infection, and appropriate treatment may be inadvertently delayed because of a delay in obtaining diagnostic biopsy. Presumably due to delayed diagnosis, this type of

Table 31.2 Cutaneous melanoma TNM staging

T classification	Thickness	Ulceration status
Tis	Not applicable	Not applicable
T1	≤1.0 mm	a: without ulceration and mitosis <1/mm^2 b: with ulceration or mitosis ≥1/mm^2
T2	1.01–2.0 mm	a: without ulceration b: with ulceration
T3	2.01–4.0 mm	a: without ulceration b: with ulceration
T4	>4.0 mm	a: without ulceration b: with ulceration

N classification	No. of metastatic nodes	Nodal metastatic mass
N1	1 node	a: micrometastasis* b: macrometastasis†
N2	2–3 nodes	a: micrometastasis* b: macrometastasis† c: in transit met(s)/satellite(s) without metastatic nodes
N3	4 or more metastatic nodes, or matted nodes, or in-transit met(s)/ satellite(s) with metastatic node(s)	

M classification	Site	Serum lactate dehydrogenase
M1a	Distant skin, subcutaneous, or nodal metastases	Normal
M1b	Lung metastases	Normal
M1c	All other visceral metastases	Normal
	Any distant metastasis	Elevated

*Micrometastases are diagnosed after sentinel or elective lymphadenectomy.
†Macrometastases are defined as clinically detectable nodal metastases confirmed by therapeutic lymphadenectomy or when nodal metastasis exhibits gross extracapsular extension.
(Reproduced from Balch CM, Gershenwald JE, Soong SJ, et al. Final version of 2009 AJCC melanoma staging and classification. *J Clin Oncol.* 2009;27:6199–6206.)

Table 31.3 Melanoma stage/prognostic groups			
Stage 0	Tis	N0	M0
Stage IA	T1a	N0	M0
Stage IB	T1b	N0	M0
	T2a	N0	M0
Stage IIA	T2b	N0	M0
	T3a	N0	M0
Stage IIB	T3b	N0	M0
	T4a	N0	M0
Stage IIC	T4b	N0	M0
Stage IIIA	T1–4a	N1a	M0
	T1–4a	N2a	M0
Stage IIIB	T1–4b	N1a	M0
	T1–4b	N1b	M0
	T1–4a	N1b	M0
	T1–4a	N2c	M0
Stage IIIC	T1–4b	N1b	M0
	T1–4b	N2b	M0
	T1–4b	N2c	M0
	Any T	N3	M0
Stage IV	Any T	Any N	M1

(Reproduced from Balch CM, Gershenwald JE, Soong SJ, et al. Final version of 2009 AJCC melanoma staging and classification. *J Clin Oncol.* 2009;27: 6199–6206.)

melanoma has the lowest 5-year survival rates of all histologic variants, generally found to be in the range of 10–20%.[22,48]

While older studies suggested that prognosis may be associated with histologic subtype (e.g., patients with nodular melanomas were thought to have a worse prognosis than patients with superficial spreading melanomas),[49] more recent multivariate analyses demonstrate that these prognostic differences are more likely due to other histologic features (i.e., tumor thickness and ulceration).[50]

Another less common clinical variant of melanoma, desmoplastic melanoma, usually does not produce pigment, and grows on the external surfaces of the skin. It may have the appearance of a hypertrophic scar *(Fig. 31.13A)* at a location where the patient does not recall having had an injury to the skin. It must be differentiated clinically from a dermatofibroma and other benign or malignant tumors of the dermis. Histologic examination reveals a cicatricial growth of the lesion with spindle cell variants of malignant melanocytes *(Fig. 31.13B)*.[51–53] This histologic subtype must be differentiated from

amelanotic melanoma *(Fig. 31.14)*, which is simply a variant of nodular or superficial spreading melanoma that is not producing sufficient pigment granules to appear as a pigmented lesion. In one series of melanomas, the incidence of amelanotic melanoma was found to be 1.8%.[54]

Histopathologic factors of prognostic significance

With respect to analysis of the primary lesion alone, the depth of invasion of melanoma into the dermis has been shown to be the most powerful determinant of outcome. In 1965, Mehnert and Heard[55] reported the earliest correlation of depth with prognosis. A few years later, Clark *et al.*[56] described the following system of levels for the classification of depth of invasion into the dermis *(Fig. 31.15)*:

Level I: *in situ* melanoma; limited to the dermis– epidermis junction

Level II: invading the papillary dermis but without expansion of this layer

Level III: invading and expanding the papillary dermis but not into the reticular dermis (to the interface of the papillary–reticular dermis)

Level IV: invading the reticular dermis, but not into the subcutaneous fat

Level V: invading the subcutaneous fat or the associated subreticular tissues.

The difficulty with this classification system is the qualitative and somewhat subjective nature of determining the depth of invasion. Various pathologists examining a histologic slide of mid-dermal invasion often disagree on the Clark level of invasion; some may call it a level III, while others call it a deep level II, and still others call it an early level IV invasion. As a result of this difficulty, Breslow[57] reported a method of quantitative measurement that employs a simple and readily reproducible system of microstaging. According to Breslow, the melanoma's depth of invasion is measured in tenths of millimeters as a thickness from the surface of the tumor in the epidermis to the deepest tumor cell identified by means of an ocular micrometer on the microscope. In a number of studies using multivariate analyses,[43,45] Breslow's method has been shown to be the most powerful prognostic indicator for survival in

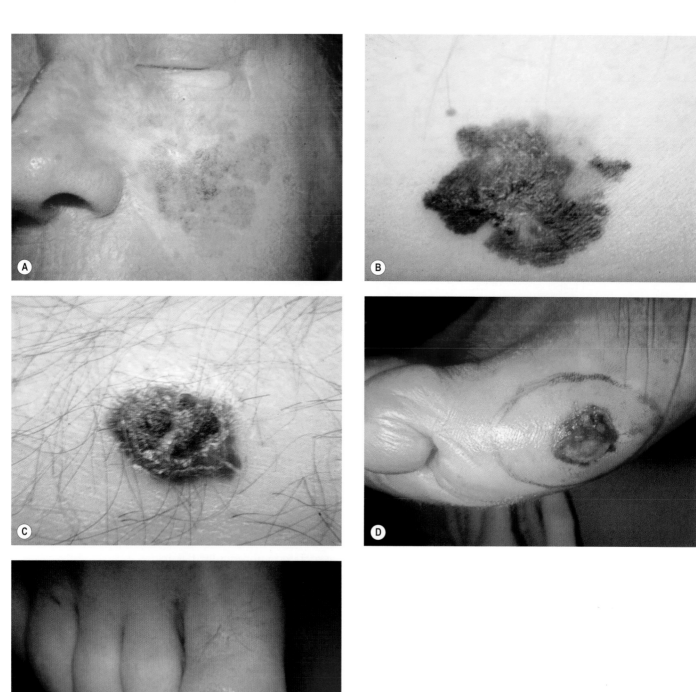

Fig. 31.12 Various morphologic types of melanoma. **(A)** Lentigo maligna melanoma: thin, flat lesion within patchy discoloration of Hutchinson freckle. **(B)** Superficial spreading melanoma: flat lesion with cells proliferating in the horizontal plane. **(C)** Nodular melanoma: thicker lesion growing in a vertical plane. **(D, E)** Acral lentiginous melanoma of the foot and nail bed.

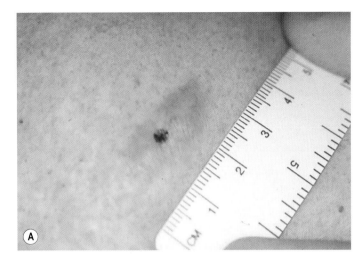

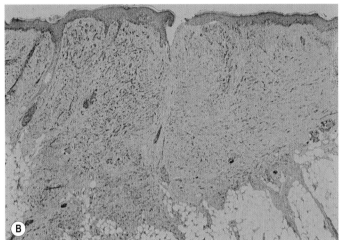

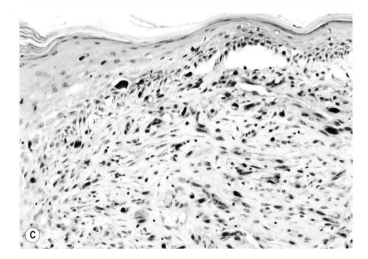

Fig. 31.13 (A) Desmoplastic melanoma is often nonpigmented and has the appearance of hypertrophic scar. **(B)** Low-power magnification of the desmoplastic melanoma shows the proliferation of the tumor in a cicatricial fashion. **(C)** High-power magnification of the lesion shows the spindle cell variant of the malignant melanocytes with the production of some pigment granules.

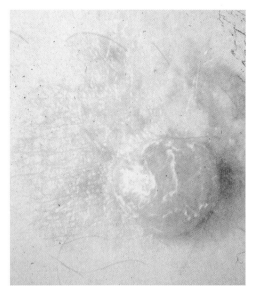

Fig. 31.14 The lack of pigment production in this amelanotic melanoma is deceptive in a lesion that is otherwise suggestive of malignancy.

early-stage melanoma (i.e., disease limited to primary tumor). Additional factors shown, in appropriate multivariate analyses of several thousand patients, to be associated with recurrence and survival include: ulceration in the lesion, the mitotic rate within the lesion, the patient's age and sex, the site of the primary lesion, and the morphologic type of melanoma.[43,58]

T category of TNM staging system

The histopathologic factors incorporated into the T category of the 2010 TNM staging system are the thickness of the primary tumor, i.e., the Breslow depth,[57] the presence or absence of ulceration of the overlying epithelium, and the mitotic rate.[43,44]

The thickness of the primary tumor (T) defines four categories *(Table 31.2)*:

T1: ≤1.0 mm

T2: 1.01–2.0 mm

T3: 2.01–4.0 mm

T4: >4.0 mm.

Increasing tumor thickness is closely correlated with poorer prognosis. The 10-year survival decreases progressively, from 96% for patients with primary lesions <0.5 mm thick to 54% for patients with lesions 4.01–6.0 mm thick.[43,44]

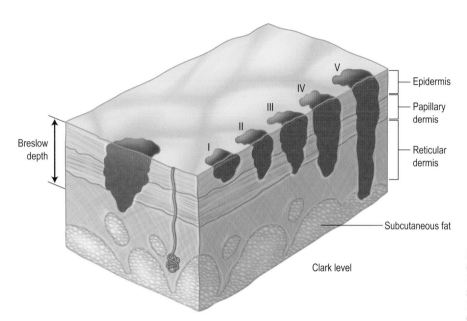

Breslow depth

I II III IV V

Epidermis

Papillary dermis

Reticular dermis

Subcutaneous fat

Clark level

Fig. 31.15 The Clark classification of melanoma is dependent on the qualitative determination of the extent of invasion into the various areas of the dermis or subcutaneous fat. The Breslow classification is determined by the micrometer reading of the depth of invasion into the dermis, measured in tenths of millimeters.

The T categories are further subdivided into "a" or "b" based upon the presence or absence of ulceration and the mitotic rate *(Table 31.2)*. Ulceration is defined as the absence of an intact epithelium over the melanoma. Outcomes in patients with ulcerated primary tumors are worse than in patients with primary melanomas of the same thickness but without ulceration. The mitotic rate was incorporated into the 2010 TNM staging system based upon the observation that it was the second most important prognostic factor in over 11 000 patients with localized melanoma analyzed in the AJCC Melanoma Staging Database. In that series, there was a highly significant correlation between increasing mitotic rate and declining survival rates ($P < 0.0001$). For instance, for melanomas less than 1.0 mm thick, the 10-year survival rate was 93% for those with <1 mitosis/mm^2 and 48% for those with >20 mitoses/mm^2.[43,44] The recommended approach to determining the mitotic rate is to identify the area of dermis containing the most mitoses (the "hot spot"), and average the number of mitoses within a 1-mm^2 area of the hot spot.[44] The substaging according to mitotic rates applies only to T1 lesions.

With respect to prognostic classification *(Table 31.3)*, stage I melanoma defines patients with low-risk melanomas (T1a–T2a) without evidence of regional or distant metastases. Further subdivision (stages IA and IB) is based upon characteristics of the primary tumor. Stage II melanoma includes primary tumors at a higher risk of recurrence or metastasis (T2b–T4b) without evidence of surgical or distant metastases. Similarly, stage II subdivision (IIA, IIB, IIC) is based upon characteristics of the primary tumor.[43,44] Details of more advanced stages of melanoma will be covered in the next section.

In-transit and regional lymph node disease

Local metastatic spread of cutaneous melanoma is known to occur through lymphatic channels in the majority – approximately 90% of cases.[59] Direct hematogenous dissemination of melanoma, more difficult to assess and treat, is another less common route of metastasis. There are a number of clinical and pathologic characteristics of regional spread of metastatic melanoma that have become incorporated into the prognostic staging system for primary melanoma, namely satellite/in-transit metastases and sentinel lymph node status.[60]

Intralymphatic spread of melanoma in the skin can present/manifest as satellite lesions, also known as microscopic satellitosis, or in-transit metastases, which are skin or subcutaneous metastases more than 2 cm from the primary lesion.[50] Microscopic satellitosis is seen in up to one-third of primary melanoma lesions greater than 3 mm thick, compared to less than 5% of thinner lesions.[60] The presence of microscopic satellitosis and in-transit metastases has been shown to carry a poorer prognosis, similar to the presence of regional lymph node metastases.[43,44] Thus, in the current AJCC system, patients with microscopic satellitosis or in-transit metastases are upstaged to the level of a patient with established lymph node metastases *(Tables 31.2 and 31.3)*.

Spread of melanoma to the regional lymph nodes portends a poorer prognosis. As melanoma is known mostly to metastasize through lymphatic channels (and the first sites of metastasis are typically regional lymph node basins), evaluation of the regional lymph node basins has become critical in the staging of melanoma. Unfortunately, clinical evaluation of the regional lymph nodes is often inaccurate: as many as 20% of clinically node-negative patients have metastatic involvement on pathologic evaluation, and up to 20% of those with clinically positive nodes are pathologically negative.[61]

Mostly of historical significance, elective lymph node dissection (ELND) has largely been supplanted by sentinel lymph node biopsy (SNLB). However, brief mention is warranted. In the setting of clinically node-negative disease, ELND involves removal of all lymph nodes in a suspected draining basin. The rationale is that removal of subclinical regional disease may provide a survival benefit over a therapeutic node resection performed after regional disease becomes clinically evident. Performance of this procedure is now controversial, in the era of lymphoscintigraphy and SNLB, especially as most melanomas are being diagnosed early (thinner and less invasive), and the morbidity associated with a completion lymphadenectomy can be quite significant. Additionally, while a few retrospective analyses suggested ELND might improve survival by 25–40%,[62] most prospective randomized trials have not demonstrated a survival benefit from ELND.[63]

Lymphoscintigraphy (lymphatic mapping) and sentinel lymph node biopsy

In the skin, as in all parts of the body, arterial blood pressure diffuses serum and nutrient material out of the vessels into the interstitial tissue to nourish the cells. The breakdown products of metabolism are then picked up by the veins and taken back into the systemic system. Because the pressure in the arteries is greater than in the veins, more of this vascular fluid is diffused into the tissue than is taken away by the vein. To avoid the consequences of edema, lymphatic vessels (the micro sump pumps of the system) draw away this excess fluid and take it to the regional lymph nodes to filter the product before returning it to the systemic vascular system. This filtering function of the lymph nodes allows detection and attack of foreign bacteria, antigens, and cancer cells. It was this principle that permitted Sappey[64] to show the lymphatic patterns of the human body in 1874 by injecting mercury into the skin. Sappey's lines are a helpful guide to determine the likely directions of lymphatic spread. Subsequent experience has shown that lesions located more than 2 cm above or below a "belt line" drawn through the umbilicus usually drain to the axillary or groin nodes, respectively. Lesions more than 2 cm on either side of the midline drain to the lymph nodes on that respective side. Lesions within 4 cm of the vertical and horizontal bands may go to any one of the pairs of options *(Fig. 31.16)*.

As a result of potentially unclear lymphatic drainage patterns, Sherman and Ter-Pogossian[65] introduced lymphoscintigraphy in 1953. They injected radiocolloid gold (^{198}Au) intradermally and used a gamma counter to detect the concentrated colloidal isotope in the filtering lymph nodes. This technique has since been modified with various other isotopes and colloids of various particle sizes for specific diagnostic purposes. The intent of each of these modifications is to identify the lymphatic vascular pattern in the tissue being evaluated.

The technique of lymphatic mapping is helpful for predicting the pattern of spread for cutaneous melanoma metastases to regional draining lymph node basins, and it may be helpful in detecting metastases in melanoma of the extremities.[66] In particular, the test may be useful in patients with T2 or thicker lesions of the lower extremity for evaluation of the iliac and pelvic lymph nodes to determine the extent of lymphadenectomy that may be indicated. The iliac nodes should certainly be removed if they appear to be involved, but a pelvic lymphadenectomy is not indicated if the para-aortic lymph nodes are involved because cure is unlikely in these cases.

The sites of lymphatic spread from melanoma at other locations, including the trunk and head and neck regions, may be also evaluated by radionuclide lymphoscintigraphy.[67] Several radiocolloids have been employed for lymphoscintigraphy, including gold, sulfur, and antimony. Antimony sulfide colloid and technetium

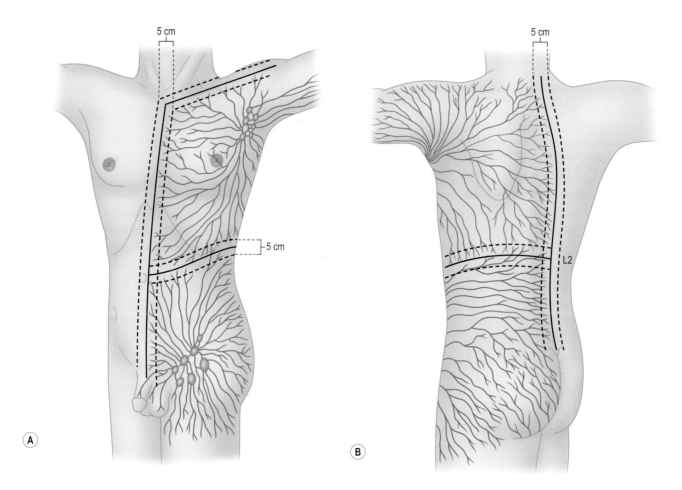

Fig. 31.16 (A, B) Lymphatic drainage as predicted by Sappey's lines. (Redrawn from Sugarbaker EV, McBride CM. Melanoma of the trunk: the results of surgical excision and anatomic guidelines for predicting nodal metastasis. *Surgery*. 1976;80:22.)

sulfur colloid have been found to be safe, and both give reliable information for determining appropriate lymph nodes for elective dissection among patients with truncal or head and neck melanomas *(Fig. 31.17)*.

A lymphoscintigram can demonstrate predicted as well as unexpected patterns of lymph node drainage from lesions at primary sites. The test has been demonstrated as a reliable predictor of the sites of nodal involvement. In a prospective study of 51 consecutive patients with primary melanomas greater than 1 mm thick and observed for a mean of 45 months, 23% of the 35 patients who chose to undergo elective lymphadenectomy were found to have micrometastases to these lymph nodes; all were in the node groups detected by the lymphoscintigram.[68] During the several years of their follow-up, 5 of the 16 patients (31%) who chose to be observed eventually developed clinical evidence of

nodal metastases; in each case, the nodes that were involved with tumor were at the very sites of drainage predicted by the lymphoscintigrams that were performed at the time of initial diagnosis *(Table 31.4)*. During the 7-year interval of follow-up, no patient in either group developed metastases to any nodes not predicted by lymphoscintigraphy.

Sentinel lymph node biopsy

As stated previously, the availability of lymphatic mapping with SLNB has obviated a possible role for ELND in the treatment of cutaneous melanoma. The concept of the sentinel lymph node is based on the principle that all lymphatic fluid from specific tissues is filtered by lymph nodes, and as such the first (or sentinel) lymph node filtering a specific site can be removed and

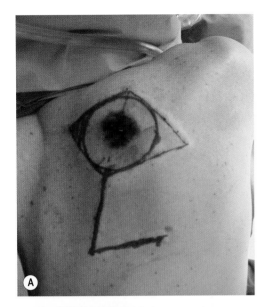

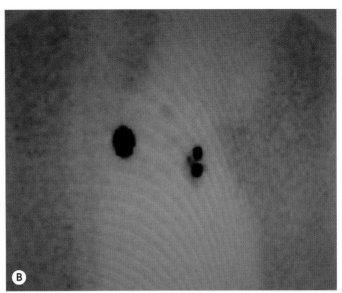

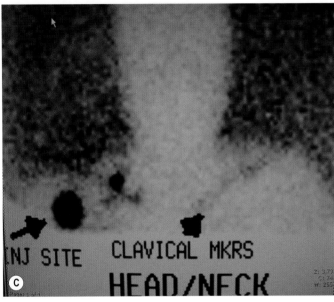

Fig. 31.17 Lymphoscintigram of a right scapular melanoma **(A)** demonstrates drainage to the right axillary lymph nodes **(B)**, as well as the right lower cervical nodes **(C)**.

Table 31.4 Reliability of lymphoscintigrams

	ELND	Observe
Number of patients*	35 (70%)	16 (30%)
Lymph node metastases	8 (23%)	–
Subsequent lymph node metastases	–	5 (31%)

ELND, elective lymph node dissection.
*51 patients with melanoma greater than 1 mm thick; 7-year follow-up (mean of 45 months).
(Data from Stephens PI, Ariyan S, Ocampo RJ, et al. The predictive value of lymphoscintigraphy for nodal metastases of cutaneous melanoma. *Conn Med.* 1999;63:387.)

evaluated for metastasis of malignant cells. The validity of this entire principle is predicated on the tenets that: finite regions drain to a specific node; the sentinel node can be found; a negative biopsy finding means no other metastases exist; and, a negative sentinel node is truly negative.

Morton et al.[59] introduced the technique of detecting the sentinel lymph node with the intraoperative injection of vital blue dyes in the dermis surrounding the site of the primary melanoma. He identified the sentinel lymph node in more than 80% of patients and reported

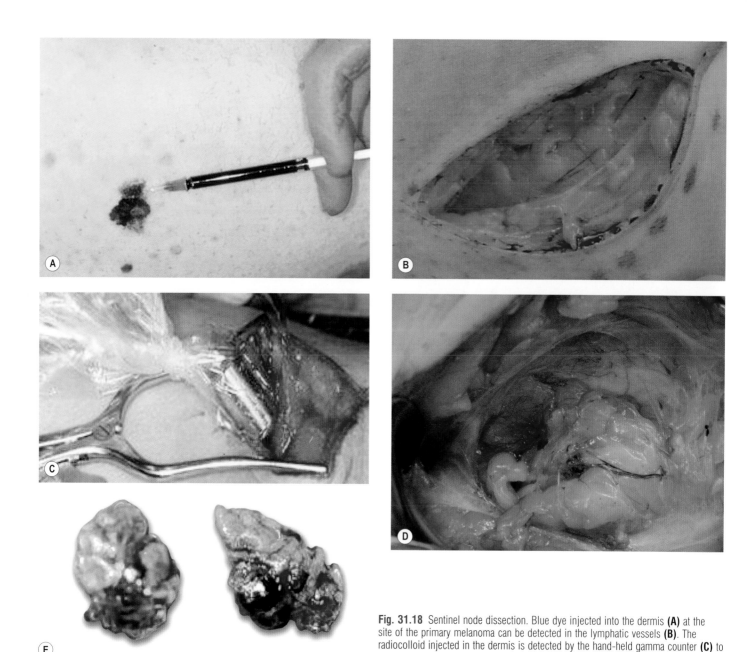

Fig. 31.18 Sentinel node dissection. Blue dye injected into the dermis **(A)** at the site of the primary melanoma can be detected in the lymphatic vessels **(B)**. The radiocolloid injected in the dermis is detected by the hand-held gamma counter **(C)** to localize the sentinel lymph node **(D)**. A second node **(E)** was also identified adjacent to the first.

Sentinel   Secondary

that the false-negative rates had been about 5%. Subsequent investigators[69–71] reported the use of preoperative lymphatic mapping and the intraoperative use of radiocolloids together with vital blue dyes with increased identification and successful removal of the sentinel lymph node to the range of 98–99% of patients with melanoma *(Fig. 31.18)*. Based on studies of melanoma patients who underwent SLNB and subsequent completion lymphadenectomy of the respective lymph node basin, it can be assumed that if the sentinel lymph nodes are not involved, the entire basin should be free of tumor in 96% of cases.[59,69,72]

N category of TNM system

SLNB has largely become the standard of care in the initial evaluation of cutaneous melanoma, particularly for patients with melanoma thicker than 1 mm in depth. The likelihood of finding nodal metastases in patients with tumors less than 1 mm in thickness is quite low

Table 31.5 Risk of detecting a positive sentinel lymph node

Breslow depth	Risk of positive sentinel lymph node
<1.0 mm	4–7%
1.01–2.0 mm	12–20%
2.01–4.0 mm	28–33%
>4.0 mm	40–44%

(Data from Rousseau DL Jr, Ross MI, Johnson MM, *et al*. Revised American Joint Committee on Cancer staging criteria accurately predict sentinel lymph node positivity in clinically node-negative melanoma patients. *Ann Surg Oncol*. 2003;10:569–574 and Morton DL, Hoon DS, Cochran AJ, *et al*. Lymphatic mapping and sentinel lymphadenectomy for early-stage melanoma: therapeutic utility and implications of nodal microanatomy and molecular staging for improving the accuracy of detection of nodal micrometastases. *Ann Surg*. 2003;238:538–549.)

(less than 10%).[73–75] However, the presence of certain high-risk features, including ulceration and/or a high mitotic rate, may justify SLNB in thin melanomas.[76–79] The likelihood of detecting metastatic deposits in an SLNB increases with the thickness of the primary lesion; for lesions <1.0 mm, 1.01–2.0 mm, 2.01–4.0 mm, and >4 mm, the risk is approximately 4–7%, 12–20%, 28–33%, and 40–44%, respectively *(Table 31.5)*.[80,81] The test is particularly useful for patients with intermediate-thickness melanomas, 1–4 mm. However, it should still be considered in the treatment algorithm of patients with very thick tumors (greater than 4 mm) because even though this group of patients has a 65–70% risk of distant metastases, the SLNB may still provide important prognostic information, and obviate a subsequent lymphadenectomy in a number of patients who would subsequently develop enlarged nodes.[82]

Based on analyses of the AJCC Melanoma Staging Database, nodal status has been demonstrated as the overriding factor predicting disease outcome.[83–85] For patients with clinically detectable nodal disease (macrometastases), the characteristics of the primary tumor essentially become irrelevant with respect to predicting 5-year survival. That is, thickness, ulceration, and mitotic rate do not maintain statistical significance on multivariate analysis.[86] As the majority of patients present without clinically apparent nodal involvement, the goal of SLNB is to identify patients with microscopic nodal metastases as early as possible so they might benefit from the early removal of these metastatic nodes before the disease can spread any further, and to consider these patients for adjuvant therapy. In patients with nodal disease (including those with nodal disease limited to micrometastases), it has been demonstrated that the most important prognostic factor is the number of involved nodes.[86]

The node (N) category of the 2010 edition of the AJCC Melanoma TNM system *(Table 31.2)* includes the following designations:

Nx: nodes are not assessable (e.g., previously resected for other reasons)

N0: no regional lymphatic metastases

N1: one involved lymph node

  N1a: micrometastasis

  N1b: macrometastasis

N2: two to three involved nodes

  N2a: micrometastases

  N2b: at least one node with macrometastasis

N2c: in-transit or satellite metastasis without lymph node involvement

N3: four or more positive nodes, matted nodes, or in-transit/satellite metastases with one or more positive nodes.

The presence of in-transit metastases, or nodal involvement, classifies the patient as stage III, with subclassification (IIIA, IIIB, or IIIC) dependent upon the extent of lymphatic disease *(Table 31.3)*.

Evaluation of systemic disease

The evaluation of the patient with malignant melanoma requires a complete physical examination of the primary site and regional draining lymph nodes to detect any clinical evidence of satellite or in-transit lesions (metastases) in the skin or of metastases to lymph nodes. The abdomen needs to be examined for evidence of an enlarged liver, enlarged spleen, or abdominal masses that would suggest intra-abdominal metastases. The extent of examination and the tests ordered for such evaluations are predicated on the stage of the primary diagnosis *(Table 31.6)*. A chest radiograph may be indicated to look for pulmonary metastases, and computed chest tomograms may add to the detection of small and early lesions. Liver enzyme function tests are simple, sensitive, and reliable for detecting liver metastases

Table 31.6 Staging evaluation: tests recommended for determination of presence and extent of tumor spread

Primary tumor (no clinical evidence of other involvement)

Physical examination
Chest radiography
Liver function tests
Lymphoscintigraphy to detect sites of sentinel nodes (if primary tumor is 1 mm or more thick)

Local and regional disease (in-transit lesions or nodal involvement)

Physical examination
Liver function tests
Computed tomography scans:
  of chest and abdomen (to examine lungs and liver)
  of pelvis if tumor involves lower extremities
  of neck if tumor involves the head and neck
Lymphoscintigraphy to detect sites of sentinel nodes
Additional scans as indicated by clinical signs or symptoms

Distant organ metastases

Physical examination
Liver function tests and serum lactate dehydrogenase level
Computed tomography scans, as indicated above
Magnetic resonance imaging scans if required to detect extent of soft-tissue invasion
Positron emission tomography scans to detect extent of tumor involvement of vital organs (lung, liver, brain)

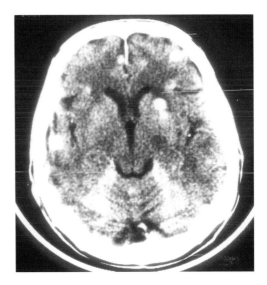

Fig. 31.19 Computed tomography scans of the brain can detect small lesions. In this patient, several lesions are identified in both hemispheres.

and, when results are negative, may serve as a baseline for later annual follow-up examinations. Serum lactate dehydrogenase (LDH) has been identified as an important independent prognostic factor in patients with disseminated melanoma. The AJCC Melanoma Staging Database included 7972 patients with distant metastases, and 1- and 2-year survival rates were significantly lower in patients with elevated serum LDH (32% versus 65% and 18% versus 40%).[43] Therefore, serum LDH must be measured at the time stage IV disease is documented, as it provides important prognostic information.

Computerized scans

Although tomographic radiographs of the lungs are helpful in detecting pulmonary metastases, computed tomographic (CT) scanning of the chest and abdomen does not offer a significant advantage as an initial screening test over chest radiographs and liver function tests.[87] Even though this imaging technique requires skillful interpretation for optimal use, analyses have shown that screening chest radiographs, a much less expensive modality, are just as useful as CT scans in detecting metastatic lesions at the time of the initial diagnosis. However, CT scans do offer the potential for superior detection of metastatic lesions in various organs, and they are quite useful for evaluating the brain (*Fig. 31.19*).

Whereas patients with primary melanomas thicker than 1 mm may be considered at moderate risk, those with lesions greater than 2 mm are considered at high risk for metastases. Patients with stage III disease are certainly candidates for intensive surveillance. These higher-risk patients should be evaluated for distant organ metastases with chest and abdominal CT scans, which enable the physician to examine the lungs, the liver, and the spleen in one test. Enhanced brain CT scans should also be considered.

On the other hand, CT scans can be helpful for staging the disease in patients who present with local or regional extension of the disease. In some patients, the extent of the disease detected from the CT scans can be elaborated by the use of magnetic resonance imaging scans (*Fig. 31.20*). Positron emission tomography (PET) scan has been found to be valuable for evaluating patients for extension of their disease and assigning stage.[88,89] The increased metabolism of the tumor is reflected in the increased uptake of radioactive-labeled glucose, which is represented by the brighter activity

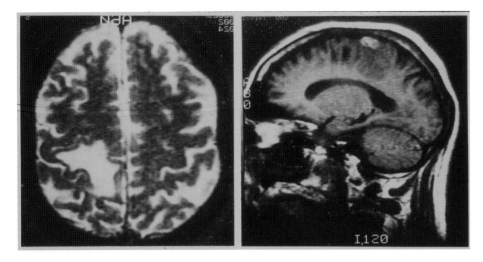

Fig. 31.20 Magnetic resonance imaging, in this case of the brain, demonstrates involvement of soft tissue by melanoma.

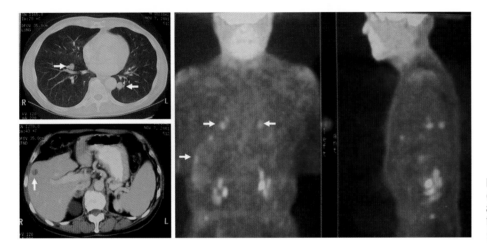

Fig. 31.21 Positron emission tomography scan of the chest and abdomen (right) confirms the increased activity of metastatic lesions seen on computed tomography scan in the lung (upper left) and liver (lower left).

at the site of the metastases *(Fig. 31.21)*. In the absence of infectious processes, the false-positive rate has been reported to be less than 5% with PET scans. The restrictions to the use of PET scans are the limited availability of the scanners and the greater expense of these studies.

M category of TNM system

The AJCC staging system categorizes patients with distant metastases according to the site(s) of disease involvement and the serum LDH level *(Table 31.2)*.[43,44] M1a, associated with the best prognosis, identifies patients with metastases limited to distant skin, subcutaneous or lymph node sites, and a normal serum LDH. M1b denotes patients with lung metastases and a normal serum LDH. M1c patients have the worst prognosis, with metastases to other visceral sites (or an elevated

serum LDH). With respect to staging *(Table 31.3)*, any M designation (i.e., the presence of any metastatic disease beyond the regional lymph nodes) places the patient in the stage IV category.

While rare, patients will occasionally present with metastatic melanoma without an identifiable primary tumor. In these situations, if the patient has isolated metastases in the lymph nodes, skin, or subcutaneous tissues and an unknown primary, the patient is considered stage III, as studies suggest there is a similar (or slightly better) survival rate compared to those with involved lymph nodes and a known primary tumor.[90–94]

Members of the AJCC Melanoma Task Force recently developed an electronic prediction tool for patients presenting with localized disease (http://www.melanomaprognosis.org). The prediction tool can be used to predict the 1-, 2-, 5-, and 10-year survival rates from initial diagnosis (with a 95% confidence interval) for an individual patient based on his/her relevant clinical and pathologic information. The predictive models were developed and validated using a combined database ($n = 28\ 047$) from 11 major institutions and study groups participating in the development of the AJCC Melanoma Staging System.[95]

Surgical considerations and treatment

Initial biopsy

Some clinicians have questioned the safety in biopsy of malignant melanoma for fear that tumor cells might be disseminated through the blood stream. To evaluate this risk, Epstein et al.[25] reviewed 170 melanoma patients from the California Tumor Registry over a 4-year period, 115 of whom underwent biopsy of the melanoma before surgical treatment and 55 of whom had not. The 5- and 10-year cure rates, as well as relative cure rates by life-table analysis to eliminate differences in the age distribution of the two groups, were more favorable for those patients who had undergone a previous biopsy. The results of this study suggest not that biopsies improve the overall cure rates but that an incomplete removal of a melanoma by a surgical biopsy followed by definitive surgery does not decrease the cure rate. Additional studies have confirmed this observation – one from the US with 230 patients[96] and a subsequent study from Denmark[97] with 225 patients followed up for a minimum of 5 years. The role of biopsy type in relation to survival was specifically analyzed by Lederman and Sober[98] in 472 patients: 119 underwent incisional biopsy (either punch or incision) and 353 had an excisional biopsy. After controlling for other factors, especially tumor thickness, no statistically significant difference was demonstrated between patients in the different biopsy type groups. Importantly, biopsy of the lesion (incisional or excisional) will make the diagnosis of melanoma as well as demonstrate the aggressiveness of the lesion by the degree of invasion into the dermis.

Our recommendation, if the lesion is small, is to perform an excisional biopsy with a 1–2-mm margin of normal-appearing skin to permit the pathologist to render a diagnosis reliably and to determine the thickest depth of invasion. However, if functional or cosmetic concerns prohibit easy removal of the entire lesion, an incisional biopsy or punch biopsy is an acceptable alternative. The only drawback of such a partial biopsy is that the final therapeutic excision may show a lesion that is classified with greater depth of invasion than had been initially discovered. In some cases, the patient would have been eligible for sentinel node biopsy if the proper depth had been assessed before wide excision and resurfacing. We do not prefer shave biopsy, though it may be acceptable when the index of suspicion is low and the lesion is broad (e.g., broad shave biopsy in some cases of lentigo maligna and melanoma *in situ* may increase diagnostic sampling), or in cases of suspected subungual melanoma.

As specific details from the biopsy specimen will dictate the next steps in management, the specimen must be assessed by a pathologist with expertise in the evaluation of pigmented lesions. Pathologic details that must be reported include: Breslow thickness in millimeters, histologic ulceration, mitotic rate per mm^2, peripheral and deep margin status, and Clark level (for lesions ≤ 1 mm in depth). Other histopathologic details of potential significance include: microscopic satellitosis, regression, tumor-infiltrating lymphocytes, neurotropism, and histologic subtype.

Wide local excision

The purpose of wide local excision (WLE) of melanoma is to decrease the incidence of local recurrence, reported in the literature to range from 3% to 20%. In large series, the highest risk of local recurrence has been documented with primary tumors on the hands and feet, with a recurrence rate of 11–12%, whereas the risk is only 5–6% for tumors on the face, scalp, and ear.[58]

It has generally been accepted that melanomas less than 0.76 mm thick are uniformly curable, as reported by Breslow.[57] Breslow and Macht[99] reported in a small series of 62 patients with lesions less than 0.76 mm that neither local recurrences nor metastases developed, regardless of the width of resection margin. Day et al.[100] reported that, although thin lesions have a good prognosis, the prognosis may be worse when the melanoma is located within the BANS area, an acronym for the upper back, upper posterior arm, posterior neck, and posterior scalp. On the other hand, Woods et al.[101] reported 11 deaths among 400 patients with melanomas less than 0.76 mm treated at the Mayo Clinic: seven of

Table 31.7 Trials comparing margin width for cutaneous melanoma

Study: author, year	n	Median follow-up	Lesion thickness	Margins	Local recurrence (%)	10-year overall survival
World Health Organization: Cascinelli, 1998[111]	612	12 years	0–1 mm	1 cm	3/186 (1.6)	87%
			1.1–2.0 mm	1 cm	5/119 (4.2)	
			0–1 mm	3 cm	1/173 (0.6)	87%
			1.1–2.0 mm	3 cm	2/134 (1.5)	
Swedish: Cohn-Cedarmark, 2000[114]	989	11 years	0.8–2 mm	2 cm	3/476 (0.6)	79%
				5 cm	5/513 (1)	76%
French Cooperative Group: Khayat, 2003[115]	326	16 years	<2.1 mm	2 cm	1/181 (0.05)	87%
				5 cm	4/185 (0.2)	86%
Melanoma Intergroup Trial: Karakousis, 1996[117]	468	8 years	1–4 mm	2 cm	(2.1)	70%
				4 cm	(2.6)	77%
British Trial: Thomas, 2004[119]	900	5 years	≥ 2 mm	1 cm	15/453 (3.3)	Not reported
				3 cm	13/447 (2.9)	Not reported

(Data from Sladden MJ, Balch C, Barzilai DA, *et al.* Surgical excision margins for primary cutaneous melanoma. *Cochrane Database Syst Rev* 2009;4:CD004835 and Stone M. Initial surgical management of melanoma of the skin and unusual sites. In: Atkins MB, Weiser M, Tsao H (eds) *UpToDate*, 18.3 ed. Waltham, MA: UpToDate, 2010.)

the melanomas were not within the BANS area at all. In a smaller series, Briggs *et al.*[102] reported that 10% of patients with melanoma less than 0.76 mm died during their 10-year experience.

The World Health Organization[103] evaluated the importance of the width of resection of the primary melanoma and the surrounding normal skin in a study of 593 patients with clinical stage I disease. Curability was not influenced by the resection margins but decreased with increasing thickness of the primary melanoma. In a large study of more than 3400 patients, Urist *et al.*[58] noted that the recurrence rate of 146 melanomas of the neck was less than 2% even though most of the patients (84–87%) were treated with resection margins of only 1–2 cm.

In a study of 598 patients with clinical stage I melanoma, the New York University–Massachusetts General Hospital Melanoma Clinical Cooperative Group noted that resection margins of 1.5 cm or less were associated with a significantly greater incidence of recurrences than were resection margins greater than 1.5 cm. However, margins greater than 3 cm did not lead to a lesser recurrence rate.[104] Indeed, for melanomas greater than 2 mm thick, retrospective data suggest that margins less than 2 cm may decrease the cure rates.[58,105–107]

The thickness of the melanoma is the key factor in determining the recommended margin of normal tissue to be excised. However, a recent systematic review and meta-analysis of randomized controlled trials of surgical excision margins in melanoma did not demonstrate a statistically significant difference in overall survival between narrow or wide excision margins.[108] Nonetheless, recommended margins have decreased progressively as a result of multiple large clinical trials that have examined the impact of margins on local recurrence *(Table 31.7)*.

With respect to *in situ* melanoma, while there are no data from randomized trials to define the optimal extent of surgical resection, retrospective data support the use of 0.5-cm margins.[16,109] For invasive melanoma, we recommend the following excision margins, based on data from multiple studies of optimal resection margins for malignant melanoma.[110–119] For patients with stage IA melanoma (≤1.0 mm in thickness), wide excision with a 1.0-cm margin is recommended. For lesions of 1.01–2.0 mm thickness, a 1–2-cm margin is recommended, recognizing that a full 2.0-cm margin may be difficult to achieve in some areas of functional or cosmetic significance.[120] For lesions >2.0 mm in thickness, a margin of at least 2.0 cm is recommended.

In determining the extent of the operation, whether on the face or on the trunk, it is important to consider the impact of the scar on the patient's self-image. The Pigment Lesion Study Group of the University of Pennsylvania evaluated the extent to which patients were distressed by scars after melanoma resection.[104] The two factors that had a negative impact were the degree of surgical depression or indentation and the

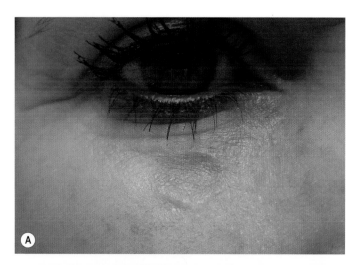

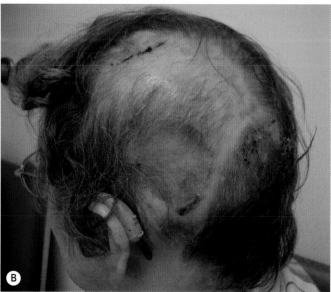

Fig. 31.22 Skin grafts provide adequate coverage for wide resections, but they can lead to significant deformities, as demonstrated in the infraorbital region **(A)** and scalp **(B)**.

patients' preoperative perception of the scar to be expected. The actual scar length did not have as much of an effect as the extent of depression of the scar. As such, skin grafts are acceptable for reconstructions of large resection sites, but they cause significant deformities *(Fig. 31.22)*, which are usually avoided with flaps for coverage. The author has previously reported on the safety of coverage of these wounds with flaps.[121]

Head and neck

Although the skin of the head and neck accounts for only 9% of total body surface area, 15–30% of all primary melanomas develop on the head and neck.[122,123] High-risk melanomas of the face should be excised as outlined above and closed with adjacent flaps. Although resurfacing the resection site with a skin graft is possible, the cosmetic results are not as acceptable as with a flap. A local or regional skin flap covers the wound with a far more satisfactory color match to the rest of the face than a distant flap *(Fig. 31.23)*.

A difficult area to resurface is a surgical defect over the chin because this area requires skin that firmly adheres to the mandible, soft tissue for contour, and a good match of the skin flap to the remainder of the face. A distant flap simply does not provide a satisfactory color match. A wide excision of this area can be resurfaced satisfactorily with an advancement flap of the neck.

On occasion, the melanoma forms on the upper part of the cheek, requiring removal of skin from the lower eyelids. This area cannot be resurfaced with a skin flap because it requires thin pliable covering. Resurfacing is best accomplished by employing a cheek advancement flap to cover most of the defect and a full-thickness skin graft to the eyelids. The best place to harvest this skin graft is from the ipsilateral or contralateral upper eyelid; the postauricular area may be an acceptable alternative.

In situations where tissue conservation is deemed necessary, frozen section analysis may be considered, but it does carry a risk of false-negative report.[124] Additionally, while investigational, Mohs micrographic surgery may be considered in these situations, or when treating superficial lesions of large diameter (e.g., lentigo maligna). Large series report that Mohs[125] may control the primary lesion, but longer follow-up is required before widespread adoption of this technique.[126] Treatment of lentigo maligna with imiquimod has also emerged as an effective therapy, but long-term comparative studies are still needed.[127–130]

Extremities

Thin melanomas of the fingertips may be excised and the defect reconstructed with volar advancement flaps *(Fig. 31.24)* to provide sensate coverage. Lesions of the finger thicker than 1 mm are more safely treated with an interphalangeal joint amputation *(Fig. 31.25)* or a ray amputation, depending on the extent of the tumor.

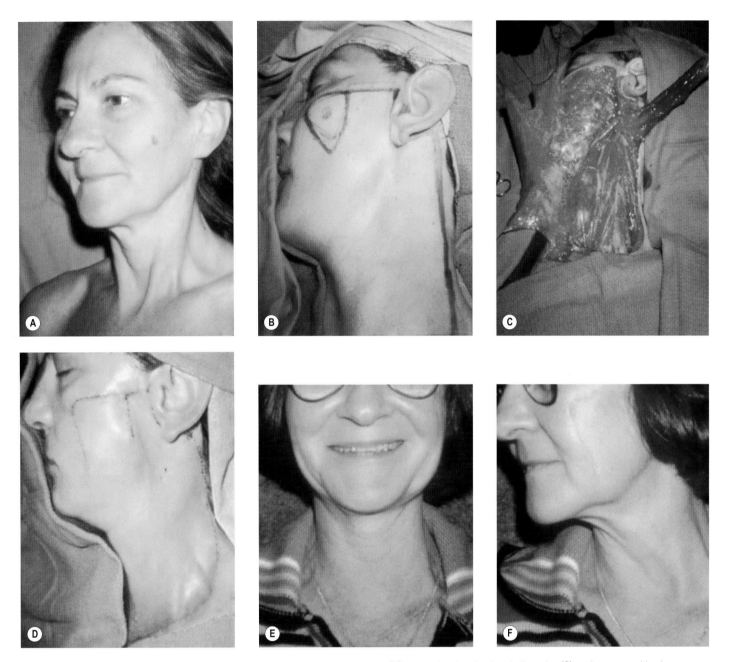

Fig. 31.23 Melanoma of the cheek **(A)** was treated with a wide excision of the primary site **(B)**, a complete functional neck dissection **(C)**, and coverage with a large cervicofacial myocutaneous flap incorporating the platysma muscle **(D)**. One-year postoperative photographs **(E and F)**.

Subungual melanoma of the fingers should be resected at the distal interphalangeal joint to preserve function.[131] Similarly, subungual melanomas involving the toes should be managed with digital amputation at the metatarsophalangeal joint.

Melanomas of the dorsum of the hand, the forearm, and the leg may be treated more readily with a wide excision. These surgical wounds have traditionally been covered with skin grafts with good success.

However, coverage of these wide excisions with local flaps *(Fig. 31.26)* has been accomplished with successful control of the primary site and a more cosmetically acceptable result.[121] Furthermore, these patients do not need to have the arm or leg immobilized, and they have a shorter hospital stay than do those who have had skin grafts.

Melanomas of the toes and feet are usually of the acral lentiginous type. These tumors spread

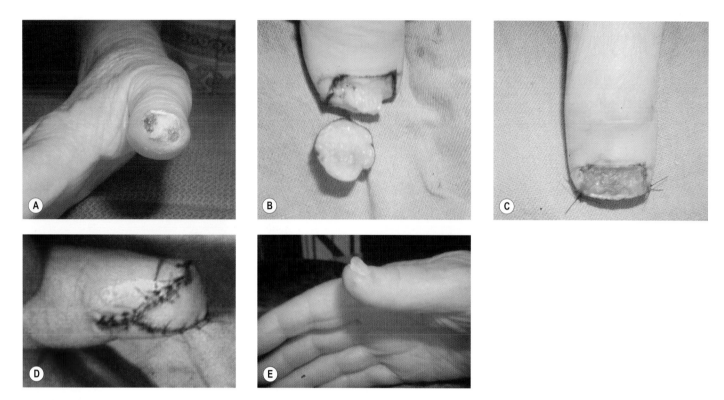

Fig. 31.24 Melanoma of the fingertip **(A)** was excised with the nail, nail matrix, and nail bed **(B)**. The wound was covered with a volar advancement flap **(C and D)**. The thumb remained free of disease 4 years postoperatively **(E)**.

aggressively and have a high incidence of local and regional recurrences. Therefore, they are best treated by aggressive resections *(Fig. 31.27)*. A significant advantage to the use of flaps in the lower extremity is that patients may be able to ambulate the day after surgery and leave the hospital much sooner than patients treated with skin grafts.

Trunk

Primary melanomas of the trunk may be excised with more liberal margins (as much as 2–4 cm if need be) and still be closed easily. Some areas may be closed by wide undermining and large advancement flaps. Otherwise, these areas may still be closed readily by one or more local flaps *(Fig. 31.28)*. Deep fascia and muscle may be preserved if not involved by tumor invasion.

Lymphadenectomy

The decision to perform a lymphadenectomy in a patient with melanoma requires further thought. In patients who present with palpable lymphadenopathy, it is appropriate to confirm diagnosis with fine-needle aspiration, core needle, or open biopsy of the clinically enlarged lymph node(s). In the absence of radiological evidence of distant metastases, wide excision of the primary site and complete dissection of the involved lymph node basin are indicated. For staging purposes, the number of positive nodes, the total number of nodes examined, and the presence or absence of extranodal tumor extension must be recorded.[120] Of note, in the lower extremities, when PET or pelvic CT scans reveal iliac and/or obturator lymphadenopathy, or if a positive Cloquet's lymph node is found, deep groin dissection should be considered.[132,133]

The majority of patients, however, will present without clinical evidence of nodal disease, and some will require SLNB (for staging purposes). The decision regarding which patients should undergo SLNB is dependent upon the pathological stage of the primary lesion. As stated previously, SLNB should be considered for patients with primary melanomas that demonstrate aggressive biology. Specifically, this includes stage IA melanomas with adverse prognostic features (i.e.,

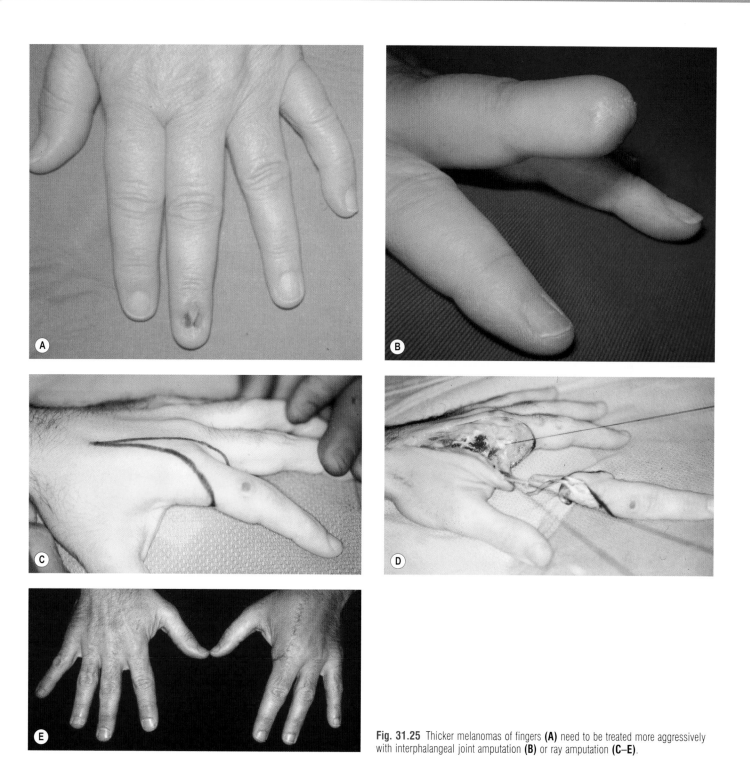

Fig. 31.25 Thicker melanomas of fingers **(A)** need to be treated more aggressively with interphalangeal joint amputation **(B)** or ray amputation **(C–E)**.

thickness ≥1.0 mm, positive deep margins, lymphovascular invasion, or young patient age), stage IB and II melanomas, as well as patients with resectable solitary in-transit stage III melanoma.[120] The decision regarding whether to proceed with SLNB is ultimately up to the patient and the treating physician, and should be performed at the time of WLE.[120]

If the sentinel lymph node is negative, regional lymph node dissection is not indicated. If the sentinel lymph node is positive, the patient should be offered complete

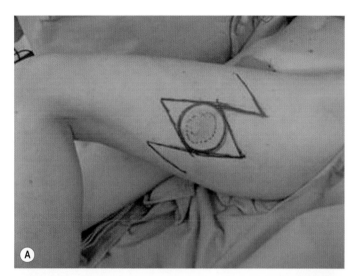

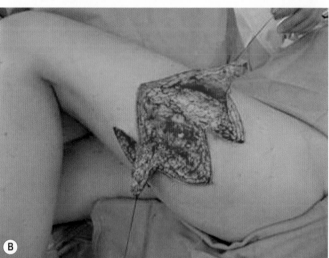

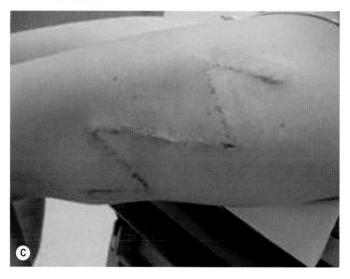

Fig. 31.26 Wide excisions of melanomas of the hands, forearms, and legs **(A)** may be treated with local transposition flaps **(B)** to allow the patient to use the extremities early in the postoperative period **(C)**.

dissection of the involved lymph node basin; 15–20% of these dissections will demonstrate melanoma in non-sentinel lymph nodes.[134,135] It has been shown that factors related to the sentinel lymph node can help predict the presence of melanoma in nonsentinel lymph nodes: size of the metastatic focus, number of metastatic foci, extracapsular extension.[136,137] Of note, these stage III patients should be considered for adjuvant treatment with interferon-alpha (IFN-α), especially if they lack any serious comorbidity and have an otherwise reasonable life expectancy.

The Multicenter Selective Lymphadenectomy Trial (MSLT) was a large trial designed to address the role of lymphatic mapping with SLNB in determining prognosis and its impact on survival.[138] The primary study group included 1347 patients with intermediate-thickness melanomas (1.2–3.5 mm) who were randomly assigned to WLE with observation or WLE with lymphatic mapping and SLNB. In the observation group, if palpable nodal metastases became evident, the patient underwent completion lymphadenectomy. Likewise, in the SLNB group, if the SLNB was histologically positive, the patient underwent immediate completion lymphadenectomy. The third of five planned interim analyses was published in 2006.[138] At a median follow-up of 60 months, the findings in the primary study group confirm the role of SLNB as a prognostic tool. A survival benefit was not demonstrated for the overall study population randomly assigned to lymphatic mapping and SLNB. However, amongst the patients who had nodal disease, the patients in the observation group who subsequently developed nodal metastases had more involved nodes at the time of lymphadenectomy (3.3 versus 1.4 nodes), and a significantly lower 5-year survival rate (52.4% versus 72.3%).

In regard to the patients with nodal metastases from melanoma of unknown origin, Reintgen *et al.*[139] reviewed 124 patients and demonstrated that regional lymphadenectomy resulted in a survival rate equal to that of lymphadenectomies in patients with known sites of primary melanoma. However, there is no place for the simple excision of the involved palpable lymph node alone because it is more than likely that additional lymph nodes have micrometastases. This question will be answered by the MSLT II trial in progress now. In the meantime, the only accepted treatment is a complete lymphadenectomy of the regional group of lymph nodes.

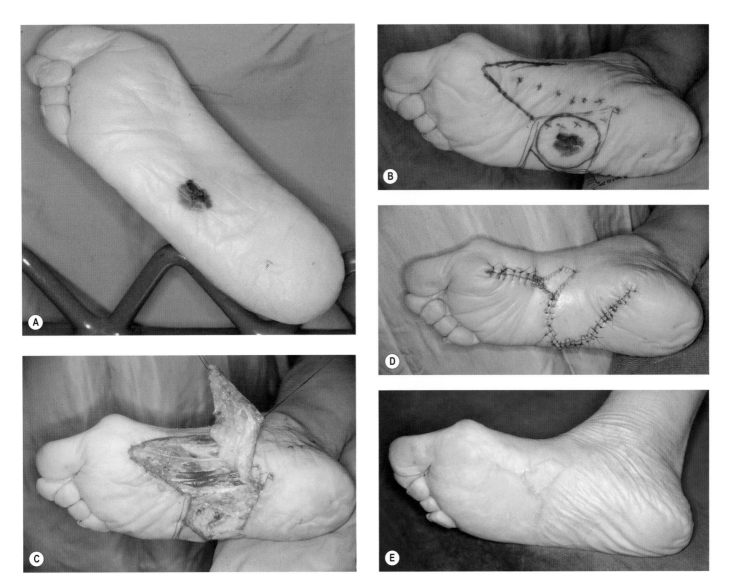

Fig. 31.27 Melanoma of the plantar area **(A)** may be resurfaced with an arterial fasciocutaneous flap **(B–E)**.

Cervical lymphadenectomy

Patients with melanoma of the face and anterior scalp *(Fig. 31.29)* who are selected for cervical lymphadenectomy because of positive sentinel lymph nodes should be also be considered for superficial parotidectomy on the ipsilateral side because the preparotid lymph nodes are the first echelon of nodal drainage. A cervical lymphadenectomy *(Fig. 31.30)* can be performed with or without preservation of the spinal accessory nerve, internal jugular vein, and sternocleidomastoid muscle to provide a more acceptable appearance and functional neck and shoulder muscles.[140]

Axillary lymphadenectomy

The patient is placed in the supine position with the arm abducted and placed freely on two arm boards. The entire arm, including the hand, is prepared for surgery and draped, so that the arm can be moved as needed during the procedure. Make a prominent S-shaped incision with the midportion placed transversely across the apex of the axilla, with one limb descending behind the anterior edge of the lateral border of the pectoralis major muscle *(Fig. 31.31)* and the second limb descending along the posterior border of the upper arm. Elevate the two opposing skin

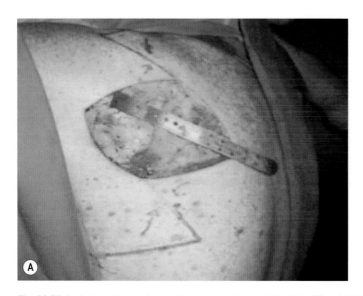
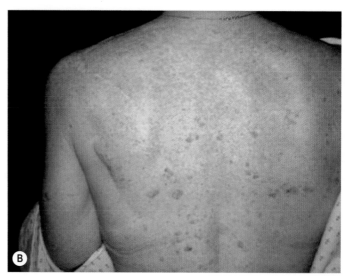

Fig. 31.28 In the truncal area, deep melanomas may be resected widely **(A)** and still be closed reliably with large transposition flaps **(B)**.

flaps at the level of Scarpa fascia to expose the axillary contents.

Identify the brachial vein along the arm and dissect proximally to the axilla, from the anterior portion of the upper arm toward the posterior portion. Dissect the entire axillary contents in this fashion, moving in a distal-to-proximal direction. Ligate and transect the branches of the brachial vein; leave the thoracodorsal artery, vein, and nerve intact, however.

Dissect the axillary contents from along the lateral border of the pectoralis major muscle, leaving the muscle fascia behind with the muscle. Free the contents from the posterior surface of the pectoralis major, which is then retracted to expose the pectoralis minor. Dissect the fat and lymphatic contents from behind both the pectoralis major and minor muscles and retract this material downward. Using a surgical sponge pad, sweep the axillary contents away from the chest wall in a caudad direction. This maneuver usually exposes the long thoracic nerve along the chest wall. Preserve this nerve.

After the axillary contents are removed, reposition the skin flaps and suture them closed over large suction catheters. These catheters remain in place for 3–10 days, depending on the amount of 24-hour drainage accumulated. The decision to remove the drain should be based on the pattern and rate of daily decrease in the drainage rather than the actual amount. The drains are most commonly ready to be removed by the fifth or sixth day. The patient is instructed to keep the arm in a sling during waking hours to decrease shearing forces on the dissected tissues and thereby lessen the drainage.

Pelvic and inguinofemoral lymphadenectomy

Excision of inguinofemoral lymph nodes is facilitated by a horizontal incision along the skin crease 2 cm above and parallel to the inguinal region and a vertical incision over the femoral vessels, beginning in the inguinal skinfold and extending inferiorly for 8–10 cm. This approach results in an "interrupted" T incision **(Fig. 31.32)**. Carry the skin incision in the inguinal area down to the fascia of the external oblique muscle and split it open to expose the internal oblique muscle. Dissect this origin of the internal oblique muscle sharply off the iliac crest to provide access to the retroperitoneal space. Pull the peritoneum away along the undersurface of the transversalis fascia from the external iliac vessels and lymph nodes. This provides an excellent view of the nodes for the pelvic lymphadenectomy.

Elevate the skin flaps on either side of the femoral incisions at the level of Scarpa fascia as well as the skin below the horizontal incision **(Fig. 31.33)**. Elevate the skin completely from the inguinal incision to the lower end of the femoral incision. Dissect the femoral fat and lymphatic tissues down to, but not including,

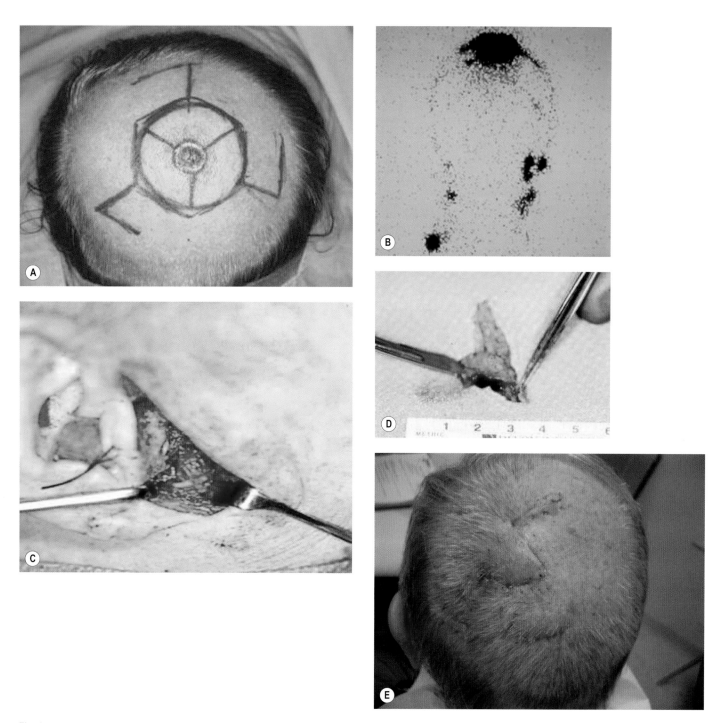

Fig. 31.29 Melanoma of the vertex of the scalp **(A)** was found to have lymphatic drainage to bilateral parotid and cervical nodes **(B)**. The parotid sentinel node **(C)** was found to be positive **(D)**. Postoperative healed flaps **(E)**.

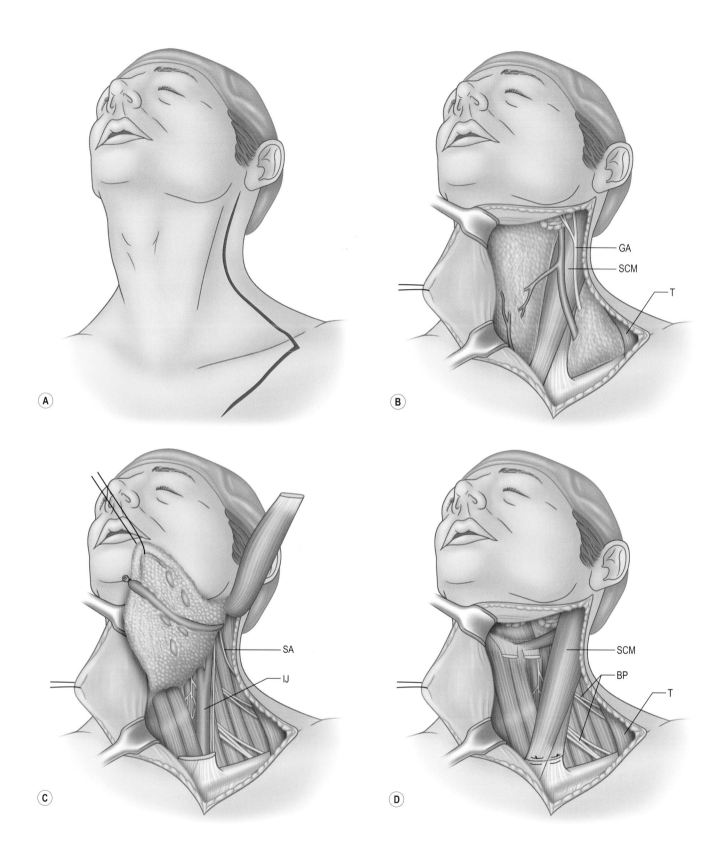

Fig. 31.30 Functional radical neck dissection can be performed while preserving the sternocleidomastoid muscle (SCM), the internal jugular vein (IJ), and the spinal accessory nerve (SA). GA, great auricular nerve; T, trapezius; BP, brachial plexus. (Reproduced from Ariyan S. Radical neck dissection. *Surg Clin North Am*. 1986;66: 133.)

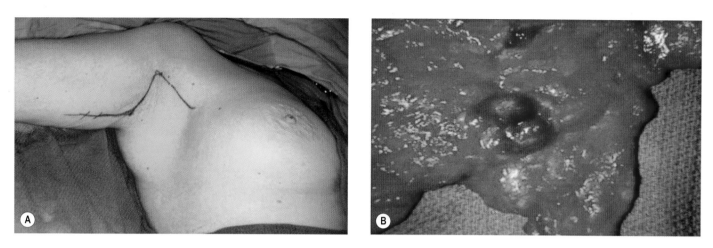

Fig. 31.31 Axillary incision is S-shaped **(A)** to provide opposing flaps for greater access to the axillary contents **(B)**. See text for details.

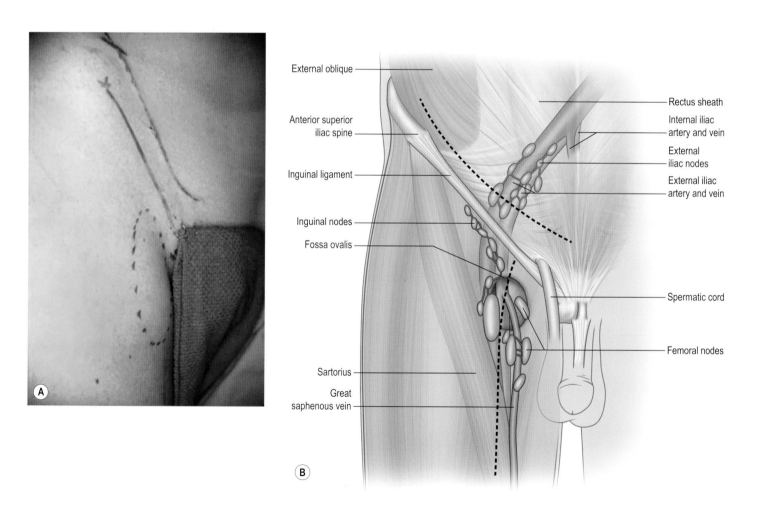

Fig. 31.32 An "interrupted" T incision **(A and B)** is used for access to both the inguinal and iliac nodes.

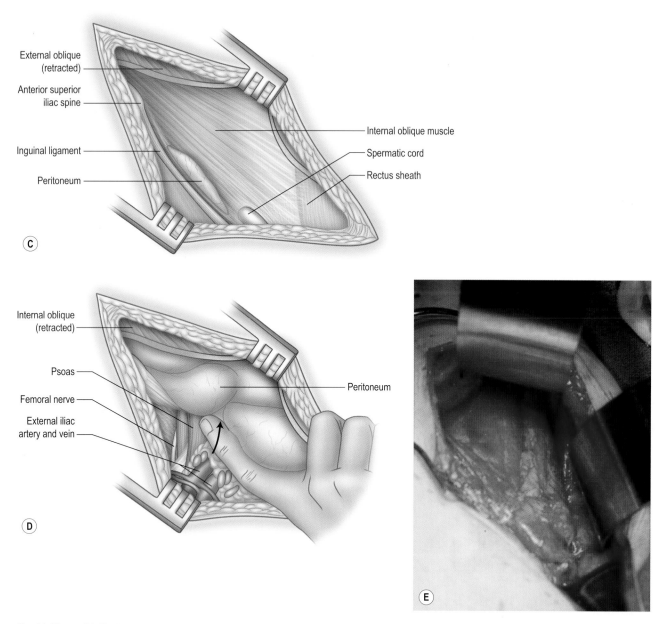

Fig. 31.32, cont'd The fascia of the external oblique muscle is split **(C)**, and the internal oblique and transversalis are dissected away from the inguinal ligament and iliac crest. The peritoneum is peeled back by finger dissection **(D)** to obtain retroperitoneal access to the iliac and obturator nodes **(E)**.

the muscle fascia. Continue the dissection cephalad on the surface of the muscle fascia until the saphenous vein and saphenous bulb are reached on the femoral vein.

Dissect the contents in the inguinal region down to the fascia of the external oblique muscle and in the caudad direction to communicate with the femoral dissection. Do not remove the muscle fascia or transpose the muscles adjacent to the femoral vessels to cover these vessels: such procedures increase the risk of lymphedema. Close the wounds over large suction catheters that remain in place for 3–10 days. Patients are

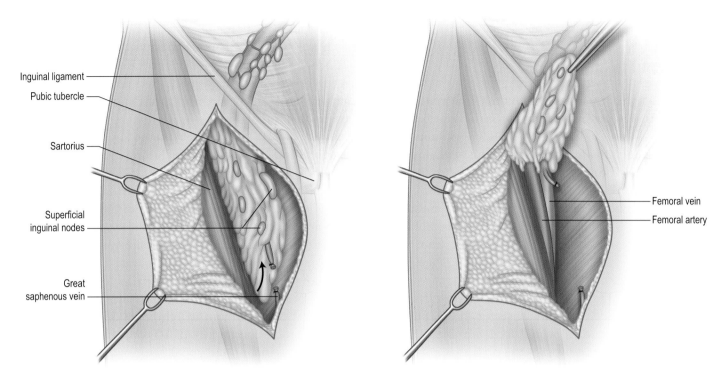

Fig. 31.33 The femoral nodes are approached through a vertical incision over the region of the femoral vessels. After the medial and lateral flaps are elevated (left), the subcutaneous fat containing the lymph nodes is dissected off the deeper muscle fascia (right).

permitted to ambulate the night of surgery or the next morning.

Adjuvant treatment for melanoma

WLE is the standard of care for early-stage melanoma, and the majority of patients present with stage I–IIA disease. However, high-risk patients with stage IIB–III disease have a generally poorer prognosis. These patients have been the primary focus in the development of adjuvant therapies for melanoma. Over the past 30 years, a number of efforts with chemotherapeutic agents (e.g., dacarbazine[141]), nonspecific immune adjuvants (e.g., bacille Calmette-Guérin (BCG) vaccine[141]), and hormonal agents (e.g., megestrol acetate), have not demonstrated a benefit over observation or placebo. The most promising results have been demonstrated with IFN-α, an immune modulator that can induce antitumor activity.

Interferon-α

Early clinical studies with IFN-α demonstrated modest antitumor activity in patients with metastatic melanoma. A series of clinical trials were then started to examine the role of adjuvant IFN-α in patients with high-risk melanoma. Each of these trials has different doses and schedules, and an optimal approach to the administration of IFN-α has not been established. Review of data combined from multiple randomized controlled trials demonstrates that IFN-α is associated with an improvement in relapse-free survival but not with overall survival.[142] The role for adjuvant IFN-α for patients with intermediate- to high-risk melanoma remains undefined.[143] Treatment with adjuvant IFN-α should be made on an individual basis, after discussion with the patient, with discussion of the potential benefits and side-effects associated with IFN-α therapy.[144] For patients with stage IIB through stage III disease which has been resected, the National Comprehensive Cancer Network (NCCN) recommends consideration of adjuvant treatment with IFN-α or enrollment in a clinical trial.[120]

Radiation therapy

When excision of a primary melanoma with appropriate margins is not possible, adjuvant radiation might be considered, though it is not generally recommended for the primary treatment of cutaneous melanoma. In exceptional circumstances, for patients who are poor candidates for surgical resection, radiotherapy may offer an acceptable alternative for control of disease.

Early studies by Barranco et al.[145] demonstrated that cultured malignant melanoma cells differ from other types of tumor cell in their radiosensitivity. They found that the relative radioresistance of melanoma could be overcome by increasing the individual dose fraction. These studies helped form the basis for clinical practice, and subsequent studies helped to determine the ideal fraction size and total therapeutic dose that effectively treats melanoma.

In patients with extensive facial lentigo maligna melanoma that precludes adequate surgical resection based on functional or cosmetic considerations, radiotherapy has been reported.[146] However, more recent advances in topical therapies such as imiquimod (Aldara) are supplanting radiation therapy in the nonsurgical treatment of lentigo maligna melanoma.

Early work by Habermalz and Fischer demonstrated some success with higher-dose radiotherapy over more frequent time intervals than conventional radiotherapy, with partial or complete regression especially seen with subcutaneous metastases.[147] Prospective nonrandomized clinical trials at the MD Anderson Cancer Center, treating high-risk groups of melanoma patients with radiation therapy, have helped establish the basis of treatment with hypofractionated radiation therapy in melanoma.[148] While locoregional control was improved with adjuvant radiation, distant metastases developed in a large number of patients (58 of 174 patients).[148] Later studies from this group evaluated the outcome of patients with clinically apparent cervical lymph node metastases from malignant melanoma managed with surgical resection and adjuvant radiation.[149] After 10-year follow-up, the group demonstrated a 94% regional control rate. Radiation-related complications for the patients were manageable.[149] The same group evaluated the utility of radiation therapy alone in the treatment of 36 patients with positive SLNB (in lieu of completion lymphadenectomy), and demonstrated 93% regional control over 5 years.[150] However, when recurrences present within radiated fields, the surgical management can be arduous and lead to breakdown and nonhealing wounds.

Recent work has been reported by groups from Australia and New Zealand, including the Trans Tasman Radiation Oncology Group. They are performing prospective trials of radiation versus observation after lymphadenectomy on patients from 16 different centers.[151] Inclusion criteria are: ≥1 parotid, ≥2 cervical or axillary, or ≥3 groin-positive nodes; extranodal spread of tumor; or minimum metastatic node diameter of 3 cm (neck or axilla) or 4 cm (groin). Radiotherapy, given as 2.4 Gy in 20 fractions over 4 weeks, demonstrates a statistically significant improvement in lymph node field control: 20 of 109 radiation and 34 of 108 observation patients relapsed regionally ($P = 0.04$). However, despite improved local regional control, overall survival appears to be better in the observation group (47 months median survival) versus the radiation group (31 months median survival), though this analysis was not statistically significant ($P = 0.14$). These data have raised concerns about possible deleterious effects of radiation as a contributor to the development of distant metastases. This question remains to be answered.

The NCCN recommends consideration of adjuvant radiation therapy for patients with multiple positive lymph nodes, lymph nodes with extracapsular spread, nodal recurrence, and in-transit metastases. Additionally, radiotherapy should be considered after excision of primary melanomas that demonstrate neurotropism (desmoplastic type),[152] as well as mucosal melanomas, which may or may not be amenable to complete excision.[153,154]

Isolated limb perfusion

Tumor recurrences correlate with the thickness of the lesion. Between 60% and 70% of recurrences appear in the first 18–24 months after surgical treatments (*Table 31.8* and *Fig. 31.34*).[155] The earliest recurrences are to local or regional lymph nodes, followed by in-transit metastases; distant metastases appear last.

Patients with local recurrences may be treated with wider surgical resections, but extensive local recurrences or in-transit metastases are more difficult to treat. In-transit metastases of extremities may be treated with isolation perfusion of that extremity with dacarbazine (DTIC),[156] cisplatin, or hypo-osmolar perfusions with carboplatin.[157] Carboplatin eradicated the lesions after perfusion in some patients *(Fig. 31.35)*, whereas the control was temporary in other patients. The advantage of DTIC is its low incidence of hepatic and systemic toxicity, which is far less than that after perfusion with L-phenylalanine mustard. Indeed, we found that such perfusions were tolerated well among our elderly patients, with no greater risk of complications in this group than in our younger patients *(Table 31.9)*.[158] In general, the major role for isolated limb perfusion is palliation of unresectable limb disease.

Treatment of metastatic melanoma

It is well established that the prognosis of patients with metastatic melanoma is poor: those with liver, brain, or bone metastasis have a median survival of only 6 months. A number of systemic therapy options are available to treat patients with metastatic disease, including single-agent or multiple-agent chemotherapy, biochemotherapy, or strategies using immune modulation. However, little consensus exists regarding standard therapy for patients with metastatic melanoma. From the surgical perspective, if the patient has metastatic disease localized to a single small focus in the lung, liver, or brain, it may be worthwhile considering resection *(Table 31.10)*. However, multiple recurrences cannot be treated by surgery and require consideration of systemic chemotherapy and/or radiation therapy. More recent advances have shown a very high response rate to gamma knife treatment of single or few metastases to brain.

Chemotherapeutic agents

Dacarbazine remains a standard of care in community practice, and has been used as a standard for comparing the efficacy of new regimens.[120,159] Combination chemotherapeutic regimens that include other cytotoxic drugs, such as *bis*(2-chloroethyl)nitrosourea (BCNU), cisplatin, lomustine, and hydroxyurea, have been reported. The trials comparing DTIC alone or in combination with other agents have shown a significant,

Table 31.8 Timing of recurrent melanoma after surgical treatment

Site	18 months	24 months	3 years	5 years	10 years
Nodal	63%	74%	86%	93%	95%
Local	55%	67%	81%	88%	95%
In-transit	55%	67%	80%	90%	97%
Systemic	40%	52%	71%	83%	95%
Overall	57%	97%	81%	90%	95%

(Modified from Fusi S, Ariyan S, Sternlicht A. Data on first recurrence after treatment for malignant melanoma in a large patient population. *Plast Reconstr Surg*. 1993;91:94.)

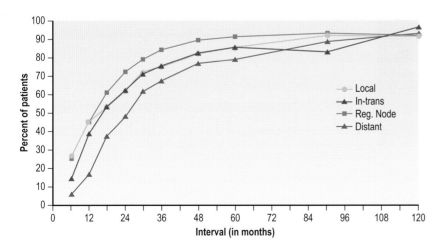

Fig. 31.34 Patterns and timing of recurrences for melanoma. The curve of the timing of local recurrence and in-transit metastases precedes that of lymph node recurrences and distant organ metastases. (From Fusi S, Ariyan S, Sternlicht A. Data on first recurrence after treatment for malignant melanoma in a large patient population. Plast Reconstr Surg 1993;91:94.)

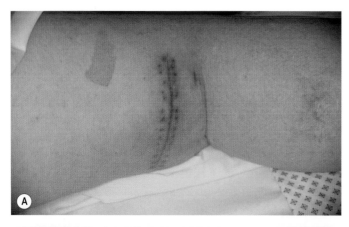

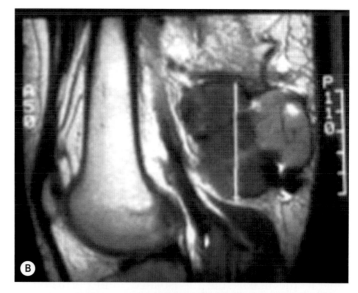

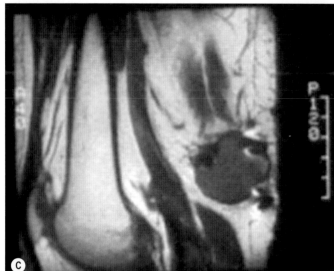

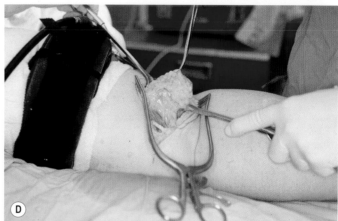

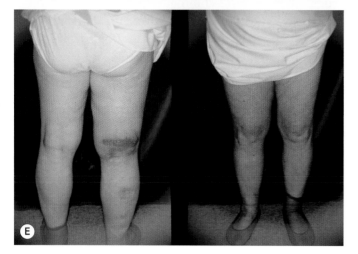

Fig. 31.35 Regional isolated perfusion of a lower extremity recurrence **(A)** led to significant response and shrinking of the tumor **(B,** before perfusion; **C,** after perfusion), permitting radical resection of the mass **(D)** without compromise to the popliteal vessels. At 1 year, there was no local recurrence **(E)**.

Table 31.9 Perfusion complications*

Age	20s	30s	40s	50s	60s	70s	80s	Total
Number	4	7	11	9	16	14	6	67
Edema (pre/post)			1		2	2	1	6
Edema (post)	1		2		2			5
Seroma	1			1	1	1		4
Wound				1	5	1	2	9
Pulmonary embolus						1		1
Total	2	0	2	2	9	2	2	19
			14/47 (32%)			4/20 (20%)		

*67 perfusions in 60 patients, 1976–1995.
(From Ariyan S, Poo WJ. The safety and efficacy of isolated perfusion of extremities for recurrent tumor in elderly patients. A 20-year experience. *Surgery*. 1998;123:335.)

Table 31.10 Surgery for metastatic melanoma: outcome

Site of first recurrence	Incidence	5-year survival	Median survival
Skin, fat, lymph node	50–60%	5–40%	8–50 months
Lung	15–35%	5–30%	8–20 months
Gastrointestinal tract	2–4%	Minority of patients	10–20 months
Small bowel (35–65%)		Mostly palliative for symptomatic relief	
Colon (10–15%)			
Stomach (5%)			
Brain (at autopsy, 50–80%)	8–15%	Unexpected (5%) 80–90% have symptomatic relief	6–8 months
Liver (rarely single metastasis)	5%	Anecdotal cases	–

(Modified from Allen PJ, Coit DG. The surgical management of metastatic melanoma. *Ann Surg Oncol*. 2002;9:762.)

though brief, improvement in survival.[160] Dacarbazine and temozolomide have been shown to have similar response rates (approximately 10–20%) and survival,[161] with median response duration averaging approximately 3–4 months.[160,161] Temozolomide can cross the blood–brain barrier, making it an attractive agent for treating melanoma, which has a propensity for metastasis to the brain.

Combination chemotherapy regimens such as CVD (dacarbazine plus cisplatin and vinblastine) or the Dartmouth regimen (dacarbazine, carmustine, cisplatin, and tamoxifen) initially reported higher response rates,[162,163] but subsequent clinical trials have not replicated these high response rates.[164] Paclitaxel, alone or in combination with carboplatin, may provide clinical benefit to some patients with metastatic melanoma, but the duration of clinical benefit is short (2–7 months).[165,166]

Tumor vaccines

The development of melanoma-specific tumor vaccines has been predicated on several clinical observations and lines of basic investigation that indicate that the immune system can eradicate melanoma cells. Although a comprehensive review of available vaccine strategies is beyond the scope of this chapter, some of the more encouraging studies are reviewed.

Ganglioside GM2, an antigen overexpressed by many melanoma cells, given in combination with BCG or other immune adjuvants, was developed as a treatment for metastatic melanoma at Memorial Sloan Kettering Cancer Center. Initial clinical trials suggested promising results[167]; however, further studies failed to show clinical benefit with this adjuvant treatment. Kirkwood et al.[168] reported their experience comparing high-dose IFN-α_{2b} and GM2 ganglioside vaccine for patients with resected melanoma, demonstrating the advantage of interferon. Additionally, a randomized phase III trial (EORTC 18961) of adjuvant GM2-KLH21 in 1314 patients with stage II melanoma was closed early by the data-monitoring committee because of inferior survival in the vaccine arm.[169]

A polyvalent melanoma cell vaccine, developed at the John Wayne Cancer Center, was shown to be capable of inducing humoral and cell-mediated immune responses to melanoma-specific antigens.[170,171] Nevertheless, this vaccine was found not to be beneficial in a clinical trial.

Dr. Steven Rosenberg and co-investigators at the surgery branch of the National Cancer Institute have identified other cancer vaccines by using specific peptide antigens recognized by autologous tumor-specific T-cell clone reactivity.[172] Peptide vaccines are most often administered with cytokine or cellular immune adjuvants such as dendritic cells. DiFronzo et al.[173] demonstrated that enhanced humoral responses in patients treated with polyvalent vaccines resulted in limited but improved disease-free survival. It is difficult to advocate any of the current vaccine strategies over another, and we recommend that patients with high-risk melanoma be enrolled into prospective trials to test these therapeutic strategies.

Interleukin-2

Interleukin-2 (IL-2) was approved by the Food and Drug Administration for treatment of metastatic melanoma in 1998. High-dose intravenous bolus IL-2 treatment resulted in overall objective response rates of about 17%.[174] In a highly selected patient population ($n = 270$), IL-2 was able to induce durable complete responses (median response duration over 59 months) in approximately 6% of patients and partial responses in 10% of patients with metastatic melanoma, albeit with high levels of toxicity.[175,176] A recent study demonstrated increased response rate in metastatic melanoma when IL-2 was given with the 210M peptide vaccine (22%) compared to IL-2 (13%) alone.[177]

Biochemotherapy

Given the individual success of chemotherapeutic agents and the biologically active agents (IFN-α and IL-2), biochemotherapy regimens were developed. By combining conventional chemotherapeutic drugs with biologically active agents, investigators were able to demonstrate modest improvement in response rates of metastatic melanoma. In single institutional phase II trials, biochemotherapy (cisplatin, vinblastine, dacarbazine, IFN-α, and IL-2) produced an overall response rate of 27–64% and a complete response rate of 15–21% in patients with metastatic melanoma.[178–180] A report of a small phase III randomized trial comparing sequential biochemotherapy (dacarbazine, cisplatin, vinblastine with IL-2, and IFN-α administered on a distinct schedule) with combined cisplatin, vinblastine, and dacarbazine (CVD) showed response rates of 48% for the biochemotherapy regimen compared to 25% for CVD alone; median survival for patients treated with biochemotherapy was 11.9 months versus 9.2 months for CVD.[181] In a phase III randomized intergroup trial (E3695), biochemotherapy (cisplatin, vinblastine, dacarbazine, IL-2, and IFN-α2b) produced a slightly higher response rate and progression-free survival than CVD alone, but it was not associated with either improved quality of response or overall survival in patients with metastatic melanoma.[182] Biochemotherapy was substantially more toxic than CVD. Additional attempts to decrease toxicity of biochemotherapy by administering subcutaneous outpatient IL-2 did not show a substantial benefit of biochemotherapy versus chemotherapy alone.[183–185] A meta-analysis demonstrated that, although biochemotherapy seemed to improve overall response rates, there was no survival benefit for patients with metastatic melanoma.[186]

Given the overall poor performance of agents in this cohort of patients, continued basic and translational research is warranted to identify active agents for these unfortunate patients. Pre-emptive strategies are also being developed. Because a majority of patients with cutaneous melanoma have some identifiable risk factor (i.e., sun exposure), chemoprevention using carotenoids and inhibitors of cyclooxygenase-2, vascular endothelial growth factor receptor, and cytochrome P-450 are actively being investigated.[187] Outcomes of this work are much anticipated.

Ipilimumab

Despite many preclinical and clinical studies evaluating multiple cytokines, vaccines, antibodies, and other types of immune modulation, alone or in combination with chemotherapy, only IL-2 for metastatic disease and IFN-α for surgical adjuvant treatment have demonstrated sufficient success to warrant approval by regulatory authorities.[142,175] Nevertheless, there has been continued optimism that immune modulation can become an effective treatment for patients with melanoma, driven largely by key advances in tumor immunobiology, including the potential to manipulate and disrupt immune activation checkpoints and tumor defense mechanisms; newer approaches to antigen presentation for immune activation; refinements to procedures for antigen-specific T-cell expansion; gene transfer to alter lymphocyte specificity and function; and the potential for discovery of improved predictive biomarkers to select patients for individual treatments.[188]

Along these lines, Hodi *et al.* induced autoimmunity in patients with metastatic melanoma using ipilimumab, an antibody directed against the cytotoxic T-lymphocyte-associated antigen CTLA-4.[189] CTLA-4 is an immune checkpoint molecule that down-regulates T-cell activation, and blocking this molecule is known to promote antitumor immunity.[189] In their multicenter clinical trial, patients with metastatic melanoma were randomly assigned to receive an anti-CTLA-4 agent (ipilimumab), a vaccine based on a melanoma antigen, or a combination of the anti-CTLA-4 agent and the vaccine. An improvement in overall survival, as well as an improvement in progression-free survival and best overall response rate, was seen in the patients who received anti-CTLA-4 therapy, as compared with the patients who received the vaccine only.[189] Of note, the side-effect profile of ipilimumab deserves mention, as 60% of patients suffered adverse events, mostly immune-related. However, this randomized controlled trial showed that there was a significant improvement in overall survival among melanoma patients treated with ipilimumab. It will likely prove useful in patients with metastatic melanoma whose disease progressed while receiving one or more previous therapies.

Molecularly targeted treatment of melanoma

Recent ground-breaking work has been reported on molecularly targeted chemotherapy in melanoma. It was demonstrated in 2002 that approximately 50% of human melanomas harbor an activating mutation in BRAF, an upstream component of the mitogen-activated protein (MAP) kinase pathway; the mutation is a substitution of glutamic acid for valine (the V600E mutation).[190] Melanoma cells containing the BRAF mutation are dependent on MAP kinase signaling for their growth and survival.[191] These findings suggested the possibility that melanoma may be amenable to targeted therapy. PLX4032 (Plexxikon; RG7204, Roche Pharmaceuticals), a potent inhibitor of BRAF with the V600E mutation, has been shown to be a remarkably successful therapeutic option in properly selected patients.[192] Eighty-one percent of patients with metastatic melanomas harboring the activating mutation in BRAF (V600E) had a response – complete or partial tumor regression – to treatment with PLX4032 in a multicenter, phase I, dose escalation trial. Responses were observed at all sites of disease, including bone, liver, and small bowel. Work is under way to determine whether treatment with PLX4032 will improve overall survival. It seems clear that melanomas can be categorized by specific molecular changes that drive their proliferation[193]; targeting the activated pathways in individual tumors may lead to tumor regression and possible cure. This type of personalized cancer therapy will likely play a prominent role in the care of patients with melanoma and other cancers in the coming decade.

Surveillance

Patients treated at the Yale Melanoma Unit are initially monitored closely *(Table 31.11)*, with increasing intervals each year. The importance of dermatologic evaluation, photo documentation, and close follow-up cannot be overstated. Education of the patient for early self-detection of recurrences together with interval physician follow-up has been most successful in maintaining

Table 31.11 Surveillance guidelines

Follow-up guidelines	
Office visits and physical examination	
Stage 0	Yearly by dermatologist or primary care physician
Stage I	Every 6 months for 5 years
Stage II–IV	Every 3 months for 2 years Every 6 months for 3 years
Metastatic surveillance	
Lactate dehydrogenase level and complete blood cell count	At each visit, at least yearly
Chest radiograph	Every other visit, at least yearly
Computed tomography scan ± positron emission tomography	With laboratory test or chest radiograph abnormality, physical findings, or symptoms

Table 31.12 Protocol for follow-up surveillance

	Physical examination	Chest radiography	Liver function tests	Imaging
Stage I, T1	Semiannual × 2 years, then annually	–	–	
Stage I–II, T2–4	Every 3 months × 3 years, then semiannually	Annual	Annual	
Stage III (lymph nodes positive)	Every 3 months × 3 years, then semiannually	Annual	Annual	Annual or as indicated

an effective monitoring program.[194] Patients are examined for local or in-transit metastases at varying intervals based on the stage of the melanoma at diagnosis *(Table 31.12)*.

Tumor recurrences correlate with the thickness of the lesion. Between 60% and 70% of recurrences appear in the first 18–24 months after surgical treatment *(Table 31.8)*.[155] The earliest recurrences are to local or regional lymph nodes, followed by in-transit metastases; distant metastases appear last. Screening is typically by physical examination, liver function serology, and chest X-ray, which will detect most recurrences. Routine screening with CT of the head, chest, and abdomen is not recommended, unless clinical suspicion for metastases is high. Chest X-rays and liver serology, despite a relatively low yield,[195] are inexpensive and useful for establishment of baseline values. The utility of PET or PET-CT imaging for the surveillance of affected patients is still under investigation. Additionally, the prospect of using specific serum screening tools such as tyrosinase mRNA, detected by reverse transcription polymerase chain reaction, is both clinically exciting and ethically challenging.[196]

The National Cancer Institute recommends that most patients without a family history and no atypical nevi should have follow-up evaluations every 6 months for the first 2 years. Thereafter, yearly follow-up is appropriate. Those with a family history or atypical nevi are followed up every 3 months.[194]

Summary

Melanoma remains a challenging and important clinical problem, with a rapidly rising yearly incidence. WLE remains the primary treatment modality for primary disease. SLNB is indicated for patients with clinically negative nodes and primary lesions with aggressive features – generally, thickness greater than 1 mm. If the sentinel lymph node is positive, completion lymphadenectomy is indicated for control of regional disease. Unfortunately, the overall cure rates for advanced melanoma have not significantly improved during the past several decades because we are unable to treat the subclinical micrometastases that are present in systemic organs at the time of the treatment of the primary melanoma. Once these metastases become evident clinically, there is little chance of cure by further surgery, chemotherapy, radiation therapy, or combinations of these treatment modalities. Adjuvant trials with chemotherapy and biochemotherapy have not demonstrated uniform success for any meaningful period of time. Therefore, we cannot overemphasize the importance of clinical trials, and patients with advanced melanoma should be encouraged to enroll in clinical trials testing different adjuvant strategies whenever possible. Recent successes in controlling metastatic lesions with molecularly targeted treatments hold promise for personalized treatments for genetic mutations in the future.

 Bonus images for this chapter can be found online at **http://www.expertconsult.com**

Fig. 31.1 Autopsy findings of patient with melanoma of right ankle spreading in a centripetal manner to right groin and remainder of body while sparing the left leg. (Redrawn from Handley WS. The pathology of melanotic growths in relation to their operative treatment. Lecture I. Lancet 1907;1:927.)

Fig. 31.2 Handley recommended removal of melanoma (a) together with 1 inch (2.5 cm) (f) of skin (b) and 2 inches (5 cm) (g) of underlying subcutaneous fat (c), muscle fascia (d), and muscle (e); (h) skin incision. (Redrawn from Handley WS. The pathology of melanotic growths in relation to their operative treatment. Lecture I. Lancet 1907;1:927.)

Access the complete references list online at **http://www.expertconsult.com**

43. Balch CM, Gershenwald JE, Soong SJ, et al. Final version of 2009 AJCC melanoma staging and classification. *J Clin Oncol.* 2009;27:6199–6206.

   The most recent melanoma staging recommendations were made on the basis of a multivariate analysis of 30 946 patients with stages I–III melanoma and 7972 patients with stage IV melanoma. For patients with localized melanoma, tumor thickness, mitotic rate, and ulceration are the most dominant prognostic factors. For patients with regional metastases, components that define the N category are the number of metastatic nodes, tumor burden, and ulceration of the primary melanoma. All patients with microscopic nodal metastases, regardless of extent of tumor burden, are classified as stage III. For patients with distant metastases, the two dominant components defining the M category continue to be the site of distant metastases and serum lactate dehydrogenase level.

57. Breslow A. Thickness, cross-sectional areas and depth of invasion in the prognosis of cutaneous melanoma. *Ann Surg.* 1970;172:902–908.

   Alexander Breslow first decribed the use of an ocular micrmeter to measure the maximal thickness of melanomas, and demonstrated a correlation of depth of invasion with patient outcome.

59. Morton DL, Wen DR, Wong JH, et al. Technical details of intraoperative lymphatic mapping for early stage melanoma. *Arch Surg.* 1992;127:392–399.

   Morton et al. first described the use of sentinel lymph node biopsy in the treatment of melanoma. This technique identifies, with a high degree of accuracy, patients with early-stage melanoma who have nodal metastases and are likely to benefit from radical lymphadenectomy.

80. Rousseau Jr DL, Ross MI, Johnson MM, et al. Revised American Joint Committee on Cancer staging criteria accurately predict sentinel lymph node positivity in clinically node-negative melanoma patients. *Ann Surg Oncol.* 2003;10:569–574.

81. Morton DL, Hoon DS, Cochran AJ, et al. Lymphatic mapping and sentinel lymphadenectomy for early-stage melanoma: therapeutic utility and implications of nodal microanatomy and molecular staging for improving the accuracy of detection of nodal micrometastases. *Ann Surg.* 2003;238:538–549; discussion 49–50.

108. Sladden MJ, Balch C, Barzilai DA, et al. Surgical excision margins for primary cutaneous melanoma. *Cochrane Database Syst Rev.* 2009(4):CD004835.

   This systematic review summarizes the evidence regarding width of excision margins for primary cutaneous melanoma. Of the five randomized controlled trials, there was no statistically significant difference in overall survival between narrow (1–2 cm) or wide (3–5 cm) excision margins. Based on the individual trials and meta-analysis, current randomized trial evidence is insufficient to address optimal excision margins for primary cutaneous melanoma.

112. Veronesi U, Cascinelli N, Adamus J, et al. Thin stage I primary cutaneous malignant melanoma. Comparison of excision with margins of 1 or 3 cm. *N Engl J Med.* 1988;318:1159–1162.

119. Thomas JM, Newton-Bishop J, A'Hern R, et al. Excision margins in high-risk malignant melanoma. *N Engl J Med.* 2004;350:757–766.

138. Morton DL, Thompson JF, Cochran AJ, et al. Sentinel-node biopsy or nodal observation in melanoma. *N Engl J Med.* 2006;355:1307–1317.

142. Kirkwood JM, Manola J, Ibrahim J, et al. A pooled analysis of eastern cooperative oncology group and intergroup trials of adjuvant high-dose interferon for melanoma. *Clin Cancer Res.* 2004;10:1670–1677.

145. Barranco SC, Romsdahl MM, Humphrey RM. The radiation response of human malignant melanoma cells grown *in vitro. Cancer Res.* 1971;31:830–833.

189. Hodi FS, O'Day SJ, McDermott DF, et al. Improved survival with ipilimumab in patients with metastatic melanoma. *N Engl J Med.* 2010;363:711–723.

   In this study, ipilimumab, which potentiates an antitumor T-cell response, demonstrated improvement in overall survial (10.0 months vs. 6.4 months) in patients with unresectable stage III or IV melanoma. Adverse events can be severe, long-lasting, or both, but most are reversible with appropriate treatment.

192. Flaherty KT, Puzanov I, Kim KB, et al. Inhibition of mutated, activated BRAF in metastatic melanoma. *N Engl J Med.* 2010;363:809–819.

   The authors conducted a multicenter, phase I, dose escalation trial of PLX4032, an orally available inhibitor of mutated BRAF, followed by an extension phase involving the maximum dose that could be administered without adverse effects. Patients received PLX4032 twice daily until they had disease progression. BRAF (v-raf murine sarcoma viral oncogene homolog B1) is a signal transduction molecule that has an activating mutation (glutamic acid for valine at amino acid 600; V600E) in half of all melanomas. In the dose escalation cohort, among the 16 patients with melanoma whose tumors carried the V600E BRAF mutation and who were receiving 240 mg or more of PLX4032 twice daily, 10 had a partial response and 1 had a complete response. Among the 32 patients in the extension cohort, 24 had a partial response and 2 had a complete response. The estimated median progression-free survival among all patients was more than 7 months. Treatment with PLX4032 in the majority of patients with tumors that carry the V600E BRAF mutation resulted in complete or partial tumor regression.

32

Implants and biomaterials

Charles E. Butler and Timothy W. King

SYNOPSIS

- What is a biomaterial? In order to discuss biomaterials, we must first define this term.
- There are many definitions of biomaterials but a widely used one from the National Institutes of Health defines a biomaterial as "any substance (other than a drug) or combination of substances synthetic or natural in origin, which can be used for any period of time, as a whole or part of a system which treats, augments, or replaces tissue, organ, or function of the body."[1]
- With the advent of tissue engineering and regenerative medicine in recent years, the definition has broadened to include "any material used in a medical device intended to interact with biological systems," allowing for structures and combination devices that actively interact with the body to be included in the field.[2]
- Biomaterials can be synthetic (i.e., those made by humans) or biological (i.e., those produced by a biological system).
- Further classifications based on development stage or material characteristics are also common but are beyond the scope of this chapter.

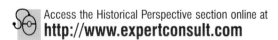

Access the Historical Perspective section online at
http://www.expertconsult.com

Metals

In order to achieve the mechanical and biophysical properties desired for applications in medicine, combinations of metals, called alloys, have been developed. These alloys are designed to be inert and withstand the corrosive environment found within the human body.

In general, these alloys have mechanical properties that exceed the properties of the natural tissue they are supporting because, unlike natural tissues, they are unable to recover from deformation.

Stainless steel

Stainless steel has been used as a biological implant since the 1920s.[6] Stainless steel was designed to prevent corrosion and consists of over 10 individual compounds which provide it with the desired chemical and mechanical properties. The stainless steel used in medical applications are iron-chromium-nickel alloys with at least 17% chromium **(Table 32.1)**. The chromium creates a protective surface, which contributes to the alloy's anticorrosive properties. The most commonly used stainless steel alloy in medical applications is "316L" which, in addition to the chromium composition, has a low carbon content to prevent carbide formation, and a high nickel content to increase the strength and hardness of the alloy. Stainless steel has a relatively high tensile strength but is easily deformed (bent). While this is useful in some applications, such as the application of arch bars for maxillomandibular fixation, overall these mechanical properties are less desirable than other currently available materials such as cobalt-chromium and titanium. In addition, stainless steel can leach metallic ions into the surrounding tissues, causing a severe inflammatory reaction and pain, which may require surgical

Table 32.1 Composition of common metal alloys

Element	Stainless steel (ASTM F138)* Weight %	Co-Cr (ASTM F90)† Weight %	Titanium (ASTM F136)‡ Weight %
Chromium	16–18	27–30	–
Nickel	10–14	2.5 max	–
Molybdenum	2–3	5–7	–
Carbon	0.03 max	0.35 max	0.08 max
Iron	Balance	0.75 max	0.25 max
Manganese	2.00 max	1.00 max	–
Phosphorus	0.045 max	–	–
Sulfur	0.03 max	–	–
Silicon	1.00 max	1.00 max	–
Nitrogen	0.10 max	–	–
Cobalt	–	Balance	–
Oxygen	–	–	0.013 max
Aluminum	–	–	5.5–6.5
Vanadium	–	–	3.5–4.5
Titanium	–	–	Balance

*ASTM. Standard specification for wrought 18chromium-14nickel-2.5molybdenum stainless steel bar and wire for surgical implants (UNS S31673). West Conshohocken, PA: ASTM International; 2008.

†ASTM. Standard specification for wrought cobalt-20chromium-15tungsten-10nickel alloy for surgical implant applications (UNS R30605). West Conshohocken, PA: ASTM International; 2009.

‡ASTM. Standard specification for wrought titanium-6 aluminum-4 vanadium ELI (extra low interstitial) alloy for surgical implant applications (UNS R56401). West Conshohocken, PA: ASTM International; 2008.

(Adapted from Holmes RE. Alloplastic materials. In: McCarthy JG, ed. *Plastic surgery*. New York: WB Saunders; 1990:698–731.)

composition), increase the chromium to 25–30% for additional corrosion resistance, and contain 5–7% molybdenum for additional strength *(Table 32.1)*. Co-Cr-Mo alloy was used in some of the early craniofacial miniplates and screws and helped to revolutionize that field. The major disadvantage of Co-Cr-Mo alloys is the scatter artifact on computed tomography (CT) imaging. Because of this, and several other benefits, titanium has essentially replaced Co-Cr-Mo alloys in most biomedical applications.[7] However, it is still used in dental applications.

Titanium

Titanium alloys were introduced into medical applications in the early 1980s.[6,8] Since that time these alloys have almost entirely replaced the other alloys in medical applications. This is because the titanium alloys are stronger, lighter, have higher resistance to corrosion, and generally cause less inflammation. Titanium also has less stress shielding (localized osteopenia secondary to the implant protecting the bone from normal loading) than other metal implants because they have less stiffness. Titanium alloys have less than 0.5% iron in them *(Table 32.1)*, which provides them with two additional beneficial properties: they do not set off metal detectors, and they do not create a significant artifact on CT or magnetic resonance imaging studies. Finally, titanium can form chemical bonds with the surrounding mineralized bone without the typical fibrous tissue forming between the implant and bone. This unique characteristic allows titanium to be used to create osteointegrated implants. Plastic surgery applications of these alloys include plates and screws for rigid fixation of bone and mesh for use in applications such as orbital wall reconstruction *(Fig. 32.1)*.

Gold

Although gold is chemically inert, in its pure form it has poor mechanical properties. Thus, when some strength is needed (for example, in dental fillings), a gold alloy is used. For applications such as eyelid weights in patients with lagophthalmos,[9] where strength is less of an issue, 24-carat gold alloy (99.9% w/w purity) is commonly used to insure chemical inertness.

removal of the implants in some patients. Stainless steel is currently used in surgical wire and in arch bars. Historically rigid fixation systems utilized stainless steel but other alloys have replaced stainless steel in this application.

Cobalt-chromium

Historically, cobalt-chromium alloys have been one of the most significant biomaterials used in humans. Vitallium, a cobalt-chromium-molybdenum (Co-Cr-Mo) alloy (ASTM 75), was first described in 1932 to address some of the problems experienced with stainless steel. These alloys replace the iron with cobalt (~60% of the

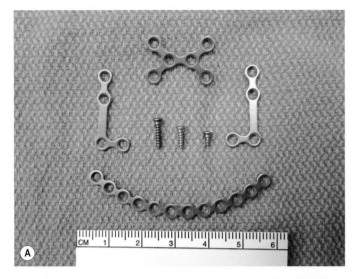

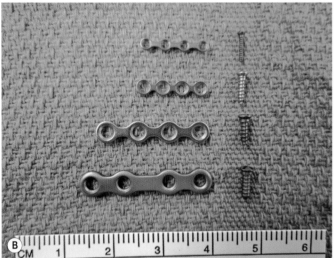

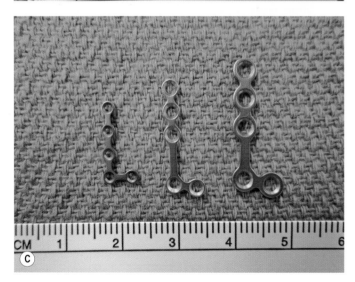

Fig. 32.1 Titanium plates for midface reconstruction. **(A)** Various 2.0-mm plates and screws. The screws are 7, 5, and 3 mm in length (left to right). **(B)** Four-hole plates and screws for the 1.0-, 1.5-, 2.0-, and 2.3-mm plating systems. **(C)** A 1.0-, 1.5-, and 2.0-mm "L" plate. The screws are all 5 mm in length. Note that, by convention, the size of the plates is based upon the screw diameter.

Platinum

Like gold, platinum is an inert metal and is the material of choice for patients with gold sensitivity who are in need of an eyelid implant for lagophthalmos. Platinum is denser than gold, thus the eyelid implants have a lower profile and are less noticeable than gold implants.

Some formulations containing platinum have been shown to be immunogenic and thus have raised concerns over long-term exposure. Because the Centers for Disease Control state that short-term exposure to platinum salts may cause irritation of the eyes, nose, and throat and long-term exposure may cause both respiratory and skin allergies, the current Occupational Safety and Health Administration standard for soluble platinum salts is 2 mcg/m^3 of air averaged over 8 hours.

Platinum is also used as a catalyst in the formation of some polymers. Platinum black, a fine powder (1 nm–1 μm) form of platinum, is used in many of these reactions.[10] Platinum black catalyzes the addition of hydrogen to unsaturated organic compounds and is used in the production of silicone gel breast implants (see below).

Platinum complexes have also been used as chemotherapy and show good activity against some tumors. Cisplatin, the best-known platinum chemotherapeutic agent, has activity against multiple types of cancer. However, it has some significant side-effects, including cumulative irreversible kidney damage and deafness.[11,12]

Polymers

Polymers are molecules composed of repeating subunits. They are typically defined as a backbone series of molecules with side chains that are covalently bound to the backbone moleclues. The physical properties of the polymer are defined by the structure of the monomer, the number of monomer units in the polymer chain, and the degree of cross-linking (the amount of bonding between two polymer chains). As polymer chains are cross-linked, the ability for them to move independently is decreased. For example, a polymer with freely flowing chains might exist as a liquid and, as the amount of cross-linking is increased, it can become a "gel" or "solid."

Silicone

Silicone is probably the most maligned and misunderstood biomaterial used in medicine today. This is likely due to the controversy revolving around the use of silicone in breast implants. Silicone gel-filled breast implants were first introduced in the US in 1962 and consisted of two shells made of thick, smooth-walled silicone elastomer, filled with a viscous silicone gel material (dimethylsiloxane) and glued together. Multiple variations and modifications to the shell and gel were made over the years in an attempt to improve the outcomes of breast augmentation and reduce the associated complications. In 1988, the US Food and Drug Administration (FDA), out of concerns from reports of implant failure and allegations of resultant complications and illness, relabeled breast implants as class III medical devices, and called for data from manufacturers showing the safety and effectiveness of these devices.[13,14]

In 1992, the FDA claimed that there was "inadequate information to demonstrate that breast implants were safe and effective" and placed a moratorium on silicone gel breast implants for cosmetic purposes but allowed their continued use for reconstruction after mastectomy, correction of congenital deformities, or replacement of ruptured silicone gel-filled implants due to medical or surgical reasons. In order to address this concern, the Department of Health and Human Services appointed the Institute of Medicine of the National Academy of Science (IOM) to begin one of the most extensive research studies in medical history. Their charge was to examine potential complications during or after silicone-based breast implant surgeries. In 1999, after reviewing years of evidence and research concerning silicone gel-filled breast implants, the IOM released a comprehensive report on both saline-filled and silicone gel-filled breast implants entitled *Safety of Silicone Breast Implants*.[15] The IOM found that "evidence suggests diseases or conditions such as connective tissue diseases, cancer, neurological diseases or other systemic complaints or conditions are no more common in women with breast implants than in women without implants." Most individual studies and all systemic review studies have also subsequently failed to find a link between silicone breast implants and disease.[13,14]

In 2006, the ban imposed by the FDA was lifted and restrictions on the use of silicone gel-filled breast

Term	Chemical formula	Description
Silicon	Si	Most abundant element on earth
		Does not occur naturally in its metallic state
Silica	SiO_2	Sand, marble, or quartz
Silicate	Na_2SiO_3	In one form, used as a desiccant (e.g., in anesthesia machines)
Siloxane	R_2SiO	Monomer of silicon and oxygen
Silicone	$|R_2SiO|_n$	Polymers of silicon and oxygen
Poly-dimethylsiloxane	$|(CH_3)_2SiO|_n$	The building block for most medical-grade silicone products, including breast implants

Table 32.2 Silicone nomenclature

(Adapted from Miller MJ, Ogunleye OT. Biomaterials. In: Guyuron B, Eriksson E, Persing JA, et al., eds. *Plastic surgery indications and practice*. New York: Saunders Elsevier; 2009:57–66.)

implants produced by the two manufacturers for breast reconstruction and for cosmetic breast augmentation ended. The FDA approval required a complete 10-year study on women who have already received the implants and a 10-year study on the safety of the devices in 40 000 women. It was also mandated that patients be given brochures explaining the risks.[13,14]

So what is silicone? It is important to understand this question in light of the history of breast implants. Silicone is a family of polymers consisting of alternating silicon (Si) and oxygen (O) molecules. *Table 32.2* shows the nomenclature of silicone. Siloxane, the basic repeating unit of silicone, consists of silicon, oxygen, and a saturated hydrocarbon (alkane) side group. Poly-dimethylsiloxane (PDMS) $|(CH_3)_2SiO|_n$ is the polymer used in most medical applications. PDMS is a very pure polymer that consists of the silicone backbone (silicon and oxygen) with two methyl side chains. It is one of the most inert biomaterials available for use in medical devices. Altering the length and molecular weight of the PDMS changes the mechanical properties and behavior of the silicone gel. PDMS molecules with less than 30 monomers are defined as low-molecular-weight formulations and have a viscosity similar to baby oil. High-molecular-weight formulations contain more than 3000 monomers and are solids. Controlling the degree of

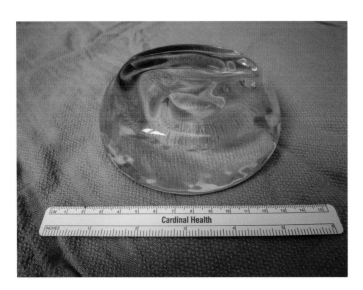

Fig. 32.2 A silicone gel-filled breast implant (Mentor).

cross-linking, changing additives, and adjusting the curing process can also modify the mechanical properties of silicone. For example, the silicone gel found in breast implants is cured in a hydrosilation reaction where some of the methyl side chains (CH_3) are replaced by vinyl side chains ($CH=CH_2$) that then allow the silicone chains to cross-link with each other. This reaction is catalyzed by platinum and some residual platinum can be found in silicone gel breast implants. The silicone shell on breast implants is made of fully polymerized silicone with an amorphous (noncrystalline) silica filler added for strength (*Fig. 32.2*).

Other plastic surgery applications of silicone include facial implants for malar, nasal, and chin reconstruction or augmentation, and orbital floor reconstruction. Hand surgeons use silicone implants for arthroplasty, flexor tendon replacement, and bone block spacers. Silicone is beneficial in these applications because it is relatively inert, malleable, and deformable. Low-molecular-weight silicone was used in the past as an injectable soft-tissue filler. However, severe tissue reaction and migration of the silicone have led many physicians to avoid this application.

Silicone is probably the most studied implantable material available today. After over 35 well-conducted studies from many countries, there is no conclusive evidence that this material causes disease. Furthermore, medical-grade silicone is ubiquitous, being found in more than 1000 medical products as either a component or as a residuum from the manufacturing process.

For example, every disposable needle and syringe, as well as intravenous tubing, is lubricated with silicone. Medications in stoppered vials contain residual silicone from its use in the manufacturing process. Silicone elastomers, in their solid form, are used for pacemaker coatings, tubing, prosthetic joints, hydrocephalus shunts, and various facial and penile implants. Like breast implants, some testicular and chin implants are made of a silicone gel in a silicone envelope.

Silicones are also found in some medications. If a medication contains an ingredient with the name "methicone" (e.g., simethicone), this is a silicone that has been modified for human consumption. Silicones are also used in household items such as lipstick, suntan/hand lotion, hairspray, processed foods, and chewing gum. Medical-grade silicones invoke a nonspecific foreign-body response, resulting in typical macrophage invasion, giant cell formation, and eventual scarring.[16]

Extensive investigations by several prestigious scientific bodies (e.g., the IOM,[17,18] and the UK Department of Health[19]) have failed to show that systemic illness is definitively attributed to silicones.

Polytetrafluoroethylene

Polytetrafluoroethylene (PTFE), also known as Teflon, was accidentally invented by Roy Plunkett in 1938 while he was trying to develop a refrigerant.[20] It consists of a carbon backbone with fluorine side chains. Expanded PTFE (ePTFE or Gore-Tex®) was created by Bob Gore in 1969 when he rapidly stretched PTFE. It is very stable chemically, cannot be cross-linked (which makes it flexible), and has a nonadherent surface. When made with a pore size of 10–30 μm it will allow some limited tissue ingrowth. It has been used for a wide variety of applications, from hiking boots to coatings on frying pans. Within the medical field it is used for vascular grafts, mesh for abdominal wall reconstruction, and implants for facial augmentation.[21] The nonadhesive properties of ePTFE have been employed in surgical meshes used for hernia repair to reduce repair site adhesion. However, there are significant limitations of ePTFE mesh used for hernia repair, including infection often requiring explantation and limited incorporation strength to the surrounding fascial edge compound to macrospores meshes such as polypropylene.

Polyester

Polyester contains an ester functional group in its main chain. Mersilene is a polyester fiber mesh knitted product for use in herniorrhaphy. Polyester mesh is softer and more hydrophilic than polypropylene, and in animal studies has shown better tissue ingrowth. Dacron is another form of polyester that has been used for vascular grafts.

Polyprolene

Polyprolene, or polypropylene, has a carbon backbone and side chains of hydrogen and methyl groups. It has been used in hernia and pelvic organ prolapse repair and is rarely rejected. However, polypropylene mesh can erode through the soft tissues over time. Therefore, the FDA has issued warnings on the use of polypropylene mesh in pelvic organ prolapse, specifically when in close proximity to the vaginal wall secondary to the number of mesh erosions reported by patients over the past few years.[22] It is also used as suture material because of its strength and low foreign-body reaction within the body. Knitted polypropylene surgical meshes are commonly used for hernia repair owing to a high ultimate tensile strength of the mesh and strong fibrovascular incorporation into the fascial defect edge. Direct placement over abdominal viscera can case dense adhesions, fistula, and erosion. Reoperation through a polypropylene mesh hernia repair is often challenging due to this generalized fibrotic scanning to adjacent intraperitoneal viscera.

Polyethylene

Polyethylene consists of a carbon backbone with hydrogen side chains (ethylene). A high-density porous form of polyethylene (Medpor) is used for facial implants *(Fig. 32.3)*. The porosity allows for tissue and vascular ingrowth. It can also be carved to customize the implant for individual patients. The implants are firmer and stiffer than the ePTFE implants and, because of the size of the pores, are more difficult to place because the soft tissues adhere to it more readily. In addition, the soft-tissue ingrowth makes the implant more difficult to remove. Porous polyethylene alone or with titanium mesh embedded within it is available for reconstruction

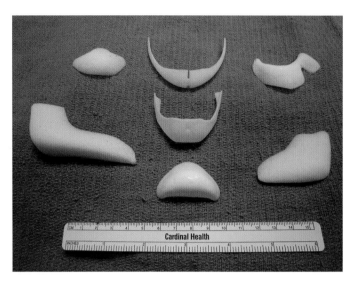

Fig. 32.3 Medpor (high-density porous form of polyethylene) implants used in facial augmentation.

of the orbital floor. One of the disadvantages of the polyethylene alone for orbital floor reconstruction is that the implant does not show up well on CT, making it difficult to diagnose a malpositioned implant.

Biodegradable polymers

Biodegradable polymers were developed to try to overcome some of the disadvantages associated with permanent implants. Most biodegradation begins through a chemical reaction such as hydrolysis or oxidation and involves some sort of biological process (e.g., enzymatic or cellular process) to eliminate the material completely. In addition to the requirement that the material itself must be biocompatible, all of the breakdown products of the material must be biocompatible as well.[23]

Although there are a multitude of materials that will degrade *in vivo*, there are only a few that are clinically relevant as biodegradable polymers. Most of these are α-hydroxy acids, specifically poly(lactic acid) (PLA), poly(glycolic acid) (PGA) and combinations, or copolymers, of these individual polymers know as poly(lactic-co-glycolic acid) (PLGA). These polymers degrade through hydrolysis, ending in lactic or glycolic acid, a common byproduct of normal biochemical pathways.

Most surgeons are familiar with this polymer as it is the polymer used to make Vicryl (polygalactin 910, Ethicon, Somerville, NJ). These polymers have also been used to create biodegradable mesh for use in abdominal wall reconstruction and plating systems for craniofacial or hand applications.

Altering the ratios of lactic to glycolic acid or adding carbon fibers or other polymers can modify the rate of degradation. In general, increasing the concentration of lactic acid decreases the rate of degradation (i.e., the polymer lasts longer). In the past 15 years manufacturers have used these polymers to develop biodegradable plates and screws for craniofacial and hand applications. Each manufacturer has modified the ratio of lactic and glycolic acid as well as the specific manufacturing protocol to optimize the degradation rate and strength of the polymer. For example, LactoSorb (Biomet, Warsaw, IN) consists of 82% PLA and 18% PGA while Resorb-X (KLS Martin, Jacksonville, FL: used in SonicWeld) is 100% poly D,L-lactic acid (PDLLA). At implantation, their strength is equal to that of titanium plating and decreases with time. Typically the structural integrity is preserved for the first 8 weeks to allow for bony healing to occur.

Vicryl knitted meshes are used as a temporary abdominofascial closure in complex abdominal wall reconstruction, particularly in a contaminated wound. The mesh helps contain the viscera initially and subsequently resolves, creating an iatrogenic hernia that is repaired in a delayed stage.

Ceramics

People have been using ceramic materials for thousands of years. However, medical applications of ceramics were not developed until the 1960s. Of the many ceramics available, only a few have been found to be suitable for implantation in humans. Ceramics have a crystalline structure and are made up of inorganic, nonmetallic molecules whose individual electrons are strongly bound to each individual atom (called heteropolar bonding; in contrast, homopolar bonding, seen in metals, allows the electrons to flow freely between atoms). The manufacturing of ceramic materials is achieved through a process called sintering, which requires the material to be fused together under high pressure and temperature. Ceramics have appealing physical properties for biomedical use, including decreased foreign-body response, resisting bacterial colonization, a high compressive strength, and tissue ingrowth into porous materials (100 μm pore size for

bone and 30 μm pore size for soft tissue). However, their benefits are overshadowed by their weaknesses; namely they are brittle and fracture easily under tensile, torsional, or bending loads. Their main uses in plastic surgery are for bone augmentation and replacement.

Calcium phosphates are the most common ceramics used in plastic surgery. In addition, calcium phosphates have been shown in the laboratory to be both osteoinductive and osteoconductive, but this has not been demonstrated in the clinical setting.

Calcium phosphates come in two formulations for medical use: hydroxyapatite ($Ca_{10}(PO_4)_6(OH)_2$) and tricalcium phosphate ($Ca_3(PO_4)_2$). Tricalcium phosphate has a faster rate of resorption and replacement by bone when compared to hydroxyapatite. They are available as granules for injection, blocks, both solid and porous, and the hydroxyapatite is also available as a cement paste. These implants are commonly used to reconstruct nonload-bearing bones of the face and cranium. The cement paste is beneficial in select cases, such as cranioplasty, because it is malleable and can be molded during the case.

Adhesives and glues

The first fibrin tissue adhesive was described in 1944 and was used to aid in the adherence of skin grafts to the recipient tissue bed. The first commercially manufactured fibrin sealant became available in 1978. Cyanoacrylate was synthesized in 1949 but this early product created a severe foreign-body reaction. Through chemical modifications to molecule, engineers were able to decrease the foreign-body reaction and create a clinically relevant product. There are several tissue adhesives available for clinical use. Most commonly, these adhesives are used to seal two tissues together or to provide hemostasis. Many of the adhesives possess both properties. Ideally, tissue adhesives should possess five characteristics (*Box 32.2*). Several classes of tissue

---

Box 32.2 **Characteristics of the ideal tissue adhesive**

Must be safe (i.e., no allergic response, disease transmission)
Must eliminate potential spaces
Must be easy to use
Must be cost-effective
Must have a clinical benefit

adhesive are available and each will be discussed in the next sections.[24]

Platelet gels

Platelet gels are derived from platelet-rich plasma (PRP). The starting material is 70 mL of whole blood that undergoes centrifugation. The platelet layer, which also contains native fibrinogen, is then combined with bovine thrombin, resulting in a gel adhesive. This product is good for individuals who do not want to use the commercially available fibrin sealant. It is also less expensive to manufacture (once the initial equipment is accounted for) than the commercially produced fibrin sealants. There are, however, some drawbacks to this product. The concentration of fibrinogen in PRP is significantly lower than in the commercially available fibrin sealants. Thus, the PRP is a less effective adhesive. In addition, the tensile strength and hemostatic capabilities of PRP are also lower than the commercially available products. The clinical applications of this product include applications where there is a large surface area that the surgeon would like to adhere together. Examples include a brow lift, a facelift, an abdominoplasty, the latissimus dorsi donor site, and deep inferior epigastric perforator/transverse rectus abdominis myocutaneous flap donor sites. Spray or mist applicators provide the best delivery method for this application.

Fibrin tissue adhesives

Fibrin sealants were the first FDA-approved tissue adhesives and consist of two parts: fibrinogen and thrombin. A small amount of factor XIII and calcium is included to catalyze the reaction and form polymerized fibrin. Screened donors provide pooled human plasma as the source of the two ingredients. The commercially available product also contains an antifibrinolytic to decrease degradation and bovine-derived aprotinin, which acts as a stabilizer. In order to prevent disease transmission, the products undergo heat pasteurization and ultrafiltration.

The product must be refrigerated and requires approximately 20 minutes to prepare. The two bottles need to be placed in a special warmer for several minutes. Once heated, the components are drawn up into individual syringes. The dual syringe delivery system is designed to mix the two ingredients immediately before they are applied. There are multiple delivery mechanisms available. The simplest delivery system is a straight blunt-tipped needle. There are also sprayer/mister applicators and applicators for endoscopic use. The misters provide the maximal mixing of the two components and produce the thinnest layer of polymerized fibrin to the wound, which has been shown to have the strongest adhesive properties.[25]

The strength of the fibrin glue is directly proportional to the concentration of fibrinogen in the mixture while the rate of polymerization is regulated by the concentration of the thrombin. Thus, in applications where the tissues need to be manipulated (e.g., a large flap), a lower concentration of thrombin should be used. Plastic surgery applications for fibrin sealants are similar to the indications for PRP described above. Fibrin sealants have also been used successfully to treat chronic seromas with percutaneous injection.[26]

Cyanoacrylate

The original cyanoacrylates were butyl-cyanoacrylate. The butyl-cyanoacrylate is a short chain with rapid breakdown, which resulted in many wounds dehiscing. In addition, the breakdown products (formaldehyde and cyanoacetate) can cause a severe inflammatory reaction if butyl-cyanoacrylate penetrates the skin. In order to address these issues, octyl-cyanoacrylates were developed. They have longer side chains, creating a stronger and longer-lasting polymer. The polymerization begins when the 2-octyl-cyanoacrylate is exposed to moisture (there is enough moisture in the air to allow polymerization to occur). Applications in plastic surgery are limited to skin closure. Because the superficial layer of the skin, where the product is applied, will not have any sutures to hold it together, it is important to make sure the deep layers are well approximated and provide a tension-free abutment of the two sides. Studies that have been done comparing traditional suturing to using octyl-2-cyanoacrylate showed that the outcomes were equivalent.[27]

Skin substitutes

Over the past 20 years, bioengineered skin substitutes have become a mainstream therapy for wound management. Originally designed to replace skin grafts for patients with severe burns, their use has broadened to include the treatment of chronic venous and chronic diabetic ulcers. As these technologies continue to advance their application will broaden even further *(Box 32.3)*.

Although the ideal skin substitute does not exist, engineers and scientists have developed, and continue to refine, several very useful products. The engineering of cultured skin substitutes has been developed on the premise that three important components are required for their formation: (1) a cell source; (2) a "tissue differentiation-inducing" substance; and (3) a matrix.[29] A variety of cells, mediators, and polymers have been tested in various combinations to engineer cultured skin substitutes. We review the most common of these below and compare them in *Table 32.3*.

Box 32.3 **Characteristics of an ideal skin substitute**

Adhere to the wound bed rapidly
Recapitulate the physiologic and mechanical properties of normal skin
Be inexpensive
Avoid immune rejection by the host
Be highly effective in accelerating tissue regeneration and wound repair.

Integra

Integra (Integra LifeSciences, Plainsboro, NJ) is a bilayer skin substitute. The "dermal" (lower) layer is a bovine collagen base with glycosaminoglycan chondroitin-6-sulfate while the upper layer is a silicone sheet that acts as a temporary epidermis.[30] As the wound heals the dermal layer is replaced with the patient's own cells.[31] A thin split-thickness skin graft is then applied on to the neodermis. Integra is indicated for the management of complex wounds such as partial- or full-thickness burns, and multiple types of ulcer. Several studies have evaluated the efficacy of Integra and have compared Integra with autograft, allograft, xenograft or Biobrane. Biobrane (Smith & Nephew, Largo, FL) is a biosynthetic dressing constructed of a silicone film with a collagen-bound nylon fabric partially embedded into the film. These studies showed that Integra has a higher rate of infection than the other tested product with regard to wound infection and graft take. However, Integra appeared to be better than autograft, allograft, or xenograft in terms of wound-healing time. Integra is also used in complex wounds to which a skin graft would not adhere.[30,32,33] The neodermis attaches to the underlying bed, vasularizes over 10–14 days, and then provides a surface for a split-thickness skin graft to adhere to.

Table 32.3 Comparison of commercially available skin substitutes

Product	Company	Tissue of origin	Layers	Uses
Integra	Integra Life Sciences Plainsboro, NJ	Synthetic	1. Silicone 2. Collagen and GAG matrix	Deep- or full-thickness soft-tissue defects for coverage Requires skin graft
Epicel	Genzyme Cambridge, MA	Autogenous	Cultured autogenous keratinocytes	Deep partial- and full-thickness burns >30% TBSA
Dermagraft	Advanced Biohealing La Jolla, CA	Allogeneic dermis	Vicryl seeded with neonatal fibroblasts	Chronic wounds Full-thickness burns with STSG
Apligraf	Organogenesis Canton, MA	Allogeneic composite	1. Neonatal keratinocytes 2. Collagen seeded with neonatal fibroblasts	Chronic wounds Excision sites Used with STSG to improve function/cosmesis
AlloDerm	LifeCell Branchburg, NJ	Allogeneic dermis	Acellular dermis	Deep partial- and full- thickness burns Soft-tissue replacement Suspensory materials Interpositional grafts Tissue patches

TBSA, total body surface area; STSG, split-thickness skin graft; GAG, glycosaminoglycan.
(Adapted from Shores JT, Gabriel A, Gupta S. Skin substitutes and alternatives: a review. *Adv Skin Wound Care*. 2007;20:493–508; quiz 509–510.)

Epicel (cultured epidermal autografts)

Epicel (Genzyme, Cambridge, MA) is a cultured epidermal autograft grown from the patient's own keratinocytes. A small skin biopsy is harvested from the patient and sent to the company for processing. The keratinocytes are grown in a co-culture using proliferation-arrested, 3T3 murine fibroblast feeder cells. Once the keratinocytes are 2–8 cell layers thick the autograft is returned to the patient for grafting. The graft is attached to petrolatum gauze backing with stainless steel surgical clips and measures approximately 50 cm².

Epicel is indicated for patients who have either deep dermal or full-thickness burns involving a total body surface area of greater than or equal to 30%. It can be used in conjunction with split-thickness skin grafts, or alone in patients for whom split-thickness skin grafts may not be an option due to the severity and extent of their burns. Epithelial cells have been combined with Integra to regenerate skin and oral mucosa successfully in animal models. This has been performed with cultured epidermal autograft placed over vascularized Integra,[34] preseeding keratinocytes into the Integra, and applied in a single stage.[35–38]

Dermagraft

Dermagraft (Advanced Biohealing, Westport, CT) is a polyglactin mesh seeded with neonatal fibroblasts. The fibroblasts produce collagen, glycosaminoglycans, fibronectin, and other growth factors. Over time the mesh is resorbed and replaced with the patient's own tissue.[31] Dermagraft has applications as both a temporary and permanent covering to increase the successful take of meshed split-thickness skin grafts on excised burn wounds and for venous ulcers and pressure ulcers.[31,39] With respect to infection, exudate, healing time, time to closure, and graft take, Dermagraft has been shown to be equivalent to allograft.[39–41]

Apligraf

Apligraf (Organogenesis, Canton, MA) is a bilayered skin-equivalent. The lower "dermal" layer consists of type I bovine collagen and fibroblasts obtained from neonatal foreskin. The upper "epidermal" layer is derived from keratinocytes. It has to be applied "fresh"

and has a shelf-life of 5 days at room temperature.[31] It has been used to cover and help heal venous ulcers and diabetic foot ulcers. It has been used as a temporary covering over meshed expanded autograft for excised burn wounds.[42]

Bioprosthetic mesh

To avoid the possible side-effects of synthetic prosthetic mesh and provide a more biocompatible material, bioprosthetic materials have been developed and used for multiple applications. Currently available bioprosthetic mesh materials are derived from decellularized mammalian tissues, either human (allogeneic) or animal (xenogeneic). Dermis is the most common source tissue for bioprosthetic meshes. Bioprosthetic mesh materials are processed to remove cells, cellular debris, and other potentially immunogeneric components optimally without disrupting the native extracellular matrix (e.g., collagen, proteoglycan) architecture. Preservation of the native extracellular matrix is important to allow these materials to remodel and regenerate (gradually being replaced with native host tissue) rather than become scarred and encapsulated by the body. An ideal mesh should possess the characteristics shown in *Box 32.4*.

There are a growing number of bioprosthetic mesh materials available from which the surgeon can select. Many of these materials are used for complex torso reconstruction, including chest wall reconstruction and ventral hernia repair.[43] They are often selected over

---

Box 32.4 Characteristics of the ideal bioprosthetic mesh

Resistance to bacterial colonization and chronic infection

Biocompatibility and noncarcinogenicity

Available readily at acceptable cost

Ability to withstand physiological stresses over a long period of time

No additional pain caused after implantation

Promotion of strong tissue ingrowth

Avoidance of substantial contraction or expansion after implementation

Limits development of adhesions to visceral structures induced

Provides cells with a supportive framework and the necessary signals for host cells to grow, differentiate, and interact, while at the same time it should become remodeled as the wound gains strength and new tissue is formed

(Adapted from Bellows CF, Alder A, Helton WS. Abdominal wall reconstruction using biological tissue grafts: present status and future opportunities. *Exp Rev Med Devices*. 2006;3:657–675.)

synthetic mesh owing to their ability to resist infection.[44] They limit repair site adhesions[45,46] and tolerate cutaneous exposure, usually without the need to remove the bioprosthetic mesh.

Small intestinal submucosa

Small intestinal submucosa (SIS or Surgisis, Cook Biotech, West Lafayette, IN) is a biomaterial created from the small intestine of pigs. After removal of the mucosal, serosal, and muscular layers of the small intestine, a strong, collagenous matrix remains. The submucosa of the small intestine provides mechanical strength to the intestine. The strong, yet biochemically rich and diverse extracellular matrix of the submucosa makes it an excellent choice for a naturally derived biomaterial. First described as a vascular graft in 1989,[47] SIS has been applied to over 20 applications in humans, including multiple types of hernia repair,[48–50] dural repair,[51] bladder reconstruction,[52,53] and stress urinary incontinence treatment.[54]

Human acellular dermal matrix

Human acellular dermal matrix (HADM) (AlloDerm, LifeCell, Branchburg, NJ; Allomax, Bard Davol, Murray Hill, NJ; and FlexHD, Ethicon360, Somerville, NJ) is made from donated allograft human dermis. Each manufacturer has a proprietary technique for producing the acellular dermal matrix. In general the epidermis and subcutaneous tissue are removed and the dermis is processed, with either freeze-drying or chemical detergents, resulting in the collagen structure of the dermal matrix. Applications of HADM include implant-based breast, abdominal wall, chest wall, and pelvis reconstruction, and lip augmentation. Micronized HADM (Cymetra, LifeCell, Branchburg, NJ) is also available and has been used for laryngoplasty and as a soft-tissue filler.

Porcine acellular dermal matrix

Porcine acellular dermal matrix (PADM) has been developed for applications similar to HADM. Porcine materials are more abundant and it is easier to control the harvesting conditions. However, because the PADM is from a xenogeneic source, additional processing must occur to prevent an adverse immunogenic reaction when implanted in humans. To inhibit immunogenicity and reduce collagenase-dependent matrix degradation, first-generation PADMs (CollaMend, Davol Bard Cranston, RI and Permacol, Covidien, Norwalk, CT) undergo intentional chemical cross-linking of collagen fibers during the manufacturing process. A secondary side-effect of the cross-linking is the alteration of the extracellular matrix structure, which has been shown to inhibit cellular infiltration, revascularization, and matrix remodeling potential.[55]

A newer generation of PADM (Strattice, LifeCell, Branchburg, NJ), is processed without chemical cross-linking. In this case, the [galactose-α(1,3)-galactose] antigen, which is the major cause of the immune response associated with acellular xenografts, is enzymatically removed.

It is not entirely clear which of these products has a better outcome; however, in a recent *in vivo* animal study comparing cross-linked PADM to noncross-linked PADM for abdominal wall reconstruction, the noncross-linked PADM was rapidly infiltrated with host cells and vessels while cross-linked PADM become encapsulated. Noncross-linked PADM had weaker adhesions to repair sites while it increased the mechanical strength of the bioprosthesis–musculofascia interface at early timepoints. Thus the study concluded that noncross-linked PADM may have early clinical advantages over cross-linked PADM for bioprosthetic abdominal wall reconstruction.[56] However, no comparative human studies have been performed to date.

Other bioprosthetic mesh products

Bovine pericardium (Veritas, Synovis, St. Paul, MN) collagen matrix is a noncross-linked bovine pericardium. The decellularization and reduction of the immunogenicity are achieved by capping free amine groups using a proprietary chemical process.

Bovine fetal dermis (Surgimend, TEI, Boston, MA) is an acellular dermal matrix derived from fetal calves. It is not cross-linked and can facilitate cell penetration, revascularization, and integration with host tissues.

Future materials

Biomaterials and implants have made huge impacts on medicine and surgery. Some implants are designed to have as little impact or interaction with the body as possible. Others are designed to interact with the body in a passive way (e.g., biodegradable PLGA polymers). The most recent biomaterials are being designed to modulate their environment to create a tissue-specific response. Furthermore, hybrid biomaterials containing cells, polymers, and growth factors are currently being developed in *in vivo* models. These biomaterials will eventually be able to "sense" their surroundings and change their biochemical and mechanical properties in response to the needs of the environment. As with the past development of biomaterials, the continued progress of the biomaterial field depends upon an interdisciplinary collaboration between engineers, scientists, clinicians, and industry. With continued cooperation between these biomaterials experts, the future use of biomaterials and implants in plastic surgery will likely change significantly in the future. The goal would be to manufacturer materials with specific properties to reconstruct site-specific defects individualized to the exact biologic, chemical, and functional needs of the reconstruction.

Access the complete references list online at **http://www.expertconsult.com**

4. Cumberland VH. A preliminary report on the use of prefabricated nylon weave in the repair of ventral hernia. *Med J Aust*. 1952;1:143–144.

5. Scales JT. Materials for hernia repair. *Proc R Soc Med*. 1953;46:647–652.

   These manuscripts offer a discussion of the ideal physical properties of synthetic surgical implants. The notion that host response can be modulated by altering these properties of the synthetic is discussed.

18. Janowsky EC, Kupper LL, Hulka BS. Meta-analyses of the relation between silicone breast implants and the risk of connective-tissue diseases. *N Engl J Med*. 2000;342:781–790.

   This report offers a meta-analysis of studies investigating a causal connection between silicone breast prostheses and connective tissue disorders. No connections between breast implants and connective tissue, rheumatic or autoimmune diseases were identified.

26. Butler CE. Treatment of refractory donor-site seromas with percutaneous instillation of fibrin sealant. *Plast Reconstr Surg*. 2006;117:976–985.

27. Toriumi DM, O'Grady K, Desai D, et al. Use of octyl-2-cyanoacrylate for skin closure in facial plastic surgery. *Plast Reconstr Surg*. 1998;102:2209–2219.

   Octyl-2-cyanoacrylate was compared to conventional sutures in 111 elective surgical procedures by a single surgeon. A significantly superior cosmetic outcome was reported at 1 year in the skin glue group.

29. Langer R, Vacanti JP. Tissue engineering. *Science*. 1993;260:920–926.

30. Pham C, Greenwood J, Cleland H, et al. Bioengineered skin substitutes for the management of burns: a systematic review. *Burns*. 2007;33:946–957.

   This review examined 20 randomized control trials to compare the safety and efficacy of bioengineered skin substitutes to biological skin replacements. The authors found that sufficient evidence was not present in the literature to draw definitive conclusions, and urged further study on this topic.

33. Heimbach D, Luterman A, Burke J, et al. Artificial dermis for major burns. A multi-center randomized clinical trial. *Ann Surg*. 1988;208:313–320.

   This series details the early use of artificial dermal grafts. The authors conclude that artifical dermal grafts coupled with epidermal grafts offer coverage comparable to conventional skin grafts with less donor site morbidiy.

44. Breuing K, Butler CE, Ferzoco S, et al. Incisional ventral hernias: review of the literature and recommendations regarding the grading and technique of repair. *Surgery*. 2010;148:544–558.

33

Facial prosthetics in plastic surgery

Gordon H. Wilkes, Mohammed M. Al Kahtani, and Johan F. Wolfaardt

SYNOPSIS

- The success of osseointegration biotechnology has revolutionized facial prosthetic reconstruction.
- Titanium is the implant material of choice as it is light, biocompatible, and resistant to corrosion.
- Implant placement technique is crucial to produce bone–implant contact with no interposed fibrous tissue and successful bone healing.
- Appropriate treatment selection requires understanding of all options available.
- Multidisciplinary team planning is required.
- Osseointegration biotechnology provides plastic surgeons with more treatment options for challenging head and neck deformities.

 Access the Historical Perspective section and Figure 33.1 online at
http://www.expertconsult.com

Deformities in the head and neck region can have a profound effect on the function, aesthetics, and psyche of an individual. Considerable time, effort, and ingenuity have been spent trying to develop meaningful reconstructive solutions to a wide variety of craniofacial defects. Autogenous reconstruction remains the gold standard, but in certain cases, autogenous reconstruction may be contraindicated, technically impossible, or have the potential to solve the reconstructive issues only partially.

Historically facial prosthetics have been of limited benefit. Retention of facial prostheses has been largely unsuccessful because of the need for adhesives or crude mechanical means of maintaining retention. The patient lacked confidence about the positioning of the prosthesis and its ability to stay in place. Often associated pain or discomfort would limit the length of time and circumstances in which the prosthesis would actually be worn. The adhesives are those used in industry and were not developed for the unique sensitive human biological environment. They often had adverse effects on the underlying skin compromised by radiotherapy, trauma, or thermal injury[1] and affected the durability and longevity of the prosthesis.

With the success of osseointegration and its ability to solve the problem of prosthetic retention,[2,3] a new treatment modality was now available.[4,5] Prosthetic longevity is increased without the need for adhesives.[6,7] Osseointegrated retained facial prosthetics now meet the necessary criteria for success: (1) aesthetic acceptability; (2) functional performance; (3) biocompatibility; and (4) desired retention.[8] The use of osseointegration biotechnology in facial prosthetic restoration has been hailed as the most significant advance in the field of facial prosthetics in the past 25 years.[9] It is estimated that more than 90000 implants have been installed extraorally in more than 45000 patients up to the year 2007.[10]

Craniofacial osseointegrated reconstruction gives the plastic surgeon another viable treatment option in many challenging head and neck defects.[11] It can provide some patients with a meaningful and enhanced quality of life when in the past other treatment options would not have been successful. Unfortunately, competing specialties or providers have presented autologous techniques and craniofacial osseointegration as unrelated technologies.[12] Osseointegrated and autogenous techniques should not be viewed as competing technologies, but rather as complementary reconstructive procedures that optimize the opportunity for success in the management of major head and neck deformities.

Why this situation has arisen is unclear. In some cases, it appears to be due to a lack of understanding of osseointegration and its benefits. It may be viewed only as a salvage procedure when all else has failed and both the patient and surgeon are desperate. It is not viewed as "real" surgery, only as throwing a few screws in the bone. Those in doubt cannot understand how patients would be satisfied with a prosthesis, "a foreign object that never becomes part of their body image." To any surgeon with experience in osseointegration, these lines of thinking are seriously flawed.

This intervention requires long-term support by both the caregiver and the funder for maintenance of the implant sites as well as future prosthetic construction. It is analogous to the time and financial commitment required in an organ transplantation program.

Advantages of craniofacial osseointegration

Craniofacial osseointegration has many advantages *(Box 33.1)*.[20] The surgical procedures are generally short with minimal morbidity and are performed on an outpatient basis. There is a short learning curve and results are predictable. The patients usually have minimal postoperative discomfort. Examination of the tumor resection site is easy and allows early diagnosis of any tumor recurrence.

Craniofacial osseointegration can successfully salvage a patient with a failed autogenous reconstruction and often offers superior aesthetics. When compared with adhesive-retained facial prosthetics, osseointegration offers predictable prosthetic retention, increased prosthetic durability and lifespan, enhanced prosthetic aesthetics, ease of displacement, no underlying skin damage, successful incorporation of the prosthesis into the body image, and a happier, more satisfied patient. Osseointegration can also be considered in diabetics and smokers.

The disadvantages of craniofacial osseointegration include the need for a larger multidisciplinary team with skills that are often not freely available. Patients also require regular maintenance visits and a new prosthesis every 2–5 years *(Box 33.2)*.[20] Lifetime ongoing costs can be an issue with some insurance companies.

Indications for craniofacial osseointegration

Craniofacial osseointegration can be of particular benefit for reconstruction of selected defects involving the ear, orbit, nose, and combined midfacial defects. The osseointegrated implants have also been used to secure hairpieces.[21] A newer application of interest to the plastic surgeon is the use of a bone-anchored hearing aid (BAHA) in children with microtia. In the past concern has been expressed combining a BAHA and an autogenous ear reconstruction. Fear of inappropriate positioning of the implant adversely affecting future autogenous ear reconstruction usually prevented patients having the benefits of both treatment modalities. This usually resulted in the BAHA being placed too far posterior or not being considered at all. Certainly the

---

Box 33.1 **Advantages of craniofacial osseointegration**[7]

Procedures short
Minimal morbidity
Minimal postoperative pain
Outpatient procedures
Short learning curve
Allows examination of tumor resection site
Salvage of autogenous failures
Use in compromised tissues
Excellent prosthetic aesthetics

Box 33.2 **Disadvantages of craniofacial osseointegration**[7]

Need for multidisciplinary team
Need for reliable, committed patient
Ongoing expense of prosthetic remakes and maintenance visits
Not one's own tissue

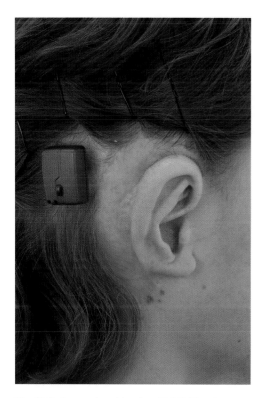

Fig. 33.2 Bone-anchored hearing aid (BAHA) and autogenous ear reconstruction for microtia.

BAHA is an excellent option for hearing restoration in bilateral microtia patients and more recently has proven of benefit in unilateral microtia patients *(Fig. 33.2)*. It is a much more straightforward, safer, and predictable way of improving hearing than previous autogenous means of canalplasty and middle-ear reconstruction.[10]

Ear reconstruction

Autogenous reconstruction of auricular defects has improved greatly in the latter half of the 20th century because of the work of pioneers such as Tanzer,[22] Brent,[23–26] Fukada and Yamada,[27] Cronin,[28] Bauer,[29] Yanai *et al.*,[30] Isshiki *et al.*,[31] Nagata,[32–34] and others. Certainly, not all reconstructive attempts are successful. The appropriate treatment selection for major ear defects continues to be controversial *(Table 33.1)*.[20] Certain auricular defects have limited autogenous options, particularly after removal of the ear for cancer with associated radiotherapy. It is our belief that these reconstructive techniques are complementary and must be presented in this manner.[8,12,20] Definite indications for osseointegrated auricular prosthetic reconstruction include:

Table 33.1 Indications for osseointegrated ear reconstruction[7]

Definitive	Relative
Major cancer resection	Microtia – most controversial
Radiotherapy	Absence of lower half of the ear
Severely compromised tissue	Calcified costal cartilage
Patient preference	
Failed autogenous reconstruction	
Potential craniofacial anomaly	
Poor operative risk	

(1) following major cancer resection; (2) radiotherapy to the proposed site of auricular reconstruction; (3) severely compromised local tissue *(Fig. 33.3)*; (4) patient preference; and (5) salvage procedure for failed autogenous reconstruction. Relative indications include: (1) microtia; (2) absence of the lower half of the ear; and (3) patients with calcified costal cartilage.

Probably the most controversial indication for osseointegrated auricular reconstruction is microtia in children. Although it is technically possible to place implants in children as young as 3 years and early results are encouraging, the follow-up in these situations is short. Because the use of craniofacial osseointegrated implants requires removal of any local ear remnants and produces scarring in the operative field, future autogenous reconstruction options are very limited. For these reasons, the use of osseointegrated auricular reconstruction in the pediatric age group requires very careful consideration by the clinician and family *(Fig. 33.4)*. A publication by Zeitoun *et al.*[35] outlines the difficulties seen using osseointegration in the pediatric population. It also showed an increased need for psychological support in many of these patients. Our approach is to offer autogenous ear reconstruction to pediatric patients with microtia. Despite the potential for difficult treatment selection decisions, we rarely find this to be the case. Patients usually decide quite quickly after the possibilities are discussed. It is rare for patients to change their mind following further discussion.

The use of an adhesive-retained auricular prosthesis is very limited and almost relegated to historical significance only. It certainly cannot be considered a "test" for an osseointegrated prosthesis. It offers none of the major advantages of implant-retained prostheses such as ease

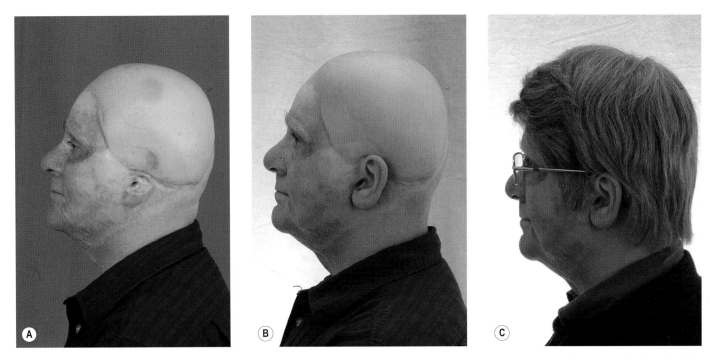

Fig. 33.3 (A–C) Reconstruction following severe electrical injury included cranioplasty, free-flap scalp coverage, and ear reconstruction with implant-retained prosthesis.

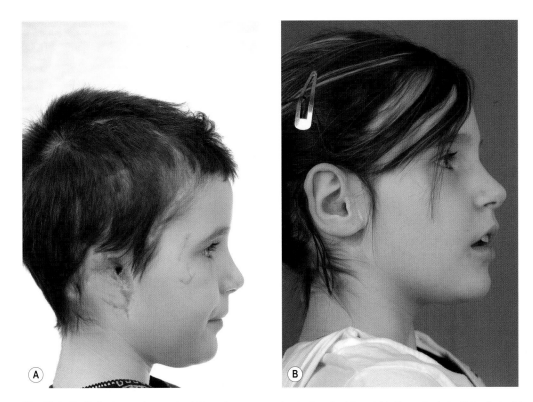

Fig. 33.4 (A, B) Ear loss and severe local tissue trauma secondary to dog attack in a child. Reconstructed with implant-retained prosthesis.

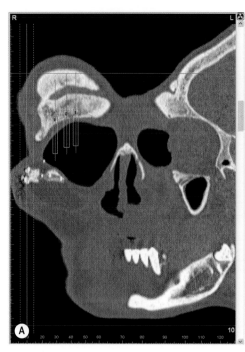

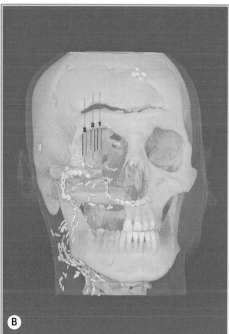

Fig. 33.5 (A, B) A Simplant™ study can be performed to determine quantity and quality of underlying bone.

Box 33.3 **Indications for osseointegrated nasal reconstruction[10]**

Failed autogenous reconstruction
Scarring at autogenous donor sites
Reconstruction following autogenous reconstruction because of
    tumor recurrence
Patient preference
Medical contraindication to multistaged autogenous reconstruction

---

Box 33.4 **Indications for osseointegrated orbital reconstruction**

Loss of orbit and orbital contents
Severe enophthalmos with compromised vision
Difficulty with an ocular prosthesis and significant eyelid distortion
    secondary to trauma or radiotherapy that is not amenable to
    autogenous correction

---

of placement, predictable retention, improved aesthetics, increased lifespan of the prosthesis, and no ongoing insult to the skin.

Osseointegrated nasal reconstruction

Indications for osseointegrated nasal reconstruction include: (1) failed autogenous reconstruction; (2) significant scarring in potential autogenous donor sites *(Fig. 33.5)*[6]; (3) tumor recurrence following initial autologous reconstruction; and (4) patient preference *(Box 33.3)*. Because of the need for multiple surgical stages and the greater variability in the ultimate result with autogenous reconstruction, many patients with total nasal loss opt for placement of implants and a nasal prosthesis *(Fig. 33.6)*. Certainly, there is less surgery involved with

less morbidity. There is no need for other donor sites, and tumor surveillance is easy with prosthesis removal.[8] The application of "nontraditional" long zygomaticus implants may be useful in difficult situations of nasal reconstruction.[36]

Osseointegrated orbital reconstruction

Patients with loss of the orbit and orbital contents have very poor autogenous reconstructive options *(Box 33.4)*. Although autogenous coverage may be necessary to cover important neurological structures, in many cases it is provided only to fill the residual orbital cavity. However, "filling the hole" does not create an aesthetic result. It is in these situations that osseointegrated orbital reconstruction clearly has advantages over

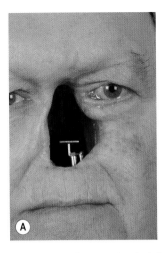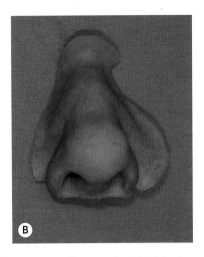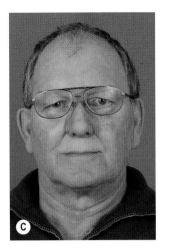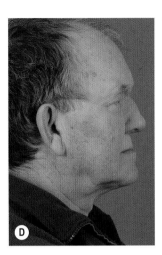

Fig. 33.6 (A–D) Nasal deformity following cancer resection reconstructed with implant-retained nasal prosthesis.

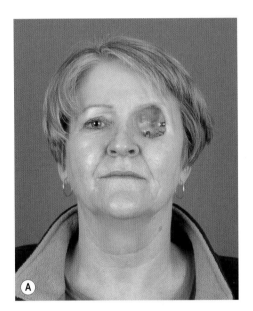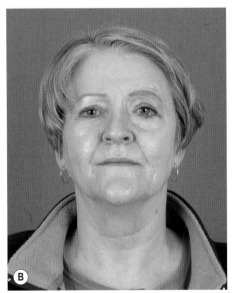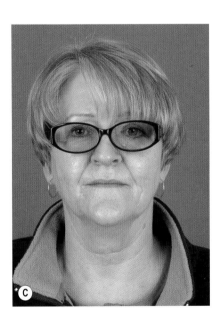

Fig. 33.7 (A–C) This patient had an orbital exenteration for a malignancy and was reconstructed with an implant-retained orbital prosthesis.

autogenous reconstruction. The aesthetic results are far superior and again allow visualization for early tumor recurrence *(Fig. 33.7)*. This approach could also be considered in patients with severe enophthalmos and significantly compromised vision. Less frequently, it can be considered in patients with an ocular prosthesis and significant eyelid distortion secondary to trauma or radiotherapy that is not amenable to autogenous correction. The hope for the future would be to create an orbital prosthesis that can mimic movement of both the lids and globe of the opposite normal eye.[13]

Midfacial reconstruction

Patients with complex facial defects that may include the orbit, nose, and maxilla again have poor autogenous options *(Fig. 33.8)*. Craniofacial osseointegration offers significant advantages. It enables examination of the posttumor defect and allows for a very acceptable aesthetic result. In the patient shown in *Figure 33.8* it allowed early detection of a recurrence on the posterior orbital wall. Treatment consisted of surgical removal and reconstruction with a temporoparietal fascial flap

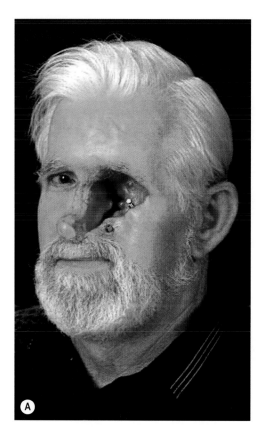

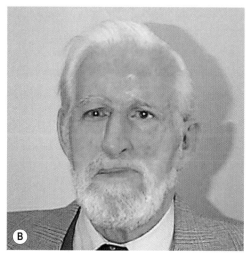

Fig. 33.8 (A, B) This patient had an extensive basal cell carcinoma invading his orbit, nasal region, and maxilla. After surgical extirpation, implants were later placed and a naso-orbital prosthesis constructed. Autogenous options were poor.

and skin graft. The patient was able to resume wearing his prosthesis again only 12 days after surgery to resect the recurrence. Extraoral osseointegration in combination with intraoral osseointegration may also result in significantly improved functional results over conventional prosthetic or autogenous techniques.

Factors important to obtain osseointegration[13,37]

Choice of implant material

Many materials have been considered for osseointegration. Although other metals such as vanadium, tantalum, aluminum hydroxide, and ceramics like hydroxyapatite are known to integrate with bone to a certain degree, titanium is currently the material of choice.[37] Titanium is relatively light but stiffer than bone. Its springiness allows it to flex with the bone. The most important factor is the ability of its titanium oxide

layer on the implant surface to react with the adjacent bone (its biocompatibility). The key to success is what happens at this implant–tissue interface. The most successful is commercially pure titanium, which is 99.75% pure. This differs from the most commonly used titanium alloy, which contains 90% titanium, 6% aluminum, and 4% vanadium, and exhibits much less satisfactory characteristics of osseointegration.

Implant–tissue interface

Except for mechanical forces, all interactions between the implant and host occur from physiochemical forces less than 1.0 mm from the surface. When the titanium implant is exposed to oxygen and comes in contact with the host, a layer of oxide is rapidly formed. It acts as a protective barrier and prevents direct contact between the metal and its environment. The titanium oxide layer continues to grow with time and creates a dynamic interface. The oxide layer is the bioactive component of the implant. The microsurface characteristics of the implant itself, including roughness, porosity, and thread design, all influence its potential for successful osseointegration. A surface roughness of 100 μm or greater is advantageous. An implant that has a very smooth surface will result in poor integration, but with minor bone resorption. A very rough surface will result in rapid integration, but secondary inflammation and resorption that can jeopardize integration later on.

The macrostructure of the implant has importance for integration. Rounding the outer edges and spaces of a threaded implant relieves stress concentration. A screw-shaped implant often shows good primary stability, whereas a cone-shaped implant might be lost because of initial micromovements and hence poor stability.

Bone bed

The bone bed into which the implant is installed is of importance. There is a difference if the implant is installed in a child with relatively soft and immature bone, compared with an adult. The older patient with osteoporosis will integrate the implant to a lesser degree, and implant failure rates have been higher. Patients who have been irradiated or sustained burns will have an altered texture of bone that will reduce the capacity to integrate implants.

Bone preparation

Meticulous, gentle surgical technique is vital for osseointegration to occur.[10] Bone preparation must result in new bone healing around the implant with no interposed fibrous tissue formation and minimal bone necrosis (*Fig. 33.9*). Proper bone healing results in bone ultimately being in intimate contact with the titanium oxide layer. Sharp drill bits, copious saline irrigation, and slower drilling speeds are required for success. Studies have shown temperatures of 89°C occurring with high-speed drilling despite cooling.[38–40] Bone exposed to temperatures greater than 47°C for 1 minute showed decreased new bone formation. Exposure to 44°C showed no negative effect. The fixture should only be handled by titanium instruments and never touched by the gloved hand. It is further important that the surgical field should be protected from fibers, powder, and other substances that might hinder osseointegration. At the junction of the titanium oxide and bone, a layer of

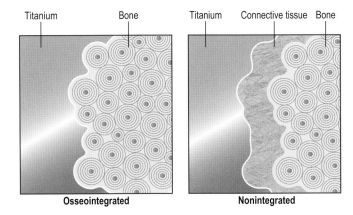

Fig. 33.9 Bone–titanium interface with only oxide layer and no interposed soft tissue.

ground substance consisting of proteoglycans and glycosaminoglycans forms. The thickness of this layer is inversely related to the strength of integration of the bone with the implant. Titanium has the thinnest ground substance layer, approximately 200 Å.

Traumatic surgery and an implant bed of low healing potential are said to be primary factors limiting successful osseointegration. Implant mobility, overloading, and poor implant biocompatibility are considered to be secondary factors in failure of osseointegration. With successful osseointegration, the weakest portion of the osseointegrated bone–implant complex is the bone itself. After successful osseointegration, attempting to remove an implant will fail within the surrounding bone, not at the implant–bone interface.

Implant load

The load of the implant should preferably be in the longitudinal direction. It is important to avoid rotational or cantilever forces once the implant has integrated. If forces are distributed in the longitudinal direction, even very high loads can be withstood by the implant during many years of function.

Treatment planning

Providing craniofacial osseointegration care requires a larger multidisciplinary team than autologous reconstruction. The core team should include appropriate surgical expertise, including plastic surgery, otolaryngology, and oral surgery, a prosthodontist, a dental technologist, an anaplastologist, and appropriate nursing and dental assistants. Careful preoperative assessment and planning are crucial for the ultimate success of this clinical endeavor. Only by having the full spectrum of team members can the patient be presented with all appropriate options to make a truly informed decision.

The treatment-planning process starts with a multidisciplinary consultation. Team members then formulate an approach to each individual patient's problem. The preoperative workup includes charting, standardized preoperative photographs, psychological profile, radiologic examination such as computed tomography (CT) scanning, including three-dimensional images and implant site planning,[41–43] impressions of the defect and the corresponding normal side, construction of surgical planning templates, and appropriate medical modeling. Preoperative assessment allows an evaluation of bony sites for implant placement, the presence of surrounding vital structures, general quality of the bone, and overlying soft tissues.

The patient should have no systemic or local factors that could significantly influence bone-remodeling capacity.[44] Age alone is not considered a contraindication. Patients as young as 3 years or in their 80s have been successfully treated. There should be no psychiatric or substance abuse conditions. Smoking is a relative contraindication,[45] as is radiotherapy,[10,46,47] or chemotherapy.[48] The literature on smoking and implant survival involves dental implants and not craniofacial osseointegrated implants.[49] A past history of radiotherapy requires assessment for hyperbaric oxygen treatment before and after implant placement to optimize the chance for successful osseointegration.[50–52] Patients must have a certain level of cognitive, visual, and dexterous ability to maintain osseointegrated implants. They must also have reasonable geographic accessibility to an osseointegration unit. Once the preoperative workup and informed consent have been obtained, treatment can begin.

In autologous reconstruction, the surgeon provides the final result. This differs from osseointegration, where the surgeon sets the stage for the final prosthetic result by the prosthodontist or anaplastologist. This makes preoperative planning and proper implant placement even more vital to ultimate treatment success. Good communication between the surgeon and prosthodontist or anaplastologist preoperatively and often intraoperatively is critical. Implants placed in the wrong position will compromise the final aesthetic and functional result or make further implant placement necessary.

Surgical technique

The surgical approach as developed by Brånemark is a meticulous multistep technique that may be performed in one or two stages, depending on the clinical situation.[53] Although titanium is used by many specialties in many clinical situations, this application resulting in osseointegration should not be confused with these other uses of titanium. Osseointegration biotechnology is very specific in terms of osseointegration fixture production and preparation, surgical technique, and final surgical result. Other implant systems (Conexcao, Otorix, Straumann, ITI, Southern) are available but are principally based on the original implant.[10]

Compared to intraoral osseointegration, the fixtures for extraoral use tend to be shorter (3–5 mm). The length used depends on the particular bone thickness. Longer fixtures can sometimes be used in the frontal bone, zygoma, and maxilla. Ideally bicortical purchase is obtained if anatomically possible. The extraoral environment tends to be a more hostile, less forgiving environment than the protected intraoral situation. The gingiva is constructed to have mucosal penetration and saliva and the cleaning action of the tongue are quite beneficial. Penetration through skin with nearby hair, muscle, and sebaceous glands lends itself to the development of more soft-tissue problems. The skin does not attach to the implant abutment and is essentially maintained as an open wound. The ability to modulate this interface better would result in less local skin problems.

Surgery can be performed in one or two stages.[1,12] The one-stage procedure is usually reserved for adult patients with good bone quality and quantity. The surgery can be performed in most instances either under general anesthesia or with sedation and local anesthesia.

A treatment template is used to choose the site for implant placement. Appropriate positioning is crucial to the ultimate prosthetic success. Advanced digital

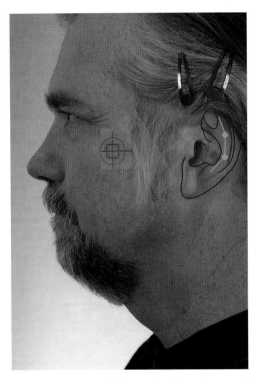

Fig. 33.10 An ear template is used to choose the appropriate site for implant placement.

technologies can be useful for this aspect of treatment planning. Adobe Photoshop or Freeform has been used successfully for this purpose *(Fig. 33.10)*. In ear reconstruction, implants need to be placed under the future site of the antihelical fold of the ear prosthesis. This is where there is maximal depth to hide the protrusion of the fixture abutment within the prosthesis.

In orbital reconstruction, the implants need to be placed well within the orbital rim rather than anteriorly, where it is technically easier to place them. Again consideration needs to be given to the space requirements of the orbital prosthesis in all three dimensions. Within the orbit, the implants should not align to a central converging point because this may make prosthetic procedures very difficult. In nasal reconstruction, better success is obtained by placing implants into the floor of the nose rather than into the glabellar region. In cases where there are concerns about the underlying bone quality or quantity, a Simplant™ study will be performed *(Fig. 33.5)*. This software in combination with a CT scan allows assessment of the bone and surgical simulation of implant placement. Appropriate

templates can then be constructed to help the surgeon with the implant surgery.

The area is infiltrated with a lidocaine (Xylocaine) and epinephrine solution and a skin flap is elevated. The periosteum is exposed and either a periosteal flap is elevated or a circular opening made in the periosteum. A surgical locating template is invaluable in difficult cases to optimize positioning of the implant, minimize the extent of surgical dissection, decrease the number of pilot drill holes needed to find adequate bone, and decrease the length of the procedure. A 3.0-mm guide drill is first used. If bone is present in the depths after drilling, it is deepened to 4.0 mm. This drilling is carried out at a speed of 2000 rpm with copious saline irrigation. The base of the guide hole is checked to determine that penetration of underlying vital structures has not occurred.

In the second step, the guide hole is then widened with a countersink. A fresh countersink drill is used, as is copious saline irrigation. This also prepares a flat countersink area on the bony surface for seating of the implant flange. In the orbit, often flangeless fixtures are placed. Issues with cleaning and accumulation of debris around the implant flange can be problematic in the orbital region.

The third step involves placing the self-tapping implant. It is placed at a drill speed of 15–20 rpm and 20–40 N-cm torque. All these precautions are taken to minimize bone necrosis. With bone necrosis, fibrous tissue will develop, compromising the tissue–implant interface, and osseointegration will not occur. All drills and countersinks are discarded after each procedure. Craniofacial implants are 3.75 mm in diameter and are available in 3.0, 4.0, and 5.5-mm lengths *(Fig. 33.11)*. A 4.0-mm implant is preferable if bony conditions allow.

At the fourth step, a cover screw or space screw is placed in the implant. This prevents soft-tissue ingrowth into the central portion of the implant where the abutment will ultimately fit. A space screw fits in the center of the implant and does not increase the profile of the implant during the healing phase. It is used if implants are placed under an area of old skin graft or thin skin flap, usually in the orbital region, The surgical incisions are then closed if a two-stage procedure is planned.

If a one-stage procedure is desired, the outer layer of the flap is elevated as an attached split-thickness graft,

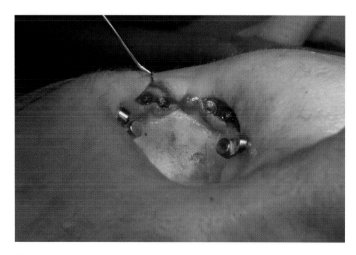

Fig. 33.11 Craniofacial implants and fixtures of commercially pure titanium.

and underlying soft tissues discarded. The edges around the outside of the flap site are aggressively thinned and the graft is replaced to take on the underlying periosteum. The commonest causes of future soft-tissue problems are tissue movement around the abutment and hair follicles left behind. In nonirradiated tissues, the implants are usually left for approximately 3 months, at which time phase II surgery can occur. In the midface or in patients with a history of radiotherapy, this time period is usually extended to 6–9 months. Usually, two implants are required for auricular reconstruction and at least three implants for orbital reconstruction. Extra implants are often placed as sleepers in the orbital region as the long-term success rates in this region are not as high as elsewhere. If an implant fails, then a sleeper can be exteriorized, and the patient can continue to wear the prosthesis uninterrupted.

Phase II surgery when necessary involves exposing the implant, radical thinning of the overlying and surrounding tissue, creation of a hairless, nonmobile zone of 1.0 cm around each abutment, and connection of an abutment to the underlying fixture. Improper soft-tissue surgery is the most common cause of ongoing tissue reaction around the abutment. Other surgical considerations include removal of any residual soft-tissue elements sufficient to produce a flat tissue surface for the ear prosthesis. More recently there has been success in the mastoid region with one-stage placement of implants under optimal local conditions.[54,55] Accepted clinical criteria for a one-stage procedure in the mastoid region of older children (>10 years) or adults include:

- no past history of irradiation
- cortical layer of bone greater than 3.0 mm in thickness
- uncomplicated surgery.

The technique is essentially the same as for phase I and II surgery, but both phases are conducted at the same operation. After one-stage surgery, the implant must be protected and not loaded for at least 3 months.

Prosthetic construction

Construction of the prosthesis generally begins 4–6 weeks after phase II surgery when local tissues have healed sufficiently to be a stable base for overlying prosthetic construction. The details of prosthetic construction have been well described elsewhere.[41] In general, a bar superstructure is individually designed and connected to the abutments. The prosthesis is first sculpted in wax and related to an acrylic resin substructure. When the prosthesis is anatomically acceptable, a mold is constructed and the prosthesis is made from silicone elastomer. Advanced digital technologies have been helpful in prosthetic construction. Capture of data from the "normal" side can be done from a moulage or laser surface scanning. With computer-aided design software (Mimics, Magic, and Freeform), the image is manipulated and the basic form of the prosthesis is easily constructed (*Fig. 33.12*). This efficiency optimizes the amount of time needed by the anaplastologist with the patient. Constructing the prosthesis using the anaplastologist's time and skills efficiently is very important, as they are in limited supply.

Another challenge to the prosthodontist and anaplastologist is color-matching based on the patient's normal pigments and extrinsic influences such as time of year and patient occupation. One of the newer solutions includes the use of spectrophotometry computer technology for color-matching of the prosthesis to the patient.[56] Patients will sometimes have summer and winter prostheses to adjust for subtle pigmentary changes. Many small details and techniques are used to add realism to the prosthesis. Clips on the undersurface of the prosthesis securely attach the prosthesis to the bar and are most commonly used for ears. Usually, two prostheses are made at a time (*Fig. 33.13*). This prevents a crisis situation if something happens to one of the

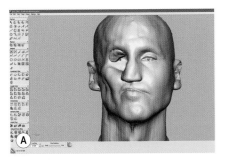
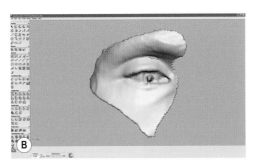
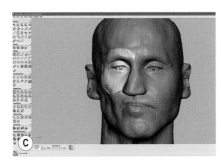
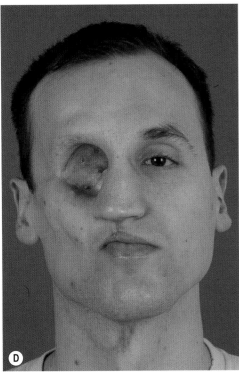
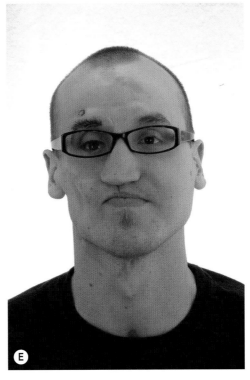

Fig. 33.12 (A–E) Advanced digital technologies were useful in prosthetic construction in this orbital defect.

prostheses. A magnetic retention system is more commonly used for orbital prostheses.

Maintenance program

The long-term success of osseointegration requires an effective ongoing maintenance regimen, analogous to the follow-up in an organ transplantation program. Strong patient commitment is required for success. In particular, conscientious care of the periabutment area is crucial. This includes gentle cleaning on a daily basis, as well as diligent application of appropriately prescribed topical agents *(Fig. 33.14)*. These can include mineral oil for general lubrication of the skin, antibiotic ointment, or topical steroid. Our patients are given a lifetime maintenance recall schedule to impress on them their commitment, which is vital to long-term success. Maintenance visits include assessing the periabutment region, measuring soft-tissue height, checking for tissue reaction, and monitoring the mechanical integrity of the implant–abutment assembly. New prostheses are constructed in the future as needed. The life of an individual prosthesis can vary from 2 to 5 years depending on extrinsic factors such as general care and exposure to sunlight or cigarette smoke.[6]

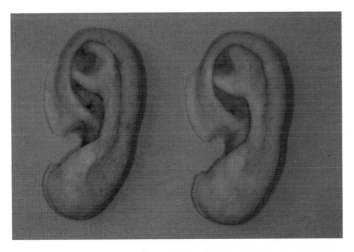

Fig. 33.13 Two prostheses are made at the same time with different coloration for different seasons and to prevent a crisis if one prosthesis is lost or damaged. There are clips on the undersurface of the prosthesis for secure attachment to the implant-retained bar superstructure.

> **Box 33.5 Ancillary soft-tissue procedures combined with craniofacial osseointegration**
>
> Soft-tissue expanders
> Scar revision
> Free vascularized bone graft
> Pedicled bone graft
> Alar repositioning
> Ectropion repair
> Eyebrow reconstruction
> Browlift
> Static facial sling
> Repositioning external auditory meatus
> Onlay cartilage graft
> Muscle flap
> Bone contouring
> Rhytidectomy
> Tragal reconstruction

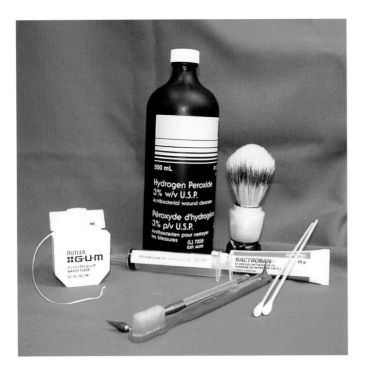

Fig. 33.14 Requirements for care at abutment sites.

Ancillary autogenous procedures

It is our belief that treatment of the patient's craniofacial defect is often best managed by a combination of osseointegration and autogenous procedures to optimize the final results (*Box 33.5* and *Figs 33.15, 33.16*).[57,58] The goal of the ancillary procedures may include decreasing the size of the facial prosthesis, placing prosthetic margins at junctions of aesthetic units, decreasing the size of the maxillary obturator, improving facial contour, improving symmetry, and bringing viable bone for implant placement into a region compromised by surgery or radiation.

Craniofacial osseointegration outcomes

To evaluate the success of craniofacial osseointegration, several parameters need to be studied.[59,60] Success from a patient's perspective is the ability to use the prosthesis on a regular basis and its positive effect on quality of life. This contributes to psychological success as much as the aesthetic and functional success. Assessment of outcomes must also include individual implant success rates and local skin response.

Individual implant success rates

Jacobsson *et al.*[18] proposed the following criteria for success of a craniofacial osseointegrated implant:

1. The unattached implant should be immobile when tested clinically.

2. Soft-tissue reactions around skin-penetrating abutments should be type 0 (reaction-free) or type 1 (slight redness), not demanding treatment in more than 95% of observations.

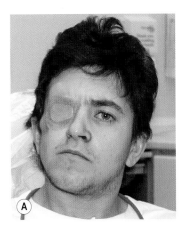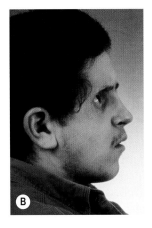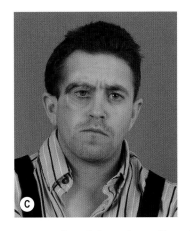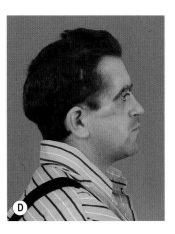

Fig. 33.15 (A–D) As a child this patient underwent enucleation of the right globe and postoperative radiotherapy for a malignant lesion. He was reconstructed with a combination of autogenous and alloplastic techniques. He had an eyebrow reconstruction, onlay cartilage graft to right zygoma, orbital revision, and an osseointegrated orbital prosthesis.

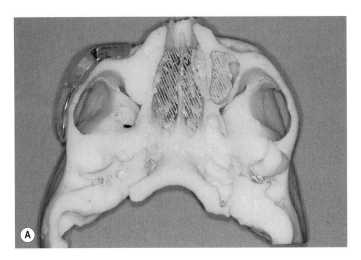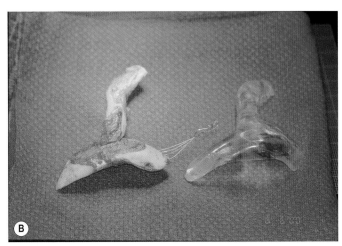

Fig. 33.16 (A, B) Medical modeling technology is used to help construct appropriate cartilage graft and to help with implant placement.

3. Individual implant performance should be characterized by the absence of persistent and/or irreversible signs and symptoms such as pain, infection, neuropathy, and paresthesia.

4. A success rate of 95% in the mastoid process and 90% in the orbital region in nonirradiated bone tissue at the end of a 5-year observation period should be a minimum criterion for success.

Many studies in the literature have documented implant success rates. A 1992 study[18] showed a success rate of 95% in the mastoid and 72% in the orbital region. It was noted that failures in the mastoid occurred within 6 months of insertion whereas failures in the orbital region tended to occur much later. Further evaluation revealed that the success rate in nonirradiated orbits within this group was 92.1% whereas that of the irradiated group was 62.7%. Subsequently, work by Granström and others has shown that hyperbaric oxygen therapy both before and after implant placement has significantly improved the success rate of craniofacial osseointegrated implants in irradiated bone. In 1994, Granström and coworkers found that, with hyperbaric oxygen therapy, no implant loss had occurred during a 5-year follow-up period in 48 implants placed in irradiated orbital, nasal, and temporal regions.[47]

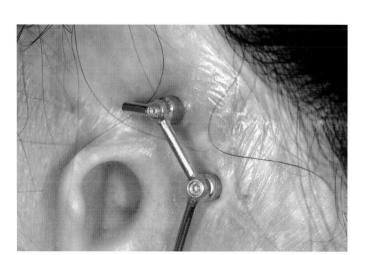

Fig. 33.17 Adverse skin reactions can intermittently be a problem requiring treatment. Lower abutment shows no soft-tissue reaction while upper abutment shows some tissue hypertrophy.

Skin response

The most common problems are related to the skin response around the percutaneous abutments. Although this does not usually threaten the long-term success of the individual implant, it uses up much of both the clinician's and patient's time to overcome this problem. Occasionally, further surgery may be indicated. Tjellström reported that 15% of his patients accounted for 70% of skin reactions.[17] He reported a grading of no skin reaction in approximately 90% of his patients. A factor contributing to adverse skin reaction was adolescence because of behavior problems and poor compliance with local hygiene *(Fig. 33.17)*.

Prosthetic success

Several studies have been published documenting prosthetic success from a patient's perspective.[17,59,61,62] In a study from 1990,[17] only 2 of 94 patients were not wearing their prosthesis at the time of assessment. Tolman and Taylor[61] evaluated patients with nonimplant-retained prostheses, and only 50% considered their prosthesis stable. After these patients had craniofacial implant prosthetic reconstruction, 93% rated their implant-retained prosthesis as stable. Of 30 patients, 19 wore the prosthesis more than 12 hours per day, 3 wore the prosthesis 8–12 hours per day, 3 wore the prosthesis 4–8 hours per day, and 5 wore the prosthesis less than

4 hours per day. Twenty-four of 30 patients viewed the prosthesis as an extension of themselves and part of their body image. Westin *et al.* found 95% of their patients wore their prosthesis every day and in most cases more than 10 hours per day.[62] In a recent study by Korus *et al.*[63] of osseointegrated ear prosthetic patients, 90% of patients rated their confidence as good with their prosthesis compared to 16% without, and 100% felt that the prosthesis felt like part of them. In regard to the implant system, 55% felt that they had a skin reaction; however 83% did not consider their reaction severe. Ultimately most patients were satisfied (97% satisfied, and 74% very satisfied). In all, 94% would ultimately undergo the same procedure again and 97% would recommend it to others.

Conclusion

Craniofacial osseointegration has an important role in the treatment of major head and neck defects. It offers treatment options in many situations where in the past only poor ones existed. Patient satisfaction is very high and they often become strong advocates for this treatment modality. Craniofacial osseointegrated prosthetic reconstruction adds another floor where the reconstructive elevator can stop.

The future of craniofacial osseointegration includes the development of new implants and implant surfaces to stimulate bone formation and remodeling to improve long-term success. Growth factors, stem cells, and new drugs will help improve success rates in compromised tissues. Further developments using advanced digital technologies such as rapid prototyping,[64,65] image acquisition technology,[66] software manipulation systems, and color-matching software,[67] will make prosthetic reconstruction more accurate, faster, and potentially cheaper. New methods of noninvasive testing will allow better evaluation of implants and better strategies to prevent implant loss will be devised.[68] Presently skin does not attach to the percutaneous abutment so the connection is maintained as essentially an open wound. Improved understanding of this soft-tissue interface will allow for more use elsewhere in the body, including the extremities, where contamination is more common.[69] Combining osseointegration technology with microelectronics could produce movable or sensory prosthetics[70–73] or some type of seeing orbital prosthesis.[74] Large titanium implants will secure large-extremity prosthetics better.[75,76] The future is exciting for a whole field of endeavor that started with the chance observation by P I Brånemark of an unusual behavior of a metal in a blood flow study in rabbits!

Bonus images for this chapter can be found online at

http://www.expertconsult.com

Fig. 33.1 Historical development of osseointegration biotechnology. Through the Brånemark experience, osseointegrated implants have been subjected to over 30 years of scientific scrutiny. Craniofacial applications were first introduced in 1977.

 Access the complete references list online at **http://www.expertconsult.com**

9. Parel SM, Brånemark PI, Tjellström A, et al. Osseointegration in maxillofacial prosthetics. *Part II: Extraoral applications J Prosthet Dent.* 1986;55:600–606.

The role of osseointegrated fixtures in facial reconstruction is discussed. Advantages over adhesive systems are highlighted.

13. Brånemark PI, Hansson BO, Adell R, et al. Osseointegrated implants in the treatment of totally edentulous jaws: experience from a 10-year period Scand J. *Plast Reconstr Surg Suppl.* 1977;1:16.

16. Albrektsson T, Brånemark P1, Jacobsson MD, et al. Present clinical applications of osseointegrated percutaneous implants. *Plast Reconstr Surg.* 1987;79:721–730.

This is a large case series cataloging outcomes in 174 patients treated with osseointegrated percutaneous implants for external hearing aids or facial epistheses.

17. Tjellström A. Osseointegrated implants for replacement of absent or defect ears. *Clin Plast Surg.* 1990;17:355–366.

20. Wilkes GH, Wolfaardt JF. Osseointegrated alloplastic versus autogenous ear reconstruction: Criteria for treatment selection. *Plast Reconstr Surg.* 1994;93:967–979.

The authors review a series of autogenous and prosthetic auricular reconstructions. Criteria for each technique were developed based on the authors' experience.

26. Brent B. Technical advances in ear reconstruction with autogenous rib cartilage grafts: personal experience with 1200 cases. *Plast Reconstr Surg.* 1999;104:319–334.

The author presents his extensive experience with rib cartilage-based auricular reconstruction. Topics from cartilage-sparing technique to tissue engineering are discussed.

32. Nagata S. A new method of total reconstruction of the auricle for microtia. *Plast Reconstr Surg.* 1993;92: 187–201.

The author presents a two-stage method for total-ear reconstruction, dividing the procedure first into designing and placing the costal cartilage framework and second into elevating the completed construct.

46. Granström G. Radiotherapy, osseointegration and hyperbaric oxygen therapy. *Periodontol.* 2000;33:145–162

57. Harris L, Wilkes GH, Wolfaardt JF. Autogenous soft tissue procedures and osseointegrated alloplastic reconstruction: their role in the treatment of complex craniofacial defects. *Plast Reconstr Surg.* 1996;98:387–392.

62. Westin T, Tjellstrom A, Hammerlid E, et al. Long-term study of quality and safety of osseointegration for the retention of auricular prostheses. *Otolayngol Head Neck Surg.* 1999;121:133–143.

34

Transplantation in plastic surgery

David W. Mathes, Peter E. M. Butler, and W. P. Andrew Lee

SYNOPSIS

- The most important antigens contributing to allograft rejection are the major histocompatibility complex (MHC) antigens.
- The immune system has two main arms that mediate both rejection and tolerance to foreign antigens: the humoral response (B cells and antibodies) and the cell-mediated response (T cells).
- T lymphocytes have a central role in coordinating the immune response, forming the cell-mediated arm of the immune response.
- Acute rejection takes place days to weeks after transplantation and occurs with rapid onset. This T-cell mediated response is characterized by fever, graft tenderness, and edema, and loss of function. Interstitial lymphocytic infiltration is seen on microscopic examination.
- Chronic rejection is characterized by fibrosis and severe organ dysfunction. This process usually occurs over years.
- Immunosuppressive medications must inhibit the body's ability to reject a transplanted organ, but not at the expense of the defense network against pathogens.
- Despite the use of powerful immunosuppressive medications most transplant patients experience episodes of acute rejection.
- Two major issues in hand transplantation are the need for maintenance immunosuppression and the evaluation of the functional outcomes of the transplants.
- Currently, clinical hand transplantation remains an experimental procedure, and the long-term outcomes of this innovative procedure are still being determined.

The fields of transplantation and plastic surgery have always been closely linked. In fact, the age of organ allotransplantation in the US began when Joseph E Murray, a plastic surgeon, transplanted a kidney between identical twin brothers in 1955.[1] Such "reconstructive surgery" using organ allografts was one of the great achievements in 20th-century medicine. Plastic surgeons often reconstruct tissue defects via transplantation of autologous tissue from other regions of the body. Nonvascularized skin, bone, and cartilage grafts alone or in combination with axial and random flaps are common everyday procedures used to reconstruct tissue defects. However, these surgical techniques all have significant limitations, often require revisions, and leave the patient with a donor site. Advances in the development of skin substitutes (prepared from allogeneic or xenogeneic sources) and the application of frozen bone allografts have shown the possibility of reconstruction without a donor site but their current application is limited. Despite advances in plastic and reconstructive surgery, including the refinement of microvascular techniques and delineation of flap vascular anatomy, many complex wounds, especially those on the central face, still remain outside the realm of possibility for restoring both form and function.

The inability to reconstruct missing tissues accurately occurs when the surgeon must deviate from the principle of replacing "like with like" due to a lack of appropriate autologous donor sources. Thus, the function of a severely injured extremity cannot be adequately restored, the appearance of a severely disfigured face cannot be satisfactorily improved, and both the function and appearance of an amputated extremity cannot be reconstructed. Understandably, the inclination toward tissue transplantation has led plastic surgery researchers to look to nonautogenous sources for reconstructive material.[2-4] However, the ability to engineer tissue from single cell sources has yet to yield a technique that can provide the complex tissue constructs needed. One technique with the potential for providing access to complex vascularized tissue constructs without the need for a donor site is through the process of allotransplantation.

The clinical feasibility of composite tissue allotransplantation (CTA) has been demonstrated by the successful transplantation of over 50 hands and nine faces.[5-9] This emerging field of reconstructive transplantation could represent a paradigm shift in the arena of reconstructive surgery. The application of these transplants to patients with complex wounds would provide the reconstructive surgeon with the opportunity to reconstruct with the exact tissues lost. However, unlike traditional solid-organ transplants (kidney, liver, and heart) that consist of relatively homogeneous parenchymal tissue, the composite tissue allograft is comprised of multiple heterogeneous tissue types (skin, bone, and muscle). Each of these distinct tissue types has been shown to exhibit varying degrees of antigenicity, with skin and mucosa the most antigenic.[10] While solid-organ transplantation is the gold standard for the treatment for end-stage organ failure, there has yet to be true consensus on the use and application of composite tissue allografts.[11,12] The survival of the hand and partial face transplants is dependent on the use of chronic immunosuppression and their application is currently limited to experimental institutionally approved protocols. In order for the field of reconstructive transplantation to expand its indications beyond the experimental arena, techniques need to be designed either to significantly reduce or eliminate the need for chronic immunosuppression. The future direction of this field is heavily dependent on the development of innovative approaches to the use of immunosuppressive agents and tolerance induction protocols.

Nomenclature

A graft is nonvascularized tissue (such as skin) that is harvested from its donor bed and transferred to a recipient site. Its survival relies on ingrowth of new vessels from the recipient bed to restore its blood supply. In contrast, a flap involves the transfer of vascularized tissue (such as muscle and skin) via either the preservation of an axial blood vessel or microvascular anastomoses of that vessel to recipient vessels located adjacent to the wound. An autograft is tissue transplanted from one location to another in the same individual. An isograft is transplanted from a genetically identical donor to the recipient, such as transplants between syngeneic mice and human monozygotic twins. An allograft is transplantation of tissues between unrelated individuals of the same species. A xenograft is transplantation between different species.

Transplantation may also be described in terms of the site into which the tissue is transplanted. Orthotopic refers to transplantation into an anatomically similar site; heterotopic refers to transplantation into an anatomic site different from the site of origin.

Transplantation immunology

Major histocompatibility complex

The most important antigens contributing to allograft rejection are the major histocompatibility complex (MHC) antigens. The MHC proteins are encoded in a gene complex on the short arm of chromosome 6 and have different nomenclature between species: human leukocyte antigen (HLA) in humans, swine leukocyte antigen (SLA) in swine, H-2 in mice, and RT1 in rat. MHC genes are expressed in a codominant fashion, with one haplotype, or set of alleles, inherited from each parent.

There are two major classes of MHC genes. Class I MHC genes encode a transmembrane glycoprotein complex with a polymorphic 44-kDa heavy chain consisting of three extracellular domains (α_1, α_2, and α_3). The α_1 domain is highly variable and contains sites for antigen binding. The heavy chain is stabilized by noncovalent binding to a lighter chain, referred to as β_2-microglobulin. There are three distinct genetic loci for the class I antigens in the human: HLA-A, HLA-B, and HLA-C. Class I antigens are expressed on nearly all nucleated cells and serve as the primary target for cytotoxic (CD8+) T lymphocytes. Class II MHC genes encode two noncovalently bound transmembrane proteins, a 34-kDa α chain and a 29-kDa β chain. There are three class II loci in humans: HLA-DR, HLA-DP, and HLA-DQ.[13] Class II antigens are expressed primarily on vascular endothelium and cells of hematopoietic stem cell origin such as lymphocytes and macrophages.

Both class I and class II molecules have a specific site at which foreign peptide antigens can be presented after they have been processed by the cell.[14–17] Tissue distribution is not the same in all species: humans, dogs, pigs, and monkeys express class II antigens on endothelial cells, whereas rodents and many species do not.[18] Matching of HLA-A, HLA-B, and HLA-DR has been found to be an important factor in determining long-term renal allograft survival.[19]

Other transplant antigens

In addition to the MHC antigens, there are three other classes of surface proteins: ABO blood group proteins, minor histocompatibility antigens, and skin-specific antigens.

The blood group antigens are important in clinical transplantation because they are expressed on vascular endothelial cells. Patients with type A or type B blood develop natural antibodies to the other protein, whereas patients with type O blood develop natural antibodies to both type A and type B proteins. Although ABO antigens will not stimulate cell-mediated rejection, a brisk antibody-mediated attack can rapidly lead to graft failure.[20]

Minor histocompatibility antigens are peptides of self origin that are not presented by the MHC complexes. Siblings (other than identical twins) with a completely matched MHC profile will still differ with respect to minor antigens because of allelic variation of the genes encoding those proteins. Although minor antigens will stimulate a cell-mediated response, they will not do so in a primary *in vitro* test. Rejection of a graft due to minor antigens alone, therefore, often proceeds at a slower rate.[21]

Skin-specific antigens (Sk antigen) are tissue-specific proteins that can cause graft rejection by a cell-mediated response. Consequently, skin is one of the most difficult tissues to which transplantation tolerance can be induced.[22]

Immunologic rejection cascade

Cells of immune response

A number of cells with varied but interconnected functions participate in the process of graft rejection. They work together to maintain the two main arms of the immune reaction, the humoral response (B cells and antibodies) and the cell-mediated response (T cells).

Macrophages

The macrophage performs the most ancient cellular defense function: phagocytosis. It is of mesenchymal origin and thought to arise from a bone marrow stem cell. It can freely circulate throughout the body, migrate through lymph nodes, or remain stationary within tissues. Kupffer cells are specialized macrophages that reside in the liver. The Langerhans cell is a specialized macrophage that is specific to the skin. The macrophage expresses class I antigens on its cell surface, and as a highly specialized immune cell, the macrophage also expresses class II MHC molecules.

Beyond simple destruction of cells, the main purpose of the macrophage is to reprocess the breakdown products of ingested cells. These fragments of foreign protein may then be bundled with a new class II antigen molecule, and during the bundling process, fragments of the foreign protein come to reside in the peptide-binding groove of the class II molecule. When the fragment is exteriorized, it faces outward and is easily recognized by the immune system as foreign. This process is known as antigen presentation. Macrophages also secrete important cytokines,[23,24] such as interleukin-1 (IL-1). This polypeptide can, in a hormonal fashion, stimulate the immunologic function of responding cells. These cells are critical to the presentation of foreign antigen.

Natural killer cells

Another primitive cell derived from the bone marrow stem cell is the lymphocyte (non-T, non-B) called the natural killer (NK) cell. NK cells are thought to be active in the antitumor response.[25] They are able to demonstrate spontaneous tumoricidal properties on exposure to tumor cells. This cell does not require recognition of MHC molecules or antigen processing (as do T cells and B cells).[26] However, the exact method this cell uses to recognize foreign cells remains unclear. They are able to kill cells by incorporating a lipophilic protein into the target cell membrane, which leads to increased permeability and cell lysis. NK cells also secrete several cytokines, including interferon-γ, interferon-α, and B-cell growth factor. They may also serve to eliminate cells that fail to express normal self-MHC proteins and thereby be self-reactive. Finally, they appear to serve as a barrier to the engraftment of donor bone marrow after non-MHC-matched bone marrow transplantation.[27]

Granulocyte

The granulocyte plays an important role in immune homeostasis. Named for their histologic staining properties, the three main cell lines are polymorphonuclear cells, eosinophils, and basophils. All of the cell lines are derived from the same bone marrow precursor. As nucleated cells, they all express class I MHC molecules; however, they do not express class II MHC antigens. In addition, these cells express a number of molecules important for their function (including adhesion and interaction with other immune cells) on their cell surface. These white blood cells carry granules of toxic substances (peroxidases) and substances that attract other white blood cells and cellular elements of the coagulation cascade. When stimulated, the granulocyte secretes these granules, initiating local inflammation in a relatively indiscriminate fashion.

B lymphocyte

Named for their site of origin in the chicken, the bursa of Fabricius, these cells play a central role in immune defense. In humans, the bursa equivalent is thought to be the fetal liver or bone marrow. Once these cells are produced, they migrate to the lymph node and spleen and appear to remain in these organs. These cells express class I and II MHC antigens. They also display a variety of B-cell-specific markers, known as B1–B8 (through which the lines of B cells can be identified). Finally, they display immunoglobulin on their surface. When stimulated, the B lymphocyte differentiates into plasma cells. These smaller cells serve as factories to produce specific antibodies. These soluble antibodies support the humoral arm of the immune response. Through rearrangement of a highly variable genetic region during immune development, antibodies are produced that can bind countless millions of different epitopes.

Immunoglobulin

Antibodies produced by B lymphocytes and plasma cells take the form of immunoglobulins. Immunoglobulins are proteins of unique structure, composed of heavy and light peptide chains. The "root" of the heavy-chain complex is called the constant fragment. The portion of an immunoglobulin molecule where light chains form complexes with heavy chains, at the site at which the antibody will bind to its target, is designated the antibody-binding fragment (Fab). Myriad possibilities exist for antigen to a specific antibody to be made because the Fab moiety is highly variable in its discrete structure. More than 100 genes code for specific segments of the variable portions of the heavy and light chains, leading to millions of potential immunoglobulin specificities.

There are five general immunoglobulin classes: IgM, IgG, IgE, IgA, and IgD. IgM is the first antibody formed after exposure to common microbial antigens, followed by the more durable IgG. IgE is involved in the hypersensitivity reaction by binding to and activating specialized eosinophils (mast cells). IgA is secreted in saliva, tears, and breast milk and thus augments resistance to infection in these fluids. IgD is found on the surface of immature B lymphocytes; its function remains unclear. Immunoglobulins may be soluble or bound to a cell's surface.

The main function of immunoglobulins is to provide opsonization and to activate complement. Opsonization occurs when the Fab fragment of an immunoglobulin binds to its associated antigen, such as an invading organism. Subsequent macrophage and monocyte phagocytosis of the antibody-coated microorganism is then markedly enhanced. Complement fixation occurs when the antibody–antigen complex triggers the complement cascade.

Complement

An antigen–antibody complex may initiate the complement cascade through a classical pathway. Substances such as endotoxin may, without immunoglobulins, initiate the cascade through the alternative pathway. Both pathways converge with the activation of C3. The sequential activation of proteases, which define the complement cascade, results in a tight cluster of proteins known as the membrane attack complex. This complex is able to rupture the membranes of foreign cells. In the normal host, this cascade is kept in check by the regulatory protein C1 inhibitor.

Dendritic cells

These cells are derived from bone marrow stem cell progenitors and are highly specialized antigen-presenting cells. They appear to have little to no effector function. They reside in the intracellular and interstitial space but migrate through the lymphatics and to the spleen when activated. There they present their antigens to T-cell-rich areas.

T lymphocytes

T lymphocytes have a central role in coordinating the immune response, forming the cell-mediated arm of the immune response. The T lymphocyte is named for its site of origin, the thymus, and is one of the central elements of the immune system. T cells derive from fetal stem cells in the thymus and undergo an extensive process of education and deletion before being released into the body. The maturing T cells are selected to recognize self MHC antigens and become tolerant to them. Those cells that demonstrate too high an affinity to self are eliminated by clonal deletion. Failure of this process appears to lead to autoimmunity.

These cells express both class I and class II antigens. In addition to HLA surface markers, lymphocytes also possess cell surface markers that serve to distinguish one subpopulation from another within the same individual. These are all glycoproteins and are described by the common determinant (CD) nomenclature (e.g., CD3).

Three broad classes of T cells are helper T (T_H) cells, cytotoxic T cells, and suppressor T cells. All T cells express CD3 on the cell surface. Cytotoxic T cells (cells that effect target cell killing) express CD8. Suppressor T cells that can buffer and down-regulate the immune response also express CD8.[28,29] T_H cell, however, expresses CD4 and serves to amplify the immune response through its interaction with other cells and secretion of critical cytokines. Each T cell expresses a T-cell receptor (TCR) capable of binding antigen. The TCR, a 90-kDa heterodimer composed of an α chain encoded on chromosome 14 and a β chain encoded on chromosome 7, is located close to the CD3 antigen and the CD28 antigen. The TCR is relatively flat and possesses an outward-facing surface. This "antigen recognition platform" is the critical interface for foreign peptide in the binding groove. As with B-cell development, T cells undergo rearrangement of genes coding for a hypervariable region on the receptor proteins. This allows a body's population of T cells to respond to a nearly limitless array of foreign antigens, with each individual T cell capable of binding one specific antigen.

T-cell binding and activation

Although the TCR is capable of binding antigen, it will not recognize the target molecule by itself.[30] The TCR can bind antigen only if it has been processed and presented by an antigen-presenting cell together with an MHC molecule; thus, it recognizes the MHC together with the target antigen. This limitation of binding is referred to as MHC restriction. CD4 (helper) T cells can only bind antigen presented with MHC class II molecules; CD8 (cytotoxic) T cells recognize antigen along with MHC class I proteins. The T_H cell is most critical to the immune response because its activation results in the production of cytokines that are necessary for the function of many other immune cells. Binding of a CD4 cell to an antigen-presenting cell that expresses target antigen together with MHC class II molecules initiates a predictable cycle of intercellular communication. The antigen-presenting cell is stimulated to produce the cytokine IL-1, a powerful chemoattractant, a primary mediator in the acute-phase reaction, and a potent activator of lymphoid cells. The T cell, in turn, secretes IL-2, which is a required stimulant for differentiation and proliferation of T cells. The IL-2 produced by the bound T cell has autocrine function by binding to newly expressed self IL-2 receptors. Secreted IL-2 also has paracrine function that affects other T cells in the region, such as CD8 cells, which require IL-2 for activation but do not produce it themselves. As CD4 cells become further activated, they secrete IL-4 and IL-5, which stimulate the maturation and proliferation of B lymphocytes. Furthermore, there is evidence that two subsets of CD4 cells, T_H1 and T_H2, function to enhance alloreactivity and stimulate antibody production by B cells, respectively. With such a central role by CD4 cells in cell signaling, it is easy to understand the severely compromised immune response from the loss of host CD4 cell function secondary to human immunodeficiency virus infection.[31-34]

Antigen recognition and graft rejection

In the case of allograft tissue, foreign antigens would be recognized by host T cells after being processed by host antigen-presenting cells and presented in the context of self MHC. This is termed indirect presentation. In addition, host T cells can directly recognize donor MHC on donor antigen-presenting cells, termed direct presentation. This mechanism helps explain the more vigorous response to allograft tissue than to foreign peptides alone.[35]

Clinically, rejection of allograft tissue can proceed at different levels of intensity for different tissues. The common component for rejection of any graft is inflammation. This may be manifested as a loss of graft function with local or systemic signs of inflammation. Several distinct clinical syndromes of graft rejection with different time courses have been noted. These syndromes differ with regard to the underlying primary immunologic process.

Hyperacute rejection occurs almost immediately after perfusion of the allograft with host blood. It is the result of preformed antibodies to either ABO blood group proteins or donor MHC molecules enacting a rapid attack on the donor tissue. Complement activation results in destruction of vascular endothelial cells and induces rapid thrombosis of vessels as well as an amplification of the inflammatory signal. Standard screening before transplantation should detect preformed antibodies, making hyperacute rejection a rare clinical entity. Many mammals possess preformed antibodies to other species that stand as a major obstacle to xenotransplantation.[36]

Acute rejection takes place days to weeks after transplantation and occurs with rapid onset. This T-cell-mediated response is characterized by fever, graft tenderness, and edema, and loss of function. Interstitial lymphocytic infiltration is seen on microscopic examination. In addition, severe forms of acute rejection may include a humoral attack on the graft, resulting in a vasculitis.[37]

Chronic rejection is an indolent process occurring months to years after transplantation. It is characterized by a progressive loss of tissue architecture with fibrosis and mononuclear cell infiltration. The etiology of chronic rejection is not well understood and may be multifactorial. The process may be slowed because of immunosuppression. It also may result from the cumulative effect of damage to the graft from ischemia during transplantation, graft infection, or drug toxicity.

Inflammatory mediators in transplantation

In addition to the direct cellular interaction observed during an immune response there are also multiple inflammatory mediators involved in immune activation and regulation. These include cell adhesion molecules (CAM), cytokines, and chemokines that are all critical to a functioning immune system. Cytokines are transient regulatory proteins that a wide variety of cells can produce in response to stimulation. These proteins can act locally by binding to a cell from the same cell line (autocrine) or to the target cell in the vicinity (paracrine).[38] The cytokines are divided into proinflammatory cytokines (IL-1α, IL-1β, IL-6; tumor necrosis factors: TNF-α, TNF-β), cytokines involved in T-cell differentiation (IL-2, IL-4, IL-5, IL-10, IL-12, IL-13, and interferon-γ), and cytokines of immunoregulatory function belonging to the transforming growth factor-β family, which primarily promotes wound healing and fibrosis.[38]

Chemokines are a subset of cytokines that are currently defined as small chemotactic cytokines. Chemokines, which are constitutively expressed, are involved in homeostatic lymphocyte trafficking to the lymphoid organs and bind to the cellular component by a specific chemokine receptor. The main role of proinflammatory chemokines (macrophage inflammatory protein-1α (MIP-1α), MIP-1β, monocyte chemoattractant protein-1 (MCP-1), and RANTES) is to attract neutrophils to an inflammatory site and trigger T lymphocytes to elicit an additional inflammatory response.[39] In humans, CCR1-positive cells increase in the peripheral blood of renal allograft recipients before acute rejection.[40] In addition, CCR1 mRNA was found to be expressed in cells derived from biopsies from renal allografts.[41] Ruster et al. described an increased number of CCR1-positive cells in glomeruli during rejection.[42] Mayer et al. reported that the mRNA expression of CCR1 was associated with the decrease of renal function in allografts with an acute rejection episode.[43] Thus, it is clear that chemokines play an important role in allograft rejection and interruption of these interactions could have an impact on allograft survival.

CAMs play a role in leukocyte migration from the circulation to tissues. Three types of CAM are involved in the transmigration process: selectins (L-, E-, and P-selectins) mediating the rolling of leukocytes along the vascular endothelium, integrins (intercellular adhesion molecule-1 (ICAM-1), vascular CAM-1 (VCAM-1), mucosal addressin cellular adhesion molecule-1 (MAd CAM-1)) leading to leukocyte adhesion to the endothelium, and finally immunoglobulin superfamily platelet endothelial CAM-1 (PECAM-1), responsible for transmigration of leukocytes.[44] The complex specific migration of leukocytes to the target tissue requires a coordinated process of proinflammatory mediators. Proinflammatory cytokines, IL-1α and TNF-α, may induce expression of proinflammatory chemokines. Chemokines play a major role in the activation of integrins needed for adhesion of rolling leukocytes to the vessel endothelium, and this process leads to leukocyte transmigration to the surrounding tissue, initiating the inflammatory process.

Immunologic screening

Methods are available to predict the compatibility of donor tissue to a particular recipient. The greatest value of these clinical tests is to exclude recipients who would be expected to manifest a hyperacute rejection to a specific donor organ.

Blood group typing is an important first step in determining transplant compatibility. An ABO mismatch will result in certain failure because of preformed antibodies.[45] Although it is possible to transplant type O donor tissue into type A or type B recipients, the limited supply of donor organs in the US makes this practice uncommon.

HLA typing is used to match organs with potential recipients. Serologic methods are employed to type HLA-A, HLA-B, and HLA-DR. A heterozygous individual with a complete match at all these loci is referred to as a six-antigen match. For renal allografts, HLA matching has been shown to affect graft survival. Kidneys transplanted from HLA-identical siblings have a 3-year success rate that well exceeds 90%, whereas parent-to-child grafts have an 82% survival. Cadaveric kidney grafts have a 70% 3-year survival rate.[46] MHC class II matching has been found to be more important than class I matching for renal transplantation; the reverse appears to be true for liver transplantation. This would suggest differences in mechanisms of graft rejection for different tissues.[47] Serologic tissue typing has certain limitations. An HLA antigen can be identified only if it is being searched for with a specific antibody. For example, if only a single HLA-DR phenotype is identified in donor tissue, the individual could be either homozygous for that allele or heterozygous with an unrecognized HLA-DR antigen. This method of testing fails to type the other class II antigens, HLA-DP and HLA-DQ.

Crossmatching is a test that detects the presence of preformed donor-specific antibodies in the serum of a particular recipient. It represents the final definitive screening measure before transplantation. In this lymphocytotoxicity assay, donor lymphocytes are incubated with recipient serum and complement. Cell viability is then assessed by a dye exclusion technique. A positive crossmatch, indicated by lysis of the donor lymphocytes, suggests that a hyperacute reaction is likely to occur. One pitfall of this test, however, is that organ-specific antibodies may be missed if those antigens are not expressed on the lymphocytes being evaluated.

Antibody screening is another modality used in clinical transplantation. Serum from prospective transplant recipients is routinely tested in a lymphocytotoxicity assay against a panel of cells from different donors with known HLA antigens. The percentage of panel cells lysed reflects the degree of panel-reactive antibody (PRA), demonstrating HLA antibodies in an individual's serum. A high PRA suggests that a patient is unlikely to have a negative crossmatch. This information is used in determining organ allocation when the tissue must be transplanted quickly. Individuals are likely to have a high PRA if they have been sensitized by previous transplantation, pregnancy, or blood transfusions.

Current immunosuppression

The multiple pathways and mechanisms employed by the immune system to defend the body against both extracellular and intracellular pathogens have presented a significant barrier to the survival of transplanted allografts. Immunosuppressive medications must inhibit the body's ability to reject a transplanted organ, but not at the expense of the defense network against pathogens. The use of several immunosuppressive agents has allowed the inhibition of the immune system that maximizes the protection of the allograft with the least cost

Table 34.1 Antibody-mediated drugs

Agent	Mechanism	Action	Side-effects
Antilymphocyte			
Antilymphocyte globulin	Antibodies directed against antigens on lymphocytes	Promotes T-cell clearance through complement-mediated lysis	Thrombocytopenia, leukopenia, increased risk of viral reactivation, serum reaction
Antithymocyte globulin	Antibodies directed against antigens on thymocytes	Promotes T-cell clearance through complement-mediated lysis	Thrombocytopenia, leukopenia, increased risk of viral reactivation, serum reaction
Alemtuzumab	Antibody against CD-52	Eliminates T cells by antibody-dependent cellular cytotoxicity	Thrombocytopenia, leukopenia, increased risk of viral reactivation, serum reaction
OKT3	Murine monoclonal antibody directed against the CD3 subunit on human T cells	Eliminates T cells by the reticuloendothelial system; blocks cytotoxic activity of activated T cells	Significant cytokine syndrome, reactivation of viruses, posttransplantation lymphoproliferative disease
Anti-IL-2			
Daclizumab, basiliximab	Blocks binding to CD25 (high-affinity chain of IL-2 receptor)	Limits T-cell expansion; acts only on activated cells	None

IL-2, interleukin-2.

to the body's overall ability to fight infection and tumors *(Table 34.1)*.

In all of the transplanted organs including the hand and face transplants, it appears that it is central to prevent allograft recognition during the peritransplantation period. This is currently achieved through so-called induction protocols. Several agents are currently used to protect the transplant during that period of cytokine excess observed after surgery *(Table 34.2)*. After the induction agents are used, "maintenance" medications are used to maintain the transplant. Finally, when ongoing rejection occurs, it is often necessary to use "rescue" agents to stop ongoing rejection and salvage a transplant that would otherwise be lost.

Corticosteroids

These agents remain a central tool for both the prevention and treatment of allograft rejection. Whereas steroids are not effective as solitary agents to prevent rejection, they have been shown to improve graft survival in combination with other agents. When used at high doses, they can also treat ongoing acute cellular rejection. Despite these uses, steroids also contribute to the morbidity associated with modern immunosuppression.

Glucocorticosteroids bind to an intracellular receptor after nonspecific uptake in the cytoplasm. The receptor–ligand complex then enters the nucleus, where it acts as a DNA-binding protein and increases the transcription of several genes.[48] The most important gene is thought to be IκBα, which binds to and prevents the function of NF-κB (a key proinflammatory cytokine that is an important transcription factor for T-cell activation). Steroids block the production of IL-1 and TNF-α by antigen-presenting cells. They also block interferon-γ production by T cells and migration and lysosomal enzyme release by neutrophils. Steroids also mute the up-regulation of the MHC and, through their diminution of the inflammatory responses, decrease the degree of costimulation in the environment. Steroids do not have an impact on the production of antibody.

Antiproliferative agents

Azathioprine

This was the first immunosuppressive agent employed in transplantation and is now largely a historical transplant medication. Azathioprine undergoes conversion in the liver to 6-mercaptopurine and then to 6-thioinosine monophosphate. These derivatives inhibit DNA synthesis by alkylating DNA precursors and inducing chromosome breaks through interference with DNA repair mechanisms. In addition, they inhibit the conversion of inosine monophosphate (IMP) to adenosine

Table 34.2 Immunosuppressive drugs

Agent	Mechanism	Action	Side-effects
Calcineurin inhibitors			
Cyclosporine	Binds to cyclophilin, blocks the NF-AT transcription factor, inhibits production of IL-2, and promotes production of TGF-β	Prevents cytokine transcription and arrests T-cell activation	Nephrotoxicity, hypertension, neurotoxicity
Tacrolimus (FK506)	Binds to FK-binding protein, blocks the NF-AT transcription factor, inhibits production of IL-2, and promotes production of TGF-β	Prevents cytokine transcription and arrests T-cell activation	Nephrotoxicity, neurotoxicity, diabetogenicity
Antiproliferative agents			
Azathioprine (Imuran)	Inhibits DNA synthesis, interferes with DNA repair mechanisms, and inhibits conversion of IMP to AMP and GMP	Blocks the proliferative response (T and B cells)	Bone marrow suppression, hepatotoxicity
Mycophenolate mofetil	Noncompetitive, reversible inhibitor of IMP dehydrogenase; interrupts production of GTP and dGTP, prevents critical step in RNA and DNA synthesis	Blocks the proliferative response (T and B cells), inhibits antibody formation, and prevents clonal expansion of cytotoxic T cells	Gastrointestinal toxicity, bone marrow suppression
Corticosteroids			
Corticosteroids	Binds to intracellular receptor, increases transcription of gene for IκBα, and prevents the transcription of NF-κB (a key activator of proinflammatory cytokines)	Blocks IL-1 and TNF-α production by antigen-presenting cells, blocks up-regulation of the MHC, inhibits production of interferon-γ by T cells and lysosomal enzymes and migration by polymorphonuclear cells	Osteonecrosis, osteoporosis, growth suppression, glucose intolerance, hypertension, central nervous system effects
Macrolide inhibitors			
Sirolimus (rapamycin)	Binds to FK-binding protein, impairs signal transduction by the IL-2 receptor, and arrests the cell cycle of lymphocytes	Interrupts T-cell activation pathway	Hypertriglyceridemia, bone marrow suppression

IL-2, interleukin-2; TGF-β, transforming growth factor-β; IMP, inosine monophosphate; AMP, adenosine monophosphate; GMP, guanosine monophosphate; GTP, guanosine triphosphate; dGTP, deoxyguanosine triphosphate; TNF-α, tumor necrosis factor-α; MHC, major histocompatibility complex.

monophosphate and guanosine monophosphate (GMP), which depletes the cell of adenosine. The effects of azathioprine are nonspecific, and it acts not only on dividing T cells but on all rapidly dividing cells. The primary toxic effect is on the bone marrow, gut, and liver cells. Azathioprine is ineffective as a single agent and cannot be used as a rescue agent. It has been used for maintenance when it is given in combination with steroids and a calcineurin inhibitor.

Mycophenolate mofetil

Mycophenolate mofetil (MMF), which was approved for use after allograft transplantation in 1995, acts through noncompetitive, reversible inhibition of IMP dehydrogenase.[49] This modification improves the bioavailability of mycophenolic acid. Physiologic purine metabolism requires that GMP be synthesized for the subsequent production of guanosine triphosphate (GTP) and deoxyguanosine triphosphate (dGTP). GTP is required for RNA synthesis and dGTP for DNA synthesis. GMP is formed from IMP by IMP dehydrogenase. MMF prevents a critical step in both RNA and DNA synthesis. However, MMF does not affect the "salvage pathway" for GMP production that is present in most cells. This pathway is not present in lymphocytes, and MMF exploits this difference and spares most other cells in the body, including neutrophils. MMF blocks the proliferative response in both T and B cells, inhibits antibody formation, and prevents clonal expansion of cytotoxic T cells.

MMF decreases biopsy-proven rejection and the need for antilymphocyte agents in rescue therapy compared with azathioprine.[50–52] MMF has replaced azathioprine in clinical transplantation. However, MMF cannot be used as a sole immunosuppressive agent and must be paired with either steroids or, more commonly, calcineurin inhibitors (tacrolimus and cyclosporine).

Calcineurin inhibitors

Cyclosporine

Cyclosporine is a cyclic endecapeptide that was isolated from the fungus *Tolypocladium inflatum gams* in 1972.[53,54] This drug acts as a T-cell-specific immunosuppressant, and its mechanism of action is primarily through its ability to bind to the cytoplasmic protein cyclophilin.[53] The cyclosporine–cyclophilin complex forms a high-affinity bond with calcineurin–almodulin complex and blocks the calcium-dependent phosphorylation and activation of NF-AT. The interference with NF-AT prevents the subsequent transcription of the gene encoding IL-2. This process also interrupts other genes critical for T-cell activation. In addition, cyclosporine increases transforming growth factor-β transcription, which appears to down-regulate T-cell activation further, decrease blood flow to the area, and activate pathways critical to wound healing.[54,55]

The effect of cyclosporine is reversible because it blocks TCR signal transduction but does not inhibit costimulatory signals.[56] If the drug is withdrawn, the T cell is not anergic but is again capable of mounting an attack on its target. The effects of cyclosporine can be overcome with the exogenous administration of IL-2. This may explain why cyclosporine is not effective once rejection is ongoing; it is only useful as a maintenance agent and is ineffective as a rescue agent.

Cyclosporine also has significant toxicity associated with its administration. It has significant vasoconstrictor effect (mediated by transforming growth factor-β) on the proximal renal arterioles and this decreases renal blood flow by 30%. Its effects on the kidney can promote fibrosis and hyperkalemia and may interfere with the resolution of acute tubular necrosis. The drug also has neurologic side-effects, such as tremors, paresthesias, headache, depression, confusion, and seizures. It may also cause hypertrichosis and gingival hyperplasia. The use of cyclosporine in solid-organ transplantation protocols has largely been replaced by tacrolimus.

Tacrolimus

Tacrolimus (FK506), a macrolide produced by *Streptomyces tsukubaensis*, was discovered in 1986. Tacrolimus, like cyclosporine, blocks the effects of NF-AT, prevents cytokine transcription, and arrests T-cell activation. The intracellular target is an immunophilin protein distinct from cyclophilin known as FK-binding protein.[56,57] The effect is additive to that of cyclosporine, and these drugs cannot be given together because of the prohibitive toxicity. Tacrolimus also increases the transcription of transforming growth factor-β and thus shares both the beneficial and toxic effects seen in the administration of cyclosporine. It is, however, 100 times more potent in its inhibition of the production of IL-2 and interferon-γ. The renal side-effects are similar to those with cyclosporine. It has more pronounced neurologic side-effects and a diabetogenic effect. The cosmetic side-effects are less than those with cyclosporine. This drug has been proved to be effective as a maintenance drug for both liver and kidney transplantation. It has only minimal use as a rescue agent.[58]

A topical preparation of tacrolimus has recently been developed and approved for use in atopic dermatitis. Its mechanism of action and local route of administration render it an attractive therapeutic alternative for the treatment of various autoimmune dermatologic conditions and could be of potential use in CTA. It has also been widely used in clinical hand and face transplant immunosuppressive protocols for both maintenance and treatment of rejection.[5] There has also been some evidence that it can be used in graft-versus-host disease (GvHD).[59] The mechanism by which topical tacrolimus may be effective in GvHD is the suppression of local cytokine secretion such as IL-2, interferon-gamma, and TNF-α in the skin.[60] The only adverse events reported in its dermatologic applications have been local irritation, pruritius, erythema, and burning.[61,62] The majority of these symptoms are reported to occur when initiating treatment and systemic effects have not been observed.

Rapamycin

Rapamycin is a macrolide antibiotic derived from *Streptomyces hygroscopicus* and is structurally similar to tacrolimus.[63,64] However, they antagonize each other's biologic activity. Both of the drugs bind to the same FK-binding protein, but rapamycin does not affect the calcineurin activity.[65,66] Instead, the interaction of rapamycin and FK-binding protein complex impairs signal transduction by the IL-2 receptor through its interaction with a cytoplasmic protein (RAFT-1). In doing so, the p70 S6 kinase cascade is interrupted and T cells are prevented from entering into the S phase of cell division.[67] Thus, rapamycin is able to interrupt T-cell activation and proliferation, even in the presence of IL-2.[68] Other receptors that are affected are IL-4, IL-6, and platelet-derived growth factor.

Rapamycin has been shown to prolong allograft survival in multiple animal models and is being used in several drug clinical regimens.[69] The drug is most commonly used after the peritransplant period to replace tacrolimus.[70] It has also been applied to the experimental human hand transplantation patients who have experienced renal toxicity secondary to tacrolimus.[71] This drug has little to no nephrotoxicity. It does, however, demonstrate some bone marrow toxicity and has been observed to cause hypertriglyceridemia. Finally, it appears to interrupt the process of wound healing and caution should be applied before using it immediately after surgery.

Antilymphocyte preparations

Antilymphocyte/antithymocyte globulin

Antilymphocyte globulin (ATG) is produced by inoculation of heterologous species with human lymphocytes, collection of the plasma, and then purification of the IgG fraction. The result is a polyclonal antibody preparation that contains antibodies against many of the antigens on human lymphocytes. When thymocytes are used as the inoculum instead of lymphocytes, the product is known as ATG. The most common ones employed in transplantation are made in the horse (ATGAM, Pharmacia & Upjohn, Kalamazoo, MI) and in the rabbit (ATG (Thymoglobulin), SangStat Medical, Fremont, CA).

The mechanism behind the effectiveness of these drugs is through the coating of the T cells by the antibodies.[72,73] These coated T cells are then eliminated by complement-mediated lysis and opsonin-induced phagocytosis. The mere presence of the antibodies on the surface of the T cell reduces its ability to express an effective TCR signal. The overall impact of the antibodies is functionally to remove the primary effector cells required for acute rejection after transplantation.

These drugs have been employed as induction agents at the time of transplantation to reduce the possibility that T-cell-mediated antigen recognition will occur when the graft is in its most vulnerable state. These drugs are also used as rescue agents, and their effectiveness is based solely on their ability to destroy cytotoxic T cells. Most of the side-effects are due to the drug's heterologous origin and the fact that it can also bind to other cells. Therefore, one can observe thrombocytopenia, anemia, and leukopenia. The most common reaction is a cytokine release syndrome. Chills and fevers occur in up to 20% of patients. A rash consisting of raised erythematous wheals on the trunk and neck is seen in 15% of patients. The use of antilymphocyte drugs has been associated with the reactivation of viral disease.

The extent of peripheral lymphocyte depletion in the blood appears to be dose-dependent. Although these agents preferentially bind to T cells, they may also bind to B cells, dendritic cells, and other nonlymphoid cell lines, especially at high doses. In fact, two pilot studies have demonstrated that high-dose ATG induction can facilitate monotherapy maintenance immunosuppression in selected patients, with graft and patient survival comparable to the current standard.[74,75] Treatment with ATG has been shown to be associated with both short- and long-term changes in T-cell populations, generating altered homeostasis characterized by expansion of specific T-cell subsets that have been shown to exhibit regulatory suppressor functions. The use of ATG induction has been demonstrated to result in a lower incidence of acute rejection and improved graft survival during the first year after transplantation. However, as has been observed with most induction agents, patient and graft survival after 20-year follow-up were not affected.[76]

OKT3

This is a murine monoclonal antibody that is directed against the signal transduction subunit on human T cells (CD3). OKT3 is thought to bind to the CD3 subunit found on all mature T cells and results in the internalization of the receptor, thus preventing antigen recognition and TCR signal transduction.[77,78] In addition, T-cell opsonization and clearance by the reticuloendothelial system occur. After the administration of OKT3, there is a rapid decrease in the circulating CD3+ T cells. There is little or no effect on those cells in the spleen and lymph nodes or thymus. After several days, there is a return to T cells that are CD4+ and CD8+ but that do not express CD3. These "blind" T cells remain incapable of binding to antigen and interfere with the process of antigen recognition and generation of cytotoxic T cells. Finally, OKT3 blocks the cytotoxic activity of already activated T cells by an inappropriate degranulation when the CD3 is bound by OKT3. This mechanism is central to its effectiveness but also to one of its most significant side-effects.

The administration of OKT3 can lead to a profound systemic cytokine response that can result in hypotension, pulmonary edema, and a fatal cardiac myodepression. In about 2% of patients, this syndrome is manifested as an aseptic meningeal inflammation. Methylprednisolone must be administered before the delivery of OKT3 to blunt this adverse reaction. This syndrome abates with subsequent doses. OKT3 has been used as a rescue agent to treat acute renal allograft rejection. OKT3 has also been employed as an induction agent. The drug is superior to steroids in halting ongoing rejection. However, it has also been shown to cause a high viral reactivation rate for cytomegalovirus, Epstein–Barr virus, and other viruses. It has been associated with high rates of posttransplantation lymphoproliferative disease. Due to its association with these significant complications, its use is far more limited now. This is especially true after the release of newer induction agents such as alemtuzumab and maintenance drugs such as rapamycin.

Anti-IL-2

Two monoclonal antibodies have become available for use in renal transplantation and have also been employed in some hand transplantations. Both of these agents (daclizumab and basiliximab) are directed against CD25, the high-affinity chain of IL-2 receptor.[79,80] These agents were designed to have the same indications for treatment as ATG and OKT3, without the significant side-effects of those agents.

The high-affinity chain on the IL-2 receptor is required for T-cell expansion and targeting. This receptor offers the advantage that the CD25 receptor is present only on those active T cells. Theoretically, this agent should affect only those cells that have been activated against a new allograft. This agent is also useful in that it does not lead to the activation of the T cell and therefore potential cytokine release, as is seen with OKT3. These agents have also had several of the murine portions of the molecule replaced with human IgG, thus eliminating much of the nonspecific reactions observed in the heterogeneous antibodies. These agents can be used in the induction phase, but because IL-2 is needed only in the initial activation of T cells, it does not appear to be useful to stop ongoing rejection. Early studies of use as induction agents demonstrated a lower incidence of acute rejection but no long-term graft prolongation in both cardiac and renal allografts.[81]

Currently it is used as induction therapy with two doses (day 0 and day 4) as part of double- or triple-immunotherapy regimens in adult renal transplant recipients and appears to reduce acute rejection episodes without increasing the incidence of biopsy-proven acute rejection than alemtuzumab induction. Basiliximab is generally associated with a tolerability profile that is similar to that reported with placebo, and better than that reported with ATG.[82] The drug does appear to allow for reduced dosage of corticosteroids or calcineurin inhibitors, while maintaining adequate immunosuppression, thereby reducing the potential for adverse effects associated with these co-administered agents. However, its use as an induction agent is usualy limited to those patients who cannot tolerate either alemtuzumab or ATG.

Alemtuzumab

Alemtuzumab is an anti-CD52 antibody that has enjoyed increased use in solid-organ transplantation as a lympho-depleting induction agent. CD52 is expressed on most T and B lymphocytes, NK cells, and monocytes.

Alemtuzumab profoundly depletes T cells from peripheral blood for several months with a somewhat reduced effect on B cells, NK cells, and monocytes (in descending order).[83–87] It has very minimal effect on CD34+ hematopoietic stem cells. The initial enthusiasm for its application in solid-organ transplantation was based on research by Calne *et al.*, where 33 kidney recipients were treated with alemtuzumab in combination with low-dose cyclosporine. These patients were then compared to the unit's historical control of patient on standard triple therapy.[88,89] The 5-year survival of these two groups was similar and this finding led to the initial suggestion that the use of this agent could lead to "prope" tolerance (graft acceptance with reduced immunosuppression).[89] However, later attempts to use the drug alone or in combination with deoxyspergualin led to 100% acute rejection, demonstrating that the drug itself was not tolerogenic. This may be due to the lack of CD52 expression on plasma cells and poor effect on memory T cells. Alemtuzumab combined with a single agent for maintenance (low-dose calcineurin inhibitors) demonstrated safety and efficacy, but has an unacceptably high rate (28%) of early cellular and humoral acute rejection. The drug is currently used as an induction agent with tacrolimus and MMF. Several groups have used it as their induction agent of choice in clinical hand transplants.

Immunologic tolerance

The ultimate goal of transplantation science is to make genetically disparate organs or tissues be accepted and regarded as self. This would make chronic immunosuppression obsolete and allow the recipient to maintain an intact immune system to protect against infections and malignant neoplasms. As true immunologic tolerance would be "functionally complete," the life expectancy of the organ would not be limited by chronic rejection. This section provides an overview of the various mechanisms of T- and B-cell tolerance and what is known about their role in models of transplant tolerance.

In the transplantation setting, it appears that T-cell-dependent immune responses are regarded as the primary cause of graft rejection. Thus, T-cell tolerance is important to the generation of tolerance to organ allografts. Mechanisms of T- and B-cell tolerance can be divided into three broad categories: clonal deletion, anergy, and suppression. Clonal deletion is the process whereby T cells with particular antigen specificity are eliminated from the repertoire. Anergy is a state in which T cells can recognize a foreign antigen but are functionally inactive and do not generate an immune response. Suppression implies the presence of cells that are capable of actively preventing other T cells from generating a response. The current thought on the mechanism of suppression is based, in part, on direct action of T-regulatory cells (T regs). These mechanisms are not mutually exclusive, and the establishment of tolerance may depend on more than one of these pathways. The application of these mechanisms for the induction of tolerance could offer the future plastic and reconstructive surgeon the transplantation of foreign tissues without the need for prolonged immunosuppression.

Clonal deletion

Clonal deletion is the process in which T cells that express a TCR specific for a certain antigen are eliminated. The deletion of these cells can occur in the thymus (central deletion) or extrathymically in the peripheral tissues (peripheral deletion). The thymus is the major site for the generation of immunocompetent T lymphocytes. T-cell progenitors migrate from the bone marrow to the thymus, where they undergo a well-defined pathway of maturation. Once the T cells express their respective TCRs, they then undergo a process of selection. During this process, cells with low-affinity TCRs are not stimulated to progress; this is called positive selection. T cells in the thymus with a high affinity for self antigen are eliminated by a process called negative selection. When this process is complete, the remaining T cells should be able to recognize self and mount a response only when they encounter foreign antigen. Extrathymic clonal deletion has been described in several experimental models using exogenous antigens[90–92] as well as self antigens,[93–95] demonstrating that elimination of self-reactive antigens can occur after maturation in the thymus. This mechanism may ensure tolerance to self antigens not expressed in the thymus. Several strategies attempt to influence this process.

The acceptance or tolerance of one's own tissues first develops *in utero* along with an immunologic ability to recognize foreign tissue. This phenomenon was successfully exploited by Medawar[95a] in his original experiments in which strain-specific neonatal rodents were injected with donor cells and went on to accept skin allografts. The production of the tolerant state in an adult can be achieved experimentally by various methods. A combination of total body irradiation to remove mature recipient T cells followed by donor bone marrow infusion before transplantation induces a state of chimerism. (The term *chimera* is derived from the Greek mythological figure composed of parts from different animals.) The chimeric host then develops an immune system that is tolerant of both donor and self antigens. A further refinement is the use of total lymphoid irradiation; the marrow cavities of long bones are protected during irradiation, thus producing a state of mixed chimerism.[96] These animals have gone on to accept donor hearts and kidney allografts. Another method of achieving transplant tolerance involves intrathymic injection of donor cells. These cells survive in the immunologically "privileged" thymus and cause production of maturing T cells that are tolerant of the donor alloantigen.[97,98] All of these methods take advantage of the central mechanism of tolerance induction and rely on the phenomenon of clonal deletion.

Anergy

For a T cell to become optimally activated, it requires a second, independent costimulatory signal in addition to the primary signal that is generated through contact between the TCR and the MHC. When T cells are stimulated in the absence of these signals, they can become functionally nonresponsive to repeated stimulation with antigen and are termed anergic.[99] Two major costimulatory interactions that take place between a T cell and antigen-presenting cell involve CD28/B7 and CD40L/CD40 pathways.[100,101] There has been considerable interest recently in trying to block these pathways. Anergy is not automatically maintained once it is induced, and the continual presence of antigen has been shown to be required to maintain tolerance.[102,103] Tolerance relying on anergy may also be

a precarious state. It can be broken by infection and inflammation.[104,105]

The blockade of these second signals uses antibodies (CD40, CTLA4) to specific receptors (CD40R, B27) to induce a peripheral form of tolerance. The concept that the presentation of antigen in certain situations could down-regulate the immune system is not new. Before the discovery of these receptors, previous investigators had noted that donor-specific blood transfusions appeared to increase graft survival, theoretically by presenting MHC antigens in a limited fashion and inducing a state of T-cell anergy rather than activation.[106] The interruption of the CD40 and CD28 pathways (costimulatory blockade) at the time of transplantation has been demonstrated to induce a state of tolerance in several rodent models without any significant infectious or malignant complications. However, the application to the primate model has not replicated these results and has demonstrated only prolongation of allograft survival rather than tolerance. Several modifications of this technique are under study and may lead to a longer-lasting state of donor-specific T-cell anergy. Other methods of peripheral tolerance induction include donor antigen-presenting cell depletion or modification and anti-CD4 antibody to block T_H-cell function.[107] These peripheral methods of tolerance induction have not been as effective as the central mechanisms.

Immune regulation by regulatory cells

A role for active suppression in inducing and maintaining tolerance had been suggested by a number of studies. However, previously there had been an inability to propagate these cells *in vitro* or to identify these cells *in vivo*. This made it difficult to identify the mechanism involved. Thus, the mechanism of suppression remained controversial, despite a number of transplantation models that provided functional evidence for the existence of such cells.[108–110] Significant progress has been achieved in the characterization of these suppressor/regulatory cells with the identification of a T-cell population that coexpresses CD4 and CD25 surface antigens.[111]

These CD4+ CD25+ T cells occur naturally in the thymus and represent a functionally distinct subpopulation of T cells. These cells have been characterized as a suppressive T-cell population that promotes tolerance to self and foreign antigens.[112] In 2003, three independent groups showed that Forkhead box protein 3 (Foxp3), a nuclear transcription factor defective in the multisystemic autoimmune disease IPEX (immune dysregulation, polyendocrinopathy, enteropathy, X-linked syndrome),[113] was expressed in CD4+ CD25+ T regs.[17–19] Foxp3 was shown to correlate with suppressive activity and appears to regulate the expression of several cell surface molecules previously used to identify T regs, such as CTLA-4, GITR, and CD25 itself.[18]

T regs can also be defined by their origin and are currently divided into two physiologically distinct groups. There are the so-called natural (n) T regs that are thought to be generated intrathymically upon presentation of self antigen by thymic epithelial cells. The other category is the adaptive or induced (i) T regs that appear to be produced in the periphery, after an encounter with either self or foreign antigens. Several groups have confirmed that mature animal and human T cells can be converted from CD25– to CD25+ or Foxp3– to Foxp3+ in different experimental settings.[28–32] Although both types of T regs share similarities, nT regs seems to have more stable expression of Foxp3.[33]

An additional finding has been that individual populations of T regs may not only have different origins, but exhibit significant plasticity in the expression of their phenotype (much like T_H cells) depending on the cytokine milieu. Recent rodent data have shown that, after *ex vivo* manipulation of CD4+ CD25+ T regs with either Th1 or Th2 cytokines, the function of the cells can be quite different.[34] In certain circumstances these T regs (CD25+Foxp3+) can not only trigger the expansion of Th17-producing T cells but can also differentiate themselves into Th17 T cells *in vitro* upon stimulation with allogeneic antigen-presenting cells.[35,36,114]

Several articles have reported a high proportion of circulating and intragraft T regs in tolerant/stable patients in renal as well as liver and lung transplantation. In contrast, recipients with chronic rejection had significantly fewer T regs and lower levels of Foxp3 transcripts than clinically tolerant patients and healthy individuals. Mechanistic studies in renal transplant recipients confirmed that donor hyporesponsiveness was abrogated by depletion of CD4+ CD25+ high T cells. Thus, a technique to produce T regs could increase the durability of tolerance and perhaps be employed along with other tolerance induction techniques.

Transplantation in plastic surgery

Skin

Skin autograft

Autologous skin grafts can be of either full or partial thickness. The full-thickness skin graft gives an excellent cosmetic result with limited graft contraction but has the disadvantage of unreliable graft "take." The amount of full-thickness skin graft is also limited by donor site availability. In cases in which large areas are to be covered, split-thickness skin grafting is used and is the most commonly practiced form of tissue transplantation in plastic surgery. It has the advantage of large available donor areas and better graft take but the disadvantage of increased graft contraction. Expansion of the split-thickness skin graft by meshing with expansion ratios from 1:1.5 to 1:9 is both useful and often essential in large burns.

Donor sites for split-thickness skin graft harvest may be limited in patients with extensive burns. This lack of available tissue has spurred the development of alternatives to conventional skin graft. Keratinocytes can be grown in culture with the ability to expand the available tissue 10 000-fold.[115] This technique has been applied in the treatment of large thermal injuries as well as leg ulcers and other benign conditions.[116] The reported disadvantages with cultured keratinocytes are that they are more sensitive to bacterial contamination than are split-thickness grafts, and take has been reported to be poorer in comparison to meshed graft.[117] They also blister spontaneously, are more susceptible to minor trauma, and contract more than split-thickness skin grafts do.[118] These effects are related to a poorly developed dermis–epidermis junction.[119] The lack of a dermal component in these autologous grafts was overcome by a combination of cultured autologous keratinocytes and allogeneic dermis.[120] The technique has had favorable reports in patients with large burns, but the problem of an allogeneic dermis remains. Development of an acellular or "artificial" skin (Integra) consisting of dermal components, collagen, and a glycosaminoglycan overlaid with a sheet of Silastic addressed this antigenic problem.[121] A disadvantage of this approach is the need to skin graft the "dermis" after removal of the outer Silastic dressing. This has been superseded by seeding the graft with keratinocytes at the time of initial application.[122]

A skin substitute containing allogeneic or xenogeneic structural proteins and ground substance seeded with autologous cells has also been described; it is composed of cultured autologous fibroblasts populating the dermis and cultured autologous keratinocytes covering the dermis.[123] These collagen gel dressings share the disadvantage of autologous cell culture in that cells require time in culture for expansion to usable numbers. An acellular dermal allograft available commercially is AlloDerm (LifeCell, Branchburg, NJ). A tissue-engineered living allogeneic dermal construct, Dermagraft (Advanced Tissue Sciences, La Jolla, CA) consists of human neonatal dermal fibroblasts seeded on to a synthetic mesh.[124] It has compared favorably with skin allograft as a temporary cover for severe burn wounds.[125] Another substitute is Graftskin (Organogenesis, Canton, MA), which is composed of a type I bovine collagen matrix seeded with allogeneic human fibroblasts and overlaid with allogeneic human keratinocytes.[126]

Skin allograft

Skin allografts have been found to be beneficial in large burns either in combination with autograft or in isolation.[127–131] Techniques such as use of widely meshed autologous split-thickness skin grafts with a meshed allograft overlay have been shown to have improved healing in comparison to autologous mesh alone. The availability of skin allografts has increased with the formation of regional tissue banks. Allogeneic skin may be frozen and banked in a manner that allows it to remain viable for a protracted period. Preservation with glycerol reduces the antigenicity of skin allografts and prolongs their survival.[132] Glycerol-treated grafts have been used in burn centers as coverage for burn wounds before autografting[133] or as composite grafts overlying widely meshed autografts.[129] However, the use of these grafts has been reported to lead to the production of antibodies that may inhibit the possibility of future CTA.

Factors that limit widespread use are that harvesting and banking services are not uniformly available, demand outstrips supply, and there is a small but significant risk of disease transmission. Cytomegalovirus infection, hepatitis, and human immunodeficiency virus infection have been reported in burn patients after cadaveric skin use.[134] Cultured allogeneic keratinocytes have also been used as a temporary covering and will survive with immunosuppressive drugs.[135] Growth in culture is possible pre-emptively in burn treatment, but skin allografts are susceptible to rejection in addition to the problems associated with cultured autografts.

Skin xenograft

Porcine xenograft has been used as a temporary dressing in large burns with seeding of autologous grafts beneath it.[136] The application of xenogeneic dermis has also been found valuable in preparing a wound for subsequent grafting by stimulation of granulation tissue formation. The acellular artificial skin described by Burke et al.[121] uses a bovine collagen dermis that recipient fibroblasts repopulate. Xenogeneic tissue has limited uses in skin grafting because its cellular components are susceptible to hyperacute rejection.

Bone

Bone autograft

A series of basic histologic events follows transplantation of a bone autograft.[137] After transplantation, the graft is surrounded by hematoma; the inflammatory cascade follows in which infiltration of inflammatory cells is followed by ingrowth of new vessels with removal and replacement of any dead or necrotic tissue. Nonvascularized grafts undergo necrosis, most of the osteocytes in the graft die, and only those on the surface that re-establish blood supply survive. The remainder of the graft is infiltrated by blood vessels from the recipient site and is repopulated by recipient osteocyte mesenchymal stem cells. Vascular ingrowth in cortical bone occurs through pre-existing haversian canals. There is an initial increase in osteoclast resorption activity, which increases the porosity and decreases the strength of the graft. Cancellous grafts are more rapidly revascularized by virtue of their open structure within 2–3 days. By comparison, revascularization of cortical grafts may take up to 2 months. The process in which vascular tissue invades the graft, bringing with it osteoblasts that deposit new bone, has been termed creeping substitution. Cortical bone shows incomplete resorption of necrotic bone, and the final graft mixture of living and dead bone does not approach the strength of a cancellous graft.[137] Vascularized bone graft obviates the reparative phase of a nonvascularized graft and does not require a well-vascularized recipient bed. Biomechanically, vascularized bone grafts are superior to nonvascularized grafts.[138]

Reconstruction of larger bone defects is limited by available autologous donor sites. An alternative being investigated experimentally is that of autologous osteocytes expanded in culture and grown in the recipient on polymer scaffolds.[29,139]

Bone allograft

The advent of well-organized tissue banks and improved methods of bone graft sterilization and preservation have allowed the clinical use of large bone allografts.[140–143] The use of frozen bone allograft has become a common practice for the reconstruction of long-bone defects, with an estimated annual volume of more than 200 000 procedures in the US.[144] MacKewen is credited with the first clinical use of allograft bone in 1881, followed by Lexer, Parrish, and others.[137,144a,145–147] Few if any of the donor cells in the nonvascularized bone graft survive. The bone remaining acts as scaffold for ingrowth of recipient mesenchymal stem cells (osteocyte precursors) that repopulate the donor scaffold by creeping substitution. The larger graft acts as a mechanical spacer; because of slow union, long-term fixation is required, and as a result, the graft is susceptible to stress fracture and loosening of metal fixation devices. Large joint replacement has been in clinical practice for some time with mixed results. Parrish reported 50% collapse with use of frozen whole bone ends in 21 cases.[146] Mixed results with use of large or smaller shell grafts for joint resurfacing or replacement after surgical excision have been reported.[148–150] In craniofacial surgery, freeze-dried bone allografts have been used in midface advancements.[151] The infection rate was high, at 22%, but osteotomies healed in all patients. Bone allograft with autogenous bone chips has been reported in mandibular reconstruction.[152,153] In hand surgery, bone allograft has been used to reconstruct defects after benign tumor removal and for traumatic or congenital defects.[154,155] No major complications were reported, such as infections, fractures, or nonunion.

Vascularized allogeneic bone is susceptible to immunologic rejection.[156–159] The humoral and cellular response generated has a time sequence similar to that generated by any other allogeneic tissue.[10] Although individual bone cells express antigens, the predominant immunogenic cell in a bone allograft is thought to be bone marrow-derived.[145] Removal of marrow as in irradiation or by replacement with recipient marrow has been shown experimentally to prolong allograft survival.[160,161] There has been a limited series of vascularized clinical allogeneic bone transplants (knee transplants) performed first under single-agent (cyclosporine) immunosuppression and later employing triple-drug immunosuppression.[162,163] All of these grafts were lost within the first 56 months, regardless of the immunosuppression chosen. One confounding factor may be the addition of a vascularized skin paddle for immune monitoring that may actually increase the immunogenicity of the transplant.

Cartilage

Autologous cartilage

Cartilage is composed of chondrocytes within lacunae dispersed throughout a water-laden matrix. There are histologically three types: hyaline cartilage, elastic cartilage, and fibrocartilage. The matrix is composed predominantly of proteoglycans and type II collagen. Cartilage has no blood supply and relies on diffusion of nutrients and oxygen through the matrix. Chondrocytes, in contrast to osteocytes, have little reparative ability and heal by forming fibrous scar tissue.[164] The viscoelastic properties of the matrix provide cartilage with a "memory" in that it returns to its original shape after deformation; the variable water content in matrix causes a balanced tension within it and thus maintains its three-dimensional shape.

Cartilage autograft is used regularly for nasal, auricular, craniofacial, and joint surface reconstruction.[165–167] There are limited potential donor sites. Development of experimental tissue-engineering techniques has allowed the expansion of chondrocytes in culture to increase their numbers. These cells are seeded on to biodegradable polymers to form new autologous cartilage.[29,139,168,169] Injectable polymer systems allow delivery of autologous cartilage by needle, transcutaneously, or arthroscopically.[170–172]

Cartilage allograft

Chondrocytes express HLA antigens on their surface and are immunogenic.[148] The matrix is only weakly antigenic.[173] Surgical scoring or dicing with resultant exposure of allogeneic cells has been shown to hasten reabsorption of allogeneic cartilage.[174] Cartilage allografts have been used for applications similar to those of autologous cartilage.[175] Allogeneic cartilage can be either preserved or fresh. Preserved cartilage has the advantage of a more abundant supply without the risk of infection that is associated with the use of fresh cartilage.[176–178] Cartilage allograft, usually with irradiation pretreatment, has been used for volume augmentation in the facial skeleton. Despite initial good results in a large number of patients,[178] long-term data suggest a high rate of resorption.[179] Whether this is immunologically based or because preserved grafts tend to contain no viable cells is a matter for debate.[180] It has also been noted that smaller grafts are less susceptible than larger ones to graft volume loss.

Cartilage xenograft

Bovine-derived cartilage xenografts are susceptible to xenogeneic mechanisms of rejection, which results in a generally poorer outcome in comparison to either allogeneic or autogenous cartilage grafts. Attempts to modify these xenogeneic responses by altering the graft's immunologic stereotactic structure have been reported as being beneficial.[181]

Nerve

Nerve autograft

The best clinical outcome after nerve transection is achieved with primary repair. Extensive injuries with a nerve gap require a nerve graft to achieve nerve repair without tension. The nerve graft undergoes the same degenerative process as in the distal recipient nerve after division.[182] What remains of the nerve graft is a myelin sheath with Schwann cells that act as a biologic conduit for the regenerating axons. The most common type of nerve graft is the interfascicular nerve graft, which joins fascicular groups to their distal matching group with an interposition nerve graft.[183] Other types in modern practice are fascicular nerve grafts (limited by matching proximal to distal fascicle) and vascularized nerve grafts, thought theoretically to be of advantage, although not of proven benefit clinically.[184] Other "conduits" have been used as nerve grafts, such[185] as silicone tubes seeded with Schwann cells, autologous vein, freeze-fractured autologous muscle, and pH tubes.[186] Artificial conduits have demonstrated improved outcome when they have been seeded with autologous Schwann cells. None of the conduits to date has been found to be superior to nerve autograft.

Nerve allograft

Nerve autograft has a limited number of donor sites. In large nerve defects, nerve allograft has been used in a small number of patients. Immunologic rejection of nerve allograft can be prevented experimentally with immunosuppressive drugs,[187,188] and immunosuppressed axons will traverse the allogeneic graft in rodents[189,190] and nonhuman primates.[191] Immunosuppression needs to be administered only while the recipient axons traverse the allograft and can then be terminated.[192–194] Mackinnon *et al.* reported a series of 7 patients who underwent nerve allografting in the upper and lower extremities.[185,195] Immunosuppression was stopped 6 months after nerve regeneration across the allografts. All but one patient demonstrated return of motor and sensory functions.

Limb and composite tissues

Microvascular autogenous tissue transfer is a well-established reconstructive modality. Available donor sites limit the autologous transplants of tissue. In addition these donor sites can be associated with potentially significant morbidity. The ability to use allogeneic limb or composite tissues such as skin, subcutaneous tissues, muscle, bone, blood vessel, and nerve would greatly broaden the realm of reconstructive surgery. Extensive skeletal and soft-tissue defects or even whole limbs could then be replaced. However, nonautogenous tissue is susceptible to immunologically mediated rejection with subsequent graft loss, and prolonged immunosuppression is the only way at present to attain long-term allograft survival. To make composite tissue transplantation clinically feasible, consideration should be given to its technical, functional, and immunologic aspects.

Technical considerations

Transplantation of vascularized limb or composite tissues was made possible by the microsurgical techniques first developed by Carrel and Guthrie in 1906.[196,197] Microvascular anastomoses and revascularization have become routine practice in large centers, with success rates in excess of 90%.[198,199] In contrast to acute traumatic cases, such as replantation, allogeneic transplantation has been performed in elective settings after appropriate preparation, such as preoperative angiography and donor selection. The operative techniques are based on the current advances in bone, tendon, and nerve repairs.

Functional considerations

Normal wound healing and bone growth occur in transplanted composite tissue allografts after experimental transplantation in various animal models.[24,200] Return of neuromuscular function has been observed in limb allografts of animals treated with immunosuppression,[201,202] including those in the primates,[203–205] while in clinical hand transplants both motor and sensory recovery have been reported.[5,206,207] Thus, functional recovery after allogeneic transplantation appears to follow the same principles as in nontransplant situations and is influenced by the recipient's age, systemic factors, and associated local injuries.

Immunologic considerations

A limb or composite tissue allograft consists of multiple discrete tissue components, such as skin, subcutaneous tissue, muscle, and bone, and each tissue has been shown to be strongly antigenic.[102] Both animal data and the current clinical human experience have confirmed the need for significant host immunosuppression to prevent allograft rejection. The potential adverse effects of indefinite, multiple-agent immunosuppression are

difficult to justify in the opinions of many for a surgical procedure aimed at improving quality of life.[12,208] This debate over the risk–benefit balance has continued since the first successful human hand transplantation. However, both the proponents and critics of the current transplants agree that significant reduction of host immunosuppression, and particularly tolerance induction to the allografts, would help achieve widespread clinical application of composite tissue allografts.

Experimental limb transplantation

Limb allograft transplantation is possible experimentally with different immunosuppressive regimens **(Table 34.3)**.[200–202,204,209–217] Immune modulation techniques that decrease the antigenicity of specific components of a limb allograft were shown to prolong survival.[161] Although sporadic incidents of tolerance have been reported after cessation of immunosuppressants,[211,218] long-term immunosuppression was generally necessary to prevent allograft rejection. Combination therapy with cyclosporine and MMF was more effective than monotherapy.[219] Although rat models provide important information on limb allograft transplantation, the rodent immune system is fundamentally different from that of the human. A large animal model such as a canine, pig, or primate offers a much closer analogy to the human immune system.

Ustuner *et al.* reported transplantation of a radial forelimb osteomyocutaneous flap between size-matched outbred swine with use of a daily cyclosporine, MMF, and prednisone oral regimen.[218] Of the eight swine, two sustained severe rejection, three demonstrated mild to moderate rejection, and three were free of rejection at the termination of the experiment at 90 days. No drug toxicity was evident in serum hematologic and chemical parameters of immunosuppressed animals. The Louisville group also examined the use of FK506, MMF, and prednisone in the same swine model.[220] Five of nine animals that survived to the study end at 90 days were noted to be free of rejection. However, this combination of immunosuppressants resulted in significant mortality and morbidity, including abscesses, diarrhea, weight loss, and pneumonia.

Lee *et al.* sought to achieve host tolerance to musculoskeletal allografts through matching of the MHC antigens between donor and host swine with only a 12-day

Table 34.3 Experimental limb allograft transplantation

Immunosuppressive agent	Animal model	Survival (days)	Author	Year
6-Mercaptopurine, azathioprine	Dog	18	Goldwyn[214]	1966
Azathioprine, hydrocortisone, antilymphocyte globulin	Dog	112	Lance[216]	1971
6-Mercaptopurine, azathioprine, prednisolone	Rat	–	Doi[212]	1979
Cyclosporine (25 mg/kg/day)	Rat	100	Black[211]	1985
Cyclosporine (8 mg/kg/day)	Rat	>400	Hewitt[272]	1985
Cyclosporine (15 mg/kg/day)	Rabbit	90	Siliski[273]	1984
15-Deoxyspirgualin	Rat	18	Walter[274]	1989
FK506	Rat	50	Kuroki[275]	1989
FK506	Rat	102	Arai[210]	1989
Cyclosporine (10 mg/kg/day)	Rat	14	Lee[10]	1991
Cyclosporine (5–10 mg/kg/day)	Rat	365	Lee[2]	1995
FK506 or cyclosporine	Rat	300	Buttemeyer[3]	1996
Cyclosporine, MMF	Rat	231–257	Benhaim[219]	1996
Cyclosporine, MMF, steroid	Swine	90	Ustuner[218]	1998
FK506, MMF, steroid	Swine	90	Jones[220]	1999
Cyclosporine + MHC match	Swine	175–329	Lee[221]	2001
Cyclosporine, steroid	Primate	304	Daniel[204]	1986
Cyclosporine (20 mg/kg/day)	Primate	296	Stark[87]	1987
Cyclosporine (25 mg/kg/day)	Primate	179	Hovius[205]	1992
FK-506 (0.5–1.0 mg/kg IV)	Primate	177	Barth[224]	2009

MMF, mycophenolate mofetil; MHC, major histocompatibility complex; IV, intravenous.

course of cyclosporine.[221] Allografts from MHC-mismatched donors treated with cyclosporine and allografts from MHC-matched (minor antigen-mismatched) donors not treated with cyclosporine were rejected. However, allografts from MHC-matched donors treated with 12 days of cyclosporine showed no evidence of rejection until sacrifice up to 47 weeks after transplantation. Thus, genetic matching may alleviate the need for immunosuppression after limb transplantation. MHC matching can be extended beyond family members, for example, as the National Bone Marrow Registry exists to match MHC of unrelated individuals.

More recently, Kuo et al. demonstrated that the use of mesenchymal stem cells combined with bone marrow transplantation, irradiation, and short-term immunosuppressant therapy could prolong CTA survival (>200 days) in a swine hind-limb model.[222] The authors suggested that the regulatory activity of the mesenchymal stem cells might be contributing to the prolongation seen in this model.

The primate model offers the closest imitation to human limb transplantation in anatomy and immune system. In the 1980s, four studies of limb allograft transplantation were performed on nonhuman primates.[204,205,217,223] All of the studies involved the transplantation of a hand or neurovascularized portion of a hand with use of high-dose cyclosporine and steroids. Many of the animals suffered multiple infectious complications, with some succumbing to fatal malignant neoplasms resulting from high levels of immunosuppression. Nonetheless, few primates demonstrated prolonged survival of their allografts. These studies confirmed the existing rodent and canine data that cyclosporine monotherapy is ineffective in preventing limb allograft rejection, even at toxic doses. Few allografts survived long enough for functional recovery to be ascertained. More recently, Barth *et al.* performed heterotopic transplants of composite facial subunits consisting of skin, muscle, and bone in mismatched *Cynomolgus* macaques.[224] They attempted to use high-dose tacrolimus monotherapy via continuous intravenous infusion for 28 days, which was then tapered to daily intramuscular doses. They had initially hoped that this limited course of high-dose tacrolimus would lead to tolerance, as had been observed in the swine kidney model. Although this protocol of tacrolimus monotherapy did provide prolonged rejection-free survival of the allografts, it was associated with the development of a high frequency of donor-derived posttransplant lymphoproliferative disorder tumors. No study has been performed in primates with combination immunosuppressant therapy. The application of such a regimen could provide insight into nerve regeneration, bone healing, and ultimate recovery of function.

Hand transplantation

Currently, clinical hand transplantation remains an experimental procedure, and the long-term outcomes of this innovative procedure are still being determined. In the current era of immunosuppression, 70 hand transplantations have been performed on 45 patients.[5,206,207,225–229] The results thus far have demonstrated that hand transplantation is technically feasible and the outcomes are promising, with patients reporting varying degrees of return of function. The support for the application of hand transplantation from hand surgeons has been strongest for those patients who have lost both hands.[12] While most programs continue to perform transplants under their local institutional review board guidelines, several programs have proposed bilateral hand transplantation as the standard for care for bilateral amputation. The support for unilateral transplantation has been much lower from the surgical community. However, patients who have undergone unilateral hand transplants have reported the restoration of self as well as return of function. Thus, while function is a critical outcome for the measurement of success, the restoration of the patient's wellbeing and sense of self must also be considered in the evaluation of hand transplantation.

The major issues in hand transplantation are the need for maintenance immunosuppression and the evaluation of the functional outcomes of the transplants.[230,231] There are well-known risks to the transplant recipient related to the use of chronic immunosuppression. These include complications such as an increased susceptibility to opportunistic infections, renal dysfunction related to the use of calcineurin inhibitor-based medications (tacrolimus and cyclosporine), and an increased incidence of malignancies. In addition, despite the use of modern immunosuppression regimens, the majority of the transplants experience episodes of acute rejection and will likely face chronic rejection. The functional outcomes have been, for the most part, favorable but the current challenge remains to improve nerve recovery and the restoration of function of the intrinsic muscles of the hand.

Immunosuppression and transplant survival

The emergence of hand transplantations and the field of reconstructive transplantation have not corresponded to any recent breakthrough in transplantation immunology. It is clear from the 1-year survival data of such highly antigenic transplants as the lung and intestine that the current potent immunosuppressant drugs can prevent the fulminant rejection of even highly antigenic tissues, as long as sufficiently high doses of different agents are used.[232,233] This has been replicated in the hand transplantation literature as there has been an excellent 1-year survival of the transplants.[5] Thus, the critical issue continues to be how much immunosuppression, and lifelong morbidity, can be justified for a nonlife-saving procedure.

The small number of current hand transplants and the variability in medications employed make it difficult to conclude the superiority of one immunosuppressive regimen over another. This type of conclusive evidence will only be derived from prospective, randomized clinical trials. Therefore, as this technique expands, it will be important to organize multicenter trials to determine the best practice for the use of immunosuppression after hand transplantation.

Currently, the majority of the transplant programs have employed the use of an induction agent such as IL-2 receptor blocker (basiliximab), ATG, or the anti-CD52 monoclonal antibody (alemtuzumab). There appears to be a recent trend towards using more anti-CD52 monoclonal antibody in hand transplant patients.[234] The Louisville group initially used the IL-2 receptor blocker (basiliximab) on its first 2 patients as the sole induction agent but then switched to alemtuzumab on all subsequent patients,[206] while the Lyons group relied solely on ATG on all its patients.[207] More recently, groups at the Johns Hopkins University and the University of Pittsburgh have implemented a program to move beyond the current three-drug regimen. They have employed alemtuzumab induction therapy as an integral part of their "Pittsburgh protocol" that uses donor bone marrow infusion in combination with tacrolimus monotherapy in an attempt to reduce the amount of chronic immunosuppression needed and thereby improve the risk–benefit balance.

The most common maintenance immunosuppressive regimen used in hand transplantation has been a continuous administration of low-dose steroid with tacrolimus, and MMF. However, over time several teams have changed from tacrolimus to sirolimus treatment to avoid the side-effects, such as hyperglycemia or renal insufficiency.[5] In some cases, the teams attempted to decrease the immunosuppressive medications and wean or eliminate steroids from the regimes. However, while such strategies have been successful in the renal transplant literature, in these hand transplants evidence of myointimal hyperplasia has been noted. In addition, one of the hand transplants in Louisville was lost due to what appeared to be chronic rejection after being maintained on reduced immunosuppression protocol.[225,235] Thus, it may not be possible simply to transfer protocols that have demonstrated results in renal transplantation directly to hand transplantation.

Measuring outcomes in hand transplantation

The accurate evaluation of the functional outcome of the hand transplant patient is critical to determining the value of this nonlife-saving transplant. Currently, there is some variation in the tools that are employed to quantify the function of the hand transplant. While the Louisville group has reported much of the functional outcomes in publications based on the Carroll test (a well-validated test that evaluates the patient's ability to perform activities of daily life that involve the upper limb),[236] the International Registry on Hand and

Composite Tissue Transplantation bases its functional outcomes on its own Hand Transplantation Score System (HTSS).[5,206] This evaluates six aspects of the hand transplant: (1) appearance (15 points); (2) sensibility (20 points); (3) motility (20 points); (4) psychological and social acceptance (15 points); (5) daily activities and work status (15 points); and (6) patient satisfaction (15 points). A total result of 81–100 points is graded as an excellent outcome, 61–80 as good, 31–60 as fair, and 0–30 as poor. The University of Pittsburgh bases its evaluation of patients on measurement of active range of motion, passive range of motion, grip strength, pinch strength, and two-point discrimination. They also use the Semmes–Weinstein evaluation to document the sensory return of the transplants. Early results from this group show that all their patients demonstrate sustained improvements in motor function and sensory return correlating with the time after transplantation and level of amputation.

All of the hand transplantation programs have used the Disabilities of the Arm, Shoulder and Hand (DASH) score to evaluate patients posttransplant.[237] The DASH Outcome Measure is a 30-item self-report questionnaire designed to measure physical function and symptoms in people with any of several musculoskeletal disorders of the upper limb. The tool is a single reliable instrument that can be used to assess any or all joints in the upper extremity.

The longest follow-up available is from the second hand transplant performed by the group in Louisville; the patient is now more than 11 years postoperative with a functioning hand. In a recent article, the group in Louisville reported detailed outcomes of the first two American hand transplant recipients at 8 and 6 years posttransplantation.[206,225] Both patients have allograft survival, with improvements in intrinsic muscle activity, total active motion, and return of functional grip, pinch strength, and sensibility. The latest Carroll test scores, which measure patients' ability to perform tasks requiring a combination of mobility, motor function, and sensation, are fair for patient 1 (72/99) and fair for patient 2 (55/99). These Carroll test scores exceed the expected results of 20–30 of 99 that would be achieved with a prosthetic hand. The first patient's Semmes–Weinstein monofilament sensation testing is in the normal range for all fingertips, and the patient has shown improvement in both static two-point discrimination and moving two-point discrimination over previous testing. Touch localization, stereognosis, and temperature and vibration sensation have also returned. The second patient has not demonstrated a similar return of sensation through year 6; however, in 2008, his protective sensation was noted to have returned. In a more recent update they reported the results of their third patient in which they stated the Carroll score was 57 at the yearly checkup. The range of motion with active digital motion was approximately 45% of normal. Sensory evaluation showed advancement of Tinel's sign to fingertips, diminished protective function, and light touch localization in the index, ring, and small fingers only.

The International Registry reported that, based on the HTSS scale, the majority of patients demonstrated good results from the hand transplant procedure.[5] They noted that from a functional point of view there was good recovery in the majority of the transplanted hands. However, the recovery of motor function was limited to the larger muscle groups but they often enabled the patients to perform most daily activities. The level of satisfaction was slightly higher in the bilateral hand-transplanted patients when compared to unilateral patients. All of the patients developed protective sensation (31 patients analyzed with a minimum of 1-year follow-up) and 90% regained tactile sensibility. The time to development of distal sensory and motor recovery was correlated to the level of amputation. It was noted that, the more distal the level of amputation, the faster the recovery of the transplanted hand. This finding has called into question the level at which to offer a hand transplant but currently there are no firm recommendations from any of the active groups.

Several of the groups included in the international registry analysis have also published individual reports. The group from Poland has recently published follow-up on two patients who have undergone successful hand transplantation.[227] The first patient was 3 years out at the time of publication and has demonstrated total active motion of fingers equal to 63% of that of his unaffected hand. His DASH score was reported as 95 and the patient returned to work 20 months after the transplant. The second patient was only 6 months posttransplant and scored 85 points on the DASH questionnaire. The surgeons reported that the Semmes–Weinstein monofilament test had documented 15 mm

two-point discrimination and the transplanted hand grip strength reached 4 kg. This patient had also returned to a full-time job.

The Lyons group documented the late results of their two bilateral hand transplant patients.[207,238] Both patients have recovered pain and cold sensations, without dysesthesia or cold intolerance. The first recipient, 6 years after transplantation when the paper was published, had a Semmes–Weinstein test that demonstrated sensitivity recovery on the right hand using 2.83–3.61 monofilaments and on the left hand using monofilaments between 3.22 and 4.08. The average two-point discrimination test was 6 mm on the right hand and 9 mm on the left hand. In contrast, the second patient's Semmes–Weinstein test demonstrated sensitivity recovery on the right side using 3.22–3.61 monofilaments and on the left side using monofilaments between 3.22 and 3.84. However, muscle strength was diminished in both patients. The first patient had bimanual grip strength of 12 kg and the second patient's grip strength was 4 kg on the right side and 8 kg on the left side.

While the authors from Lyons comment that manual dexterity evaluated using the Minnesota and Caroll test demonstrated a normal capacity of reaching, grasping, moving, positioning, and turning the objects, they did not provide scores for these tests. They did comment that the first recipient continued to have impairment to lateral pinch and bimanual grasp. The patients were, according to the authors, able to perform the majority of daily activities by the first year after transplantation. One of the two patients had returned to work.

Finally, the Innsbruck group has published 8-year follow-up after hand transplantation.[239] One of the most significant findings from this group is that patients can continue to observe improvement of their function and sensation even at year 4 and 5 after transplant. Their first patient demonstrated excellent recovery after bilateral hand transplantation. Eight years after transplantation, hand function in this patient was outstanding. He is able to use his hands symmetrically, performing all activities of daily life. The current DASH score is 34. The second patient was a forearm transplant who has experienced continuous improvement of motor function during the first 3 years and, according to the authors, has satisfactory hand function. The patient noted that the hand function is superior to that he had achieved with myoelectric prostheses. While the patient has noted recovery of hot and cold discrimination (at 6 months after transplantation), his overall sensitivity remains poor with no detectable two-point discrimination. Grip strength measured 6.8 kg on the right side and 5.5 kg on the left side. However, compared with results after hand transplantation, fine motor skills were slightly inferior in our forearm transplant patient. The third patient was still in the process of undergoing intensive outpatient therapy at the time of the publication.

The world experience in hand transplantation demonstrates the clinical utility of this emerging technique. However, there are many questions that are currently unanswered. These questions surround the best use of immunosuppression and immunosuppressive regimens. It highlights the importance for future colorations between centers to address best practice in the immunosuppression regimen. This review also reveals the need for continued collaborations between groups to standardize the way in which functional outcomes are measured so that case outcomes can be compared more easily.

Future of transplantation in plastic surgery

The current strategy for the posttransplant management of composite tissue allograft is to treat them with well-established regimens of immunosuppression used in solid-organ transplantation. The majority of CTA transplant patients have been treated with an induction agent (such as ATG or alemtuzumab) and then maintained with up to three immunosuppressive (tacrolimus, MMF, and steroids) medications. This has led to a high level of success in terms of initial graft survival. It has not prevented episodes of acute rejection. However, in order for the field of reconstructive transplantation to expand its indications beyond the experimental arena, techniques need to be designed either to significantly reduce or eliminate the need for chronic immunosuppression. The future direction of this field is heavily dependent on the development of innovative approaches to the use of immunosuppressive agents and tolerance induction protocols.

Many regard the use of chronic high-dose immunosuppression to achieve transplantation of limb allograft difficult to justify clinically.[240] Development of effective regimens to induce host tolerance without long-term immunosuppression, therefore, is essential to alter the risk–benefit balance. Such regimens may involve site-specific immunosuppression directed at the graft, possible matching of MHC antigens between donor and recipient, monoclonal antibodies that block a particular step in the process of antigen recognition, or exposure to donor antigen with the introduction of hematopoietic stem cells either before or at the time of transplantation to establish a state of mixed chimerism.[241]

T-cell-depleting therapies have been effective at promoting graft acceptance and tolerance in several animal models.[242,243] However, clinical translation of these protocols had not yielded significant progress until the introduction of the anti-CD52 monoclonal antibody, alemtuzumab (Campath-1H). CD52 is expressed on most T and B lymphocytes, NK cells and monocytes, and alemtuzumab rapidly depletes these cells with varying kinetics of repopulation. The initial clinical reports by Calne et al.[88,89] suggested that the use of alemtuzumab in combination with low-dose cyclosporine in kidney transplantation could achieve a state of "prope" tolerance (graft acceptance with reduced immunosuppression). However, the use of alemtuzumab alone or in combination with deoxyspergualin led to 100% acute rejection.[244,245] This demonstrated that alemtuzumab was not in itself tolerogenic. It use as an induction agent has recently been demonstrated to significantly reduce the episodes of biopsy-proven acute rejection (14% versus 26%) when compared against thymoglobulin. However, there was no difference in survival, initial length of stay, and maintenance immunosuppression (including early steroid elimination).[246]

Attempts to use T-cell depletion agents such as alemtuzumab or ATG in the field of CTA have yielded similar results and highlight the need for additional strategies to allow for the reduction of immunosuppression.

Regarding the opportunity to develop innovative treatment protocols, CTA also offers some unique advantages, such as continuous monitoring and adequate biopsy sampling of the graft by simple visual inspection of the skin, allowing for a timely intervention, treatment, and precise adjustments of immunosuppression on an individualized basis. In addition, some CTAs may contain varying amounts of donor bone marrow and a vascularized bone marrow niche, which could serve as a continuous source of donor cells, including bone marrow-derived stem cells. This has been demonstrated in certain experimental animal models to modulate the host immune response favorably. Hence, novel cell-based strategies to minimize immunosuppression or induce immune tolerance are particularly appealing in CTA.

Recently, the group from the University of Pittsburgh has introduced a strategy that takes advantage of the cellular depletion provided by alemtuzumab, combining it with a donor bone marrow cell infusion. This technique has had some reported success with living related kidney transplants; it has also enabled minimization of the maintenance of immunosuppression after liver, pancreas, heart and lung transplantation and even enabled weaning of some patients entirely from long-term immunosuppression. Thus far, they have provided early reports on 8 hand/forearm transplants performed in 5 patients who are under the protocol. Currently, all recipients are maintained on a single immunosuppressive drug (tacrolimus) at low levels and continue to have increased motor and sensory function of their transplanted hands. Despite the combination of alemtuzumab induction and the donor bone marrow cell infusion all of the transplants have experienced at least one episode of acute rejection that required additional treatment. However, acute episodes of skin rejection observed with this protocol were responsive to topical therapy alone in about 50% of cases or short courses of steroids. Both superficial and deep tissue biopsies as well as high-resolution ultrasound did not show any evidence of vascular myointimal proliferation as an indirect sign of chronic rejection. This bone marrow cell-based immunomodulatory protocol has been proven to be well tolerated and efficacious and has allowed hand/forearm transplantation with low-dose tacrolimus monotherapy but does not appear to allow for the complete withdraw of all immunosuppression. Long-term data and follow-up, however, are still needed to confirm these findings.

The use of a single antibody may not have the ability to lead to tolerance to donor antigen. Thus the addition of other monoclonal antibodies such as CD40 ligand may be needed to produce a state of T-cell anergy to these antigens. It has been observed that full activation of T cells requires both cell–cell interaction and simultaneous delivery of costimulatory signals. A T cell that encounters foreign antigen in the absence of necessary cytokines fails to activate, which may lead to a state of tolerance.[247] This mechanism is based on the blockade of CD28/CTLA4-CD80 and the CD40-CD40 ligand (CD154) pathways.[248,249] Several nonhuman primate tolerance models to evaluate the effect of interrupting these critical pathways have demonstrated prolonged survival of renal allografts.[250,251] It remains to be seen whether such strategies could allow limb transplantations to be performed with the ultimate cessation of immunosuppression.

However, it currently appears that T-cell depletion alone (with or without bone marrow) or the reliance of other antibodies is unlikely to lead to tolerance to organ allografts. Regimens that lead to the induction of mixed hematopoietic chimerism, however, have been shown to lead to tolerance to organ allografts in multiple preclinical studies.[96,252–254] The strategy involves the use of bone marrow or stem cells to induce a state of mixed chimerism. Owen observed more than a half-century ago that it is possible to induce tolerance by exposing the donor's bone marrow to the recipient's immune system before its maturity.[255] Such fetal or neonatal induction of tolerance for musculoskeletal allografts has been achieved in experimental swine and rodent models, respectively.[256–258] Successful adaptation of this approach could even have therapeutic potential for congenital conditions. Similar application of mixed chimerism protocols could also lead to tolerance induction in adults.[96,259] Foster *et al.* demonstrated that rodent mixed chimeras would accept syngeneic donor limb allografts.[260] Huang *et al.* have used a minimally toxic protocol to generate mixed chimeras in the miniature swine with *in vitro* donor-specific tolerance while preserving immunocompetence to third-party antigens.[261,262] Employing a similar strategy in the same model, Hettiaratchy *et al.* demonstrated tolerance to the muscle and bone portions of a CTA allografts across a major MHC barrier.[263] In addition, case reports have shown tolerance to a kidney allograft in patients who received a bone marrow transplant from the same donor, sometimes years apart.[264–266] However, the combination of most conditioning regimens combined with the infusion of bone marrow often results in GvHD. The greater the genetic disparity between the bone marrow recipient and the donor, the more likely the recipient will develop GvHD.

These findings led Sachs and colleagues to embark on a clinical trial using this approach to attempt to induce tolerance in patients with end-stage renal disease and advanced multiple myeloma using HLA-identical sibling donors.[267] Six patients received cyclophosphamide, ATG, and thymic irradiation as well as cyclosporine (which was tapered off after 2 months) and subsequently followed by donor leukocyte infusions to improve graft-versus-tumor effects.[268,269] All patients demonstrated initial engraftment of the donor marrow but the donor cell chimerism was lost in all of the patients except 2. These 2 patients converted to full donor chimerism and had to be treated for GvHD. The other 4 patients maintained long-term renal function (up to >9 years) in the absence of immunosuppression. One of the 4 patients did have a single rejection episode that was controlled by the transient use of immunosuppression.

The group recently modified its protocol to address the induction of tolerance in recipient kidneys from HLA-mismatched living donors. To reduce the risk of GvHD they now use an anti-CD2 monoclonal antibody (siplizumab or MEDI-507) for its T-cell depletion rather than ATG. Five patients received cyclophosphamide, MEDI-507, thymic irradiation, and cyclosporine.[270] Occurrences of humoral rejection and engraftment syndrome led to the addition of rituximab and corticosteroids for the last 2 patients.[271] Mixed chimerism was transiently achieved in all patients but donor cells could not be detected after day 21 and GvHD did not develop. One patient lost his kidney graft as a result of an early and irreversible antibody-mediated rejection. In the other 4 patients, immunosuppression was successfully withdrawn during the first year posttransplant and normal renal function has been sustained for more than 3–6 years to date. The mechanisms underlying this operational tolerance are not fully elucidated. This model is also designed for living related transplants and in its current form would not be possible for CTA transplants.

Composite tissue transplantation offers potential solutions for many reconstructive problems, including, but not limited to, limb amputation. Whereas the current hand transplant recipients have demonstrated survival of allografts while receiving chronic immunosuppression, the risk–benefit balance remains precarious for transplantations aimed toward improving the quality of the recipient's life. Successful adaptation of tolerance induction modalities reducing or eliminating the need for chronic immunosuppression may launch another transplantation frontier in reconstructive surgery.

 Access the complete references list online at http://www.expertconsult.com

1. Harrison JH, Merrill JP, Murray JE. Renal homotransplantation in identical twins. *Surg Forum.* 1956;6:432–436.

   This is the senior author's report of his landmark human renal transplant. In addition to a detailed case report, a background discussion of considerations in renal transplantation is offered.

5. Petruzzo P, Lanzetta M, Dubernard JM, et al. The International Registry on Hand and Composite Tissue Transplantation. *Transplantation.* 2010;90:1590–1594.

   Follow-up on all cases recorded in the International Registry on Hand and Composite Tissue Transplantation through July 2010 is included in this publication. Demographics, complications, and outcomes are discussed.

6. Siemionow M, Papay F, Alam D, et al. Near-total human face transplantation for a severely disfigured patient in the USA. *Lancet.* 2009;374:203–209.

   A case of near-total (80%) human facial transplantation is reported with dramatic functional improvements and free from major complications. The authors posit that facial transplantation should be considered as an early reconstructive option for patients with severely disfiguring facial injuries.

7. Lantieri L, Meningaud JP, Grimbert P, et al. Repair of the lower and middle parts of the face by composite tissue allotransplantation in a patient with massive plexiform neurofibroma: a 1-year follow-up study. *Lancet.* 2008;372:639–645.

8. Dubernard JM, Lengele B, Morelon E, et al. Outcomes 18 months after the first human partial face transplantation. *N Engl J Med.* 2007;357:2451–2460.

   The authors performed the first partial human face transplant in 2005. This report reviews the procedure's outcomes from functional, immunologic, and psychosocial perspectives.

61. Guo S, Han Y, Zhang X, et al. Human facial allotransplantation: a 2-year follow-up study. *Lancet.* 2008;372:631–638.

89. Calne R, Friend P, Moffatt S, et al. Prope tolerance, perioperative campath 1H, and low-dose cyclosporin monotherapy in renal allograft recipients. *Lancet.* 1998;351:1701–1702.

252. Kawai T, Poncelet A, Sachs DH, et al. Long-term outcome and alloantibody production in a nonmyeloablative regimen for induction of renal allograft tolerance. *Transplantation*. 1999;68:1767–1775.

266. Sayegh MH, Fine NA, Smith JL, et al. Immunologic tolerance to renal allografts after bone marrow transplants from the same donors. *Ann Intern Med*. 1991;114:954–955.

270. Kawai T, Cosimi AB, Spitzer TR, et al. HLA-mismatched renal transplantation without maintenance immunosuppression. *N Engl J Med*. 2008;358:353–361.

    Five patients with end-stage renal disease were treated with HLA single-haplotype mismatched living related combined bone marrow and kidney transplants. Four of these patients have sustained renal function after complete discontinuation of immunosuppression.

272. Hewitt CW, Black KS, Fraser LA, et al. Composite tissue (limb) allografts in rats. I. Dose-dependent increase in survival with cyclosporine. *Transplantation*. 1985;39:360–364.

273. Siliski JM, Simpkin S, Green CJ. Vascularized whole knee joint allografts in rabbits immunosuppressed with cyclosporin A. *Arch Orthop Trauma Surg*. 1984;103:26–35.

274. Walter P, Menger MD, Thies J, et al. Prolongation of graft survival in allogeneic limb transplantation by 15-deoxyspergualin. *Transplant Proc*. 1989;21:3186.

275. Kuroki H, Ikuta Y, Akiyama M. Experimental studies of vascularized allogeneic limb transplantation in the rat using a new immunosuppressive agent, FK-506: morphological and immunological analysis. *Transplant Proc*. 1989;21:3187–3190.

35

Technology innovation in plastic surgery: A practical guide for the surgeon innovator

Leila Jazayeri and Geoffrey C. Gurtner

SYNOPSIS

- Plastic surgeons have historically been distinguished by their ability to innovate and should continue to maintain this competitive advantage.
- This chapter will familiarize the surgeon-innovator with a systematic approach to innovation. This process includes idea formation, valuation, funding, intellectual property, institutional technology transfer, the FDA regulatory process, and conflicts of interest.
- Negative pressure wound therapy, acellular dermal matrix, and noninvasive body contouring are used to discuss the impact of innovation within plastic and reconstructive surgery.

Introduction

Innovation drives the advancement of medicine. Recent medical innovations, from evidence-based medicine to robotic and endoscopic surgery, have revolutionized the practice of medicine. In the surgical arena, innovation has lead to increasingly effective and less invasive therapies resulting in better patient care.

What separates invention from innovation? Invention is the formulation of new ideas for products or processes, while innovation creates the application of new inventions. In business, invention uses cash to create a product and innovation takes a product and creates cash. In medicine, invention is an attempt to create a solution to a clinical problem and innovation drives the solution to the bedside – analogous to the process by which translational research applies basic science to clinical problems.[1]

Plastic surgeons, by trade, are innovators. We devise innovative solutions to difficult problems. Our competitive advantage lies in innovation. Unlike the neurosurgeon or cardiologist, we do not lay claim to any one part of the body.[2] In the hospital we are called upon for our creative solutions to the neurosurgeon's need for calvarial reconstruction; the cardiac surgeon's need for chest wall reconstruction, and the orthopedic surgeon's need for hardware coverage. Our innovative spirit transcends beyond innovative surgical methods and encompasses innovation of novel technologies as well. Historically, microsurgery, distraction osteogenesis, tissue expansion, endoscopic plastic surgery, liposuction and laser technology have all served as platforms to expanding the scope of our practice, as well as expanding the scope of what we can offer our patients.[3]

The expansive breath of plastic surgery exposes our field to multiple competing subspecialists. Dermatologists, otolaryngologists, ophthalmologists, obstetricians and internists are increasingly involved in aesthetic surgery. Similarly, general surgeons are competing for abdominal wall reconstruction, breast reconstruction, and wound healing. Otolaryngologists compete for head and neck reconstruction. Orthopedic surgeons compete for hand cases. Each of these fields involves important new innovations, and subsequently opportunities for patient care, research, and revenue. Aesthetic surgery is riddled with novel technologies including skin resurfacing techniques, noninvasive body contouring, injectables, and laser therapy. The attractive revenue stream in this cash-based field is obvious and draws in more and more competition. Similarly, abdominal wall reconstruction has been revolutionized by the introduction of new biomaterials. Breast reconstruction is changing with the introduction of new breast implants. The field of wound healing has dramatically changed with negative pressure wound therapy. Head and neck reconstruction has seen the introduction of bioabsorbable plates, screws and alloplastic bone substitutes, while PyroCarbon arthroplasty and artificial nerve conduits continue to expand the offerings of hand surgery. Innovation is the sustainable competitive advantage for plastic surgeons in this competitive clinical reality.

Today, however, the arena of medical innovation is far more complex than it was 50 years ago. There is more scrutiny from the US Food and Drug Administration, an exponential growth in the number of patents filed and more complexity in regulatory pathways for new medical products. In the setting of a healthcare and economic crisis, it is harder to justify increased development expenses with increased competition for limited investment funds. When the surgeon is asked to innovate, he/she also faces a plethora of challenges unique to the surgeon innovator including conflict of interest concerns and navigating within the confines of the intellectual property claims of universities.[4] The challenges faced by today's surgeon innovator are captured well by Machiavelli's *The Prince*: "There's nothing more difficult to plan, nor more dubious of success, nor more dangerous to manage than the creation of a new order of things. Whenever his enemies have the ability to attack the innovator, they will do so with a passion of partisans while others defend him sluggishly so that the innovator and his party are likely to be vulnerable." The enterprise of surgical innovation may receive little support and face many barriers, however it can create new technologies that may revolutionize a field and impact millions of patients. To overcome today's barrier's to surgical innovation, we must create and use a systematic approach to translate ideas based on a human problem into a product that can change clinical practice.[5] This chapter sets out to discuss a systematic approach to surgical innovation and gives a few examples of new technologies in our field.

The idea

Mark Twain said, "The name of the greatest of all inventors is accident." In 1957, Mason Sones accidently injected the right coronary artery with dye, he immediately recognized the problem and pulled the catheter out while the injection of dye continued. He later said, "That day I realized that I had discovered something very important." He then went on to refine the technique that led to coronary angiography. On the other hand, Plato's frequently cited proverb, "necessity in the mother of invention" hints that innovation certainly does not need to rely on an accidental discovery.

Today, there are calculated and systematic innovation paradigms that start with the identification of a clinical problem. The problem should be an unmet clinical need. The scientific knowledge in the arena and the limitations of the current solutions should then be explored. The clinical problem can be taken to the laboratory or into multidisciplinary think boxes where a solution is systematically developed, with the hope of translating it back to the operating room. Robert Frost thought that ideas are feats of association, "Having what is in front of you brings up something in your mind that you almost didn't know you knew." This paradigm of discovery may describe why the majority of surgical devices are rooted in the ideas of observant surgeons. The timeless story of Dr Thomas Fogarty's development of the Fogarty catheter started with a defined clinical problem and was assisted with "feats of association". Fogarty was a scrub technician and witnessed acute limb loss as a result of surgery to remove blood clots. As a medical student of the University of Cincinnati, he started to work on a solution to the clinical problem he had identified years previously. In his garage, he developed a balloon on the tip of a catheter that could be inserted through a small access incision and passed through the artery beyond the blockage. Once past the blockage, the balloon could be inflated and the clot dragged out of the artery. His ability to invent and prototype this novel device was perhaps facilitated by his prior association with surgical tools as a scrub technician. He met much criticism from his mentors but went on to patent the balloon catheter, built the device in his garage, and worked tirelessly to have the catheter adapted by vascular surgeons. The Fogarty catheter has since revolutionized vascular surgery and led to a platform for innovations in minimally invasive techniques.

Whether accidental or systemically created, the idea behind an innovation can lead to the development of two broad categories of innovations: a novel method or a novel device. Because the majority of the chapter discusses medical devices, we will briefly discuss the innovation of novel methods. Delos Cosgrove describes his idea for a novel surgical method: "Several years ago, in preparation to perform aortic valve replacement, I found the ascending aorta entirely calcified and both femoral arteries occluded. Recognizing the danger of cannulating either one of these vessels, I raised the patient's arm to expose the axillary artery, which I used as the cannulation site. The aortic valve replacement was successfully performed."[6] Bruce Lytle expanded this idea and refined the process of cannulating the subclavian artery for this problem. Substantial changes to a surgical intervention are reviewed by the Institutional Review Board (IRB), funded through academic sources, and described in new academic publications and presentations. The surgical community generally shares new methods without recovering royalties for the benefit of patients, even though novel surgical methods can be patented if desired.[7]

Determining the value

Value is the subjective relationship between the perceived benefit and perceived cost of a product or service.

$$\text{Value} = \frac{\text{perceived benefit}}{\text{perceived cost}}$$

As physicians, we are constantly assigning value to our therapies as a means of deciding how to provide medical care. We define the value of a given therapeutic intervention as the potential benefit to the patient in relation to the potential risk. Based on the risk–benefit ratio, we decide to precede or abandon a given therapy. Similarly, as surgeons we define the value of a surgical innovation as the potential benefit to the patient in relation to the potential risk. Based on the risk–benefit ratio, we decide to adopt or not adopt an innovation. In today's healthcare arena, before any novel surgical device is even available for use at the patient's bedside,

its commercial value must be demonstrated. The commercial return on a device must outweigh its development risks in order to have a realistic chance of having the device available for patient use. To understand the value of an innovation, it is important to understand the perceived benefit the innovation has on (1) patient care, (2) technology, and (3) commercial impact. We will review some of the terms used to describe an innovation's perceived benefit in these arenas.

The impact an innovation has on *patient care* can be described as revolutionary or incremental. A *revolutionary innovation* has a significant impact on patient care where an *incremental innovation* has a smaller affect. Consider the revolutionary impact of the endograft for repair of abdominal aortic aneurysms (AAA). The technique of using a transfemoral intraluminal graft for repair of AAA was first published by Balko and associates in 1986, the first published human experience was by Parodi in 1991, and the first device manufactured was designed by Harrison M. Lazarus and developed by Endovascular Technologies Company.[8–10] In September 1999, two devices were granted FDA approval for marketing. Now endovascular repair of AAA offers shorter hospital stays, decreased operative mortality and morbidity and an undisputed advantage to patients with multiple or significant comorbidities. On the other hand, consider the reiterations of multiple laparoscopic dissectors. These instruments have been developed in the attempt to improve laparoscopic dissection, but none with a significant impact on patient outcomes or care.

The impact an innovation has on *technology* can be defined as enabling or refining. An *enabling technology* is an innovation that serves as a platform for further developments within a field. In 1976, the Fischers introduced the modern era of liposuction, which is now one of the most commonly performed cosmetic surgery procedures.[11] This innovation has served as a platform for many further developments including ultrasound and power-assisted liposuction. Both ultrasound and power-assisted liposuction represent refining technologies. A *refining technology* is an innovation that marginally improves upon available technology and does not lead to a significant technology change.

Finally, to help describe the *commercial impact* of an innovation, the market-based terms "disruptive technology" and "sustaining technology" are used

Disruptive technology

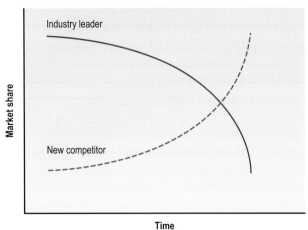

Sustaining technology

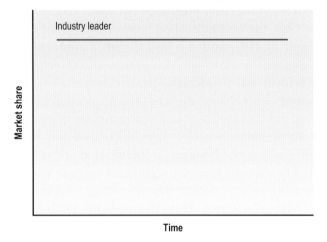

Fig. 35.1 Disruptive versus sustaining technology change.

(Fig. 35.1). A *disruptive technology* is an innovation that supersedes industry leaders and takes over their market share. When disruptive technologies are introduced they are often inferior to the existing leading device and ignored by the incumbent industry leader. In surgery, the device's inferiority is usually secondary to the device's learning curve, lack of safety information, and inferior technology. However, as clinicians learn to use the device, as its safety profile expands and as the technology improves, its market share surpasses that of its leading competitor. The "industry leader" can be applied to the corporation that produces the leading technology, or more broadly the subspecialty that uses the technology. For example, when percutaneous transluminal balloon angioplasty was introduced, its safety profile was not well understood and it was inferior to open coronary artery bypass. Over time, it proved to be a disruptive technology that shifted the market share of patients away from cardiothoracic surgeons (the incumbent industry leaders) to interventional cardiologists. The coronary stent, on the other hand, was a *sustaining technology*. A sustaining technology change is an improvement, usually made by the current industry leader, to maintain growth in the market. The technology can still be enabling (leading to further technology changes) or revolutionary (leading to significant improvements in patient care) but by definition it is not disruptive to market forces. In this case, the coronary stent led to further technologic advancement and improved patient outcomes but did not supersede industrial or clinical leaders. The interventional cardiologist used this technology to maintain their growth in the market.[1]

Generally, the larger the perceived benefit of an innovation, the larger the potential for financial return, however there also tends to be more risk involved in all stages of its development. With a revolutionary innovation, there is significant risk in developing the unproven technology, a riskier FDA approval pathway usually requiring Pre-market Approval, and more resources needed to create a large and experienced development team that can handle the challenges involved in developing a revolutionary technology. A revolutionary innovation, such as the endograft for AAA repair, will also have a large patient impact and large potential market that will justify the increased resources and risk required to develop the device. An incremental innovation, such as the "bullet" endoscopic dissector, has a smaller patient impact and ultimately less potential revenue. To justify its value, there must be less risk and resources involved in its development. Indeed there is less risk in the technologic feasibility of incremental technologies because they generally rely on proven technologies, the FDA regulatory pathway general falls in a "510(k) pathway", with faster approval based on predicate devices, and the development team can be a small group of focused individuals. It is important to understand what general category a new innovation falls in so that the risks and subsequently expected benefits can generally be understood.

Funding

An innovative idea develops from concept, to product, to patient use in a stepwise manner. As each milestone is met, the innovation builds value and reduces risk *(Fig. 35.2)*. Funding throughout this process is acquired based on progress towards building value. The initial smaller investment used to prove the innovative concept is termed *seed money*. This smaller investment is generally $50 000–$500 000 and can come from a variety of sources: Friends and family, angel investors, device company grants, small business innovation research (SBIR) and technology transfer (STTR) grants. Angel investments come from affluent individuals or a group of individuals, often with industry expertise, usually in exchange for ownership equity in the company. Angel investments in 2009 were estimated at $17.6 billion from 259 480 active investors, with a total of 57 225 entrepreneurial ventures receiving angel funding. Healthcare services and medical devices and equipment accounted for 17% of the investments second only to software, which accounted for 19%.[12] Small business technology transfer grants (STTR) reserve a specific percentage of federal R&D funding for partnerships between small businesses and nonprofit research institutions. The idea is to combine the innovative ideas that tend to come out of small businesses or academic centers that lack the means to support serious R&D, with the ability of non-profit research laboratories to develop high-tech innovations. The goal of these partnerships is to transfer the technologies from the laboratory to the marketplace, with small businesses profiting from the commercialization and thus stimulating the US economy. Each year, the Department of Defense, Department of Energy, Department of Health and Human Services, National Aeronautics and Space Administration, and the National Science Foundation are required by STTR to reserve a portion of the R&D funds towards these partnerships.

Larger investments can come from venture or corporate funding. Venture capital funds pool together investments from institutional investors and high net worth individuals. These investors become limited third party investors in the venture fund. The fund then invests in novel technologies that have the potential to generate high commercial returns at the expense of risks too high for the standard capital markets. In exchange for the high risk, venture capital funds buy a significant amount of control and ownership of the company. To ensure realization of the high risk investments, firms look for companies with an innovative technology with the potential for rapid growth with a well-developed business model, impressive management team, and markets valued at greater than $500 million.

Venture capital is offered in stages, the funding stages parallel the growth of the company. As the new enterprise moves from concept, to company, to product, and finally acquisition, buyout or IPO it gains value and sheds risk. Venture capitalists require a detailed analysis of the development pathway with a focus on reducing risk and building value at critical growth milestones. Examples of critical milestones are securing IP, building a working prototype, successful animal testing, FDA approval and first in man use. Paralleling each of these growth milestones are funding benchmarks. The first funding benchmark is the seed stage, as discussed above this can come from friends and family or angel investors. Many venture capital funds may not invest at the seed stage because the risks are very high and the concept has not been fully realized at this point. The second benchmark is known as start-up stage where the venture is ready to launch; these funds are required for company development, marketing, and product development. The third benchmark, which can be further divided into several rounds, is the expansion stage.

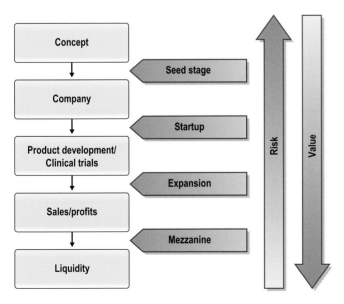

Fig. 35.2 Stages of funding.

Funds here are used for manufacturing, sales, and getting a company to a stage where it starts to turn profits. Often the final financing round is the mezzanine or bridge round which is prior to the final acquisition, buyout, or IPO. In this stage, short-term debt is usually used to support growth opportunities while preparing for an acquisition, a buyout or an IPO.

The first round of external funds is generally called "Series A" and the second round "Series B". The investment vehicle is generally "Series A Preferred Stock" or "Series B Preferred". This is preferred equity share in the company, meaning in exchange for their investment, the VC group will have first right to dividends in the case of success and liquidated assets in the case of failure. The equity share in each round is determined by the value of the company at that stage or the "pre-money valuation" in relation to the investment of the VC firm.

Intellectual property

The US Patent and Trademark Office (USPTO) issues several different types of patent documents covering different types of subject matter. Medical devices are most often protected by *utility patents*. Approximately 90% of the patent documents issued by the PTO in recent years have been utility patents. Utility patents protect any new invention or functional improvements on existing inventions. This can be to a product, machine, a process, a method of making things, or composition of matter. A patent does not grant the *right to use* or sell an invention, rather it grants the *right to exclude* others from making, using, selling, offering for sale, or importing the invention in the United States for up to 20 years from the date of patent application filling. Thus, if an inventor takes a patented laparoscopic grasper and adds a design to make it more ergonomic, and then obtains a new patent on that improvement, he or she can exclude others from using their improvement. However, the new inventor needs the permission of the original laparoscopic grasper, to manufacture theirs.

To be considered for patent, an invention must be novel, unobvious, and useful. To be novel, the invention cannot have been known or used by others or even described in a printed publication. Specifically, a US patent cannot be obtained after 1 year from the time an invention has been revealed through public use or publication. In many countries, the 1 year grace period is not granted. Thus, inventors in the academic environment should obtain intellectual property prior to publishing their work and surgeon inventors should likewise obtain intellectual property prior to public use. The invention must also be unobvious to those involved in the relevant field. Finally, it must be useful, in the case of a surgeon innovator, it must meet a patient or surgeon need.

To make sure an invention or idea is novel, the surgeon innovator can search the literature and the US Patent and Trademark Office database. One can begin by using keyword searches to find a similar device on any publically available search engines.[13,14] Once the closest device or invention is found, the existing patent should be intimately explored to understand which aspects of the innovation are protected and which are not.

There are three main parts of a patent: the figures, the written specifications, and the claims. The patent figures or drawings are required of almost all utility patents. The drawings must show every feature of the invention specified in the claims, and are required by the US patent office rules to be in a particular form. The written specifications are a written description of the invention, how to make it, and how to use it. The USPTO states that the specifications should be, "in such full, clear, concise, and exact terms as to enable any person skilled in the art to which it pertains, or with which it is most nearly connected, to make and use the same, and shall set forth the best mode contemplated by the inventor of carrying out his invention." Finally, the claims section is used to describe the scope of protection the applicant is requesting. This section is critical and forms the bases for litigation and prosecuting infringement. Here, technical language should be used to really define the embodiments of your innovation that differentiate it from inventions that came before. In patent language, prior inventions are referred to as prior art. The claims section really defines the invention. Most patents contain about 10–20 claims, though there are some patents with only one claim and others with hundreds of claims. There are two types of claims: independent claims and dependent claims. Independent claims standalone. Dependent claims, on the other hand, refer to another claim on which it depends, and it has to be read in conjunction with that claim to understand the scope of the claim.

A *full utility patent application* includes the figures, written specifications, and claims as detailed above. Legal counsel, specializing in intellectual property is advisable at this stage, as the surgeon inventor usually does not have the expertise to ensure that the utility patent meets both the inventors and the USPTO's expectations. Since June 8, 1995, the USPTO has offered inventors the option of filing a *provisional patent application* to provide a lower cost ($110–220) first patent filing in the United States. A provisional patent protects an invention in its early stages. This document describes the inventions with relevant drawings, without making any claims. Once it is submitted, the USPTO files the information but does not review it until a full utility patent application is ready for review. The provisional patent is valid for a year while the inventor perfects the invention and the utility patent application. Patentability is then evaluated as though filed on the earlier provisional application filing date, however the 20-year patent term would be measured from the later nonprovisional application filing date.

While a provisional patent offers documented protection of an invention in its early stages, patents in the United States are theoretically issued to the *"First-to-Invent"* as opposed to the *"First-to-File"* approach taken by other countries. It is thus very important to have adequate proof of the date of inventions through a laboratory notebook that is dated, signed, and witnessed on a regular basis. This documentation of an invention can ultimately alter a patent's recipient. A surgeon inventor should thus carefully document all inventions, once an invention is deemed novel, unobvious, and useful; perform an initial patent search and then file a provisional patent. Beyond the provisional patent, additional counsel should be obtained. At an academic institution this counsel can be obtained through the technology licensing office.

Institutional technology transfer

In 1980, the Bayh-Dole Act enabled small businesses as well as public and nonprofit organizations, including universities, to retain intellectual property developed during the pursuit of federally sponsored research and development. Since then, there has been an explosion of new relationships between universities, industry, and the federal government. Research universities have not only developed increasingly close ties to industry, but through licensing and other forms of technology transfer, universities have become an important force in the development of technology which has ultimately contributed significantly to local regional economic development.[15–18] In the last two decades, institutional prestige for research universities has been increasingly defined in terms of commercial success, in addition to academic sciences.[16]

Most universities have created technology-licensing offices (TLO) to manage their patent portfolios. Surgeon innovators should become familiar with the IP policies of their specific institution. Most universities have employee contract that claims IP on any invention created with university resources. Under the Bayh-Dole Act, however, universities are also required to share a portion of new technology revenues with the inventor. The surgeon innovator thus generally begins the process of invention with disclosure of the invention to the TLO. The TLO then evaluates the technology and almost invariably chooses to retain the intellectual property. At this point, depending on the competencies and culture of the TLO, an active or passive role is taken to market a technology to industry and potential developers with the initial goal of understanding the invention's true value. Once the technology and its financial potential are understood, again depending on the culture of the TLO, various steps are taken to develop and license the technology. A fair opportunity to license the technology is generally given to the inventor. There is a huge spectrum of licensing agreements and stipulations that can or cannot be included in a licensing agreement. Some general licensing terms are outlined in *Table 35.1*.

FDA regulatory approval process

In the United States, medical devices are regulated by the Center for Devices and Radiological Health (CDRH), a branch of the FDA. The CDRH is responsible for promoting and protecting the public health by making safe and effective medical devices available in a timely manner. To determine the safety and efficacy of a medical device, the CDRH has developed three

Table 35.1 **Basic licensing terms**

Issue fee	The fee paid to the licensing body for issuance of the license
Exclusivity	A stipulation guaranteeing that no other group may license the technology for the term of the license
Term	The length of a license
Field of use	Granted use of the patent is specific fields, i.e., medical, industrial, educational
Licensed territory	The specific region granted to the licensee
Annual royalty payment	The annual fee for use of the license
Equity	Equity in the licensee company can be granted as part of the payment for a license
Earned royalty	A percentage of the revenues from products that rely on the licensed patent, paid to the licensing body
Sublicensing fee	The fee paid to the licensing body, if the licensee sublicenses

Table 35.2 **Basic licensing terms**

Device classification	FDA regulatory approval process	Examples
Class I	Exemption: subject to general controls	Hand-held surgical instruments
Class II	510(k) premarket notification: demonstrates equivalency to class I or class II devices with existing 510(k) approval	Suture materials
Class III	Pre-market approval (PMA): extensive data with pre-clinical studies and human clinical trials	Breast implants

main approval pathways: Exemption, 510(k) pre-market notification, and pre-market approval application (PMA) *(Table 35.2)*. The approval pathway is determined by the degree of risk associated with the device and the extent to which it poses new safety and efficacy concerns. Devices are also classified according to their perceived risk and the extent of control needed to ensure safety and effectiveness with a 3-tiered system: class I, class II, or class III. Regulatory control increases from class I to class III.

In general, device class loosely correlates with corresponding FDA approval pathways. Most class I devices are exempt from pre-market notification (PMN) or pre-market approval (PMA); most class II devices require pre-market notification 510(k); and most class III devices require pre-market approval. Class I devices are considered the lowest risk devices. They are subject to general controls. General controls are published standards regarding labeling, manufacturing, pre-market surveillance, and reporting. Devices are placed in this class when general controls alone are sufficient to assure safety and efficacy. Examples of class I devices are hand-held surgical instruments. A total of 47% of medical devices fall under this category and 95% of class I devices are exempt from pre-market notification (PMN) and 510(k) FDA approval pathways.[19]

Class II devices are higher-risk devices. General controls alone are insufficient to provide assurance of safety and effectiveness. There is, however, enough information available to ensure safety and efficacy with special controls including performance standards, design controls, and post-market surveillance. Most medical devices are considered class II devices. Examples of class II devices include: powered wheelchairs, surgical drapes, surgical needles and suture material, and some pregnancy-test kits. A total of 43% of medical devices fall under this category. Approval of most class II devices requires pre-market notification 510(k). There are about 60 generic class II devices that are exempt from pre-market notification, as long as they meet the requirements of General Controls and Special Controls.

Class I and II devices that require more than General and Special Controls require pre-market review by the FDA with PMN or 510(k). Under 510(k), a manufacturer must demonstrate that a medical device is substantially equivalent in intended use, technology, safety and efficacy to: (1) a class I or II device with existing 510(k) approval or (2) a device marketed prior to the Medical Device Amendments of 1976, giving it 'grandfather marketing' status. One can search the FDA's 510(k) database for devices already on the market or with grandfather marketing status.[20] Once a PMN is submitted, the FDA has 90 days to respond. If the FDA agrees that the device is "substantially equivalent", the manufacturer can market the device. The FDA, on the other hand, can require further data or determine the device is not substantially equivalent and re-classify the device as a class III device.

Class III devices pose the highest potential risk. These devices usually sustain or support life, are implanted, or present significant risk of illness or injury. Furthermore, they have a new intended use or technology that is not equivalent to a prior device. Given the potential safety concerns of class III devices, general and special controls alone will not provide enough assurance of safety and effectiveness. Examples include implantable pacemakers and breast implants. A total of 10% of medical devices fall under this category and these devices will usually require pre-market approval (PMA) from the FDA before they can be legally marketed. The PMA application is significantly more involved than the 510(k). Pre-market approval requires extensive data with preclinical studies, human clinical trials, and a full description of the device, including the details of manufacturing and labeling. Once a PMA is submitted, the FDA has 180 days to perform a detailed review. The FDA can grant the PMA, require more data, deny the claim, or accept with the requirement of post-market surveillance. Any substantial change to a PMN or PMA device requires new clearance.

Clinical testing of an unapproved device that poses a significant risk, or approved devices used for a purpose distinct from its approved indication, requires FDA approval in the form of an Investigational Device Exemption (IDE). The IDE application includes information of the device and the proposed study protocol.[21] Both IRBs and the FDA can make the determination of whether a device will require an IDE. If an IRB determines that the device's risk is not significant, FDA notification is not required and the IRB will oversee the trials. If the request for determination is initially submitted to the FDA, the result is binding.[21] The applications and approval leading to First Clinical Use are important, because first clinical use is a key milestone for a new device company. In many cases, if a company fails to reach this milestone within a reasonable amount of time, its funding and viability will be threatened. FDA approval to initiate clinical studies in the United States is estimated to take 3–6 months, with review by IRBs adding an additional 3–6 months. Because of this time delay, many companies choose to perform their initial clinical testing outside the United States. When initial clinical testing is performed within the United States,

only about one quarter of the trials are performed at academic institutions, largely attributed to bureaucracy associated with IRBs and contract negotiations at large academic institutions.[22]

Conflict of interest

There is an obvious conflict of interest when a surgeon also becomes an innovator of surgical devices. The surgeon innovator serves to benefit the rewards of both improved patient care and financial gains as the inventor and possible developer of a given innovation. However, to help bring an invention to the bedside, the clinical inventor often becomes integrally involved in designing and developing the innovation, performing the majority of early animal studies, and eventually taking a leadership role and holding an equity position in the company developing the device. These conflicts of interests must be addressed to ensure patient safety.

There is no one comprehensive regulatory process to address all the conflicts of interest present in the process of surgical innovation. However, there are some processes that help assure third party checks and balances in human trials. Studies required for PMA approval are typically large multicenter randomized trials. The study's sponsor typically must utilize a contract research organization (CRO), core laboratories, a data safety monitoring board (DSMB), and an executive committee, to help resolve potential conflicts of interest. The CRO helps recruit, qualify, and audit sites. Core laboratories evaluate primary data in a blinded manner. The DSMB is composed of a group of senior clinical investigators and statisticians with no other involvement in the study. They review the data at specified intervals with a mandate to stop or modify the study if harm to study participants, including an obvious benefit in one arm of the study, becomes evident. Ultimately, it is incumbent on the surgeon innovator to advance the technology they feel may benefit their patients. To do so, he/she should try to separate themselves, as much as feasible, from activities where financial gain will bias objective analysis. To help identify and avoid conflicts of interest, the surgeon innovator should also provide colleagues and patients with full disclosure of industry relationships.

Innovations in plastic surgery

Innovation in plastic surgery continues to advance our field. There is a large list of recent innovations that spans every field within plastic surgery. The impact of the various new technologies is as diverse as the technologies themselves. Negative pressure wound therapy (NPWT) is continuing to emerge as *revolutionary innovation* that introduced a new approach to wound care. Acellular dermal matrix (ACM) is being used in more and more applications within plastic surgery and may become a *disruptive technology* that replaces prior synthetic or living tissue substitutes. Finally, liposuction was an *enabling technology* that served as a platform for further *refining technologies*, including noninvasive body sculpting. This small sampling of recent innovations is discussed below and we briefly touch on the spectrum of their impact on patient care, the market, and further innovation.

Negative pressure wound therapy

In the late 1980s, Drs Louis Argenta, MD and Michael Morykwas, PhD, both professors of plastic surgery at the university of Wake Forest, developed an innovative approach to the treatment of acute and chronic wounds through the use of sub-atmospheric pressure known today as negative pressure wound therapy (NPWT). In 1993, a partnership between KCI and Wake Forest allowed KCI to commercialize what became KCI's proprietary VAC Therapy system. Two years later, the system was approved by the FDA and launched. Then in 2000, KCI received approval for Medicare Part B reimbursement for VAC Therapy, making it available to elderly and disabled homecare patients in the United States. This revolutionary technology has changed the way many acute and chronic wounds are treated. Today KCI's wound VAC has served more than 3 million patients worldwide, in 21 000 hospitals and skilled nursing facilities and 11 000 home health agencies, and now more than 1 million Americans have in-home access to the VAC device.

NPWT, also referred to as vacuum-assisted wound closure, is the wound dressing system that applies continuous intermittent sub-atmospheric pressure to

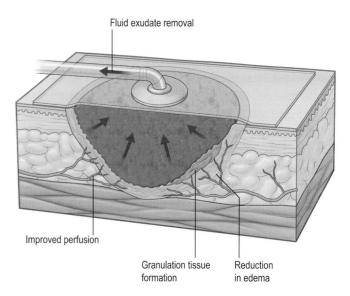

Fluid exudate removal

Improved perfusion

Granulation tissue formation

Reduction in edema

Fig. 35.3 Negative pressure wound therapy.

the surface of a wound *(Fig. 35.3)*. NPWT works through a combination of mechanisms. The closed system reduces wound edema by generating a pressure gradient between the wound and suction canister that promotes fluid transport from the wound bed and interstitial space. By removing this transudative and exudative fluid, NPWT improves oxygenation to cells. NPWT also diminishes mediators of the inflammatory response. In humans, it has been shown to decrease matrix metalloproteinase. MMPs inhibit angiogenesis by generating inhibitors such as angiostatin and endostatin.[23] NPWT is also thought to act via mechanotransduction; the conversion of mechanical stimulus into chemical activity. *In vitro*, the mechanical deformation increases human fibroblast growth and migration and in animal models of wound closure, the mechanical deformation correlates to increased collagen organization and expression of vascular endothelial growth factor and fibroblast growth factor.[24,25] These modifications of a wound's microenvironment make it more conducive to wound healing.

NPWT is being used to treat a spectrum of wounds including acute wounds, diabetic wounds, open abdominal and sternal wounds, pressure ulcers, and in conjunction with grafts and flaps. However, high quality evidence supports its use over conventional techniques, most clearly in the setting of diabetic foots wounds. When compared with wet to dry dressing changes in diabetic foot ulcers, NPWT reduces time to wound closure, length of hospitalization, complication rates, and costs.[26–34]

There are lower levels of evidence to show that NPWT has superior wound healing efficacy when compared with traditional moist saline dressings in the setting of acute wounds, skin grafts and flap fixation, decubitus ulcers, and open abdominal and sternal wounds. In these settings, NPWT meets additional surgeon-user needs and illustrates the importance of need-based innovation in adaptation. In a prospective randomized study of 54 patients with both acute and chronic wounds, NPWT was associated with healthier-appearing wounds and significantly faster reduction of wound surface area, however no significant difference was found in the time needed to reach surgical intervention for healing by tertiary intention.[35] In the traumatic setting, there are observational studies that show its efficacy is comparable, but not superior, to standard dressings changes,[36] however the frequently cited advantages, in the trauma population, are: ease of application, decreased number of dressing changes, and reduction in the complexity of subsequent reconstructive surgery.[37,38] In the treatment of pressure ulcers, no statistically significant differences have been shown in wound surface area, however the cited advantages have been improved patient comfort and less labor intensity.[39,40] In the setting of skin graft fixation, NPWT observational studies and randomized trials have improved skin graft take when compared to bolster dressings, with the additional benefit of ease of application and removal.[41–43]

High-level evidence showing the superiority of NPWT compared with traditional moist saline dressings is still lacking, however it is clear that NPWT meets very specific needs of the surgeon user. NPWT is easy to use; it decreases the number of dressing changes for both the patient and the medical caregiver and ultimately prepares the wound for surgical closure by tertiary intention. By understanding and meeting the needs of the surgical community, the plastic surgeon and engineer that developed NPWT changed the armamentarium of the general surgeon's approach to the open abdomen, the cardiothoracic surgeons' approach to post-sternotomy mediastinitis, the vascular surgeons approach to groin wounds and ultimately, the plastic surgeon's approach to all of these wounds as well as graft and flap reconstruction. NPWT is an example of quick adaptation of a technology developed with the assistance of a surgeon ultimately addressing multiple clinical needs.

Acellular dermal matrix

In recent years, acellular dermal matrix (ADM) is emerging as a *disruptive technology* in both reconstructive and aesthetic surgery. ADM is a dermal graft in which the dermis is separated from the epidermis and all cellular elements, to avoid tissue rejection and graft failure *(Fig. 35.4)*. These bioprosthesis are harvested from human cadavers, porcine or bovine donors. The dermal matrix then acts as a scaffold that permits tissue regeneration with revascularization and repopulation with fibroblasts. The ADM is thought to incorporate into

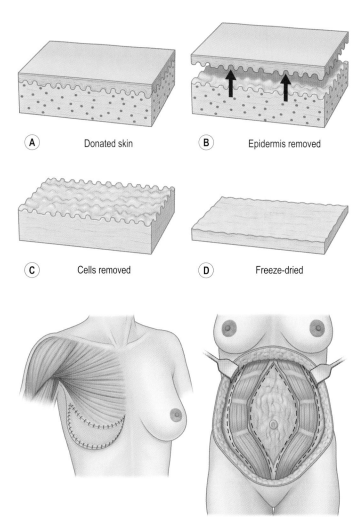

Ⓐ   Donated skin   Ⓑ   Epidermis removed

Ⓒ   Cells removed   Ⓓ   Freeze-dried

Fig. 35.4 Acellular dermal matrix.

surrounding tissue and eventually be replaced with host collagen.[44,45]

Its use has been described in the burn literature for over 20 years; initially as a substitute, and now as a compliment to skin grafting. Beyond the use of ADM as a skin graft, ADM provides a tissue substitute that is pliable, easy to shape and suture, and can be used in the setting of infection. These properties make it a desirable tool in plastic surgery. An early ACM, AlloDerm®, was placed on the market in 1994 and has now been used in over 1 million cases. Recently, innovative plastic surgeons have popularized the use of ACM in implant-based breast reconstruction. ACM is used to provide additional coverage of implant-based reconstructions, support for faster inferior pole expansion, as well as assistance with precise placement of the inframammary fold.[46,47] Overall, studies still conflict on its risk profile for postoperative complications. A retrospective analysis of 415 immediate implant-based breast reconstructions showed that ADM is associated with high rates of postoperative seromas and infection.[48] However, because acellular dermal matrix enhances surgical options in implant-based reconstruction, plastic surgeons have quickly adapted this technology.

Similarly, ADM is largely replacing the use of synthetic meshes in contaminated abdominal wall defects. These bioprosthesis are thought to incorporate into contaminated tissue without becoming infected.[49] This is an important competitive advantage when compared to synthetic mesh, which is contraindicated in this setting. There still remains a question of the longevity of mechanical integrity ACM provides in abdominal wall reconstruction. However, because ACM has met the need for a large fascial substitute that can be used in the setting of a contaminated wound, many plastic surgeons quickly adapted this new technology, despite these unanswered questions. Interestingly, by embracing ACM-based abdominal wall reconstruction, plastic surgeons are expanding their role among general surgeons in this arena.

Like other disruptive technologies, this emerging technology lacks long-term follow-up, familiarity, and a complete safety profile. However, it is a soft tissue substitute that needs not be harvested, thus fills a principle need of the reconstructive surgeon. This technology may thus go on to expand its indications, supersede other synthetic technologies, and replace more invasive reconstructive options of the present.

Noninvasive body contouring

The push towards noninvasive medical interventions is an important force driving the patient–consumer market for medical intervention. At its inception over three decades ago, liposuction itself was a large step in a less invasive form of body contouring compared with traditional surgical approaches. The introduction of liposuction, like other *enabling technologies* served as a platform for the continued introduction of *refining innovations*. The Fischers first introduced sharp suction techniques for fat removal in 1974.[50] Illouz then refined the technique with the introduction of high power negative pressure suction connected to blunt tip cannulas as well as the development of the "wet technique" used for hydro dissection to assist with fat removal.[51] In the 1980s, Dr Jeffrey Klein introduced the tumescent technique that had an important impact on the safety and efficacy of liposuction. The high volumes of diluted

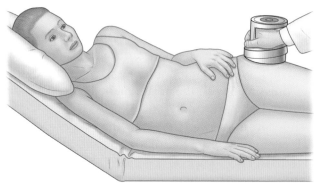

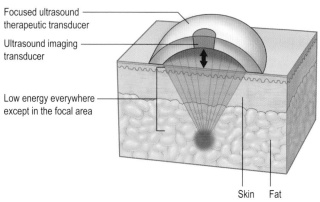

Focused ultrasound
therapeutic transducer

Ultrasound imaging
transducer

Low energy everywhere
except in the focal area

Skin   Fat

Fig. 35.5 Noninvasive body contouring.

lidocaine and epinephrine decreased the need for general anesthesia minimized blood loss.[52]

To address the issues of surgeon fatigue and improved effectiveness, especially in more fibrous areas several *refining innovations* have been introduced, none of which have made a significant change in this field.[53] Ultrasound assisted liposuction was developed by Zocchi in the 1980s. Ultrasonic waves were introduced to rupture adipocytes creating microcavitations of liquefied fat. Controversy exists as to whether UAL reduces complications or improves efficacy when compared with traditional techniques.[54,55] Similarly, power and laser-assisted lipolysis were refinements to traditional liposuction that have not shown significant differences in clinical outcomes.[53] Focused ultrasound body contouring is a recent innovation that introduces a potentially new frontier in body contouring that may or may not prove to be efficacious. This technology uses focused ultrasound energy delivered through a hand-held probe *(Fig. 35.5)*. The ultrasonic waves are focused in the subcutaneous fat, causing permanent disruption of fat cells with the aim of not damaging the epidermis, dermis, or underlying tissues and organs. The disrupted adipocytes are then supposed to be metabolized by the liver. The procedure is a change from prior refinements, as it requires no incisions or injections. This technology is not FDA approved for use in the United States. Small preliminary clinical trials and use outside of the United States have demonstrated safe and effective treatment in small areas.[56–58] Since its inception in the 1970s, liposuction has proven to be an enabling technology that continues to serve as a platform for numerous refining technologies. Noninvasive transdermal focused ultrasound offered by products like LipoSonix and UltraShapr Contour I systems may prove to be another refinement in liposuction technology or new frontier in this field.

 Access the complete references list online at **http://www.expertconsult.com**

1. Riskin DJ, Longaker MT, Gertner M, et al. Innovation in surgery: a historical perspective. *Ann Surg.* 2006;244(5): 686–693.

2. Gurtner GC, Rohrich RJ, Longaker MT. From bedside to bench and back again: technology innovation in plastic surgery. *Plast Reconstr Surg.* 2009;124(4):1355–1356.

    In 2005 Dr Longaker and Dr Rorich highlighted innovation as the competitive advantage of the plastic surgeon. We then expanded on this concept by discussing the adaption of new technologies as an important determinant of the advancement of various fields within surgery.

3. Longaker MT, Rohrich RJ. Innovation: a sustainable competitive advantage for plastic and reconstructive surgery. *Plast Reconstr Surg.* 2005;115(7):2135–2136.

5. Zenios S, Makower J, Yock P, et al. *Biodesign: The Process of Innovating Medical Technologies.* Cambridge, New York: Cambridge Univesity Press; 2010.

    These authors designed their textbook as a template to teach innovation and entrepreneurship. They detail the Biodesign process used by Stanford University's interdisciplinary Biodesign group. This three-phase approach involves identifying a medical need, inventing a device or service, and implementing its use.

6. Cosgrove DM. Developing new technology. *J Thorac Cardiovasc Surg.* 2001;121(suppl 4):S29–S31.

13. United States Patent and Trademark Office Official Site. Available from: www.uspto.gov/patft/index.html.

    Publically available resources for searching patents, free of charge, include the United States Patent and Trademark

Office Official Site. Online. Available at: www.uspto.gov/patft/index.html. Additional resources include, but are not limited to, the searchable databases of all published US patents. Online. Available at: www.freepatentsonline.com and www.google.com/patents

20. U.S. Food and Drug Administration database of devices with existing 510(k) approval. Online. Available at: www.accessdata.fda.gov/scripts/cdrh/cfdocs/cfPMN/pmn.cfm

    The U.S. Food and Drug Administration has an informative and publically available website at: www.fda.gov/MedicalDevices/default.htm. The FDA's 510(k) database is available at: www.accessdata.fda.gov/scripts/cdrh/cfdocs/cfPMN/pmn.cfm

22. Kaplan AV, Baim DS, Smith JJ, et al. Medical device development: from prototype to regulatory approval. *Circulation.* 2004;109(25): 3068–3072.

    Thomas Fogarty's expert opinion is provided in this review of medical device development. The complexity of device approval in the United States is discussed and identified as a delay in the introduction of new devices into clinical practice in contrast to the process in Europe.

46. Spear SL, Parikh PM, Reisin E, et al. Acellular dermis-assisted breast reconstruction. *Aesthetic Plast Surg.* 2008;32(3):418–425.

50. Fischer A, Fischer G. First surgical treatment for molding body's cellulite with three 5-mm incisions. *Bull Int Acad Cosmet Surg.* 1976;3:35.

36

Robotics, simulation, and telemedicine in plastic surgery

Joseph M. Rosen, Todd E. Burdette, Erin Donaldson, Robyn Mosher, Lindsay B. Katona, and Sarah A. Long

SYNOPSIS

- This chapter describes the latest innovations in nonbiological technologies – robotics, simulation, and telemedicine – and their integration into plastic surgery practice.
- Robotics provides plastic surgeons with custom prostheses and robotic limbs, both of which help patients achieve cosmesis and function; it also provides surgical tools that reduce human error and increase surgical visibility, precision, and safety.
- Simulation is used to train plastic surgery residents and fellows in all procedures, and to train senior surgeons on new procedures. Like robotics, simulation provides an increase in safety and reduction in medical errors, since trainees will effectively "make mistakes" on a simulator, rather than on live patients.
- Telemedicine can make use of both robotics and simulation to deliver medical care to a distant population, whether during everyday life, in wartime, or following a disaster.
- This chapter will provide plastic surgeons with a basic understanding of how to apply current technologies to enhance their armamentarium with solutions to clinical and surgical problems.

 Access the Historical Perspective section and Fig. 36.1 online at **http://www.expertconsult.com**

Introduction

Medical technology can help doctors to diagnose, heal, and transcend traditional limitations of the human body, via tools like pacemakers, ventilators, artificial hips, three-dimensional (3D) body imaging, and even robotic arms. Plastic surgery, a specialty that prides itself on approaching complex problems with innovative solutions, has an opportunity to lead the medical community in the responsible and creative use of new technology.

Surgeons can enhance their practice with biological technologies, such as transplantation and tissue engineering, covered in Chapters 13, 19, 32, 34, 35, or with nonbiological technologies. This chapter discusses the latest innovations in nonbiological technologies – robotics, simulation, and telemedicine – and their widespread integration into plastic surgery practice. Plastic surgeons can implant custom prostheses that are fabricated by robots; outfit amputee patients with robotic limbs; and employ surgical robots that reduce human error and increase surgical visibility, precision, and safety. Simulation is used to train plastic surgery residents in common procedures, and to train senior surgeons on new procedures. Like robotics, simulation promotes safety, as trainees will make initial errors on a simulator before operating on live patients. Finally, telemedicine can utilize both robotics and simulation to deliver medical care to a distant population, whether during everyday life, in wartime, or following a disaster.

This chapter will provide plastic surgeons with a basic understanding of how to apply current technologies to enhance their armamentarium with solutions to clinical and surgical problems. Technological tools can resolve needs that are not met with current standards of care (for example, a robotic limb that restores function following an amputation with suboptimal limb salvage). However, it is critical that both outcomes and costs be considered whenever we evaluate new technology; the outcomes should be demonstrable, and the cost–benefit ratio considerable. (See section on robotic surgery: the evidence base for improved outcomes, below, and also Ch. 10.)

Robotics

Introduction

Definition of a robot

1. *A machine that looks like a human being and performs various complex acts … of a human being.*
2. *A device that automatically performs complicated, often repetitive tasks.*
3. *A mechanism guided by automatic controls.*[16]

In the past half-century, robots have evolved from a science fiction concept into a reality. Today, they perform basic operations in daily life (vacuuming homes, assembling cars) and carry out highly specialized tasks (space exploration and repairs, military operations with unmanned recovery of injured victims, and medical drug delivery and surgery).

The role of robotics in plastic surgery: planning and performance

Robots are now used in plastic surgery in three applications, all of which involve planning and performance. First, industrial robots can fabricate medical products using computer-aided design and manufacturing (CAD/CAM),[17] including custom prosthetics for contouring and filling cranial defects. In the future, robots may fabricate an entire prosthetic face. Second, high-end artificial arms and hands[18–25] contain enough intelligence and autonomy to be considered robots themselves. Third, surgical robots are now used in endoscopic and image-guided surgery such as transoral partial glossectomy, and may be adapted for future use in minimally invasive plastics procedures.

The use of robotics in plastic surgery: surgical tools and prosthetics

Surgical robots in the operating room

Robot-assisted surgery is routinely practiced across specialties in the operating rooms of large hospitals and centers of excellence. Intuitive Surgical's da Vinci® system, the first US Food and Drug Administration (FDA)-cleared robotic surgical system, is now cleared for use in cardiac, general, thoracic, urologic, gynecologic, pediatric and transoral otolaryngologic surgery *(Fig. 36.2)*.[26] The US FDA has not cleared the da Vinci system for use in plastic surgery. As this system is cleared for ear, nose, and throat (ENT) surgery, we believe it may have potential future application in plastics procedures. The da Vinci system's tremor filtration feature, for example, would make it very useful in ultra-microsurgery, allowing plastic surgeons to sew together even smaller vessels than we can now achieve. Plastic surgeons have begun preliminary studies to investigate the use of robotic surgery for two techniques. Patel et al. tested robotic rectus abdominus muscle harvest, first on 2 cadavers and then on one 30-year-old woman.[26a] They found the technique possible and said that it may also "provide an approach to minimally invasive transperitoneal reconstruction." Also, Selber tested robotic latissimus dorsi muscle harvest using 10 cadavers, and concluded that, "robotic harvest of the latissimus dorsi muscle is feasible and reproducible. It offers technical advantages over endoscopic harvest and cosmetic advantages over the open technique".[26b]

Design features and usage of robotic surgery

In robotic surgery, the surgeon does not directly manipulate the endoscopic tools, but instead remotely controls a robot that manipulates the tools. In the da Vinci system, the surgeon holds on to a device that mimics his or her hand motions – like a highly precise version of the Wii™ home video game. The da Vinci system provides surgeons with: (1) the range of motion and fine tissue control available in open surgery; (2) many advantages of endoscopic surgery, including small incisions and less blood loss; and (3) improvements, such as tremor filtration, and 3D magnified vision of the operative field via paired stereoscopic robotic eyes. Among

Fig. 36.2 da Vinci Si high-definition robotic surgical system, showing two surgeon consoles, patient cart, and vision cart. (Courtesy of Intuitive Surgical and ©2012 Intuitive Surgical, Inc.)

surgical robots, da Vinci is the market leader, with over 2000 systems installed worldwide.[26]

Another surgical robot system, the ViKY™, is made by EndoControl Medical in France.[27] The ViKY, compared to da Vinci, is "simpler, smaller and specialized" according to its manufacturer's chief executive officer, and costs under $200 000 for four components, including a compact robotic endoscope holder and a uterus manipulator.[28] One surgeon performed a hysterectomy single-handedly, using two ViKY components to control a camera and support the uterus, effectively replacing the function of two surgical assistants.[28] In plastic surgery, a similar application might be a breast reconstruction with a transverse rectus abdominis myocutaneous flap, which uses an assistant. Recently a surgeon used both the da Vinci and ViKY systems in a total laparoscopic hysterectomy and bilateral salpingo-oophorectomy, which required only four incisions.[29]

Advantages and disadvantages of robotic surgery versus endoscopic surgery

Robotic surgery has many benefits, including 3D viewing at high magnification, filtering of involuntary hand tremors, digitized recording, improved surgical ergonomics, and (in the case of da Vinci) miniature articulating instruments with seven degrees of freedom.

(According to da Vinci literature, there are three external degrees of freedom – external yaw, external pitch, and external insertion (moving the instrument up or down along the vertical axis) – and four internal degrees of freedom – internal yaw, internal pitch, roll, and grip.) In contrast, endoscopic surgery suffers from a reduced range of motion, two-dimensional viewing, and the fulcrum effect. These robotic features provide greater precision and dexterity; smaller incisions; easier tissue dissection, suturing and tumor resection; less trauma and blood loss; and improved quality and safety. A robotic blade can be programmed to cut only a certain depth into tissue, and to avoid wrong-side surgery. Thus, robots reduce human error and promote "slower but safer" surgery. Note Isaac Asimov's first law of robotics: "a robot may not harm a human being."[30,31]

Drawbacks of surgical robots include high price and maintenance costs; uncertain outcomes and litigation; and suitability of the systems for surgeons, including training curve and lack of tactile or force feedback (i.e., the surgeon can't feel how deep he or she is penetrating into tissue, or how tight a stitch is).[32–34] Also, surgical robots are designed to work on single small regions, and the current instruments are too large for plastic surgery. As with any new technology, the benefit–risk ratio should improve with time, experience, and new designs.

Future use of surgical robots in plastic surgery

Surgical robots are not often used in plastic surgery, in large part because of their cost. Most plastic surgery is performed in private clinics, few of which can afford a $1.0–2.3 million surgical robot. However, with increasing use, the cost of surgical robots may decrease; vendors may develop robotic instruments at all price levels; and existing systems may be customized and approved for plastic surgery procedures.

The fact that robots save on human labor may be controversial (as was the case when robots replaced workers on assembly lines), but ultimately, such savings might offset and justify the purchase of such robots. Surgical robots are available 24/7; and while they need periodic maintenance, they do not require sleep, food, or vacation. They enhance human abilities: one surgeon likened the da Vinci system to operating with four arms simultaneously.[35]

Robotics in limb and hand surgery

In general, the goal of reconstructive plastic surgery is to maximize both function and cosmesis. Although autologous flaps and grafts are the usual raw materials for these endeavors, robotic parts may sometimes yield better function and cosmesis, while minimizing both convalescence and psychosocial trauma. When salvaging a limb, there may be several expensive operations, after which the patient may be left with a minimally functional limb, multiple donor site morbidities, and months of lost work.[36] Therefore, surgeons may consider robotic parts along with reconstructive options from the beginning of a clinical evaluation to ensure the best outcome.

Robotics as a rung on the reconstructive ladder: upper limb example

Plastic surgeons use the concept of a "reconstructive ladder" to describe surgeries of increasing complexity *(Fig. 36.3)*. For example, following an amputation, autogenous tissue reconstruction progresses from secondary healing and primary closure to skin grafting, local flap coverage, distant flap coverage, and free tissue transfer. A robotic prosthesis can be added at any point in the reconstructive ladder. A limb stump may require

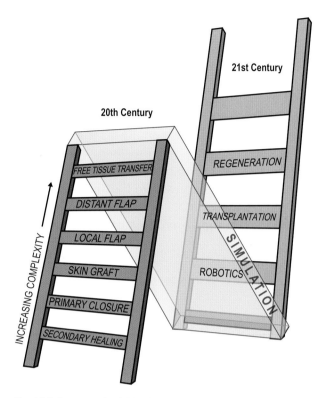

Fig. 36.3 Reconstructive ladder, 21st century. New technologies of robotics, transplantation, and regeneration enhance the reconstructive ladder in the 21st century. Simulation provides the bridge from the 20th-century plastic surgery training and techniques to the 21st-century ones. (Courtesy of Joseph Rosen, MD.)

simple closure or skin grafting for soft-tissue coverage before fitting the patient with a prosthesis. Or the surgeon might perform a free-tissue transfer with vascularized bone for limb lengthening to optimize the final function of a robotic prosthesis.

Current upper extremity prosthetic options

There are seven categories of arm prostheses that vary by complexity and function *(Figs 36.4, 36.5)*:

1. A passive arm prosthesis serves a cosmetic role, and may provide a passive function such as stabilizing, pulling, wedging, and balancing *(Fig. 36.5A)*.

2. A body-powered arm prosthesis has a cable-and-pulley system driven by the patient's muscle movements to provide active grip and release *(Fig. 36.5B,C)*. Body-powered devices can provide elbow control as well.

An externally powered (robotic) arm prosthesis can be one of three types:

3. A robotic/fully myoelectric arm – in this arm, the user contracts muscles in the residual limb, causing surface electromyogram electric signals that are translated into controlled movements of the elbow, wrist, or hand.

4. A robotic arm based on a surgical technique called targeted muscle reinnervation (TMR) is currently the most modern attempt at prosthetic control. Surgeons (plastic, general, or neurological) transplant residual nerves from the amputated arm to alternative muscle sites, which then produce electromyogram signals on the surface of the skin

that can be computer-processed to control prosthetic arms *(Fig. 36.5D)*.[19]

5. A robotic, neurally controlled arm – in this design, the user thinks to initiate movement, as with a biological arm, and the brain's neural signals travel from implants placed in the patient's brain to external computer software that translates them into controlled movements of the elbow, wrist, or hand *(Fig. 36.5E–G)*. This is a future robotic arm design, now in development.

6. A hybrid arm prosthesis typically combines a lightweight, inexpensive, body-powered proximal arm and elbow with distal robotic components for the wrist and hand to articulate and grasp objects precisely *(Fig. 36.5H,I)*. New robotic prostheses can perform advanced, active functions, such as wielding a fishing rod by flexing the arm while rotating the wrist and grasping with the hand. However, robotic prostheses do not replace the need for the sixth category of prosthesis:

7. An "activity-specific" nonrobotic arm can allow the user to hold a guitar pick, release a bowling ball, or participate in sports such as surfing, golf, swimming, and rock climbing *(Fig. 36.5J–L)*. For example, a surfing prosthesis looks like an arm fin, and can be completely submerged in water.

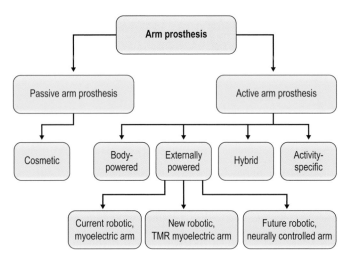

Fig. 36.4 There are seven categories of prostheses that vary by complexity and function. (1) Passive arm prostheses serve a cosmetic role. The 6 types of active arm prostheses include the following: (2) body-powered arm prostheses. (3–5) Externally powered arms, including: (3) current robotic arms with myoelectric control; (4) current robotic arms with targeted muscle reinnervation; (5) future robotic arms with neural control; (6) hybrid arm prostheses, typically combining body-powered and robotic components; and (7) activity-specific arm prostheses. For photos of the prostheses classified here, see Fig. 36.5. (Courtesy of Joseph Rosen, MD and Erin Donaldson, MS.)

Robotic hand prostheses and neural arm–hand prostheses

The current state of the art for robotic hands is the i-LIMB ultra, made by Touch Bionics, a myoelectric prosthetic hand with five individually powered digits

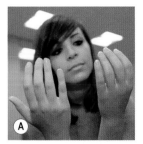
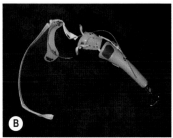
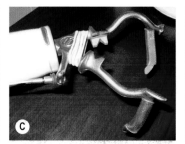
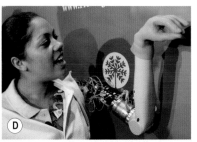

Fig. 36.5 Images showing examples of the six major types of prosthetic arm/hand. **(A)** Passive/cosmetic prosthetic arm and hand. In this image, the prosthetic arm and hand are on the viewer's right (patient's left). (Touch Bionics, livingskin.) **(B)** Body-powered prosthetic arm with body attachments at left, and custom farm/working hook at right. **(C)** Close-up of custom farm/working hook attachment. (Reproduced from Burdette TB, Long SA, Ho O, et al. Early delayed amputation: A paradigm shift in the limb salvage time line for patients with major upper-limb injury. J Rehabil Res Dev 2009; 46:38–94.) **(D)** Active, externally powered, myoelectric prosthetic arm that is used in a patient who has had targeted muscle reinnervation. (Courtesy of the Chicago Rehabilitation Institute.)

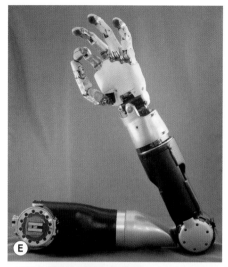

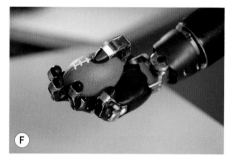

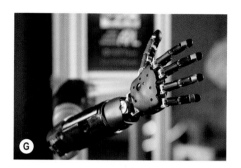

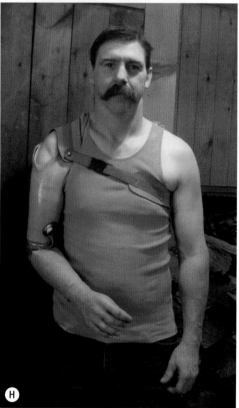

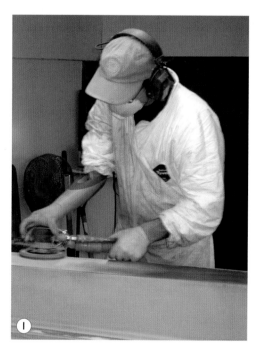

Fig. 36.5, cont'd (E–G) The robotic arm of the future: an active, externally powered, neural prosthetic arm. Robotic, neurally controlled (or "brain-controlled") arms are currently in development and Food and Drug Administration phase III testing in human subjects. In such a design, the user thinks to initiate movement, as with a biological arm, and the brain's neural signals are collected from implants placed in the patient's brain, and translated into controlled movements of the elbow, wrist, or hand. The photos shown here are prototypes of the modular prosthetic limb (MPL), which gives users 22 degrees of motion plus independent control of all five fingers, and weighs the same as a natural human arm (about 9 lb or 4 kg). It may even allow quadriplegic patients to recapture the use of limbs, potentially bypassing spinal cord injury. **(E)** Earliest MPL prototype. **(F,G)** Current MPL prototypes undergoing human testing. (Courtesy of DARPA/JHUAPL/HDT Engineered Technologies (Defense Advanced Research Projects Agency, Johns Hopkins University Applied Physics Laboratory, and HDT Engineered Technologies.) **(H,I)** Active, hybrid prosthetic arm. A hybrid arm prosthesis typically combines a lightweight, inexpensive, body-powered proximal arm and elbow, with distal robotic components for the wrist and hand to articulate and grasp objects precisely. The arm shown here, a DynamicArm® by Otto Bock, has a hybrid control scheme where the elbow is controlled by servo with body movement across the back of the shoulders, and the hand is controlled by myoelectric signals from the bicep and triceps. This patient has two attachments. **(H)** A forearm/hand made of a silicone cosmetic prosthesis that fits on the hybrid arm and is active as the hand opens and closes on command. **(I)** A working hand attachment that is bare for work use and is also active.

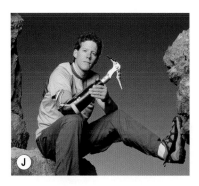
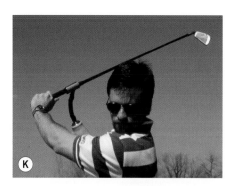
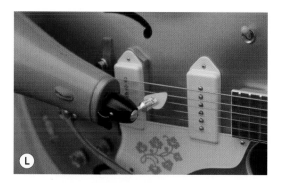

Fig. 36.5, cont'd (J–L) Active, activity-specific prosthetic arm. An 'activity-specific' nonrobotic arm can allow the user to participate actively in sports such as surfing, rock climbing, golfing, swimming, biking, and more; and to play musical instruments. **(J)** Photo of Aron Ralston taken from the cover of the book, *Between a Rock and a Hard Place*, published by Atria Books. (Courtesy of Atria Books.) Prosthetic arms/hands used for **(K)** golfing and **(L)** playing a guitar. (Courtesy of TRS, Inc.)

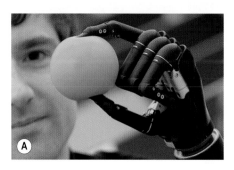
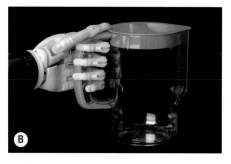
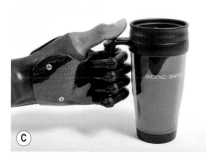

Fig. 36.6 (A) Touch Bionics i-LIMB ultra hand is the current state of the art for robotic hands: a myoelectric prosthetic hand with five fully articulating, individually powered digits. Because of the independent motors, the hand has six gripping patterns. The grasp of the robotic hand is like that of a human hand, with a thumb that can rotate, and articulating fingers able to close tightly around objects. **(B)** A slightly older version of the I-LIMB hand gripping a cup. **(C)** Touch Bionics i-LIMB digits contains up to four individually powered (myoelectric) fingers that provide greater grasping ability for partial-hand patients (those who have experienced a midhand amputation) or those who have lost several fingers. (Courtesy of Touch Bionics, www.touchbionics.com.)

(Fig. 36.6).[20] Because of the independent motors, the hand has six gripping patterns – an advance over the single-grip pattern available in its immediate predecessors. The i-LIMB ultra hand looks and acts like a real human hand in many ways; is lightweight, robust and appealing to both patients and clinicians; and represents a generational advance in bionics and patient care.[20] When a partial hand is needed due to a midhand amputation, or several missing fingers, Touch Bionics has a product called i-LIMB digits which contains up to five individually powered (myoelectric) fingers that provide greater grasping ability for partial-hand patients *(Fig. 36.6C)*.[20] Touch Bionics also provides a very lifelike cosmetic hand, with functional aesthetic restoration and precise skin-tone matching, called livingskin™ *(Figs 36.5A and 36.7)*. Another bionic hand on the market is the bebionic prosthesis, a fully articulating myoelectric hand with compliant surface and multiple grip patterns that allow precise grasping. The bebionic glove product is a realistic cosmetic cover for the hand *(Figs 36.8)*.[21]

The Defense Advanced Research Projects Agency (DARPA) undertook a 6-year, $49 million collaborative research project, called Revolutionizing Prosthetics, whose goal was to produce two extremely advanced arm prostheses that would restore motor and sensory capabilities to upper extremity amputees, and would look, feel and perform like the native limb. One device could involve invasive technology, and one had to be completely noninvasive.[22] The noninvasive design task was assigned to DEKA Research and Development[23] and the invasive task went to a consortium led by Johns Hopkins University Applied Physics Laboratory (APL). DEKA's "Luke" arm, now in clinical trials, is modular in design, and contains a hand that is similar in function to the i-LIMB, with six grip patterns, and myoelectric (not neural) control.[23] The Johns Hopkins consortium collaborated with many academic and corporate partners in the difficult task of extracting motor neural signals and sensory feedback to control an arm and hand solely by the intent of the user.[24] The project

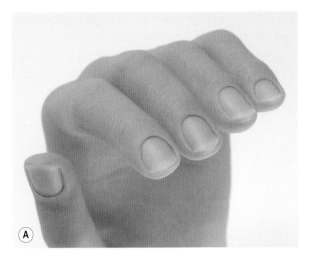

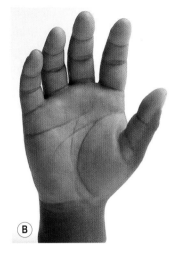

Fig. 36.7 Touch Bionics livingskin cosmetic hand with functional aesthetic restoration. A livingskin aesthetic restoration provides "a high-definition silicone prosthesis that is created to resemble human skin by mimicking the three dermal layers of natural human skin. To ensure proper color matching and fit, every prosthetic device is custom crafted for each individual." (Courtesy of Touch Bionics, www.touchbionics.com.)

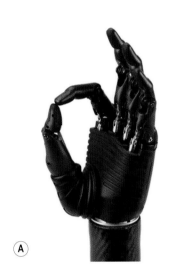

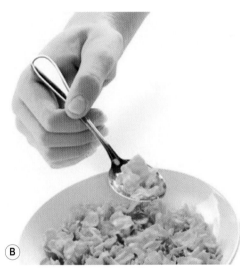

Fig. 36.8 (A) The bebionic fully articulating myoelectric hand and **(B)** bebionic glove, a cosmetic cover modeled after the anatomy of the human hand.

specified a five-fingered hand, an opposable thumb, a wrist, elbow, and shoulder, which together could generate over 22 ranges of motion, and resulted in the modular prosthetic limb (MPL) design *(Fig. 36.5E–G)*. Following the Revolutionizing Prosthetics program, DARPA, APL and consortium members have continued the research, and the arm is now in FDA Phase III testing in human subjects. This arm may even allow quadriplegic patients to recapture the use of limbs, potentially bypassing spinal cord injury by connecting their thoughts directly to a bionic limb.[25]

Choosing a robotic arm: benefits and limitations

A robotic limb will benefit a patient when it provides more function and cosmesis than a surgically reconstructed limb. Generally, for an injury that is more severe,

and closer to the midarm, a robotic arm will be an appropriate choice *(Fig. 36.9)*. In the appropriate patient, a prosthetic arm can be the difference between a dependent existence and an independent return to society.

The advantages of a robotic arm include: saving the patient the time, cost and complications of replantation surgery, rehabilitation, and lost work; more function and cosmesis than a replanted arm; and specialized functions. The disadvantages of a robotic arm include weight, power supply, susceptibility to the elements, the need for frequent repairs, and lack of feedback and control. Robotic arms also have no stereognosis (i.e., no ability to know where the limb is in space, which would allow use of the arm in the dark, for example). Robotic arms are not suitable for all patients; plastic surgeons must consider the patient's goals, intelligence, maturity, motivation, and physical constraints, such as strength,

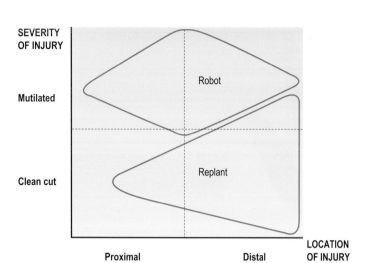

Fig. 36.9 Choice of robotic prosthetic limb versus replantation, based on severity and location of limb injury. Robots are the appropriate choice for midarm amputations, but they fail when the injury occurs at either the extreme proximal or distal ends. Replants are the best choice for clean-cut wounds at the distal end. If the amputation is at the midshoulder, there are no good solutions for robotic replacement – the prosthesis is hard to mount in this area. A replant will not work in this area either. (Courtesy of Joseph Rosen, MD.)

dexterity, joint mobility, stump quality, and pain management. A robotic arm is an adjustment, and for many it requires a shift in self-image, control, and expectations.

The plastic surgeon's role, besides helping the patient choose and order the right prosthesis, is to follow the patient through rehabilitation, with the help of an anaplastologist and/or prosthetist, who can be found via the International Anaplastology Association and the American Academy of Orthotists and Prosthetists.[37,38] The surgeon should contact a prosthetist soon after the trauma, before final wound closure, to discuss socket and terminal device design and fabrication. The prosthetist will inform the surgeon that sometimes more length is a detriment to including prosthetic components, but not enough length will conversely hurt suspension of the socket. The surgeon will need to give the prosthetist a prescription for the prosthesis, and they will discuss the patient's treatment plan together. If the patient needs a replacement limb with a lifelike covering, an anaplastologist will collaborate with the prosthetist to provide cosmesis as well as function, creating a lifelike skin to cover the prosthesis.

Lower limb prostheses

Lower limb prostheses that employ computerized, robotic, or active technology are in development,

including both leg and foot designs.[39] The Massachusetts Institute of Technology has designed a myoelectric ankle–foot prosthesis that can walk on level ground or climb stairs; in the future they hope to have neural signals automatically trigger terrain-appropriate, local prosthetic leg behaviors.[40] The C-leg® by Otto Bock Healthcare has a robotic knee that employs a microprocessor, software, and feedback from 50 sensors to anticipate the user's movements and adjust motion in real time, to keep the knee stable as the user walks and maintain support even if he or she stumbles.[41]

Robotics in craniofacial surgery and ear, nose, and throat surgery

Dr. Paul Tessier of France pioneered craniofacial reconstruction surgery, developing many operations to correct mid-facial defects in children in the 1900s.[42,43] The field was reinvented in 2005, when Dr. Jean-Michel Dubernard in France performed the first partial face transplant. Dr. Maria Siemionow and a surgical team at Cleveland Clinic performed the first US near-total human facial transplant in 2008;[44] Dr. Bohdan Pomahac and a team at Brigham and Women's Hospital conducted the second US facial transplant in 2009;[45] and others have followed around the world, progressing to full facial transplants in 2010. Composite tissue transplantation advances the craniofacial surgeon's skill set, and robotics has the potential to advance the field further. Major craniofacial remodeling operations might be done in a minimally invasive fashion, using only a few small incisions, if the miniature, articulated, remotely controlled instruments from the da Vinci system were adapted to perform such procedures.

Other surgical specialists are exploring this area. Selber et al. conducted a preclinical investigation to explore the feasibility of robotic reconstruction of oropharyngeal defects; they stated that, "transoral robotic free flap reconstruction is the next logical step in transoral robotic surgery."[46] Otolaryngologists now perform thyroidectomy via incisions in the axillae to avoid obvious neck scars. And oncologic otolaryngologists use the da Vinci system's articulated instruments to reach deep into the mouth and throat for ENT surgeries. According to Dr. Joseph Paydarfar (personal communication), an ENT surgeon at Dartmouth-Hitchcock Medical Center:

The da Vinci is quite exciting and I think it will result in a paradigm shift in how we manage cancers of the throat … The robot, with its 3D-high definition camera, allows us to see up close in the throat in ways that were really not possible before. In addition, the manipulator arms of the robot allow for significantly improved ability to manipulate tissues and work around corners – with our older technologies, sometimes we could see what it was we wanted to manipulate, but because we were limited to [the] linear nature of our instruments [we] would not be able to reach the tissue. The learning curve is steep (i.e., easy to learn) especially for the video game generation. We use the 5 mm instruments [that] are slightly smaller than the standard 8 mm. However, as the specialty of robotic ENT surgery advances, more instruments will become available that will be specialty-specific.

In a case series of 17 patients, Aubry et al. studied the use of transoral robotic surgery (TORS) for head and neck cancer. They concluded that TORS "(extended) the indications for endoscopic resection for selected cases of head and neck cancers" and allowed "effective cancer resection under excellent operating conditions with low morbidity and improved functional recovery." They did caution that more studies should be done to compare this new surgical modality with open surgery, endoscopic laser and chemoradiotherapy techniques.[46a] In a systematic review of the literature on the use of robotics for otolaryngology-head and neck surgery (OHNS), Maan et al. concluded that the evidence base suggests that the benefits of OHNS robotic surgery include access, precision, and operative time; but suggested that more controlled, prospective studies with objective outcome measures should be done, and that cost is still the biggest drawback of robotic surgery for OHNS.[46b]

When it is not possible to reconstruct the face surgically, facial prostheses are used that include prosthetic eyes, ears, and full prosthetic faces.[47,48] The current facial prostheses are inanimate, with passive functions that may: (1) restore passive cosmesis and appearance, to improve psychosocial quality of life; (2) protect a trauma or resection site; (3) improve hearing, by restoring the helix of the ear; and/or (4) provide a structure for support, such as a prosthetic ear in which to place a hearing aid, or a prosthetic nose or eye on which to place glasses. We can imagine facial prostheses becoming active and animated in the future – using robotic

components to restore function, and to help patients actually see, smell, eat, and speak.[49] A bionic eye (retinal prosthesis) made by Second Sight[49a] elicits visual perception in blind subjects with severe to profound retinitis pigmentosa. Argus® II is currently being evaluated in a clinical study conducted in the US and Europe, and has received marketing clearance in 2011 in Europe.

Robotics in chest and abdominal (trunk) surgery

In the trunk, some plastic surgeons treat large ventral hernias with endoscopic component separation procedures.[50] This operation could potentially be done entirely via minimally invasive techniques with the use of surgical robots. Also, to treat congenital, posttraumatic or postablative chest anomalies, robotic fabricating systems use CAD/CAM technology and 3D imaging to mill a custom prosthesis that precisely fits the defect. Such technology minimizes operative time and cost by reducing the adjustments of the implant's fit during the procedure.[17,51]

Robots in urologic (prostate) surgery

Plastic and urologic surgeons correct congenital urologic defects and reconstruct anatomy after trauma or disease. Robotics could play a role in fabricating urologic implants that restore function; for example, penile implants to correct birth defects, trauma, or erectile dysfunction, or for sexual reassignment surgery.

Any urologic or gynecologic operation that is done endoscopically can be a candidate for robotic surgery. Radical prostatectomy (RP) was first done laparoscopically in 1997. Today, about half of prostate cancer is treated via surgery, whether open, laparoscopic, or robotic. Roughly 85% of the 81 000 American men who choose surgery to treat their prostate cancer choose da Vinci surgery, according to Intuitive Surgical.[26] Robotic-assisted surgery of the prostate, kidney, and ureter has increased rapidly.[52] These procedures are highly marketed and concerns about the true benefits of the robotics have been raised.[53] This problem illustrates one of the dilemmas surrounding robotic-assisted surgery, which is the cost–benefit ratio. It is important to avoid utilizing technology that is not proven to improve outcomes, unless one is studying and comparing the technology with the current standard of care.

Robotic surgery: the evidence base for improved outcomes

There is some evidence for improved outcomes in robotic surgery as compared to endoscopic surgery and open surgery, but to date there are no randomized controlled trials, only population-based studies, and studies that are often based on a single institution and/or practice.

Robotic prostate surgery is often used as a benchmark to examine outcomes. For RP surgery, the primary goal is to remove cancer. Secondary concerns include potency and urinary continence, although potency is impacted by factors outside of surgical method (i.e., if there are tumors on the nerve, it cannot be spared). Blood loss, mean operating times, and other factors are also measurable outcomes.

Berryhill et al.[54] conducted a population-based review of 22 studies, of 40 patients or more, comparing robotic RP (RRP) using da Vinci, to laparoscopic radical prostatectomy (LRP) and open RP. They found that robotic surgery had the least blood loss, better cancer control, and fewer overall complications. For mean operating times, RRP (164 min) beat LRP (227 min) but not open RP (147 min). Urinary continence and potency were hard to assess, because of different measuring methods among the reviewed studies and the lack of a randomized controlled trial.

In September 2009, a meta-analysis of more than 100 studies, which included over 30 000 patients, was published by the Institute for Clinical Economic Review. It concluded that, while robotic-assisted laparoscopic prostatectomy (RALP) was still unproven, it may potentially offer a small to substantial net benefit over traditional forms of treatment, including open surgery.[55] The main reason it was determined to be unproven was because of the smaller number of RALP patients included. The graphs and the data table from this study led to two reasonable conclusions:

1. RALP was potentially superior to both open surgery and conventional laparoscopy.

2. There was a greater consistency in outcomes among RALP patients. The average outcomes were superior for RALP, and the ranges of results reported in the studies examined were tighter.

Coelho et al.[56] reviewed 16 studies with at least 100 patients from 2006 to 2009. They reported that robotic-assisted surgery was likely comparable and possibly superior to open surgery; and that studies have shown the safety and efficacy of RALP, with outcomes of decreased blood loss and transfusion risk compared with open radical prostectomy. However they concluded that high-quality trials have not been done, so definitive conclusions cannot be made.

As with any new technology, robotic surgery will improve over time. Expected system improvements, more training, more centers of excellence, and better simulation should improve outcomes, which can then be measured with larger prospective randomized studies.

Next-generation robotic devices and the future of robotics in surgery

In summary, robotics impacts plastic surgery in two major areas – surgical tools and prosthetic design. In the future, advanced prostheses will include active robotic faces with intelligent animation; there will be bionic eyes and complete ear implants.[49] Almost any human part might be aided or replaced by a robotic counterpart that could transcend the limitations of its biological function. Surgical robots will evolve to possess tactile sense; they may become cheaper, smaller, and customized for plastics procedures with small incisions and limited scope. Robotic components will become miniaturized, including smaller telemanipulator systems, freely mobile intracorporeal robots[33] and even nanoscale devices. Centers of excellence will expand, as will simulation and training, making surgical robot technology more available and likely improving outcomes across all procedures. Data fusion and patient-specific models[57] will allow surgeons to view computed tomography (CT) and magnetic resonance images overlaying the actual anatomy during surgery. Surgical robots may become more active and autonomous, and increasingly serve as medical assistants, delivering supplies or holding retractors.

Passive surgical tools will also become active and robotic. Drs. Court Cutting and Barry Grayson of New York University (NYU) conduct nasoalveolar molding, using a device that molds the jaw and teeth prior to cleft lip surgery.[58] This device might conceptually evolve into a smart robotic device, programmed to move the anatomy from the wrong configuration to the right one over time.

Working with biomedical engineers and computer experts, plastic surgeons will be at the forefront of technological changes, shaping the future for the benefit of their patients.

Simulation

 Access the Historical Perspective section online at
http://www.expertconsult.com

Introduction and definition of simulation

Simulation is increasingly utilized in surgery, as the field reacts to continued pressure to standardize training. The main push for standardization comes from the desire to improve patient safety. Simulation can be defined as "the imitative representation of the functioning of one system or process by means of the functioning of another."[63] This includes the use of a model, whether physical or logical, over time, to gain insight into the way the system or process operates in order to evaluate and analyze it.[64] This chapter's focus is on computer-based simulators that engage the learner and test cognitive knowledge. Animation is a new feature that accompanies some computer-based simulators. Trainees first watch animated computer films, to view the specific procedure and become familiar with the relevant anatomy, before they practice the procedure on the computer-based simulator. This is analogous to the "see one, do one" approach for traditional surgical training.

Simulation can be implemented in three phases, based on the American College of Surgeons (ACS) plan for general surgery trainees: it can be used to learn skills; to practice and understand procedures; and to practice team training in the operating room.[64] Simulators, physical devices which manifest simulation in the medical area, can take various forms, including bench models, animal models, cadavers, mannequins, and computer simulators.[64] Specialized surgical skills workshops have reduced the rate of complications in endoscopic carpal tunnel procedures.[65] Thus, when applied to medical procedures, ethically and practically, simulation provides an effective tool for both education and planning in a variety of surgical specialties. In plastic surgery, simulation has applications in residency training, maintenance of certification, and patient-specific planning of procedures. Simulation provides a safe and consistent way for plastic surgeons to improve and verify technical skills, cognitive knowledge, and teamwork.

Rationale for using simulation for plastic surgery and evidence of its utility in surgical training paradigms

Both the Accreditation Council for Graduate Medical Education and American Board of Medical Specialties sanction the common six core competencies for all surgeons: (1) medical knowledge; (2) patient care; (3) interpersonal and communication skills; (4) professionalism; (5) practice-based learning and improvement; and (6) systems-based practice.[66] Despite these aims, the Institute of Medicine reported that roughly 44000–98000 deaths in the US occur each year as a result of medical errors – significant enough to deem it a public health risk.[67] These staggering statistics have prompted greater concern for patient safety across the field. Furthermore, the rising cost of healthcare has put pressure on medical centers to alleviate costs. While operating room time has real costs up to thousands of dollars per hour,[68] simulation provides a safe way for surgeons to practice procedures at a significantly reduced cost.[64]

Using virtual reality and simulation, residents and attending surgeons can practice skills and procedures without risk to the patient; it is a supplement to the "see one, do one, teach one" paradigm. If a trainee can practice certain skills and procedures on a simulator, operating room times can be reduced, and potentially fewer mistakes made by trainees, thereby increasing patient safety.

The role of simulation in plastic surgery

Training simulators

Simulation for training is growing in pervasiveness in plastic surgery, with early use in residency programs.

While the ACS has pioneered the foundational structure for using simulators for training through its Accredited Educational Institutes (AEIs) consortium, the plastic surgery community has primarily focused on developing procedural simulators specific to the field. Technical skills are usually taught in general surgery training; the AEIs aid this process with skills simulators such as box trainers for suturing.[69]

As minimally invasive robotic surgery gains traction, simulators are likewise utilized to train on specific operating tools, such as the da Vinci system. The Mimic Technologies dV-Trainer™, a simulator for the da Vinci system, is a tabletop virtual environment with a two-handed haptic device with force feedback and tracking *(Fig. 36.10)*. A study by Kenney et al. revealed that the dV-Trainer had content, construct, and face validity, which is a positive assessment of the simulator's realism by the novice user.[70] Intuitive Surgical also offers the da Vinci Skills Simulator™, introduced in 2011. Designed to offer an immersive virtual experience via the surgeon console, the da Vinci simulator enables users to measure and track skills assessment without the need for additional system components, instruments, or skills models. Intuitive's da Vinci simulator and Mimic's dV-Trainer are complementary products, developed collaboratively by the companies and targeted for different customer needs. The dV-Trainer is for use as a standalone product – it is not dependent on the console – and the da Vinci simulator is for use on the console. The da Vinci simulator uses the Mimic simulation software, but it houses it in hardware that is directly compatible with an existing da Vinci system.

The American Council of Academic Plastic Surgeons (ACAPS) *Ad Hoc* Committee on Virtual Reality and Simulation for Plastic Surgery Education is committed to helping develop and distribute simulators to educate residents on plastic surgery procedures. The Committee is divided into groups of experts in four plastic surgery subspecialties: (1) craniofacial; (2) cosmetic; (3) reconstructive; and (4) hand procedures. A survey completed by 85 ACAPS members in February 2009 indicated that 93% were interested in using a 3D surgical simulator system for training residents in plastic surgery.

The Committee's goals are to adapt this advanced virtual surgery simulation technology for standardized teaching, and for procedures in the four aforementioned areas of expertise. Using a process called cognitive task

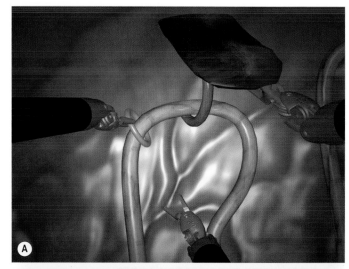
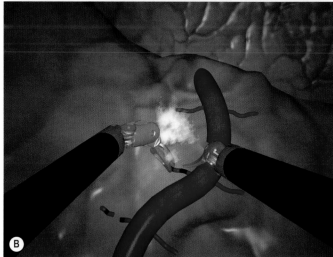

Fig. 36.10 The Mimic dV-Trainer simulator for robotic surgery is designed to train surgeons how to use the da Vinci surgical system and to teach system awareness, instrument manipulation, and basic skills such as needle handling and energy management. **(A)** The Ring Walk exercise assists in refining dexterity, moving an object with a linear constraint, using the camera to navigate around the surgical field, and learning how to use the clutch with the instruments. **(B)** The Energy dissection exercise instructs the user in applying the use of cautery and coagulation as part of dissection, as well as controlling blood loss. (Courtesy of Jeff Berkley, PhD, and Gordon Nealy; copyright 2012 Mimic Technologies, Inc.)

analysis, procedures such as open carpal tunnel release and reduction mammaplasty are broken into steps which are weighted according to their relevance to the outcome of the procedure. For instance, in the latissimus dorsi procedure, flap positioning and chest closure are weighted at 20%, while dressing is 5%. In this way, key teaching points are emphasized in the developed simulator.

BioDigital Systems and the NYU Institute of Reconstructive Plastic Surgery have undertaken the

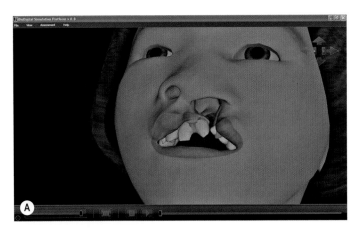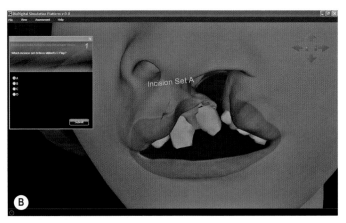

Fig. 36.11 BioDigital/SmileTrain cleft lip and palate simulator showing a simulated patient's appearance **(A)** before and **(B)** during surgery. (Courtesy of SmileTrain, Court Cutting, MD, and BioDigital Systems, LLC. ©2012 BioDigital Systems.)

Table 36.1 **Completed surgical animations for various surgical procedures**

Procedure	Animated procedure	
Genoplasty	Genoplasty-sliding	
Prognathia	Bilateral sagittal split osteotomy Vertical ramus osteotomy	
Micrognathia	Mandibular distraction:	V-vector H-vector O-vector
Temporomandibular joint ankylosis	Transport distraction	
Maxillary hypoplasia	Le Fort I	
Midface hypoplasia	Le Fort III	
Upper two-thirds hypoplasia	Monobloc	
Craniosynostosis	Cranial vault/frontal orbital advancement	
Breast reconstruction	Pedicle TRAM reconstruction DIEP flap reconstruction Latissimus dorsi flap reconstruction Free TRAM reconstruction Tissue expander	

TRAM, transverse rectus abdominis myocutaneous; DIEP, deep inferior epigastric perforator.

development of animators and simulators to educate residents in plastic surgery procedures. Using a multidisciplinary team of plastic surgeons as medical experts, artists to provide realism, and computer scientists for technical development, the team has created a library of training programs to teach craniofacial and breast reconstruction procedures. ***Table 36.1*** summarizes the procedures for which animations have already been completed.

The BioDigital cleft lip and palate simulator, developed under the leadership of Court Cutting, MD, is currently available as a beta version, and is presently being ported to the web-based BioDigital Human™ online *(Fig. 36.11)*. Its CT-based patient model enables the trainee to practice, record, and review surgery in real time; to explore the anatomy at every tissue layer; and to cut surfaces, create flaps, and transpose tissue.[71,72] Simulators in the *Interactive Craniofacial Surgical Atlas*, created under the direction of Joseph McCarthy, MD, include the frontal orbital advancement simulator, the Monoblock advancement/distraction simulator, and the Le Fort III advancement/distraction simulator. These new simulators include features such as videos of live surgeries, to help illustrate the procedure being simulated; audio voiceover, to facilitate learning as the trainee practices; and 3D visualization.

Simulators for other specialized procedures include a simulator for latissimus dorsi myocutaneous flap with tissue expander for breast reconstruction following mastectomy *(Fig. 36.12)*.

The cleft lip, Le Fort II monobloc simulator, developed under the leadership of Alexes Hazen, MD, with the cognitive task analysis defined by the ACAPS Committee, includes features such as those in the Interactive Craniofacial Surgical Atlas.

NYU and members of the ACAPS *Ad Hoc* committee tested the efficacy of the latissimus dorsi trainer (version 1) in a four-institute pilot study in the US. The simulator is now actively being used at New York University, Case

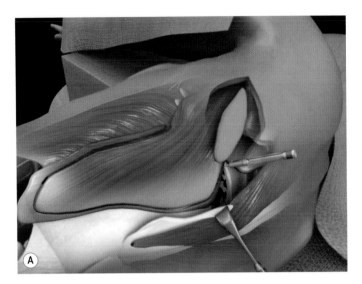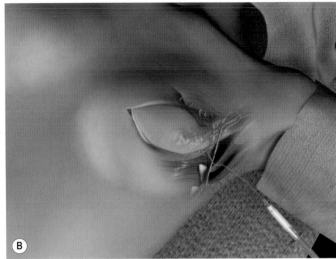

Fig. 36.12 BioDigital latissimus dorsi simulator. (Courtesy of BioDigital Systems, LLC. ©2012 BioDigital Systems.)

Western Reserve University, the University of Wisconsin, and Dartmouth-Hitchcock Medical Center, while the committee plans to conduct phases II and III testing at other institutions as well. The benefit of simulators for training has been demonstrated in other surgical disciplines, and the objective of this pilot study is to provide such data for plastic surgery. Residents and medical students will be tested on their knowledge of the procedure, before and after exposure to the simulator.

Plans to incorporate virtual reality and simulation for training in plastic surgery resident curricula are currently underway. The American Society of Plastic Surgeons and ACAPS are immersed in a joint effort to develop a novel online "standardized and comprehensive plastic surgery educational vehicle" (J Locee, chair, personal communication). The field of plastic surgery was divided into seven sections ((1) head and neck; (2) upper extremity; (3) trunk; (4) lower extremity; (5) breast; (6) aesthetic surgery; and (7) nonclinical competencies). Each module will comprise various learning tools, including didactic reading, oral board cases, and multimedia components, such as simulated procedures. In this manner, simulation will complement other educational instruments to provide residents with the fundamentals of all plastic surgery procedures outside the operating room.

Investigators at Dartmouth's Thayer School of Engineering are currently conducting team-training research to help enhance communication and ensure safe patient handoffs between operating room personnel and other hospital staff. The envisioned system – a computational team-training simulation – will seamlessly monitor medical operations to reduce or prevent catastrophic medical errors and to improve patient safety (E Santos, personal communication). One simulated scenario includes a breast reduction case in which a patient's nipple is mistakenly discarded, due to either her plastic surgeon's inexperience or his misunderstanding of her preferences. Using this case, and other scenarios, the Santos team will model reasoning among doctors, nurses, and patients,[73] and will simulate the team's clinical decision-making and reasoning prior to, during, and after surgical procedures, to analyze inconsistencies or gaps in the procedure – a key indicator of medical errors – with the goal of alerting the team when any discrepancy occurs.

Surgical planning simulators

Plastic surgeons can use simulation not only to practice new procedures on a virtual patient, but also for patient-specific surgical planning. Prior to the first US near-total face transplant procedure, performed by a surgical team led by Dr. Maria Siemionow at Cleveland Clinic in 2008, the surgeons used stereolythic anatomical models made from the patient's CT scans, showing the facial defect, as part of their surgical planning *(Fig. 36.13)*[44] (M Siemionow, personal communication).

Prior to the second US facial transplant, performed by microsurgeons at Brigham and Women's Hospital in

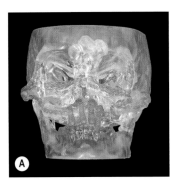 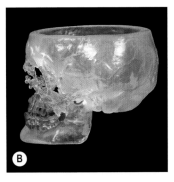 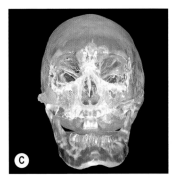 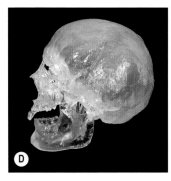

Fig. 36.13 (A, B) The stereolithic anatomical model based on the computed tomographic scan of the patient who had the first US facial transplant, performed by a team of surgeons led by Dr. Maria Siemionow at the Cleveland Clinic in 2008. **(A)** Frontal view of the craniofacial defect after gunshot injury to the patient's face, indicating damage of the frontal and midface skeleton including the infraorbital floor and the nasal, zygomatic, and maxillary bones mixed with the metal pieces. **(B)** The left side of the defect, with a significant tridimensional defect showing missing nose and nasal bones and upper jaw bony support. **(C)** Frontal view at 6 months after transplantation, demonstrating complete restoration of the craniofacial defect by replacement of all missing bony components of the facial skeleton and soft tissues of the patient with the composite facial allograft from the donor. **(D)** Left-side view after transplantation confirming restoration of the tridimensional defect of the craniofacial skeleton, including nose and bony structures supporting the upper and midface skeleton. (Reproduced with permission from Siemionow MZ, Papay F, Djohan R, et al. First U.S. near-total human face transplantation: a paradigm shift for massive complex injuries. Plast Reconstr Surg 2010;125: 111–122.)

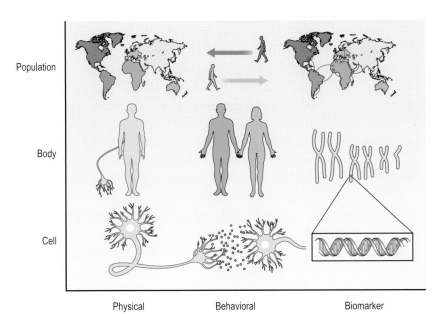

Fig. 36.14 Physical–behavioral–genomics model. No model yet exists that encompasses the physical body, behavior, and biomarkers of an individual, but Dr. Joseph Rosen and colleagues are developing such a model. A full human model could include a person's cells, tissues, and organs, vital signs, biomechanics, physiology, behavior and genetic traits, combined with the epidemiology of a larger population. Such a comprehensive model might simulate and predict the individual's behavior and health. (Courtesy of Joseph Rosen, MD.)

2009 under the leadership of Dr. Bohdan Pomahac, the team also used CT scans of the recipient's head and facial defect to generate a life-sized 3D model of the cranium, built in acrylic. The team then generated a second 3D facial model, based on a CT scan of normal facial anatomy, from which parts were removed and transferred to the recipient's model. This allowed the surgeons to plan how much bone was needed from the donor, as well as to anticipate the anatomical logistics of the donor recovery procedure (B Pomahac, personal communication).

Future applications of simulation

A future vision must include simulation trainers in plastic surgery plans universally, and also provide training for new procedures as part of continuing education, in a safe, efficient, and effective manner. The ACAPS *Ad Hoc* Committee on Virtual Reality and Simulation for Plastic Surgery Education, in partnership with BioDigital Systems and NYU, plans to release a procedure simulator for craniofacial and reconstructive procedures in 2012. As simulation centers are developed at increasing numbers of medical centers, and surgery curricula continue to incorporate simulation as a beneficial tool for training, simulation will become more ingrained in the field of plastic surgery for resident training, maintenance of certification, and patient-specific practice. As simulators become more advanced, they will be used at various levels in practice, and may even incorporate a physical–behavioral–genomics model of a human being, one that combines information about a person's cells, tissues, and organs, vital signs, biomechanics, physiology, behavior and genetic traits, combined with the epidemiology of a larger population. Such a comprehensive model might simulate and predict the individual's behavior and health *(Fig. 36.14)*.

Telemedicine

 Access the Historical Perspective section online at
http://www.expertconsult.com

Introduction

In the future, telemedicine will extend robotics and simulation to make plastic surgery safer, simpler, more successful, and more accessible. The patient–provider relationship and delivery of care will be transformed by telemedicine, as doctors will not need to be physically present in order to care for their patients. This section of the chapter defines telemedicine as a clinical tool, explains the role of social networks in telemedicine, presents potential challenges in its utilization for plastic surgery, and explains current and future applications in plastic surgery.

Definition and methods

Telemedicine refers to the application of telecommunications technologies to a medical context. Telemedicine may be defined as an "exchange of medical information from one site to another via electronic communications" with the overall goal of improving patient care.[83] Telemedicine may be as simple as faxing a copy of an X-ray, or as complicated as multipoint video conferencing across several continents with high-resolution image transfer. A resident can ask an attending physician for advice; one physician can ask another physician for advice; or a patient can ask advice of a doctor. Many components of current plastic surgery consultation can be converted to a digital format, including long-distance triage, remote consultation, telesurgery,[84,85] postoperative assessments, patient education, continuing medical education for providers, and public health education.

Worldwide, the need for telemedicine has only increased as the gap in access to technology broadens between those living in rural and urban areas. People living in rural areas have less access to medical care generally, and in many cases, to specialty care, with the exception of medical volunteerism groups such as ReSurge International (formerly Interplast).[86] ReSurge International is one of a number of groups that provide temporary specialty care to remote areas on international surgical humanitarianism trips, and supplement this with visiting educators who provide direct, hands-on training for local medical personnel. The interaction with local providers is such that surgeons in host countries can post cases on a secure website to receive advice when ReSurge International teams are not in country. Specialist physicians, such as plastic surgeons, are often a small percentage of the overall physician workforce and tend to be concentrated in urban centers. Through this networked-care mechanism, we are moving toward more efficient use of specialists as their time and expertise are available anywhere, anytime.

Several technologies are commonly used in telemedicine applications. The first, called store-and-forward, is used to transfer digital images from one location to another. The locations can be in the same village or city, or many miles or oceans apart. An image is taken with a digital camera (store) and then sent (forward) to another location for interpretation and analysis. This method is used for nonemergent situations, when a consultation can be provided in the next day or few days, and a patient's well-being is not dependent on an immediate response from a physician.

Another technology often used in telemedicine applications is called two-way interactive television. This technology is used when a face-to-face interaction is desired, and is used between a patient/provider in one location and a specialist in another location. In most

Table 36.2 Two telemedicine technologies and comparison		
Type	Store-and-forward	Two-way interactive
Situations used	Nonemergent	Face-to-face, often urgent
Present uses	Teleradiology, ultrasonography, telepathology, teleanesthesia, teledermatology	Real-time videoconferencing for patient consultations using otoscopes, stethoscopes
Advantages	Requires less bandwidth	Real-time
Disadvantages	Takes longer	More expensive, requires more bandwidth

cases, the patient/provider pair is located in a rural environment and the specialist is located in an urban center. Video conferencing equipment at both locations enables a live, real-time consultation for the patient without having to travel (*Table 36.2*).

Social networking

The future delivery of healthcare will not be limited to face-to-face interactions. Online social networks, such as PatientsLikeMe.com and CarePlace.com, already link patients with similar conditions. Clayton Christensen, in his book *The Innovator's Prescription*, discusses facilitated networks as an important part of a future healthcare system.[87] Facilitated networks can exist specifically for plastic surgeons, creating a space where they can share best practices and support each other in their lines of work. They can also exist for patients, where people with similar conditions are able to share which therapies or surgeries worked for them, or how they are coping with a specific condition. In the plastic surgery realm, obesity.com is a website where patients can find resources on weight loss surgery, including a body mass index calculator, research, forums, insurance assistance, pictures, providers, and stories.

Plastic surgery and telemedicine

Plastic surgeons have used telemedicine predominantly in communicating about individual cases in the international medical arena. Telemedicine can be used in the preoperative, operative, and postoperative phases of a given plastic surgical operation. Through organizations such as ReSurge International, plastic surgeons anywhere in the world receive daily updates about cases in developing nations where consultations are requested. These surgeons can choose to log on to the online system to provide their expertise on the case. They can view patient diagnostics and past medical history, and write a case report. This is a prime example of medical care at a distance.

The other major area in which telemedicine impacts plastic surgery is in telesurgery. Using telesurgery, surgeons can operate on patients who are geographically remote: for example, a patient who cannot physically or financially afford to travel to the doctor.[84] In the future, surgeons might remotely operate on an injured soldier on a battlefield,[85] or a victim of an earthquake, hurricane, pandemic, or other disaster (*Figs 36.15, 36.16*). One major advantage of telesurgery, like other forms of telemedicine, is that patients can remain in their own environment, where they can receive care and support from community or family members.

A brief description of the specific "tele" terms relating to telesurgery may help the reader. The term teleoperation means doing work at a distance. Telesurgery refers to doing surgery across a distance. For example, a surgeon, in one location, can control a surgical robot at a remote location (known as telerobotics). Telerobotics is depicted in *Figure 36.15* with a schematically drawn robotic surgeon; though in practice, a telerobotics system might look more like the da Vinci system (*Fig. 36.2*), with the surgeon using a control console and viewing system at his or her site, directing the actual operating robot at a remote site, which must also have a camera to send back images to the surgeon of the robot's-eye view. Telepresence is the feeling of being somewhere one is not physically present: the best current example is videoconferencing, which makes one "present" via 2 senses: sight and sound. In the surgical example, telepresence could mean an expert surgeon projecting his or her image into a remote operating room, via two-way videoconferencing, to be a mentor assisting the other surgeons in real time. The OR surgeon(s) would see the remote mentor "appearing" on a monitor in the OR, and the mentor would likewise see an image of the OR and surgical field. Virtual telepresence could also be employed, in which a computer-generated surgical mentor (perhaps from an animation or a simulator)

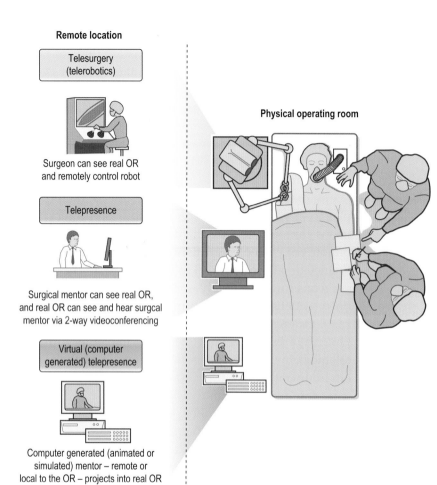

Fig. 36.15 Telesurgery and telepresence are two ways in which a remote surgeon can assist in, and/or direct procedures in, an operating room (OR) anywhere else in the world. In telesurgery, the remote surgeon controls a robot that actually conducts the surgery. In telepresence, the remote surgeon serves as a mentor to instruct the surgeons in the actual OR, using two-way videoconferencing (alternately, a computer-generated, animated or simulated surgical mentor is projected into the actual OR). In both telepresence and telesurgery, the remote surgeons see a view of the actual OR with images collected by camera and transmitted in real time.

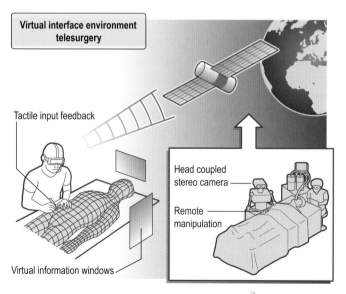

Fig. 36.16 Telesurgery via satellite using haptics and robotics. Image depicting conceptualization of how surgeons might someday conduct surgery from Earth to space. (Courtesy of Joseph Rosen, MD.)

would project into the actual OR to help instruct the surgeons (*Fig. 36.15*).

Ubiquitous mobile telemedicine

There are tremendous barriers to overcome before telemedicine can be incorporated ubiquitously. We must demonstrate its cost-effectiveness; resolve insurance reimbursement issues; resolve legal issues regarding licensing of physicians working across state and international lines; and provide sufficient internet connectivity and bandwidth. Telemedicine technology will be important in the ongoing healthcare debate, as it promises to provide a potentially higher quality of care at a decreased cost.

Telemedicine has the potential to transform the role of the plastic surgeon as a provider, by making access to care both cheaper and faster as part of a networked healthcare system.[88] Providers will not have to receive teleimages over email or be physically present in a room with expensive video conference equipment, but will be connected to a network through mobile handheld devices that allow them to acquire data and diagnostics about a case, formulate a patient plan, supervise surgery, and perform consultations in real time.

Technological convergence

The reconstructive ladder for the 21st century is one in which the plastic surgeon is able to weigh the risks and benefits associated with fixing a deformed limb or face with many choices: through reconstructive surgery, using microsurgical techniques; or through replacement using either robotic prostheses, a human tissue transplant, regenerative medicine, or tissue engineering.

Diagnostics, therapeutics, and networking are all being supported by robotics, simulation, and telemedicine. These technologies depend on information technology/information management bandwidth, speed and processor power, all of which will become better, faster, and cheaper. We will be able to make diagnostic decisions from smaller and smarter devices, linked to a larger network, and these devices' capabilities will increasingly converge. It is now possible to access the *Plastic and Reconstructive Surgery Journal* from a desktop computer, laptop computer, and even an iPhone. In the future, we will be able to put simulators on an iPhone and remotely view and participate in telesurgery over this or another handheld device.

Conclusion

The information revolution is transforming medicine, surgery, and ultimately plastic surgery in three important areas – robotics, simulation, and telemedicine. This chapter's objective has been to provide a basic understanding of currently available and future technologies in all three areas, to help plastic surgeons enhance their armamentarium with the widest variety of solutions to clinical and surgical problems. Robots bring new technology to surgery, and accelerate the introduction of surgical innovations. Simulation trains surgeons to use robotics; it enables doctors to translate new surgical technology and innovations into procedural skills and expertise. Telemedicine provides simulation at a distance, and uses robotics to perform telerobotics and telesurgery. All of these areas are mutually empowering, and in the future, these three technologies will increasingly converge and blend with newly invented technologies, in the continual attempt to minimize costs and risks, while maximizing outcomes and quality of life.

Acknowledgments

The authors wish to thank Carolyn L Kerrigan MD MSc and Phoebe Arbogast BA for their expert assistance in reviewing and editing this chapter. We also wish to extend thanks to the various doctors and product developers who helped review the chapter and provided comments, content, and images.

Bonus images for this chapter can be found online at **http://www.expertconsult.com**

Fig. 36.1 Mechanical hand from suit of armor. (Reproduced from Paré A. Instrumenta chyrurgiae et icones anathomicae, 1564. Published in Arnold K, Olsen D. Medicine Man, The Forgotten Museum of Henry Wellcome. London, British Museum Press, 2003:236.)

 Access the complete references list online at **http://www.expertconsult.com**

25. Hopkins Applied Physics Lab Awarded DARPA Funding to Test Thought-Controlled Prosthetic Limb System. July 14, 2010 Press Release of The Johns Hopkins University Applied Physics Laboratory. Available online at: http://www.jhuapl.edu/newscenter/pressreleases/2010/100714.asp. Accessed 17/11/11.

26. da Vinci System robotic surgical system. Available online at: http://www.davincisurgery.com/davinci-surgery/ Also at http://www.intuitivesurgical.com/products/. Accessed 17/11/11.
   These websites describe what robotic surgery is, and describe the leading robotic surgery system, the da Vinci system,

including surgeons' perspectives, types of procedures, and clinical outcomes.

36. Burdette TB, Long SA, Ho O, et al. Early delayed amputation: A paradigm shift in the limb salvage timeline for the patient with major upper extremity injury. *J Rehabil Res Dev.* 2009;46:385–394. Available online at: http://www.rehab.research.va.gov/jour/09/46/3/pdf/burdette.pdf. Accessed 17/11/11.

   This paper describes a timeline for helping the plastic surgeon decide whether to amputate a limb, versus salvaging the limb, and provides information on limb prostheses.

54. Berryhill Jr R, Jhaveri J, Yadav R, et al. Robotic prostatectomy: a review of outcomes compared with laparoscopic and open approaches. *Urology.* 2008;72:15–23.

   This is a population-based review of 22 studies, of 40 patients or more, comparing robotic radical prostatectomy (RRP) using da Vinci, to laparoscopic radical prostatectomy (LRP), and open radical prostatectomy (RP).

64. Rosen JM, Long SA, McGrath DM, et al. Simulation in Plastic Surgery Training and Education: The Path Forward. *Plast Reconstr Surg.* 2009;123:729–738.

   This paper describes the American College of Surgeons' resident training program for simulation in general surgery and how it might be applied to plastic surgery training programs.

66. Sachdeva AK, Pellegrini CA, Johnson KA. Support for Simulation-based Surgical Education through American College of Surgeons-Accredited Education Institutes. *World J Surg.* 2008;32(2):196–207.

72. BioDigital SmileTrain Cleft and Palate Viewer. Available online at: http://www.biodigital.com/smiletrain/download.html. Accessed 17/11/11.

84. Marescaux J, Leroy J, Gagner M, et al. Transatlantic robot-assisted telesurgery. *Nature.* 2001;413:379–380.

87. Christensen CM, Grossman JH, Hwang J. *The Innovator's Prescription: A Disruptive Solution for Health Care.* New York: McGraw Hill; 2009:24.

88. Koop CE, Mosher R, Kun L, et al. Future delivery of health care: Cybercare. *IEEE Eng Med Biol Mag.* 2008;27:29–38.

   This paper describes how many of the problems associated with the current US healthcare system might be solved by providing medical care across distributed networks ("Cybercare") based on telemedicine and related technologies.

Index

Note: **Boldface** roman numerals indicate volume. Page numbers followed by f refer to figures; page numbers followed by t refer to tables; page numbers followed by b refer to boxes.

Note: **Boldface** roman numerals indicate volume. Page numbers followed by f refer to figures; page numbers followed by t refer to tables; page numbers followed by b refer to boxes.

Note: **Boldface** *roman numerals indicate volume. Page numbers followed by f refer to figures; page numbers followed by t refer to tables; page numbers followed by b refer to boxes.*

Note: **Boldface** *roman numerals indicate volume. Page numbers followed by f refer to figures; page numbers followed by t refer to tables; page numbers followed by b refer to boxes.*

Note: **Boldface** *roman numerals indicate volume. Page numbers followed by f refer to figures; page numbers followed by t refer to tables; page numbers followed by b refer to boxes.*

Note: **Boldface** roman numerals indicate volume. Page numbers followed by f refer to figures; page numbers followed by t refer to tables; page numbers followed by b refer to boxes.

*Note: **Boldface** roman numerals indicate volume. Page numbers followed by f refer to figures; page numbers followed by t refer to tables; page numbers followed by b refer to boxes.*

*Note: **Boldface** roman numerals indicate volume. Page numbers followed by f refer to figures; page numbers followed by t refer to tables; page numbers followed by b refer to boxes.*

Note: **Boldface** *roman numerals indicate volume. Page numbers followed by f refer to figures; page numbers followed by t refer to tables; page numbers followed by b refer to boxes.*

*Note: **Boldface** roman numerals indicate volume. Page numbers followed by f refer to figures; page numbers followed by t refer to tables; page numbers followed by b refer to boxes.*

*Note: **Boldface** roman numerals indicate volume. Page numbers followed by f refer to figures; page numbers followed by t refer to tables; page numbers followed by b refer to boxes.*

Note: **Boldface** *roman numerals indicate volume. Page numbers followed by f refer to figures; page numbers followed by t refer to tables; page numbers followed by b refer to boxes.*

*Note: **Boldface** roman numerals indicate volume. Page numbers followed by f refer to figures; page numbers followed by t refer to tables; page numbers followed by b refer to boxes.*

Note: **Boldface** *roman numerals indicate volume. Page numbers followed by f refer to figures; page numbers followed by t refer to tables; page numbers followed by b refer to boxes.*

Note: **Boldface** roman numerals indicate volume. Page numbers followed by f refer to figures; page numbers followed by t refer to tables; page numbers followed by b refer to boxes.

Note: **Boldface** roman numerals indicate volume. Page numbers followed by f refer to figures; page numbers followed by t refer to tables; page numbers followed by b refer to boxes.

Note: **Boldface** *roman numerals indicate volume. Page numbers followed by f refer to figures; page numbers followed by t refer to tables; page numbers followed by b refer to boxes.*

*Note: **Boldface** roman numerals indicate volume. Page numbers followed by f refer to figures; page numbers followed by t refer to tables; page numbers followed by b refer to boxes.*

Note: **Boldface** roman numerals indicate volume. Page numbers followed by f refer to figures; page numbers followed by t refer to tables; page numbers followed by b refer to boxes.

*Note: **Boldface** roman numerals indicate volume. Page numbers followed by f refer to figures; page numbers followed by t refer to tables; page numbers followed by b refer to boxes.*

Note: **Boldface** roman numerals indicate volume. Page numbers followed by f refer to figures; page numbers followed by t refer to tables; page numbers followed by b refer to boxes.

Note: **Boldface** roman numerals indicate volume. Page numbers followed by f refer to figures; page numbers followed by t refer to tables; page numbers followed by b refer to boxes.

Note: **Boldface** roman numerals indicate volume. Page numbers followed by f refer to figures; page numbers followed by t refer to tables; page numbers followed by b refer to boxes.

Note: **Boldface** roman numerals indicate volume. Page numbers followed by f refer to figures; page numbers followed by t refer to tables; page numbers followed by b refer to boxes.

*Note: **Boldface** roman numerals indicate volume. Page numbers followed by f refer to figures; page numbers followed by t refer to tables; page numbers followed by b refer to boxes.*

*Note: **Boldface** roman numerals indicate volume. Page numbers followed by f refer to figures; page numbers followed by t refer to tables; page numbers followed by b refer to boxes.*

Note: **Boldface** roman numerals indicate volume. Page numbers followed by f refer to figures; page numbers followed by t refer to tables; page numbers followed by b refer to boxes.

Note: **Boldface** roman numerals indicate volume. Page numbers followed by f refer to figures; page numbers followed by t refer to tables; page numbers followed by b refer to boxes.

Note: **Boldface** *roman numerals indicate volume. Page numbers followed by f refer to figures; page numbers followed by t refer to tables; page numbers followed by b refer to boxes.*

Note: **Boldface** *roman numerals indicate volume. Page numbers followed by f refer to figures; page numbers followed by t refer to tables; page numbers followed by b refer to boxes.*

Note: **Boldface** *roman numerals indicate volume. Page numbers followed by f refer to figures; page numbers followed by t refer to tables; page numbers followed by b refer to boxes.*

*Note: **Boldface** roman numerals indicate volume. Page numbers followed by f refer to figures; page numbers followed by t refer to tables; page numbers followed by b refer to boxes.*

Note: **Boldface** *roman numerals indicate volume. Page numbers followed by f refer to figures; page numbers followed by t refer to tables; page numbers followed by b refer to boxes.*

Note: **Boldface** *roman numerals indicate volume. Page numbers followed by f refer to figures; page numbers followed by t refer to tables; page numbers followed by b refer to boxes.*

*Note: **Boldface** roman numerals indicate volume. Page numbers followed by f refer to figures; page numbers followed by t refer to tables; page numbers followed by b refer to boxes.*

*Note: **Boldface** roman numerals indicate volume. Page numbers followed by f refer to figures; page numbers followed by t refer to tables; page numbers followed by b refer to boxes.*

Note: **Boldface** *roman numerals indicate volume. Page numbers followed by f refer to figures; page numbers followed by t refer to tables; page numbers followed by b refer to boxes.*

*Note: **Boldface** roman numerals indicate volume. Page numbers followed by f refer to figures; page numbers followed by t refer to tables; page numbers followed by b refer to boxes.*

Note: **Boldface** *roman numerals indicate volume. Page numbers followed by f refer to figures; page numbers followed by t refer to tables; page numbers followed by b refer to boxes.*

Note: **Boldface** roman numerals indicate volume. Page numbers followed by f refer to figures; page numbers followed by t refer to tables; page numbers followed by b refer to boxes.

Note: **Boldface** roman numerals indicate volume. Page numbers followed by f refer to figures; page numbers followed by t refer to tables; page numbers followed by b refer to boxes.

*Note: **Boldface** roman numerals indicate volume. Page numbers followed by f refer to figures; page numbers followed by t refer to tables; page numbers followed by b refer to boxes.*

Note: Boldface roman numerals indicate volume. Page numbers followed by f refer to figures; page numbers followed by t refer to tables; page numbers followed by b refer to boxes.

*Note: **Boldface** roman numerals indicate volume. Page numbers followed by f refer to figures; page numbers followed by t refer to tables; page numbers followed by b refer to boxes.*

*Note: **Boldface** roman numerals indicate volume. Page numbers followed by f refer to figures; page numbers followed by t refer to tables; page numbers followed by b refer to boxes.*

Note: **Boldface** roman numerals indicate volume. Page numbers followed by f refer to figures; page numbers followed by t refer to tables; page numbers followed by b refer to boxes.

*Note: **Boldface** roman numerals indicate volume. Page numbers followed by f refer to figures; page numbers followed by t refer to tables; page numbers followed by b refer to boxes.*

*Note: **Boldface** roman numerals indicate volume. Page numbers followed by f refer to figures; page numbers followed by t refer to tables; page numbers followed by b refer to boxes.*

*Note: **Boldface** roman numerals indicate volume. Page numbers followed by f refer to figures; page numbers followed by t refer to tables; page numbers followed by b refer to boxes.*

*Note: **Boldface** roman numerals indicate volume. Page numbers followed by f refer to figures; page numbers followed by t refer to tables; page numbers followed by b refer to boxes.*

Note: **Boldface** roman numerals indicate volume. Page numbers followed by f refer to figures; page numbers followed by t refer to tables; page numbers followed by b refer to boxes.

Note: **Boldface** *roman numerals indicate volume. Page numbers followed by f refer to figures; page numbers followed by t refer to tables; page numbers followed by b refer to boxes.*

Note: **Boldface** roman numerals indicate volume. Page numbers followed by f refer to figures; page numbers followed by t refer to tables; page numbers followed by b refer to boxes.

Note: **Boldface** roman numerals indicate volume. Page numbers followed by f refer to figures; page numbers followed by t refer to tables; page numbers followed by b refer to boxes.

Note: **Boldface** roman numerals indicate volume. Page numbers followed by f refer to figures; page numbers followed by t refer to tables; page numbers followed by b refer to boxes.

Note: **Boldface** *roman numerals indicate volume. Page numbers followed by f refer to figures; page numbers followed by t refer to tables; page numbers followed by b refer to boxes.*

Note: **Boldface** roman numerals indicate volume. Page numbers followed by f refer to figures; page numbers followed by t refer to tables; page numbers followed by b refer to boxes.

Note: **Boldface** *roman numerals indicate volume. Page numbers followed by f refer to figures; page numbers followed by t refer to tables; page numbers followed by b refer to boxes.*

Note: **Boldface** roman numerals indicate volume. Page numbers followed by f refer to figures; page numbers followed by t refer to tables; page numbers followed by b refer to boxes.

Note: **Boldface** roman numerals indicate volume. Page numbers followed by f refer to figures; page numbers followed by t refer to tables; page numbers followed by b refer to boxes.

Note: **Boldface** roman numerals indicate volume. Page numbers followed by f refer to figures; page numbers followed by t refer to tables; page numbers followed by b refer to boxes.

Note: **Boldface** roman numerals indicate volume. Page numbers followed by f refer to figures; page numbers followed by t refer to tables; page numbers followed by b refer to boxes.

Note: **Boldface** roman numerals indicate volume. Page numbers followed by f refer to figures; page numbers followed by t refer to tables; page numbers followed by b refer to boxes.

*Note: **Boldface** roman numerals indicate volume. Page numbers followed by f refer to figures; page numbers followed by t refer to tables; page numbers followed by b refer to boxes.*

*Note: **Boldface** roman numerals indicate volume. Page numbers followed by f refer to figures; page numbers followed by t refer to tables; page numbers followed by b refer to boxes.*

*Note: **Boldface** roman numerals indicate volume. Page numbers followed by f refer to figures; page numbers followed by t refer to tables; page numbers followed by b refer to boxes.*

Note: **Boldface** *roman numerals indicate volume. Page numbers followed by f refer to figures; page numbers followed by t refer to tables; page numbers followed by b refer to boxes.*

Note: ***Boldface*** *roman numerals indicate volume. Page numbers followed by f refer to figures; page numbers followed by t refer to tables; page numbers followed by b refer to boxes.*

Note: **Boldface** *roman numerals indicate volume. Page numbers followed by f refer to figures; page numbers followed by t refer to tables; page numbers followed by b refer to boxes.*

Note: Boldface roman numerals indicate volume. Page numbers followed by f refer to figures; page numbers followed by t refer to tables; page numbers followed by b refer to boxes.